T0206099

# Principles of Animal Nutrition

# Principles of Animal Nutrition

Guoyao Wu

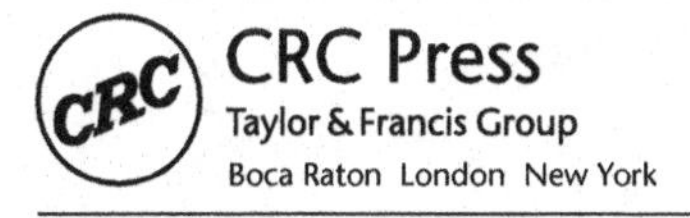


CRC Press is an imprint of the
Taylor & Francis Group, an **informa** business

Cover image prepared by Dr. Gregory A. Johnson.

CRC Press
Taylor & Francis Group
6000 Broken Sound Parkway NW, Suite 300
Boca Raton, FL 33487-2742

First issued in paperback 2021



ISBN 13: 978-1-03-209599-8 (pbk)
ISBN 13: 978-1-4987-2160-8 (hbk)



Publisher's Note
The publisher has gone to great lengths to ensure the quality of this reprint but points out that some imperfections in the original copies may be apparent.

**Library of Congress Cataloging-in-Publication Data**

Names: Wu, Guoyao, 1962- , author.
Title: Principles of animal nutrition / Guoyao Wu.
Description: Boca Raton : Taylor & Francis, 2018.
Identifiers: LCCN 2017036706 | ISBN 9781498721608 (hardback)
Subjects: LCSH: Animal nutrition. | Metabolism.
Classification: LCC SF95 .W8 2017 | DDC 636.08/52--dc23
LC record available at https://lccn.loc.gov/2017036706

**Visit the Taylor & Francis Web site at**
**http://www.taylorandfrancis.com**

**and the CRC Press Web site at**
**http://www.crcpress.com**

# Contents

Preface ........ xxiii
Acknowledgments ........ xxv
Author ........ xxvii

**Chapter 1** Physiological and Biochemical Bases of Animal Nutrition ........ 1

Fundamental Concepts of Animal Nutrition ........ 2
Definition of Nutrients and Diets ........ 2
Definition of Nutrition ........ 2
Composition of Feedstuffs ........ 2
Composition of Animals ........ 4
Proximate or Weende Analysis of Feedstuffs ........ 4
Modified Methods for Analysis of Feedstuffs and Animals ........ 6
Biochemistry as the Chemical Basis of Nutrition ........ 6
Physiology as the Foundational Basis of Nutrition ........ 7
Integration of Systems Physiology in Nutrient Utilization ........ 8
Structure of the Animal Cell ........ 8
Definitions of Cell, Tissue, Organ, and System ........ 8
Composition and Function of the Animal Cell ........ 8
Transport of Substances across the Biological Membrane ........ 10
Overview of the Animal System ........ 13
The Nervous System ........ 14
The Neuron ........ 14
Neurotransmitters ........ 15
The Central Nervous System ........ 16
The Peripheral Nervous System ........ 16
The Circulatory System ........ 16
Blood Circulation ........ 16
Blood–Brain Barrier ........ 20
The Lymphatic System ........ 21
The Digestive System ........ 22
The Stomach in Nonruminants ........ 22
The Stomach in Ruminants ........ 26
The Small Intestine ........ 28
The Large Intestine ........ 31
The Pancreas ........ 31
The Liver ........ 32
The Musculoskeletal System ........ 34
The Respiratory System ........ 34
The Urinary System ........ 35
The Male Reproductive System ........ 35
The Female Reproductive System ........ 37
The Endocrine System ........ 38
The Immune System ........ 39
Sense Organs ........ 42
Overview of Metabolic Pathways ........ 42

Major Metabolic Pathways and Their Significance ........ 42
Characteristics of Metabolic Pathways ........ 45
Enzyme-Catalyzed Reactions ........ 45
Intracellular Compartmentalization of Metabolic Pathways ........ 48
Cell-, Zone-, Age-, and Species-Dependent Metabolic Pathways ........ 49
Biological Oxidation in Mitochondria ........ 50
The Krebs Cycle in Mitochondria ........ 50
The Electron Transport System in Mitochondria ........ 53
Uncouplers of Oxidative Phosphorylation and Inhibitors of the Electron Transport System ........ 57
Summary ........ 58
References ........ 61

**Chapter 2** Chemistry of Carbohydrates ........ 67

General Classification of Carbohydrates ........ 67
Overview ........ 67
D- and L-Configuration of Carbohydrates ........ 68
Cyclic Hemiacetals (Aldoses) and Hemiketals (Ketoses) ........ 69
Monosaccharides ........ 70
Definition ........ 70
Chemical Representation of Monosaccharide Structures ........ 70
Open-Chain Form ........ 70
Cyclic Hemiacetal or Hemiketal Form ........ 70
Glucose and Fructose in Plants ........ 73
Glucose and Fructose in Animals ........ 73
Other Monosaccharides in Plants and Animals ........ 75
Simple Aminosugars as Monosaccharides in Plants and Animals ........ 75
Disaccharides ........ 76
Definition ........ 76
Cellobiose ........ 79
Lactose ........ 79
Maltose and Isomaltose ........ 80
Sucrose ........ 81
α,α-Trehalose ........ 82
Oligosaccharides ........ 82
Definition ........ 82
Trisaccharides ........ 82
Tetrasaccharides ........ 82
Pentasaccharides ........ 82
Homopolysaccharides ........ 84
Homopolysaccharides in Plants ........ 84
Definition ........ 84
Arabinan ........ 85
Cellulose ........ 85
Galactan ........ 85
β-D-Glucans ........ 85
Levans ........ 87
Mannans ........ 87
Starch ........ 87
Homopolysaccharides in Animals ........ 88

Definition ... 88
Chitin ... 88
Glycogen ... 88
Homopolysaccharides in Microbes and Other Lower Organisms ... 89
Cellulose ... 89
Chitin ... 90
Dextrans ... 90
Glycogen ... 90
Levans ... 91
Mannans ... 91
Pullulan ... 92
Heteropolysaccharides ... 92
Heteropolysaccharides in Plants ... 92
Definition ... 92
Arabinogalactan ... 92
Exudate Gums ... 93
Hemicelluloses ... 93
Inulins ... 93
Mannans as Glucomannans, Galactomannans, or Galactoglucomannans ... 93
Mucilages ... 94
Pectins ... 94
Heteropolysaccharides in Animals ... 94
Definition ... 94
Hyaluronic Acid ... 94
Sulfated Heteropolysaccharides ... 95
Heteropolysaccharides in Microbes ... 96
Arabinogalactan ... 96
Lipopolysaccharides ... 96
Murein ... 97
Xanthan ... 97
Heteropolysaccharides in Algae and Seaweeds (Marine Plants) ... 97
Agar (or Agar–Agar) ... 97
Algin (Alginic Acid) ... 97
Carrageenans ... 98
Phenolic Polymers in Plants ... 98
Lignins ... 98
Tannins ... 98
Non-Starch Polysaccharides in Plants, Algae, and Seaweeds ... 98
Chemical Reactions of Carbohydrates ... 99
Monosaccharides ... 99
Epimerization ... 99
Reduction ... 100
Oxidation ... 100
Dehydration of Aldoses and Ketoses ... 100
Formation of Glycosides ... 101
Esterification ... 101
Nonenzymatic Glycation ... 101
Disaccharides and Polysaccharides ... 102
Oxidation ... 102
Reacting with Iodine ... 102
The Molisch Test for Nearly All Carbohydrates ... 102

Summary ... 102
References ... 104

Chapter 3 Chemistry of Lipids ... 109

Classification and Structures of Lipids ... 109
Fatty Acids ... 111
Definition of Fatty Acids ... 111
Nomenclature of Fatty Acids ... 112
Short-Chain Fatty Acids ... 112
Medium-Chain Fatty Acids ... 113
Long-Chain Fatty Acids ... 114
Simple Lipids ... 119
Fats ... 119
Waxes ... 119
Compound Lipids ... 121
Glycolipids (Glycerol–Glycolipids) ... 121
Phospholipids (Phosphatides) ... 123
Sphingolipids ... 123
Ether Glycerophospholipids ... 124
Lipoproteins ... 126
Derived Lipids ... 127
Definition ... 127
Steroids ... 128
Eicosanoids ... 134
Terpenes ... 137
Chemical Reactions ... 139
Hydrolysis of TAG and Saponification of Fatty Acids ... 139
Esterification with Alcohols ... 140
Substitution of the Hydroxyl Hydrogen ... 140
Hydrogenation of Unsaturated Fatty Acids ... 140
Iodination and Bromination of the Double Bonds of Unsaturated Fatty Acids .. 141
Peroxidation of Unsaturated Fatty Acids ... 141
Reaction of the Hydrogen Atom in Methylene and Carboxyl Groups with Halogens ... 142
Summary ... 142
References ... 143

Chapter 4 Chemistry of Protein and Amino Acids ... 149

Definition, Chemical Classification, and Properties of AAs ... 149
Definition of AAs ... 149
α-, ß-, γ-, δ-, or ε-AAs ... 149
Imino Acids ... 151
Differences in the Structures of AAs ... 151
Naming and Chemical Expression of AAs ... 153
The Zwitterionic (Ionized) Form of AAs ... 153
D- or L-Configurations of AAs ... 155
Definition of L- and D-AAs ... 155
Optical Activity of L- and D-AAs ... 155
L- and D-AAs in Nature ... 155

*R/S* Configurations of AAs 158
Allo-Forms of AAs 158
Modified AA Residues in Proteins or Polypeptides 159
Free AAs and Peptide (Protein)-Bound AAs 161
Physical Appearance, Melting Points, and Tastes of AAs 163
Solubility of AAs in Water and Solutions 164
Chemical Stability of AAs 164
Stability of Crystalline AAs 164
Stability of AAs in Water and Buffers 164
Stability of AAs in Acid and Alkaline Solutions 165
Definition, Chemical Classifications, and Properties of Peptides and Protein 165
Definitions of Peptides and Proteins 165
Major Proteins in Animals 166
Actin and Myosin 166
Proteins in Connective Tissues 167
Separation of Peptides from Proteins 168
Protein Structures 168
The Concept of Crude Protein and True Protein 170
Crystalline AAs, Protein Ingredients, and Peptide Additives for Animal Diets 172
Crystalline AAs 172
Protein Ingredients 174
Peptides Used as Feed Additives 175
Chemical Reactions of Free AAs 177
Chemical Reactions of the Amino Group in α-AAs 177
Reaction of the α-Amino Group of AAs with a Strong Acid 177
Acetylation of the α-Amino Group of AAs 177
Conjugation of the α-Amino Group in AAs with a Reagent 178
Deamination of AAs 178
Transamination of AAs with α-Ketoacids 179
Oxymethylation of AAs 179
Chemical Reactions of the Carboxyl Group in α-AAs 179
Reaction of the Carboxyl Group of AAs with an Alkaline 179
Decarboxylation of AAs 179
Chemical Reactions of the Side Chains in α-AAs 180
Amidation 180
Deamidination 180
Iodination of the Phenol Ring in Tyrosine 180
Chemical Reactions Involving the ε-$NH_2$ Group of Lysine 180
Condensation of Two AAs 181
Chemical Reactions Involving Both the Amino and Carboxyl Groups of the Same α-AA 181
Chelation of AAs with Metals 182
Esterification and $N^{\alpha}$-Dehydrogenation of α-AAs 182
Oxidative Deamination (Decarboxylation) of AAs 182
Intramolecular Cyclization Reactions Involving the Side Chain Group and the α-Amino Group of α-AAs 183
Peptide Synthesis 183
Chemical Reactions of Proteins and Polypeptides 185
Hydrolysis of the Peptide Bond in Protein and Polypeptides 185
Dye-Binding of Protein and Polypeptides 185
Biuret Assay of Protein and Peptides 185

Lowry Assay of Protein and Peptides ... 185
Maillard Reaction of Protein and Peptides ... 186
Buffering Reactions of Proteins ... 187
Binding of Hemoglobin to $O_2$, $CO_2$, CO, and NO ... 187
Protein Solubility in Water ... 188
Summary ... 188
References ... 189

**Chapter 5** Nutrition and Metabolism of Carbohydrates ... 193

Digestion and Absorption of Carbohydrates in Nonruminants ... 194
Digestion of Starch and Glycogen in Nonruminants ... 194
Roles of α-Amylase in the Mouth and Stomach ... 194
Roles of Pancreatic α-Amylase and Apical Membrane Disaccharidases in the Small Intestine ... 194
Effects of the Structure of Starches on Their Digestion in the Small Intestine ... 195
Digestion of Milk- and Plant-Source Di- and Oligosaccharides in Nonruminants ... 196
Substrate Specificity of Carbohydrases in Nonruminants ... 196
Developmental Changes of Carbohydrases in Nonruminants ... 196
Nonruminant Mammals ... 196
Avian Species ... 197
Absorption of Monosaccharides by the Small Intestine in Nonruminants ... 197
Role of Glucose and Fructose Transporters in the Apical Membrane of Enterocytes ... 197
Role of Basolateral Membrane GLUT2 in the Exit of Monosaccharides from Enterocytes into the Lamina Propria ... 199
Trafficking of Monosaccharides from the Lamina Propia into the Liver ... 199
Developmental Changes of Intestinal Monosaccharide Transport in Nonruminants ... 200
Digestion and Absorption of Carbohydrates in Pre-Ruminants ... 201
Digestion of Carbohydrates in Pre-Ruminants ... 201
Absorption of Monosaccharides in Pre-Ruminants ... 201
Digestion and Absorption of Carbohydrates in Ruminants ... 201
Fermentative Digestion of Carbohydrates in Ruminants ... 201
Major Dietary Complex Carbohydrates in the Rumen ... 201
Retention Times of Feed Particles and Carbohydrates in the Rumen ... 202
Extracellular Hydrolysis of Complex Carbohydrates into Monosaccharides by Ruminal Microbes ... 202
Intracellular Hydrolysis of Complex Carbohydrates into Monosaccharides Ruminal Protozoa ... 203
Intracellular Degradation of Monosaccharides in Ruminal Microbes ... 203
Generation and Utilization of NADH and NADPH in the Rumen ... 203
Production of SCFAs in the Rumen ... 204
Entry of SCFAs from the Rumen into Blood ... 206
Production of Methane in the Rumen ... 207
Ruminal Metabolic Disorders ... 209
Species Differences in Carbohydrate Digestion among Ruminants ... 210
Absorption of Monosaccharides by the Small Intestine in Ruminants ... 210
Fermentation of Carbohydrates in the Large Intestine of Nonruminants and Ruminants ... 210

Digestion and Absorption of Carbohydrates in Fish ........ 211
Dietary Carbohydrates for Fish ........ 211
Digestion of Carbohydrates in Fish ........ 212
Digestion of Starch and Glycogen ........ 212
Digestion of β-(1-4)-Linked Carbohydrates ........ 212
Overall Digestibility of Starch ........ 212
Absorption of Monosaccharides by the Intestine of Fish ........ 213
Glucose Metabolism in Animal Tissues ........ 213
Glucose Turnover in the Whole Body ........ 213
Pathway of Glycolysis ........ 214
Definition of Glycolysis ........ 214
Entry of Glucose into Cells via Different Transporters ........ 215
Pathway of Glycolysis ........ 215
Energetics and Significance of Glycolysis ........ 218
Conversion of Pyruvate into Lactate and the Cori Cycle ........ 219
Conversion of Pyruvate into Lactate or Ethanol ........ 219
Cytosolic Redox State in Animal Cells ........ 219
Glycolysis and Cell Proliferation ........ 219
Pasteur Effect in Animal Cells ........ 220
Warburg Effect ........ 220
Quantification of Glycolysis in Animal Cells ........ 220
Regulation of Glycolysis ........ 220
Transfer of NADH from the Cytosol into Mitochondria ........ 220
Mitochondrial Oxidation of Pyruvate to Acetyl-CoA ........ 222
Oxidation of Acetyl-CoA via the Mitochondrial Krebs Cycle and ATP Synthesis ........ 223
Overall Reaction of the Krebs Cycle ........ 223
Production of ATP and Water in Mitochondria ........ 224
Energetics of Acetyl-CoA Oxidation ........ 225
Energetics of Glucose Oxidation in Aerobic Respiration ........ 225
Nutritional and Physiological Significance of the Krebs Cycle in Animals ... 225
Metabolic Control of the Krebs Cycle ........ 226
Isotopic Tracing of the Krebs Cycle ........ 227
Mitochondrial Redox State ........ 228
Crabtree Effect in Animal Cells ........ 228
Cytosolic Pentose Cycle ........ 229
Reactions of the Pentose Cycle ........ 229
Activity of the Pentose Cycle in Animal Tissues and Cells ........ 229
Physiological Significance of the Pentose Cycle ........ 231
Quantification of the Pentose Cycle ........ 232
Regulation of the Pentose Cycle ........ 233
Metabolism of Glucose via the Uronic Acid Pathway ........ 233
Gluconeogenesis ........ 234
Definition of Gluconeogenesis ........ 234
Pathway of Gluconeogenesis ........ 235
Physiological Substrates for Gluconeogenesis ........ 238
Regulation of Gluconeogenesis ........ 240
Quantification of Gluconeogenesis ........ 245
Nutritional and Physiological Significance of Gluconeogenesis ........ 246
Glycogen Metabolism ........ 248
Glycogen as a Hydrophilic Macromolecule ........ 248

Pathway of Glycogen Synthesis ........ 248
Pathway of Glycogen Degradation (Glycogenolysis) ........ 249
Regulation of Glycogenesis ........ 250
Regulation of Glycogenolysis ........ 252
Determination of Glycogenesis and Glycogenolysis ........ 253
Nutritional and Physiological Significance of Glycogen Metabolism ........ 253
Fructose Metabolism in Animal Tissues ........ 253
Synthesis of Fructose from Glucose in a Cell-Specific Manner ........ 253
Pathways for Fructose Catabolism ........ 254
Nutritional, Physiological, and Pathological Significance of Fructose ........ 256
Beneficial Effects of Fructose in Reproduction ........ 256
Pathological Effects of Excess Fructose ........ 256
Galactose Metabolism in Animal Tissues ........ 256
Pathway of UDP-Galactose Synthesis from D-Glucose in animal Tissues ........ 256
Pathway of Galactose Catabolism ........ 257
Physiological and Pathological Significance of Galactose ........ 258
Nutritional and Physiological Effects of Dietary NSPs in Animals ........ 259
Nonruminants ........ 259
Effects of NSPs on Feed Intake by Animals ........ 259
Effects of NSPs on Nutrient Digestibility, Growth, and Feed Efficiency ........ 259
Effects of NSPs on Intestinal and Overall Health ........ 260
Ruminants ........ 261
Effects of NDF on Rumen pH and Environment ........ 261
Effects of NDF on Intestinal Health ........ 261
Effects of NDF on Lactation and Growth Performance ........ 261
Effects of NDF on Feed Intake ........ 261
Summary ........ 262
References ........ 263

**Chapter 6** Nutrition and Metabolism of Lipids ........ 271

Digestion and Absorption of Lipids in Nonruminants ........ 272
Overall View ........ 272
Digestion of Lipids in the Mouth and Stomach ........ 272
Digestion of Lipids in the Small Intestine ........ 272
General Process ........ 272
Formation of Lipid Micelles ........ 273
Digestion of TAGs, Phospholipids, and Cholesterol Esters ........ 274
Digestibility of Dietary Lipids ........ 275
Absorption of Lipids by the Small Intestine ........ 276
General Process ........ 276
Absorption of Lipids into Enterocytes ........ 276
Resynthesis of TAGs in Enterocytes ........ 277
Assimilation of Wax Esters ........ 278
Assembly of Chylomicrons, VLDLs, and HDLs in Enterocytes ........ 278
Diurnal Changes in Intestinal Lipid Absorption ........ 280
Digestion and Absorption of Lipids in Preruminants ........ 280
Digestion of Lipids in the Mouth and Small Intestine ........ 280
Limited Digestion by Salivary Lipase in Mouth, Forestomaches, and Abomasum ........ 280
Extensive Digestion of Lipids in the Small Intestine ........ 281

Absorption of Lipids by the Small Intestine ....... 281
Digestion and Absorption of Lipids in Ruminants ....... 281
Digestion of Lipids in the Rumen ....... 282
Roles of Microorganisms ....... 282
Products of Lipid Hydrolysis ....... 282
Biohydrogenation of Unsaturated Fatty Acids ....... 283
Digestion of Lipids in the Abomasum ....... 283
Digestion of Lipids in the Small Intestine ....... 284
Digestibility of Dietary Lipids in the Small Intestine ....... 284
Absorption of Lipids by the Small Intestine ....... 285
Absorption of Lipids into Enterocytes ....... 285
Resynthesis of TAGs in Enterocytes ....... 285
Assembly of Chylomicrons and VLDL in Enterocytes ....... 285
Digestion and Absorption of Lipids in Fish ....... 285
Digestion of Lipids in the Intestine ....... 285
Absorption of Lipids in the Intestine ....... 286
Lipoprotein Transport and Metabolism in Animals ....... 287
Release of Lipoproteins from the Small Intestine and Liver ....... 287
Overall View ....... 287
Metabolism of Chylomicrons, VLDLs, and LDLs ....... 287
Metabolism of HDLs ....... 293
Important Role for HDLs in Cholesterol Metabolism ....... 294
Species Differences in Lipoprotein Metabolism ....... 294
Fatty Acid Synthesis in Tissues ....... 295
Synthesis of Saturated Fatty Acids from Acetyl-CoA ....... 295
Formation of Malonyl-CoA from Acetyl-CoA by Acetyl-CoA Carboxylase ....... 295
Formation of $C_4$ Fatty Acid Chain from Acetyl-CoA and Malonyl-CoA by Fatty Acid Synthase ....... 296
Addition of Malonyl-CoA to the $C_4$ Fatty Acid to Form $C_{16}$ Fatty Acids ....... 296
Metabolic Fate of Palmitate ....... 297
Synthesis of Saturated Fatty Acids from Propionyl-CoA or Butyryl-CoA plus Acetyl-CoA ....... 299
Synthesis of Short-Chain Fatty Acids ....... 299
Synthesis of MUFAs in Animals ....... 299
Synthesis of $\Delta^9$ MUFAs ....... 299
Introduction of Double Bonds between $\Delta^9$ Carbon and $\Delta^1$ Carbon ....... 300
Failure of Animals to Introduce Double Bonds beyond $\Delta^9$ Carbon ....... 301
Differences between *Trans* Unsaturated Fatty Acids and PUFAs in Animal Nutrition ....... 301
Measurements of Fatty Acid Synthesis ....... 302
Species Differences in the Use of Substrates for *De Novo* Fatty Acid Synthesis ....... 302
Tissue Differences within the Same Animal in the Use of Substrates for *De Novo* Fatty Acid Synthesis ....... 303
Nutritional and Hormonal Regulation of Fatty Acid Synthesis ....... 304
Short-Term Mechanisms ....... 304
Long-Term Mechanisms ....... 306
Cholesterol Synthesis and Cellular Sources ....... 306
Cholesterol Synthesis from Acetyl-CoA in Liver ....... 306
Sources of Cellular Cholesterol and the Regulation of Its Homeostasis ....... 308
TAG Synthesis and Catabolism in Animals ....... 308
TAG Synthesis in Animals ....... 308

MAG Pathway for TAG Synthesis ... 310
G3P Pathway for TAG Synthesis ... 310
Additional Pathways for TAG Synthesis ... 310
Function of DAG in Protein Kinase C Signaling ... 310
Storage of TAGs in WAT and Other Tissues ... 310
Mobilization of TAGs from Tissues to Release Glycerol and Fatty Acids ... 311
Intracellular Lipolysis by HSL in Animal Tissues ... 311
Tissue Distribution and Function of HSL ... 311
Regulation of HSL Activity in Animal Tissues ... 312
Intracellular Lipolysis by Adipose Triglyceride Lipase ... 312
Tissue Distribution and Function of Adipose Triglyceride Lipase ... 312
Regulation of ATGL Activity ... 312
Intracellular Lipolysis by Diacylglyceol Lipase and Monoacylglycerol Lipase in Animal Tissues ... 313
Functions of Diacylglyceol Lipase and Monoacylglycerol Lipase ... 313
Regulation of DGL and MGL Activities ... 313
Intracellular Lipolysis by Lysosomal Acid Lipase (LAL) ... 313
Oxidation of Fatty Acids in Animals ... 314
Metabolic Fate of Fatty Acids: $CO_2$ Production and Ketogenesis ... 314
Mitochondrial β-Oxidation of Fatty Acids to $CO_2$ and Water ... 314
Pathway of Mitochondrial β-Oxidation of Fatty Acids ... 314
Energetics of Fatty Acid β-Oxidation ... 318
Oxidation of Long-Chain Unsaturated Fatty Acids ... 318
Oxidation of Short- and Medium-Chain Fatty Acids ... 318
Regulation of Mitochondrial Fatty Acid β-Oxidation ... 320
Peroxisomal β-Oxidation Systems I and II ... 321
Activation of Very-Long-Chain Fatty Acids into Very-Long-Chain Acyl-CoA ... 321
Transport of Very-Long-Chain Acyl-CoA from the Cytosol into the Peroxisome ... 322
Shortening of Very-Long-Chain Fatty Acyl-CoA ... 322
Regulation of Peroxisomal β-Oxidation ... 323
Role of Peroxisomal β-Oxidation in Ameliorating Metabolic Syndrome ... 324
Production and Utilization of Ketone Bodies in Animals ... 324
Production of Ketone Bodies Primarily by Liver ... 324
Regulation of Hepatic Ketogenesis ... 325
Utilization of Ketone Bodies by Extrahepatic Tissues ... 327
α-Oxidation of Fatty Acids ... 328
ω-Oxidation of Fatty Acids ... 329
Measurements of Fatty Acid Oxidation and Lipolysis ... 329
Metabolism and Functions of Eicosanoids ... 329
Synthesis of Bioactive Eicosanoids from PUFAs ... 329
Degradation of Bioactive Eicosanoids ... 330
Physiological Functions of Eicosanoids ... 332
Phospholipid and Sphingolipid Metabolism ... 333
Phospholipid Metabolism ... 333
Synthesis of Phospholipids ... 333
Sources of Ethanolamine and Choline in Animals ... 333
Sphingolipid Metabolism ... 335
Metabolism of Steroid Hormones ... 336
Synthesis of Progesterone and Glucocorticoids ... 336

Synthesis of Testosterone and Estrogen ..... 336
Fat Deposition and Health in Animals ..... 338
Summary ..... 340
References ..... 341

**Chapter 7** Nutrition and Metabolism of Protein and Amino Acids ..... 349

Digestion and Absorption of Protein in Nonruminants ..... 349
Digestion of Protein in the Stomach of Nonruminants ..... 350
Secretion of Gastric Hydrochloric Acid ..... 350
Digestive Function of Gastric HCl and Gastric Proteases ..... 352
Developmental Changes of Gastric Proteases in Nonruminant Mammals ..... 353
Developmental Changes of Gastric Proteases in Avian Species ..... 354
Regulation of the Secretion of Gastric Proteases in Nonruminants ..... 354
Digestion of Proteins in the Small Intestine of Nonruminants ..... 354
Flow of Digesta from the Stomach into the Small Intestine for Proteolysis ..... 354
Release of Pancreactic Pro-Proteases into the Lumen of the Duodenum ..... 355
Release of Proteases and Oligopeptidases from the Small-Intestinal Mucosa into the Intestinal Lumen ..... 356
Extracellular Hydrolysis of Proteins and Polypeptides in the Small Intestine ..... 356
Developmental Changes in Extracellular Proteases in the Small Intestine of Nonruminant Mammals ..... 357
Developmental Changes in Extracellular Proteases in the Small Intestine of Avian Species ..... 358
Regulation of the Activities of Small-Intestinal Proteases in Nonruminants 359
Protein Digestibility versus Dietary AA Bioavailability in Nonruminants ..... 359
Catabolism of Free AAs and Small Peptides by the Luminal Bacteria of the Small Intestine in Nonruminants ..... 359
Absorption of Small Peptides and AAs by the Small Intestine of Nonruminants ..... 360
Transport of Di- and Tri-Peptides by Enterocytes ..... 360
Transport of Free AAs by Enterocytes ..... 361
Polarity of Enterocytes in AA and Peptide Transport ..... 364
Metabolism of AAs in Enterocytes ..... 365
Digestion and Absorption of Protein in Preruminants ..... 366
Digestion of Proteins in the Abomasum and the Small Intestine in Preruminants ..... 366
Absorption of Protein Digestion Products by the Small Intestine in Preruminants ..... 366
Digestion and Absorption of Protein in Ruminants ..... 367
Degradation of Dietary Protein in the Rumen ..... 368
Extracellular Proteolysis by Bacterial Proteases and Oligopeptidases ..... 368
Extracellular and Intracellular Degradation of NPN into Ammonia in the Rumen ..... 368
Intracellular Protein Synthesis from Small Peptides, AAs, and Ammonia in Microbes ..... 371
Role of Ruminal Protozoa in Intracellular Protein Degradation ..... 372
Role of Ruminal Fungi in Intracellular Protein Degradation ..... 374
Major Factors Affecting Protein Degradation in the Rumen ..... 374
Effects of Type of Dietary Protein on Its Degradation in the Rumen ..... 374

Effects of Type of Carbohydrate on Microbial Protein Synthesis in the Rumen....375
Effects of Dietary Concentrate and Forage Intake on Proteolytic Bacteria in the Rumen....376
Nutritional Importance of Protein Digestion in the Rumen....377
Protecting High-Quality Protein and Supplements of AAs from Rumen Degradation....378
Heating....378
Chemical Treatments....379
Polyphenolic Phytochemicals....379
Physical Encapsulation of Protein or AAs....379
Inhibition of AA Degradation....379
Flow of Microbial Protein from the Rumen into the Abomasum and Duodenum....379
Digestion of Microbial and Feed Proteins in the Abomasum and Small Intestine....381
Digestion and Absorption of Nucleic Acids in the Small Intestine....382
Nitrogen Recycling in Ruminants and Its Nutritional Implications....382
Fermentation of Protein in the Large Intestine of Nonruminants and Ruminants....384
Nonruminants....384
Ruminants....384
Digestion and Absorption of Protein in Fish....384
Developmental Changes of Gastric Proteases in Fish....384
Developmental Changes in Extracellular Proteases in the Intestine of Fish....385
Bioavailability of Dietary AAs to Extra-Digestive Organs....385
Net Entry of Dietary AAs from the Small Intestine into the Portal Vein....385
Extraction of AAs from the Portal Vein by the Liver....385
Endogenous Synthesis of AAs in Animals....387
Needs for Endogenous Synthesis of AAs in Animals....387
EAAs as Precursors for Synthesis of NEAAs....388
Cell- and Tissue-Specific Syntheses of AAs....390
Species Differences in Syntheses of AAs....392
Synthesis of AAs from Their α-Ketoacids or Analogs in Animal Cells and Bacteria....392
Syntheses of D-AAs in Animal Cells and Bacteria....394
Regulation of AA Syntheses in Animals....394
Degradation of AAs in Animals....395
Partition of AAs into Pathways for Catabolism and Protein Synthesis....395
Cell- and Tissue-Specific Degradation of AAs....396
Compartmentalization of AA Degradation in Cells....401
Interorgan Metabolism of Dietary AAs....402
Intestinal–Renal Axis for Arg Synthesis....402
Renal Gln Utilization for Regulation of Acid–Base Balance....402
Gln and Ala Synthesis from BCAAs....402
Conversion of Pro to Gly through Hydroxyproline....404
NO-Dependent Blood Flow....404
Regulation of AA Oxidation to Ammonia and $CO_2$....405
Detoxification of Ammonia as Urea via the Urea Cycle in Mammals....406
The Urea Cycle for Disposal of Ammonia in Mammals....406
Energy Requirement of Urea Synthesis....407
Regulation of the Urea Cycle....408
Detoxification of Ammonia as Uric Acid in Birds....408

Uric Acid Synthesis for Disposal of Ammonia in Birds ........ 408
Energy Requirement of Uric acid Synthesis ........ 410
Species Differences in Uric Acid Degradation ........ 410
Regulation of Uric Acid Synthesis ........ 411
Comparison between Urea and Uric Acid Synthesis ........ 411
Species-Specific Degradation of AAs ........ 412
Major Products of AA Catabolism in Animals ........ 413
Intracellular Protein Turnover ........ 414
Intracellular Protein Synthesis ........ 414
Gene Transcription to form mRNA ........ 417
Initiation of mRNA Translation to Generate Peptides at Ribosomes ........ 417
Peptide Elongation to Produce Protein ........ 418
Termination of Peptide Chain Elongation ........ 418
Posttranslational Modifications of Newly Synthesized Proteins ........ 418
Protein Synthesis in Mitochondria ........ 420
Energy Requirement of Protein Synthesis ........ 420
Measurement of Protein Synthesis ........ 421
Intracellular Protein Degradation ........ 422
Proteases for Intracellular Protein Degradation ........ 422
Intracellular Proteolytic Pathways ........ 422
Biological Half-Lives of Proteins ........ 423
Energy Requirement for Intracellular Protein Degradation ........ 423
Measurements of Intracellular Protein Degradation ........ 423
Nutritional and Physiological Significance of Protein Turnover ........ 424
Nutritional and Hormonal Regulation of Intracellular Protein Turnover ........ 426
Dietary Provision of AAs and Energy ........ 426
MTOR Cell Signaling ........ 426
Physiological and Pathological Stresses ........ 427
Dietary Requirements for AAs by Animals ........ 428
Needs for Formulating Dietary AA Requirements of Animals ........ 428
General Considerations of Dietary Requirements of AAs ........ 428
Qualitative Requirements of Dietary AAs ........ 429
Quantitative Requirements of Dietary AAs ........ 430
Factors Affecting Dietary Requirements of AAs ........ 432
The "Ideal Protein" Concept ........ 432
Evaluation of the Quality of Dietary Protein and AAs ........ 433
Analysis of AAs in Diets and Feed Ingredients ........ 433
Determination of Protein Digestibility ........ 434
Apparent vs. True Digestibility of Dietary Protein ........ 434
Measurement of $AA_{EIb}$ in the Small Intestine with the Use of an Indicator Technique ........ 436
Measurement of Protein Digestibility of a Feed Ingredient Added to a Basal Diet ........ 436
Animal Feeding Experiments to Determine the Quality of Dietary Protein ........ 437
Summary ........ 438
References ........ 439

**Chapter 8** Energy Metabolism ........ 449

Basic Concepts of Energy ........ 449
Definition of Energy ........ 449

Unit of Energy in Animal Nutrition ........ 450
Gibbs Free Energy ........ 451
ATP Synthesis in Cells ........ 452
Partition of Food Energy in Animals ........ 453
Gross Energy ........ 453
Digestible Energy ........ 454
Definition of Digestible Energy ........ 454
Losses of Fecal Energy in Various Animals ........ 454
Measurements of the Digestibility of Feeds ........ 456
Metabolizable Energy ........ 457
Net Energy and Heat Increment ........ 458
Energetic Efficiency of Metabolic Transformations in Animals ........ 462
Determination of Heat Production as an Indicator of Energy Expenditure by Animals ........ 468
Total Heat Production by Animals ........ 468
Direct Calorimetry for Measurement of Heat Production ........ 469
Indirect Calorimetry for Measurement of Heat Production ........ 470
Closed-Circuit Indirect Calorimetry ........ 470
Open-Circuit Indirect Calorimetry ........ 471
Comparative Slaughter Technique for Estimating Heat Production ........ 471
Lean Tissues and Energy Expenditure ........ 472
Usefulness of RQ Values in Assessing Substrate Oxidation in Animals ........ 473
Caution in the Interpretation of RQ Values ........ 474
Summary ........ 475
References ........ 476

**Chapter 9** Nutrition and Metabolism of Vitamins ........ 479

Chemical and Biochemical Characteristics of Vitamins ........ 479
General Characteristics of Vitamins ........ 479
General Sources of Vitamins for Animals ........ 480
Water-Soluble Vitamins ........ 481
Thiamin (Vitamin $B_1$) ........ 482
Riboflavin (Vitamin $B_2$) ........ 486
Niacin (Vitamin $B_3$) ........ 488
Pantothenic Acid (Pantothenate) ........ 491
Pyridoxal, Pyridoxine, and Pyridoxamine (Vitamin $B_6$) ........ 494
Biotin ........ 497
Vitamin $B_{12}$ (Cobalamin) ........ 500
Folate ........ 503
Ascorbic Acid (Vitamin C) ........ 507
Lipid-Soluble Vitamins ........ 511
Vitamin A ........ 512
Vitamin D ........ 518
Vitamin E ........ 522
Vitamin K ........ 526
Quasi-Vitamins ........ 530
Choline ........ 531
Carnitine ........ 534
*myo*-Inositol ........ 535
Lipoic Acid ........ 537

Pyrroloquinoline Quinone ... 538
Ubiquinones ... 539
Bioflavonoids ... 541
*para*-Aminobenzoic Acid ... 542
Summary ... 543
References ... 545

**Chapter 10** Nutrition and Metabolism of Minerals ... 553

Overall Views of Minerals ... 555
Chemistry of Minerals ... 555
Overall View of Absorption of Dietary Minerals ... 556
General Functions of Minerals ... 559
Macrominerals ... 561
Sodium ... 561
Potassium ... 565
Chloride ... 567
Calcium ... 569
Phosphorus ... 572
Magnesium ... 574
Sulfur (S) ... 576
Microminerals ... 578
Iron ($Fe^{2+}$ and $Fe^{3+}$) ... 578
Zinc (Zn) ... 585
Copper (Cu) ... 589
Manganese (Mn) ... 594
Cobalt ... 596
Molybdenum ... 597
Selenium ... 599
Chromium ... 602
Iodine ... 602
Fluorine ... 604
Boron ... 605
Bromine ... 607
Nickel ... 608
Silicon ... 609
Vanadium ... 610
Tin (Sn) ... 612
Toxic Metals ... 613
Aluminum (Al) ... 613
Arsenic (As) ... 615
Cadmium (Cd) ... 617
Lead (Pb) ... 618
Mercury (Hg) ... 618
Summary ... 621
References ... 623

**Chapter 11** Nutritional Requirements for Maintenance and Production ... 633

Nutritional Requirements for Maintenance ... 634
Energy Requirements for Maintenance ... 634
Additional Factors Affecting the BMR ... 635

Metabolic Size of Animals ........ 635
Age and Sex of Animals ........ 635
Normal Living Conditions of Animals ........ 636
Protein and AA Requirements for Maintenance ........ 636
Fatty Acid Requirements for Maintenance ........ 637
Vitamin Requirements for Maintenance ........ 638
Mineral Requirements for Maintenance ........ 638
Water Requirements for Maintenance ........ 638
Use of Energy and Its Substrates for Maintenance ........ 641
Nutritional Requirements for Production ........ 641
Suboptimal Efficiencies of Animal Protein Production in Current Agricultural Systems ........ 642
Nutritional Requirements for Reproduction of Females ........ 643
Early Developmental Events of Conceptuses ........ 645
Effects of Nutrients and Related Factors on Reproductive Performance of Females ........ 648
Intrauterine Growth Restriction ........ 650
Determination of Nutrient Requirements by Gestating Dams ........ 650
Nutritional Requirements for Reproduction of Males ........ 651
Overall Undernutrition or Overnutrition ........ 651
Protein and Arginine Intake ........ 651
Deficiencies of Minerals and Vitamins ........ 651
Diseases, Toxins, Stress, and Excess Minerals ........ 652
Fetal and Neonatal Programming ........ 652
Nutritional Requirements for Postnatal Growth of Animals ........ 652
Components of Animal Growth ........ 652
Absolute versus Relative Rate of Animal Growth ........ 653
Regulation of Animal Growth by Anabolic Agents ........ 654
Compensatory Growth ........ 656
Critical Role of Dietary AA Intake in Animal Growth ........ 657
Nutritional Requirements for Milk Production ........ 658
Mammary Gland ........ 658
Milk Synthesis by MECs ........ 662
Release of Milk Proteins, Lactose, and Fats from MECs to the Lumen of the Alveoli ........ 668
Efficiency of Energy Utilization for Milk Production ........ 669
Nutritional Requirements for Production of Muscular Work ........ 669
Energy Conversion in Skeletal Muscle ........ 669
High Requirements for Dietary Energy, Protein, and Minerals for Muscular Work ........ 670
Nutritional Requirements for Production of Wool and Feathers ........ 672
Wool Production in Sheep and Goats ........ 672
Nutritional Requirements for Production of Eggs in Poultry ........ 672
Composition of the Egg ........ 672
Formation of the Egg ........ 673
High Requirements for Dietary Energy, Protein, and Calcium for Egg Production ........ 674
Feather Growth and Color of Birds ........ 675
Summary ........ 676
References ........ 679

**Chapter 12** Regulation of Food Intake by Animals ..... 687

Regulation of Food Intake by Nonruminants ..... 687
Control Centers in the Central Nervous System ..... 687
Hypothalamus, Neurotransmitters, and Neuropeptides ..... 687
Leptin and Insulin ..... 689
Ghrelin ..... 691
Peptide YY ..... 691
Cholecystokinin ..... 691
Glucagon-Like Peptide-1 ..... 692
Control of Food Intake by Nutrients and Metabolites ..... 692
Dietary Energy Content ..... 692
Dietary Content of Sweet Sugars ..... 692
Glucose Concentrations in the Plasma ..... 692
Protein and AAs ..... 694
Fatty Acids and Ketone Bodies ..... 697
Nitric Oxide ..... 698
Serotonin ..... 698
Norepinephrine ..... 698
Other Chemical Factors ..... 699
Regulation of Food Intake by Ruminants ..... 699
Physical Limits of the Rumen ..... 699
Control of Food Intake by Nutrients and Metabolites ..... 700
Dietary Energy Content ..... 700
Dietary Nitrogen Content ..... 700
Glucose ..... 700
Short-Chain Fatty Acids ..... 701
Diet Selection in Nonruminants and Ruminants ..... 701
Nonruminants ..... 701
Ruminants ..... 702
Economic Benefits of Feed Efficiency Improvement ..... 702
Summary ..... 703
References ..... 704

**Chapter 13** Feed Additives ..... 709

Enzyme Additives ..... 709
Overview ..... 709
Special Thermozymes for Feeds ..... 710
Enzyme Additives for Nonruminants ..... 711
β-Glucanases ..... 711
Pentosanases (Arabinase and Xylanase) ..... 712
Other Enzymes ..... 715
Enzyme Additives for Ruminants ..... 716
Nonenzyme Additives ..... 718
Nonruminants ..... 718
Antibiotics ..... 719
Direct-Fed Microbials (Probiotics) ..... 721
Prebiotics ..... 722
Agents to Remove or Absorb Mycotoxins in Feeds ..... 722
Ruminants ..... 723

Ionophore Antibiotics ........ 724
Direct-Fed Microbials........ 725
Other Substances for Ruminants and Nonruminants........ 725
Amino Acids and Related Compounds ........ 725
Anti-Mold Feed Additives and Antioxidants ........ 726
*Yucca schidigera* Extract (BIOPOWDER)........ 726
Summary ........ 728
References ........ 729

**Index**........ 735

# Preface

Animals are biological transformers of dietary matter and energy into high-quality foods (e.g., meats, eggs, and milk) for human consumption, as well as raw materials (e.g., wool and leather) for clothing and accessories for humans. Through biotechnological techniques, animals are also employed to produce enzymes and proteins to treat a wide array of human diseases. Mammals, birds, fish, and shrimp possess both common and divergent metabolic pathways for their maintenance and adaptations, but all of them need food to survive, grow, develop, and reproduce. Thus, animal nutrition is a foundational subject of great importance to the production of livestock (e.g., cattle, goats, pigs, rabbits, and sheep), poultry (e.g., chickens, ducks, geese, and turkeys), and fish (e.g., common carp, large-mouth bass, salmon, and tilapia), as well as the health and well-being of companion animals (e.g., cats, dogs, ferrets, gerbils, horses, and parrots). As an interesting, dynamic, and challenging discipline in biological sciences, animal nutrition spans an immense range of topics, from chemistry, biochemistry, anatomy, and physiology to reproductive biology, immunology, pathology, and cell biology. Knowledge of these subjects is necessary for an adequate understanding of the principles of animal nutrition.

There is a rich history of research on laboratory, farm, and companion animals. *The Principles of Animal Nutrition*, with Special Reference to the Nutrition of Farm Animals was published by H.P. Armsby in 1902, which summarized the knowledge of animal nutrition gained in the nineteen century. In the past 56 years, since I.E. Coop wrote *The Principles and Practice of Animal Nutrition* in 1961, the field of animal nutrition and metabolism has developed rapidly because of great advances in biochemistry, physiology, and analytical techniques. Of particular note, many species differences in the digestion, assimilation, and excretion of nutrients were illustrated in: *Animal Nutrition (6th ed., 1979)* by L.A. Maynard and J.K. Loosli, *Comparative Animal Nutrition and Metabolism* by P.R. Cheeke and E.S. Dierenfeld (2010), and *Principles of Companion Animal Nutrition* (2nd ed., 2010) by J.P. McNamara. Additionally, more applied books include: *Basic Animal Nutrition and Feeding* (5th ed.) by W.G. Pond, D.C. Church, K.R. Pond, and P.A. Schoknecht (2004); *Animal Nutrition* by P. McDonald, R.A. Edwards, J.F.D. Greenhalgh, C.A. Morgan, and L.A. Sinclair (2011); and *Animal Feeding and Nutrition* by M.H. Jurgens, K. Bregendahl, J. Coverdale, and S.L. Hansen (2012). While those publications highlighted the feeds and practical feeding of livestock and poultry, a comprehensive and systematic coverage of the biochemical and physiological bases of animal nutrition is warranted to better understand the "black box" of the animal systems. With this in mind, and with the support of CRC Press, a project to write a new, well-organized book entitled *Principles of Animal Nutrition* was launched in June 2014.

*Principles of Animal Nutrition* consists of 13 chapters. This book begins with an overview of the physiological and biochemical bases of animal nutrition (Chapter 1), which is followed by a detailed description of chemical properties of carbohydrates (Chapter 2), lipids (Chapter 3), and protein/amino acids (Chapter 4). The text then advances to the current understanding of the digestion, absorption, transport, and metabolism of carbohydrates (Chapter 5), lipids (Chapter 6), protein/amino acids (Chapter 7), energy (Chapter 8), vitamins (Chapter 9), and minerals (Chapter 10) in animals, as well as interactions among nutrients (Chapters 5 through 10). To integrate the basic knowledge of nutrition with practical animal feeding, the monograph continues with a discussion on nutritional requirements of animals for maintenance and production (Chapter 11), as well as the regulation of food intake by animals (Chapter 12). Finally, this book ends with information on feed additives, including those used to enhance animal growth and survival, improve feed efficiency for protein production, and replace feed antibiotics. While the classical and modern concepts of animal nutrition are emphasized throughout this book, every effort has been made to include the most recent progress in this ever-expanding field so that readers in various biological disciplines can integrate biochemistry and physiology with nutrition, health, and disease in mammals, birds, and other animal species (e.g., fish and shrimp). At the end of each chapter, selected references are listed to provide readers with both comprehensive reviews of the chosen topics and original experimental data. Reading the scientific literature is essential for: (a) a thorough understanding of the history of the field, (b) creative thinking, and (c) rigorous development as a productive scientist. In the Index section, a list of key words, phrases, and abbreviations is provided to help readers quickly find information presented in all chapters.

This book owes its origin to the lecture notes of four graduate courses (ANSC/NUTR 601 "General Animal Nutrition," ANSC/NUTR 603 "Experimental Nutrition," ANSC/NUTR 613 "Protein Metabolism," and NUTR 641 "Nutritional Biochemistry") that the author has taught at Texas A&M University as a faculty member over the past 25 years. This book can be used as a reference or textbook by both senior undergraduates and graduate students majoring in animal science, biochemistry, biomedical engineering, biology, human medicine, food science, kinesiology, nutrition, pharmacology, physiology, toxicology, veterinary medicine, and other related disciplines. In addition, all chapters provide useful references to general and specific knowledge about the principles of animal nutrition for researchers and practitioners in biomedicine, agriculture (including animal science and plant breeding), and aquaculture, and for government policymakers.

Animal agriculture plays an important role in improving human nutrition, growth, and health, as well as economic and social developments worldwide. The global population was 7.4 billion in 2016 and has been projected to be 9.6 billion in 2050. With the increases in global population and human consumption of meats, milk, and eggs per capita, demands for animal-source protein and other animal products are expected to increase by 70% between 2016 and 2050 worldwide. With a daunting task to fully understand the biology of animals, maximally enhance the efficiency of metabolic transformations of feed into animal products, and continuously sustain animal agriculture, animal nutritionists face tremendous challenges to produce livestock, poultry, and fish for feeding the growing population in our world. *Principles of Animal Nutrition* is expected to guide and transform the practice of animal nutrition to greatly facilitate the achievement of this noble goal in the coming years.

The sciences of animal nutrition have been built on the shoulders of many giants and pioneers worldwide. Their seminal contributions to the field have made this book possible. The author must apologize to those whose published works are not cited in the text due to space limitations. Finally, sincere thanks are extended to the author's past and current students for constructive comments on his courses and for helpful discussions to improve the classroom presentations on the subject matter of animal nutrition.

**Guoyao Wu**

*June 2017*
*College Station, Texas, USA*

# Acknowledgments

This book was initiated at the invitation of Ms. Randy L. Brehm, a senior editor at CRC Press, and completed with the patience and guidance of its editorial staff. The author would like to thank Ms. Ruthann M. Cranford, Mr. Sudath Dahanayaka, Mr. B. Daniel Long, Mr. Kaiji Sun, and Mr. Neil D. Wu for their assistance in drawing the structures and metabolic pathways of nutrients, as well as preparing all chapters of the manuscript text. The help of Dr. Gregory A. Johnson in illustrating urea recycling in ruminants and the cell structure and of Dr. Zhaolai Dai in preparing a table of major gastrointestinal bacteria is gratefully appreciated. Sincere thanks also go to the following accomplished scientists for critically reviewing various chapters and providing constructive suggestions for improvement:

- Prof. Fuller W. Bazer, Department of Animal Science, Texas A&M University, College Station, TX;
- Prof. Werner G. Bergen, Department of Animal Science, Auburn University, Auburn, AL;
- Prof. John T. Brosnan, Department of Biochemistry, Memorial University of Newfoundland, St. John's, Canada;
- Prof. Margaret E. Brosnan, Department of Biochemistry, Memorial University of Newfoundland, St. John's, Canada;
- Prof. Jeffrey L. Firkins, Department of Animal Science, Ohio State University, Columbia, OH;
- Prof. Catherine J. Field, Faculty of Medicine, University of Alberta, Edmonton, Canada;
- Prof. Nick E. Flynn, Department of Chemistry and Physics, West Texas A&M University, Canyon, TX;
- Prof. Wayne Greene, Department of Animal Science, Auburn University, Auburn, AL;
- Prof. Chien-An Andy Hu, Department of Biochemistry and Molecular Biology, University of New Mexico, Albuquerque, NM;
- Prof. Shengfa F. Liao, Department of Animal and Dairy Sciences, Mississippi State University, MS;
- Prof. Timothy A. McAllister, Agriculture and Agri-Food Canada, Lethbridge, Alberta, Canada;
- Prof. Cynthia J. Meininger, Department of Medical Physiology, Texas A&M University, College Station, TX;
- Prof. Steven Nizielski, Department of Biomedical Sciences, Grand Valley State University, Allendale, MI;
- Prof. James L. Sartin, Department of Anatomy, Physiology, and Pharmacology, Auburn University, Auburn, AL;
- Prof. Stephen B. Smith, Department of Animal Science, Texas A&M University, College Station, TX;
- Prof. Luis O. Tedeschi, Department of Animal Science, Texas A&M University, College Station, TX;
- Prof. James R. Thompson, Animal Science Program, University of British Columbia, Vancouver, Canada;
- Prof. Nancy D. Turner, Department of Nutrition and Food Science, Texas A&M University, College Station, TX;
- Prof. Rosemary L. Walzem, Department of Poultry Science, Texas A&M University, College Station, TX;
- Prof. Hong-Cai Zhou, Department of Chemistry, Texas A&M University, College Station, TX.

The author is appreciative of the important contributions of his former and current students, postdoctoral fellows, visiting scholars, and technicians to the conduct of research and valuable discussions. He is also very grateful to his graduate advisors, Prof. Sheng Yang and Dr. James R. Thompson, as well as postdoctoral mentors Dr. Errol B. Marliss and Dr. John T. Brosnan for training in animal biochemistry, nutrition, and physiology, as well as their enthusiastic support and inspiration for a lifelong pursuit of these disciplines. Productive and enjoyable collaborations with colleagues at Texas A&M University (particularly Drs. Fuller W. Bazer, Robert C. Burghardt, R. Russell Cross, Harris J. Granger, Gregory A. Johnson, Darrell A. Knabe, Catherine J. McNeal, Cynthia J. Meininger, Jayanth Ramadoss, M. Carey Satterfield, Jeffrey W. Savell, Stephen B. Smith, Thomas E. Spencer, Carmen D. Tekwe, Nancy D. Turner, Shannon E. Washburn, Renyi Zhang, and Huaijun Zhou), as well as at other institutions (particularly David H. Baker, Makoto Bannai, Francois Blachier, Douglas G. Burrin, Zhaolai Dai, Teresa A. Davis, Catherine J. Field, Susan K. Fried, Yongqing Hou, Shinzato Izuru, Zongyong Jiang, Sung Woo Kim, Xiangfeng Kong, Defa Li, Ju Li, Peng Li, Shengfa Liao, Gert Lubec, Wilson G. Pond, Peter J. Reeds, J. Marc Rhoads, Ana San Gabriel, Bie Tan, Nathalie L. Trottier, Binggen Wang, Genhu Wang, Xiaolong Wang, Fenglai Wang, Junjun Wang, Malcolm Watford, Zhenlong Wu, Shixuan Zheng, Weiyun Zhu, Kang Yao, and Yulong Yin), are gratefully acknowledged. Furthermore, the author is indebted to the past and current heads of the Department of Animal Science at Texas A&M University for their support of his research and teaching programs.

Work in the author's laboratory was supported, in part, by funds from Ajinomoto Inc. (Tokyo, Japan), American Heart Association, The Chinese Academy of Science, Gentech Inc. (Shanghai, China), Guangdong Yuehai Feeds Group Co., Ltd. (Zhanjiang, China), Houston Livestock Show and Rodeo, Henan Yinfa Animal Industries Co. (Zhengzhou, China), the Hubei Hundred-People Talent Program at Wuhan Polytechnic University, International Council of Amino Acid Science (Brussels, Belgium), International Glutamate Technical Committee (Brussels, Belgium), JBS United (Sheridan, Indiana), Juvenile Diabetes Research Foundation (USA), National Institutes of Health (USA), National Natural Science Foundation of China, Pfizer Inc., Scott & White Hospital (Temple, TX), Texas A&M AgriLife Research, Texas A&M University, the Thousand-People Talent Program at China Agricultural University, United States Department of Agriculture, U.S. National Corn Growers Association, U.S. National Watermelon Promotion Board, and U.S. Poultry & Egg Harold E. Ford Foundation.

Special thanks are extended to thousands of scientists who have made great contributions to our understanding of the principles of animal nutrition. The author has enjoyed reading their articles and acquired a great deal of knowledge from the published work. Finally, the professional typesetting of the entire manuscript by Mr. Ragesh K. Nair and his staff of Nova Techset at Techset Composition is gratefully acknowledged.

# Author

**Dr. Guoyao Wu** is a University Distinguished Professor, University Faculty Fellow, and Texas A&M AgriLife Research Senior Faculty Fellow at Texas A&M University. He received his BS in Animal Science from South China Agricultural University in Guangzhou, China (1978–1982), MS in Animal Nutrition from China Agricultural University in Beijing, China (1982–1984), and MSc (1984–1986) and PhD (1986–1989) in Animal Biochemistry from the University of Alberta in Edmonton, Canada. Dr. Wu completed his postdoctoral training in diabetes, nutrition, and biochemistry at McGill University Faculty of Medicine in Montreal, Canada (1989–1991) and Memorial University of Newfoundland Faculty of Medicine in St. John's, Canada (1991). He joined the Texas A&M University faculty in October 1991. Dr. Wu's sabbatical leave was to study human obesity at the University of Maryland School of Medicine in Baltimore, USA (2005).

Dr. Wu has taught graduate (experimental nutrition, general animal nutrition, protein metabolism, and nutritional biochemistry) and undergraduate (problems in animal science, nutrition, and biochemistry) courses at Texas A&M University over the past 25 years. He has given numerous lectures at other institutions in the U.S., Canada, Mexico, Brazil, Europe, and Asia. His research focuses on the biochemistry, nutrition, and physiology of amino acids and related nutrients in animals at genetic, molecular, cellular, and whole-body levels. Research interests include: (1) functions of AAs in gene expression (including epigenetics) and cell signaling; (2) mechanisms that regulate intracellular synthesis and catabolism of proteins and AAs; (3) hormonal and nutritional regulation of homeostasis of metabolic fuels; (4) biology and pathobiology of nitric oxide and polyamines; (5) key roles of AAs in preventing metabolic diseases (including diabetes, obesity, and intrauterine growth restriction) and associated cardiovascular complications; (6) essential roles of AAs in survival, growth, and development of embryos, fetuses, and neonates; (7) dietary requirements of AAs and proteins in the life cycle; and (8) animal models (e.g., pigs, rats, and sheep) for studying human metabolic diseases.

Dr. Wu has published 540 papers in peer-reviewed journals, including *Advance in Nutrition, Amino Acids, American Journal of Physiology, Annals of New York Academy of Sciences, Annual Review of Animal Biosciences, Annual Review of Nutrition, Biochemical Journal, Biology of Reproduction, British Journal of Nutrition, Cancer Research, Clinical and Experimental Immunology, Comparative Biochemistry and Physiology, Diabetes, Diabetologia, Endocrinology, Experimental Biology and Medicine, FASEB Journal, Food & Function, Frontiers in Bioscience, Frontiers in Immunology, Gut, Journal of Animal Science, Journal of Animal Science and Biotechnology, Journal of Agricultural and Food Chemistry, Journal of Biological Chemistry, Journal of Chromatography, Journal of Nutrition, Journal of Nutritional Biochemistry, Journal of Pediatrics, Journal of Physiology (London), Livestock Science, Molecular and Cellular Endocrinology, Molecular Reproduction and Development, Proceedings of National Academy of Science USA*, and *Reproduction*, and 58 book chapters. Dr. Wu's work has been extensively cited in Google Scholar over 38,000 times, with an H-index of 100. Three of his papers have each been cited more than 2,200 times. He was a Most Cited Author and a Most Influential Scientific Mind (2014–2016) in the Web of Science (Institute for Scientific Information), and was among the 10 most cited scientists in the field of agricultural sciences (2016) worldwide.

Dr. Wu has received numerous prestigious awards from China, Canada, and the United States, which include the China National Scholarship for Graduate Studies Abroad (1984), The University of Alberta Andrew Stewart Graduate Prize (1989), Medical Research Council of Canada Postdoctoral Fellowship (1989), American Heart Association Established Investigator Award (1998), Texas A&M AgriLife Faculty Fellow (2001), Texas A&M University Faculty Fellow (2002), Nonruminant Nutrition Research Award from the American Society of Animal Science (2004), Outstanding Young Investigator Award from the National Science Foundation of China (2005), Texas A&M

Agriculture Program Vice Chancellor's Award for Excellence in Team (2006) and Individual (2008) Research, and in Diversity (2011), Changjiang Scholar Award from China (2008), Texas A&M University Distinguished Research Achievement Award (2008), Texas A&M Agrilife Research Senior Faculty Fellow Award (2008), Chutian Scholar Award from Hubei Province of China (2008), FASS-AFIA New Frontiers in Animal Nutrition Research Award from the Federation of Animal Science Societies and American Feed Industry Association (2009), Dingying Scholar Award from South China Agricultural University (2009), the Thousand-People-Talent Award from China (2010), the Samburu Collaboration Award from the International Association of Giraffe Care Professionals (2010), Distinguished Scientist of Sigma Xi Honor Society—Texas A&M University Chapter (2013), and the Hundred Talent Award from the Hubei Province of China (2014).

Dr. Wu is a member and elected Fellow of the American Association for the Advancement of Science, as well as a member of the American Heart Association, American Society of Animal Science, American Society of Nutrition, and Society for the Study of Reproduction. He has served on Editorial Advisory Boards for *Biochemical Journal* (1993–2005), *Journal of Animal Science and Biotechnology* (2010–Present), *Journal of Nutrition* (1997–2003), and *Journal of Nutritional Biochemistry* (2006–present), as well as being an editor of *Amino Acids* (2008–present), an editor of *Journal of Amino Acids* (2009–Present), editor-in-chief of *SpringerPlus—Amino Acids Collections* (2012–2016), and as the managing editor (2009–2016) and editor (2017–present) of *Frontiers in Bioscience*.

# 1 Physiological and Biochemical Bases of Animal Nutrition

The word "animal" is derived from the Latin word *animalis*, meaning "having breath," "having soul," and "living being." All animals are multicellular, eukaryotic, and motile organisms of the kingdom *Animalia* (Dallas and Jewell 2014). With adequate intake of nutrients, they survive, grow, develop, and reproduce as important parts of the ecosystem. Animals can be divided into two broad groups: vertebrates (animals with a backbone; e.g., amphibians, birds, fishes, mammals, and reptiles) and invertebrates (animals without a backbone; e.g., corals, clams, crabs, insects, lobsters, oysters, shrimp, spiders, and worms). On the basis of the types of food they consume, animals are classified as (1) carnivores (e.g., cats, dogs, ferrets, minks, and tigers) whose diets consist mainly of nonplant materials (e.g., meat, fish, and insects); (2) herbivores (ruminants [e.g., cattle, deer, goats, sheep, cervids, and New World camelids], horses, and rabbits) whose diets are composed primarily of plant materials; or (3) omnivores (e.g., humans, pigs, poultry, rats, and mice) whose diets include both plant and animal materials (Bondi 1987; Dyce et al. 1996). Among companion animals, cats are obligate carnivores, whereas dogs are facultative carnivores, and these two members of the order Carnivora have very different patterns of nutrient metabolism and requirements.

Wilson (1992) estimated that there were 1,032,000 animal species in nature, including 18,800 species of fish and lower chordates, 9,000 species of birds, 6,300 species of reptiles, 4,200 species of amphibians, and 4,000 species of mammals. Despite the vast diversity among vertebrates and invertebrates, animals exhibit greater similarities in physiology, metabolism, and nutrition than differences (Baker 2005; Beitz 1993; Wu 2013). To date, our understanding of animal nutrition is based primarily on practical feeding and scientific studies of a limited number of terrestrial vertebrate species (including cats, cattle, chickens, dogs, ducks, ferrets, goats, guinea pigs, horses, humans, mice, minks, pigs, rabbits, rats, sheep, and turkeys), and other aquatic and terrestrial species, including fish, shrimp, insects, and *Caenorhabditis elegans* (Cheeke and Dierenfeld 2010; McDonald et al. 2011; NRC 2002). In recent years, tremendous progress in the nutrition of wild animals has been made (Barboza et al. 2009).

Human civilization has a rich history of studies investigating the nutrient requirements of livestock, poultry, and fish during their life cycle under various physiological and pathological conditions (Baker 2005; Bergen 2007). This is because these agriculturally important animals are the major source of high-quality proteins, as well as vitamins and minerals, for consumption by humans and their companion animals to sustain their optimal growth, development, reproduction, and health (Davis et al. 2002; Reynolds et al. 2015; Wu et al. 2014b). Animal production accounts for 50%–75% and 25%–40% of the total amount of agricultural output in industrialized and developing nations, respectively (Wu et al. 2014a). Thus, research on farm animals has great scientific, social, and economic significance. In addition, rats and mice have long been used as animal models to discover dietary requirements for nutrients and metabolic diseases resulting from their deficiencies. Furthermore, elucidation of metabolic pathways has been facilitated by the occurrence of inherited diseases (knockdown or knockout of genes) in humans and animals (Brosnan et al. 2015; Vernon 2015). Therefore, extensive knowledge exists in the literature regarding the physiological and biochemical bases of nutrition in farm and laboratory animals (Asher and Sassone-Corsi 2015; Dellschaft et al. 2015; Rezaei et al. 2013), as well as humans (Bennett et al. 2015; Meredith 2009). Integration of these large databases provides a strong foundation for this book.

## FUNDAMENTAL CONCEPTS OF ANIMAL NUTRITION

### Definition of Nutrients and Diets

A nutrient is defined as a compound or substance needed to support the maintenance, growth, development, lactation, reproduction, and health of animals. A list of known nutrients required by animals is given in Table 1.1. Food is an edible material that contains nutrients. Food for farm animals (e.g., livestock, poultry, fish, and shrimp) is commonly known as feed. On the basis of their composition and use, feeds are classified as (1) dry forages (e.g., dried pasture, leaves, stems, green chop, and hay) and roughages (e.g., hay, straws, and hulls with >18% crude fiber); (2) green pasture, range plants, and freshly fed green forages (e.g., forage feeds); (3) silages (e.g., ensiled corn, alfalfa, and grass); (4) energy feeds (e.g., corn, wheat, barley, and rice); and (5) protein feeds (e.g., soybean meal, meat and bone meal, blood meal, poultry meal, fish meal, and milk replacer). Synthetic amino acids (AAs), mineral supplements, vitamin supplements, and other additives (e.g., antibiotics, coloring materials, flavors, phytochemicals, hormones, and medicines) may be included with feeds to prepare complete diets for animals.

Feedstuff is any material used for feed. An ingredient in feed is a component or constituent that comprises the feed. Thus, feedstuff and feed ingredient are interchangeable terms. Feed ingredients may be grains, milling byproducts, animal byproducts, vitamin premix, mineral premix, fats, oils, and other nutritional sources (McDonald et al. 2011). A diet is a mixture of feedstuffs that supplies nutrients to an animal. The ration is the daily allowance or amount of feed provided to an animal. A meal is the feed consumed by an animal on regular occasions (e.g., morning and evening). The sources of feedstuffs vary among animal species. For example, grazing ruminants consume pasture, whereas wild fish may ingest phytoplankton, zooplankton, microalgae, macroalgae, aquatic plants, insects, crustaceans, mollusks, shellfish, fish, birds, and mammals (Wilson and Castro 2011).

### Definition of Nutrition

According to the Merriam-Webster's dictionary (Merriam-Webster 2005), nutrition is "the act or process of nourishing or being nourished; specifically, the sum of the processes by which an animal takes in and utilizes food substances." Nutrition is also defined as the science that interprets the interaction of nutrients and other substances in food that influence the maintenance, growth, development, reproduction, and health of animals. Thus, nutrition includes: (1) food intake; (2) digestion, absorption, assimilation, biosynthesis, and catabolism of nutrients; and (3) excretion of metabolites. This definition implies that nutritional science is a cluster of scientific disciplines related to biology, which include biochemistry, food chemistry, immunology, molecular biology, pediatrics, pharmacology, physiology, public health, reproductive biology, and toxicology. Thus, animal nutrition includes essentially every biological science that can be applied to the study of nutrient utilization and nutritional problems in livestock, poultry, fish, and other species. Animal nutrition, like medicine, is a field for both scientists and practitioners, and it can be considered a unique discipline because of its specific objective: improving the survival, growth, and health of animals by understanding their metabolism and the roles of dietary nutrients (Dai et al. 2015; Ford et al. 2007; Hou et al. 2015; NRC 2002; Pond et al. 1995).

### Composition of Feedstuffs

All animals depend on feed for survival, growth, and reproduction. Thus, it is important to understand its basic components, which are dry matter (DM) and water (Figure 1.1). DM consists of organic and inorganic substances. Organic matter consists of carbohydrates, lipids, proteins, small peptides, free AAs, nucleic acids, other nitrogenous substances (e.g., urea, ammonia, nitrite, and nitrate), organic acids, and vitamins. Inorganic matter (ash) is composed of minerals and cannot be burned in a furnace (e.g., 400°C). Ash includes macrominerals and microminerals (Table 1.1). Some

## TABLE 1.1
## Nutrients Required by Animals

| Water and Macro Organic Nutrients | Vitamins and Minerals |
|---|---|
| Water | Vitamins |
| Glucose and fructose | Water-soluble vitamins |
| Protein or amino acids[a] | Thiamin (vitamin $B_1$) |
| Proteinogenic amino acids | Riboflavin (vitamin $B_2$) |
| Alanine | Niacin (nicotinic acid and nicotinamide; vitamin $B_3$) |
| Arginine | |
| Asparagine | Pantothenic acid (vitamin $B_5$) |
| Aspartate | Pyrodoxine, pyridoxal, and pyridoxamine (vitamin $B_6$) |
| Cysteine | |
| Glutamate | Cobalamin (vitamin $B_{12}$) |
| Glutamine | Biotin |
| Glycine | Folate (pteroylglutamic acid) |
| Histidine | Ascorbic acid (vitamin C) |
| Isoleucine | Choline |
| Leucine | Myo-inositol |
| Lysine | Lipid-soluble vitamins |
| Methionine | Vitamin A |
| Phenylalanine | Vitamin D |
| Proline | Vitamin E |
| Serine | Vitamin K |
| Threonine | Macrominerals |
| Tryptophan | Sodium |
| Tyrosine | Potassium |
| Valine | Chlorine |
| Nonproteinogenic amino acids | Calcium |
| Taurine | Phosphorus |
| Fatty acids | Magnesium |
| Linoleic acid (ω6, 18:2) and arachidonic acid[b] | Sulfur |
| α-Linolenic acid (ω3, 18:3), EPA,[b] and DHA[b] | Microminerals[c] |
| Fibers of plant source (for healthy intestine) | Possibly essential ultratrace elements[d] |

*Source:* Adapted from Pond, W.G. et al. 1995. *Basic Animal Nutrition and Feeding*, 4th ed. John Wiley & Sons, New York, NY; Rezaei, R. et al. 2013. *J. Anim. Sci. Biotechnol.* 4:7.

*Note:* DHA, 5,8,11,14,17,20-docosahexaenoic acid; EPA, 5,8,11,14,17-eicosapentaenoic acid.

[a] Animals may not be able to sufficiently synthesize all amino acids to meet the needs for maximal growth and production performance or for optimal health and well-being (Hou et al. 2016; Wu 2013).

[b] Small amounts in diets may be necessary for maximal growth and production performance or for optimal health and well-being.

[c] Including iron ($Fe^{2+}$ and $Fe^{3+}$), $zinc^{2+}$, copper ($Cu^{+}$ and $Cu^{2+}$), cobalt (Co), iodide ($I^{-}$), manganese ($Mn^{2+}$), selenium (Se), chromium ($Cr^{3+}$), molybdenum (Mo), silicon ($Si^{2+}$ and $Si^{4+}$), fluoride (F), vanadium (V), boron (B), nickel (Ni), and tin (Sn).

[d] Possibly essential ultratrace elements in animal nutrition include barium (Ba), bromine (Br), rubidium (Rb), and strontium (Sr).

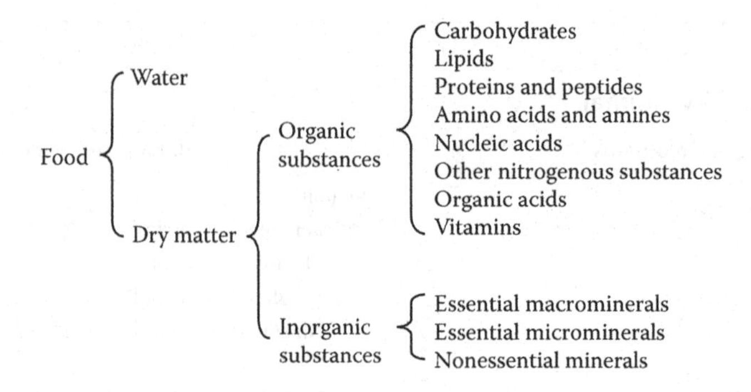


**FIGURE 1.1** Composition of foods from plants and animals. Foods consist of plant- and animal-source materials. Both plants and animals contain organic and inorganic substances. However, the types of proteins, carbohydrates, and lipids differ markedly between plants and animals, whereas nucleotides and minerals are the same in foods derived from both types of organisms. Animals contain vitamins A, C, D, E, and K, B-series vitamins, and cholecalciferol as the precursor of vitamin $D_3$. The structures of vitamins C and E and B-series vitamins in animals are the same as those in plants.

of the minerals are nutritionally nonessential and can even be toxic to animals. Note that arsenic (As), cadmium (Cd), mercury (Hg), and lead (Pb) are highly toxic to animals and humans (Pond et al. 1995). The composition of nutrients in some feedstuffs is given in Table 1.2. Comparison of nutrient content among diets should be made on a DM basis (Li et al. 2011).

## Composition of Animals

Like feed, an animal is also composed of water, nitrogenous compounds (e.g., protein, peptides, AA, and their nitrogen-containing metabolites), lipids, carbohydrates (e.g., glycogen, glucose, and fructose), water- and lipid-soluble vitamins, and macro- and microminerals (McDonald et al. 2011). Amounts of vitamins in the body are very small, but vital to metabolism and life. The composition and chemistry of proteins, lipids, and carbohydrates differ remarkably between feedstuffs and animals. Animals contain vitamins A, B series, C, D, E, and K, and cholecalciferol as the precursor of vitamin $D_3$ (Bondi 1987). The structures of vitamins C, B series, and E in animals are the same as those in plants (NRC 2012). Likewise, the chemistry of nucleotides and minerals is the same in feedstuffs and animals. The chemical composition of pigs, expressed on a fresh carcass basis, is given in Table 1.2. The percentages of fats in animals increase with increased age, but the opposite is true for body water content (Hu et al. 2015). This is because fats are hydrophobic and, therefore, their deposition reduces the water-holding capacity of the body. Of note, the percentage of proteins in animals increases moderately between birth and a young age and decreases thereafter (Pond et al. 1995). Knowledge about changes in the composition of animals with age helps nutritionists design balanced diets to maximize protein gain and minimize fat accretion in the body.

## Proximate or Weende Analysis of Feedstuffs

The traditional method used to determine the nutrient composition in feedstuffs and animals is known as the proximate or Weende analysis, which was devised in 1865 by Henneberg and Stohmann at the Weende Experiment Station in Germany. This scheme is outlined in Figure 1.2. The proximate methods readily provide information on (1) crude protein (CP), which is determined by the Kjeldahl analysis of total nitrogen (CP % = 6.25 × N %; Yin et al. 2002); (2) carbohydrates, which are separated into crude fiber and nitrogen-free extract (NFE); (3) NFE, which is a misnomer in that no extract is involved; indeed, NFE is measured by the difference between the original sample weight and the sum of the weights of water, crude fat, CP, crude fiber, and ash, rather than by

**TABLE 1.2**
**Composition of Nutrients in Feedstuffs and Pigs[a]**

| Feedstuffs or Pigs | Water | Crude Protein | Crude Fat | Minerals | Carbohydrates |
|---|---|---|---|---|---|
| **Composition of Nutrients in Feedstuffs (%, As-Fed Basis)** | | | | | |
| Blood meal | 6.74 ± 0.03 | 89.3 ± 0.14 | 1.43 ± 0.06 | 2.48 ± 0.07 | 0.05 ± 0.00 |
| Corn grain | 10.9 ± 0.05 | 9.20 ± 0.09 | 3.80 ± 0.12 | 1.40 ± 0.03 | 74.7 ± 1.3 |
| Fish meal | 7.95 ± 0.04 | 63.3 ± 0.33 | 9.70 ± 0.51 | 16.2 ± 1.2 | 2.85 ± 0.19 |
| Meat and bone meal | 4.53 ± 0.04 | 51.8 ± 0.28 | 9.24 ± 0.63 | 31.9 ± 1.5 | 2.53 ± 0.16 |
| Soybean meal | 11.0 ± 0.03 | 43.7 ± 0.12 | 1.24 ± 0.05 | 6.36 ± 0.11 | 37.7 ± 0.94 |
| Sorghum meal | 10.9 ± 0.03 | 9.98 ± 0.10 | 3.47 ± 0.18 | 1.65 ± 0.13 | 74.0 ± 1.6 |
| **Composition of Nutrients in Pigs (% of Wet Weight)** | | | | | |
| 1-day-old pigs (1.5 kg)[b] | 82.1 ± 0.07 | 12.7 ± 0.39 | 1.38 ± 0.07 | 3.16 ± 0.07 | 0.66 ± 0.04 |
| 14-day-old pigs (4.2 kg)[b] | 69.6 ± 0.82 | 14.9 ± 0.57 | 12.0 ± 0.88 | 3.07 ± 0.06 | 0.43 ± 0.03 |
| 60-day-old pigs (20 kg)[c] | 68.2 ± 0.70 | 14.7 ± 0.51 | 13.7 ± 0.76 | 2.98 ± 0.05 | 0.40 ± 0.02 |
| 120-day-old pigs (60 kg)[c] | 66.1 ± 0.75 | 14.4 ± 0.64 | 16.3 ± 0.82 | 2.85 ± 0.06 | 0.35 ± 0.03 |
| 180-day-old pigs (110 kg)[c] | 49.7 ± 0.52 | 12.3 ± 0.79 | 35.0 ± 2.04 | 2.71 ± 0.08 | 0.29 ± 0.02 |

[a] Values are means ± SEM, n = 6. The composition of nutrients in feedstuffs and pigs was determined as described by Wu et al. (1999). Data on crude protein content in feedstuffs were taken from Li et al. (2011). The pigs were the offspring of Yorkshire × Landrace dams and Duroc × Hampshire sires and weaned at 21 days of age to a milk replacer (Kim and Wu 2004). After a 10-day period of feeding, pigs were fed corn- and soybean-based diets to meet National Research Council nutrient requirements (NRC 2012). Gastrointestinal contents of pigs were excluded from chemical analyses of the bodies, which were performed as described by Li et al. (2011).

[b] Nursed by sows.

[c] Barrows (castrated male pigs).

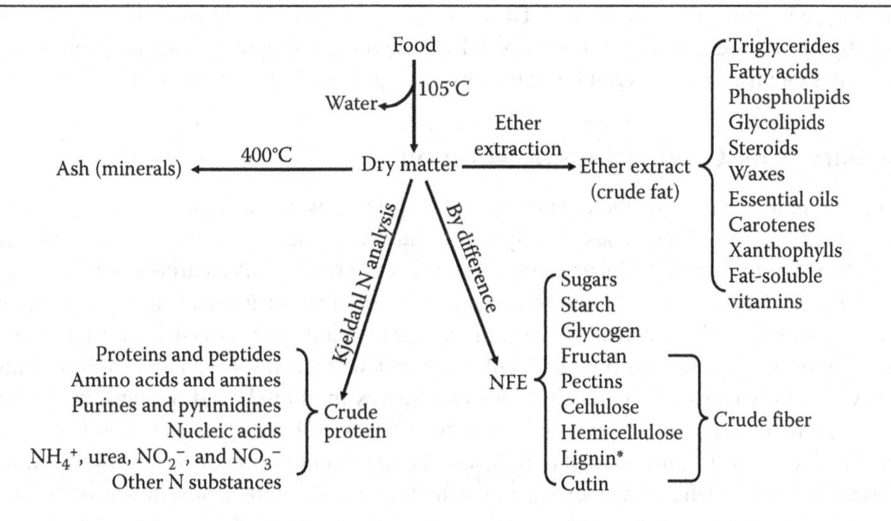


**FIGURE 1.2** Proximate analysis of nutrients in feedstuffs and animals tissues. This method provides useful information about the composition of water and dry matter (including crude protein [CP], crude fats [diethyl ether extracts], crude fiber, and other carbohydrates) in feedstuffs and animal tissues. Cutin is a plant cell wall material consisting of water-insoluble polyester polymers of long-chain hydroxyl acids (e.g., $C_{16}$- and $C_{18}$-carbon chains) and their derivatives. CP % = 6.25 × N %. Nitrogen-free extract (NFE) consists primarily of carbohydrates; it is calculated by difference and is not actually extracted from food. *Lignin is a class of cross-linked complex phenolic polymers that form important structural materials in plant cell walls.

direct analysis; and (4) volatile compounds (e.g., short-chain fatty acids [SCFAs; acetate, propionate, and butyrate] and essential oils [such as menthol and camphor]), which may be lost when DM is determined at 100–105°C for 12–24 h (Pond et al. 1995).

In proximate analysis, CP includes protein and other nitrogenous substances, including peptides, AAs, amines, polyamines, carnitine, creatine, purine and pyrimidine nucleotides, nucleic acids, ammonia, urea, nitrite, and nitrate (Wu 2013). Crude fat includes triglycerides, fatty acids, phospholipids, steroids, waxes, carotenes, and xanthophylls. Crude fiber includes cellulose, hemicellulose (partial), lignin (partial), and cutin. NFE consists of sugars, starches, glycogen, fructan, pectins, hemicellulose (partial), and lignin (partial) (Pond et al. 1995).

## Modified Methods for Analysis of Feedstuffs and Animals

The proximate analysis procedure has been criticized as being imprecise for quantifying protein, lipids, ash, and carbohydrates. AAs in food and animal proteins can now be routinely determined by high-performance liquid chromatography after acidic, alkaline, and enzymatic hydrolysis (Dai et al. 2014). Atomic absorption spectrophotometry is widely available for the analysis of individual minerals. Furthermore, procedures for the determination of plant fiber were developed by Peter Van Soest and coworkers at the USDA laboratories in the 1960s (Van Soest and Wine 1967). This scheme divides the nutrients in plants into cell walls and cell contents through the extraction of the test material with a boiling neutral detergent solution (3% sodium lauryl sulfate, 1.86% disodium ethylenediaminetetraacetate [EDTA], and 0.68% sodium tetraborate; pH = 7.0). Cell contents are soluble in a neutral detergent, whereas cell wall materials are insoluble in a neutral detergent and called neutral detergent fiber (NDF) (Table 1.3). NDF consists mainly of lignin, cellulose, and hemicellulose and is the most common measurement of plant fibers in the diets of ruminants and horses (Van Soest 1967). NDF is fractionated further by extraction with an acid detergent which solubilizes hemicellulose and fiber-bound protein. The acid detergent fiber (ADF) is the residue obtained after refluxing with 0.5 M sulfuric acid and cetyltrimethylammonium bromide and represents cellulose, lignin, acid- and heat-damaged protein, and silica (Van Soest and Wine 1967). The acid-soluble polysaccharide is hemicellulose. Thus, NDF is comprised of ADF and hemicellulose. The ADF is the least digestible fiber portion of forage or other roughage. The precise composition of complex carbohydrates can then be analyzed by liquid chromatography–mass spectrometry.

## Biochemistry as the Chemical Basis of Nutrition

Biochemistry is the science of the chemistry of living organisms, including microorganisms, animals, and plants (Devlin 2011). Thus, this dynamic and diverse field is also a foundation of nutrition. Biochemists study the synthesis, degradation, and roles of protein, AAs, carbohydrates, lipids, vitamins, and nucleic acids, as well as the function and metabolism of minerals at molecular, cellular, organ, and systemic levels. Biochemists have made significant progress in our understanding of how enzymes catalyze reactions and how molecules interact with each other. These professionals also play a key role in elucidating the mechanisms of diseases in animals and humans, such as inborn metabolic disorders (e.g., ammonia toxicity due to the lack of urea cycle enzymes and sickle-cell anemia), diabetes, cancer, cardiovascular diseases, *acquired immune deficiency syndrome*, and nutritional diseases due to a deficiency or excess of nutrients (e.g., AAs, fatty acids, minerals, or vitamins).

There is a significant overlap between nutrition and biochemistry. These two disciplines are interdependent and closely related. Biochemistry is the basis for studying the utilization of nutrients by animals and humans, whereas nutritional studies can provide observations that often lead to exciting biochemical studies. For example, the discovery of the Krebs cycle in 1937 was based on the nutritional question of how the chemical energy in ingested food or dietary protein, carbohydrates, and fats was converted into biological energy in animals. Also, the discovery of the hepatic urea cycle was prompted by the nutritional observation that urinary excretion of urea was elevated when

**TABLE 1.3**
**Classification of Forage Fractions Using the Van Soest Method**

| Fraction | Components | Nutritional Availability | |
|---|---|---|---|
| | | Ruminants | Nonruminants |
| Cell contents (soluble in neutral detergent)[b] | Sugars, soluble carbohydrates, starch | Complete | Complete |
| | Pectin | Complete | High[a] |
| | Nonprotein nitrogen | High | High |
| | Proteins | High | High |
| | Lipids | High | High |
| | Other solubles (e.g., amino acids) | High | High |
| Cell walls | | | |
| Soluble in acid detergent | Hemicelluloses[c] | Partial | Low |
| | Fiber-bound protein | Partial | Low |
| Insoluble in acid detergent (ADF)[d] | Cellulose | Partial | Low |
| | Lignin | Partial | Indigestible |
| | Heat-damaged protein | Indigestible | Indigestible |
| | Silica | Not available | Not available |

*Source:* Adapted from Van Soest, P.J. 1967. *J. Anim. Sci.* 26:119–128.

[a] High fermentation in the large intestine to provide short-chain fatty acids for colonocytes.

[b] The materials which are soluble in a neutral detergent solution are highly digestible in animals. The materials which are insoluble in the neutral detergent solution are called neutral detergent fiber (NDF) and include hemicellulose, cellulose, and lignin. The NDF is indigestible in nonruminants, while hemicellulose and cellulose are partially digestible in ruminants.

[c] Hemicellulose, cellulose, and lignin can be determined as NDFs. They are cell wall materials that are insoluble in a neutral detergent.

[d] Acid detergent fiber (ADF) is the residue (e.g., plant cell wall material) remaining after boiling a plant-source sample in an acid detergent solution.

dietary intake of protein was increased in humans. Nutritional and biochemical studies are often indistinguishable because both are intended to understand how organic and inorganic molecules interact to support animal metabolism. In essence, biochemistry helps us understand how animals act as transformers of DM and energy into molecules that are required for all physiological functions.

## Physiology as the Foundational Basis of Nutrition

The word *physiology* originated from the Greek *phusiología*, meaning "natural philosophy." It is the study of how living organisms perform their vital functions through the integration of activities among individual cells, tissues, organs, and systems (Guyton and Hall 2000). Physiologists study the physical and chemical processes in the body, including: (1) sensations, motility, and function of the gastrointestinal tract; (2) blood and lymph circulation; (3) interorgan transport of inorganic and organic molecules; (4) respiration; (5) central and peripheral nervous systems; (6) excitation and contraction of skeletal muscle and smooth muscle; (7) male and female fertility; (8) hormone secretion; and (9) excretion of metabolites. Thus, knowledge of *physiology* helps us understand how ingested food is digested, absorbed, and assimilated in animals to sustain homeostasis in the body (maintenance of static or constant conditions in the internal environment) and support growth, development, reproduction, physical activity, and health.

Physiological research is based, in part, on nutritional observations. For example, the discovery of the synthesis of nitric oxide (a major vasodilator and regulator of hemodynamics) from L-arginine in 1988 was based on nutritionists' observation of a marked increase in urinary excretion of nitrate from lipopolysaccharide-challenged rats. In addition, the discovery of the vitamin K-dependent mechanism for blood coagulation was based on nutritional findings that (1) a hemorrhagic disease occurred in cattle after they had consumed spoiled sweet clover containing dicumarol (an inhibitor of 2,3-epoxide reductase) or in rats fed a lipid-deficient diet which impairs intestinal absorption of vitamin K; and (2) bleeding in rats could be treated with spoiled fish meal that contains menaquinone (vitamin $K_2$). The interaction between nutrition and physiology has given rise to a research area known as nutritional physiology, which is the study of how nutrients influence physiological processes in the body and vice versa.

## INTEGRATION OF SYSTEMS PHYSIOLOGY IN NUTRIENT UTILIZATION

### Structure of the Animal Cell

#### Definitions of Cell, Tissue, Organ, and System

The word *cell* comes from the Latin "cella," meaning "a small chamber." The cell is the basic unit of the animal, plant, and microorganism (Cooper and Hausman 2016). This chapter focuses on cells in animals. Each type of cell (e.g., enterocyte, hepatocyte, myocyte, and red blood cells [RBCs]) performs one or more particular functions. Many different but similarly specialized cells are held together by intercellular supporting structures to form a tissue (e.g., connective tissue, white adipose tissue, and brown adipose tissue [BAT]). A group of tissues are joined in structural units to form an organ (e.g., small intestine, liver, and skeletal muscle) that serves specific functions. A number of different organs work together to form a system (e.g., digestive system, musculoskeletal system, and reproductive system) that carries out a common function, such as the breakdown of food to provide nutrients through the digestive system, milk production, immune response, muscle movement through the coordination of the musculoskeletal system, and the production of eggs and offspring through the female reproductive system (Baracos 2006; Dyce et al. 1996; Lu 2014).

#### Composition and Function of the Animal Cell

Most animal cells contain the plasma membrane, cytoplasm, and nucleus (Figure 1.3). The cytoplasm is separated from the nucleus by the nuclear membrane, and the plasma membrane (also known as the cell membrane) separates the intracellular components from the extracellular environment (Guyton and Hall 2000). The different substances that make up the cell are collectively known as protoplasm and include water, proteins, lipids, carbohydrates, minerals, and vitamins.

The majority of biochemical reactions for nutrient synthesis and degradation take place inside the cell (Brosnan 2005). Also, the transport of nutrients into the cell is the first step in the utilization of nutrients by animals. Thus, it is important to understand the composition and function of cells. Although different cells in the body differ in many aspects (e.g., shape, morphology, protein expression, metabolites, anatomical location, and functions), all of them have common basic characteristics. Except for mammalian RBCs, all cells in the animal kingdom are divided internally by membranes into compartments. Intracellular compartmentalization is an important feature of animal metabolism (Watford 1991).

The cell membrane is a structure made of phospholipid bilayers with embedded proteins and cholesterol (Devlin 2011). The fluid nature of the cell membrane permits its integral proteins to move laterally along the plane of the bilayers. The selective permeability of the cell membrane allows the cell to control and maintain its internal environment. The cytoplasm (a thick jellylike solution) consists of cytosol (fluid fraction), organelles, the cytoskeleton, and various other particles. Organelles are subcellular entities enclosed by lipid-bilayer membranes, which are similar to the plasma membrane in structure. The organelles include the mitochondria, rough endoplasmic reticulum, centrioles, smooth endoplasmic reticulum, ribosomes, Golgi apparatus, lysosomes, and peroxisomes (Cooper and Hausman 2016). The nucleus is the largest organelle in the nucleated cell. Of note, the mammalian mature RBCs contain no DNA, nucleus, mitochondria, or other organelles (Barminko et al.

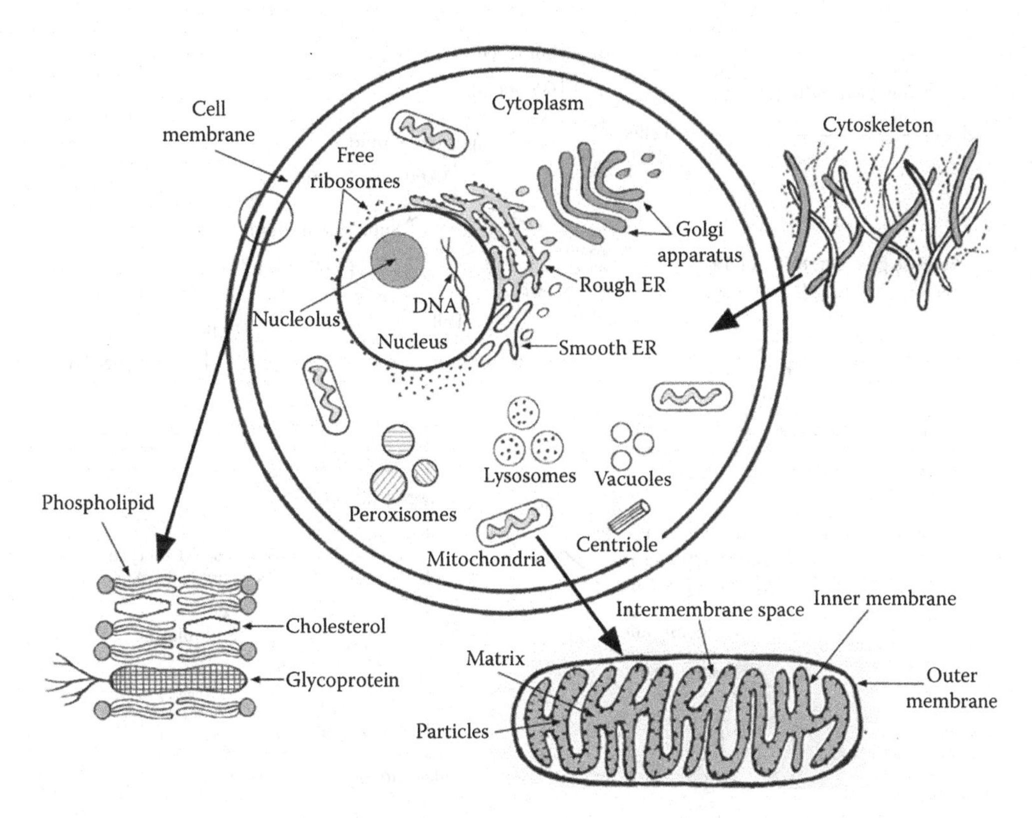


**FIGURE 1.3** The structure of the animal cell. The animal cell (except for the red blood cell in mammals) contains all of the following components: plasma membrane, cytoplasm, and organelles, including the mitochondria, nucleus, endoplasmic reticulum (ER, smooth and rough), centriole, ribosomes, Golgi apparatus, lysosomes, peroxisomes, vacuoles, and cytoskeletal elements. Note that the mammalian red blood cell does not contain mitochondria or other organelles. The avian red blood cell possesses a nucleus and a limited number of mitochondria. The organization of phospholipids, cholesterol, and glycoproteins to form the lipid-bilayer cell membrane, as well as the organization of mitochondrial components, is also presented. The stalked particles contain the $F_0$ and $F_1$ domains of ATP synthase.

2016). In contrast, avian RBCs possess a nucleus and a limited number of mitochondria (Campbell 1995), whereas RBCs of fish (e.g., rainbow trout [Ferguson and Boutilier 1989] and zebrafish [Laale 1977]) contain nuclei and metabolically active mitochondria. Note that microsomes are not cellular organelles, but rather are formed artificially from the endoplasmic reticulum when cells are disrupted during homogenization. A scheme of cell fractionation through centrifugation is outlined in Figure 1.4. The biological functions of the cell fractions and the organelles are summarized in Table 1.4.

As the powerhouse of the cell, the mitochondrion consists of a simple outer membrane (a lipid-bilayer structure), a more complex inner membrane (also a lipid-bilayer structure), the intermembrane space (the space between these two membranes), and the matrix (the space inside the inner mitochondrial membrane) (Cooper and Hausman 2016). The inner mitochondrial membrane is invaginated into folds or cristae to augment its surface area. The outer mitochondrial membrane is composed of 30%–40% lipid and 70%–60% protein, including a high concentration of the integral protein called porin (also called voltage-dependent anion channel) (Devlin 2011). Each porin protein is composed of 1 transmembrane α-helix and 13 transmembrane β-strands and has a molecular cutoff size of ~5 kDa for nonelectrolytes (Lemasters and Holmuhamedov 2006). The outer mitochondrial membrane has little to no permeability barrier to substrates (e.g., ADP, succinate, and phosphate) or products (e.g., ATP and GTP) of mitochondrial energy metabolism and helps to import proteins and nucleic acids (RNA and DNA) from the cytosol into the mitochondria (Weber-Lotfi et al. 2015).

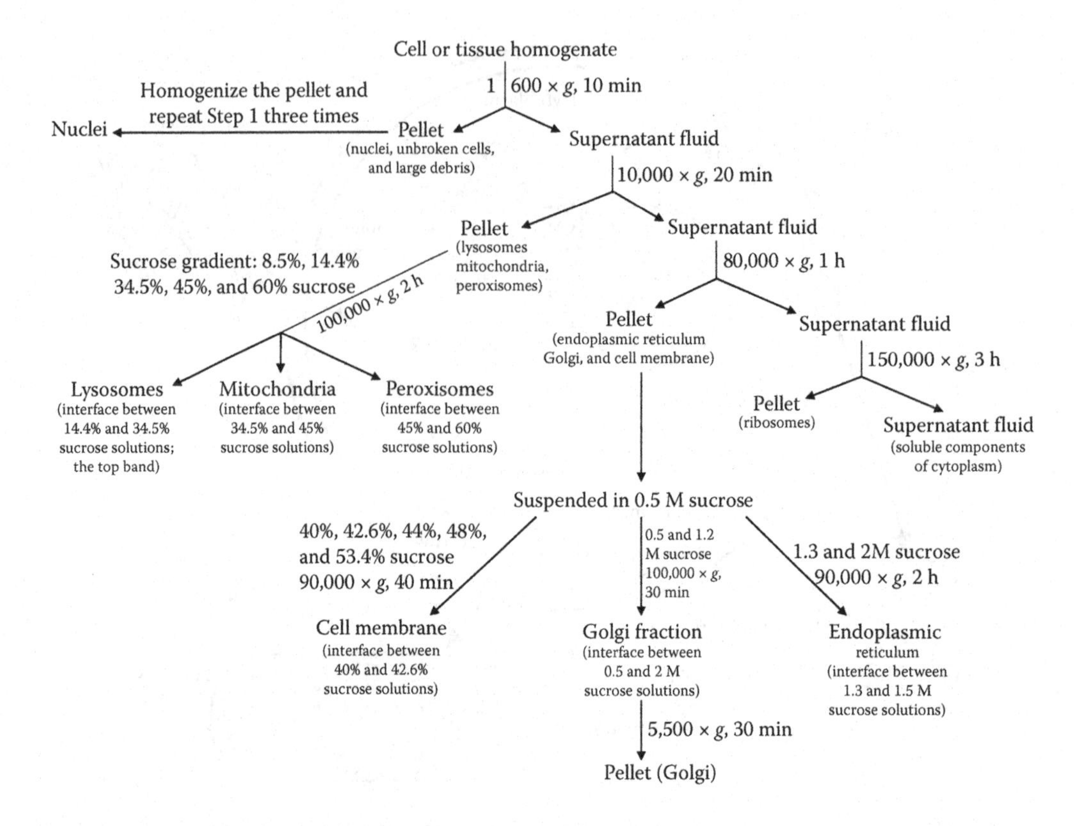


**FIGURE 1.4** A scheme for sucrose-based cell or tissue fractionation. Cells or a tissue is homogenized in 250 mM sucrose, 5 mM imidazole-HCl (pH 7.4), 1 mM EDTA-$Na_2$, and protease inhibitors. The homogenate is centrifuged at 600 × *g* to separate nuclei (pellet) from other cell components (supernatant). High-speed centrifugation of the latter at 10,000 × *g* yields a pellet (mitochondria, lysosomes, and peroxisomes) and the supernatant (cytosolic fraction, cell membranes, and endoplasmic reticulum). These two fractions are subject to ultrahigh-speed centrifugation on sucrose gradients, yielding cytoplasm, peroxisomes, mitochondria, lysosomes, Golgi, and endoplasmic reticulum. (Adapted from Cooper, G.M. and R.E. Hausman. 2016. *The Cell: A Molecular Approach.* Sinauer Associates, Sunderland, MA; De Duve, C. 1971. *J. Cell Biol.* 50:20D–55D; Croze, E.M. and D.J. Morré. 1984. *J. Cell Physiol.* 119:46–57.)

The inner mitochondrial membrane contains 80% protein and 20% lipid, including unsaturated fatty acids and cardiolipin (diphosphatidylglycerol) (Palmieri and Monné 2016). This membrane limits the types of substrates and intermediates that can diffuse from the cytosol into the mitochondrial matrix and vice versa. Specific transporters are responsible for the movement of select substances (e.g., pyruvate ↔ $OH^-$, phosphate ↔ L-malate, L-malate ↔ citrate, L-malate ↔ α-ketoglutarate, ADP ↔ ATP, glutamate ↔ aspartate, glycerol-3-phosphate ↔ dihydroxyacetone phosphate, and phosphate and $H^+$) across the inner mitochondrial membrane from either side (Devlin 2011). The mitochondrial matrix contains enzymes for the β-oxidation of fatty acids, the whole Krebs cycle, some reactions of AA metabolism, part of the urea cycle, and the components for mitochondrial protein synthesis. The mitochondria are also essential for cells to synthesize steroid hormones that affect many aspects of the endocrinology and metabolism of animals (Stocco 2000).

## Transport of Substances across the Biological Membrane

Substances cross the cell membrane and the membranes of organelles through simple diffusion (passive diffusion), facilitated diffusion (passive transport), or active transport (Figure 1.5). The mode of transport of nutrients depends on their chemical properties and concentrations across the membrane (Cooper and Hausman 2016). Rates of nutrient transport increase with the increase

**TABLE 1.4**
**Major Functions of the Plasma Membrane, Cytoplasm, and Organelles of the Cell**

| Cellular Organelle or Fraction | Marker | Major Functions |
|---|---|---|
| Plasma membrane | $Na^+/K^+$ ATPase<br>5′-Nucleotidase | Separation of the interior of the cell from the outside environment; transport of molecules into and out of cells; intercellular adhesion and communication; receptor for hormones, certain AA, and other molecules; cell signaling; endocytosis; exocytosis; passive osmosis and diffusion |
| Cytosol | Lactate dehydrogenase | Control of cell volume, shape, and pH (pH 7.0); suspension of organelles; storage of cellular components; intracellular transport of substances; enzymes for glycolysis, fatty acid and glucose synthesis, and pentose cycle; some enzymes for AA metabolism |
| Nucleus[a] | DNA | Site of DNA synthesis and storage; site of chromosomes; site of DNA-directed RNA synthesis (in nucleolus); control of protein synthesis and cell growth |
| Mitochondrion | Cytochrome oxidase | Cellular respiration; ATP production through oxidative phosphorylation; contribution to thermogenesis; enzymes for the Krebs cycle, as well as the oxidation of fatty acids, much glucose, and some AAs to $CO_2$ and $H_2O$; regulation of apoptosis, stress response, and cell growth |
| Rough endoplasmic reticulum | Ribosomal RNA | Site for synthesis of secretory and membrane proteins in cells; protein sorting, processing (e.g., folding and glycosylation), and trafficking |
| Smooth endoplasmic reticulum | Cytidylyl transferase<br>Glucose 6-phosphatase | Protein sorting, processing, and transport; oxidation of xenobiotics via cytochrome P450; synthesis of many lipids (including cholesterol and steroids) and glucose |
| Ribosomes | High content of RNA | Site for synthesis of endogenous cellular proteins |
| Golgi apparatus | Galactosyl transferase | Modification (e.g., glycosylation), sorting, and packaging of proteins for secretion; sulfation reactions; transport of lipids; creation of lysosomes |
| Lysosome | Acid hydrolases | Site of many hydrolases (optimum pH = 4–5); protein degradation via proteases and autophagy |
| Peroxisome | Catalase<br>Uric acid oxidase | Production and degradation of hydrogen peroxide; initiation of degradation of very long-chain fatty acids through β-oxidation; contain D-amino acid oxidases |
| Cytoskeleton | Relevant proteins | Microtubules, microfilaments, and intermediate filaments |
| Centrosome[b] | Ninein protein | Interact with chromosomes to build mitotic spindles in mitosis; facilitate cell division |

*Source:* Cooper, G.M. and R.E. Hausman. 2016. *The Cell: A Molecular Approach.* Sinauer Associates, Sunderland, MA; Devlin, T.M. 2011. *Textbook of Biochemistry with Clinical Correlations.* John Wiley & Sons, New York, NY.

[a] Containing nuclear membrane, nucleolus, and chromatin.

[b] Consisting of two centrioles (self-replicating organelles made up of nine bundles of microtubules) surrounded by an amorphous mass of protein.

in their extracellular concentrations for influx or in their intracellular concentrations for efflux. Both passive transport and active transport processes require transmembrane proteins.

*Simple Diffusion*

Simple diffusion refers to the movement of molecules into and out of the cell or its organelles along high-to-low concentration gradients (Friedman 2008). For example, in animals, many small uncharged molecules (e.g., $O_2$, $CO_2$, CO, NO, $N_2$, $H_2S$, glycerol, and ethanol) can diffuse freely through the cell membrane via simple diffusion (Cooper and Hausman 2016). Another example of simple diffusion is osmosis, which refers to the movement of water across a semipermeable

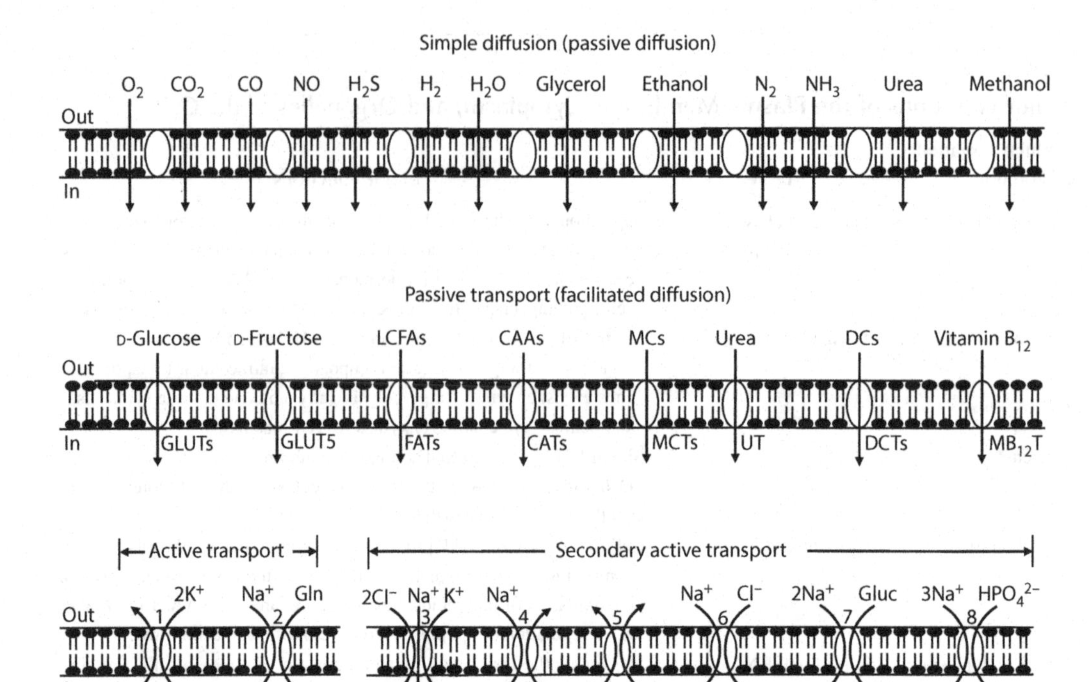


**FIGURE 1.5** Transport of substances across the biological membranes. Gases, nutrients, and their metabolites are transported through the plasma membrane or the membranes of organelles via simple diffusion or carrier-mediated transporters. Note that the rate of glycerol transport by animal cells is very low via simple diffusion but is relatively high via the passive transport of facilitated carriers (e.g., aquaporins 3, 7, and 9). CAAs, cationic amino acids; CATs, cationic amino acid transporters; DCs, dicarboxylates; DCTs, dicarboxylate transporters; FATs, fatty acid transporters; GLUTs, glucose transporters; LCFAs, long-chain fatty acids; $BM_{12}T$, membrane-bound vitamin $B_{12}$ transporter; MCs, monocarboxylates; MCTs, monocarboxylate transporters; UT, urea transporters. Active transport or secondary active transport is indicated by a number: 1, $Na^+$–$K^+$ pump; 2, glutamine (Gln) transporters; 3, $Na^+$–$K^+$–$Cl^-$ cotransporter; 4, $Na^+/H^+$ exchanger; 5, $Na^+$–bicarbonate cotransporter; 6, $Na^+$–$Cl^-$ cotransporter; 7, SGLT1 (sodium–glucose-linked transporter 1); and 8, $Na^+$–phosphate cotransporter.

membrane (e.g., the animal cell membrane) from the solution with a lower osmolarity (osmol/L solution) or osmolality (osmol/L water) toward the solution with a higher osmolarity or osmolality (Reece 1993). This tends to equalize solute concentrations on the two sides of the membrane. Excess flow of water from the extracellular space into cells (e.g., RBCs) can lyse the cells.

### *Carrier-Mediated Transport*

Large polar molecules (e.g., vitamin $B_{12}$, glucose, and AAs) and ions (e.g., $H^+$, $Na^+$, and $Cl^-$) cannot cross a lipid-bilayer membrane (e.g., the plasma membrane and the mitochondrial membrane) by simple diffusion, and instead they cross the cell membrane through specific transmembrane proteins called transporters, channel proteins, or protein pores (Friedman 2008). On the basis of the requirement of ATP or electrochemical potential, carrier-mediated transport is classified as facilitated diffusion, active transport, or secondary (coupled) active transport (Cooper and Hausman 2016).

### *Facilitated Diffusion*

Facilitated diffusion refers to the energy-independent, transporter (carrier protein)-mediated movement of substances across the membrane in the direction of their concentration or electrochemical gradients. Examples of facilitated diffusion are the intestinal absorption of long-chain fatty acids, basic AAs (e.g., arginine and lysine), small peptides (di- and tripeptides), monocarboxylates (e.g., pyruvate and lactate), and dicarboxylates (e.g., α-ketoglutarate and succinate) from the lumen of the small intestine into the enterocytes. The transport of these substances requires fatty acid transporters, cationic AA transporters, the $H^+$-driven peptide transporter 1 (PepT1), monocarboxylate transporters, and dicarboxylate transporters, respectively (Beitz 1993; Friedman 2008). Other examples of facilitated diffusion are the aquaporin-mediated rapid movement of water and glycerol across some cell membranes, as well as glucose transport by glucose transporter-4 in mammalian skeletal muscle. For example, aquaporin 7 transports glycerol out of adipocytes, and aquaporin 9 takes up glycerol from the extracellular space into hepatocytes (Lebeck 2014). Of note, protein channels for ion transport (also known as ion channels) provide passive transport of large numbers of ions down their electrochemical gradient when the channels are open.

*Active Transport*

Active transport refers to the energy-dependent, carrier protein–mediated movement of substances through the biological membrane against their concentration or electrochemical gradients. An example of active transport is the uptake of glutamine from the plasma (0.5–1 mM) into skeletal muscle (10–20 mM) by transporter N (Xue et al. 2010). The energy required for active transport is almost exclusively provided by ATP hydrolysis.

Secondary active transport refers to a form of active transport where a substance crossing the biological membrane is coupled with the movement of an ion (typically $Na^+$ or $H^+$) down its electrochemical potential (Friedman 2008). Secondary active transport requires a carrier protein and is commonly referred to as ion-coupled transport. On the basis of the direction of movement of coupled solutes, transporters of secondary active transport are known as either symporters (cotransporters) for the same direction of solute movement or antiporters (exchangers or counter-transporters) for the opposite direction of solute movement. An example of secondary active transport is the transport of glucose from the lumen of the small intestine into the enterocyte through sodium–glucose-linked transporter-1 (SGLT1; a symporter) on the apical membrane (brush-border membrane) (Boron 2004). SGLT1 utilizes the co-movement of $Na^+$ down its electrochemical gradient to drive the complete uptake of glucose from the intestinal lumen. In contrast, the $Na^+/H^+$ exchanger, which plays a major role in regulating the intracellular pH and $Na^+$ homeostasis, is an antiporter. Secondary active transport does not directly require energy (ATP, GTP, or UTP) (Cooper and Hausman 2016).

## OVERVIEW OF THE ANIMAL SYSTEM

An animal is composed of nine systems (nervous, digestive, circulatory, musculoskeletal, respiratory, urinary, reproductive, endocrine, and immune systems) and five sense organs (Dyce et al. 1996). Utilization of dietary nutrients by animals involves the cooperation of all the organs in the body. For example, the nervous system controls the food intake and behavior of animals; the digestive system is required for the digestion and absorption of enteral nutrients in diets; the circulatory system is needed for the transport of absorbed nutrients from the stomach and intestine into the general circulation; the respiratory system is responsible for the supply of oxygen to oxidize fatty acids, glucose, and AAs into $CO_2$ and water; the endocrine system regulates nutrient metabolism under physiological and pathological conditions; the immune system protects the animal from infection and ensures a healthy state; the urinary system excretes metabolites from the body; the musculoskeletal system provides the structure, support, and movement (e.g., walking, chewing, swallowing, and breathing) of the organism, with skeletal muscle being the major component of growth (Davis et al. 2002; Field et al. 2002; Scanes 2009); and the reproductive system ensures the continuous propagation of the animal species (Guyton and Hall 2000). Thus, it is important for nutritionists to understand the complexity and interactions of all the anatomical systems in animals. Figure 1.6 provides an overview of the utilization of food by animals through digestion, absorption, transport via lymphatic vessels and blood circulation, metabolism, and excretion.

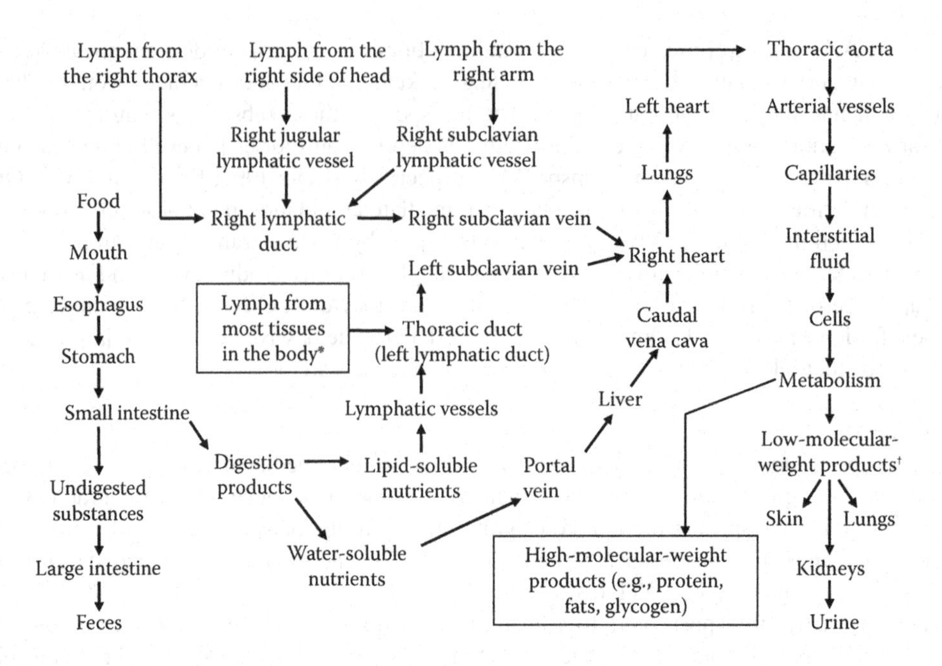


**FIGURE 1.6** An overview of the utilization of food by animals. Ingested food is digested in the stomach and the small intestine to form water-soluble and lipid-soluble products. The water-soluble digestion products enter the portal vein and then the liver. The substances that escape hepatic catabolism are transported to the right atrium of the heart. In contrast, the lipid-soluble digestion products enter lymphatic vessels, the left subclavian vein, and then the right atrium of the heart. The lymphatic system also provides a route for both fluid and large-molecular-weight substances (e.g., proteins, lipoproteins, and large particular matter) in the extracellular interstitial space to return to the blood. Through microcirculation, nutrients are transported to the cells for metabolism. Metabolic products are either deposited in the body or excreted through the skin, lungs, and kidneys. Undigested food is fermented in the large intestine and its metabolites are excreted in the feces. * Including parts of the chest region, the lower part of the body, as well as the left side of the head and the left arm. † Including water, $CO_2$, $NH_3$, $NH_4^+$, urea, nitrate, and sulfate.

## The Nervous System

The nervous system includes the central nervous system and the peripheral nervous system (Figure 1.7) and is the commander of the body by controlling its voluntary and involuntary actions. The neuron (also known as the nerve cell) is the basic unit of the nervous system. The complex neural network includes neurons, neurotransmitters, and glial cells (meaning "glue" in Greek). The glial cells (non-neuronal cells) support and nourish neurons, produce myelin, and participate in signal transmission in the nervous system (Brodal 2004).

### The Neuron

The neuron has all the components of the animal cell. In addition, the neuron has specialized parts: a cell body, dendrites (thin, branching structures from the cell body), and an axon (also known as a nerve fiber). The types of neurons include: (1) sensory neurons in the sense organs; (2) motor neurons, which are efferent *neurons* that originate in the spinal cord and form synapses with skeletal muscle to control muscle contraction; and (3) interneurons that connect neurons within the central nervous system (Sporns et al. 2004).

As an electrically excitable cell, the neuron maintains an electrochemical potential across the plasma membrane through ion pumps to control the flux of ions (e.g., sodium, potassium, chloride, and calcium). The electrochemical pulse travels along the neuron's axon to the synapse (a junction between two neurons), and then onto the synapse of another nerve cell, or the receptor

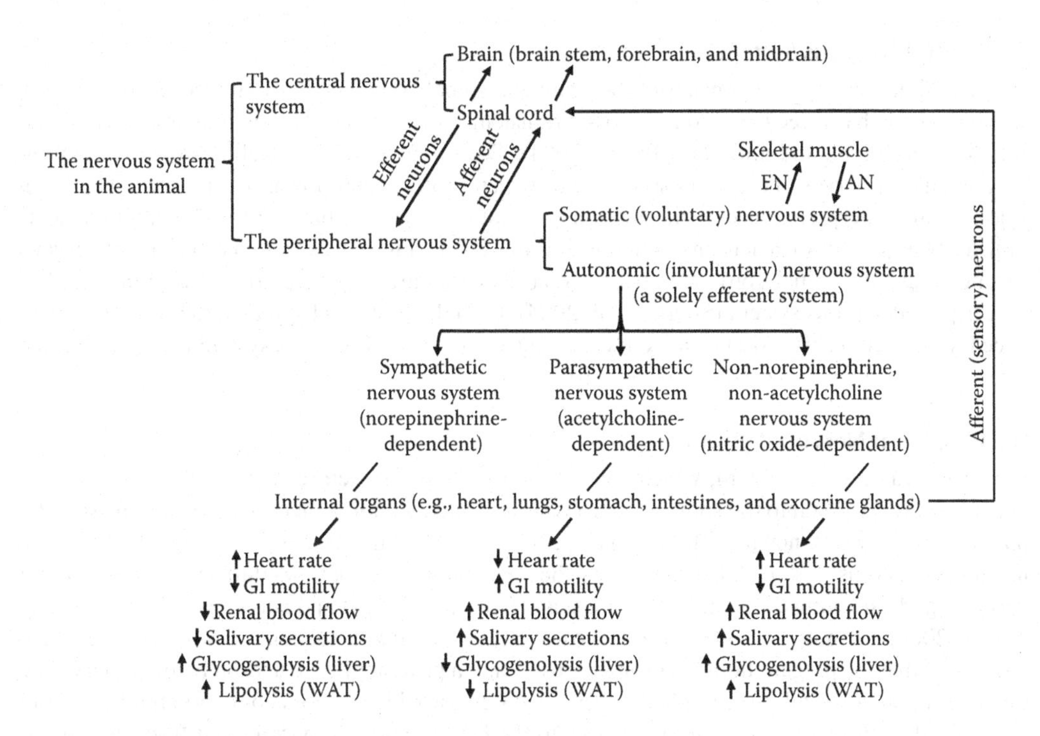


**FIGURE 1.7** The nervous system in animals. The nervous system is composed of the central nervous system (the brain and spinal cord) and the peripheral nervous system. The brain processes and interprets sensory information transmitted from the spinal cord. Afferent neurons conduct impulses from the peripheral nervous system toward the spinal cord, whereas efferent neurons carry impulses from the spinal cord to the peripheral nervous system. AN, afferent neurons; EN, efferent neurons; GI, gastrointestine; WAT, white adipose tissue; ↑, increase; ↓, decrease.

site of a muscle or gland cell (Kaeser and Regehr 2014). Upon stimulation by the electrical signal, the synapse of the transmitting neuron releases chemical neurotransmitters into the synaptic cleft (the extracellular space between two neurons). These neurotransmitters (e.g., acetylcholine) bind to their receptors (e.g., acetylcholine receptor, a ligand-gated sodium channel) on the postsynaptic membranes of the recipient cell and transmit an action potential to the next cell. The neurotransmitters may then be inactivated by uptake and destruction, depending on the neurotransmitter and tissue (Brodal 2004). Thus, neurons process and transmit information through electrical and chemical signals through synapses or to the receptor site of other target cells (e.g., muscle and gland cells). Neurons connect each other to form complex and well-integrated neural networks.

## Neurotransmitters

Neurotransmitters are the signals released by neurons at the synapses. These molecules are released from the neuron on the presynaptic side of the synapse into the synaptic cleft and then bind to specific receptors on the cell membrane of the neuron in the postsynaptic side of the synapse (Brodal 2004). Some AAs are neurotransmitters, such as L-glutamate, L-aspartate, glycine, D-serine, and γ-aminobutyric acid (GABA). Most of the other neurotransmitters are either AA metabolites or peptides formed from AAs, which include: (1) gasotransmitters (nitric oxide, carbon monoxide, and hydrogen sulfide [$H_2S$]); (2) monoamines (dopamine, norepinephrine [noradrenaline], epinephrine [adrenaline], histamine, agmatine, melatonin, and serotonin); (3) peptides (substance P, cocaine, opioid peptides, *N*-acetylaspartylglutamate, gastrin, cholecystokinin [CCK], oxytocin, vasopressin, peptide YY, and neuropeptide Y); and (4) acetylcholine (Kaeser and Regehr 2014).

### The Central Nervous System

The central nervous system consists of the brain and spinal cord. The brain, the commander of the neural network, has three main components: brainstem, forebrain (containing thalamus, hypothalamus, and cerebrum), and midbrain (Brodal 2004). The spinal cord is a tubelike structure containing a bundle of nerves and cerebrospinal fluid, which protects and nourishes the cord. The brain processes and interprets sensory information transmitted from the spinal cord. The latter connects with peripheral tissues via neurons. Afferent neurons conduct impulses from the peripheral nervous system toward the spinal cord, whereas efferent neurons carry impulses from the spinal cord to the peripheral nervous system (Sporns et al. 2004). Both the brain and spinal cord are protected by three layers of connective tissue called the meninges. The central nervous system is responsible for processing information received from all parts of the body.

### The Peripheral Nervous System

The peripheral nervous system, which consists of all nervous structures outside the brain and the spinal cord, is divided into the somatic nervous system and autonomic nervous system. The somatic *nervous system* (also known as the voluntary nervous system) innervates the *skeletal muscle*. The autonomic nervous system (also known as the involuntary nervous system) innervates internal organs (e.g., heart, lungs, stomach, intestines, and exocrine glands) and acts largely unconsciously (Brodal 2004). Of note, the autonomic nervous system requires a sequential two-neuron efferent pathway in that the preganglionic neuron synapses onto a postganglionic neuron before innervating the target organ. Overall, the peripheral nervous system provides a means of communication from the external environment and internal tissues to the central nervous system, and from the central nervous system to the proper effector organs in the body (e.g., skeletal muscle, smooth muscle, the small intestine, and glands).

On the basis of the type of neurotransmitter, the autonomic nervous system can be divided into (1) the norepinephrine-dependent sympathetic nervous system ("fight or flight"), (2) the acetylcholine-dependent parasympathetic nervous system ("rest and digest"), and (3) NO-dependent, non-norepinephrine and non-acetylcholine nervous system (McCorry 2007). One tissue (e.g., the small intestine, heart, renal tubules, or the vasculature) can be innervated by both sympathetic and parasympathetic nervous systems, which often have opposite and complementary effects. For example, the sympathetic nervous system (1) increases the heart rate and the contractility of cardiac myocytes, (2) relaxes the bladder wall for urine storage, (3) reduces renal blood flow (and glomerular filtration rate), (4) inhibits salivary gland secretion, (5) decreases the motility of the gastrointestinal tract, and (6) promotes hepatic glycogenolysis and adipose tissue lipolysis (McCorry 2007). In contrast, the parasympathetic nervous system (1) decreases the heart rate and the contractility of cardiac myocytes, (2) constricts the bladder wall for urine emptying, (3) enhances renal blood flow (and glomerular filtration rate), (4) stimulates salivary gland secretion, (5) increases the motility of the gastrointestinal tract, and (6) inhibits hepatic glycogenolysis and adipose tissue lipolysis (Brodal 2004).

## The Circulatory System

### Blood Circulation

#### *Blood*

Blood is a tissue. It accounts for 6%–8% of the body weight, depending on species, age, and physiological state (Fox et al. 2002). Blood consists of cells and intercellular material. However, unlike other tissues, the intercellular material in blood is a fluid called plasma and the cells move within the vascular system. Some blood cells, such as the leukocytes, may migrate through vessel walls to combat infections. Serum is defibrinated plasma (i.e., without fibrin and cellular components). Normally, the pH of blood is 7.4 (Guyton et al. 1972). Blood, plasma, and serum are often used for the analysis of physiological compounds (e.g., AAs, urea, lipids, glucose, and hormones). Plasma is obtained when a sample of fresh blood is treated with an anticoagulant (e.g., heparin or EDTA) to prevent clotting, followed by centrifugation to remove cells (i.e., the pellet). In contrast, serum is collected after a sample of fresh blood (without anticoagulant treatment) is permitted to clot and is then centrifuged. One milliliter of blood contains 0.70–0.75 mL plasma or 0.58–0.62 mL serum, depending on species, age, and physiological state. For example, in the 20 kg pig that has 1.4 L blood, 1 mL blood contains 0.735 mL plasma or 0.616 mL serum.

#### *The Heart and Blood Vessels*

The circulatory system consists of the heart, as well as a system of arterial and venous vessels for the circulation of blood (Guyton et al. 1972). The heart has four chambers (upper left and right atria plus lower left and right ventricles) in mammals and birds, two chambers (an atrium and a ventricle) in fish, or three chambers (two atria and one ventricle) in amphibians and most reptiles (Dyce et al. 1996). Except for the pulmonary artery and the umbilical artery (see below), arteries supply oxygenated blood to a tissue, whereas veins carry low-oxygen blood (referred to as deoxygenated blood herein) away from the tissue. Blood flow in the major veins of the lower extremities depends, in part, on the contractions of leg skeletal muscle. There are *valves* in most *veins* to prevent backflow of venous blood and ensure its return to the heart.

#### *Direction of Blood Flow in Postnatal Animals*

Understanding blood circulation is important for understanding the utilization of food nutrients, designing physiologically sound experiments, and interpreting experimental data. A general scheme of the circulation in postnatal mammals and birds is shown in Figure 1.8. In these species, the venous deoxygenated blood from the body enters the right atrium and then the right ventricle of the heart and subsequently is pumped through the pulmonary artery into the lungs for gas exchange. Thereafter, the oxygenated blood flows through the pulmonary vein to the left atrium and then to the left ventricle of the heart and ultimately is pumped through the thoracic aorta and its branches to the rest of the body via small arteries and then arterioles (Dyce et al. 1996). In fish, the venous deoxygenated blood from the body enters the atrium via the sinus venosus, flows into the ventricle, and is then pumped through the bulbus arteriosus into the gills for gas exchange, after which the oxygenated blood flows to the rest of the body (Guyton and Hall 2000). In amphibians and most reptiles, the left atrium and the right atrium receive the oxygenated blood and deoxygenated blood from the lungs and the body, respectively; both types of the blood are mixed in the ventricle and pumped through pulmonary and skin circulations into the lungs and skin, respectively, for gas exchange (Farmer 1997). It is important to note that, in all species studied, the hepatic portal circulation is an important exception to the usual arrangement of the systemic circulation, in that the liver receives much more blood from the portal vein than from the hepatic artery. For example, in mammals, the hepatic artery and portal vein supply 25%–30% and 70%–75% of blood to the liver, respectively (Dyce et al. 1996). Venous blood drained from the stomach, spleen, small intestine, pancreas, and large intestine enters the liver via the portal vein before entering the general circulation.

#### *Direction of Blood Flow in Fetuses*

While postnatal animals receive enteral nutrients from the small intestine, growing mammalian fetuses are nourished by their mothers through the umbilical vein (Figure 1.9). Similarly, nutrients required for avian embryonic growth are derived from the yolk sac of the fertilized egg via blood vessels. Understanding fetal circulation is essential to understanding fetal nutrition and metabolism. Fetal circulation differs from the adult circulation in several respects (Dyce et al. 1996; Guyton and Hall 2000). First, the maternal uterine artery supplies oxygenated blood to the uterus, and this blood enters the placenta through its microvasculature. Subsequently, the umbilical vein carries oxygenated blood from the placenta to the fetal liver and heart. Second, much of the blood from the caudal end of the fetal aorta is transported to the placenta by two umbilical arteries. Metabolic

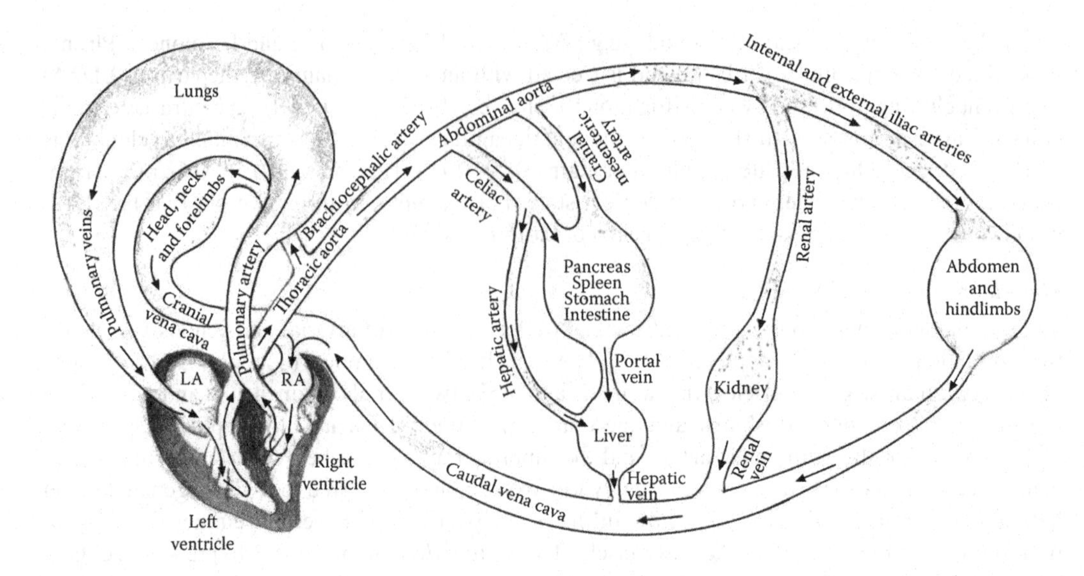


**FIGURE 1.8** Blood circulation in postnatal mammals and birds. The arteries supply oxygen-rich blood to tissues, and the veins drain low-oxygen blood from the tissues. Most veins contain valves to prevent the retrograde flow of venous blood and ensure its return to the heart. The hepatic portal vein drains blood from the stomach, small intestine, pancreas, spleen, and large intestine (collectively known as the portal-drained viscera) to the liver. The caudal (inferior) vena cava carries the venous blood from the abdomen, internal organs, and hindlimbs to the right atrium of the heart. The cranial (superior) vena cava carries the venous blood from the head, neck, and forelimbs to the right atrium of the heart. The venous blood enters the right atrium and then the right ventricle of the heart, and, through the pulmonary artery, flows to the lungs for gas exchange. The oxygen-rich arterial blood flows through the pulmonary vein to the left atrium and then the left ventricle of the heart, and ultimately is pumped to the thoracic aorta for flow to the various parts of the body. (Adapted from Dyce, K.M. et al. 1996. *Textbook of Veterinary Anatomy*. W.B. Saunders Company, Philadelphia, PA.)

wastes in the fetal umbilical arteries enter the maternal circulation sequentially through the placenta and uterine vein. Furthermore, blood from the fetal umbilical arteries undergoes gas and nutrient transfer through the placental capillaries and then returns to the fetal heart through the umbilical vein. Third, because the fetal lungs are nonfunctional, a relatively small amount of the total blood volume is present in the pulmonary circulation at any given time. There are two bypasses, or shortcuts, between the right side and the left side of the fetal heart and between the pulmonary artery and the aorta. These bypasses are (1) the foramen ovale that connects the right atrium and the left atrium of the fetal heart and (2) the ductus arteriosus that connects the pulmonary artery and the aorta of the fetus (Dyce et al. 1996).

### *Microcirculation*

Within the microcirculation, blood flows from arterioles (with an internal diameter between 10 and 20 μm) to capillaries and then to venules. The capillaries with an internal diameter of 4–9 μm are the site for the transport of nutrients from arterial blood to tissues, and the venules are the site for the removal of metabolites from the tissues to the general circulation (Figure 1.10). Blood capillaries are extremely thin tubular structures with a single layer of semipermeable endothelial cells (Granger et al. 1988). Each capillary is surrounded by a basement membrane. Between two adjacent endothelial cells, there is a thin intercellular junction, which allows fluid and small solutes to leave the circulation and enter the interstitial space (the extracellular space between cells) of the perfused tissue. The intercellular junction varies in size, with its diameter ranging from <1 nm in the brain and spinal cord (so-called tight junctions) to 15 nm in the kidney glomerulus and to ~180 nm in hepatic sinusoids (blood capillaries in the liver) (Sarin 2010).

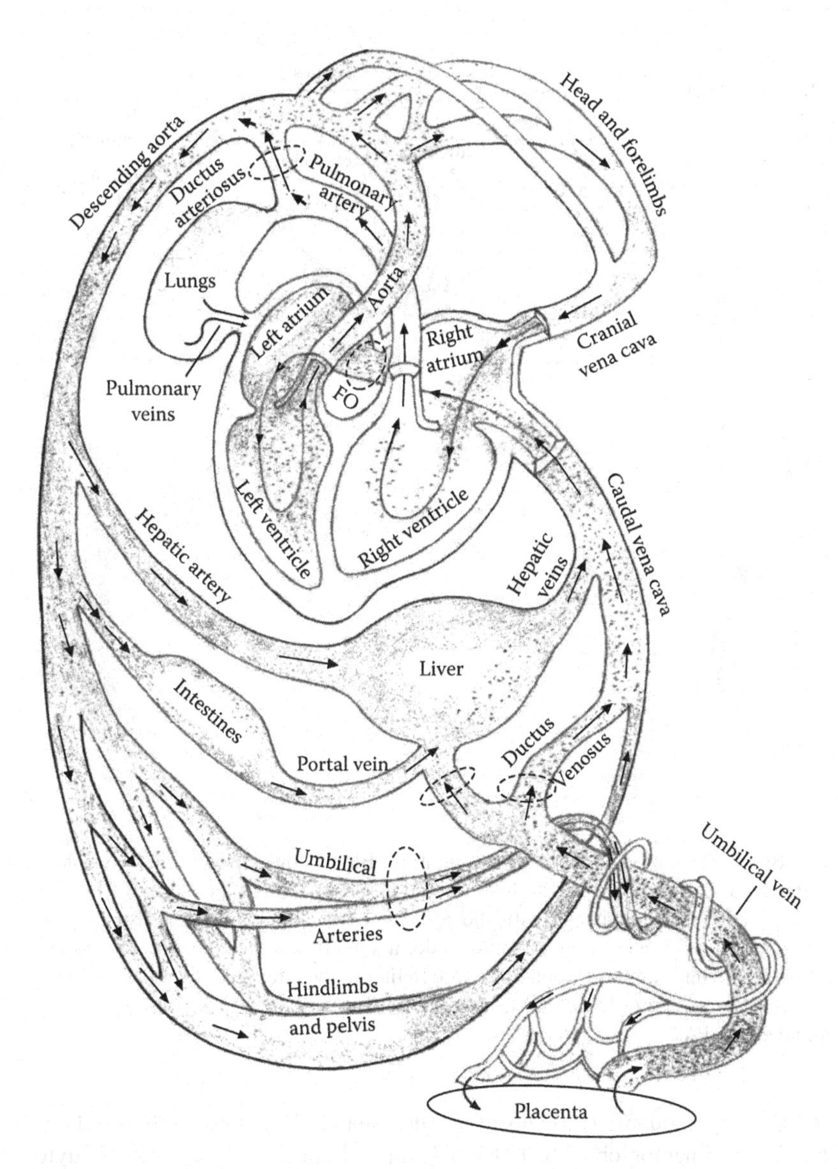


**FIGURE 1.9** Blood circulation in the fetal–placental tissues. The umbilical vein supplies oxygenated blood from the placenta to the fetus. More than two-thirds of the umbilical venous blood enters the fetal liver through the fetal portal vein, while the remainder bypasses the liver and flows through the ductus venosus to the caudal vena cava for delivery to the fetal right atrium. Because fetal lungs are nonfunctional, two bypasses (shortcuts) carry blood to the fetus: (1) the foramen ovale that connects the right atrium and the left atrium of the fetal heart; and (2) the ductus arteriosus that connects the pulmonary artery and the aorta of the fetus. Fetal low-oxygen blood returns to the placenta via two umbilical arteries by way of the internal iliac arteries. (Adapted from Dyce, K.M. et al. 1996. *Textbook of Veterinary Anatomy.* W.B. Saunders Company, Philadelphia, PA.)

At the capillaries, continual exchanges of fluid and low-molecular-weight substances (<10,000 Da) between the arterial plasma and the extracellular interstitial fluid occur by either transcellular diffusion and transport or intercellular diffusion (Guyton et al. 1972). The capillaries are permeable to most molecules (e.g., $O_2$, $CO_2$, AAs, glucose, fatty acids, triglycerides, minerals, vitamins, ammonia, and urea) in the plasma except for large plasma proteins. For example, when compared with water (100% permeable), the permeability of the following molecules is as follows: NaCl (58.5 Da),

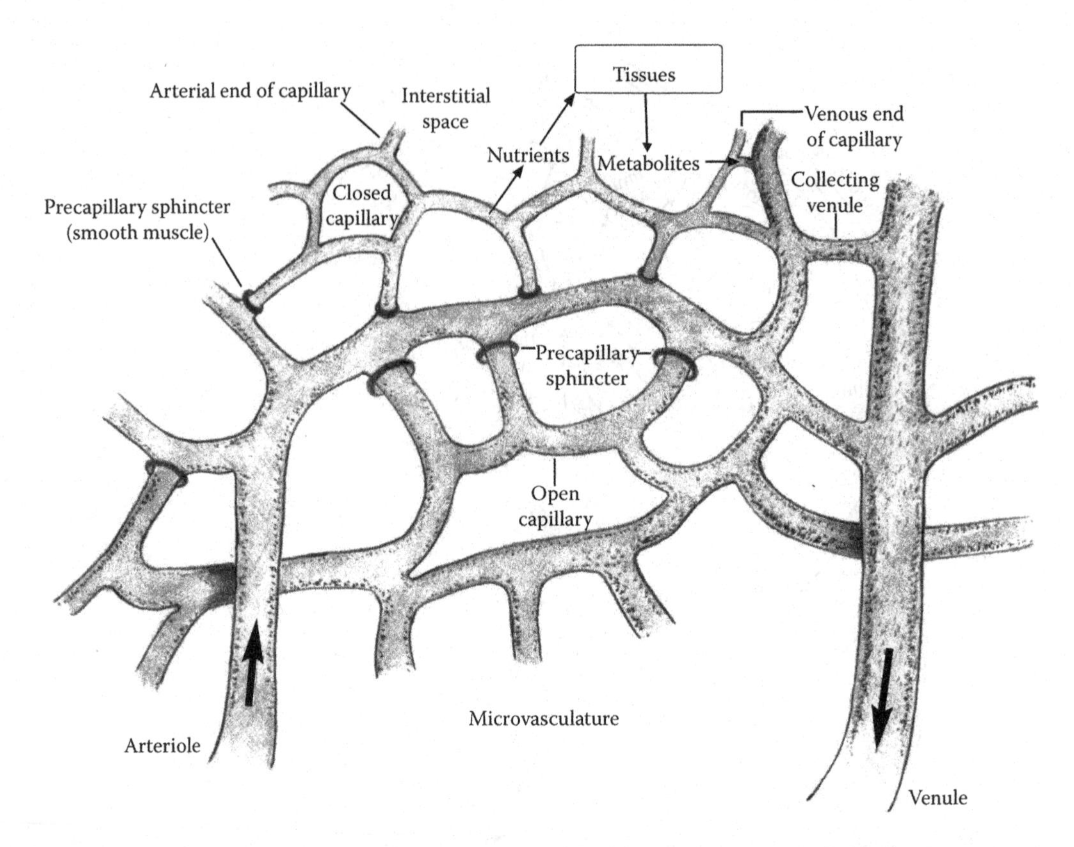


**FIGURE 1.10** Blood circulation in the microvasculature. Blood flows through the arterioles and then the metarterioles (terminal branches of the arteriole) to the capillaries. Nutrients and gases in the lumen of the capillaries undergo continuous exchange with those in the extracellular interstitial space of a tissue. At a point where a capillary originates from a metarteriole, a smooth muscle ring (the precapillary sphincter) encircles the capillary to open or close blood flow. Metabolites in the interstitial fluid may also be taken up into lymphatic vessels. (Adapted from Dyce, K.M. et al. 1996. *Textbook of Veterinary Anatomy.* W.B. Saunders Company, Philadelphia, PA.)

96%; urea (60 Da), 80%; glucose (180 Da), 60%; sucrose (342 Da), 40%; inulin (5 kDa), 20%; myoglobin (17.6 kDa), 3%; hemoglobin (68 kDa), 1%; and albumin (69 kDa), 0.1% (Guyton and Hall 2000). After passing through the capillaries, blood enters the venule (a very small vein with an internal diameter of 7–50 μm) and then a large vein. The driving forces for the venous return are (1) the pressure gradient provided by the heart and (2) the contraction of skeletal muscles. Thus, the major function of the microcirculation is to transport nutrients and $O_2$ to tissues and to remove cellular metabolites (including $CO_2$) from the tissues.

## Blood–Brain Barrier

A unique feature of the brain's vasculature is the blood–brain barrier. It refers to a structure in the endothelium of cerebral capillaries and the choroid plexus epithelium that prevents the exchange of certain substances (e.g., saturated long-chain fatty acids) between the microvasculature and brain. There is evidence that a small amount of polyunsaturated fatty acids (e.g., linoleic acid [$C_{18:2}$ ω6] and linolenic acid [$C_{18:3}$ ω3]) can cross the blood–brain barrier from the blood into the brain (Moore et al. 1990). Understanding this blood–brain barrier is essential to understanding why long-chain fatty acids serve as an important energy source for peripheral, extraintestinal organs (e.g., skeletal muscle, heart, and liver), but not for the brain.

### The Lymphatic System

In animals, including mammals, birds, and fish, the lymphatic system provides a route for both fluid and large-molecular-weight substances (e.g., proteins, lipoproteins, and large particulate matter) in the extracellular interstitial space to return to the blood circulation. These large-molecular-weight substances cannot be removed by absorption directly into the blood capillaries. The return of proteins from the extracellular interstitial space of tissues into the general circulation helps maintain blood osmolality and, therefore, is essential to life. For example, ~50% of plasma proteins are filtered by the blood capillaries into the interstitial space each day, and these extracellular proteins must be returned to the blood through lymphatic vessels (Gashev and Zawieja 2010). While ~90% of the fluid filtered from the blood capillaries into the interstitial space is reabsorbed into the venous ends of the blood capillaries, 10% of the blood-derived interstitial fluid initially enters the lymphatic capillaries as a component of lymph (Guyton and Hall 2000). The lymphatic capillaries merge to form larger lymphatic vessels, which are similar to veins in structure, but have an intrinsic pumping ability to propel lymph. Two major lymphatic vessels, the thoracic duct (also known as the left lymphatic duct; the largest lymphatic duct in the body) and the right lymphatic duct (also known as the *right thoracic* duct), merge with the blood circulation vessels at the level of the left and right subclavian veins, respectively, to return the contents of lymph into the blood (Figure 1.6). Thus, lymph vessels collect tissue fluid or lymph and transport it to large veins.

The lymphatic system consists of (1) lymphatic vessels, including: (a) lymphatic capillaries (10–60 μm in internal diameter) permeable to proteins, other large molecules, and microorganisms, and (b) larger lymphatic collecting ducts (~100–200 μm in internal diameter) resembling a vein in structure; and (2) a variety of widely scattered aggregations of lymphoid tissues (e.g., lymph nodes and tonsils) (Scallan et al. 2010). A lymph node is an oval or kidney-shaped organ, which is distributed widely throughout the body and linked by lymphatic vessels. Lymph nodes are the major sites of B-cells, T-cells, and other immune cells, filtering foreign particles. Like the blood capillaries, the lymphatic capillaries are composed of a single layer of endothelial cells. However, unlike the blood capillaries, the lymphatic capillaries either have no basement membrane or have only a discontinuous basement membrane and are not associated with pericytes. In addition, although there is an intercellular cleft (junction or pore) between two adjacent endothelial cells in the lymphatic capillaries, the diameter of this junction is relatively large (~2 μm), allowing the fluid and large solutes in the extracellular interstitial space to easily enter the lymphatic vessels (Scallan et al. 2010).

Larger lymphatic collecting ducts are lined with a layer of endothelial cells and have endothelial valves (consisting of two endothelial cell leaflets inside the vessel lumen) (Dyce et al. 1996). The lymphatic ducts also have a basement membrane, a thin layer of smooth muscle cells, pericytes, and adventitia (binding the lymph vessels to the surrounding tissue). The endothelial valves prevent retrograde lymph flow. Phasic contractions of lymphatic smooth muscle (modulated by nitric oxide) propel a unidirectional flow of lymph along the intervalvular segment of lymphatic vessels (Gashev and Zawieja 2010). In contrast to the lymphatic capillaries, the lymphatic collecting ducts have a very low permeability to plasma proteins (e.g., <3% for albumin) (Scallan et al. 2010). The lymphatic vascular tree eventually converges with major veins at the junction of the neck and thorax. Nearly all the lymph from the lower part of the body, as well as lymph from the left side of the head, the left arm, and parts of the chest region, enters the thoracic duct and then empties into the large vein at the juncture of the left internal jugular vein and the left subclavian vein. Lymph from the right side of the neck and head, the right arm, and parts of the chest region enters the right lymph duct and then empties into the large vein at the juncture of the right internal jugular vein and the right subclavian vein (Guyton and Hall 2000). Overall, the flow of lymph is as follows: lymph capillaries (taking up water, other nutrients, proteins, and metabolites from interstitial fluid) → lymph collecting vessels → lymph trunks → lymph ducts → subclavian veins (Figure 1.6). Lymphatics play an essential role in transporting, eventually into the right atrium of the heart, dietary lipids and lipid-soluble substances absorbed from the mammalian small intestine.

The lymphatic system functions to (1) drain interstitial fluid and large molecules from tissues back into the blood circulation; (2) transport long-chain fatty acids, cholesterol, and lipid-soluble vitamins absorbed from the small intestine into the blood circulation; and (3) maintain whole-body fluid homeostasis. Total flow of lymph into the lymphatics in a healthy adult man is 2–4 L/day (Guyton and Hall 2000). Thus, the lymphatic capillaries take up any excess extracellular fluid in the body tissues (mainly fluid filtrated out of the blood capillaries) and the lymphatic vessels return this fluid to the heart. Impairment of the formation and circulation of lymph results in edema, that is, the accumulation of interstitial fluid in abnormally large amounts (Gashev and Zawieja 2010).

## The Digestive System

The digestive system includes the mouth, teeth, tongue, pharynx, esophagus, stomach, small intestine and large intestine, as well as accessory digestive organs (salivary glands, pancreas, liver, and gallbladder) (Dyce et al. 1996). The mouth plays an important role in the physical breakdown of feeds or prey animals. Besides the mouth and stomach, the intestine harbors various kinds of microbes with high metabolic activities (Table 1.5). This system is responsible for the prehension and digestion of feed and the absorption of its products into the circulation. Digestion is defined as the chemical breakdown of food by enzymes in the lumen or the brush-border (luminal) membrane of the stomach, small intestine, and large intestine into smaller molecules. This process is simply the enzymatic hydrolysis of chemical bonds in the ingested proteins, lipids, and carbohydrates. Absorption refers to the movement of substances (e.g., nutrients) across the mucosal cells of the stomach, small intestine, and large intestine into the interstitial fluid, from which they enter the capillaries (into the blood) or lacteals (into the lymph) (Guyton and Hall 2000). Digestion and absorption are regulated by neural control and gastrointestinal hormones (e.g., gastrin, secretin, cholecystokinin, somatostatin, and glucagonlike peptide-1), which affect gastric emptying, the distention and motility of the gastrointestinal tract, as well as salivary, gastric, pancreatic, and intestinal secretions (including digestive enzymes and ions) (Brodal 2004; Bondi 1987).

The gastrointestinal tract differs markedly among many animal species (Figures 1.11 and 1.12). For example, pigs and chickens (nonruminants) all have a single stomach. In contrast, the stomachs of ruminants consist of four parts: rumen, reticulum, omasum, and abomasum (true stomach), with each having different functions (Cheeke and Dierenfeld 2010). Due to the presence of large populations of microorganisms in the rumen, dietary proteins and carbohydrates are extensively fermented there before entering the small intestine in ruminants. Fish have morphologically diverse gastrointestinal tracts (Wilson and Castro 2011); channel catfish, rainbow trout, salmonids, and most of the fin fishes have true stomachs, tilapias have a modified stomach, and the common carp has no stomach. Unlike mammals, birds and most fish which have a spiral small intestine, the intestine of shrimp is straight in shape and has no turns. The diverse structures of the digestive systems among animal species provide a physiological basis for the efficient use of different sources of the food available to them in the ecosystem (McDonald et al. 2011; Liao et al. 2010). In all but agastric animals, the stomach, small intestine, liver, and pancreas are required for the efficient digestion of nutrients, such as fats, proteins, and carbohydrates (Figure 1.13). The digestive apparatus is qualitatively similar among the animal organisms. The mean retention time (h) of food in the digestive tract of animals is: water shrew, 2; mink, 4; fish, 5–7; chicken, 5–9; cat, 13; rabbit, 15; dog, 23; rat, 28; horse, 29; elephant, 33; pig, 43; goat, 43; man, 46; sheep, 47; and cattle, 60 (Blaxter 1989).

### The Stomach in Nonruminants

In all animals (e.g., nonruminants), the stomach is located between the esophagus and the duodenum. The stomach consists of four regions: cardia, fundus, body, and pyloric antrum. Relaxation of the stomach stimulates the appetite. Ingested food enters the stomach through the junction between the esophagus and the stomach and leaves the stomach through the pyloric sphincter (the junction between the stomach and the duodenum). Gastric contractions propel the ingested food and chyme

**TABLE 1.5**
**Major Bacterial Species in the Digestive Tract and Feces of Animals**

| Phylum | Species | Primary Origin | Location in GI Tract |
|---|---|---|---|
| Firmicutes | Lactobacilli | Human, baboon, swine, rat, mouse, chicken, ruminant | Stomach/rumen, small intestine, large intestine, feces |
| | Streptococci | Human, baboon, swine, rat, mouse, ruminant | Mouth, stomach/rumen, small intestine, large intestine, feces |
| | Clostridia | Human, baboon, swine, rat, mouse, chicken, ruminant | Stomach/rumen, small intestine, feces |
| | *Veillonella* | Human, swine, rat, chicken | Mouth, stomach, small intestine, large intestine, feces |
| | *Peptostreptococcus* | Human, swine, rat, ruminant | Stomach/rumen, feces |
| | Staphylococci | Human, baboon, swine, rat, mouse | Stomach, small intestine, large intestine, feces |
| | *Eubacterium* | Human, mouse, ruminant | Rumen, large intestine, feces |
| | *Bacillus* | Human, swine, rat, mouse | Large intestine, feces |
| | *Peptococcus* | Human | Feces |
| | *Ruminococcus* | Human, swine, ruminant | Rumen, small intestine, large intestine, feces |
| | *Acidaminococcus* | Human | Large intestine, feces |
| | *Butyrivibrio* | Human, ruminant | Rumen, feces |
| | *Megasphaera* | Human, swine, ruminant | Mouth, rumen, large intestine, feces |
| | *Faecalibacterium* | Swine | Large intestine, feces |
| | *Selenomonas* | Ruminant | Rumen |
| | *Lachnospira* | Ruminant | Rumen |
| | *Anaerovibrio* | Ruminant | Rumen |
| Bacteroidetes | *Bacteroides* | Human, baboon, swine, rat, mouse, chicken | Mouth, stomach, small intestine, large intestine, feces |
| | *Prevotella* | Human, swine, ruminant | Mouth, rumen, large intestine, feces |
| Proteobacteria | *Actinobacillus* | Human, baboon, swine, rat, mouse | Mouth, stomach, small intestine |
| | *Escherichia* | Human, baboon, swine, rat, mouse, chicken, ruminant | Stomach, small intestine, large intestine, feces |
| | *Succinivibrio* | Human, ruminant | Rumen, feces |
| | *Salmonella* | Chicken | Large intestine, feces |
| | *Ruminobacter* | Ruminant | Rumen |
| | *Succinimonas* | Ruminant | Rumen |
| | *Wolinella* | Ruminant | Rumen |
| Actinobacteria | Bifidobacteria | Human, swine, rat | Stomach, small intestine, large intestine, feces |
| | *Propionibacterium* | Human, mouse | Large intestine, feces |
| Fusobacteria | *Fusobacterium* | Human, swine, mouse | Mouth, large intestine, feces |
| Fibrobacteres | *Fibrobacter* | Ruminant | Rumen |

*Source:* Booijink, C.C.G.M. 2009. PhD Thesis. Wageningen University, Wageningen, The Netherlands; Dai, Z.L. et al. 2015. *Mol. Hum. Reprod.* 21:389–409; Robinson, C.J. et al. 2010. *Microbiol. Mol. Biol. Rev.* 74:453–476; Russell, J.B. and J.L. Rychlik. 2001. *Science* 292:1119–1122; Savage, D.C. 1977. *Annu. Rev. Microbiol.* 31:107–133.

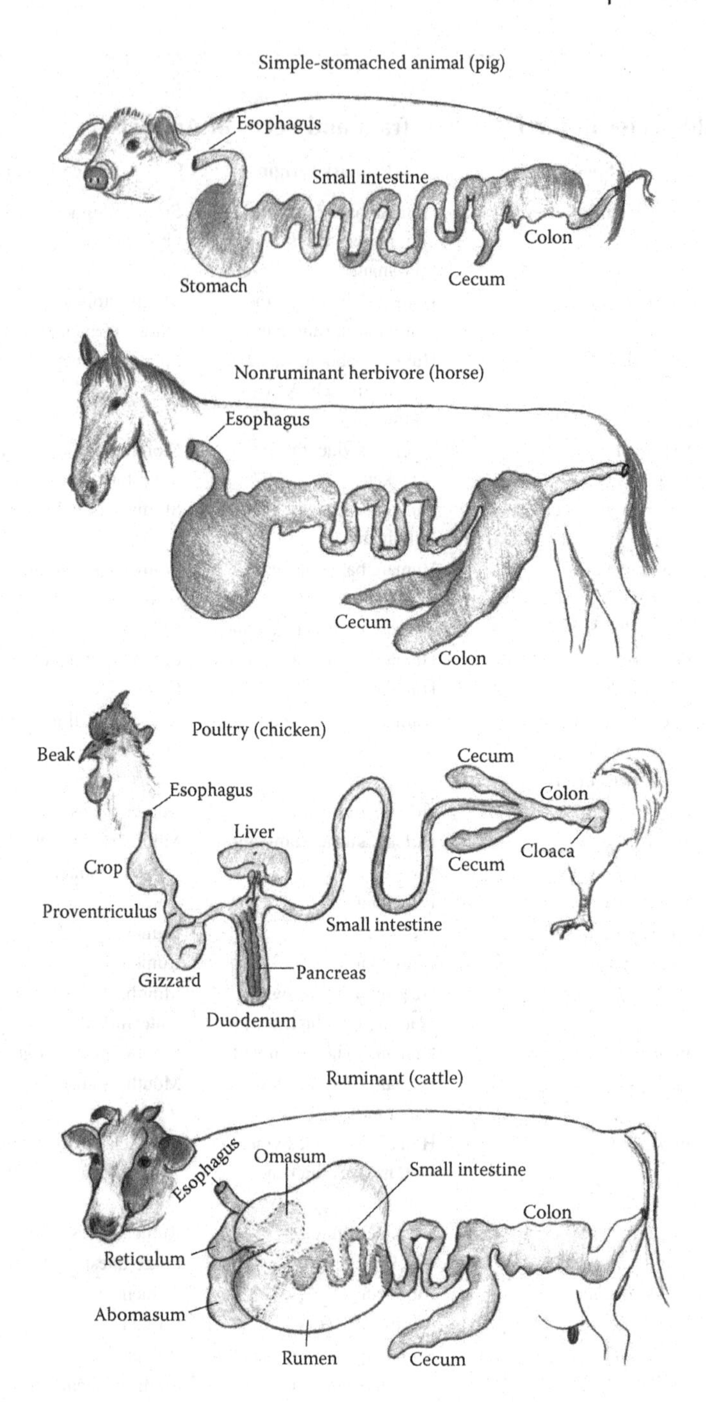


**FIGURE 1.11** Comparative aspects of the digestive systems in mammals and birds. Nonruminants (e.g., pigs, horses, and chickens) have a single stomach, the small intestine (duodenum, jejunum, and ileum), and the large intestine (colon and cecum). The digestive system of birds differs markedly from that of nonruminant mammals in that birds have the crop (a temporary storage pouch), the proventriculus (also known as the "true stomach"), and the gizzard (ventriculus; also known as the mechanical stomach). In ruminants, the stomach consists of four compartments: rumen, reticulum, omasum, and abomasum, with the first three parts being called the forestomach. The rumen contains large amounts of bacteria to ferment dietary fibers, other carbohydrates, and proteins. The abomasum in ruminants acts like the stomach in nonruminants. (Adapted from Bondi, A.A. 1987. *Animal Nutrition*. John Wiley & Sons, New York, NY.)

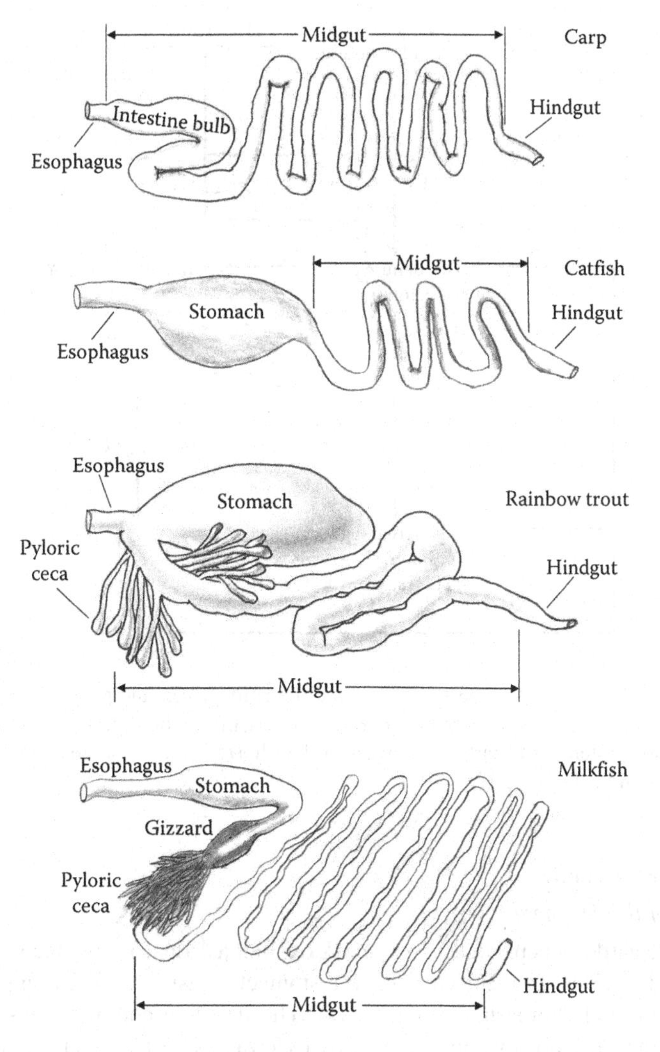


**FIGURE 1.12** Comparative aspects of digestive systems in fish. Depending on the species, fish have very different digestive tract morphologies. Some fish have a stomach, but some do not. The intestine of fish is not divided into the small and large intestine.

into the duodenum. The stomach secretes digestive enzymes and gastric acid to facilitate food digestion. The pH of the luminal fluid of the stomach is ~2.0 in adults, 2–3 in the young mammals (e.g., 2.5 in 7-day-old pigs), and 7.0 in the fetus (Pond et al. 1995; Yen 2000). The gastric acidity helps to kill the ingested pathogens and to reduce the susceptibility of animals to outbreaks of gastrointestinal disease. Of note, rabbits have an enlarged stomach to store large meals because they are crepuscular (i.e., eating primarily at dawn and dusk) (McDonald et al. 2011). Thus, the stomach functions primarily in both nutrient digestion and health protection.

The stomach of birds differs markedly from that of nonruminant mammals (Hill 1971). In birds (e.g., chickens, ducks, geese, and turkeys), ingested feed passes through the esophagus into the crop, which is a temporary storage pouch before digestion starts in the proventriculus (also known as the "true stomach"). Within the proventriculus, feed is mixed with hydrochloric acid (HCl) and digestive enzymes as in mammals to initiate the hydrolysis of proteins and fats. Subsequently, the digesta enters the gizzard (ventriculus; also known as the mechanical stomach) for grinding, mixing, and mashing, which helps to facilitate further digestion in the small intestine.

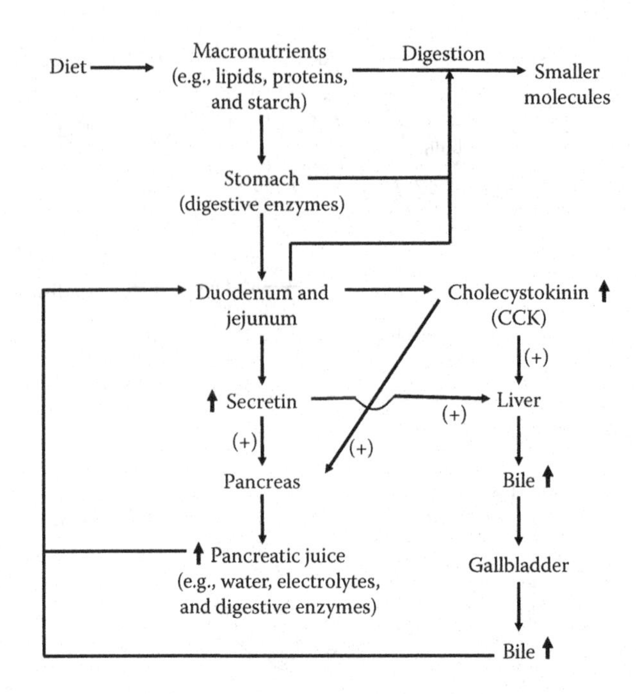


**FIGURE 1.13** Coordination among the stomach, small intestine, liver, and pancreas for efficient digestion of nutrients, such as fats, proteins, and carbohydrates. The organs of the digestive tract release enzymes to hydrolyze dietary fats, proteins, and carbohydrates, as well as hormones to regulate nutrient digestion, absorption, and metabolism in the body.

## The Stomach in Ruminants

### *Compartments of the Stomach*

Ruminants include cattle, sheep, goats, oxen, musk ox, llamas, alpacas, guanacos, deer, bison, antelopes, camels, and giraffes. In these animals, the stomach consists of four compartments: rumen, reticulum, omasum, and abomasum (Figure 1.14). The first two compartments are incompletely separated but distinct structurally and functionally (Vieira et al. 2008), and are collectively known as the reticulorumen. The rumen, reticulum, and omasum are also called the forestomach.

The rumen is the first compartment of the forestomach and is divided into cranial, dorsal, ventral, caudodorsal blind, and caudoventral blind sacs by muscular pillars. The rumen wall of ruminants has small and extensive fingerlike projections called papillae, which increase the rumen surface area and function to absorb some nutrients and fermentation products from the rumen into the blood (Cheeke and Dierenfeld 2010). Under normal feeding conditions, the rumen exhibits several characteristics: a mean temperature of 39°C (38–40°C); pH 5.5–6.8 (depending on the type of feedstuffs); a mean redox potential of −350 mv (a strong reducing environment without $O_2$); and the presence of $CO_2$ and methane as the major gases. The extreme anaerobic environment in the rumen is responsible for its unique features of digestion. In particular, ruminal pH greatly affects microbial fermentation and growth (Hungate 1966). When a large amount of monosaccharides or starch (highly fermentable carbohydrates) is added to forage diets, fiber digestion is impaired (Wickersham et al. 2009). Reductions in ruminal organic-matter digestibility due to a drop in ruminal pH are not equal for all nutrients in that the fermentation of fiber and protein is severely depressed but the catabolism of monosaccharides and starches remains very active.

The reticulum is the second and the most cranial compartment of the forestomach. Of note, in camelids (camels, llamas, alpacas, vicunas), the reticulum has glandlike cells and the omasum has a tubular structure that is almost indistinct (Tharwat et al. 2012); therefore, these animals are

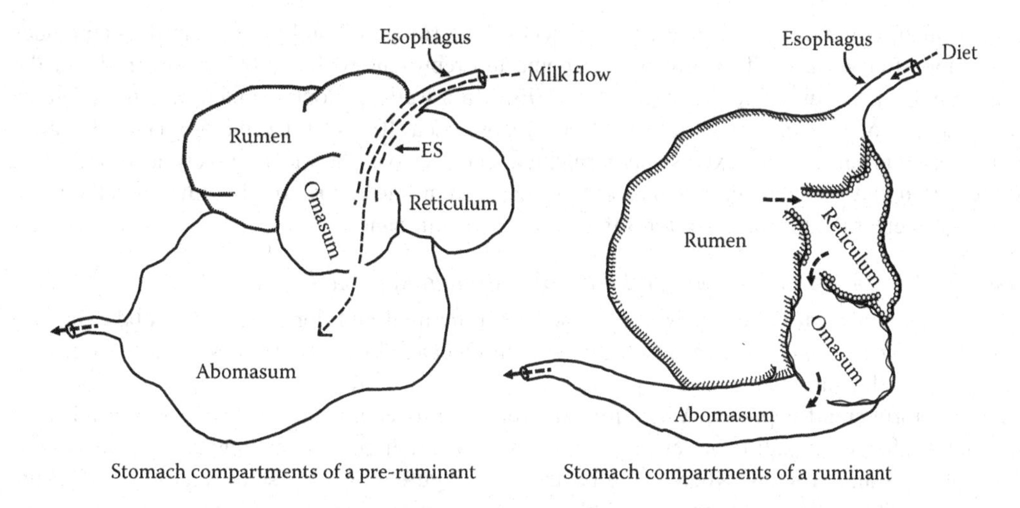


**FIGURE 1.14** The stomachs of preruminants and ruminants. These animals have rumen, reticulum, omasum, and abomasum as four-compartment stomachs. In preruminants, ingested liquid milk enters the abomasum through the esophageal groove (ES). In both preruminants and ruminants, solid feedstuffs enter, sequentially, the esophagus, rumen, reticulum, omasum, and abomasum for digestion. The rumen has cranial and dorsal sacs for solids, and the ventral sac for liquid. In preruminants, the walls of the rumen, reticulum, and omasum are underdeveloped. In contrast, in well-developed ruminants, the rumen wall has small and extensive finger-like projections called papillae to increase the rumen surface area, the reticulum has folds in the mucosa that appear like honeycomb, and the omasum has many longitudinal folds called laminae. Digesta flows out of the abomasum (which is similar to the stomach in nonruminants) into the duodenum.

occasionally incorrectly said to have a three-compartment stomach. In all ruminants, the abomasum is the true stomach, similar to that in nonruminants.

*Rumen Development*

The development of the rumen as a fermentation chamber for forages and grains is fundamentally important for ruminant nutrition (Hungate 1966). At birth, the rumen is undeveloped and has a limited amount of microbes. The rumen and abomasum represent 25% and 60%, respectively, of the total stomach mass in the newborn and increase with age. Rumen development depends on the consumption of fibrous diets and the establishment of microorganisms, including anaerobic bacteria (prokaryotes), fungi (primarily multicellular eukaryotes), and protozoa (unicellular eukaryotes). The microbes which colonize the rumen are obtained from the housing environment, dams and other animals with which the neonates come into contact, and bacteria found in milk or other feeds. The development of the rumen wall and the papillae is also primarily stimulated by butyrate and, to a lesser extent, propionate. Preruminants are animals with a rumen that is not anatomically or functionally mature. The preruminants are functionally similar to simple-stomached animals and are almost solely dependent on their own digestive enzymes. The preruminants have an esophageal groove, which is a muscular fold extending downwards from the opening of the esophagus to the omasum on the wall of the reticulum. Because of neural stimulation, the act of natural suckling or voluntary consumption of a liquid diet induces reflex closure of the esophageal groove into a tubular structure, directing milk into the abomasum for efficient utilization of nutrients and animal growth. Incomplete closure of the groove, primarily due to the lack of suckling reflex, as in force feeding, results in the initial entry of milk or any liquid food into the rumen or reticulum, which causes indigestion in neonates. Dry feed, such as grain mixtures or forage, does not pass through the esophageal groove, and, therefore, flows from the esophagus into the reticulorumen to further stimulate its development. The rumen and abomasum represent 65% and 20%, respectively, of the total stomach mass at 3 months of age. By the time of weaning (e.g., 3–8 months of age), the rumen is more mature and is able to digest fibrous feeds. The rumen (including the papillae) continues to develop after weaning. The rumen and abomasum represent 80% and 8%, respectively, of the total stomach mass in the adult (Steele et al. 2016). In a well-developed rumen, its fluid contains large amounts of anaerobic bacteria ($10^{10}$–$10^{11}$/mL), protozoa ($10^5$–$10^6$/mL), and fungi ($10^3$–$10^4$/mL), dietary organic nutrients are extensively fermented, and each papilla can effectively absorb ruminal fermentation end-products (e.g., SCFAs). After absorption into the ruminal epithelial cells, these metabolites enter the bloodstream for utilization by the ruminant.

*Digestive Function of the Rumen and the Abomasum in Ruminants*

Feed passes first from the esophagus into the rumen (cranial and dorsal sacs for solids, and the ventral sac for liquids) and then into the reticulum (McDonald et al. 2011). Within the reticulorumen, the following reactions take place. First, proteins are hydrolyzed by proteases and peptidases to form small peptides, AAs, ammonia, other nitrogenous metabolites, carbon skeletons, and SCFAs. Second, small peptides, AAs, and ammonia are used primarily by bacteria to synthesize new AAs and proteins, whereas the bacteria are engulfed and digested by protozoa (Firkins et al. 2007). Third, dietary fibers and soluble carbohydrates are fermented to pyruvate, lactate, and large amounts of SCFAs. Fourth, all vitamins are synthesized from the appropriate precursors by microbes. Fifth, unsaturated long-chain fatty acids undergo biohydrogenation to form saturated long-chain fatty acids and conjugated fatty acids, whereas oxidation of fatty acids to $CO_2$ and water is limited (Bauman et al. 2011). The feed and its fermented products are mixed freely within the reticulorumen before entering the omasum. Finally, the digesta moves into the abomasum for further digestion, mostly as in nonruminants. Thus, ruminants can convert low-quality roughages into high-quality protein (e.g., milk and meat) for human consumption.

The rumen contains high urease activity to hydrolyze urea into ammonia and $CO_2$. Some of the ammonia is utilized locally for the synthesis of AAs and proteins by microbes; the remaining ammonia enters the blood through the ruminal epithelium and the portal vein, and then reaches the liver, where ammonia is converted into urea (Wu 2013). Through circulation, this urea becomes part of the saliva and reenters the rumen for utilization by microbes (Wickersham et al. 2009). This pathway of urea metabolism within the digestive system is called urea recycling. Its role is to maximize efficiency of the utilization of dietary nonprotein nitrogen (NPN) and protein nitrogen for AA synthesis in ruminants. A unique characteristic of ruminants is rumination, which refers to the process whereby digesta is regurgitated from the forestomach into the esophagus, remasticated by the animal, and reswallowed into the forestomach for further digestion.

There are positive relationships among feed intake, the turnover rates of ruminal liquid, particles and bacteria, and microbial fermentation efficiency (Hungate 1966). First, the number of ruminal microbes depends on their ability to reproduce at a rate equal to or greater than their losses from the rumen. Second, the survival of ruminal microbes is enhanced by their attachment to feed particles. Third, the efficiency of ruminal microbes to digest feedstuffs is increased when the transit of the feed particles through the rumen is prolonged. Ruminal organic-matter digestion will be reduced when the total number of ruminal microbes is lowered. Microbial fermentation efficiency is very important for the ruminant, because the host requires both SCFAs and microbial protein for survival, growth, and reproduction (Stevens and Hume 1998).

### The Small Intestine

The intestine of mammals and birds is divided into the small intestine (the portion of the digestive tract between the pylorus and the ileocecal valve) and the large intestine (the portion of the digestive tract between the ileocecal valve and the anus), but the intestine is not separated into small and large intestines in fish. The small intestine of mammals and birds is divided into three parts: duodenum (the portion of the digestive tract between the pylorus and the jejunum; e.g., 10 cm in length in young pigs), jejunum, and ileum. The jejunum and ileum constitute 40% and 60%, respectively, of the small intestine length below the duodenum (Madara 1991). Inside the lumen of the small intestine, there is an aqueous diffusion layer (known as the *unstirred water layer*) that is adjacent to the *intestinal* mucosal membrane. This unstirred water layer can affect the efficiency of nutrient absorption and drug delivery. Mechanisms for the digestion and absorption of nutrients in the small intestine are similar between ruminants and nonruminants (Beitz 1993; Bergen and Wu 2009; Liao et al. 2010).

The small intestine is a highly differentiated and complex organ (Figure 1.15). The wall of the small intestine consists of four main layers: (1) the mucosa, (2) the submucosa, (3) the muscularis externa, and (4) the serosa. The epithelium of the small intestine rests on the underlying lamina propria, which is a connective tissue layer containing blood and lymphatic capillaries, as well as mononuclear cells (e.g., lymphocytes, mast cells, plasma cells, and macrophages), polymorphonuclear leukocytes, and nerve fibers (Madara 1991). The blood and lymphatic capillaries carry the absorbed water- and lipid-soluble nutrients to the portal vein and lymphatic vessels, respectively. The lamina propria is covered with an amorphous sheet called the basal lamina on which the epithelium directly rests. The lamina propria is supported by the underlying muscularis mucosa (two thin layers of smooth muscle together with varying amounts of elastic tissue). The epithelium, the lamina propria,

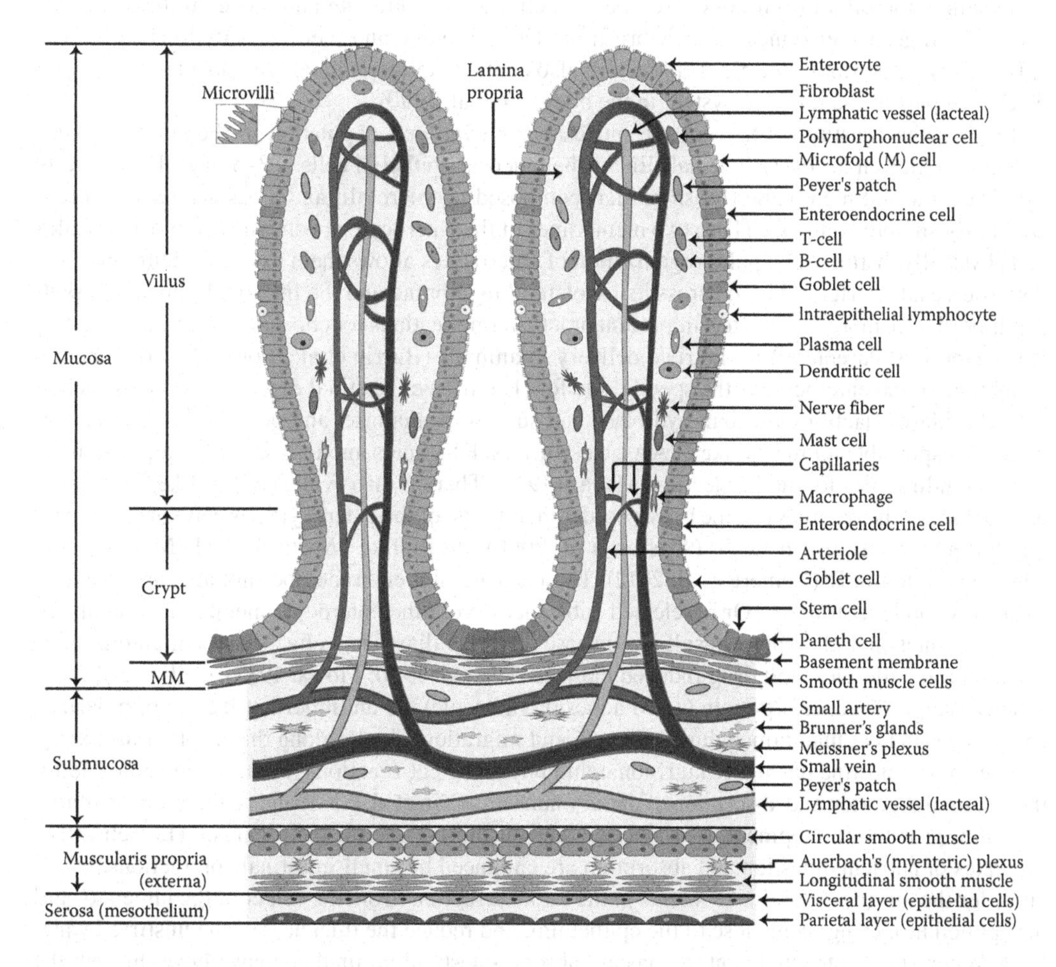


**FIGURE 1.15** The structure of the wall of the small intestine. The wall of the small intestine consists of the epithelium in the crypt and villus regions, as well as the supporting connective tissue of lamina propria, smooth muscle cells, the vasculature, nerves, and basolateral epithelial cells. The lamina propria contains blood capillaries, lymph capillaries, and various types of cells (including lymphocytes and macrophages). Stem cells in the crypt differentiate into four major types of cells: the enterocyte, goblet cell, enteroendocrine cell, and Paneth cell.

and the muscularis mucosa are collectively termed as the mucosa (Barrett 2014). The mucosa is supported by the submucosa, which is a connective tissue layer containing the plexuses of larger blood vessels. The submucosa is underlain by the muscularis externa (two fairly substantial layers of smooth muscle; inner circular and outer longitudinal for contractions), which propels intestinal luminal contents downward from the duodenum into the cecum. The fourth and outermost layer of the wall of the intestine is the serosa, which is a layer of mesothelial cells.

The small-intestinal epithelium consists of two compartments: the villus and the crypt of Lieberkühn. The crypt–villus junction is defined as the point at which the distance between opposing epithelial layers suddenly begins to widen (Madara 1991). The crypt is divided into the Paneth cell zone, stem cell zone, proliferation compartment, and maturation zone. The undifferentiated stem cell of the crypt is the progenitor cell from which intestinal epithelial cells originate. During migration from the crypt to the villus tip via the intestinal crypt–villus axis, stem cells differentiate into one of at least four mature cell types: the villus columnar absorptive cell (enterocyte), the mucin-producing and mucin-secreting goblet cell, the enteroendocrine cell secreting a variety of substances, and the Paneth cell that likely plays a role in the secretion of molecules for protection against microflora (Yen 2000). As the epithelial cells proliferate and move up the villus, the activity of digestive enzymes on their brush-border membrane and their capacity to absorb nutrients increase. The small-intestinal epithelium also contains intraepithelial lymphocytes and Peyer's patches as part of the immune system in the body (Li et al. 1990).

Enterocytes constitute >85% of the mucosal epithelial cell population in the small intestine (Klein and McKenzie 1983). The half-life of the mucosal epithelial cells is 3–5 days. Each enterocyte has an apical membrane (brush border) composed of microvilli and a basolateral membrane with fairly smooth contours. These two membranes of the enterocyte are chemically, biochemically, and physically distinct. The polar organization of enterocytes allows them to receive nutrients from both sources: the arterial blood across its basolateral membrane and the intestinal lumen across its brush-border membrane. This has important practical implications for choosing the route of feeding (e.g., enteral vs. parenteral) for nutrient delivery to animals (Burrin et al. 2000). The brush-border membrane of the enterocyte is the specific site for (1) intrinsic intestinal digestive enzymes such as disaccharidases (lactase-phlorizin hydrolase and sucrase-isomaltase) and peptidases; (2) transport proteins responsible for the uptake of AAs, electrolytes, fatty acids, monosaccharides, and vitamins; and (3) binding sites for dietary lectins (Madara 1991). There is also evidence that, like the basolateral surface of the enterocytes, the brush-border membrane of the enterocyte has cell-surface receptors for epidermal growth factor (Avissar et al. 2000), insulinlike growth factor-I (Morgan et al. 1996), and vitamin D (Nemere et al. 2012). The basolateral membrane does not appear to contain sugar or peptide hydrolases. Only selected substances cross the enterocyte membrane, and abnormality of intestinal absorption results in diseases such as diarrhea, celiac sprue (an autoimmune disease), food allergies, and drug-induced damage (Li et al. 1990; Mowat 1987). Cell-to-cell interactions via the E cadherin protein (a cell adhesion molecule) are an important feature of polarized enterocytes and are maintained during growth and migration of cells along the crypt–villus axis.

The small intestine has many nutritional and physiological functions. First, it is responsible for the terminal digestion and absorption of dietary nutrients (Yin et al. 2002) and is, therefore, essential to health, growth, development, reproduction, and sustaining life for the organism (Barrett 2014). The rates of nutrient digestion and absorption are enhanced by small-intestinal contractions, which allow for the mixing of luminal contents in the radial direction (from the center of the lumen toward the epithelium), bring them close to the epithelium, and reduce the thickness of the unstirred water layer. When small-intestinal contractions are absent, intestinal luminal contents move through the small intestine as a laminar flow just like that occurring in a pipe. Second, in mammalian neonates, the small intestine can absorb immunoglobulins from milk before the "*gut closure*" (e.g., 24 h after birth in calves and goat kids; 24–36 h after birth in piglets and lambs; 24–28 h after birth in foals, cats, and dogs). This is important for the immunity of the newborns. Third, the gut is the barrier separating the internal milieu of the organism from the external environment; therefore, it is critical for the exclusion of food-borne pathogens and preventing the translocation of luminal microorganisms into the circulation. Finally, as the largest lymphoid organ in the body, the small intestine participates in immune surveillance of the intestinal epithelial layer and regulation of the mucosal response to foreign antigens (Mowat 1987). This is of enormous immunological importance, because (1) the normal intestinal tract encounters enormous amounts of dietary antigenic loads, (2) ingested dietary antigens need to be processed and recognized without inducing harmful hypersensitivity reactions, and (3) the integrity of intestinal mucosa must be protected against the invasion of exogenous pathogenic microorganisms.

### The Large Intestine

The large intestine, also called the hindgut or large bowel, is the last part of the digestive system in vertebrates. The large intestine is defined as the combination of the cecum, colon, rectum, and anal canal (Barrett 2014). Like the small intestine, the lumen of the large intestine also has an *unstirred water layer.* The relative capacities of large intestines differ markedly among animal species (Table 1.5). The hindgut harbors large amounts of microorganisms (e.g., bacteria, protozoa, and fungi) that also ferment carbohydrates, proteins, and AAs to form SCFAs, $H_2S$, ammonia, indoles, skatole, and other AA metabolites just like ruminal bacteria (Bondi 1987; Yang et al. 2014). In all animals, the numbers of bacteria in the large intestine are several magnitudes greater than those in the small intestine (Table 1.5). For example, bacterial counts of $10^7$–$10^{12}$/g feces have been reported in the hindgut of mammals, birds, and reptiles. In addition, substantial amounts of protozoa ($10^3$–$10^8$/g feces) have also been found in the large intestine of these species. Colonocytes have a high capacity to absorb SCFAs, electrolytes, and water, but these cells take up only a limited amount of AAs and nitrogenous metabolites from the lumen of the large intestine (Bergen and Wu 2009). In contrast to enterocytes, colonocytes use butyrate as their major energy source and, to a lesser extent, glutamine, acetate, and propionate as their metabolic fuels (Barrett 2014; Wu 2013). Because dietary fibers stimulate intestinal motility and generate SCFA production in the large intestine, consumption of adequate amounts of these plant-source substances is beneficial for the optimal gut health, longevity, and productivity of animals, particularly lactating dams and breeding stock.

Some nonruminant herbivores, such as horses (Coverdale et al. 2004) and rabbits (Brewer 2006), have a particularly high capacity to digest dietary fiber and plant-source protein in the large intestine, which allows them to graze on pasture and consume roughages. They are called "hindgut fermenters," which are subdivided into cecal fermenters and colonic fermenters. Cecal fermenters are those hindgut fermenters whose cecum is the primary site of fermentation and include the rabbit, guinea pig, ostrich, goose, and duck (Cheeke and Dierenfeld 2010; Clemens et al. 1975). These animals are generally small as adults (e.g., 3–6 kg) with the exceptions of the koala (~10 kg) and the capybara (~50 kg) (Cheeke and Dierenfeld 2010). Of note, the rabbit directly ingests soft fecal pellets (cecotrophs) from its rectum as a result of a neurologic licking response (Davies and Davies 2003). Colonic fermenters use the proximal colon as the primary site of fermentation and are usually large as adults. Examples of colonic fermenters include the horse, zebra, donkey, elephant, rhinoceros, monkey, lemur, and beaver. Because of their relatively high capacities to utilize plant cell wall materials and dietary fibers, hindgut fermenters (particularly rabbits, geese, and ducks) contribute greatly to sustainable animal agriculture just like ruminants.

### The Pancreas

The pancreas is an organ with both endocrine and exocrine roles. It is present in all vertebrates, but the shape is very different depending on the species, with a soft and *diffuse* organization in rodents as opposed to a firm and pear-shaped structure in pigs (Dyce et al. 1996). As an endocrine organ, the pancreas synthesizes and releases insulin and glucagon to regulate blood glucose levels. The autoimmune destruction of insulin-producing β-cells results in insulin-dependent diabetes mellitus in animals (Beitz 1993). Insulin-independent (resistant) diabetes mellitus occurs in obese animals as in obese humans. As an exocrine organ, the pancreas synthesizes and releases (1) proteases, co-lipase, and pro-phospholipase $A_2$ as proenzymes that are activated in the small-intestinal lumen; and (2) α-amylase, lipases, cholesteryl ester hydrolase, ribonuclease (RNAase), and deoxy ribonuclease (RNAase) in active forms. These digestive enzymes hydrolyze dietary protein, starch, glycogen, lipids, and nucleic acids. Pancreatic juice also contains sodium carbonate and sodium bicarbonate to neutralize acid from the stomach and increase the alkalinity in the lumen of the small intestine (Guyton and Hall 2000). Because of these important digestive and metabolic functions, rapid weight loss often occurs in animals with pancreatic diseases. Likewise, young mammals exhibit growth depression during the first week postweaning when the secretion of pancreatic lipase, α-amylase, and proteases is substantially reduced (Yen 2000).

### The Liver

The liver is a central organ in the digestion, metabolism, transport, and storage of nutrients, as well as detoxification and immunity. On the basis of gross anatomy, the liver has four lobes of unequal size and shape: left, right, caudate, and quadrate (Dyce et al. 1996). In the porcine liver, the right lobe is subdivided into the main lobe and a caudate process. The gallbladder, which is present in most vertebrates as a small pouch sitting under the liver, stores bile (a mixture of water, bile salts, cholesterol, and bilirubin) produced by the liver and then releases the bile into the duodenum in response to feeding (e.g., 46 and 38 mL/kg body weight per day in 45- and 60-kg pigs, respectively; Yen 2000). The animals with a gallbladder are bears, cats, cattle, channel catfish, chickens, dogs, geese, goats, guinea pigs, hawks, humans, mice, monkeys, owls, pigs, rabbits, sheep, and zebrafish (Oldham-Ott and Gilloteaux 1997). On the contrary, some species of mammals (i.e., horses, deer, rats, seals, and laminoids), birds (e.g., pigeons, parrots, and doves), and fish (e.g., lampreys), as well as all invertebrates, lack a gallbladder (Oldham-Ott and Gilloteaux 1997). In the species without a gallbladder, bile flows directly from the liver into the lumen of the duodenum through the bile duct.

As a highly perfused organ, the liver receives 20%–25% of blood output from the heart (Dyce et al. 1996). The nutrients that are absorbed into the portal vein and those that are carried within the hepatic artery enter the liver for extraction by hepatocytes and other types of cells. The nutrients that bypass the liver without uptake and metabolites released from the liver enter the inferior vena cava for utilization (including metabolism) in extrahepatic tissues or for excretion through the kidneys. Of note, the porous endothelium of the liver allows hepatocytes to extract both small and large molecules from the blood and to release large molecules (e.g., lipoproteins and cholesterol) into the blood (Guyton et al. 1972). However, RBCs do not cross the hepatic sinusoidal endothelium. Kupffer cells (macrophages) in the liver play an important role in fighting pathogens and in the local immune response.

At the histological level, each lobe of the liver is composed of many lobules, with the center of each lobule being the hepatic central vein. At the periphery of the lobules are portal triads (portal tracts), which contain five different structures: the hepatic artery, hepatic portal vein, common bile duct, lymphatic vessels, and branches of the vagus nerve (Argenzio 1993). Hepatic lobules are composed of the parenchymal cells (the functional parts of an organ) of the liver (i.e., hepatocytes; 80% of the liver volume, 60% of cells) and nonparenchymal cells (6.5% of the liver volume but 40% of cells) (Guyton and Hall 2000). Each hepatic lobule is hexagonal in shape and consists of plates of hepatocytes, branches of the portal vein and the hepatic artery, sinusoids (very small blood vessels), hepatic central vein, hepatic vein, bile ducts, and associated nonparenchymal cells (e.g., hepatic stellate cells and Kupffer cells). As noted previously, the portal vein and hepatic artery supply blood to the liver. These two sources of blood mix in the hepatic sinusoids where nutrients and gases are exchanged with hepatocytes and associated cells through the extracellular interstitial space. Thereafter, the blood flows sequentially into the venule end of the hepatic sinusoids, the hepatic central vein, and the hepatic vein and then leaves the liver through the inferior vena cava (also known as caudal vena cava) into the right atrium of the heart (Dyce et al. 1996).

On the basis of oxygen supply and metabolism, the functional unit of the liver is the hepatic acinus, which is oriented around the afferent vascular system (Rappaport 1958). The acinus is divided into three zones. Zone I (periportal hepatocytes) is nearest to the venules of the portal vein and the arterioles of the hepatic artery and is the most oxygenated. Zone III (perivenous hepatocytes), which is farthest from the microvasculature of the entering blood vessels, is around the hepatic central vein and is poorly oxygenated (Figure 1.16). Zone II (midzone) is the transition zone located between zones I and III. Periportal, midzone, and perivenous hepatocytes represent ~80%, 10%–15%, and 5%–10% of total hepatocytes, respectively. These three different types of cells have very different metabolic patterns (Schleicher et al. 2015). Such a concept of metabolic zonation helps us understand how nutrients are utilized and synthesized in the liver.

Hepatocytes do not possess all the transporters needed for the uptake of physiological substances from the blood, nor do they express all the enzymes for nutrient metabolism (Häussinger et al. 1992). For example, mammalian hepatocytes lack transporters for some molecules (e.g., citrulline), as well as enzymes for (1) initiating the catabolism of some AAs (e.g., branched-chain AAs) under

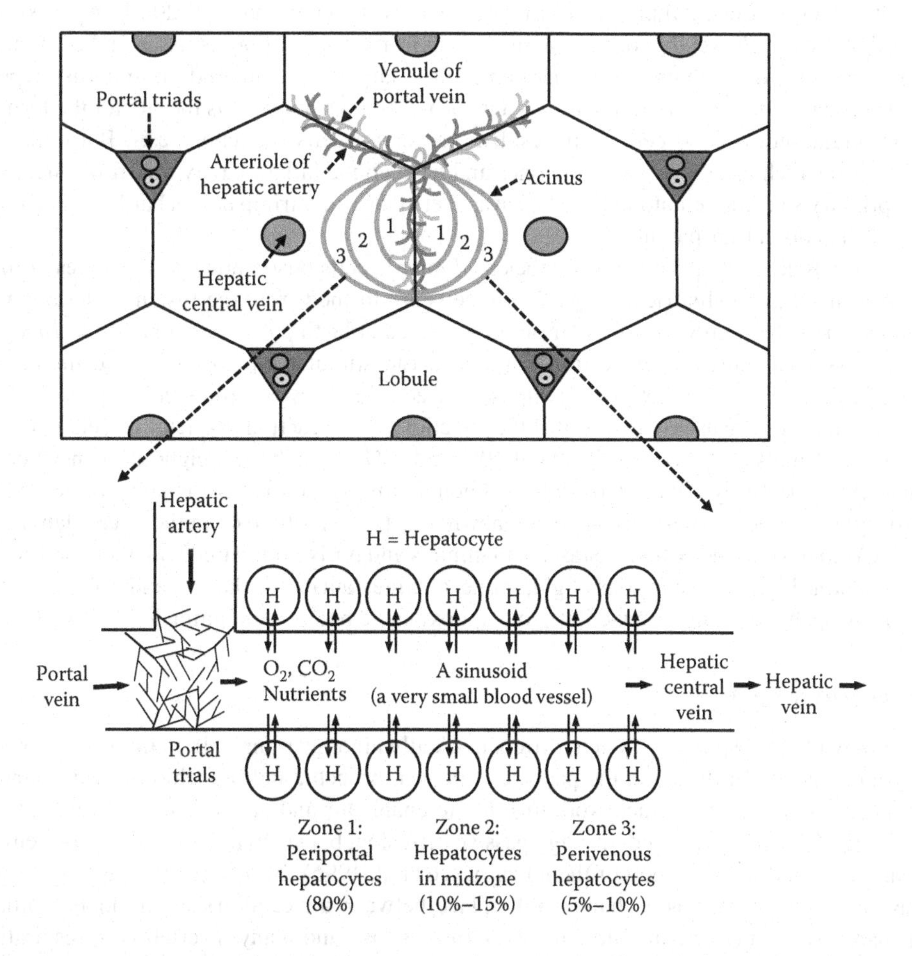


**FIGURE 1.16** The hepatic acinus and nutrient exchange through the hepatic sinusoid in the liver. The liver is composed of many lobules (hexagonal structures), with the center of each lobule being the hepatic central vein. At the periphery of the lobules are portal triads, which contain the hepatic artery and the portal vein to supply blood to the liver. The hepatic acinus, which is oriented around the afferent vascular system, is the functional unit of the liver. The acinus consists of hepatocytes aligned around the arterioles of the hepatic artery and the venules of the portal vein. Their microvasculatures anastomose into sinusoids, which are the sites for the exchange of nutrients, $O_2$, and $CO_2$ with hepatocytes. On the basis of the distance from the portal venules and hepatic arterioles, the acinus is divided into three zones: Zone 1 (periportal hepatocytes, the best oxygenated), Zone 2 (mid-acinar hepatocytes), and Zone 3 (perivenous hepatocytes, poorly oxygenated). Blood leaves the liver through the hepatic central vein.

physiological conditions, (2) the net synthesis of some AAs (e.g., arginine), and (3) the oxidation of some metabolites (e.g., ketone bodies, urea, and uric acid) (Roach et al. 2012; Wu 2013). However, hepatocytes have a high capacity to oxidize fatty acids and the α-ketoacids of AAs to $CO_2$ and $H_2O$ and play an important role in the interorgan metabolism of nutrients in animals. Furthermore, the hepatocytes are capable of synthesizing glucose, glycogen, fats, plasma proteins (e.g., albumin, ferritin, and fibrinogen), lipoproteins, cholesterol, and bile, as well as storing glycogen, vitamins (e.g., vitamins A and $B_{12}$), and minerals (e.g., iron and copper) (Jungermann and Keitzmann 1996).

## The Musculoskeletal System

The *musculoskeletal system* is the combination of skeletal muscles as well as their associated bones, cartilage, attached tendons, ligaments, joints, and other connective tissue. Bones are living structures with blood vessels, lymphatic vessels, and nerves (Guyton and Hall 2000). Approximately one-third of the bone's weight consists of an organic framework of fibrous tissue and cells, and the remaining two-thirds is composed of inorganic salts (largely calcium and phosphorus) deposited within the organic framework. In mammals and birds, the bone marrow is the site for the formation and differentiation of blood cells from resident progenitor cells (hematopoiesis; Barminko et al. 2016). In fish which usually possess no bones and have no medullary cavity (marrow), the kidneys are the primary sites for hematopoiesis (Kobayashi et al. 2016). Shrimp have a hard exoskeleton (the shell) which is often transparent.

Skeletal muscle is composed of multinucleated muscle cells (also known as myocytes or muscle fibers) organized in a cylindrical shape. These cells are formed from the fusion of developmental myoblasts during fetal growth, and their number is fixed at birth (Oksbjerg et al. 2013). Myogenin, which is a skeletal muscle-specific transcription factor, stimulates myogenesis and the repair of muscles from injury. The myofibrils (composed of actin and myosin filaments, repeated in units called sarcomeres) in muscle fibers fulfill the function of contraction. Skeletal muscle is the largest tissue in animals and accounts for about 40% and 45% of the body weight in the newborn and young adult, respectively (Dyce et al. 1996). Although this organ was traditionally considered to be a relatively inert protein reservoir, it is now known to actively participate in the interorgan metabolism of AAs and whole-body homeostasis in mammals and birds. Compared with the blood, skeletal muscle contains high concentrations of glutamine, alanine, taurine, β-alanine, and carnosine to support gluconeogenesis, immune functions, and antioxidative reactions in animals (Wu 2013).

## The Respiratory System

The anatomy of the respiratory system differs markedly among animals. In mammals, the respiratory system consists of the nose, the passages (trachea, bronchi, and bronchioles), lungs, and diaphragm (a skeletal muscle), which work together to enable air and gases to get into and out of the lungs; $O_2$ and $CO_2$ are exchanged, through passive diffusion, between the external gaseous environment and the blood in the alveoli of the lungs (Dyce et al. 1996). Birds lack the diaphragm muscle but have air sacs, where gas exchanges take place between air capillaries and blood capillaries, rather than in alveoli (King and Molony 1971). In most fish and many invertebrates, respiration is accomplished through the gills; however, lungfish have one or two lungs. In amphibians, the skin plays a vital role in gas exchange. In reptiles, which lack the diaphragm muscle, gas exchange still occurs in the alveoli of the lungs.

Supplying $O_2$ to the tissues and removing $CO_2$ from the tissues are the two major functions of the respiratory system (Dyce et al. 1996). Secondary functions include temperature control, elimination of water, and voice production. In addition, the exhalation of $CO_2$ helps regulate the acid–base balance in the blood. The physiological importance of the respiratory system is epitomized by the very fact that $O_2$ is vital to animals. An animal may survive for days without water consumption, for weeks without food, but its life without $O_2$ inhalation is measured only in minutes.

## The Urinary System

In mammals and birds, the urinary system consists of two kidneys, two ureters, the bladder, and the urethra. The kidneys are located at the rear of the abdominal cavity in mammals, birds, and reptiles and are surrounded by a tough fibrous tissue called the renal capsule (Boron 2004). The kidney is divided into two parts: the outer renal cortex and the inner renal medulla. The kidneys receive blood from a pair of renal arteries, and the blood leaves the kidneys through a pair of renal veins. The rate of blood flow through the kidneys is very high, representing ~20% of the blood output from the left ventricle of the heart (Dyce et al. 1996).

The functional unit of each kidney is the nephron, which spans the length of the cortex and medulla (Figure 1.17). The number of nephrons in several species is as follows: cattle, $4 \times 10^6$; pigs, $1.25 \times 10^6$; dogs, $0.415 \times 10^6$; and cats, $0.19 \times 10^6$ (Reece 1993). The first process in urine formation is glomerular filtration. Namely, filtration takes place when components of blood pass through the glomerular capillary endothelium, the basement membrane, and Bowman's capsule epithelium into the luminal space of Bowman's capsule in the renal cortex. The glomerular filtrate is an ultrafiltrate of the blood and includes water, ions, and small molecules that easily pass through the filtration membrane. However, larger molecules such as proteins and blood cells are essentially prevented from passing through the filtration membrane. The amount of filtrate produced every minute (the glomerular filtration rate) is high (e.g., 4 mL/min/kg body weight in a 9.5 kg dog) (Reece 1993). The second process of urine formation is tubular reabsorption of nutrients, which occurs primarily in the proximal tubule (e.g., 65% Na), followed by the loop of Henle (25% Na), the distal tubule (5% Na), and the collecting duct (5% Na). In this process, water, AAs, glucose, metabolites, vitamins, and minerals inside the tubular lumen pass through the brush-border membrane and the basolateral membrane of the tubular epithelium into peritubular blood capillaries (Figure 1.18). The remaining portion is called tubular fluid. About 99% of this filtrate is reabsorbed as it passes through the nephron and the remaining 1% becomes urine. The final process of urine formation is tubular secretion, which involves the transport of some substances (e.g., $H^+$, minerals, and some waste products) from the peritubular blood capillaries into the interstitial fluid and then to the tubular lumen via tubular epithelial cells (Weiner and Verlander 2011). The final urine is collected into the ureters, stored in the bladder, and discharged through the urethra.

The primary function of the urinary system is to eliminate water and metabolites (e.g., ammonia, urea, creatinine, nitrite, nitrate, sulfates, and conjugated drugs) from the animal. In healthy animals, the kidneys do not excrete a significant amount of glucose or ketone bodies (Boron 2004). At elevated concentrations in the blood, they exceed the renal tubular transport capacity and are lost from the body as parts of the urine (e.g., diabetic ketoacidosis). In addition, the kidneys play important roles in regulating (1) whole-body water balance and blood volume; (2) blood pressure; (3) concentrations of electrolytes and metabolites in the blood and urine; and (4) blood pH. The kidneys also participate in interorgan metabolism of AAs, for example, through the endogenous synthesis of arginine from citrulline in adult mammals and glycine production from hydroxyproline in animals (Wu 2013).

## The Male Reproductive System

The mammalian male reproductive system consists of (1) two testes (producing sperm and male reproductive hormones); (2) the scrotum (enclosing and protecting the testes); (3) the epididymis (the site for maturation and storage for sperm before they pass into the vas deferens); (4) the vas deferens (the sperm duct) that carries mature sperm from the epididymis to the ejaculatory ducts; (5) the penis (whose erection is dependent on nitric oxide-induced vasodilation of blood vessels in the corpora cavernosa); and (6) accessory sex glands (seminal vesicles, the prostate, the Cowper glands, and the urethral glands) that produce fluids to lubricate the reproductive tract and nourish the sperm cells (Dyce et al. 1996). Semen is composed of spermatozoa suspended in fluid from the

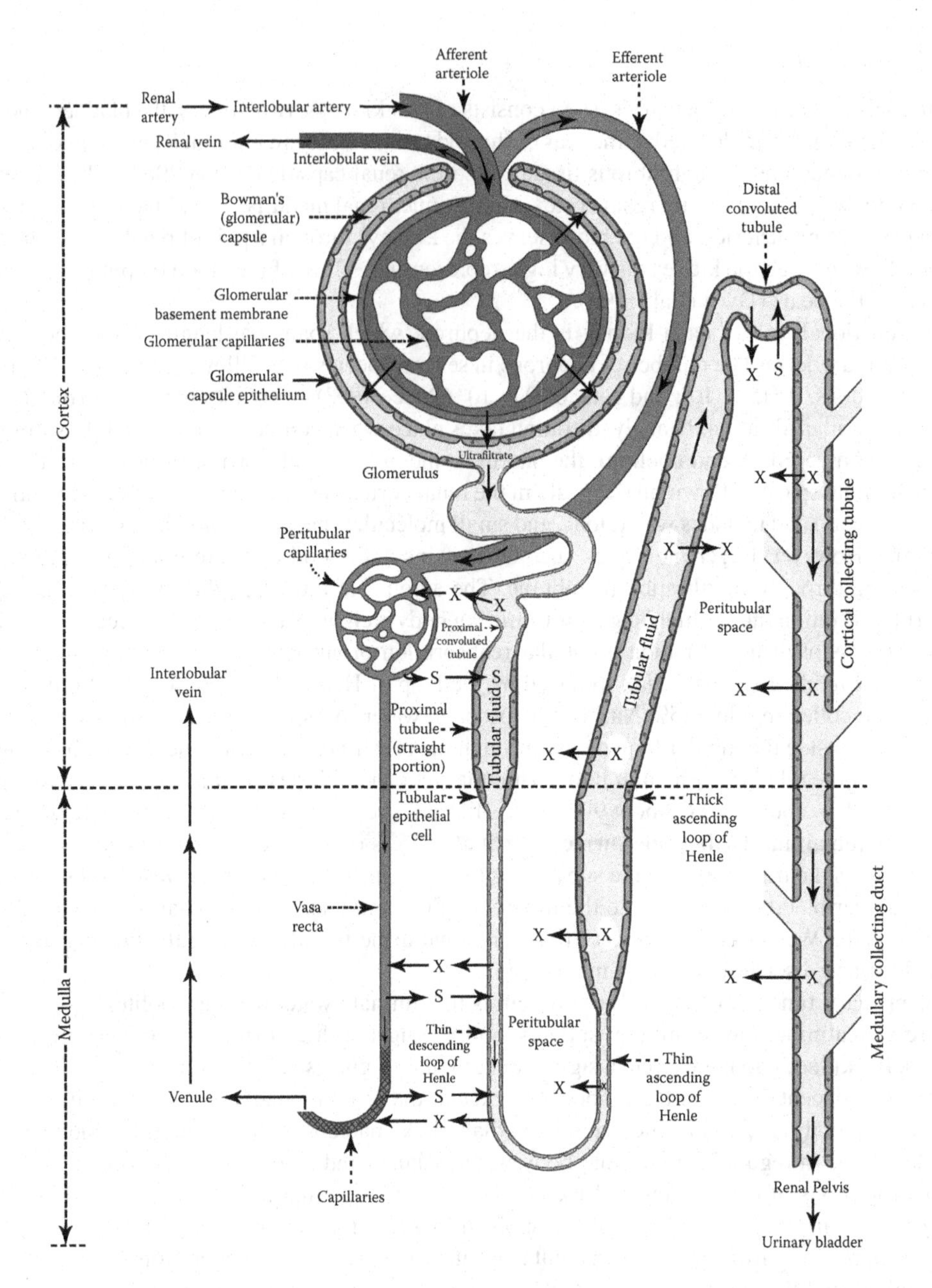


**FIGURE 1.17** The structure of the kidney. The kidney consists of the outer renal cortex and the inner renal medulla. A pair of renal arteries supply blood to the kidneys and venous blood leaves the kidneys through a pair of renal veins. The functional unit of the kidney is the nephron, which spans the cortex and medulla. Urine formation involves three processes: (1) glomerular filtration of arterial blood; (2) tubular reabsorption of the filtrates into peritubular blood capillaries; and (3) tubular secretion into the interstitial fluid and then to the tubular lumen via tubular epithelial cells. Metabolites are excreted from the body mainly through urine, which is collected into the ureters, stored in the bladder, and discharged through the urethra. The letter "X" represents nutrients being reabsorbed from the renal tubule into the blood in a segment-dependent manner: primarily AAs, glucose, vitamins, $H_2O$, NaCl, $K^+$, and $HCO_3^-$ in the proximal tubule; $H_2O$ in the loop of Henle; NaCl in the thick ascending limb; $H_2O$, NaCl, and $HCO_3^-$ in the distal tubule; and NaCl, some urea, and $H_2O$ in the collecting duct. The letter "S" represents substances entering the renal tubule from the blood in a segment-dependent manner: primarily $H^+$ and $NH_3$ in the proximal tubule; and $H^+$ and $K^+$ in the distal tubule. (Adapted from Dyce, K.M. et al. 1996. *Textbook of Veterinary Anatomy*. W.B. Saunders Company, Philadelphia, PA.)

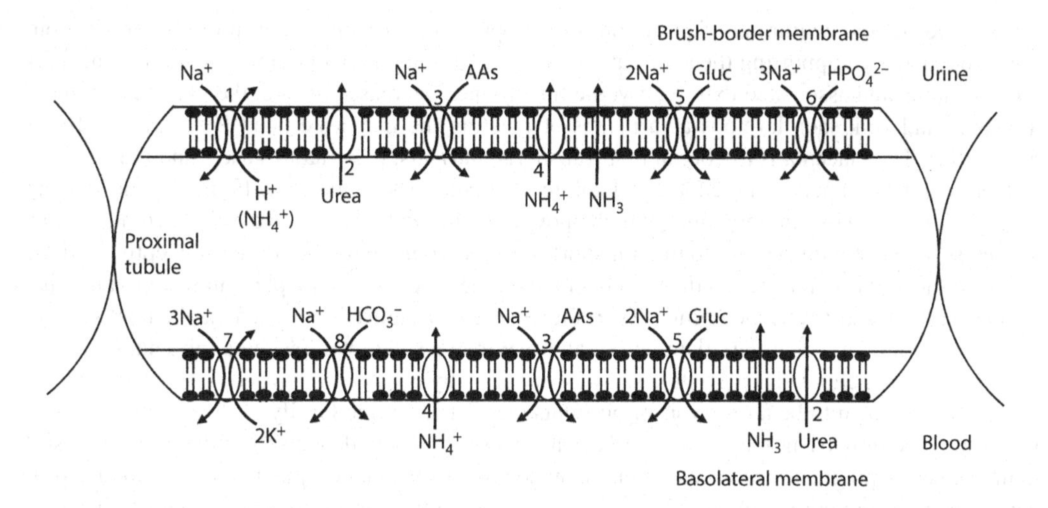


**FIGURE 1.18** Transport of sodium, glucose, AAs, $NH_3$, and $NH_4^+$ by proximal renal tubules. Active transport or secondary active transport is indicated by a number: 1, $Na^+/H^+$ ($NH_4^+$) exchanger; 2, urea transporters; 3, sodium-dependent amino acid transporters; 4, $NH_4^+$ transporter; 5, SGLT1 (sodium–glucose-linked transporter 1); 6, $Na^+$–phosphate cotransporter; 7, $Na^+$–$K^+$ pump; 8, $Na^+$–bicarbonate cotransporter. $NH_3$ is transported across the cell membrane through simple diffusion. AAs, amino acids. (Adapted from Weiner, I.D. and J.W. Verlander. 2011. *Am. J. Physiol. Renal Physiol.* 300:F11–F23; Reece, W.O. 1993. *Dukes' Physiology of Domestic Animals.* Edited by M.J. Swenson and W.O. Reece. Cornell University Press, Ithaca, NY, pp. 573–628.)

accessory sex glands called seminal plasma. This fluid has high concentrations of arginine and polyamines that are essential for DNA and protein syntheses. Collectively, these male reproductive organs produce mature sperm and deliver them to enable the fertilization of eggs produced by the ovaries of females.

The male reproductive system in birds is similar to that in mammals (Lake 1971), with the exception of the following aspects. First, the avian testes are located within the body cavity (the anterior abdomen), in contrast to most mammals, whose testes are located outside the abdomen and protected in the scrotum. Second, the ductus epididymis in birds is very short, compared with that in mammals. Third, spermatozoa are stored mainly in the ductus deferens in birds but in the epididymis in mammals. Fourth, the accessory sex glands noted previously for mammals are absent in birds. These characteristics of the anatomy of the avian male reproductive system may help birds to adapt to their behaviors (e.g., long-distance flights) and living environment. Fifth, after ejaculation, the avian spermatozoa have a longer survival period than their mammalian counterpart. For example, within the vaginal pouch (uterovaginal gland) and the oviduct, avian sperm cells can remain viable for up to two weeks.

### The Female Reproductive System

The mammalian female reproductive system consists of the vagina, the uterus, two oviducts, and two ovaries (Dyce et al. 1996). The vagina connects with the cervix (neck portion) of the uterus, while the uterus connects with the oviducts that are in intimate contact with the ovaries. The uterus selectively transports or synthesizes and secretes substances into the uterine lumen that are collectively known as histotroph. Its components include nutrient-transport proteins, ions, mitogens, cytokines, interleukins, enzymes, hormones, growth factors, proteases and protease inhibitors, AAs and their derivatives, fatty acids and their derivatives, glucose, fructose, vitamins, and minerals (Bazer et al. 2015). Cervical and uterine secretions help regulate the passage of sperm from the vagina to the oviduct in which fertilization of the ovum occurs.

Before fertilization, the ovum (egg) is expelled from the ovary, received by the fimbria of the oviduct (fallopian tube) and moved to the midportion of the oviduct where fertilization normally takes place. At the beginning of gestation, histotroph in the uterine lumen provides an environment conducive to supporting the survival, growth, and development of embryos. As the conceptus (embryo/fetus and associated extraembryonic membranes) increases in size, the placenta (amnion, allantois, and yolk sac) develops as a means of meeting the increased need for nutrients (Bazer et al. 2014). The placenta is the organ that transports nutrients, respiratory gases, and the products of their metabolism between the maternal and fetal circulations (Dyce et al. 1996). The developing fetus is surrounded by amniotic fluid, which buoys the fetus and allows it to develop symmetrically. Allantoic fluid accumulates due to the transport of water from the mother to the conceptus, and the allantoic sac is also connected to the fetal bladder via the urachus and the placental vasculature that resides within the allantoic membrane. Therefore, in the fetus, nutrients cleared via the fetal kidneys into the bladder can reach the allantoic sac and then reenter the fetal–placental circulation across the allantoic epithelium. The allantoic sac was traditionally considered a reservoir for fetal wastes, but it is now known to be a reservoir of nutrients (e.g., the arginine family of AAs) and to play an important role in nutrient metabolism (Wu et al. 2006). Much evidence shows that the successful maintenance of pregnancy requires (1) maintenance of a functional corpus luteum to produce progesterone (a steroid hormone) and (2) interactions between the conceptus and various uterine cells (e.g., uterine luminal, superficial, and glandular epithelia, as well as stromal cells) (Bazer et al. 2010). Coordination among these cells ensures adequate provision of nutrients and oxygen from mother to fetus, as well as conceptus survival, growth, and development.

The avian female reproductive system consists of the vagina, uterus, oviduct, and ovary (Dyce et al. 1996). Birds have a very short uterus known as the shell gland or pouch, in which the egg (the largest cell ever known in the animal kingdom) produced by the ovary is retained during the entire period of shell formation. Interestingly, female birds in most families (including domestic fowl) have only one functional ovary (the left one), which is covered by the fimbria of the oviduct. The right ovary is present at the embryonic stage but is vestigial thereafter. The mature ovarian follicle, containing all deposited yolk, ruptures to release the ovum, which falls into the trumpetlike fimbria at the upper end of the oviduct. The ovum remains in the oviduct for 15–20 min, which is the only time it can be fertilized and then traverses to the magnum where the ovum remains for ~4 h to acquire the deposition of albumen (egg white) around the yolk (Gilbert 1971). Next, the ovum passes to the isthmus and remains there for 15 min to acquire the shell membrane to protect the embryo. Then, the ovum migrates further to the uterus to acquire the shell and shell pigments during a period of 18–20 h and finally is expelled via the vagina. The production effort of a hen is remarkable, as it produces a large number of eggs (e.g., 275 eggs each weighing 58 g) per year. In contrast to mammals, avian fertilized eggs are hatched outside the mother. In birds, as in most reptiles, the embryo and its *extraembryonic membranes* develop within a shelled egg.

## The Endocrine System

The endocrine system consists of glands and organs that synthesize and secrete hormones into the body to be carried toward target organs where they will exert their effects. Endocrine glands in animals include the hypothalamus, pituitary gland (anterior lobe and posterior lobe), pineal gland, adrenal gland (cortex and medulla), thyroid gland, parathyroid gland, pancreas, gonads (testes and ovaries), placenta, gastrointestinal tract, and white adipose tissue (Devlin 2011). Hormones (e.g., insulin and glucagon) were traditionally defined as substances that are secreted by specialized endocrine cells and carried through the circulation to target cells at distant body sites (Dyce et al. 1996). Hormones are now more broadly defined as chemical messengers that elicit biological effects in the body (Cooper and Hausman 2016). Thus, paracrine hormones (e.g., fibroblast growth factors and transforming growth factor-β) are substances that are produced and released by cells and then act on neighboring cells. Autocrine hormones (e.g., interleukin-1 and vascular endothelial growth factor) are substances produced by the cell that bind to membrane receptors on the same cell.

Let us use secretin (a 27-AA polypeptide which was the first hormone to be discovered in 1902) as an example to illustrate how a hormone acts. It is produced and released by the S cells of the duodenum and jejunum and regulates secretions in the stomach, pancreas, and liver. In the stomach, secretin augments HCl production by enhancing the release of somatostatin and inhibiting the secretion of gastrin. In the pancreas, secretin increases the formation of bicarbonate by the centroacinar cells and the intercalated ducts of the pancreas, as well as the production of bile by the liver. Furthermore, in coordination with cholecystokinin, secretin stimulates the gallbladder to contract to release its stored bile into the lumen of the duodenum. In all the target tissues, secretin binds to its receptors on the plasma membrane, leading to the activation of adenylyl cyclase for the generation of cAMP (a cellular secondary messenger) from ATP. Thus, secretin plays an important in the digestion of nutrients, particularly lipids, protein, and vitamins.

Understanding the endocrine system is important for studying nutrition because animal metabolism is regulated by hormones, whose concentrations in plasma are affected by their developmental stage, diets, disease, toxins, and housing conditions. In general, the hypothalamus secretes releasing and release-inhibiting hormones that control the activity of the anterior pituitary, whose trophic hormones act on target glands or tissues to modulate the release of ultimate hormones in the cascade (Guyton and Hall 2000). In contrast, hormones of the posterior pituitary are synthesized by the hypothalamus and transported to the posterior pituitary for storage prior to their release. Hormones secreted by the various endocrine glands and cell types are summarized in Table 1.6.

### The Immune System

The immune system has two components: the innate immune system (nonspecific) and the adaptive immune system (acquired and specific), which act together to prevent and/or respond to the invasion of various pathogens (Dyce et al. 1996). The innate immune system consists of several integral components: (1) physical barriers (e.g., skin, epithelial cell layer in respiratory tract, and gastrointestinal tract); (2) mononuclear phagocytes (e.g., monocytes and macrophages), dendritic cells, polymorphonuclear granulocytes (e.g., neutrophils, eosinophils, and basophils), mast cells, natural killer (NK) cells, and platelets; (3) humoral factors, including collectins, complements, lysozymes, C-reactive proteins, and interferons; (4) antimicrobial peptides in the mucosa and lumen of the small intestine; and (5) neutrophil extracellular traps, composed of DNA and proteins as major structural components (Iyer et al. 2015; Li et al. 2007). The innate immune system can rapidly respond to invading microbes and is the first line of defense against infections. However, the major disadvantages of this immune system include nonspecificity and a lack of memory.

The adaptive immune system consists of T-lymphocytes, B-lymphocytes, and humoral factors. At birth, this immune system is largely present, but functionally immature (Mowat 1987). The bone marrow is primarily responsible for hematopoiesis and lymphopoiesis, while the thymus is required for T-cell development. Secondary lymphoid organs include the spleen, lymph nodes, and the mucosa-associated lymphoid tissues in the gastrointestinal, respiratory, and reproductive tracts. In contrast to the innate immune system, the acquired immune response is highly specific because each lymphocyte carries surface receptors only for a single antigen. In addition, the adaptive immune system becomes effective over several days after initial stimulation and possesses immunological memory through the production of specific antibodies by B-lymphocytes (Wu 2013). When pathogens escape humoral immunity, they are targeted by cell-mediated immunity that involves cytokines (e.g., interferon-$\gamma$ [IFN$\gamma$]) and other cytotoxic proteins produced by T-lymphocytes. Extracellular pathogens are neutralized effectively by antibodies, whereas intracellular pathogens (e.g., viruses and certain bacteria) in infected host cells are generally cleared by cytotoxic T lymphocytes (Iyer et al. 2015).

Innate and acquired immune systems are regulated by an interactive network of chemical communications, which includes the synthesis of the antigen-presenting machinery, immunoglobulins,

**TABLE 1.6**
**Secretion of Hormones and Their Major Functions in Animals**

| Endocrine Gland or Exocrine Organ | Hormone | Major Functions |
|---|---|---|
| Hypothalamus | Thyrotropin-releasing hormone | ↑ Thyroid-stimulating hormone release from anterior pituitary |
| | Corticotropin-releasing hormone | ↑ Release of adrenocorticotropic hormone from anterior pituitary |
| | GH-releasing hormone | ↑ Release of growth hormone from anterior pituitary |
| | Gn-releasing hormone | ↑ Release of FSH and LH from anterior pituitary |
| | Somatostatin | ↓ Secretion of growth hormone and thyroid-stimulating hormone |
| | Prolactin-releasing hormone | ↑ Lactotropes to release prolactin |
| | Dopamine | ↓ Prolactin release from the anterior pituitary gland |
| Anterior pituitary | Growth hormone | ↑ Protein synthesis and whole-body lean tissue growth |
| | Prolactin | ↑ Milk synthesis (including protein and fat synthesis) |
| | Thyroid-stimulating hormone | ↑ Thyroxine ($T_4$) and triiodothyronine (T3) synthesis by thyroid gland |
| | LH | ↑ Ovulation and development of the corpus luteum in females; ↑ testosterone production by Leydig cells in males; LH acts synergistically with FSH |
| | FSH | Regulates growth and development of reproductive organs in males and females; acts synergistically with LH |
| | Adrenocorticotropic hormone | ↑ Production and release of glucocorticoids by adrenal cortex |
| | ß-Lipotropin | ↑ Production of melanin by melanocytes in skin and hair |
| | β-Endorphin | Acts on cells and neurons to produce analgesic effects |
| | MSH | ↑ Production of melanin by melanocytes in skin and hair; actions in brain regulate food intake and sexual arousal |
| | Activin (gonadotrope cells) | ↑ FSH secretion; has no effect on LH secretion |
| Posterior pituitary | Vasopressin (ADH)[a] | ↑ Water reabsorption in renal tubules and arterial blood pressure |
| | Oxytocin[a] | ↑ Contractions of uterus; causes milk letdown from mammary glands |
| Pineal | Melatonin | Controls circadian rhythms; an antioxidant |
| Adrenal cortex | Glucocorticoids[b] | Regulates glucose, protein and lipid metabolism, and gene expression; plays an important role in anti-inflammatory reactions |
| | Aldosterone[c] | ↑ Renal reabsorption of sodium and water |
| | Adrenal androgens[d] | Regulates the development of sexual organs and characteristics in both males and females |
| Adrenal medulla | Dopamine | Affects emotion, locomotor activity, and neuroendocrine secretion |
| Adrenal medulla and noradrenergic neurons in brain | Epinephrine and NEP | Functions as hormones to enhance glucose metabolism, heart rate, muscle strength, and blood pressure, and as neurotransmitters in brain |
| Kidneys | Erythropoietin | ↑ Hemoglobin synthesis and bone marrow differentiation |
| | Renin | Acts as an enzyme that converts angiotensinogen to angiotensin I |
| Heart atria | Atrial natriuretic factor | ↓ Aldosterone release |
| Thyroid gland | $T_3$ and $T_4$ | ↑ Whole-body energy metabolism |
| | Calcitonin | ↑ Calcium deposition in bone and reduce blood calcium |
| Parathyroid gland | Parathyroid hormone | ↑ Renal 1α-hydroxylase activity and blood calcium concentration |
| Thymus | Thymopoietin (α-thymosin) | ↑ T-cell development; Stimulate phagocytes |

(*Continued*)

**TABLE 1.6 (*Continued*)**
**Secretion of Hormones and Their Major Functions in Animals**

| Endocrine Gland or Exocrine Organ | Hormone | Major Functions |
|---|---|---|
| Pancreas | Insulin (β-cells) | ↑ Glucose oxidation, protein synthesis, fatty acid synthesis, triacylglycerol synthesis and storage, and glycogen synthesis |
| | Glucagon (α-cells) | ↑ Glycogen breakdown, glucose synthesis, and lipolysis |
| | Somatostatin (D-cells) | ↓ Secretion of insulin and glucagon in pancreas (a paracrine effect) |
| | Pancreatic polypeptide (F-cells) | Regulates pancreatic secretion activity (both endocrine and exocrine); serves as an antagonist of cholecystokinin; reduces food intake |
| Liver | Insulinlike growth factor I | ↑ Muscle protein synthesis; anabolism |
| Gastrointestinal tract | Various hormones[e] | Regulates pancreatic secretion, as well as gut motility, secretion, and function |
| WAT | Various hormones[f] | Regulates fat and glucose metabolism, inflammation, and food intake |
| Various organs | Prostaglandins | Regulates vasodilation, metabolism, inflammation, and reproduction |
| Embryo | Chorionic gonadotropin[g] | Pregnancy recognition in some species |
| Placenta[h] | Placental lactogen[i] | ↑ Mammary gland growth and development; act like GH |
| Testes | Testosterone (sex hormone) | ↑ Development of male reproductive organs and protein synthesis |
| | Inhibin (from Sertoli cells) | Inhibits FSH secretion by antagonizing activin |
| Ovary | Progesterone (corpus luteum) | Required for embryogenesis and maintenance of pregnancy; stimulate DNA and protein synthesis, as well as growth in the uterus; ↓ myometrial contractions; maintain uterine quiescence |
| | 17-β-Estradiol (sex hormone) | ↑ Development of female reproductive organs and protein synthesis; regulates the estrus and mammary gland development |
| | Relaxin | ↓ Myometrial contractions; maintain uterine quiescence |
| | Inhibin (from granulosa cells) | Inhibits FSH secretion by antagonizing activin |
| | Follistatin | Inhibits FSH secretion by acting as an activin-binding protein |
| Various organs[j] | 1,25-Dihydroxycholecalciferol | ↑ Intestinal absorption of calcium and phosphorus |

*Source:* Cooper, G.M. and R.E. Hausman. 2016. *The Cell: A Molecular Approach*. Sinauer Associates, Sunderland, MA; Devlin, T.M. 2011. *Textbook of Biochemistry with Clinical Correlations*. John Wiley & Sons, New York, NY.

*Note:* ADH, antidiuretic hormone; FSH, follicle-stimulating hormone; GH, growth hormone; Gn, gonadotropin; LH, luteinizing hormone; MSH, melanocyte-stimulating hormone; NEP, norepinephrine; WAT, white adipose tissue; ↑, enhance; ↓, inhibit.

[a] Synthesized in the hypothalamus and stored in the posterior pituitary gland.

[b] Cortisol is the predominant glucocorticoid in humans and pigs, but corticosterone is the predominant glucocorticoid in rats.

[c] An example of mineralocorticoids.

[d] Including dehydroepiandrosterone (DHEA), dehydroepiandrosterone sulfate, and androstenedione.

[e] Including gastrin (stimulating HCl secretion by parietal cells), cholecystokinin (CCK; stimulating gallbladder contraction and release of pancreatic enzymes), secretin (stimulating pancreatic acinar cells to release bicarbonate and water), somatostatin, glucagonlike peptide-I (increasing insulin release and decreasing glucagon release), and substance P (a vasodilator).

[f] Hormones released from white adipose tissue include leptin, adiponectin, resistin, and adipokines.

[g] Present in some species (e.g., horse and humans) but absent in others (e.g., pigs and ruminants).

[h] Placenta is also a source of progesterone and estrogens (estradiol, estrone, and estriol).

[i] Absent in pigs and rabbits.

[j] Predominantly in kidney and also in other tissues, such as the bone, placenta, and skin.

and cytokines (Calder 2006). Both immune systems are highly dependent upon an adequate availability of AAs for the synthesis of these proteins and polypeptides and other molecules (e.g., NO, superoxide, hydrogen peroxide, histamine, glutathione, and anthranilic acid), which are of enormous biological importance. AAs affect immune responses either directly or indirectly through their metabolites (Wu 2013). Furthermore, fatty acids, minerals, and vitamins also play an important role in regulating the production of immunomodulatory substances. Although the immune system is vital to health, it can be dysfunctional under certain conditions (e.g., insulin-dependent diabetes mellitus, rheumatoid arthritis, and asthma), resulting in the development of autoimmune and hypersensitivity diseases. Nutrients (e.g., glycine, tryptophan, and polyunsaturated fatty acids) can be beneficial to prevent and treat immune-related disorders (Li et al. 2007, 2016).

### SENSE ORGANS

There are five senses: sight (eye), hearing (ear), taste (tongue), smell (nose), and touch (skin). These organs send information from the external environment (including food) to the brain through the peripheral nervous system, thereby allowing the animals to react in a timely manner (Dyce et al. 1996). These sense organs have specialized sensory neurons (also called receptors) for specific stimuli. Examples of these receptors are photoreceptors (vision receptors), mechanoreceptors (hearing and touch receptors), and chemoreceptors (taste receptors and smell receptors or olfactory sensory neurons). When sensory receptors are activated, the electrical potential causes the depolarization of the membrane to transduce their respective stimuli across the cell membrane to an attached neuron (Sporns et al. 2004). The electrochemical information is collected by the dendrites of the neuron, transferred through its cell body, and then brought to the axon. This allows the electrochemical signal to be transmitted toward the brain for processing and integration.

The integumentary system is composed of the skin (the soft outer covering) and its associated structures (including hair, scales, feathers, hooves, nails, nerve receptors, and exocrine glands) (Dyce et al. 1996). The skin consists of multiple layers of ectodermal tissues (e.g., epidermis, basement membrane, and dermis in mammals) to guard the underlying muscles, bones, ligaments, and internal organs (Guyton and Hall 2000). Thus, the integumentary system protects the body from damage, infection, and loss of internal water. The skin also plays a role in thermoregulation and preventing external water from entering the animal. As noted previously, nerve endings in the *skin* and other parts of the body transmit sensations to the brain.

## OVERVIEW OF METABOLIC PATHWAYS

### MAJOR METABOLIC PATHWAYS AND THEIR SIGNIFICANCE

In all animals, dietary macronutrients undergo oxidation to form $CO_2$ and $H_2O$ with the concomitant release of chemical energy to support various biological processes. Of note, the French chemist Antoine Lavoisier (1743–1794) is often considered as the founder of nutritional sciences because of his seminal contribution to the development of modern chemistry and his discovery of the role of oxygen in oxidation of nutrients. It is now known that many series of biochemical reactions are responsible for both the oxidation and catabolism of nutrients. These metabolic pathways are complex, but are the foundation of life (Brosnan 2005; Srere 1987; Watford 1991). Thus, it is important that nutritionists understand the features and physiological significance of the major metabolic pathways, as well as their interrelationships, in organisms.

A metabolic pathway can be defined as a series of enzyme-catalyzed reactions in which a substance is either degraded to simpler products or synthesized from simpler precursors. A pathway can be linear (such as proline synthesis), cyclic (such as the Krebs cycle), or spiral (fatty acid synthesis). Major metabolic pathways and their physiological significance are summarized in Table 1.7. A physiologically useful definition of a metabolic pathway is a series of enzyme-catalyzed reactions,

**TABLE 1.7**
**Major Pathways for Nutrient Metabolism and Their Physiological Significance**

| Nutrient | Pathway | Sites | Major Functions |
|---|---|---|---|
| All | Krebs cycle | Mitochondria | Oxidation of glucose-, fatty acid-, and AA-derived acetyl-CoA to produce $CO_2$, water, NADH, ATP, and GTP; bridge the metabolism of glucose, fatty acids, and AAs; anaplerosis[a] |
| | Respiration chain | Mitochondria | Major source of energy in mitochondrion-containing cells |
| | Glucose–alanine cycle | Cytosol of liver and skeletal muscle | Skeletal muscle synthesizes alanine from glucose-derived pyruvate and AAs, and releases alanine, which is taken up by liver for glucose production; transports nitrogen in a nontoxic form from skeletal muscle to the liver |
| | One-carbon metabolism | Cytosol and Mit in most cells | Provides the methyl group for the methylation of DNA, RNA, protein, and AAs, and for the conversion of homocysteine into methionine; produces thymidine and purines for nucleic acid synthesis |
| Glucose | Glycolysis | Cytosol of all cells | Converts glucose into pyruvate and lactate; produces 3-phosphoglycerol to provide glycerol backbone for triglycerides, glycolipids, and phospholipids; generates ATP under anaerobic conditions in all cells; sole source of energy in mitochondrion-free cells |
| | Glycogen synthesis | Cytosol of most cells (particularly liver, heart, and skeletal muscle) | Converts glucose into glycogen for storage in the fed state; helps to regulate blood glucose concentration; helps to control osmolality in cells by converting monomers to polymers |
| | Glycogen degradation | Cytosol of most cells (particularly liver, heart, and skeletal muscle) | Provides glucose rapidly in response to needs; muscles: convert glucose into glucose-1-P, which enters glycolysis as glucose-6-P; liver: provides free glucose to enter the blood |
| | Gluconeogenesis | Liver and kidneys (mainly cytosol but also Mit in some species) | Converts noncarbohydrate substances into glucose; regulates glucose homeostasis (particularly in neonates, strict carnivores, and ruminants, and in all animals during starvation)[b]; helps to regulate blood pH by consuming $H^+$ |
| | Pentose cycle | Cytosol of all cells | Serves as the major source of cellular NADPH; provides ribose 5-phosphate for purine and pyrimidine synthesis |
| | Hexosamine | Cytosol of all cells | Converts fructose-6-P and glutamine into glucosamine-6-P, a precursor for synthesis of all aminosugars and glycoproteins |
| Fatty acids | Fatty acid synthesis | Cytosol of most cells[c] | Converts excess glucose and AAs into fatty acids, which serve as precursors for synthesis of TAG; prevents loss of water-soluble energy substrates from the body |
| | TAG synthesis | Cytosol and Mit of most cells[c] | Converts fatty acids and glycerol to fats for storage; prevents the toxicity of free fatty acids |

(*Continued*)

**TABLE 1.7 (*Continued*)**
**Major Pathways for Nutrient Metabolism and Their Physiological Significance**

| Nutrient | Pathway | Sites | Major Functions |
|---|---|---|---|
| | TAG–fatty acid cycle | Most cells; mainly in white adipose tissue | Regulates the balance of TAG in the body |
| | Cholesterol synthesis | Cytosol and Mit of liver | Synthesize cholesterol from acetyl-CoA to form cell membranes and to synthesize bile acids, bile alcohols, and steroid hormones |
| | Lipoproteins | Small intestine and liver | Synthesize chylomicrons in the small intestine, VLDL in the liver, and HDL in peripheral tissues |
| | β-Oxidation | Mitochondria primarily in liver, heart, and skeletal muscle | Converts fatty acids into acetyl-CoA for oxidation via the Krebs cycle; provides acetyl-CoA for ketogenesis under fasting, lactation, and late pregnancy, and for the activation of hepatic pyruvate carboxylase in liver |
| | HMG-CoA cycle | Mit of hepatocytes in liver; rumen epithelium | Formation of acetoacetate (a ketone body) from acetyl-CoA; helps to regulate the availability of acetyl-CoA in cells |
| | Ketogenesis | Mit of liver, colonocytes, and ruminal epithelium | Converts acetyl-CoA into ketone bodies as metabolic fuels for the brain and other extrahepatic tissues when blood glucose concentration is low |
| AAs | Urea cycle | Mit and cytosol of liver, enterocytes in mammals | Converts ammonia and bicarbonate into urea for detoxification of ammonia |
| | Protein synthesis | Mainly the cytosol and Mit of all cells except for mature RBCs | Synthesizes secretory and membrane proteins in RER, cellular proteins on ribosomes, and some (~13) proteins in Mit; helps to control osmolality in cells by converting monomers to polymers |
| | Proteolysis | Mainly the cytosol and lysosomes of all cells | Degrades proteins to release AAs |
| | Protein turnover | Most cells except for the lack of protein synthesis in mature RBCs | Regulates the balance of proteins in cells, the release of secretory proteins from cells, and endogenous provision of AAs; regulates metabolism, immune response, and cell growth |
| | Ubiquitin cycle | Cytosol of all cells | Protein degradation by ubiquitin-dependent proteasomes |
| | AA synthesis | Cytosol and/or Mit of cells | Synthesizes AAs in a cell-dependent manner to compensate for a deficiency of AAs in diets; fulfills specific physiological needs (e.g., glucose–alanine cycle and malate–aspartate shuttle) |
| | AA degradation | Cytosol and/or Mit of cells | Degradation of AAs in a cell-dependent manner to regulate the homeostasis of AAs in the body |
| | Uric acid synthesis | Mainly the liver of most animals (e.g., birds and mammals) | Converts ammonia and carbons (from formate, glycine, and bicarbonate) into uric acid for detoxification of ammonia in birds; purine degradation in mammals |
| | Synthesis of nucleotides | Liver and other tissues | Production of RNA and DNA for protein synthesis; component of genetic material |
| | Synthesis of other substances | Liver and kidney, and many types of cells | Provides carnitine, carnosine, glutathione, creatine, inositol, acetylcholine |

(*Continued*)

**TABLE 1.7 (*Continued*)**
**Major Pathways for Nutrient Metabolism and Their Physiological Significance**

| Nutrient | Pathway | Sites | Major Functions |
|---|---|---|---|
| Vitamin (Vit) | Production of Vit $B_3$ and D | Liver, kidney, skin, bone, and/or small intestine | Synthesizes vitamins $B_3$ and D from precursors in a species-dependent manner |
| | Vit A formation from β-carotene | Enterocytes of all species except for cats | Converts β-carotene to retinol for supporting the functions of the eyes, epithelial cells, and reproductive systems |
| | Vit C synthesis | Liver of most species[d] | Converts glucose to Vit C for supporting antioxidative function as well as the activity of prolyl oxidase and lysyl oxidase |
| | Vit K cycle | Cytosol of the liver | Regenerates a reduced form of Vit K from oxidized Vit K |

*Note:* AAs, amino acids; HMG, 3-hydroxy-3-methylglutaryl-CoA; Mit, mitochondria; P, inorganic phosphate; RBCs, red blood cells; TAG, triacylglycerol; VLDL, very-low-density lipoprotein; HDL, high-density lipoprotein.

[a] The Krebs cycle provides (1) oxaloacetate for gluconeogenesis; (2) succynyl-CoA for heme synthesis; (3) α-ketoglutarate for the synthesis of glutamate and glutamine; and (4) citrate for the transport of acetyl-CoA from the mitochondria to the cytosol for fatty acid synthesis.

[b] Carnivores ingest a limited amount of carbohydrates from their diets, whereas ruminants absorb little or no glucose in the small intestine.

[c] Major sites of lipogenesis are livers in chickens, humans, and adult rats; white adipose tissues in pigs and ruminants; and both livers and white adipose tissues in cats, dogs, mice, rabbits, and young rats.

[d] Humans and other primates, as well as guinea pigs and fruit bats, cannot synthesize vitamin C.

initiated by a flux-generating step and ending with the formation of products. Such a definition indicates that a metabolic pathway may span more than one tissue. This is graphically illustrated by the interorgan metabolism of AAs. For example, the pathway for arginine synthesis in most adult mammals could be considered to be initiated in the small intestine by converting glutamine into citrulline and to end in the kidneys and other cell types (e.g., endothelial cells and macrophages) by converting citrulline into arginine (glutamine → → citrulline → → arginine) (Wu 2013). The central role of the Krebs cycle to bridge glucose, fatty acid, and AA metabolism is illustrated in Figure 1.19.

## Characteristics of Metabolic Pathways

### Enzyme-Catalyzed Reactions

Enzymes are biological catalysts. They are responsible for nearly all reactions in cells. An example is the conversion of D-glucose into D-glucose-6-phosphate by hexokinase:

$$\text{D-Glucose} + \text{ATP} \rightarrow \text{D-Glucose-6-phosphate} + \text{ADP (hexokinase)}$$

Most enzymes are proteins in nature, while a few of them are now known to be RNA (Devlin 2011). The significance of enzymes in living organisms is not just their roles in making biochemical reactions possible. The existence of enzymes not only enhances the rates of metabolic pathways but also enables their precise regulation to meet physiological needs. As a result of this regulation, individual reactions and metabolic pathways can be integrated into an exquisite metabolic system that functions effectively in the whole organism to maintain its homeostasis (Brosnan 2005; Schimke and Doyle 1970). It should be borne in mind that most, but not all, of enzyme-catalyzed reactions follow Michaelis–Menten kinetics in a hyperbolic relationship (Figure 1.20). The mathematical

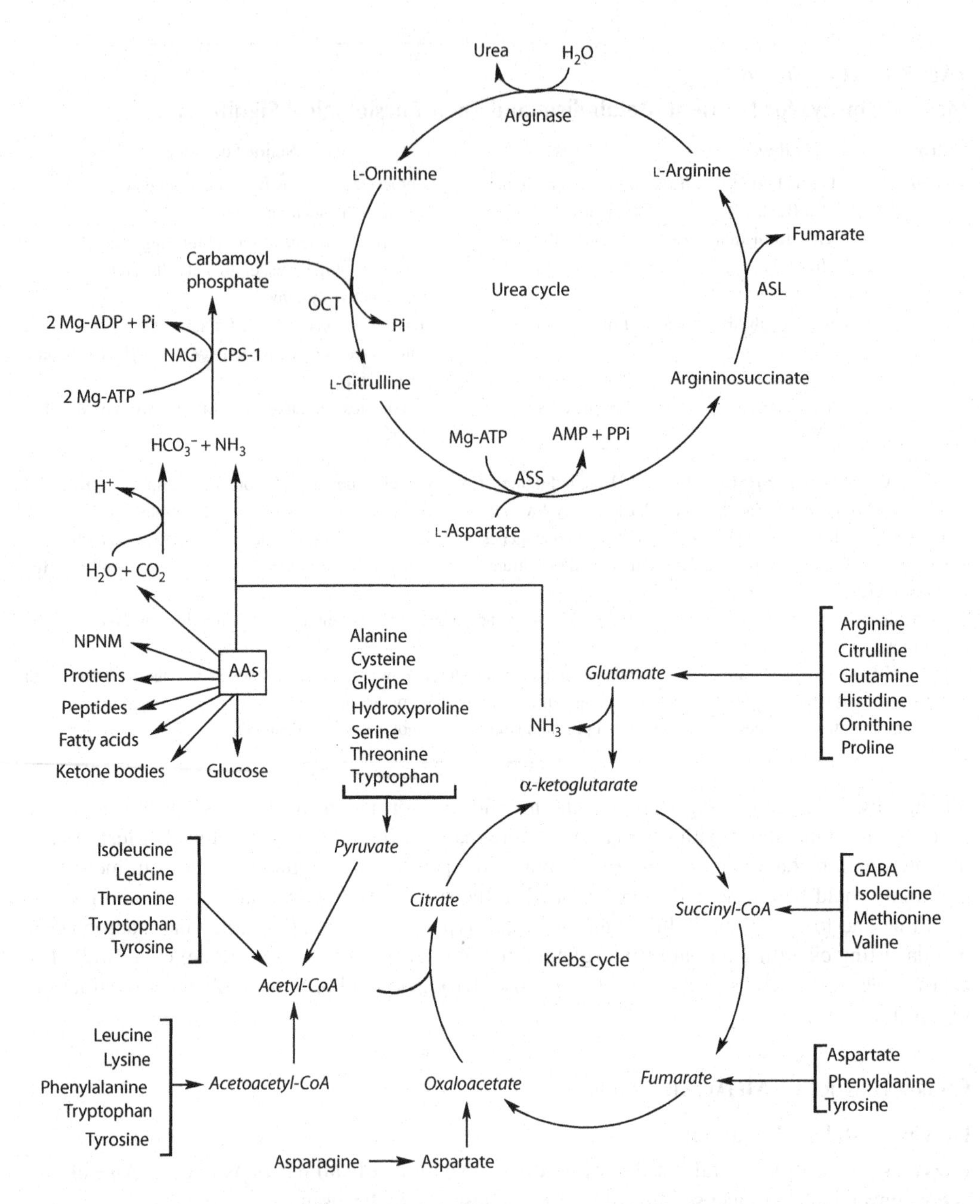


**FIGURE 1.19** Interrelationships among the metabolism of glucose, amino acids, and fatty acids in animals. The Krebs cycle plays a central role in bridging the pathways for nutrient metabolism. In animals, amino acids are utilized to produce proteins (including enzymes), small peptides, other nitrogenous metabolites (e.g., nitric oxide, creatine, carnitine, and ammonia), fatty acids, and glucose. Ammonia plays an important role in bridging the Krebs cycle with the urea cycle. AAs, amino acids; ASL, argininosuccinate lyase; ASS, argininosuccinate synthase; CPS-1, carbamoylphosphate synthetase-I; GABA, γ-aminobutyrate; NAG, *N*-acetylglutamate; NPNM, nonpeptide nitrogenous metabolites; OCT, ornithine carbamoyltransferase. (Adapted from Rezaei, R. et al. 2013. *J. Anim. Sci. Biotechnol.* 4:7.)

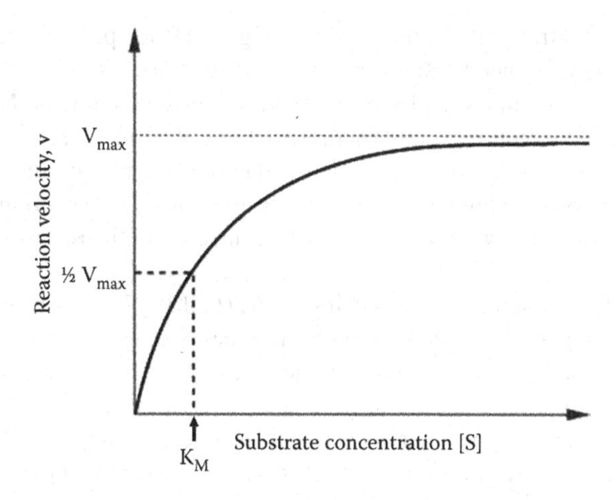


**FIGURE 1.20** A hyperbolic relationship exists between the substrate concentration and velocity in an enzyme-catalyzed reaction. Most enzymes exhibit Michaelis–Menten kinetics. The initial velocity of the reaction increases with increasing substrate concentration and reaches the maximum value ($V_{max}$) when the enzyme is saturated with the substrate. The equation $v = V_{max}$ $[S]/(K_M + [S])$ is known as the Michaelis–Menten equation, where v is reaction velocity and $K_M$ is the substrate concentration [S] at which the velocity of the reaction is one-half the maximum value (i.e., 1/2 $V_{max}$). A $K_M$ value may indicate the physiological relevance of an enzyme-catalyzed reaction in animals.

relationship between initial rate (i.e., catalytic activity) and substrate concentration can be described by the following equation:

$$V_i = \frac{V_{max}[S]}{K_M + [S]} \qquad \frac{1}{V_i} = \frac{K_M + [S]}{V_{max}[S]} \qquad \frac{1}{V_i} = \frac{K_M}{V_{max}} \times \frac{1}{[S]} + \frac{[S]}{V_{max}[S]}$$

where $V_{max}$ is the maximum rate of reaction, $K_M$ is the Michaelis constant, and [S] is the substrate concentration. Some enzymes may show an allosteric behavior which has more complex sigmoid kinetics than the Michaelis–Menten kinetics (Devlin 2011).

Catabolism of a substrate is enhanced with an increase in its concentrations until the reaction velocity reaches a maximum. A high capacity for the degradation of a nutrient in animals is a biochemical basis for a high, safe level of its dietary supplementation. Similar principles apply to the formation of a product from its precursors in animals. This also means that there are limits to nutrient catabolism and synthesis in animals. For example, substrate availability and enzyme activity limit AA synthesis in pigs and, therefore, their growth, development, lactation, and reproduction (Hou et al. 2016). Therefore, providing sufficient amounts of preformed nutrients or their immediate precursors in diets may be necessary for maximum growth and production performance of farm animals, as well as their optimal health and well-being.

Enzymes are classified as (1) oxidoreductases that catalyze oxidation–reduction reactions (e.g., lactate dehydrogenase and glyceraldehyde-3-phosphate dehydrogenase); (2) transferases that catalyze the transfer of a chemical group from one molecule to another (e.g., hexokinase and aminotransferase); (3) hydrolases that catalyze essentially irreversible hydrolysis reactions (e.g., arginase and glutaminase) in which a bond is broken by water; (4) lyases that usually catalyze carbon–carbon bond cleavage (e.g., aldolase and decarboxylases); (5) isomerases that catalyze the intramolecular transfer of functional groups (e.g., AA racemases and glucose-6-phosphate isomerase); and (6) ligases that catalyze the joining of two molecules by forming a new chemical bond (e.g., argininosuccinate synthetase and aminoacyl tRNA synthetase) (Devlin 2011). Regardless of the types of reactions, enzymes contain substrate-binding sites. Allosteric enzymes also have additional sites (allosteric sites) for the binding of an activator or inhibitor. In a catalytic reaction, an enzyme may utilize a coenzyme, cosubstrate (a second substrate; e.g., ATP for protein kinase), or cofactor. A coenzyme is a small organic molecule that is often a derivative of a vitamin (e.g., NADH and FAD), whereas a cofactor is an inorganic metal ion that binds to the enzyme (e.g., $Mn^{2+}$ or $Mg^{2+}$). In all enzyme-catalyzed reactions, an important kinetic variable is $K_M$, which refers to the substrate concentration [S] at which the velocity of the reaction is one-half the maximum value ($V_{max}$). The $K_M$ value may suggest the physiological relevance of an enzyme-catalyzed reaction, such as the affinity of the enzyme toward its substrate(s) and the possible occurrence of the reaction under physiological conditions.

Metabolic control of nutrient utilization is cell specific (Fell 1997). However, biochemical studies have revealed the following general mechanisms for regulating enzyme activity in animals: (1) concentrations of substrates and cofactors: based on the Michaelis–Menten kinetics noted previously; (2) allosteric regulation: the regulation of enzyme activity by an effector molecule which binds to a regulatory site on the enzyme other than its active (substrate-binding) site; effectors that enhance or decrease enzyme activity are referred to as allosteric activators or inhibitors, respectively; (3) covalent modifications: enzyme-catalyzed alterations of an enzyme through the addition or removal of chemical groups; an example is the phosphorylation and dephosphorylation of protein; the phosphorylation and dephosphorylation mechanism does not involve a change in the amount of the enzyme protein, and allows for rapid activation or inactivation of an enzyme; (4) concentrations of activators and inhibitors: allosteric activators or inhibitors, as well as competitive, uncompetitive, or noncompetitive inhibitors; (5) reduction–oxidation (i.e., redox) potential: ratios of NADH/$NAD^+$, NADPH/$NADP^+$, or reduced glutathione/oxidized glutathione; (6) acyl-CoA potential: ratios of acyl-CoA/CoA; (7) amounts of enzymes: long-term regulation of enzyme activity through changes in protein synthesis or degradation, or both protein synthesis and degradation; (8) pH and temperature: factors that affect the chemical structures of enzymes; each enzyme has its optimal pH and temperature; and (9) ion concentrations: factors that affect the chemical structures of enzymes; some ions are cofactors for specific enzyme. Nutrients and hormones can affect one or more of the factors listed above and, therefore, metabolic pathways in the body.

Animals contain endogenous inhibitors or activators of enzymes under both physiological and pathological conditions. Inhibitors reduce enzyme activity through one of the following modes: (1) competitive inhibition (an inhibitor with a structure similar to that of the substrate binds to the enzyme) in which $K_M$ is increased, but $V_{max}$ is not altered; (2) noncompetitive inhibition (an inhibitor binds both the free enzyme and the enzyme–substrate complex) in which $K_M$ is not altered but $V_{max}$ is decreased; (3) uncompetitive inhibition (an inhibitor binds only the enzyme–substrate complex) in which both $K_M$ and $V_{max}$ are decreased; this kind of enzyme inhibition is very rare. Knowledge of enzyme inhibition can greatly facilitate the development of a means to overcome the inhibition. For example, L-$N^G$-monomethylarginine inhibits NO synthase in cells through competitive inhibition, which can be alleviated by increasing the concentration of the enzyme substrate, L-arginine (Alderton et al. 2001). In contrast, L-lactate inhibits proline oxidase in pig enterocytes through noncompetitive inhibition, which is ameliorated by removing extracellular L-lactate (Dillon et al. 1999).

Although it has long been stated that a metabolic pathway is limited by a single enzyme, a concept of distributed metabolic control has gained growing recognition over the past three decades (Fell 1997). Accordingly, metabolic control is distributed throughout the metabolic sequence or resides in one or more of the reactions. For example, control points for glycolysis can be plasma glucose concentration, ATP needs, glucose transport, hexokinase, 6-phospho-fructokinase-1, enolase, and pyruvate kinase, but not 6-phospho-fructokinase-1 alone. This ensures that metabolic chaos will not occur in animals (Brosnan 2005).

### Intracellular Compartmentalization of Metabolic Pathways

Enzymes and, therefore, metabolic pathways are localized in different organelles of the cell. An excellent example of the intracellular compartmentalization of a metabolic pathway is the urea cycle. It involves both mitochondria and the cytosol. Within a compartment, enzymes are either loosely or closely associated, and they sequentially pass intermediates along the pathway (Ovadi and Saks 2004). In the hepatic urea cycle, the physiological significance of the intracellular compartmentalization is evident in that the ammonia produced in the mitochondrion and ornithine are locally converted to citrulline, a nontoxic product, for export to the cytosol, where citrulline and aspartate are efficient substrates for the formation of arginine, the hydrolysis of which yields urea and ornithine. When such a metabolic pathway is well organized in a sequential association, it is called a metabolon (Srere 1987). Advantages of a metabolon include: (1) the facilitation of the transfer of intermediates between enzymes to maintain a high concentration of substrate in the catalytic site to enhance the efficiency of product formation; and (2) fewer side reactions (chemical or enzymatic) when intermediates are not free within cells.

### Cell-, Zone-, Age-, and Species-Dependent Metabolic Pathways

Another feature of metabolism is its occurrence in a cell-, age-, or species-specific manner. For example, in mammals, gluconeogenesis occurs only in the liver and kidney. Even within the same organ, cells do not have the same metabolic pathways, as graphically illustrated by the metabolic zonation of the liver (Häussinger et al. 1992). Specifically, the liver exhibits remarkable heterogeneity of its hepatocytes along the porto-central axis in the ultrastructure and expression of enzymes, resulting in different metabolic patterns within different zones of the liver lobules (Table 1.8). This

**TABLE 1.8**
**Primary Localization of Metabolic Pathways in Periportal or Perivenous Hepatocytes of the Liver[a]**

| Periportal Hepatocytes | Perivenous Hepatocytes |
|---|---|
| Amino acid (AA) metabolism | Amino acid (AA) metabolism |
| AA uptake and degradation (except glutamate, aspartate, and histidine) | Glutamate and α-ketoglutarate uptake[b] |
| | Ornithine aminotransferase |
| Glutaminase[b] | Glutamine synthetase[b] |
| Histidine degradation[b] | Aspartate uptake |
| Urea cycle | Glutathione synthesis |
| Lipid metabolism | Lipid metabolism |
| ATP-citrate lyase | Bile acid synthesis[b] |
| Cholesterol synthesis | Esterification of free fatty acids |
| Fatty acid oxidation | Fatty acid synthesis |
| Ketogenesis[c] | Triacylglycerol synthesis |
| Hepatic lipase | Very-low-density lipoprotein synthesis |
| Glucose metabolism | Glucose metabolism |
| Glucose release | Glucose uptake |
| Gluconeogenesis | Glycolysis |
| Glycogen degradation to glucose | Glycogen degradation to pyruvate |
| Glycogen synthesis from lactate and AAs | Glycogen synthesis from glucose |
| Other pathways | Other pathways |
| Carbonic anhydrase V | Carbonic anhydrase II and III |
| Oxidative energy metabolism | Xenobiotic metabolism and detoxification |

*Source:* Schleicher, J. et al. 2015. *Biochim. Biophys. Acta* 1851:641–56; Häussinger, D. et al. 1992. *Enzyme* 46:72–93.

[a] Except for those pathways indicated with a superscript letter b, most pathways are unequally distributed along the acinus (metabolic zonation), with highest activities in the indicated hepatocytes.

[b] Exclusively located in the indicated hepatocytes.

[c] This pathway is highly active in most animals during starvation but is limited in pigs.

spatial organization of various metabolic pathways and functions provides the biochemical basis for (1) adaptation of the liver to changes in nutritional, physiological, and pathological conditions; and (2) prevention of futile cycles (Schleicher et al. 2015). Temporal differences in the expression of enzymes are also notable within the same animals, as indicated by the finding that intestinal arginine degradation is extensive in postweaning pigs, but is negligible in preweaning pigs (Wu and Morris 1998).

A well-known difference in species-dependent metabolism is that the conversion of ammonia and $CO_2$ into urea takes places in mammals, but not in birds. In addition, cows synthesize large amounts of glucose from propionate in the liver (Thompson et al. 1975), but this pathway of gluconeogenesis is insignificant in nonruminants (Bondi 1987). Furthermore, in sheep, which possess high arginase activity to degrade arginine in the placentomes, citrulline is unusually abundant in allantoic fluid during early and mid-gestation (e.g., up to 10 mM) as a result of increased transfer from mother to fetus to conserve the arginine carbons (Kwon et al. 2003). In contrast, in pigs which express little arginase activity in placentae, arginine is particularly abundant in allantoic fluid primarily due to its direct transport from mother to fetus (Wu et al. 1996). These examples illustrate the complexity of metabolism among animal species in their strategies to maximize survival and the efficiency of nutrient utilization. Understanding cell- or tissue-specific metabolic pathway is essential in appreciating the coordination of fuel utilization for the precise regulation of homeostasis in animals.

Disturbance of homeostasis for a prolonged period of time may result in disease and even death. For example, a reduction in blood pH from 7.4 to 7.1 is fatal, as shown in untreated insulin-dependent diabetic animals and humans (Marliss et al. 1982). This is because low pH denatures protein, is deleterious to cell structure, and inhibits enzyme activity. The severe, adverse outcomes are the dysfunction of multiple organs, such as the impaired function of the respiratory center in the brain, as well as cardiac and renal failure.

## Biological Oxidation in Mitochondria

In chemistry, oxidation is defined as the removal of electrons from an electron donor (called the reductant), and reduction as the gain of electrons by an electron acceptor (the oxidant). In an oxidation–reduction reaction, an oxidant and its reductant form a redox couple. For example, in the following reaction catalyzed by L-lactate dehydrogenase, L-lactate is oxidized to pyruvate and $NAD^+$ is reduced to NADH:

$$\text{L-Lactate} + NAD^+ \leftrightarrow \text{Pyruvate} + NADH + H^+$$

In animal cells containing mitochondria, the conversion of food energy (i.e., chemical energy in AA, lipids, and carbohydrates) into biological energy (primarily as ATP and, to a lesser extent, GTP and UTP) occurs through well-coordinated metabolic pathways. The major reactions are (1) generation of acetyl-CoA from glucose via glycolysis (pyruvate production), fatty acids via β-oxidation, and AAs via oxidation, which will be discussed in other chapters; (2) oxidation of acetyl-CoA via the Krebs cycle to form GTP, $CO_2$, $H_2O$, NADH + $H^+$, and $FADH_2$; (3) oxidation of NADH + $H^+$ and $FADH_2$ in the presence of $O_2$ to produce $H_2O$ in the electron transport system (respiratory chain); and (4) synthesis of ATP from ADP and inorganic phosphate (Pi) by ATP synthase via the proton gradient in the mitochondrial respiration chain (Devlin 2011). As noted previously, the Krebs cycle and the electron transport system are two major metabolic pathways for biological oxidation in animals.

### The Krebs Cycle in Mitochondria

In 1937, Hans A. Krebs published a landmark paper describing the role of citric acid in the oxidation of acetate (as acetyl-CoA) in homogenates of pigeon breast muscle. This pathway was named "the Krebs cycle" after Dr. Krebs and is also known as the citric acid cycle or the tricarboxylic acid cycle. In this cycle, acetyl-CoA combines with oxaloacetate (OAA) to form citrate, which is then converted sequentially into isocitrate, α-ketoglutarate, succinate, fumarate, L-malate, and OAA (Figure 1.21). L-malate, citrate, and α-ketoglutarate are the intermediates of the Krebs cycle that can exit the mitochondrial matrix into the cytosol. In animal cells, the mitochondrial matrix contains all the enzymes of the Krebs cycle with the exception of succinate dehydrogenase, which is bound to the inner mitochondrial membrane. In prokaryotic cells (e.g., bacteria), which lack mitochondria, enzymes of the Krebs cycle are present in the cytosol. A series of eight enzyme-catalyzed

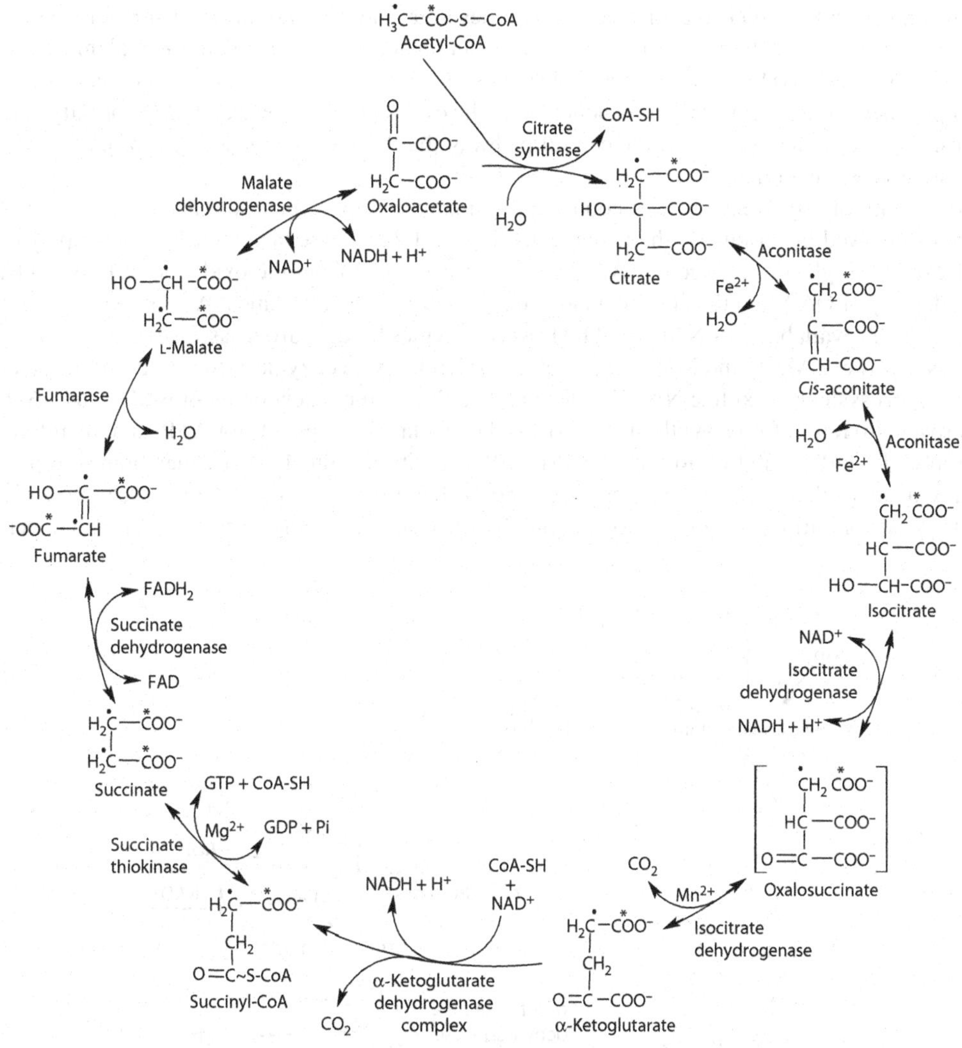

**FIGURE 1.21** The Krebs cycle for oxidation of acetyl-CoA to $CO_2$, water, NADH + $H^+$, and $FADH_2$. The carboxyl and methyl carbons of acetyl-CoA are shown with labels designated by symbols "*" and "•," respectively. In the first turn of the cycle, two molecules of $CO_2$ are produced, which are derived from the oxaloacetate portion of citrate but not the acetyl-CoA that immediately enters the cycle. Because succinate is a symmetrical compound and because succinate dehydrogenase does not differentiate between its two carboxyl groups, the "randomization" of labeling occurs at this step such that all four carbons of succinate, fumarate, malate, and oxaloacetate are labeled after one turn of the cycle. The carboxyl and methyl carbons of acetyl-CoA are completely lost as $CO_2$ after 2 and 15 turns of the cycle, respectively. (From Wu, G. 2013. *Amino Acids: Biochemistry and Nutrition*. CRC Press, Boca Raton, FL. With permission.)

reactions in the cycle generate GTP (equivalent to ATP in high-energy phosphate bonds), $CO_2$, water, NADH + $H^+$, and $FADH_2$. These two reducing equivalents (NADH + $H^+$ and $FADH_2$) are then fed into the electron transport system in the inner mitochondrial membrane for oxidation, producing ATP from ADP and Pi, as well as $H_2O$ from $2H^+$ and $0.5O^-$.

It should be borne in mind that the Krebs cycle oxidizes acetyl-CoA only, with no net changes in any intermediates of the cycle. Net oxidation of these intermediates occurs through their conversion into L-malate, which exits the mitochondrion into the cytosol to produce pyruvate. Pyruvate is then transported into the mitochondrial matrix for oxidation to acetyl-CoA by pyruvate dehydrogenase. In addition to its functions of oxidizing acetyl-CoA (a common metabolite of fatty acids, AAs, and glucose) and generating ATP, the Krebs cycle provides four- and five-carbon precursors for the synthesis of glucose and certain AAs (e.g., aspartate, glutamate, asparagine, glutamine, alanine, and proline), as well as NADH + $H^+$ for many biochemical reactions. Under metabolic conditions that favor lipogenesis, citrate exits the mitochondrion to the cytosol to provide acetyl-CoA for fatty acid synthesis. Thus, the Krebs cycle is the central pathway that bridges the metabolism of fatty acids, AAs, and glucose in animals.

The activity of the Krebs cycle is controlled by many factors to meet the needs for ATP and substrates involved in various synthetic reactions (Figure 1.22). These factors include: (1) supply of acetyl-CoA from glucose-, glycerol-, AA-derived pyruvate, and from the oxidation of fatty acids; (2) availability of OAA and thus its precursors (e.g., glucose and glucogenic AAs) for reacting with acetyl-CoA; (3) availability of $NAD^+$ and FAD as coenzymes for dehydrogenases; (4) availability of minerals (e.g., $Fe^{2+}$, $Mg^{2+}$, and $Mn^{2+}$) as cofactors for Krebs cycle enzymes; (5) activity of the electron transport system to oxidize NADH + $H^+$ and $FADH_2$ for the regeneration of $NAD^+$ and FAD, respectively; (6) rates of ATP synthesis (determined by metabolic demands for ATP) and, therefore, the supply of ADP, Pi, and $O_2$ to mitochondria; (7) integrity of mitochondrial membranes to prevent any uncontrolled exchange of substances across them; (8) amounts of Krebs cycle enzymes and the phosphorylation state of α-ketoglutarate dehydrogenase; (9) concentrations of iron, copper,

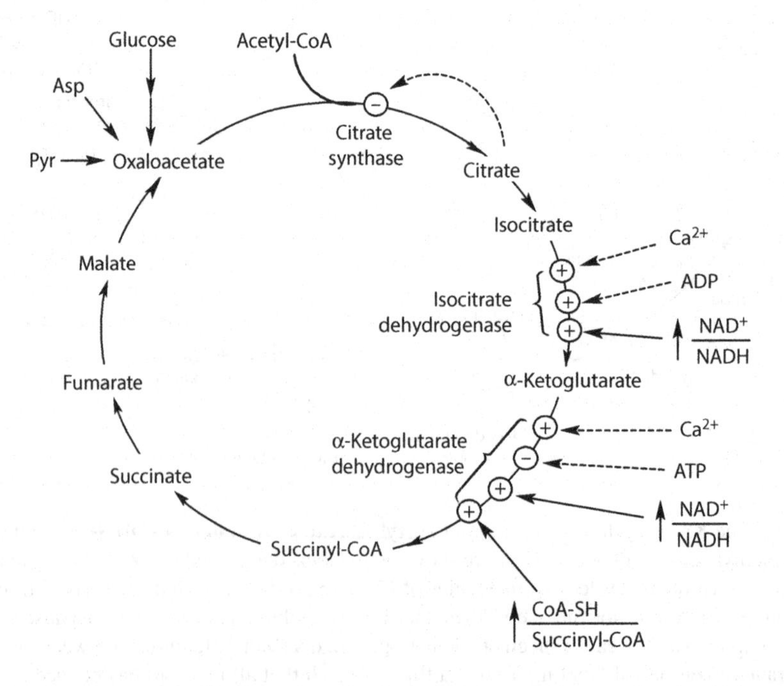


**FIGURE 1.22** Regulation of the Krebs cycle by intrinsic and extrinsic factors. The intrinsic factors include components of the cycle itself. The extrinsic factors include the supply of acetyl-CoA and the activity of the electron transport system, as well as associated enzymes and substrates (e.g., oxygen and phosphate provision).

and $Ca^{2+}$, as well as the ratio of ATP/ADP and GTP/GDP; and (10) numerous endogenous and exogenous inhibitors of Krebs cycle enzymes (e.g., inhibition of aconitase by $H_2O_2$, nitric oxide, and fluoroacetate; of α-ketoglutarate dehydrogenase complex by arsenite; and of succinate dehydrogenase by malonate) and the electron transport system (e.g., inhibition of complexes I, III, and IV by oligomycin and uncouplers, and additional inhibition of complex IV by $H_2S$, CO, and cyanide; Devlin 2011). Thus, the Krebs cycle is regulated by both intrinsic and extrinsic factors.

## The Electron Transport System in Mitochondria

The NADH and $FADH_2$ generated from the oxidation of fatty acids, AAs, and glucose in the mitochondrial matrix are oxidized to $NAD^+$ and FAD via the electron transport system (Figure 1.23). The discovery of respiratory-chain enzymes led to the award of the Nobel Prize in Physiology or Medicine to Otto H. Warburg in 1931. Note that the $NAD^+$ molecule has one net negative charge, and the superscript "+" denotes the positive charge on the nitrogen atom in its nicotinamide ring. The reduction–oxidation reactions involving quinone, $NAD^+$, FAD, and $Fe^{2+}$ are shown in Figure 1.24. This respiration chain is localized in the inner mitochondrial membrane and consists of complexes I through IV. Complexes I, III, and IV also act as proton pumps to translocate four electrons from

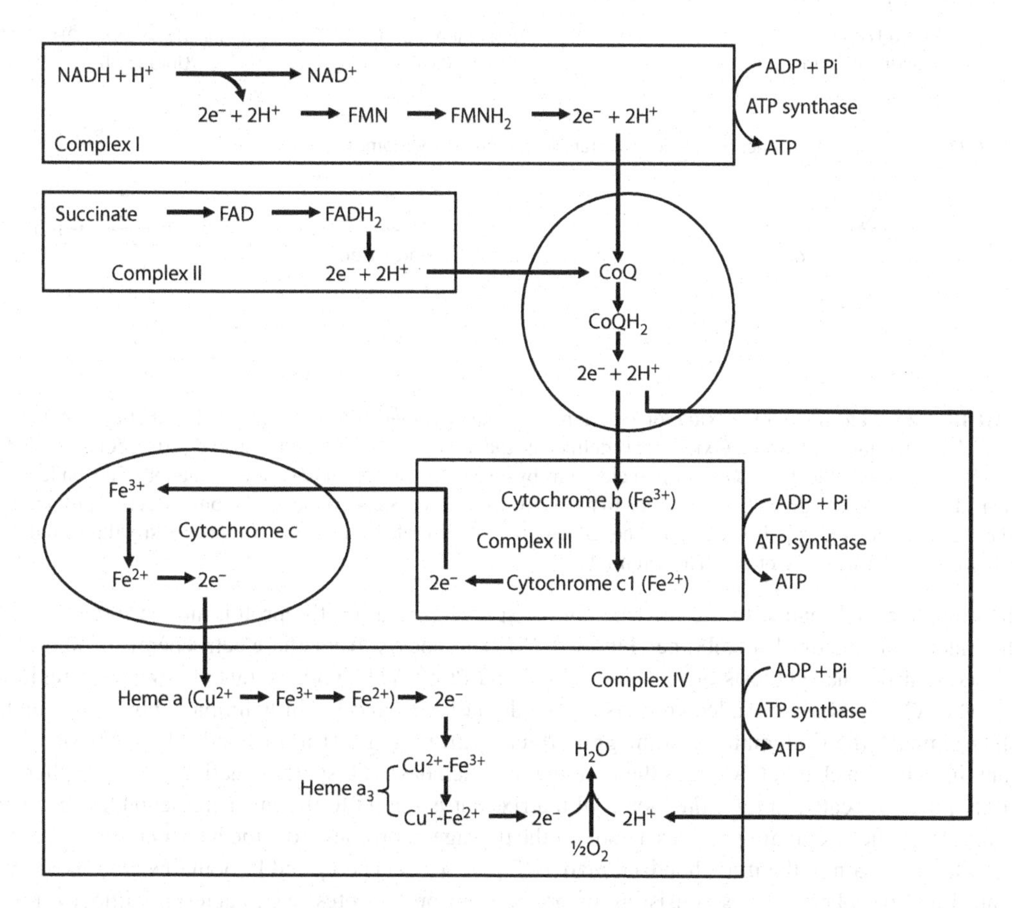


**FIGURE 1.23** The mitochondrial electron transport system (the respiration chain). NADH and $FADH_2$ are generated from the oxidation of fatty acids, amino acids, and glucose in the mitochondrial matrix. These reducing equivalents are oxidized to $NAD^+$ and FAD with the formation of $H_2O$ via the electron transport system, which is localized in the inner mitochondrial membrane and consists of complexes I–IV. The energy released from the oxidation reactions is used in the formation of the proton gradient which drives the synthesis of ATP from ADP and Pi by ATP synthase (also known as complex V). (Adapted from Dai, Z.L. et al. 2013. *BioFactors* 39:383–391.)

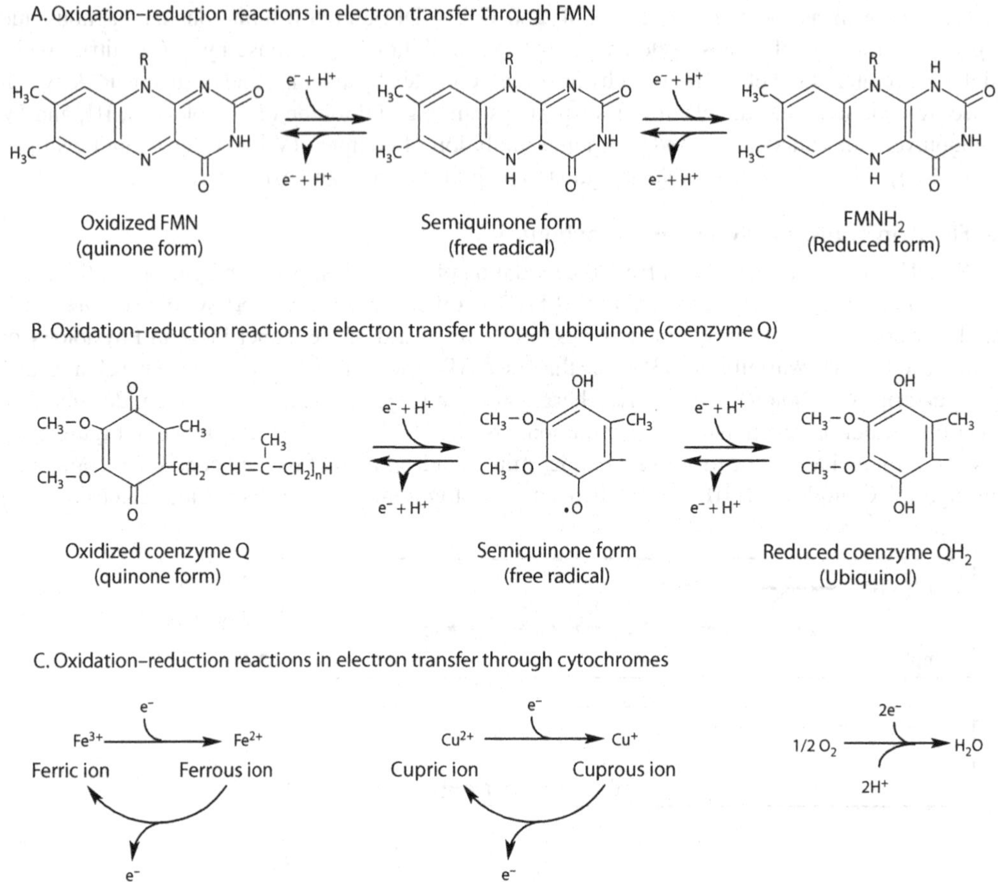

A. Oxidation–reduction reactions in electron transfer through FMN

Oxidized FMN (quinone form) ⇌ Semiquinone form (free radical) ⇌ $FMNH_2$ (Reduced form)

B. Oxidation–reduction reactions in electron transfer through ubiquinone (coenzyme Q)

Oxidized coenzyme Q (quinone form) ⇌ Semiquinone form (free radical) ⇌ Reduced coenzyme $QH_2$ (Ubiquinol)

C. Oxidation–reduction reactions in electron transfer through cytochromes

$Fe^{3+}$ Ferric ion → $Fe^{2+}$ Ferrous ion

$Cu^{2+}$ Cupric ion → $Cu^{+}$ Cuprous ion

$1/2\ O_2$ + $2e^-$ + $2H^+$ → $H_2O$

**FIGURE 1.24** The reduction–oxidation reactions involving quinone, $NAD^+$, FAD, and $Fe^{2+}$ in the mitochondrial electron transport system. Oxidation is defined as the removal of electrons from an electron donor (called the reductant), and reduction as the gain of electrons by an electron acceptor (called the oxidant). The tendency of an electron donor to give up its electrons to an electron acceptor is called the oxidation–reduction potential. The reductant of a redox pair with a large negative potential will release its electrons more easily than a redox pair with smaller negative or positive potentials.

the mitochondrial matrix to the intermembrane space, generating the proton-motive force across the inner mitochondrial membrane (Figure 1.25). The energy from the electrochemical gradient is used to drive the synthesis of ATP from ADP and Pi by ATP synthase (also known as complex V). The ATP synthase complex consists of two domains: $F_0$ and $F_1$. In mammals, birds, fish, and other animals, the $F_0$ domain is an integral protein within the inner mitochondrial membrane and contains a proton channel, whereas the $F_1$ domain (which has ATP synthase activity) is a peripheral protein that is located in the mitochondrial matrix, but is bound to the inner mitochondrial membrane. Thus, the $F_0$ domain provides a pore for the passage of protons from the intermembrane space into the $F_1$ domain in the mitochondrial matrix (Figure 1.23). The $F_0$ and $F_1$ domains are linked by central and peripheral stalks consisting of proteins. In prokaryotes (e.g., bacteria) without mitochondria, ATP synthase is localized in the cell membrane. The discovery of enzymatic mechanisms for ATP synthesis led to the award of the Nobel Prize in Chemistry to Paul D. Boyer and John E. Walker in 1997.

Complex I (NADH dehydrogenase) is also known as NADH-CoQ reductase and contains iron–sulfur (FeS) centers. This complex uses NADH + $H^+$ as substrates, as well as FMN and coenzyme Q (CoQ, a lipid-soluble mobile carrier) as its coenzymes. Note that NADH + $H^+$ are generated

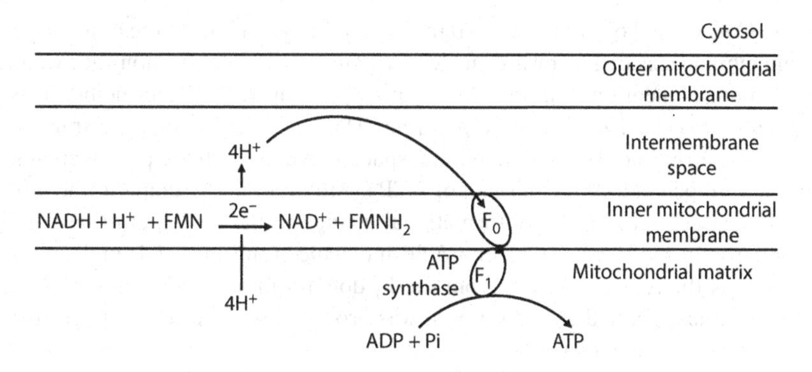


**FIGURE 1.25** Translocation of protons in complex I of the mitochondrial electron transport system and mitochondrial ATP synthesis in animals. During the oxidation of NADH + $H^+$ and $FADH_2$, complex I acts as a proton pump to translocate four electrons from the mitochondrial matrix to the intermembrane space. This generates the proton-motive force across the inner mitochondrial membrane to drive synthesis of ATP from ADP and Pi by ATP synthase (also known as complex V). The ATP synthase complex consists of two domains: $F_0$ (an integral protein containing a proton channel) and $F_1$ (a peripheral protein containing ATP synthase activity). Electrons pass through the $F_0$–$F_1$ complex, resulting in ATP synthesis. (Adapted from Devlin, T.M. 2011. *Textbook of Biochemistry with Clinical Correlations*. John Wiley & Sons, New York, NY.)

from $NAD^+$ and a reductant (e.g., succinate) by an enzyme (e.g., succinate dehydrogenase) in the mitochondrion (Figure 1.26). Complex I transfers two electrons and two protons from NADH + $H^+$ to FMN and then from $FMNH_2$ (one electron and one proton at a time) to CoQ, forming the reduced form of CoQ ($CoQH_2$), ubiquinol (Figure 1.20). Thus, FMN is a two-electron acceptor and $FMNH_2$ is a one-electron donor. The energy released during the transfer of electrons and protons from

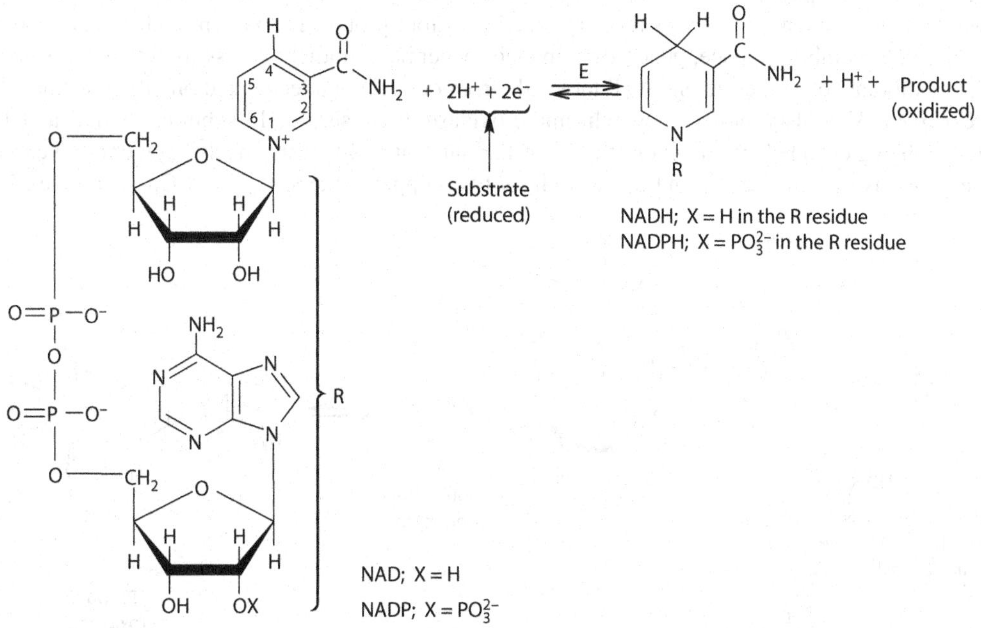

**FIGURE 1.26** The role of $NAD^+$ and $NADP^+$ in reduction–oxidation reactions. $NAD^+$ or $NADP^+$ accepts a proton to be reduced to NADH or NADPH, respectively. The $NAD^+$ molecule has one net negative charge, and the superscript "+" denotes the positive charge on the nitrogen atom in its nicotinamide ring. Likewise, the $NADP^+$ molecule has three net negative charges, and the superscript "+" denotes the positive charge on the nitrogen atom in its nicotinamide ring.

NADH + $H^+$ to CoQ is used by complex I to pump four protons ($H^+$) from the mitochondrial matrix into the intermembrane space, generating an electrochemical gradient (proton-motive force) across the inner mitochondrial membrane, as noted previously. This makes the intermembrane space more acidic and the mitochondrial matrix more alkaline. The four protons that are translocated from the mitochondrial matrix into the intermembrane space move through the proton channel in the $F_0$ domain (the inner mitochondrial membrane) of ATP synthase to the $F_1$ domain (the mitochondrial matrix) of ATP synthase, causing a conformational change in the $F_1$ domain (Devlin 2011). This results, sequentially, in the synthesis of one ATP molecule from one ADP molecule and one Pi molecule, as well as the release of ATP from the $F_1$ domain into the mitochondrial matrix. This process of ATP synthesis, called chemiosmosis, was proposed by Peter D. Mitchell in 1961 and is now widely accepted in biochemistry.

Complex II (succinate dehydrogenase) is also known as succinate-CoQ reductase, and it contains FeS centers and covalently bound FAD. This enzyme oxidizes succinate to fumarate, with the transfer of two electrons and two protons to FAD to form $FADH_2$ (Figure 1.27). The $FADH_2$ donates the electrons and protons to CoQ via the FeS centers, producing ubiquinol. The free energy released during these oxidative reactions is not sufficient to pump protons from the mitochondrial matrix into the intermembrane space. Thus, complex II is not a proton pumper, does not generate an electrochemical gradient across the inner mitochondrial membrane, and does not synthesize ATP.

Complex III is also known as cytochrome c reductase (CoQ-cytochrome c reductase or cytochrome $bc_1$ complex). This complex contains cytochrome b, cytochrome $c_1$ (a water-soluble, mobile electron carrier), and a Rieske FeS protein with a heme group that can bind an electron. Complex III is a dimer of cytochrome b and cytochrome $c_1$, with the globular head of the Rieske protein moving between cytochromes b and $c_1$. Because cytochromes can accept only one electron at a time, the two electrons from ubiquinol are transferred sequentially to cytochrome c through a series of reactions involving an iron–sulfur cluster and a heme, called the Q-cycle. Overall, complex III transfers two electrons and two protons from ubiquinol to cytochrome $c_1$. As in complex I, the energy released from the oxidative reactions drives the translocation of four protons from the mitochondrial matrix into the intermembrane space, generating an electrochemical gradient across the inner mitochondrial membrane to synthesize one ATP molecule from one ADP molecule and one Pi molecule.

Complex IV is also known as cytochrome c oxidase. It consists of 13 subunits, with 3 and 10 subunits being encoded by mitochondrial DNA and nuclear DNA, respectively. Cytochrome c oxidase contains cytochromes a and $a_3$, as well as two copper centers, $C_{UA}$ and $C_{UB}$. Complex IV

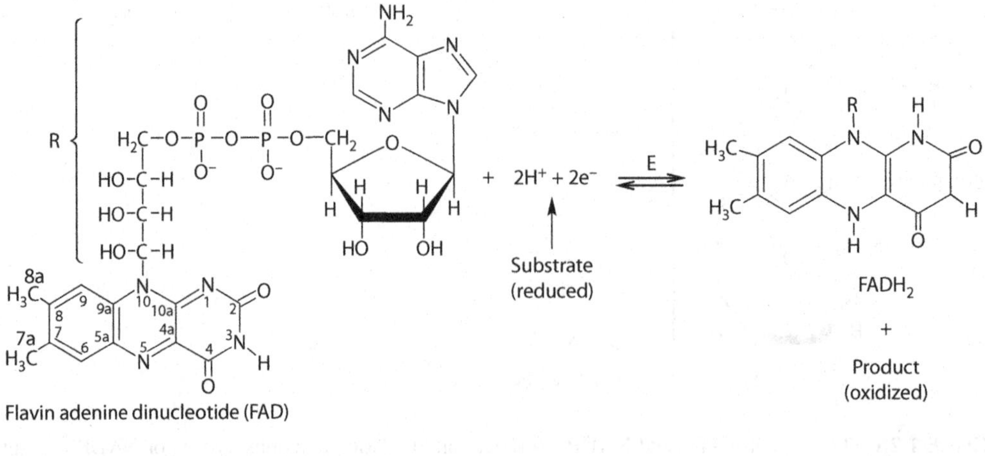

Flavin adenine dinucleotide (FAD)

+ $2H^+ + 2e^-$ ⇌ (E)

Substrate (reduced)

$FADH_2$ + Product (oxidized)

**FIGURE 1.27** The role of FAD in reduction–oxidation reactions. FAD accepts two protons and two protons from a reductant (e.g., succinate) to be reduced as $FADH_2$. The β-oxidation of fatty acids and the oxidation of acetyl-CoA in the mitochondrion produce $FADH_2$. This reducing equivalent is oxidized via the respiration chain to FAD, with the generation of $H_2O$ and ATP.

transfers 2 electrons and 2 protons from the reduced cytochrome c to 0.5 $O_2$ as the final oxidant of NADH + $H^+$ and $FADH_2$ (i.e., the terminal acceptor of the two electrons from NADH + $H^+$ or $FADH_2$) to produce $H_2O$. The energy released during the oxidative reactions is used by complex IV to pump four protons from the mitochondrial matrix to the intermembrane space. However, two of the four protons leak from the intermembrane space into the cytosol to generate superoxide anion ($O_2^-$), and the remaining two protons form an electrochemical gradient across the inner mitochondrial membrane. Thus, only two protons translocate from the intermembrane space into the $F_0$–$F_1$ complex of ATP synthase, and the electrochemical potential is sufficient to synthesize only 0.5 ATP molecule from 0.5 ADP molecule and 0.5 Pi molecule. Note that due to the release of two electrons from the mitochondrion to the cytosol, the rate of superoxide production (and hence oxidative stress) is positively correlated with the rate of ATP production in cells (and hence dietary energy intake).

The energetic efficiency of electron transport for ATP production is approximately 80%. Specifically, oxidation of 1 NADH + $H^+$ molecule produces 2.5 ATP molecules from 2.5 ADP molecules and 2.5 Pi molecules through the mitochondrial electron transport system (1, 1, and 0.5 ATP molecules at complexes I, III, and IV, respectively). This gives a P/O ratio of 2.5 (the number of ATP molecules synthesized per atom of oxygen consumed) for the transport of 2 electrons and 2 protons from NADH + $H^+$ to 0.5 $O_2$, rather than a theoretical P/O ratio of 3. Oxidation of 1 $FADH_2$ molecule does not involve complex I and produces 1.5 ATP molecules from 1.5 ADP molecules and 1.5 Pi molecules through the electron transport system (1 and 0.5 ATP molecules at complexes III and IV, respectively). This gives a P/O ratio of 1.5 for the transport of 2 electrons and 2 protons from $FADH_2$ to 0.5 $O_2$, rather than a theoretical P/O ratio of 2. Oxidation of 1 mol acetyl-CoA via the Krebs cycle and the respiration chain generates a total of 10 mol ATP in cells with mitochondria from the production of 3 mol NADH + $H^+$ (equivalent to 7.5 mol ATP), 1 mol $FADH_2$ (equivalent to 1.5 mol ATP), and 1 mol ATP (catalyzed by succinate thiokinase).

### Uncouplers of Oxidative Phosphorylation and Inhibitors of the Electron Transport System

Uncoupling protein-1 (UCP-1) uncouples oxidative reactions from ATP synthesis. This protein is uniquely expressed in BAT (Wu et al. 2012). UCP-1 is localized exclusively in the inner mitochondrial membrane and provides a pore for the movement of electrons from the intermembrane space to the mitochondrial matrix, such that the electrons will not pass through the $F_0$–$F_1$ complex of ATP synthase. As a result, the mitochondrial electron transport is uncoupled from ATP synthesis, and the energy from the oxidation of NADH + $H^+$ and $FADH_2$ is released as heat. Thus, mitochondrial electron transport may proceed without ATP production although $O_2$ is consumed by cells. In many mammals (including humans, rats, mice, cattle, and sheep), BAT starts to develop in fetuses during the mid- or last-trimester of gestation and is abundant in newborns, with most BAT being located near the kidneys, heart, and neck. Fatty acid oxidation in BAT plays a major role in nonshivering thermogenesis in the newborn of these species to keep them warm, particularly during exposure to a cold environment (Cannon and Nedergaard 2004). BAT can also oxidize glucose (Pravenec et al. 2016), glutamine, and leucine (Xi et al. 2010). Of note, some animal species (e.g., pigs and chickens) do not contain BAT at any stage of their life cycle (Satterfield and Wu 2011).

Besides UCP-1, mammals also express UCP-2 in the WAT, stomach, spleen, and lung, as well UCP-3 in the skeletal muscle, heart, liver, WAT, BAT, spleen, and thymus (Mailloux and Harper 2011). The major function of UCP-2 and UCP-3 (mitochondrial membrane transporters) in these tissues appears to inhibit the mitochondrial production of reactive oxygen species, but not to promote thermogenesis. In addition, some chemicals (e.g., proton ionophores) can serve as uncouplers of the mitochondrial oxidative phosphorylation by reducing proton concentration in the inner mitochondrial membrane (Table 1.9). Specifically, these substances, which are lipophilic (e.g., 2,4-dinitrophenol-$O^-$), accept protons from the intermembrane space (where proton concentration is relatively high) to form protonated molecules (e.g., 2,4-dinitrophenol-OH). The protonated molecules rapidly diffuse into the mitochondrial matrix, where the protons that have been picked up within the intermembrane space are dissociated due to a relatively low $H^+$ concentration. Through the addition of a

**TABLE 1.9**
**Uncouplers of Oxidative Phosphorylation and Inhibitors of the Electron Transport System Block ATP Synthesis from ADP and Inorganic Phosphate in Mitochondria**

| Substance | Action | Comment |
|---|---|---|
| UCP-1 | Uncoupler of oxidative phosphorylation | Uniquely expressed in BAT in many animals |
| DNP | Uncoupler of oxidative phosphorylation | Synthetic substance |
| Dicumarol | Uncoupler of oxidative phosphorylation | Naturally occurring anticoagulant |
| Rotenone | Inhibitor of complex I | Common insecticide found in roots of plants |
| Ptericidin | Inhibitor of complex I | Synthetic substance |
| Amobarbital | Inhibitor of complex I | Synthetic substance |
| Mercurials | Inhibitor of complex I | Mercury derivatives (toxic substances) |
| Demerol | Inhibitor of complex I | Also known as meperidine, synthetic substance |
| Malonate | Inhibitor of complex II | Binds to the active site of the target enzyme |
| Carboxin | Inhibitor of complex II | A synthetic pesticide |
| TTFA | Inhibitor of complex II | A synthetic chelating substance |
| Antimycin | Inhibitor of complex III | Produced by *Streptomyces* bacteria |
| Dimercaprol | Inhibitor of complex III | Treatment of metal toxicity through chelation |
| Cyanide | Inhibitor of complex IV | Synthetic substance |
| Azide | Inhibitor of complex IV | Synthetic substance |
| $H_2S$ | Inhibitor of complex IV | A metabolite of cysteine; synthetic substance |
| CO (high dose) | Inhibitor of complex IV | A metabolite of heme; synthetic substance |
| NO (high dose) | Inhibitor of complexes I, II, III, and IV | A metabolite of arginine; synthetic substance |
| DCCD | Inhibitor of ATP synthase | Covalent bonding to carboxyl groups of protein |
| Oligomycin | Inhibitor of ATP synthase | Binds $F_0$ and blocks movement of $e^-$ into $F_0$–$F_1$ |

*Source:* Cooper, G.M. and R.E. Hausman. 2016. *The Cell: A Molecular Approach*. Sinauer Associates, Sunderland, MA; Devlin, T.M. 2011. *Textbook of Biochemistry with Clinical Correlations*. John Wiley & Sons, New York, NY.

*Note:* BAT, brown adipose tissue; CO, carbon monoxide; DCCD, dicyclohexylcarbodiimide; DNP, 2,4-dinitrophenol; $H_2S$, hydrogen sulfide; NO, nitric oxide; TTFA, 2-thenoyltrifluoroacetone; UCP-1, uncoupling protein-1.

proton to an uncoupler in the inner mitochondrial membrane (known as protonation), the electrons that are translocated from the mitochondrial matrix into the intermembrane space during the oxidation of NADH + $H^+$ and $FADH_2$ do not enter the $F_0$–$F_1$ complex of ATP synthase, resulting in no ATP production.

In addition to the endogenous and exogenous uncouplers of oxidative phosphorylation, some toxic substances can also block ATP synthesis from ADP and Pi by directly inhibiting enzymes or proteins in the electron transport system. These substances are listed in Table 1.9. Caution should be taken to ensure that such toxic chemicals will not be part of any diets for animals. Note that while physiological levels of CO and NO stimulate energy metabolism in organisms, high concentrations of these gases reduce ATP production by inhibiting complexes I–IV (Dai et al. 2013). This further highlights the importance of a balanced diet in the health and well-being of mammals, birds, fish, and other species.

## SUMMARY

Nutrients are substances required by animals to maintain life, grow, develop, lactate, and reproduce. Proximate analysis of feedstuffs traditionally provides useful information on their content of water and DM, including CP, crude fat, minerals, crude fiber, and other carbohydrates. Modern analytical methods have made it possible to determine AA composition in protein, free fatty acids and their

**TABLE 1.10**
**Metabolic Diseases or Disorders Resulting from Nutrient Deficiencies or Imbalances in Animals**

| Metabolic Disease | Cause |
|---|---|
| | **Nonruminants** |
| Ascite-pulmonary hypertension (poultry) | Deficiency of arginine and inadequate NO synthesis |
| Hyperkalemic periodic paralysis (HYPP, horses) | Elevated levels of potassium in blood and Na-channel defect |
| Hypoglycemia (pigs) | Low concentrations of glucose in blood |
| Porcine stress syndrome (heat stress and PSE) | Deficiencies of antioxidative nutrients; presence of oxidative stress |
| | **Ruminants** |
| Grass tetany (pastoral hypomagnesemia) | Deficiency of magnesium (Mg) cattle; sheep are also susceptible |
| Ketosis in lactating cows | Excess fat mobilization due to an inadequate intake of dietary energy |
| Milk fever (parturient paresis, lactating cows) | Calcium deficiency |
| Pregnancy toxemia (most commonly in sheep) | Excess fat mobilization due to an inadequate intake of dietary energy |
| Low-fat milk syndrome (milk fat depression) | Excess production of *trans*-10, *cis*-12 CLA (dairy cows) |
| Ruminal bloat (ruminal tympany) | Excess gas accumulation in the rumen |
| Ruminal acidosis | Excess accumulation of lactic acid in the rumen |
| | **Both Ruminants and Nonruminants** |
| Abnormal wool (sheep) | Copper deficiency |
| Alopecia (loss of hair or feathers; baldness) | Deficiencies of vitamins, particularly niacin, riboflavin, biotin, and pantothenic acid; deficiencies of protein/AAs |
| Anemia | Deficiencies of vitamins E, $B_{12}$, and K, folate, iron, and protein/AAs |
| Beriberi | Caused by thiamin deficiency (leg disorders, including weakness, edema, pain and paralysis) |
| Capillary fragility | Deficiencies of vitamin C and iron |
| Cardiomyopathy and skeletal muscle myopathy | Deficiencies of vitamin E, taurine, and protein/AAs |
| Cheilosis[a] and angular stomatitis[b] (both occurring) | Riboflavin deficiency |
| Diabetes | Elevated concentrations of glucose in blood due to insulin deficiency or insensitivity of tissues (e.g., skeletal muscle) to insulin |
| Edema (abnormal fluid accumulation) | Deficiencies of protein/AAs and thiamin |
| Goiter (enlargement of the thyroid gland) | Iodine deficiency |
| Gout | Excessive uric acid accumulation due to arginine deficiency |
| Hartnup disease | Impaired absorption of dietary tryptophan by the small intestine |
| Hemorrhage (loss of blood) | Deficiencies of iron, vitamins K, E, and C, and protein/AAs |
| Homocysteinemia | Deficiencies of vitamins $B_6$ and $B_{12}$, folate; excess intake of SAAs |
| Hyperammonemia | Deficiencies of arginine and Mn; excess intake of AAs |
| Hypertension | Deficiency of arginine; excess dietary intake of sodium |
| Impaired blood clotting | Vitamin K deficiency |
| Impaired fertility in males and females and fetal death | Deficiencies of nutrients, especially vitamins A and E, zinc, arginine, and phosphorus |
| Impairment of growth and development and general weakness | Deficiencies of all nutrients, particularly protein/AAs, n3 and n6 polyunsaturated fatty acids, vitamins, and essential minerals |
| Keshan disease | Selenium deficiency to cause oxidative stress |
| Kwashiorkor | Primarily a severe deficiency of dietary protein and AAs |

*(Continued)*

**TABLE 1.10 (*Continued*)**
**Metabolic Diseases or Disorders Resulting from Nutrient Deficiencies or Imbalances in Animals**

| Metabolic Disease | Cause |
|---|---|
| Liver cirrhosis (degeneration of parenchymal cells) | Deficiencies of choline and arginine; excess ammonia accumulation |
| Liver and kidney steatosis | Excess fat accumulation to cause tissue degeneration |
| Low appetite | Deficiencies of nutrients, particularly protein/AAs, n3 and n6 polyunsaturated fatty acids, vitamins (e.g., niacin), and essential minerals |
| Marasmus | Primarily severe deficiencies of both protein and energy in diets |
| Neural tube defects | Folate deficiency and accumulation of homocysteine |
| Pellagra | Niacin deficiency (the four-D's syndromes: dermatitis, diarrhea, dementia and death) |
| Photophobia | Riboflavin deficiency |
| Rickes and osteomalacia | Vitamin D and calcium deficiencies |
| Scurvy (bleeding gum) | Vitamin C deficiency |
| Xerophthalmia and keratomalacia | Vitamin A deficiency |

*Note:* AAs, amino acids; CLA, conjugated linoleic acid; PSE, pale soft exudative pork muscle; SAAs, sulfur-containing amino acids (methionine and cysteine).

[a] Cracks and fissures at the corners of the mouth.

[b] Inflammation of the oral mucosa.

derivatives, simple and complex sugars, macro- and microelements, as well as water- and lipid-soluble vitamins. To date, more than 40 nutrients are known to be essential for mammals, birds, fish, and shrimp. Under the control of the nervous system and the influence of sense organs, animals consume feed and water to meet their nutrient requirements. In addition, the physiological state of the animal (e.g., pregnant, lactating, suckling, and weanling) must be considered when classifying a nutrient as nonessential, conditionally essential, or essential.

Utilization of dietary nutrients (including biological oxidation of nutrients for ATP production via the Krebs cycle and the electron transport system in the mitochondria) depends on well-coordinated biochemical and physiological processes. They include: (1) digestion and absorption in the gastrointestinal tract; (2) transport of absorbed nutrients through the circulatory system (including the blood capillaries); (3) uptake of excess interstitial fluid by the lymphatic capillaries and its transfer to the lymphatic vessels for return to the blood circulation; (4) provision of oxygen by the respiratory system; (5) enzyme-, coenzyme-, and cofactor-dependent metabolism of nutrients via a series of complex pathways (e.g., glycolysis, gluconeogenesis, the Krebs cycle, the urea cycle, intracellular protein turnover, β-oxidation, ketogenesis, hexosamine synthesis, one-carbon unit transfer, and the mitochondrial electron transport system); (6) tubular reabsorption of nutrients and bicarbonate from the lumen of renal tubules (e.g., proximal tubule) into the blood in the kidneys; and (7) excretion of metabolites through the kidneys, lungs, and skin. Of note, the metabolic pathways are compartmentalized (e.g., cytosol, nucleus, mitochondrion, ribosome, and lysosome) in a cell-, tissue-, species-, and age-specific manner. Their regulation by various hormones (e.g., insulin, glucagon, growth factors, thyroid hormones, glucocorticoids, progesterone, estrogen, and adiponectin) is essential to animal growth (primarily musculoskeletal growth and fetal growth), immunity, health, and survival. In animals, deficiencies of nutrients cause a wide array of metabolic diseases, and examples are given in Table 1.10. Therefore, adequate knowledge of principles of animal nutrition is required for the development of balanced diets that enhance the efficiency of global livestock, poultry, and fish production, as well as the health and well-being of all animals.

## REFERENCES

Alderton, W.K., C.E. Cooper, and R.G. Knowles. 2001. Nitric oxide synthases: Structure, function and inhibition. *Biochem. J.* 357:593–615.

Argenzio, R.A. 1993. General functions of the gastrointestinal tract and their control and integration. In: *Dukes' Physiology of Domestic Animals.* Edited by M.J. Swenson and W.O. Reece. Cornell University Press, Ithaca, NY, pp. 325–348.

Asher, G. and Sassone-Corsi P. 2015. Time for food: The intimate interplay between nutrition, metabolism, and the circadian clock. *Cell* 161:84–92.

Avissar, N.E., H.T. Wang, J.H. Miller, P. Iannoli, and H.C. Sax. 2000. Epidermal growth factor receptor is increased in rabbit intestinal brush border membrane after small bowel resection. *Dig. Dis. Sci.* 45:1145–1152.

Baker, D.H. 2005. Comparative nutrition and metabolism: Explication of open questions with emphasis on protein and amino acids. *Proc. Natl. Acad. Sci. USA* 102:17897–17902.

Baracos, V.E. 2006. Integration of amino acid metabolism during intense lactation. *Curr. Opin. Clin. Nutr. Metab. Care* 9:48–52.

Barboza, P.S., K.L. Parker, and I.D. Hume. 2009. *Integrative Wildlife Nutrition.* Springer, New York, NY.

Barminko, J., B. Reinholt, and M.H. Baron. 2016. Development and differentiation of the erythroid lineage in mammals. *Dev. Comp. Immunol.* 58:18–29.

Barrett, K.E. 2014. *Gastrointestinal Physiology.* McGraw Hill, New York, NY.

Bauman, D.E., K.J. Harvatine, and A.L. Lock. 2011. Nutrigenomics, rumen-derived bioactive fatty acids, and the regulation of milk fat synthesis. *Annu. Rev. Nutr.* 31:299–319.

Bazer F.W., G.A. Johnson, and G. Wu. 2015. Amino acids and conceptus development during the peri-implantation period of pregnancy. *Adv. Exp. Med. Biol.* 843:23–52.

Bazer, F.W., G. Wu, G.A. Johnson, and X. Wang. 2014. Environmental factors affecting pregnancy: Endocrine disrupters, nutrients and metabolic pathways. *Mol. Cell. Endocrinol.* 398:53–68.

Bazer, F.W., G. Wu, T.E. Spencer, G.A. Johnson, R.C. Burghardt, and K. Bayless. 2010. Novel pathways for implantation and establishment and maintenance of pregnancy in mammals. *Mol. Hum. Reprod.* 16:135–152.

Beitz, D.C. 1993. Carbohydrate metabolism. In: *Dukes' Physiology of Domestic Animals.* Edited by M.J. Swenson and W.O. Reece. Cornell University Press, Ithaca, NY, pp. 437–472.

Bennett, B.J., K.D. Hall, F.B. Hu, A.L. McCartney, and C. Roberto. 2015. Nutrition and the science of disease prevention: A systems approach to support metabolic health. *Ann. N.Y. Acad. Sci.* 1352:1–12.

Bergen, W.G. 2007. Contribution of research with farm animals to protein metabolism concepts: A historical perspective. *J. Nutr.* 137:706–710.

Bergen, W.G. and G. Wu. 2009. Intestinal nitrogen recycling and utilization in health and disease. *J. Nutr.* 139:821–825.

Blaxter, K.L. 1989. *Energy Metabolism in Animals and Man.* Cambridge University Press, New York, NY.

Bondi, A.A. 1987. *Animal Nutrition.* John Wiley & Sons, New York, NY.

Booijink, C.C.G.M. 2009. Analysis of diversity and function of the human small intestinal microbiota. *Ph.D. Thesis.* Wageningen University, Wageningen, the Netherlands.

Boron, W.F. 2004. *Medical Physiology: A Cellular and Molecular Approach.* Elsevier, New York, NY.

Brewer, N.R. 2006. Biology of the rabbit. *J. Am. Assoc. Lab. Anim. Sci.* 45:8–24.

Brodal, P. 2004. *The Central Nervous System: Structure and Function.* Oxford University Press, Cambridge, UK.

Brosnan, J.T. 2005. Metabolic design principles: Chemical and physical determinants of cell chemistry. *Adv. Enzyme Regul.* 45:27–36.

Brosnan, M.E., L. MacMillan, J.R. Stevens, and J.T. Brosnan. 2015. Division of labour: How does folate metabolism partition between one-carbon metabolism and amino acid oxidation? *Biochem. J.* 472:135–146.

Burrin, D.G., B. Stoll, R.H. Jiang, X.Y. Chang, B. Hartmann, J.J. Holst, G.H. Greeley, and P.J. Reeds. 2000. Minimal enteral nutrient requirements for intestinal growth in neonatal piglets: How much is enough? *Am. J. Clin. Nutr.* 71:1603–1610.

Calder, P.C. 2006. Branched-chain amino acid and immunity. *J. Nutr.* 136:288S–233S.

Campbell, T.W. 1995. *Avian Hematology and Cytology.* Iowa State University Press, Ames, IA.

Cannon, B. and J. Nedergaard. 2004. Brown adipose tissue: Function and physiological significance. *Physiol. Rev.* 84:277–359.

Cheeke, P.R. and E.S. Dierenfeld. 2010. *Comparative Animal Nutrition and Metabolism.* CABI, Wallingford, UK.

Clemens, E.T., C.E. Stevenes, and M. Southworth. 1975. Site of organic acid production and pattern of digesta movement in gastrointestinal tract of geese. *J. Nutr.* 105:1341–1350.

Cooper, G.M. and R.E. Hausman. 2016. *The Cell: A Molecular Approach.* Sinauer Associates, Sunderland, MA.

Coverdale, J.A., J.A. Moore, H.D. Tyler and P.A. Miller-Auwerda. 2004. Soybean hulls as an alternative feed for horses. *J. Anim. Sci.* 82:1663–1668.

Croze, E.M. and D.J. Morré. 1984. Isolation of plasma membrane, Golgi apparatus, and endoplasmic reticulum fractions from single homogenization of mouse liver. *J. Cell Physiol.* 119:46–57.

Dai, Z.L., Z.L. Wu, S.Q. Hang, W.Y. Zhu, and G. Wu. 2015. Amino acid metabolism in intestinal bacteria and its potential implications for mammalian reproduction. *Mol. Hum. Reprod.* 21:389–409.

Dai, Z.L., Z.L. Wu, S.C. Jia, and G. Wu. 2014. Analysis of amino acid composition in proteins of animal tissues and foods as pre-column o-phthaldialdehyde derivatives by HPLC with fluorescence detection. *J. Chromatogr.* B. 964:116–127.

Dai, Z.L., Z.L. Wu, Y. Yang, J.J. Wang, M.C. Satterfield, C.J. Meininger, F.W. Bazer, and G. Wu. 2013. Nitric oxide and energy metabolism in mammals. *BioFactors* 39:383–391.

Dallas, S. and E. Jewell. 2014. *Animal Biology and Care.* Wiley-Blackwell, London, UK.

Davies, R.R. and J.A.E.R. Davies. 2003. Rabbit gastrointestinal physiology. *Vet. Clin. Exot. Anim.* 6:139–153.

Davis, T.A., M.L. Fiorotto, D.G. Burrin, P.J. Reeds, H.V. Nguyen, P.R. Beckett, R.C. Vann, and P.M. O'Connor. 2002. Stimulation of protein synthesis by both insulin and amino acids is unique to skeletal muscle in neonatal pigs. *Am. J. Physiol. Endocrinol. Metab.* 282:E880–E890.

De Duve, C. 1971. Tissue fractionation: Past and present. *J. Cell Biol.* 50:20D–55D.

Dellschaft, N.S., M.R. Ruth, S. Goruk, E.D. Lewis, C. Richard, R.L. Jacobs, J.M. Curtis, and C.J. Field. 2015. Choline is required in the diet of lactating dams to maintain maternal immune function. *Br. J. Nutr.* 113:1723–1731.

Devlin, T.M. 2011. *Textbook of Biochemistry with Clinical Correlations.* John Wiley & Sons, New York, NY.

Dillon, E.L., D.A. Knabe, and G. Wu. 1999. Lactate inhibits citrulline and arginine synthesis from proline in pig enterocytes. *Am. J. Physiol.* 276:G1079–G1086.

Dyce, K.M., W.O. Sack, and C.J.G. Wensing. 1996. *Textbook of Veterinary Anatomy.* W.B. Saunders Company, Philadelphia, PA.

Farmer, C. 1997. Did lungs and the intracardiac shunt evolve to oxygenate the heart in vertebrates? *Paleobiology* 23:358–372.

Fell, D. 1997. *Understanding the Control of Metabolism.* Portland Press, London, UK.

Ferguson, R.A. and R.G. Boutilier. 1989. Metabolic-membrane coupling in red blood cells of trout: The effects of anoxia and adrenergic stimulation. *J. Exp. Biol.* 143:149–164.

Field, C.J., I.R. Johnson, and P.D. Schley. 2002. Nutrients and their role in host resistance to infection. *J. Leukoc. Biol.* 71:16–32.

Firkins, J.L., Z. Yu, and M. Morrison. 2007. Ruminal nitrogen metabolism: Perspectives for integration of microbiology and nutrition for dairy. *J. Dairy Sci.* 90 (Suppl. 1):E1–E16.

Ford, S.P., B.W. Hess, M.M. Schwope, M.J. Nijland, J.S. Gilbert, K.A. Vonnahme, W.J. Means, H. Han, and P.W. Nathanielsz. 2007. Maternal undernutrition during early to mid-gestation in the ewe results in altered growth, adiposity, and glucose tolerance in male offspring. *J. Anim. Sci.* 85:1285–1294.

Fox, J.G., L.C. Anderson, F.M. Loew, and F.W. Quimby. 2002. *Laboratory Animal Medicine.* Academic Press, New York, NY.

Friedman, M. 2008. *Principles and Models of Biological Transport.* Springer, New York, NY.

Gashev, A.A. and D.C. Zawieja. 2010. Hydrodynamic regulation of lymphatic transport and the impact of aging. *Pathophysiology* 17:277–287.

Gilbert, A.B. 1971. Transport of the egg through the oviduct ad oviposition. In: *Physiology and Biochemistry of the Domestic Fowl.* Edited by D.J. Bell and B.M. Freeman. Academic Press, London, UK, pp. 1345–1352.

Granger, H.J., M.E. Schelling, R.E. Lewis, D.C. Zawieja, and C.J. Meininger. 1988. Physiology and pathobiology of the microcirculation. *Am. J. Otolaryngol.* 9:264–277.

Guyton, A.C., T.G. Coleman, and H.J. Granger. 1972. Circulation: Overall regulation. *Annu. Rev. Physiol.* 34:13–46.

Guyton, A.C. and J.E. Hall. 2000. *Textbook of Medical Physiology.* W.B. Saunders Company, Philadelphia, PA.

Häussinger, D., W.H. Lamers, and A.F. Moorman. 1992. Hepatocyte heterogeneity in the metabolism of amino acids and ammonia. *Enzyme* 46:72–93.

Hill, K.J. 1971. The structure of the alimentary tract. In: *Physiology and Biochemistry of the Domestic Fowl.* Edited by D.J. Bell and B.M. Freeman. Academic Press, London, UK, pp. 91–169.

Hou, Y.Q., K. Yao, Y.L. Yin, and G. Wu. 2016. Endogenous synthesis of amino acids limits growth, lactation and reproduction of animals. *Adv. Nutr.* 7:331–342.

Hou, Y.Q., Y.L. Yin, and G. Wu. 2015. Dietary essentiality of "nutritionally nonessential amino acids" for animals and humans. *Exp. Biol. Med.* 240:997–1007.

Hu, S.D., X.L. Li, R. Rezaei, C.J. Meininger, C.J. McNeal, and G. Wu. 2015. Safety of long-term dietary supplementation with L-arginine in pigs. *Amino Acids* 47:925–936.

Hungate, R.E. 1966. *The Rumen and Its Microbes.* Academic Press, New York, NY.

Iyer, A., L. Brown, J.P. Whitehead, J.B. Prins, and D.P. Fairlie. 2015. Nutrient and immune sensing are obligate pathways in metabolism, immunity, and disease. *FASEB J.* 29:3612–3625.

Jungermann, K. and T. Keitzmann. 1996. Zonation of parenchymal and nonparenchymal metabolism in liver. *Annu. Rev. Nutr.* 16:179–203.

Kaeser, P.S. and W.G. Regehr. 2014. Molecular mechanisms for synchronous, asynchronous, and spontaneous neurotransmitter release. *Annu. Rev. Physiol.* 76:333–363.

Kim, S.W. and G. Wu. 2004. Dietary arginine supplementation enhances the growth of milk-fed young pigs. *J. Nutr.* 134:625–630.

King, A.S. and V. Molony. 1971. The anatomy of respiration. In: *Physiology and Biochemistry of the Domestic Fowl.* Edited by D.J. Bell and B.M. Freeman. Academic Press, London, UK, pp. 91–169.

Klein, R.M. and J.C. McKenzie. 1983. The role of cell renewal in the ontogeny of the intestine. I. Cell proliferation patterns in adult, fetal, and neonatal intestine. *J. Pediatr. Gastroenterol. Nutr.* 2:10–43.

Kobayashi, I., F. Katakura, and T. Moritomo. 2016. Isolation and characterization of hematopoietic stem cells in teleost fish. *Dev. Comp. Immunol.* 58:86–94.

Kwon, H., T.E. Spencer, F.W. Bazer, and G. Wu. 2003. Developmental changes of amino acids in ovine fetal fluids. *Biol. Reprod.* 68:1813–1820.

Laale, H.W. 1977. The biology and use of zebrafish, *Brachydanio rerio*, in fisheries research: A literature review. *J. Fish Biol.* 10:121–173.

Lake, P.E. 1971. The male in reproduction. In: *Physiology and Biochemistry of the Domestic Fowl.* Edited by D.J. Bell and B.M. Freeman. Academic Press, London, UK, pp. 1411–1447.

Lebeck, J. 2014. Metabolic impact of the glycerol channels AQP7 and AQP9 in adipose tissue and liver. *J. Mol. Endocrinol.* 52:R165–178.

Lemasters, J.J. and E. Holmuhamedov. 2006. Voltage-dependent anion channel (VDAC) as mitochondrial governator—Thinking outside the box. *Biochim. Biophys. Acta* 1762:181–190.

Li, D.F., J.L. Nelssen, P.G. Reddy, F. Blecha, J.D. Hancock, G.L. Allee, R.D. Goodband, and R.D. Klemm. 1990. Transient hypersensitivity to soybean meal in the early-weaned pig. *J. Anim. Sci.* 68:1790–1799.

Li, X.L., R. Rezaei, P. Li, and G. Wu. 2011. Composition of amino acids in feed ingredients for animal diets. *Amino Acids* 40:1159–1168.

Li, Y.S., W.F. Xiao, W. Luo, C. Zeng, W.K. Ren, G. Wu, and G.H. Lei. 2016. Alterations of amino acid metabolism in osteoarthritis: Its implications for nutrition and health. *Amino Acids* 48:907–914.

Li, P., Y.L. Yin, D.F. Li, S.W. Kim, and G. Wu. 2007. Amino acids and immune function. *Br. J. Nutr.* 98:237–252.

Liao, S.F., D.L. Harmon, E.S. Vanzant, K.R. McLeod, J.A. Boling, and J.C. Matthews. 2010. The small intestinal epithelia of beef steers differentially express sugar transporter messenger ribonucleic acid in response to abomasal versus ruminal infusion of starch hydrolysate. *J. Anim. Sci.* 88:306–314.

Lu, D.X. 2014. Systems nutrition: An innovation of A scientific system in animal nutrition. *Front. Biosci.* 6:55–61.

Madara, J.L. 1991. Functional morphology of epithelium of the small intestine. In: *Handbook of Physiology: The Gastrointestinal System.* Edited by S.G. Shultz. American Physiological Society, Bethesda, MD, pp. 83–120.

Mailloux, R.J. and M.E. Harper. 2011. Uncoupling proteins and the control of mitochondrial reactive oxygen species production. *Free Radic. Biol. Med.* 51:1106–1115.

Marliss, E.B., A.F. Nakhooda, P. Poussier, and A.A. Sima. 1982. The diabetic syndrome of the "BB" Wistar rat: Possible relevance to type 1 (insulin-dependent) diabetes in man. *Diabetologia* 22:225–232.

McCorry, L.K. 2007. Physiology of the autonomic nervous system. *Am. J. Pharm. Educ.* 71(4):78.

McDonald, P., R.A. Edwards, J.F.D. Greenhalgh, C.A. Morgan, and L.A. Sinclair. 2011. *Animal Nutrition*, 7th ed. Prentice Hall, New York, NY.

Meredith, D. 2009. The mammalian proton-coupled peptide cotransporter PepT1: Sitting on the transporter-channel fence? *Philos. Trans. R. Soc. Lond. B Biol. Sci.* 364:203–207.

Merriam-Webster. 2005. *The Merriam-Webster Dictionary.* Merriam-Webster Inc., Springfield, MA.

Moore, S.A., E. Yoder, and A.A. Spector. 1990. Role of the blood-brain barrier in the formation of long-chain omega-3 and omega-6 fatty acids from essential fatty acid precursors. *J. Neurochem.* 55:391–402.

Morgan, C.J., A.G.P. Coutts, M.C. McFadyen, T.P. King, and D. Kelly. 1996. Characterization of IGF-I receptors in the porcine small intestine during postnatal development. *J. Nutr. Biochem.* 7:339–347.

Mowat, A.M. 1987. The cellular basis of gastrointestinal immunity. In: *Immunopathology of the Small Intestine.* Edited by M.N. Marsh. John Wiley, London, UK, pp. 41–72.

National Research Council (NRC). 2002. *Scientific Advances in Animal Nutrition.* National Academies Press, Washington, DC.

National Research Council (NRC). 2012. *Nutrient Requirements of Swine.* National Academies Press, Washington, DC.

Nemere, I., N. Garcia-Garbi, G.J. Hämmerling, and Q. Winger. 2012. Intestinal cell phosphate uptake and the targeted knockout of the 1,25$D_3$-MARRS receptor/PDIA3/ERp57. *Endocrinology* 153:1609–1615.

Oksbjerg, N., P.M. Nissen, M. Therkildsen, H.S. Møller, L.B. Larsen, M. Andersen, and J.F. Young. 2013. In utero nutrition related to fetal development, postnatal performance, and meat quality of pork. *J. Anim. Sci.* 91:1443–1453.

Oldham-Ott, C.K. and J. Gilloteaux. 1997. Comparative morphology of the gallbladder and biliary tract in vertebrates: Variation in structure, homology in function and gallstones. *Microsc. Res. Tech.* 38:571–597.

Ovadi, I. and V. Saks. 2004. On the origin of intracellular compartmentalization and organized metabolic systems. *Mol. Cell. Biochem.* 256:5–12.

Palmieri, F. and M. Monné. 2016. Discoveries, metabolic roles and diseases of mitochondrial carriers: A review. *Biochim. Biophys. Acta* 1863:2362–2378.

Pond, W.G., D.C. Church, and K.R. Pond. 1995. *Basic Animal Nutrition and Feeding*, 4th ed. John Wiley & Sons, New York, NY.

Pravenec, M., P. Mlejnek, V. Zídek, V. Landa, M. Šimáková, J. Šilhavý, H. Strnad et al. 2016. Autocrine effects of transgenic resistin reduce palmitate and glucose oxidation in brown adipose tissue. *Physiol. Genomics* 48:420–427.

Rappaport, A.M. 1958. The structural and functional unit in the human liver (liver acinus). *Anat. Rec.* 130:673–689.

Reece, W.O. 1993. Water balance and excretion. In: *Dukes' Physiology of Domestic Animals.* Edited by M.J. Swenson and W.O. Reece. Cornell University Press, Ithaca, NY, pp. 573–628.

Reynolds, L.P., M.C. Wulster-Radcliffe, D.K. Aaron, and T.A. Davis. 2015. Importance of animals in agricultural sustainability and food security. *J. Nutr.* 145:1377–1379.

Rezaei, R., W.W. Wang, Z.L. Wu, Z.L. Dai, J.J. Wang, and G. Wu. 2013. Biochemical and physiological bases for utilization of dietary amino acids by young pigs. *J. Anim. Sci. Biotechnol.* 4:7.

Roach, P.J., A.A. Depaoli-Roach, T.D. Hurley, and V.S. Tagliabracci. 2012. Glycogen and its metabolism: Some new developments and old themes. *Biochem. J.* 441:763–787.

Robinson, C.J., B.J.M. Bohannan, and V.B. Young. 2010. From structure to function: The ecology of host-associated microbial communities. *Microbiol. Mol. Biol. Rev.* 74:453–476.

Russell, J.B. and J.L. Rychlik. 2001. Factors that alter rumen microbial ecology. *Science* 292:1119–1122.

Sarin, H. 2010. Physiologic upper limits of pore size of different blood capillary types and another perspective on the dual pore theory of microvascular permeability. *J. Angiogenes. Res.* 2:14.

Satterfield, M.C. and G. Wu. 2011. Growth and development of brown adipose tissue: Significance and nutritional regulation. *Front. Biosci.* 16:1589–1608.

Savage, D.C. 1977. Microbial ecology of the gastrointestinal tract. *Ann. Rev. Microbiol.* 31:107–133.

Scallan, J., V.H. Huxley, and R.J. Korthuis. 2010. *Capillary Fluid Exchange: Regulation, Functions, and Pathology.* Morgan & Claypool Life Sciences, San Rafael, CA.

Scanes, C.G. 2009. Perspectives on the endocrinology of poultry growth and metabolism. *Gen. Comp. Endocrinol.* 163:24–32.

Schimke, R. and D. Doyle. 1970. Control of enzyme levels in animal tissues. *Annu. Rev. Biochem.* 39:929–976.

Schleicher, J., C. Tokarski, E. Marbach, M. Matz-Soja, S. Zellmer, R. Gebhardt, and S. Schuster. 2015. Zonation of hepatic fatty acid metabolism—The diversity of its regulation and the benefit of modeling. *Biochim. Biophys. Acta* 1851:641–656.

Sporns, O., D.R. Chialvo, M. Kaiser, and C.C. Hilgetag. 2004. Organization, development and function of complex brain networks. *Trends Cogn. Sci.* 8:418–425.

Srere, P.A. 1987. Complexes of sequential metabolic enzymes. *Annu. Rev. Biochem.* 56:89–124.

Steele, M.A., G.B. Penner, E. Chaucheyras-Durand, and L.L. Guan. 2016. Development and physiology of the rumen and the lower gut: Targets for improving gut health. *J. Dairy. Sci.* 99:4955–4966.

Stevens, C.E. and I.D. Hume. 1998. Contributions of microbes in vertebrate gastrointestinal tract to production and conservation of nutrients. *Physiol. Rev.* 78:393–427.
Stocco, D.M. 2000. Intramitochondrial cholesterol transfer. *Biochim. Biophys. Acta* 1486:184–197.
Tharwat, M., F. Al-Sobayil, A. Ali, and S. Buczinski. 2012. Transabdominal ultrasonographic appearance of the gastrointestinal viscera of healthy camels (*Camelus dromedaries*). *Res. Vet. Sci.* 93:1015–1020.
Thompson, J.R., G. Weiser, K. Seto, and A.L. Black. 1975. Effect of glucose load on synthesis of plasma glucose in lactating cows. *J. Dairy Sci.* 58:362–370.
Watford M. 1991. The urea cycle: A two-compartment system. *Essays Biochem.* 26:49–58.
Wilson, E.O. 1992. *The Diversity of Life*. Harvard University Press, Cambridge, MA.
Van Soest, P.J. 1967. Development of a comprehensive system of feed analyses and its application to forages. *J. Anim. Sci.* 26:119–128.
Van Soest, P.J. and R.H. Wine. 1967. Use of detergents in the analysis of fibrous feeds. IV. Determination of plant cell-wall constituents. *J. Assoc. Off. Anal. Chem.* 50:50–55.
Vernon, H.J. 2015. Inborn errors of metabolism: Advances in diagnosis and therapy. *JAMA Pediatr.* 169:778–782.
Vieira, R.A., L.O. Tedeschi, and A. Cannas. 2008. A generalized compartmental model to estimate the fibre mass in the ruminoreticulum: 2. Integrating digestion and passage. *J. Theor. Biol.* 255:357–368.
Weber-Lotfi, F., M.V. Koulintchenko, N. Ibrahim, P. Hammann, D.V. Mileshina, Y.M. Konstantinov, and A. Dietrich. 2015. Nucleic acid import into mitochondria: New insights into the translocation pathways. *Biochim. Biophys. Acta* 1853:3165–3181.
Weiner, I.D. and J.W. Verlander. 2011. Role of $NH_3$ and $NH_4$ transporters in renal acid-base transport. *Am. J. Physiol. Renal Physiol.* 300:F11–F23.
Wickersham, T.A., E.C. Titgemeyer, and R.C. Cochran. 2009. Methodology for concurrent determination of urea kinetics and the capture of recycled urea nitrogen by ruminal microbes in cattle. *Animal* 3:372–379.
Wilson, J.M. and L.F.C. Castro. 2011. Morphological diversity of the gastrointestinal tract in fishes. *Fish Physiol.* 30:1–55.
Wu, G. 2013. *Amino Acids: Biochemistry and Nutrition*. CRC Press, Boca Raton, FL.
Wu, G., F.W. Bazer, and H.R. Cross. 2014a. Land-based production of animal protein: Impacts, efficiency, and sustainability. *Ann. N.Y. Acad. Sci.* 1328:18–28.
Wu, G., F.W. Bazer, W. Tuo, and S.P. Flynn. 1996. Unusual abundance of arginine and ornithine in porcine allantoic fluid. *Biol. Reprod.* 54:1261–1265.
Wu, G., F.W. Bazer, J.M. Wallace, and T.E. Spencer. 2006. Intrauterine growth retardation: Implications for the animal sciences. *J. Anim. Sci.* 84:2316–2337.
Wu, G., J. Fanzo, D.D. Miller, P. Pingali, M. Post, J.L. Steiner, and A.E. Thalacker-Mercer. 2014b. Production and supply of high-quality food protein for human consumption: Sustainability, challenges and innovations. *Ann. N.Y. Acad. Sci.* 1321:1–19.
Wu, G., and S.M. Morris, Jr. 1998. Arginine metabolism: Nitric oxide and beyond. *Biochem. J.* 336:1–17.
Wu, G., T.L. Ott, D.A. Knabe, and F.W. Bazer. 1999. Amino acid composition of the fetal pig. *J. Nutr.* 129:1031–1038.
Wu, Z.L., M.C. Satterfield, F.W. Bazer, and G. Wu. 2012. Regulation of brown adipose tissue development and white fat reduction by L-arginine. *Curr. Opin. Clin. Nutr. Metab. Care* 15:529–538.
Xi, P.B., Z.Y. Jiang, Z.L. Dai, X.L. Li, K. Yao, W. Jobgen, M.C. Satterfield, and G. Wu. 2010. Oxidation of energy substrates in rat brown adipose tissue. *FASEB J.* 24:554.5.
Xue, Y., S.F. Liao, K.W. Son, S.L. Greenwood, B.W. McBride, J.A. Boling, and J.C. Matthews. 2010. Metabolic acidosis in sheep alters expression of renal and skeletal muscle amino acid enzymes and transporters. *J. Anim. Sci.* 88:707–717.
Yang, Y.X., Z.L. Dai, and W.Y. Zhu. 2014. Important impacts of intestinal bacteria on utilization of dietary amino acids in pigs. *Amino Acids* 46:2489–2501.
Yen, J.T. 2000. Digestive system. In: *Biology of the Domestic Pig*. Edited by W.G. Pond and H.J. Mersmann. Cornell University Press, Ithaca, NY, pp. 390–453.
Yin, Y.L., R.L. Huang, H.Y. Zhong, T.J. Li, W.B. Souffrant, and C.F. de Lange. 2002. Evaluation of mobile nylon bag technique for determining apparent ileal digestibilities of protein and amino acids in growing pigs. *J. Anim. Sci.* 80:409–420.

# 2 Chemistry of Carbohydrates

Carbohydrates are widely distributed organic substances in nature (Sinnott 2013). Plants capture sunlight energy to convert water and $CO_2$ into glucose ($6CO_2 + 6H_2O + 2870\ kJ \rightarrow C_6H_{12}O_6 + 6O_2$). Glucose is then used to form starch and other complex carbohydrates. This transformation of energy from sunlight into carbohydrates is essential for food production, and the released oxygen molecule is vital for animal life (Demura and Ye 2010). In the ecosystem, animals consume plants as their major sources of monosaccharides, disaccharides, starch, and cellulose to produce meat (containing glycogen) and milk (the source of lactose). Lactose is the principal carbohydrate for preweaning mammals.

In the nineteenth century, chemists thought that carbohydrates were the hydrates of carbon and had the empirical formula of $C_m(H_2O)_n$, where $m$ is ≥3 and $m$ may be different from $n$. This was found to be true for the simple sugars known at that time and for their covalently linked dimers and polymers. In 1891, Emil Fisher established the structures of monosaccharides (glucose, fructose, mannose, and arabinose) and discovered that these compounds contain hydroxyl and carbonyl groups. Between 1920 and 1930, W. Norman Haworth discovered that a hexose primarily formed a six-membered ring (pyranose), but could also form a five-membered ring (furanose), with each ring structure containing an oxygen atom. Subsequently, it was observed that some substances (e.g., deoxyribose [$C_5H_{10}O_4$] and pyruvic acid [$C_3H_4O_3$]) with the chemical properties of carbohydrates could be derived from polyhydroxy aldehydes or ketones but they did not have the formula of $C_m(H_2O)_n$. To date, carbohydrates are defined as polyhydroxy aldehydes, polyhydroxy ketones, or their derivatives (Sinnott 2013). Examples of carbohydrates are hexoses, starch, cellulose, glycogen, chitins (in the exoskeletons of animals), and murein (in the bacterial cell wall), as well as sugar alcohols (alditols), deoxy sugars, aminosugars, and sugar phosphates (Robyt 1998). Therefore, on the basis of modern definitions, not all carbohydrates contain hydrogen and oxygen in the ratio of 2:1, and some of them even contain nitrogen, sulfur, or phosphorus.

Carbohydrates comprise up to 75% of the dry matter (DM) in plant-source feedstuffs and constitute the greatest proportion of the diets consumed by animals other than carnivores (Pond et al. 2005). In contrast, relatively small amounts of glucose and glycogen are present in the bodies of animals, where they fulfill essential functions as metabolic fuels and synthetic precursors. Complex carbohydrates also occur in the membranes of microbes, plants, and animals. In plants, water-insoluble carbohydrates, particularly cellulose and hemicellulose are responsible for their structural stability and mechanical firmness, whereas the water-soluble carbohydrates (e.g., glucose and starch) serve as energy reserves (Robyt 1998). This chapter highlights the chemistry of carbohydrates relevant to animal nutrition.

## GENERAL CLASSIFICATION OF CARBOHYDRATES

### OVERVIEW

In nutrition, carbohydrates are classified into five groups: (1) monosaccharides (also known as simple sugars); (2) disaccharides (containing 2 monosaccharide units); (3) oligosaccharides (containing 3–10 monosaccharide units); (4) polysaccharides (containing more than 10 monosaccharide units); and (5) conjugated carbohydrates. The latter substances are covalently bound to lipids or proteins to form glycolipids or glycoproteins, respectively. Polysaccharides are subdivided into homopolysaccharides (containing only one type of monosaccharide) and heteropolysaccharides (containing more than one type of monosaccharide). Upon hydrolysis by strong acids or specific enzymes,

**TABLE 2.1**
**Classification of Carbohydrates**

| Classification | Examples |
|---|---|
| Monosaccharides | |
| Trioses ($C_3H_6O_3$) | Glyceraldehyde and dihydroxyacetone |
| Tetroses ($C_4H_8O_4$) | Erythrose |
| Pentoses ($C_5H_{10}O_5$) | Aarabinase, xylose, xylulose, ribose, ribulose, and 5-deoxyribose |
| Hexoses ($C_6H_{12}O_6$) | Glucose, fructose, galactose, and mannose |
| Heptoses ($C_7H_{14}O_7$) | Sedoheptulose, mannoheptulose (in avocados), and L-*glycero*-D-*manno*-heptose |
| Disaccharides | Sucrose (D-α-glucose and D-α-fructose), lactose (milk sugar; D-α-glucose and D-α-galactose), maltose, isomaltose, cellobiose, α,α-trehalose, α,β-trehalose, and β,β-trehalose) |
| Oligosaccharides[a] | |
| Trisaccharides | Raffinose, kestose, maltotriose (three units of glucose), planteose, and melezitose (in sweet exudates of many trees and in insects), and panose (synthesized by microbes) |
| Tetrasaccharides | Stachyose and lychnose (1-α-galactosyl-raffinose) |
| Polysaccharides[b] | |
| Homoglycans[c] | Pentosans $(C_5H_8O_4)_n$, for example, arabans and xylans<br>Hexosans $(C_6H_{12}O_6)_n$, for example, starch, cellulose, mannans, levans, and glycogen |
| Heteroglycans[d] | Hemicelluloses, pectins, exudate gums, seaweed polysaccharides (algin, carrageenans, agar, aminopolysaccharides [e.g., chondroitin and hyaluronic acid], and sulfated polysaccharides [e.g., chondroitin sulfate]) |
| Conjugated carbohydrates | |
| Glycolipids[e] | Glyceroglycolipids and sphingolipids |
| Glycoproteins[f] | Mucins, immunoglobulins, and membrane-bound hormone receptors |

[a] Containing 2–10 units of monosaccharides.
[b] Containing more than 10 units of monosaccharides.
[c] Containing more than 10 units of a single type of monosaccharides.
[d] Containing more than 10 units of different types of monosaccharides.
[e] Monosaccharides or oligosaccharides covalently bound to a lipid moiety.
[f] Monosaccharides or oligosaccharides covalently bound to a protein moiety.

oligosaccharides and polysaccharides are broken down into monosaccharides. Carbohydrates of nutritional interest are summarized in Table 2.1.

### D- and L-Configuration of Carbohydrates

The smallest carbohydrate has three carbons. If a carbohydrate has at least one asymmetric carbon or chiral center, it will have D- and L-configurations according to the absolute configuration of glyceraldehyde, as defined by Emil Fischer in 1885. If there is more than one chiral center in the molecule, the arrangement at the highest number chiral center (e.g., the carbon attached to the –OH group in the monosaccharide shown here) is used to specify the configuration. The D- and L-structures are the mirror images of each other and therefore are called enantiomers. Most naturally occurring carbohydrates have only the D-configuration, but some of them have both the D- and L-structures. The absolute D- and L-configuration should not be confused with "*d*" (for *dextrorotatory*) if the compound rotates plane-polarized light to the right or "*l*" (for *levorotatory*) if the compound rotates plane-polarized light to the left. For example, although D-glucose rotates plane-polarized light to the right, D-fructose rotates plane-polarized light to the left.

CHO | HO–C–H | $CH_2OH$
L-glyceraldehyde

CHO | H–C–OH | $CH_2OH$
D-glyceraldehyde

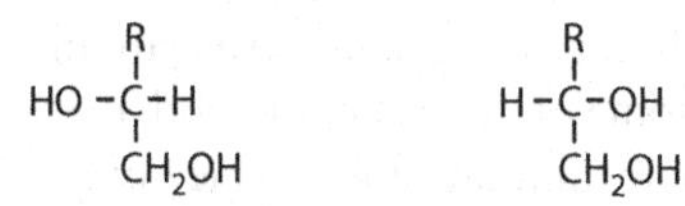

R | HO–C–H | $CH_2OH$
L-monosaccharide

R | H–C–OH | $CH_2OH$
D-monosaccharide

R = Remaining part of a monosaccharide; R ≠ H.

## Cyclic Hemiacetals (Aldoses) and Hemiketals (Ketoses)

Carbohydrates contain important functional groups: aldehyde (–CHO), hydroxyl (–OH), and carbonyl (–C=O). They exist mainly as cyclic hemiacetal, acetal, ketal, or hemiketal compounds. A hemiacetal (*hemi* meaning "half" in Greek) contains a hydroxyl group (–OH) and an alkoxyl group ($-OCH_3$). In an acetal, two alkoxyl groups ($-OCH_3$) are bonded to the same carbon atom. When an aldehyde (e.g., acetaldehyde) reacts with methanol in the presence of HCl, a hemiacetal (e.g., 1-methoxy-1-ethanol), an acetal (1,1-dimethoxy-ethane), and water are produced. However, when the carbonyl compound is a ketone instead of an aldehyde, the products are a hemiketal, a ketal, and water. Thus, hemiacetals and hemiketals are compounds that are derived from aldehydes and ketones, respectively (Ege 1984).

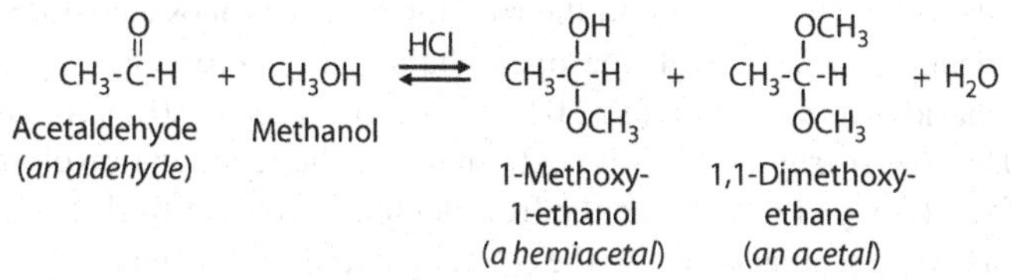

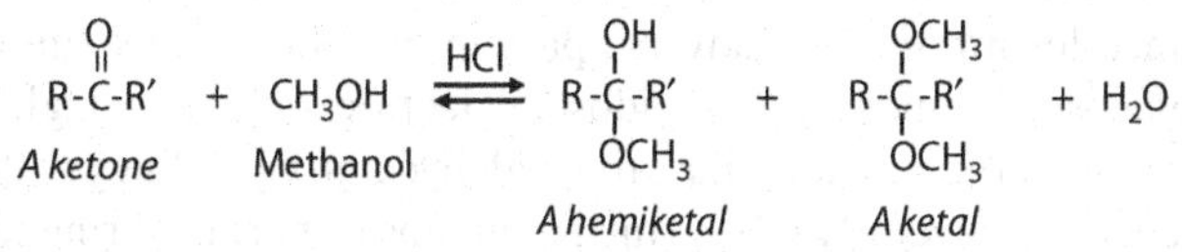

$$CH_3\text{-}\overset{O}{\overset{\|}{C}}\text{-}H + CH_3OH \overset{HCl}{\rightleftharpoons} CH_3\text{-}C(OH)(OCH_3)\text{-}H + CH_3\text{-}C(OCH_3)(OCH_3)\text{-}H + H_2O$$

Acetaldehyde (*an aldehyde*) + Methanol ⇌ 1-Methoxy-1-ethanol (*a hemiacetal*) + 1,1-Dimethoxy-ethane (*an acetal*) + $H_2O$

$$R\text{-}\overset{O}{\overset{\|}{C}}\text{-}R' + CH_3OH \overset{HCl}{\rightleftharpoons} R\text{-}C(OH)(OCH_3)\text{-}R' + R\text{-}C(OCH_3)(OCH_3)\text{-}R' + H_2O$$

*A ketone* + Methanol ⇌ *A hemiketal* + *A ketal* + $H_2O$

(R may be equal to R′. However, R or R′ cannot be a hydrogen atom.)

These concepts of hemiacetals and hemiketals can be explained with aldose and ketose sugars (Bruice 2011). In an aldose sugar (e.g., D-glucose), a stable cyclic hemiacetal is formed by an attack from the –OH group bonded to the fifth carbon (C-5) on the aldehyde carbon (C-1), leading to intramolecular cyclization (pyranose with a 6-member ring). The cyclic form of D-glucose is called D-glucopyranose. In a ketose sugar (e.g., D-fructose), a stable cyclic hemiketal is formed by an attack from the –OH group bonded to the sixth carbon (C-6) on the ketone carbon (C-2), resulting in intramolecular cyclization (pyranose with a 6-member ring). However, when the ketone carbon of D-fructose is attacked by the –OH group bonded to the fifth carbon (C-5), a stable cyclic furanose (a 5-member ring) is generated. Thus, the cyclic form of D-fructose is called either D-fructopyranose or D-fructofuranose. In an aqueous solution, the ratio of fructopyranose to fructofuranose is 3:1. Note that aldoses and ketoses undergo these transformations spontaneously without enzyme catalysis.

## MONOSACCHARIDES

### Definition

Monosaccharides are divided into aldoses (also known as polyhydroxy aldehydes) and ketoses (also known as polyhydroxy ketones) according to whether they contain an aldehyde or ketone group (Sinnott 2013). In organisms, most monosaccharides exist only in the D-configuration (e.g., D-glucose, D-fructose, and D-ribose), but some of them occur in both the D- and L-configurations (e.g., lactate, arabinose, and galactose). Of note, animal cells produce only L-lactate (a 3-carbon metabolite) from D-glucose and other substrates. In contrast, bacteria synthesize both D-lactate and L-lactate, depending on the cell type. L-Arabinose and L-galactose are constituents in plants. A monosaccharide with a free aldehyde group or a free ketone group is a reducing sugar which reduces another compound, with itself being oxidized, such that the carbonyl carbon of the reducing sugar is converted into a carboxyl group. Ketoses (e.g., D-fructose) are not reducing sugars unless they are isomerized to their aldose form (e.g., the isomerization of D-fructose to D-glucose under alkaline conditions). All monosaccharides are highly soluble in water. Monosaccharides commonly present in plant cell walls are hexoses (D-glucose, D-galactose, and D-mannose), pentoses (L-arabinose and L-xylose), 6-deoxyhexoses (L-rhamnose and L-fucose), and uronic acids (glucuronic and galacturonic or their 4-*o*-methyl ethers).

### Chemical Representation of Monosaccharide Structures

#### Open-Chain Form

A monosaccharide can be present in a linear (open-chain) form, a Haworth projection, or a chair form (Figure 2.1). The open-chain form and the ring forms of a monosaccharide can be spontaneously interconverted in water. Although the open-chain form represents only small amounts of nearly all monosaccharides in a solution (e.g., 0.002% for D-glucose, 0.02% for D-galactose, 0.05% for D-ribose, and 0.8% for D-fructose) (Table 2.2), many of the reactions involving C-1 take place in the open-chain form (Robyt 1998). Since the free aldehyde group of D-glucose in the open-chain form is chemically active (e.g., reactive with the $\varepsilon$-$NH_2$ group of lysine, either free or protein-bound to form a covalent bond), the minute concentration of the monosaccharide in this configuration is of physiological importance for minimizing adverse protein glycation. Thus, among all the aldohexoses (allose, altrose, glucose, mannose, gulose, idose, galactose, and talose), glucose has the lowest proportion of straight-chain structure and, thus, free aldehyde groups (Angyal 1984). This may be a major reason why glucose was favored as the principal monosaccharide during the evolution of both plants and animals (Brosnan 2005).

#### Cyclic Hemiacetal or Hemiketal Form

When a hemiacetal or hemiketal ring is formed spontaneously by intramolecular cyclization in a solution, anomerization occurs at C-1 through acid and base catalysis, forming an $\alpha$- or $\beta$-isomer (called an anomer). In the $\alpha$-isomer, the –OH group at C-1 will be facing down in a six- or five-membered ring. For the $\beta$-isomer, the –OH group at C-1 will be facing up in the six-membered ring. At equilibrium in water, the $\beta$-isomer is more abundant than the $\alpha$-isomer for D-glucose, D-fructose, D-galactose, D-xylose, or D-ribose, but the opposite is true for D-mannose and D-rhamnose (Table 2.2). Of note, the equilibrium of hexoses between the $\alpha$- and $\beta$-pyranose forms in water is not affected by changes in temperature of the solution, but the proportion of furanose forms is increased with the increasing temperature (Angyal 1984). A hemiacetal is in chemical equilibrium with the open-chain aldehyde, and a hemiketal is in chemical equilibrium with the open-chain ketone. A monosaccharide with a hemiacetal or a free aldehyde is a reducing sugar.

According to the Haworth projection, a monosaccharide can exist as a six-membered ring (pyranose) or a five-membered ring (furanose) structure (Figure 2.2). Monosaccharides exist primarily

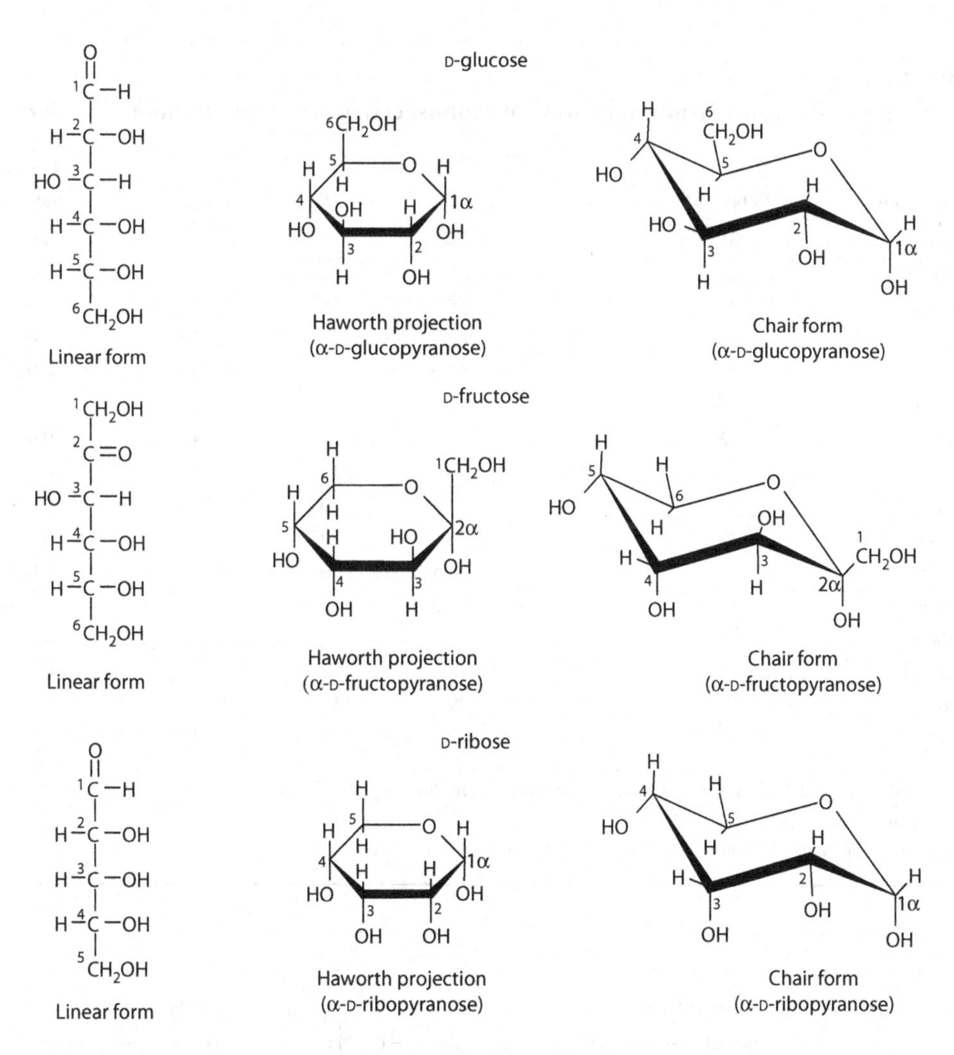


**FIGURE 2.1** Chemical structure of a monosaccharide in a linear (open-chain) form, a Haworth projection, or a chair form. The open-chain form represents only small amounts of monosaccharides compared with the ring forms, but participates in many of the reactions involving C-1. When a hemiacetal or hemiketal ring is formed, anomerization (also known as mutarotation) occurs at C-1 to form an α- or β-isomer (called an anomer). In the α-isomer, the –OH group at C-1 is facing down in the six-membered ring. In the β-isomer, the –OH group at C-1 is facing up in the six-membered ring.

in the pyranose form, rather than the furanose form (Table 2.2). For example, D-fructose (which has a ketone group) in solution forms a six-membered cyclic hemiketal called D-fructopyranose, with its hydroxyl group on the C-6 carbon attacking the C-2 ketone carbon to form an oxygen-linked bridge. When the hydroxyl group on the C-5 carbon of the open-chain D-fructose attacks its C-2 ketone carbon, D-fructofuranose with a five-membered ring is formed. In contrast to D-fructose, D-glucose (which has an aldehyde group) in solution forms a six-membered cyclic hemiacetal called D-glucopyranose, when its hydroxyl group on the C-5 carbon attacks the C-1 aldehyde carbon to form an oxygen-linked bridge. In the conversion of the open-chain D-glucose into D-glucofuranose with a five-membered ring, the hydroxyl group on its C-4 carbon attacks the C-1 aldehyde carbon. For both D-fructose and D-glucose, the pyranose form is thermodynamically more stable than the furanose form. Thus, in an aqueous solution, D-glucopyranose (or D-fructopyranose) is much more abundant than D-glucofuranose (or D-fructofuranose) (Table 2.2).

**TABLE 2.2**
**Distributions of Various Structural Forms of Monosaccharides at Equilibrium in Water[a]**

| | | Pyranose Form | | Furanose Form | | |
|---|---|---|---|---|---|---|
| **Carbohydrate** | **Temp (°C)** | α | β | α | β | **Open-Chain Form** |
| D-Allose | 31 | 14 | 77.5 | 3.5 | 5 | 0.01 |
| D-Arabinose | 31 | 60 | 35.5 | 2.5 | 2 | 0.03 |
| D-Fructose | 31 | 2.5 | 65 | 6.5 | 25 | 0.8 |
| D-Galactose | 31 | 30 | 64 | 2.5 | 3.5 | 0.02 |
| D-Glucose | 31 | 38 | 62 | 0.5 | 0.5 | 0.002 |
| Glycero-D-Gal | 22 | 28 | 67 | 2 | 3 | 0.01 |
| Glycero-L-Gal | 22 | 36 | 57 | 3 | 4 | 0.02 |
| D-Idose | 31 | 38.5 | 36 | 11.5 | 14 | 0.2 |
| D-Mannose | 44 | 65.5 | 34.5 | 0.6 | 0.3 | 0.005 |
| D-Psicose | 27 | 22 | 24 | 39 | 15 | 0.3 |
| D-Rhamnose | 44 | 65.5 | 34.5 | 0.6 | 0.3 | 0.005 |
| D-Ribose | 31 | 21.5 | 58.5 | 6.5 | 13.5 | 0.05 |
| D-Sorbose | 31 | 93 | 2 | 4 | 1 | 0.25 |
| D-Tagatose | 31 | 71 | 18 | 2.5 | 7.5 | 0.3 |
| D-Talose | 22 | 42 | 29 | 16 | 13 | 0.03 |
| D-Xylose | 31 | 36.5 | 63 | 0.3 | 0.3 | 0.002 |

*Source:* Adapted from Angyal, S.J. 1984. *Adv. Carbohydr. Chem. Biochem.* 42:15–68.
Gal, galactose; Temp, temperature.
[a] The distribution values of monosaccharides are expressed as % (mol/mol).

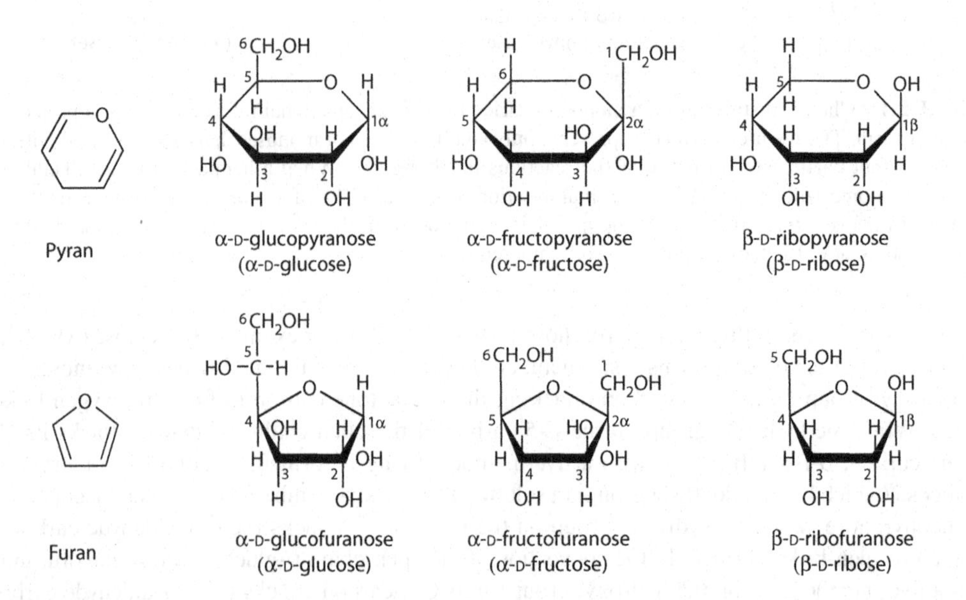


**FIGURE 2.2** The Haworth projection of a monosaccharide as a six-membered ring (pyranose) or a five-membered ring (furanose) structure. For a monosaccharide, the pyranose form is more stable than the furanose form. Examples are α-D-glucose, α-D-fructose, and β-D-ribose.

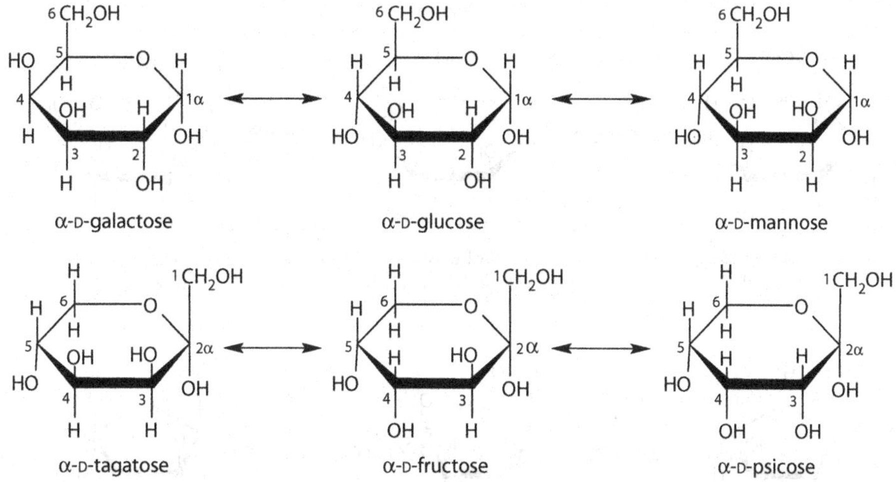

α-D-galactose ⟷ α-D-glucose ⟷ α-D-mannose

α-D-tagatose ⟷ α-D-fructose ⟷ α-D-psicose

**FIGURE 2.3** Epimerization of monosaccharides in solution. In carbohydrates, this reaction refers to the formation of isomers at a carbon other than C-1, resulting in the generation of a different substance. Epimerization can be either spontaneous (generally a very slow process) or catalyzed by enzymes (epimerases). For example, α-D-galactose and α-D-mannose are formed from α-D-glucose in animal and plant cells.

Epimerization of monosaccharides refers to the formation of stereoisomers at a carbon other than C-1 and, therefore, different substances (Figure 2.3). For example, D-mannose and D-galactose are formed from the epimerization of D-glucose at carbon 2 and carbon 4, respectively, and these three sugars are epimers. Epimerization can be spontaneous (generally a slow process) or catalyzed by enzymes (epimerases) and bases (e.g., in alkaline solution). Epimerization differs from mutarotation (generally a fast process) not only in the rates of spontaneous reactions but also in the chemical mechanisms. Specifically, epimerization is the formation of stereoisomers (called epimers) at one chiral center of a monosaccharide. In contrast, mutarotation involves the formation of a hemiacetal or hemiketal ring and anomers from the intramolecular cyclization of a monosaccharide and a subsequent change in its specific rotation (Figure 2.4).

## Glucose and Fructose in Plants

Glucose and fructose have different chemical structures but the same molecular formula of $C_6(H_2O)_6$ (Robyt 1998). Glucose and fructose are usually the two most abundant monosaccharides in plants, with the amount of glucose generally being greater than that of fructose. Glucose is the basic unit of starch, which is usually the main storage form of monosaccharides in plants. Of note, fructose is the only widely spread ketohexose of nutritional and physiological significance in nature, and it occurs in many plants (particularly green plants), honey, trees, vine fruits, flowers, berries, tubers, and most root vegetables (Rumessen 1992). In addition, fructose is a component of the sweet disaccharide (sucrose) and polysaccharides called fructosans or fructans in plants.

Total amounts of glucose or fructose differ markedly among plants and with their developmental stage (Table 2.3). Forage plants contain 1%–3% glucose plus fructose on DM basis. In contrast, green plants contain much smaller amounts of free hexoses (glucose and fructose) than starch, because hexoses are linked to form polysaccharides (starch, cellulose, and hemicellulose) that are quantitatively the most important constituents of plant-source feeds (McDonald et al. 2011).

## Glucose and Fructose in Animals

α-D-Glucose is the main product of starch digestion in the gastrointestinal tract of nonruminants, and is produced from glucogenic substrates in both ruminants and nonruminants. Glucose is the predominant

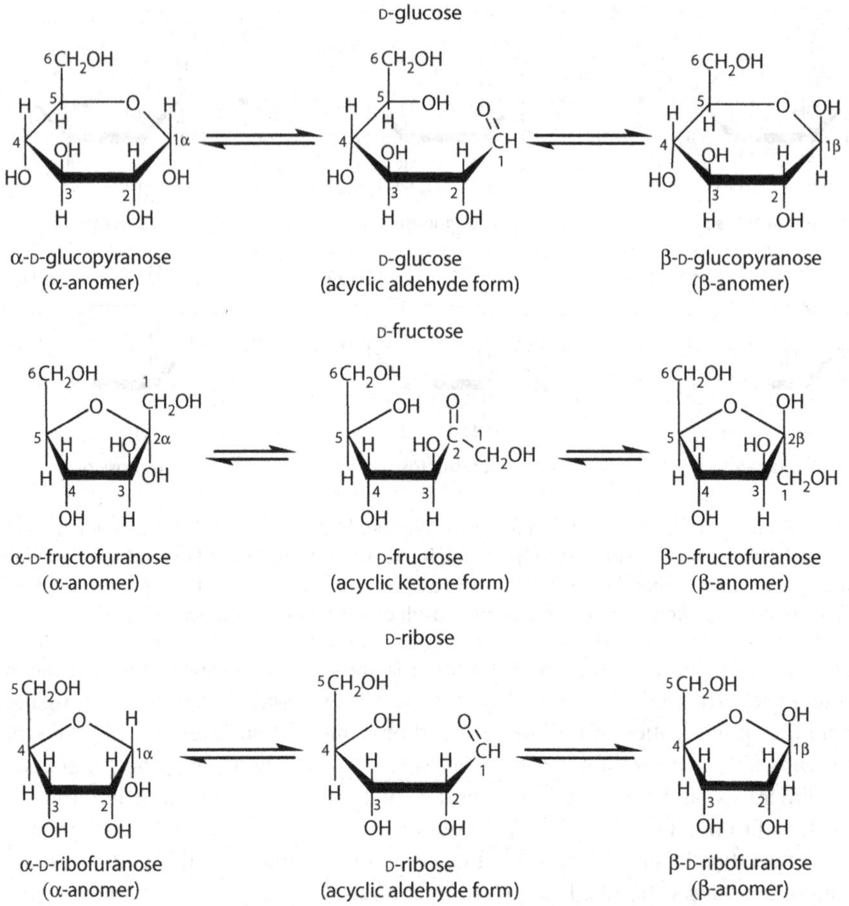

D-glucose

α-D-glucopyranose (α-anomer) ⇌ D-glucose (acyclic aldehyde form) ⇌ β-D-glucopyranose (β-anomer)

D-fructose

α-D-fructofuranose (α-anomer) ⇌ D-fructose (acyclic ketone form) ⇌ β-D-fructofuranose (β-anomer)

D-ribose

α-D-ribofuranose (α-anomer) ⇌ D-ribose (acyclic aldehyde form) ⇌ β-D-ribofuranose (β-anomer)

**FIGURE 2.4** Mutarotation of monosaccharides (e.g., D-glucose, D-fructose, and D-ribose) in a solution. Intramolecular cyclization of an open-chain monosaccharide results in the generation of a ring structure and an α- or β-anomer. This reaction spontaneously proceeds rapidly at pH 7.0 and can also be catalyzed by mutarotase. The α- or β-anomers are at chemical equilibrium in the solution. In the case of D-glucose, the aldehyde group (–CHO) reacts with the hydroxyl group (alcohol) at C-5 to form a hemiacetal at C-1. In the case of D-fructose, the ketone group (–C=O) reacts with the hydroxyl group (alcohol) at C-5 to form a hemiketal. The hydroxyl group at the hemiacetal or hemiketal carbon is most reactive in monosaccharides.

hexose in the blood of healthy gestating mammals and postnatal animals, which ranges from 2 to 15 mM, depending on the species, developmental stage, and nutritional state (Bergman 1983b). When dietary intake of fructose and its disaccharides or polymers is low or negligible, fructose is virtually absent from the plasma of postnatal mammals, birds, or fish. Likewise, D-fructose is present only as a minor sugar in fetal fluids of humans (e.g., 0.05–0.08 mM; Trindade et al. 2011), dogs, cats, guinea pigs, rabbits, rats, and ferrets (Wang et al. 2016). In contrast, large amounts of fructose are present in the semen of males (Akhter et al. 2014; Baronos 1971) and in the fetal fluids (including fetal blood) of ungulates (such as cattle, sheep, and pigs) and whales (Table 2.4). For example, the concentrations of fructose in the semen of cattle and sheep are 29 and 14 mM, respectively, in comparison with 3 mM glucose. In sheep, the concentration of fructose (up to 32 mM) is 30 times that of glucose in the allantoic fluid during pregnancy (Kim et al. 2012). Different distributions of glucose and fructose in the fluids of livestock species and other mammals likely have important physiological significance.

Wang et al. (2013) reported that the free aldehyde group of glucose (22.6 mM) in the open-chain form nonenzymatically glycated serum albumin (1.5 mM, close to the physiological concentration

**TABLE 2.3**
**Composition of Monosaccharides, Disaccharides, Oligosaccharides, and Starch in Plant-Source Feedstuffs**

| Feedstuffs | DM | Glucose | Fructose | Sucrose | Raffinose | Stachyose | Verbascose | Starch | β-Glucan |
|---|---|---|---|---|---|---|---|---|---|
| | | | | % (As-Fed Basis) | | | | | |
| Barley | 89.0 | 0.15 | 0.10 | 2.0 | 0.23 | 0.002 | – | 60.5 | 5.0 |
| Corn grain | 88.3 | 0.35 | 0.25 | 1.4 | 0.20 | 0.01 | 0.01 | 63.7 | – |
| Oats | 89.0 | 0.05 | 0.09 | 0.64 | 0.19 | 0.03 | – | 55.8 | 5.4 |
| Peas (field) | 88.1 | – | – | 0.19 | 0.04 | 0.23 | 0.32 | 43.5 | – |
| Rice (milled) | 90.0 | 0.04 | 0.03 | 0.14 | 0.02 | – | – | 73.5 | 0.11 |
| Rye | 88.0 | 0.08 | 0.10 | 1.90 | 0.40 | 0.002 | – | 58.7 | 2.4 |
| SBM (48% CP) | 90.0 | – | – | 4.30 | 3.78 | 7.33 | 0.00 | 1.89 | – |
| SBM (45% CP) | 93.9 | – | – | 7.10 | 0.77 | 4.88 | 0.00 | 1.89 | – |
| Sorghum | 89.0 | 0.09 | 0.09 | 0.85 | 0.11 | – | – | 67.1 | 1.0 |
| SPC | 92.6 | – | – | 0.67 | 0.46 | 0.91 | 0.00 | 1.89 | – |
| Wheat | 89.0 | 0.03 | 0.03 | 0.79 | 0.62 | 0.01 | – | 58.6 | 1.4 |

*Source:* Adapted from Henry, R.J. and H.S. Saini. 1989. *Cereal Chem.* 66:362–365; Koehler, P. and H. Wieser. 2013. *Handbook of Sourdough Biotechnology*. Edited by M. Gobbetti and M. Gänzle. Springer, New York, pp. 11–45; Shelton, D.R. and W.J. Lee. 2000. *Handbook of Cereal Science and Technology*. Edited by K. Kulp and J.G. Ponte, Jr. Marcell Dekker, New York, pp. 385–414; National Research Council (NRC). 2012. *Nutrient Requirements of Swine*. National Academy Press, Washington, DC.

SBM (48% CP), soybean meal (47.7% crude protein, dehulled); SBM (45% CP), soybean meal (44.6% crude protein, expelled); SPC, soy protein concentrate.

in blood) via the covalent bond, as occurs in diabetic patients. Interestingly, fructose (a ketose, 22.6 mM) did not react with the protein. Much of the evidence shows that nonenzymatic glycation, which is driven by high glucose concentrations, can result in the abnormal structure and function of proteins (Cao et al. 2015). Thus, the presence of much larger amounts of fructose than glucose in fetal fluid and blood helps to minimize protein glycation in the conceptus. This protective mechanism would be of physiological importance for embryonic and fetal survival and growth. Thus, D-fructose has been added to the culture medium of embryos (Barceló-Fimbres and Seidel 2008).

## Other Monosaccharides in Plants and Animals

The structures of select monosaccharides in nature, trioses, tetroses, pentoses, and hexoses (e.g., galactose), are illustrated in Figures 2.5 and 2.6. They are all present in plants for the synthesis of polysaccharides. Some of these monosaccharides (the trioses, D-sorbitol, and myoinositol) also occur in animals. Of particular note, D-sorbitol (2.2 mM) is much more abundant than D-fructose or D-glucose in horse semen, whereas inositol (a metabolite of D-glucose) has a concentration of 29 mM in boar semen (Table 2.5) and 50 mM in the epididymal luminal fluid of male rats (Hinton et al. 1980). Ribose is present in all living cells as a component of ribonucleic acid, certain vitamins, and energy-rich compounds (e.g., ADP and ATP). Xylose and arabinose (aldopentoses), which contains an aldehyde (–CHO) functional group, occur in a polymerized form in xylans (xylose), arabinans (arabinose), and hemicellulose. Furthermore, both plants and animals contain heptoses with seven carbon atoms.

## Simple Aminosugars as Monosaccharides in Plants and Animals

Some monosaccharides (2-amino-2-deoxysugar) are amidated by the amino group from glucosamine-6-phosphate, which is formed from L-glutamine and D-fructose-6-phosphate. Examples

**TABLE 2.4**
**Concentrations of D-Glucose and D-Fructose in the Semen of Males and in Fetal Blood and Fluids[a]**

| | Volume (mL) | D-Glucose (mM) | D-Fructose (mM) |
|---|---|---|---|
| | **Cattle** | | |
| Semen | 5.0 | 3.0 | 29 |
| Fetal blood (Day 260) | 13% of FW | 1.5 | 3.5 |
| Fetal allantoic fluid (Day 100) | 480 | 1.7 | 18 |
| Fetal amniotic fluid (Day 100) | 1025 | 2.2 | 3.7 |
| | **Pigs** | | |
| Semen | 300 | 0.17 | 0.72 |
| Fetal blood (Day 103) | 11% of FW | 2.1 | 4.6 |
| Fetal allantoic fluid (Day 30) | 200 | 1.8 | 6.5 |
| Fetal amniotic fluid (Day 30) | 1.5 | 1.7 | 4.2 |
| | **Sheep** | | |
| Semen | 1.5 | 3.0 | 14 |
| Fetal blood (Day 76) | 13% of FW | 1.1 | 5.6 |
| Fetal allantoic fluid (Day 80) | 115 | 1.1 | 32 |
| Fetal amniotic fluid (Day 80) | 432 | 0.56 | 9.0 |
| | **Human** | | |
| Semen | 3.4 | 5.7 | 15 |
| Fetal blood (full term) | 11% of FW | 3.6 | 0.08 |

*Source:* Adapted from Bacon, J.S.D. and D.J. Bell. 1948. *Biochem. J.* 42:397–405; Baronos, S. 1971. *J. Reprod. Fertil.* 24:303–305; Bazer, F.W. et al. 1988. *J. Reprod. Fertil.* 84:37–42; Bazer, F.W. et al. 2012. *J. Anim. Sci.* 90:159–170; Bearden, H.J. and J.W. Fuquay. 1980. *Applied Animal Reproduction.* Reston Publishing Company, Reston, Virginia; Britton, H.G. 1962. *Biochem.* J. 85:402–407; Hitchcock, M.W.S. 1949. *J. Physiol.* 108:117–126; Li, N. et al. 2005. *Biol. Reprod.* 73:139–148; Schirren, C. 1963. *J. Reprod. Fertil.* 5:347–358; Trindade, C.E. et al. 2011. *Early Hum. Dev.* 87:193–197.

FW, fetal body weight.

[a] The day of gestation is indicated in parentheses. The numbers of spermatozoa in 1 mL of semen from cattle, pigs, sheep and humans are 1.2, 0.20, 2.0 and 0.10 billion, respectively. Trace amounts of fructose are present in maternal blood or adult-male blood.

of simple aminosugars are shown in Figure 2.7. Among over 60 aminosugars present in nature, *N*-acetyl-D-glucosamine (the main component of chitin) is the most abundant (Denzel and Antebi 2015). Glucosamine-6-phosphate, which is synthesized from L-glutamine and fructose-6-phosphate, is an important aminosugar in the metabolism and physiology of both plants and animals. Other significant aminosugars include *N*-acetyl-glucosamine, sialic acid, and aminoglycosides. Some aminoglycosides are also antimicrobial compounds.

## DISACCHARIDES

### Definition

Disaccharides consist of two units of monosaccharides, which link together via a glycosidic bond and the elimination of one water molecule: $2C_6H_{12}O_6 \rightarrow C_{12}H_{22}O_{11} + H_2O$. The linkage may involve: (1) the α- or β-hydroxyl group at C-1 of the hemiacetal or at C-2 of the hemiketal; and (2) the α-hydroxyl group in C-2, C-3, C-4, or C-6 of a monosaccharide. In forming

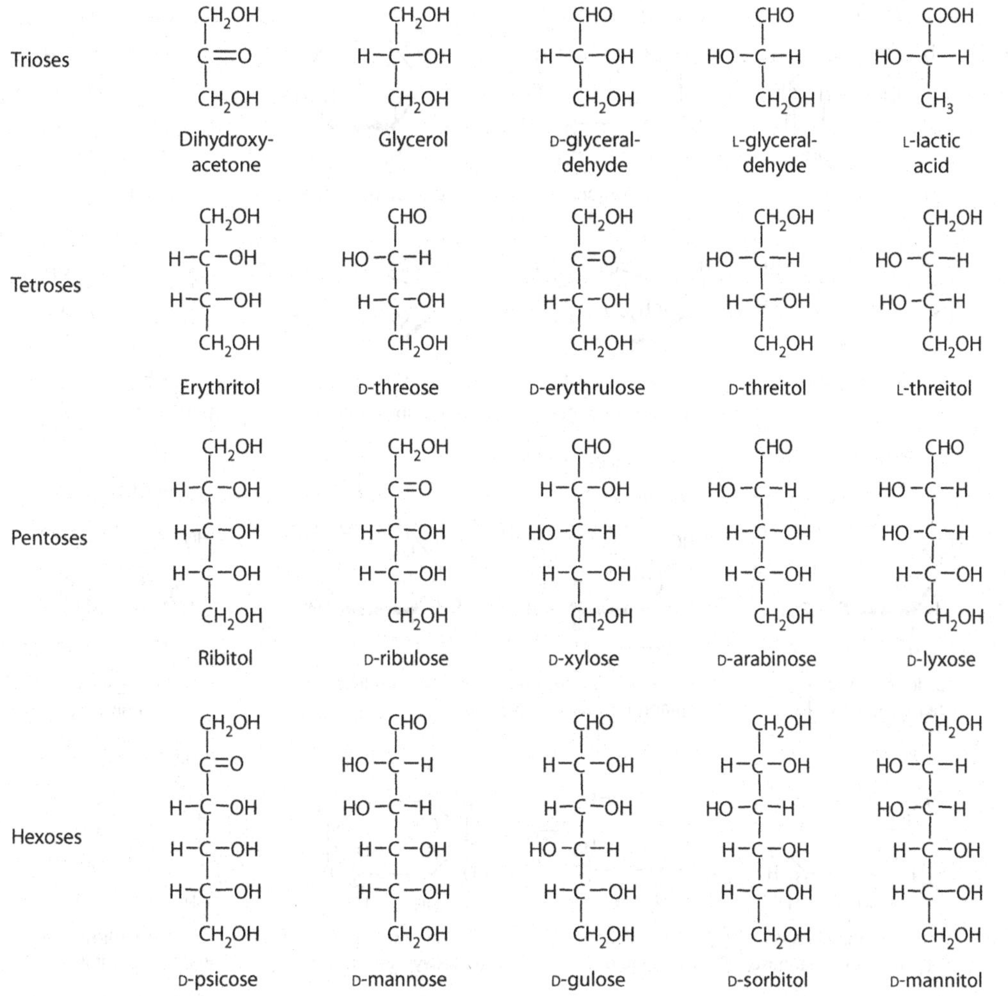

| | | | | | |
|---|---|---|---|---|---|
| Trioses | $CH_2OH$<br>C=O<br>$CH_2OH$<br>Dihydroxy-acetone | $CH_2OH$<br>H–C–OH<br>$CH_2OH$<br>Glycerol | CHO<br>H–C–OH<br>$CH_2OH$<br>D-glyceral-dehyde | CHO<br>HO–C–H<br>$CH_2OH$<br>L-glyceral-dehyde | COOH<br>HO–C–H<br>$CH_3$<br>L-lactic acid |
| Tetroses | $CH_2OH$<br>H–C–OH<br>H–C–OH<br>$CH_2OH$<br>Erythritol | CHO<br>HO–C–H<br>H–C–OH<br>$CH_2OH$<br>D-threose | $CH_2OH$<br>C=O<br>H–C–OH<br>$CH_2OH$<br>D-erythrulose | $CH_2OH$<br>HO–C–H<br>H–C–OH<br>$CH_2OH$<br>D-threitol | $CH_2OH$<br>HO–C–H<br>HO–C–H<br>$CH_2OH$<br>L-threitol |
| Pentoses | $CH_2OH$<br>H–C–OH<br>H–C–OH<br>H–C–OH<br>$CH_2OH$<br>Ribitol | $CH_2OH$<br>C=O<br>H–C–OH<br>H–C–OH<br>$CH_2OH$<br>D-ribulose | CHO<br>H–C–OH<br>HO–C–H<br>H–C–OH<br>$CH_2OH$<br>D-xylose | CHO<br>HO–C–H<br>H–C–OH<br>H–C–OH<br>$CH_2OH$<br>D-arabinose | CHO<br>HO–C–H<br>HO–C–H<br>H–C–OH<br>$CH_2OH$<br>D-lyxose |
| Hexoses | $CH_2OH$<br>C=O<br>H–C–OH<br>H–C–OH<br>H–C–OH<br>$CH_2OH$<br>D-psicose | CHO<br>HO–C–H<br>HO–C–H<br>H–C–OH<br>H–C–OH<br>$CH_2OH$<br>D-mannose | CHO<br>H–C–OH<br>H–C–OH<br>HO–C–H<br>H–C–OH<br>$CH_2OH$<br>D-gulose | $CH_2OH$<br>H–C–OH<br>HO–C–H<br>H–C–OH<br>H–C–OH<br>$CH_2OH$<br>D-sorbitol | $CH_2OH$<br>HO–C–H<br>HO–C–H<br>H–C–OH<br>H–C–OH<br>$CH_2OH$<br>D-mannitol |

**FIGURE 2.5** Structures of select trioses, tetroses, pentoses, and hexoses in nature. All of these monosaccharides are present in plants, but the trioses and D-sorbitol also occur in animals as glucose metabolites. Compounds that have a plane of symmetry in their structure (e.g., erythritol, ribitol, and galactitol) or have no asymmetric carbon (e.g., dihydroxyacetone, glycerol, and pyruvate) are optically inactive and do not have D- or L-configurations.

a disaccharide from two monosaccharides, when the C1 of the first monosaccharide is α-D-glucose, the resulting glycosidic bond has a prefix of glucosyl "α-1." The word "glucosyl" is often omitted in writing. For example, the C1 of α-D-glucose (the first monosaccharide) and the C2 of β-D-fructose (the second monosaccharide) form an α-1,2 glycosidic linkage in the resulting disaccharide (sucrose).

A glycoside is usually a nonreducing carbohydrate, but a few disaccharides (e.g., cellobiose, melibiose, and turanose) still have reducing abilities. Most naturally occurring disaccharides are found in plants, but lactose is synthesized in the mammary glands of lactating mammals (Rezaei et al. 2016). The structures of select disaccharides are shown in Figure 2.8. Chemically, a glucosyl β-1,4 linkage is very different from a galactosyl β-1,4 linkage, and holds important nutritional implications. For example, the small intestine of mammals produces lactase to hydrolyze lactose (a disaccharide with galactosyl β-1,4 linkage), but its mucosal cells do not express enzymes to break down glucosyl β-1,4-linked disaccharides. Likewise, all animal cells do not metabolize disaccharides

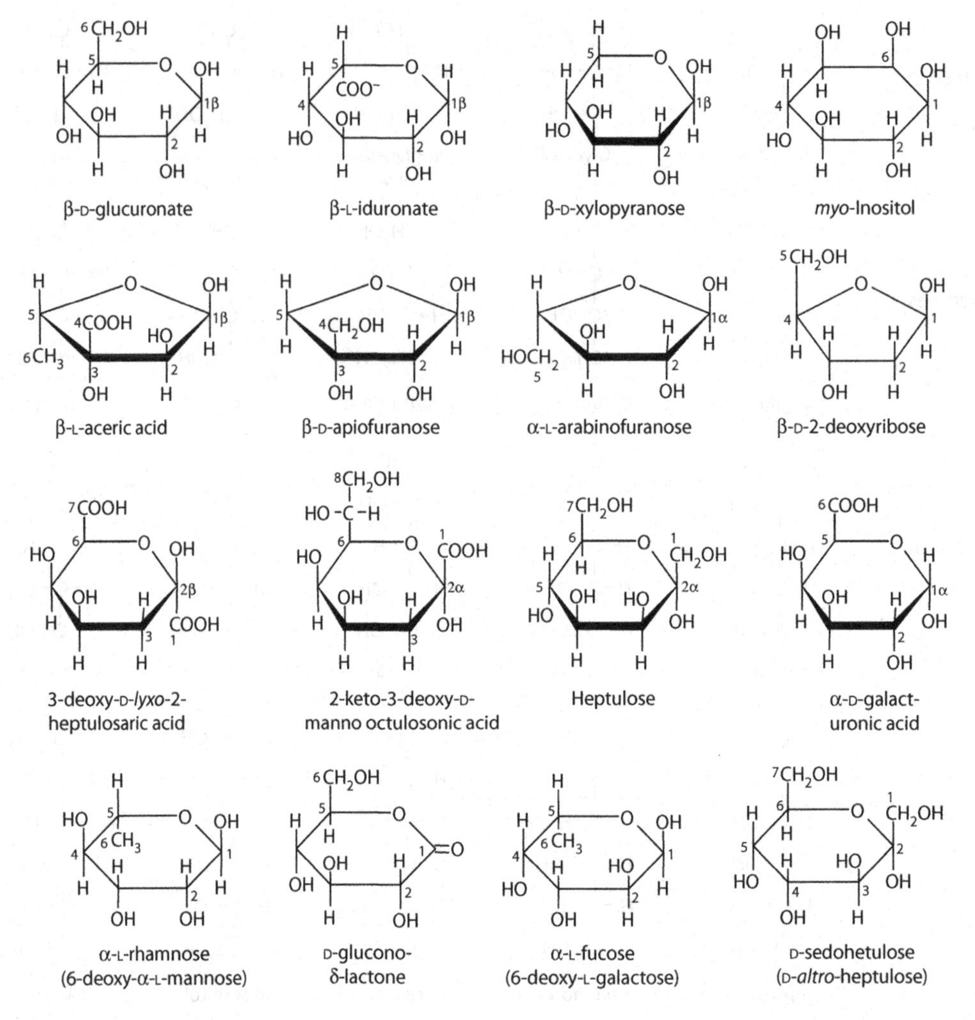


**FIGURE 2.6** Haworth structures of select hexoses (6-carbon molecules) and heptoses (7-carbon molecules) in nature. All of these monosaccharides are present in plants. Myoinositol also occurs in animals and microbes as a glucose metabolite.

**TABLE 2.5**
**Concentrations of D-Sorbitol, Inositol, Glycerylphosphorylcholine (GPC), and Citric Acid in Livestock Semen**

| Animal | D-Sorbitol (mM) | Inositol (mM) | GPC (mM) | Citric Acid (mM) |
|---|---|---|---|---|
| Cattle | 4.1 | 2.0 | 14 | 38 |
| Sheep | 4.0 | 0.67 | 64 | 7.3 |
| Pig | 0.66 | 29 | 6.8 | 6.8 |
| Horse | 2.2 | 1.7 | 2.7 | 1.4 |

*Source:* Adapted from Bearden, H.J. and J.W. Fuquay. 1980. *Applied Animal Reproduction*. Reston Publishing Company, Reston, Virginia.

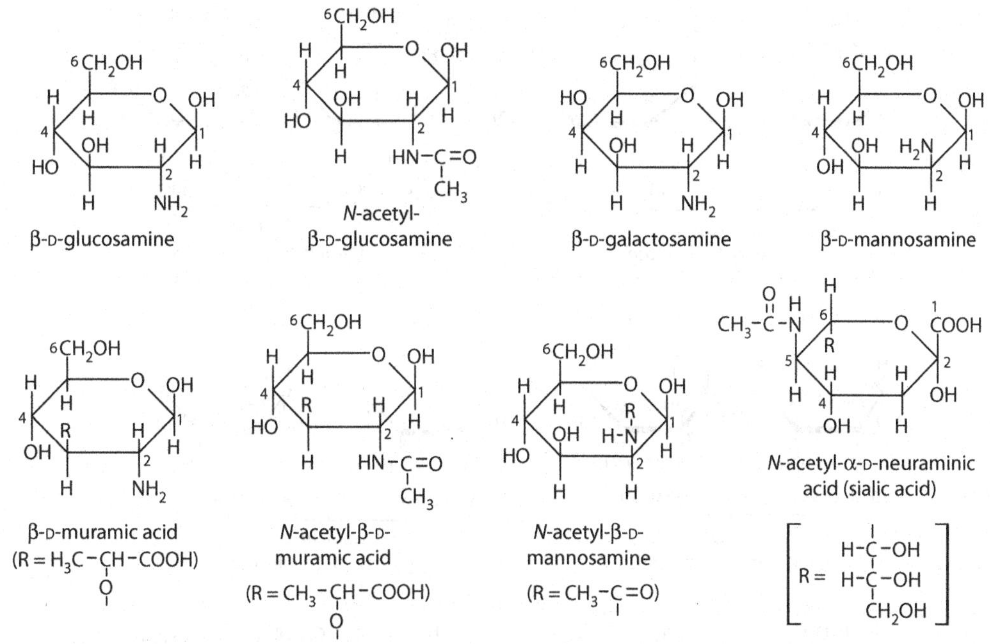

β-D-glucosamine

N-acetyl-β-D-glucosamine

β-D-galactosamine

β-D-mannosamine

β-D-muramic acid ($R = H_3C-CH(O-)-COOH$)

N-acetyl-β-D-muramic acid ($R = CH_3-CH(O-)-COOH$)

N-acetyl-β-D-mannosamine ($R = CH_3-C(=O)-$)

N-acetyl-α-D-neuraminic acid (sialic acid) [$R = H-C-OH$, $H-C-OH$, $CH_2OH$]

**FIGURE 2.7** Structures of select simple and complex aminosugars in nature. All of these aminosugars are present in plants. Sialic acids, as well as α-anomers of D-glucosamine and *N*-acetyl-D-glucosamine, also occur in animals and microbes as metabolites of fructose-6-phosphate and L-glutamine.

with glucosyl β-1,4 linkages. In contrast, bacteria in the digestive tract of animals possess enzymes to degrade disaccharides with α-1,4 or β-1,4 linkages.

## Cellobiose

Cellobiose (the fundamental repeating unit of cellulose) is a reducing sugar and consists of two β-D-glucose molecules linked by the β-1,4 glycosidic bond. The nomenclature of this glycosidic bond refers to the configuration of the anomeric carbon of the first monosaccharide (i.e., β-D-glucose); the number of the anomeric carbon (C-1) of the first monosaccharide; and the number of the carbon (C-4) of the second monosaccharide (i.e., β-D-glucose) to which the first monosaccharide is linked. Cellobiose can be synthesized from two units of β-D-glucose or obtained by enzymatic or acidic hydrolysis of cellulose and cellulose-rich materials (e.g., cotton and paper). Cellobiose has eight hydroxyl (–OH) groups, one acetal linkage, and one hemiacetal linkage, which provide strong intermolecular and intramolecular hydrogen bonds (Robyt 1998).

## Lactose

Lactose is a disaccharide formed from β-D-galactose and α-D-glucose via a galactosyl β-1,4-linkage, which is different from a glucosyl β-1,4-linkage in cellobiose and dietary fiber. Lactose was first isolated in 1633 and identified as a sugar in 1780. This disaccharide is present only in the milk of mammals (Table 2.6) and is the most abundant carbohydrate in the milk of most land-based animals, including cats, cows, dogs, goats, horses, mice, pigs, rats, and sheep (Rezaei et al. 2016). Of note, the milk of most marine mammals contains little or no lactose, and these animals may have no tolerance to this disaccharide (Geraci 1981). However, lactose is the predominant sugar in dolphin milk at mid-lactation. Lactose is present at very low concentrations in the milk of bears and monotremes (e.g., platypus and echidna). Globally, most adults also exhibit lactose maldigestion due to their reduced capacity to hydrolyze lactose in the gastrointestinal

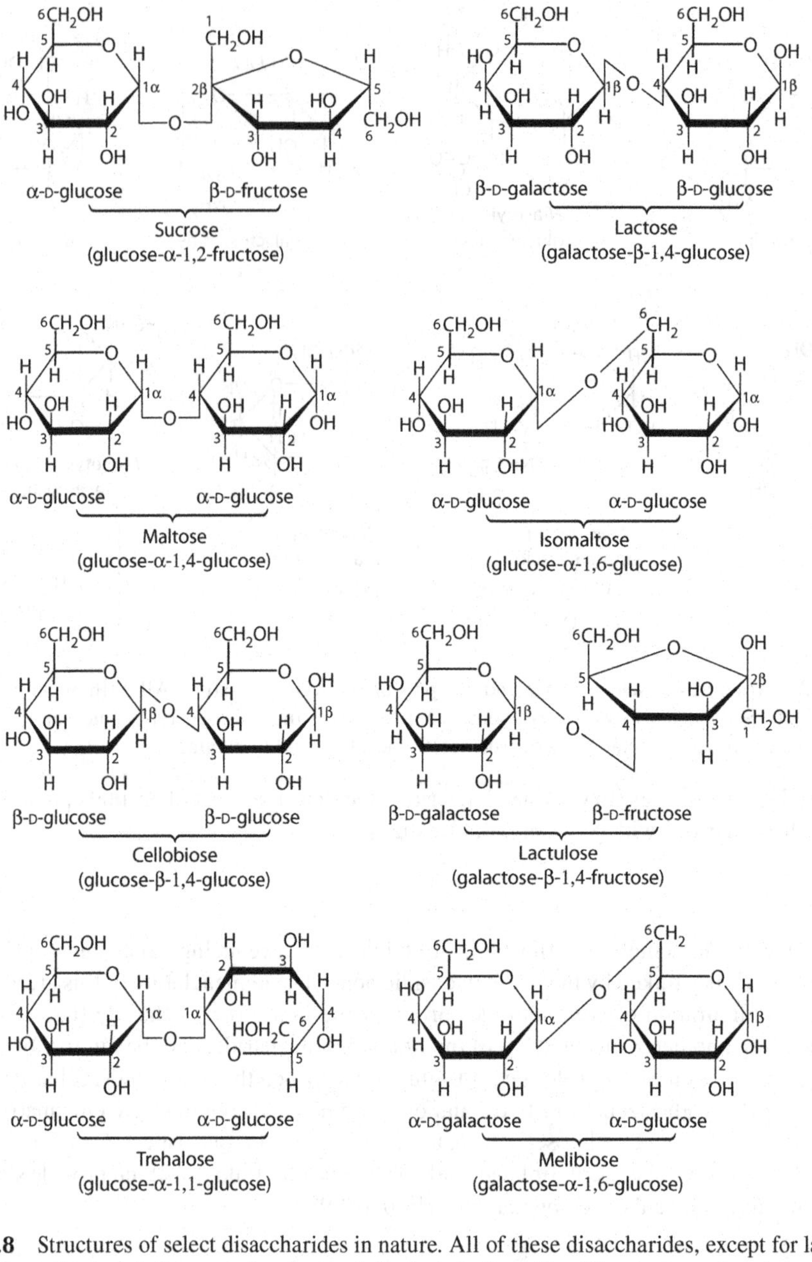

α-D-glucose β-D-fructose
Sucrose
(glucose-α-1,2-fructose)

β-D-galactose β-D-glucose
Lactose
(galactose-β-1,4-glucose)

α-D-glucose α-D-glucose
Maltose
(glucose-α-1,4-glucose)

α-D-glucose α-D-glucose
Isomaltose
(glucose-α-1,6-glucose)

β-D-glucose β-D-glucose
Cellobiose
(glucose-β-1,4-glucose)

β-D-galactose β-D-fructose
Lactulose
(galactose-β-1,4-fructose)

α-D-glucose α-D-glucose
Trehalose
(glucose-α-1,1-glucose)

α-D-galactose α-D-glucose
Melibiose
(galactose-α-1,6-glucose)

**FIGURE 2.8** Structures of select disaccharides in nature. All of these disaccharides, except for lactose, are present in plants. Lactose is the most abundant carbohydrate in the milk of livestock species, dogs, rats, mice, and humans.

tract, but they have greater tolerance for the consumption of fermented dairy products than those that are unfermented (Heaney 2013). This digestive problem can also occur in some laboratory, companion, or farm animals, such as monkeys, dogs, cats, calves, foals, and goats (Gaschen and Merchant 2011).

### Maltose and Isomaltose

Maltose consists of two α-D-glucose joined together via α-1,4 linkage. This disaccharide is the fundamental repeating unit of starch and glycogen (Lu and Sharkey 2006). The difference in the

**TABLE 2.6**
**Composition of Lactose and Total Carbohydrates (Carb) in the Mature Milk of Mammals[a]**

| Species | Lactose | Total Carb | Species | Lactose | Total Carb | Species | Lactose | Total Carb |
|---|---|---|---|---|---|---|---|---|
| Antelope | 42 | 47 | Fox | 47 | 50 | Rabbit | 18 | 21 |
| Baboon | 60 | 77 | Giant panda | 12 | 15 | Rat (Lab) | 30 | 38 |
| Bat | 34 | 40 | Giraffe | 34 | 40 | Reindeer | 28 | 35 |
| Bear (black) | 3.0 | 27 | Goat (domestic) | 43 | 47 | Rhesus monkey | 70 | 82 |
| Bear (grizzly) | 4.0 | 32 | Goat (mountain) | 28 | 32 | Rhinoceros | 66 | 72 |
| Bear (polar) | 4.0 | 30 | Gorilla | 62 | 73 | Sea lion | 0.0 | 6.0 |
| Beaver | 17 | 22 | Guinea pig | 30 | 36 | Seal (fur) | 1.0 | 24 |
| Bison | 51 | 57 | Hamster | 32 | 38 | Seal (gray) | 1.0 | 26 |
| Buffalo | 40 | 47 | Horse (domestic) | 62 | 69 | Seal (harp) | 8.9 | 23 |
| Blue whale | 10 | 13 | Human | 70 | 80 | Seal (hooded) | 0.0 | 10 |
| Camel | 49 | 56 | Kangaroo | <0.01 | 47 | Sheep (domestic) | 48 | 55 |
| Cat (domestic) | 42 | 49 | Lion | 27 | 34 | Sperm whale | 20 | 22 |
| Chimpanzee | 70 | 82 | Llama | 60 | 66 | Squirrel (gray) | 30 | 34 |
| Cow (domestic) | 49 | 56 | Mink | 69 | 76 | Tree shrew | 15 | 20 |
| Coyote | 30 | 32 | Moose | 33 | 38 | Water buffalo | 48 | 55 |
| Deer | 26 | 30 | Mouse (lab) | 30 | 36 | Water shrew | 1.0 | 30 |
| Dog (domestic) | 33 | 38 | Mule | 55 | 62 | White whale | 2.0 | 18 |
| Dolphin | 10 | 11 | Musk ox | 27 | 33 | Wolf | 32 | 35 |
| Donkey (Ass) | 61 | 68 | Opossum | 16 | 20 | Yak | 50 | 54 |
| Elephant | 51 | 60 | Peccary | 66 | 71 | Zebra | 74 | 82 |
| Ferret | 38 | 44 | Pig (domestic) | 52 | 58 | | | |
| Fin whale | 2.0 | 26 | Pronghorn | 40 | 43 | | | |

*Source:* Adapted from Rezaei, R. et al. 2016. *J. Anim. Sci. Biotechnol.* 7:20.
[a] Values are g/kg whole milk.

configuration of the glycosidic link between maltose and cellobiose (the β-1,4 bond) is responsible for their different digestibilities in nonruminants. Isomaltose, a product of the hydrolysis of starch and glycogen, is similar to maltose but has an α-(1-6)-linkage, instead of the α-(1-4)-linkage in maltose.

## Sucrose

The word "sucrose" was coined in 1857 by the English chemist William Miller from the French *sucre* and the generic chemical suffix *-ose* for sugars in English. Sucrose is composed of α-D-glucose and β-D-fructose with an α-1,2-glycosidic linkage. The nomenclature of this covalent bond indicates: the configuration of the anomeric carbon (α) of the first monosaccharide (i.e., α-D-glucose); the number of the anomeric carbon (C-1) of the first monosaccharide; and the number of the carbon (C-2) of the second monosaccharide (i.e., β-D-fructose) to which the first monosaccharide is linked. The correct specification of the configuration of the anomeric carbon is critical. Amounts of sucrose vary markedly among feedstuffs (Table 2.3). Sucrose is very abundant in sugar beets and sugarcane (Sinnott 2013). Indeed, sucrose is present in larger amounts (2%–8% of DM) than monosaccharides in herbage. The amount of disaccharides increases during the day as a result of photosynthesis and decreases during the night (Ruan 2014). Success in conserving herbage as silage depends on the presence of readily fermentable carbohydrates (sugars, starch, or fructosans).

### α,α-Trehalose

Trehalose (also known as mycose or tremalose) is a disaccharide of two α-D-glucose molecules formed by an α,α-1,1 glucoside bond (Lunn et al. 2014). The nomenclature of this glycosidic bond refers to the configuration of the anomeric carbon (α) of the first monosaccharide (i.e., α-D-glucose) and the second monosaccharide (i.e., α-D-glucose); the number of the anomeric carbon (C-1) of the first monosaccharide; and the number of the carbon (C-1) of the second monosaccharide to which the first monosaccharide is linked. α,α-Trehalose was originally discovered in 1832 in an ergot of rye and subsequently isolated from trehala manna. This disaccharide is produced by fungi, yeast, plants, and invertebrate animals (e.g., insects). Of note, it is also a major energy source for insects, as it is typically their primary "blood" (hemolymph) sugar.

## OLIGOSACCHARIDES

### Definition

Oligosaccharides consist of 3–10 units of monosaccharides, which are linked via glycosidic bonds. The formation of each glycosidic linkage results in the elimination of one water molecule, as noted for the formation of a disaccharide. Nearly, all naturally occurring oligosaccharides are found in plants. However, human, elephant, and bear milk are exceptions, as they contain relatively high levels of oligosaccharides. Examples of oligosaccharides in corn grain, peas, and soybean meal are provided in Table 2.3. Bacteria in the digestive tract of animals possess enzymes to hydrolyze all oligosaccharides with α-1,4 or β-1,4 linkages. However, animal cells do not produce the enzymes necessary to hydrolyze either α-1,6-galactosyl oligosaccharides (e.g., stachyose, raffinose, and verbascose) or β-1,4-glucosyl oligosaccharides (e.g., products of microbial cellulose hydrolysis).

### Trisaccharides

Trisaccharides are composed of three units of monosaccharides with two glycosidic bonds for linkages. These compounds most often occur in plants and are negligible in animals. Similar to disaccharides, each glycosidic bond in a trisaccharide is formed between any hydroxyl groups of monosaccharides, with the removal of one water molecule per glycosidic linkage (Robyt 1998). Raffinose (also called melitose) [α-D-galactopyranosyl-(1,6)-α-D-glucopyranosyl-(1,2)-β-D-fructofuranoside] is a nonreducing trisaccharide present in plants, particularly sugar beets and beans, such as soybeans and green beans (Sengupta et al. 2015). Melezitose is a nonreducing trisaccharide in the sweet exudates of many trees. Of note, a trisaccharide (3′-galactosyl-lactose), which consists of β-D-galactopyranosyl-(1,3)-β-D-galactopyranosyl-(1,4)-β-D-glucose, is a major oligosaccharide in the milk of some mammals, such as the tammar wallaby and the grey kangaroo (Messer et al. 1980). The structures of select trisaccharides are shown in Figure 2.9.

### Tetrasaccharides

Plants also contain tetrasaccharides and pentasaccharides. A tetrasaccharide consists of four units of monosaccharides with three glycosidic bonds connecting them. Stachyose [α-D-galactopyranosyl-(1,6)-α-D-galactopyranosyl-(1,6)-α-D-glucopyranosyl-(1,2)-β-D-fructofuranoside] is a tetrasaccharide (Figure 2.10) which is widely present in plants, including green beans, soybeans, and other beans (Hagely et al. 2013). It is composed of two α-D-galactose units, one α-D-glucose unit, and one β-D-fructose unit, which are linked sequentially as galactose(α-1,6)galactose(α,1-6)glucose (α,1-2)fructose.

### Pentasaccharides

A pentasaccharide consists of five units of monosaccharides with four glycosidic bonds for linkages. Verbascose [α-D-galactopyranosyl-(1,6)-α-D-galactopyranosyl-(1,6)-α-D-galactopyranosyl-α-D-glucose β-D-fructose α-D-glucose

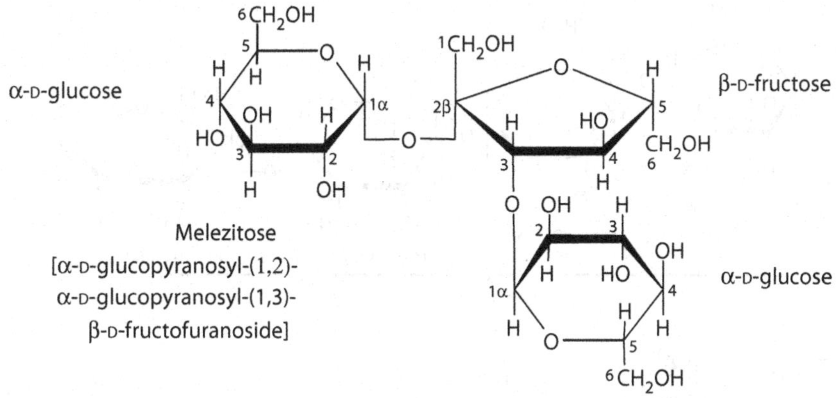

Melezitose
[α-D-glucopyranosyl-(1,2)-
α-D-glucopyranosyl-(1,3)-
β-D-fructofuranoside]

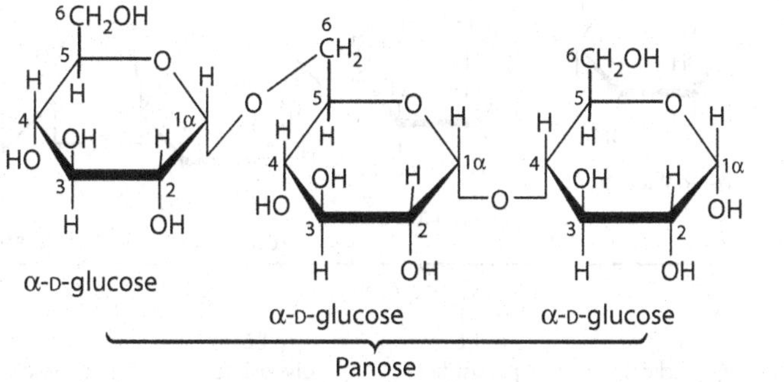

α-D-glucose α-D-glucose α-D-glucose

Panose
[α-D-glucopyranosyl-(1,6)-α-glucopyranosyl-(1,4)-α-D-glucopyranoside]

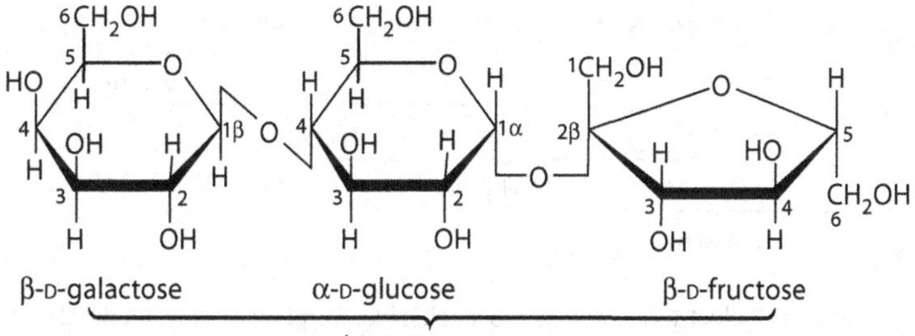

β-D-galactose α-D-glucose β-D-fructose

Lactosucrose
[β-D-galactopyranosyl-(1,4)-α-glucopyranosyl-(1,2)-β-D-fructofuranoside]

α-D-galactose α-D-glucose β-D-fructose

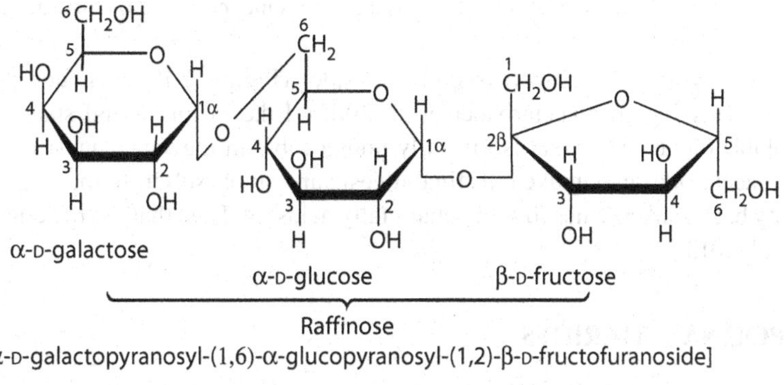

Raffinose
[α-D-galactopyranosyl-(1,6)-α-glucopyranosyl-(1,2)-β-D-fructofuranoside]

**FIGURE 2.9** Structures of select trisaccharides in plant-source feedstuffs. All of these trisaccharides occur in plants. Raffinose (nondigestible in the small intestine) is an important component of carbohydrates in legumes. Except for melezitose, these substances are not present in animals. Melezitose is also produced by many species of insects as part of their honeydew.

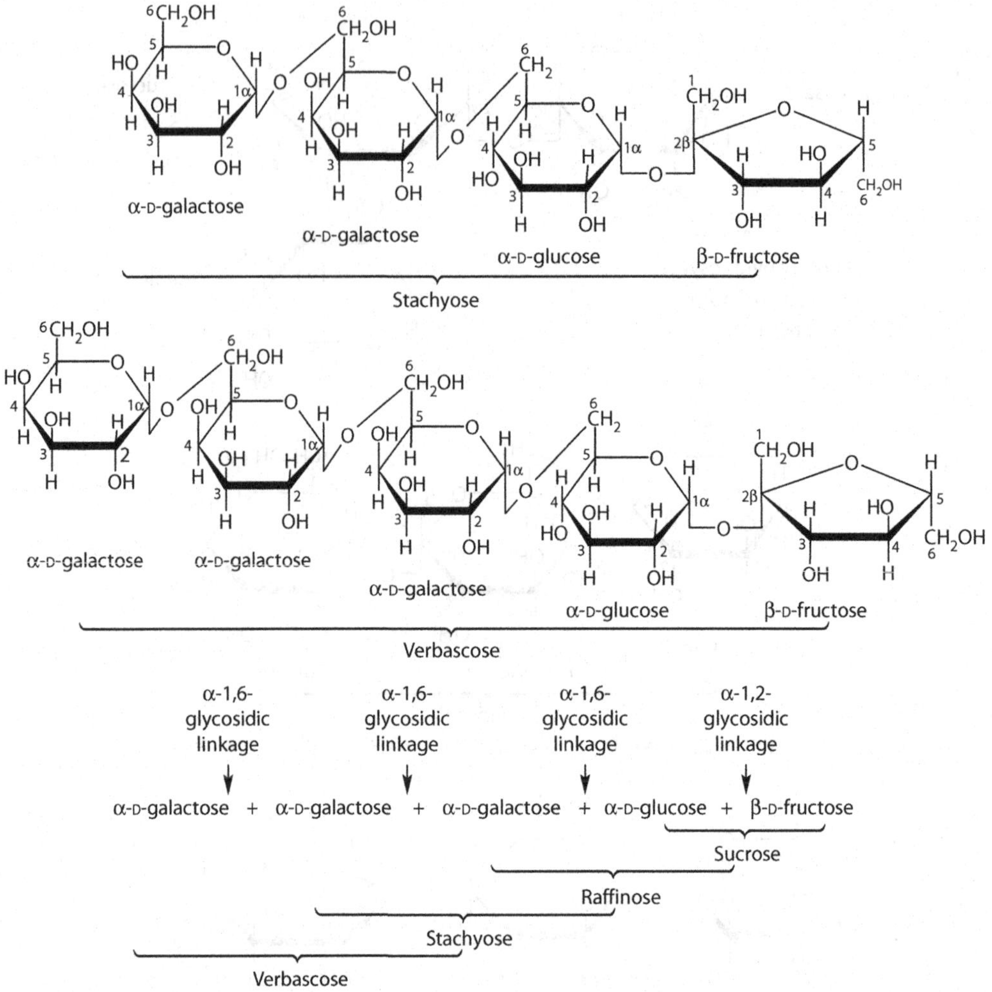

**FIGURE 2.10** Structures of select tetra- and pentasaccharides in plant-source feedstuffs. Stachyose (a tetrasaccharide) and verbascose (a pentasaccharide) are soluble dietary fibers that are indigestible in the small intestine. These oligosaccharides are widely present in plants, particularly legumes, but are absent in animals. Bacterial enzymes can hydrolyze tetra- and pentasaccharides into constituent monosaccharides.

(1,6)-α-D-glucopyranosyl-(1,2)-β-D-fructofuranoside] (Figure 2.10), a major pentasaccharide, is common in many legumes (Peterbauer et al. 2002). Like raffinose and stachyose, verbascose is a water-soluble dietary fiber that is virtually undigestible in the small intestine of animals. All of these oligosaccharides may make intestinal digesta and stools softer. In the large intestine, they are degraded by bacterial enzymes to short-chain fatty acids (SCFAs) that are beneficial for colon health (Turner et al. 2013).

## HOMOPOLYSACCHARIDES

### Homopolysaccharides in Plants

#### Definition

Homopolysaccharides (homoglycans) are polysaccharides consisting of a single type of many monosaccharide molecules joined together through glycosidic linkages. Depending on the monosugar, a homopolysaccharide may be called a: glucan (consisting of D-glucose); fructan (consisting of fructose); galactan (consisting of galactose); arabinan (consisting of arabinose); or xylan (consisting of xylose). Plant-source homopolysaccharides include starch, cellulose, levans, galactans, and β-D-glucans (Robyt 1998). Glycogen serves to store glucose and energy in animals, whereas other homopolysaccharides fulfill structural functions in the cell wall of plants. Animal cells can hydrolyze homopolysaccharides with an α-1,4 linkage but not those with a β-1,4 linkage. However, cellulose, levans, galactans, and β-D-glucans can be extensively degraded by enzymes released from bacteria present in the rumen of ruminants and in the large intestine of all animals (Pond et al. 2005).

### Arabinan

Arabinan has a complex branched structure consisting of D-arabinose residues linked via α-1-3, α-1-5, and β-1-2 glycosidic bonds (Chandrasekaran 1998). Pure arabinan is present in the plant cell wall at a very low concentration. Highly purified linear 1,5-α-L-arabinan can be obtained from sugar beets.

### Cellulose

Cellulose is the major structural component of cell walls in higher plants and the most abundant biopolymer on the planet. This homopolysaccharide amounts to approximately 20%–40% of the DM in green plants (including grasses and bamboo), and constitutes the bulk of flax (80%), jute (60%–70%), and wood (40%–50%) (Robyt 1998). Cellulose is a linear polymer of β-1,4-linked D-glucose units and there is no evidence of branching in this polysaccharide (Figure 2.11). The numbers of polymerized glucose molecules in cellulose may range from 900 to 2000. Cellulose is present in plant tissues to form fibers, which are composed of crystalline microfibrils held together by strong hydrogen bonds (Li et al. 2015). The crystalline microfibrils in cellulose are encircled by a largely amorphous matrix of hemicellulose, lignin (cross-linked phenol polymers with a high molecular weight), and some proteins on the cell walls. The different types of polysaccharides, lignin, and proteins are held together on the plant cell walls by hydrogen bonding and van der Waals forces (Li et al. 2015). This chemical structure contributes most to the rigidity and strength of higher plants. In addition, the β-1,4-linkages of its glucose molecules make cellulose virtually insoluble in water and indigestible to animal-source digestive enzymes.

### Galactan

Pure galactan (also called galactosan) is a linear chain of β-D-galactose residues linked via the β-1,4-glycosidic bond in plants (Arifkhodzhaev 2000). This homopolysaccharide is present in plant cell walls at a very low concentration. Interestingly, the galactose residues of galactan are primarily linked via the α-1-6-glycosidic bond in *Anogeissus latifolia* and via the α-1-3-glycosidic bond in acacia trees.

### β-D-Glucans

β-D-Glucans are homopolysaccharides containing linear backbones of β-D-glucose linked via β-1,3 glycosidic bonds and possibly branch chains consisting of β-1,4 or β-1-6 glycosidic bonds. They are present in cereal grains (Table 2.3). Examples of β-D-glucans are callose and lichens. Some β-D-glucans have branch chains consisting of various β-D-glucose linkages. They are often called soluble fibers or β-glucans. β-D-Glucans are present in the cell walls of plants (e.g., barley, oat, and wheat), yeast, bacteria, fungi, and algae (Farrokhi et al. 2006). Different sources of β-glucans differ in their backbone linkages, branch chains, molecular mass, and solubility in water. For example, cereal β-glucans have both β-1,3 and β-1,4 glycosidic linkages on their backbones, whereas lichens contain both β-1,3 and β-1,6 glycosidic linkages on their backbones. Besides the common β-1,3 glycosidic linkages on their backbones as a major feature, yeast and fungal β-glucans contain β-1,6 side branches. In contrast, barley and oat β-D-glucans have no branch chains, and cereal β-D-glucans are generally well fermented in the large intestine (Robyt 1998).

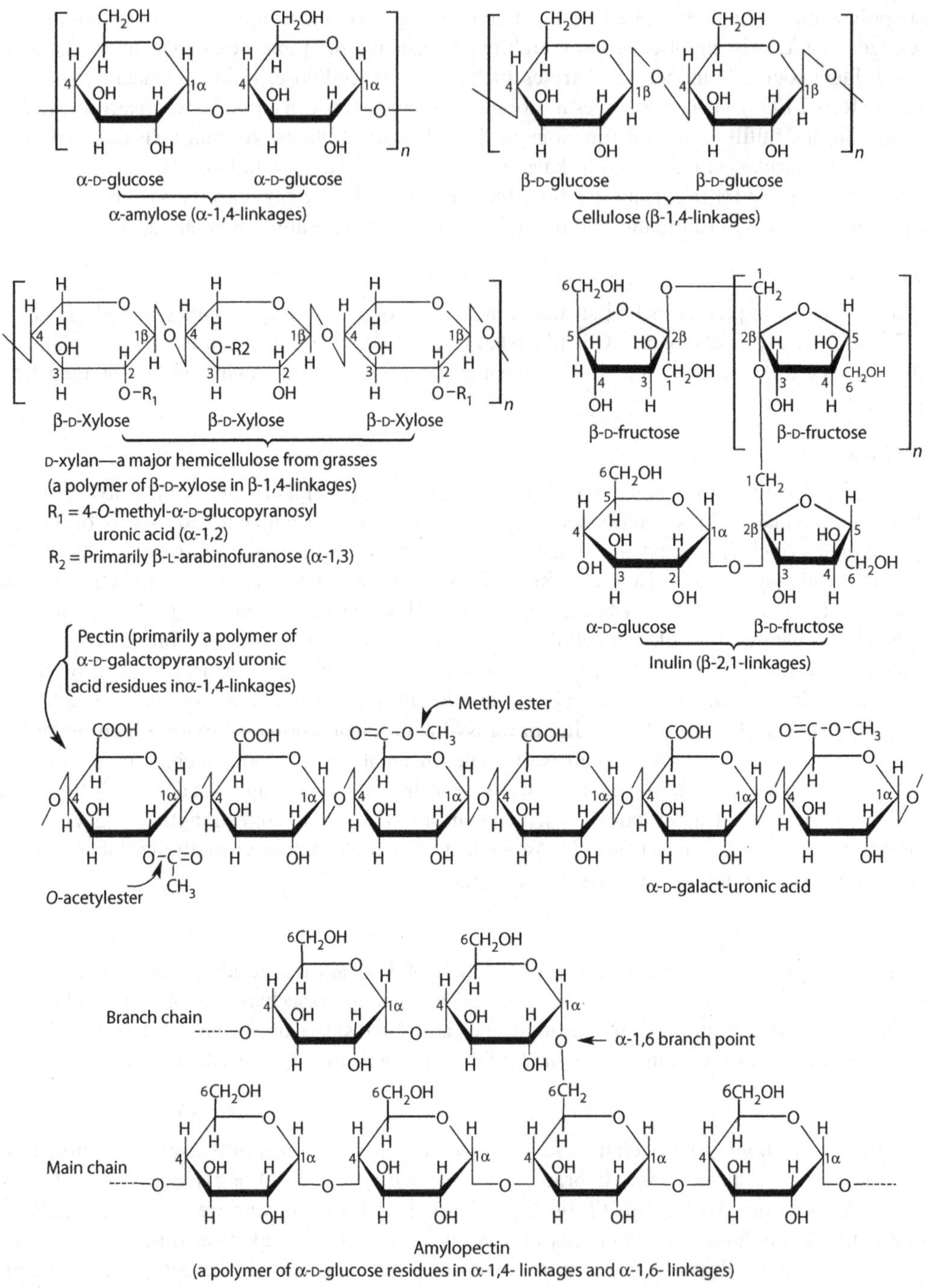

α-D-glucose α-D-glucose

α-amylose (α-1,4-linkages)

β-D-glucose β-D-glucose

Cellulose (β-1,4-linkages)

β-D-Xylose β-D-Xylose β-D-Xylose

D-xylan—a major hemicellulose from grasses
(a polymer of β-D-xylose in β-1,4-linkages)
$R_1$ = 4-*O*-methyl-α-D-glucopyranosyl uronic acid (α-1,2)
$R_2$ = Primarily β-L-arabinofuranose (α-1,3)

β-D-fructose β-D-fructose

α-D-glucose β-D-fructose

Inulin (β-2,1-linkages)

Pectin (primarily a polymer of α-D-galactopyranosyl uronic acid residues inα-1,4-linkages)

Methyl ester

*O*-acetylester

α-D-galact-uronic acid

Branch chain

α-1,6 branch point

Main chain

Amylopectin
(a polymer of α-D-glucose residues in α-1,4- linkages and α-1,6- linkages)

**FIGURE 2.11** Structures of select homopolysaccharides and heteropolysaccharides in plants. Amylose is a polymer of α-1,4-linked glucose residues without any branch, and amylopectin is a polymer of α-1,4-linked glucose residues branched by α-1,6-linkages. Starch is a mixture of amylose and amylopectin. In contrast, cellulose is a polymer of β-D-glucose with β-1,4-linkages. Starch and cellulose are homopolysaccharides. In contrast, D-xylan and inulin (heteropolysaccharides) consist of more than 10 units of different types of monosaccharides. None of these polysaccharides are produced by animals.

### Levans

Levan is a homopolysaccharide consisting of D-fructose molecules and is a type of fructan present in many plants, including grasses, herbage, tubers, and sugar beets (Benkeblia 2013). By definition, fructans are a group of fructose-based oligo- and polysaccharides (Bali et al. 2015). Levans contain main chains of 100–200 D-fructofuranose units in β-2,6 glycosidic linkages. These homopolysaccharides also have branch chains of D-fructofuranose residues in β-2,1 glycosidic linkages. The number of D-fructofuranoses ranges from one to four. Levans can serve as storage for carbohydrates instead of starch in some special species of plants and are indigestible to animal-source digestive enzymes (van Arkel et al. 2013).

### Mannans

Mannans exist as linear homopolysaccharides of D-mannose linked via the β-1,4 glycosidic bond in plants. They are called pure mannans and are an important part of hemicellulose in the plants. Of interest, mannans account for as much as 60% of palm seeds, including the ivory nut (*Phytelephas macrocarpa*) (Melton et al. 2009). Mannans bind to cellulose in the plant cell wall, serve to store free carbohydrates in plants, and modulate plant growth and development.

### Starch

Starch is synthesized by all plants (Keeling and Myers 2010). It is the major homopolysaccharide in plants, particularly in grains, seeds (which may contain up to 70% on an as-fed basis), cereal by-products, and tubers (with ~30% starch on the DM basis), but its content differs markedly among feedstuffs (Tables 2.3 and 2.7). The starch is generally a mixture of amylose and amylopectin, both of which consist of α-D-glucose residues (Smith et al. 2005). Amylose is a long linear chain in which 250–300 units of D-glucose are joined by α-1,4 linkage and generally has no branches. In contrast, amylopectin is a short chain of various α-D-glucose molecules joined together via α-1,4 linkages in the main chain and a relatively high content of α-1,6 branching chains, with branching occurring every 24–30 units of α-D-glucose. The ratio of amylose to amylopectin varies with the sources of starch, but it is usually 1:3 (g/g).

**TABLE 2.7**
**Composition of Nonfiber Carbohydrates and SCFAs in Selected Feedstuffs**

| Feedstuff | Sugars | Starch | Pectin | SCFAs |
|---|---|---|---|---|
| | % of Nonfiber Carbohydrates Plus SCFAs[a] | | | |
| Alfalfa silage | 0 | 24.5 | 33.0 | 42.5 |
| Grass hay | 35.4 | 15.2 | 49.4 | 0 |
| Corn silage | 0 | 71.3 | 0 | 28.7 |
| Barley | 9.1 | 81.7 | 9.2 | 0 |
| Corn grain | 20.0 | 80.0 | 0 | 0 |
| Beet pulp | 33.7 | 1.8 | 64.5 | 0 |
| Soyhulls | 18.8 | 18.8 | 62.4 | 0 |
| Soybean meal, 48% CP | 28.2 | 28.2 | 43.6 | 0 |

*Source:* Adapted from National Research Council. 2001. *Nutrient Requirements of Dairy Cattle*, 7th Revised ed. National Academy Press, Washington, DC.

SCFAs, short-chain fatty acids.

[a] Nonfiber carbohydrates consist of simple sugars, starch, and soluble fiber.

Starches from different sources of plants have different structures (Figure 2.11). On the basis of the rates of their *in vitro* enzymatic digestion, there are three types of starch: (1) rapidly digested starch (with high amylopectin content and high digestibility, such as the starch in the waxy corn (found in China in 1909) containing 100% amylopectin and 0% amylose), freshly cooked starch, and white bread; (2) slowly digested starch (with a certain weight ratio of amylose to amylopectin of, e.g., 45:55 [more amylopectin than amylose] and low digestibility), such as starch in most raw cereals (dent corn varieties, barley, wheat, and rice), whose semicrystalline structure renders it less accessible to digestive enzymes; and (3) resistant starch (with high-amylose content and limited digestibility), such as high-amylose corn, high-amylose wheat, legumes, and bananas (Zhang and Hamaker 2009). Resistant starch is further classified as physically inaccessible (RS1; e.g., partially milled grain), resistant starch granule (RS2; e.g., raw potato and banana starch), retrograded starch (RS3; e.g., cooked potato after cooling), and chemically modified starch (RS4; many types of starch with different cross-linking). The rate of digestion of the RS4 starch in the small intestine is relatively low (Yin et al. 2010). In its natural state, tuber and grain starch (e.g., in potatoes) exist in a water-insoluble granular form (Sinnott 2013), which resists digestion in the small intestine of nonruminants (Pond et al. 2005). Such starch-containing foods must be cooked before they can be more efficiently utilized by chickens and pigs. The cooking of foods markedly aids in their digestion by animals through breaking down (gelatinizing) and solubilizing starch granules. In general, amorphous or completely dispersed starches are highly susceptible digestive enzymes.

## Homopolysaccharides in Animals

### Definition

As in plants, homopolysaccharides in animals are homoglycans composed of a single type of monosaccharide molecule joined through glycosidic linkages. In contrast to plants, the monosaccharide unit can be either D-glucose or its derivative *N*-acetyl-glucosamine. To date, glycogen and chitin are the only homopolysaccharides known to be present in animals.

### Chitin

Animal-source chitin is a water-insoluble long-chain polymer of primarily *N*-acetyl-glucosamine molecules in β-1,4 glycosidic linkages. Chitin occurs in the exoskeletons of crustaceans (e.g., crabs, lobsters, and shrimps), insects, the radulae of molluscs, as well as the beaks and internal shells of squid and octopuses (Younes and Rinaudo 2015). The structure of animal-source chitin is the same as that of cellulose in plants, except that the C-2 of the D-glucopyranose residue in cellulose is substituted with an *N*-acetyl-amino group (Figure 2.12). Chitin also has the same structural and protective functions in animals as cellulose does in plants. In the presence of a strong alkali (e.g., sodium hydroxide), chitin undergoes partial deacetylation to form water-soluble chitosan composed of *N*-acetyl-D-glucosamine (also called 2-amino-2-deoxy-β-D-glucose; Sinnott 2013).

### Glycogen

Glycogen is a polymer of α-D-glucose in α-1,4 glycosidic linkages on the main chain with α-1,6 branch linkages (Roach et al. 2012). It has a molecular weight of approximately $10^8$, a mass equivalent to $6 \times 10^5$ glucose residues. However, the precise molecular weight of glycogen is not known. Glycogen resembles amylopectin in structure (Figure 2.12) but has a higher degree of branching than amylopectin. Specifically, branching occurs in glycogen approximately every 8–12 glucose residues.

Glycogen occurs in all animal cells (Table 2.8). It is the only homopolysaccharide in mammals, the principal homopolysaccharide in birds and fish, and a quantitatively significant homopolysaccharide in insects and crustaceans (e.g., crabs, lobsters, and shrimps) with extensive exoskeletons. In mammals, birds, and fish, glycogen is present primarily in the liver, as well as skeletal and cardiac muscles. For example, the liver of animals contains approximately 1.5%–8% glycogen; calves, 2%–5%; adult cattle, 1.5%–4%; hens, 3%–4%; geese, 4%–6%; and skeletal muscle, 0.5%–1%

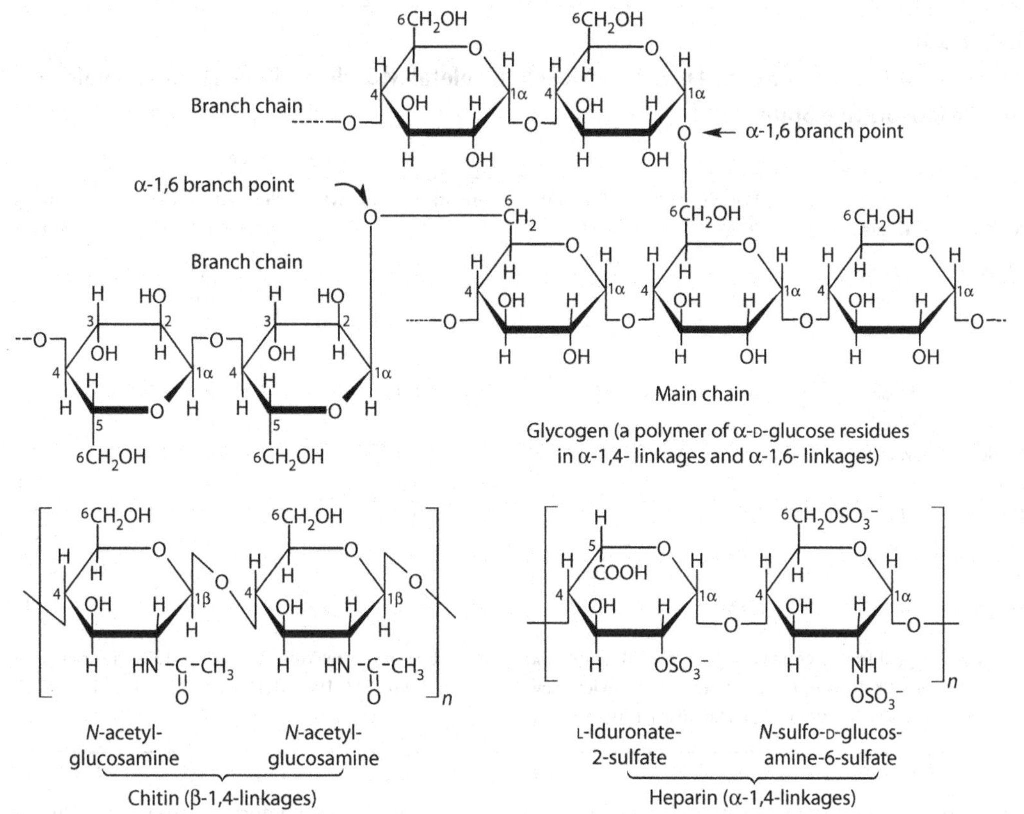

**FIGURE 2.12** Structures of select homopolysaccharides and heteropolysaccharides in animals. Glycogen is the major homopolysaccharide in mammals, birds, and fish, and it is also present in shrimp and insects. It is a polymer of α-D-glucose with α-1,4-linkages in the main chain and α-1,6-branching linkages. Chitin, which is a polymer of α-D-glucosamine molecules, is the main homopolysaccharide in many aquatic animals. Heparin is a heteropolysaccharide in animals and contains α-1,4- and β-1,4-linkages.

(Bergman 1983a,b; McDonald et al. 2011). In resting and well-nourished horses, skeletal muscle contains up to 4% glycogen. In animals, approximately 80% of total glycogen is present in skeletal and cardiac muscles, approximately 15% in the liver, and approximately 5% in other tissues.

Glycogen serves as the major form of glucose storage in animals, which helps to minimize the negative impacts of high glucose concentrations on osmolarity. However, excess storage of glycogen in the liver and muscle causes abnormalities in their structure and function. Owing to its limited reserve in the body, glycogen can only provide enough glucose to sustain a starving animal for up to 12 h. However, glycogen is the immediate source of glucose when animals have an urgent need for glucose under physiological and stressful conditions (e.g., exercise and exposure to a cold environment).

## Homopolysaccharides in Microbes and Other Lower Organisms

### Cellulose

Some bacteria contain cellulose, which is a linear polymer of β-1,4-linked D-glucose units as in plants (Römling and Galperin 2015). These bacteria belong primarily to the genera *Acetobacter*, *Sarcina ventriculi*, and *Agrobacterium*, including: (1) the nitrogen-fixing plant symbiont *Rhizobium leguminosarum*, (2) soil bacteria *Burkholderia* spp. and *Pseudomonas putida*, (3) plant pathogens *Dickeya dadantii* and *Erwinia chrysanthemi*, (4) tumor-producing *Agrobacterium tumefaciens*,

**TABLE 2.8**
**Amounts of Glycogen in the Liver and Muscle (Skeletal Muscle and Heart) of Animals in the Postabsorptive State**

| Animal | Tissue | Tissue Weight (wt) (kg) | Glycogen in Tissue Amount (g) | Percent of Tissue wt (%) | Percent of Body wt (%) | Energy (kcal) |
|---|---|---|---|---|---|---|
| Chicken | Muscle | 0.96 | 11.5 | 1.2 | 0.58 | 47 |
| (2 kg) | Liver | 0.04 | 1.8 | 4.5 | 0.09 | 7.4 |
| Pig | Muscle | 35 | 263 | 0.75 | 0.38 | 1078 |
| (70 kg) | Liver | 1.5 | 71 | 4.7 | 0.10 | 291 |
| Sheep | Muscle | 26 | 260 | 1.0 | 0.47 | 1066 |
| (55 kg) | Liver | 0.83 | 38 | 4.6 | 0.07 | 156 |
| Cattle | Muscle | 240 | 4800 | 2.0 | 0.96 | 19,680 |
| (500 kg) | Liver | 7.5 | 375 | 5.0 | 0.075 | 1538 |
| Human | Muscle | 35 | 245 | 0.70 | 0.35 | 1005 |
| (70 kg) | Liver | 1.5 | 72 | 4.8 | 0.10 | 295 |
| Horse | Muscle | 212 | 4452 | 2.1 | 1.05 | 18,253 |
| (425 kg) | Liver | 6.8 | 370 | 5.4 | 0.087 | 1517 |

*Source:* Adapted from Bergman, E.N. 1983a. *World Animal Science*. Elsevier, New York, Vol. 3, pp. 137–149; Bergman, E.N. 1983b. *World Animal Science*. Elsevier, New York, Vol. 3, pp. 173–196; McDonald, P. et al. 2011. *Animal Nutrition*, 7th ed. Prentice Hall, New York.

*Escherichia coli*, and (5) *Salmonella enterica*. In natural habitats, the bacteria synthesize cellulose to form protective envelopes or biofilms.

### Chitin

In addition to animals, chitin is also present in fungi (including yeasts), green algae, as well as brown and red seaweeds (types of algae). As in animals, chitin is a long-chain linear polymer of *N*-acetyl-glucosamine in β-1,4 glycosidic linkages (Egusa et al. 2015). Owing to its intermolecular hydrogen bonding, chitin is insoluble in water. In these lower organisms, chitin functions to support their cell structures and facilitate biomineralization in the cell membrane.

### Dextrans

Dextrans are synthesized from sucrose by many different bacteria (Sinnott 2013). These carbohydrates have continuous α-1-6-linked D-glucopyranose units in the main chains, as well as branch linkages of α-D-glucopyranose residues via α-1-2, α-1-3, or α-1-4 bonds (Figure 2.13). The length of the branch chains varies with the species of bacteria. Dextrans are soluble in water and can reduce blood viscosity when fed to animals.

### Glycogen

Besides animals, glycogen is also present in bacteria, fungi (including yeasts [single cell-organisms] and multicellular species of the fungi kingdom), protozoa, and the blue–green algae (Roach et al. 2012). In these lower organisms, glycogen is also composed of D-glucose linked via α-1,4-glycosidic bonds on the main chain, as well as branch points where D-glucose molecules are joined to the main chain via α-1,6-linkage. The average length of the chain is 8–12 and 11–12 glucose units in bacteria and yeasts, respectively. Glycogen biosynthesis in non-animal species is a major strategy for the storage of glucose in response to excess nutrient supply and for coping with starvation.

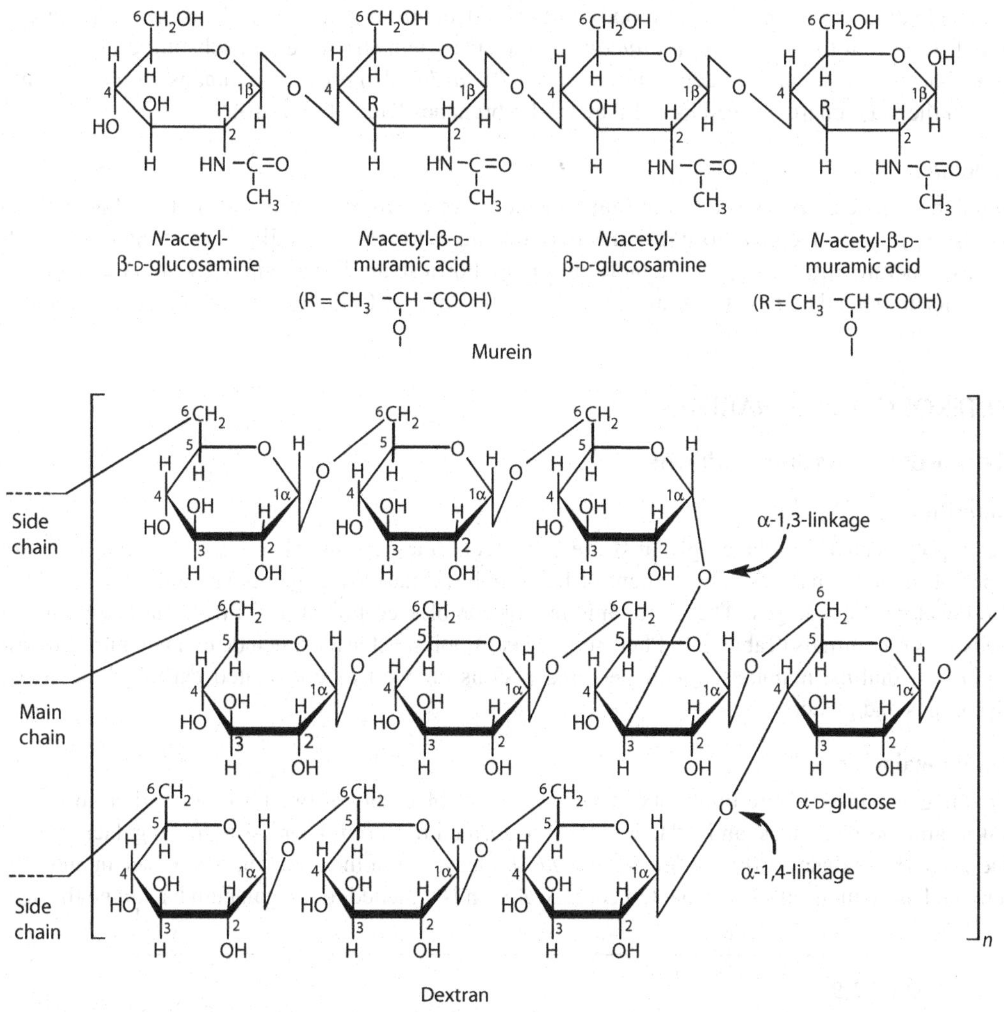

**FIGURE 2.13** Structures of select homopolysaccharides and heteropolysaccharides in microbes. Dextrans are homopolysaccharides made by many different bacteria, whereas murein is a heteropolysaccharide in the cell walls of all known bacteria.

## Levans

Levans are fructose polymers (fructans) containing mainly β-2,6 linkages in microbes, as in plants (Srikanth et al. 2015). Bacterial levans also have branch chains of D-fructofuranose residues in β-2,1 glycosidic linkages. These polysaccharides are synthesized from sucrose by two Gram-positive bacteria genera, *Bacillus* and *Streptococcus*. Bacterial levans have the same chemical structures as plant levans. In microbes, levans contribute to the formation of the extracellular polysaccharide matrix.

## Mannans

Mannans in microbes and other lower organisms are homopolysaccharides of D-mannose, and their structures vary by microbial species (Chandrasekaran 1998). For example, the monosaccharide molecules are linked via the β-1,4 bond as a linear polymer in green algae, which belong to the *Codiaceae and Dasycladaceae* families (Frei and Preston 1968). In yeasts, mannan has α-1,6 linkages in the main chain as well as α-1,2 and α-1,3 branches, and these structures are similar to those of carbohydrates in mammalian glycoproteins. The structure of mannan in *Saccharomyces cerevisiae* differs from that of *Candida albicans* by the side-chain structure and substitution frequency. Some bacteria (e.g., marine bacterium *Edwardsiella tarda*) also produce mannans with α-1,3 linkages in the main chain, as well as α-1,2 and β-1,6 branches (Guo et al. 2010).

### Pullulan

Pullulan is made by many species of fungi, including yeasts (Cheng et al. 2011). It is a linear chain consisting of α-D-glucopyranose residues in α-1,4 and α-1,6 glycosidic linkages in the ratio of 2:1. In this structure, three α-D-glucose molecules in maltotriose are linked via α-1,4, and the maltotriose units are joined end to end by an α-1,6 glycosidic linkage. Pullulan has no branch chains and is highly soluble in water (Robyt 1998).

## HETEROPOLYSACCHARIDES

### Heteropolysaccharides in Plants

#### Definition

Heteropolysaccharides (heteroglycans) are polysaccharides consisting of two or more different types of monosaccharides. The content of heteropolysaccharides in plants varies by their species and developmental stages. Therefore, amounts of complex carbohydrates differ markedly among feedstuffs for animals (Table 2.9). Plant-source heteropolysaccharides include exudate gums, hemicelluloses, inulins, mannans, mucilages, and pectins, as well as conjugated carbohydrates (e.g., glycolipids and glycoproteins).

#### Arabinogalactan

Arabinogalactan is a heteropolysaccharide consisting of arabinan (which is formed from α-1-5-linked arabinose residues) and galactan (which is formed from α-1,4- or β-1,4 linked galactose residues) (Arifkhodzhaev 2000). In *Stevia rebaudiana* leaves, arabinogalactan, which has an antiviral activity, has an unusual β-1,6-galactan core. Arabinan is attached to the galactan backbone through

**TABLE 2.9**
**Composition of Complex Carbohydrates in Selected Feedstuffs**

| Feedstuff | Neutral Detergent Fibers (NDF) | Nonfiber Carbohydrates | Nonstructural Carbohydrates |
|---|---|---|---|
| | % of Dry Matter | | |
| Alfalfa silage | 51.4 | 18.4 | 7.5 |
| Alfalfa hay | 43.1 | 22.0 | 12.5 |
| Mixed hay, mainly grass hay | 60.9 | 16.6 | 13.6 |
| Corn silage | 44.2 | 41.0 | 34.7 |
| Ground corn | 13.1 | 67.5 | 68.7 |
| Beet pulp | 47.3 | 36.2 | 19.5 |
| Whole cottonseed | 48.3 | 10.0 | 6.4 |
| High moister shelled corn | 13.5 | 71.8 | 70.6 |
| Barley | 23.2 | 60.7 | 62.0 |
| Corn gluten meal | 7.0 | 17.3 | 12.0 |
| Soybean hulls | 66.6 | 14.1 | 5.3 |
| Soybean meal, 48% CP | 9.6 | 34.4 | 17.2 |

*Source:* Adapted from The National Research Council. 2001. *Nutrient Requirements of Dairy Cattle*, 7th Revised ed. National Academy Press, Washington, DC.

β-1,3, β-1,6 glycosidic bonds (Arifkhodzhaev 2000). Arabinogalactans are water soluble and have been obtained from apple fruit, aquatic moss, broad-bean leaves, coffee beans, coniferous woods, rapeseed, saguaro cactus cortex, siratro leaves, soybean seeds, sycamore, and tomato (Fincher et al. 1974). In plants, arabinogalactan is a major component of many gums (including gum arabic and gum ghatti), and is usually attached to proteins (8% of the proteoglycan by weight) to form an arabinogalactan–protein complex (Fincher et al. 1974). The proteoglycan, which contains 90% of glycan, acts as an intercellular signaling molecule and a glue to heal plant wounds.

### Exudate Gums

Exudate gums are produced by plants to seal wounds in their bark. Most of these heteropolysaccharides are soluble in water and they all have complex structures with emulsifying, stabilizing, thickening, and gel-forming properties. Their main chains are composed of D-galactopyranosyl units linked with β-1,3 and β-1,6 bonds, as well as D-glucopyranosyl uronic acid units linked with β-1,6 bonds (Aspinall 1967). The main chains carry three kinds of branched trisaccharides consisting of α-L-rhamnopyranose, β-D-glucuronic acid, β-D-galactopyranose, and α-L-arabinofuranose with 1,3-, 1,4-, and 1,6-glycosidic linkages. Exudate gums also contain α-L-rhamnopyranosyl units at the nonreducing ends. Chemical breakdown of exudate gums is limited in the small intestine of nonruminants (Pond et al. 2005). Thus, gums are indigestible to animal-source enzymes, but are fermented to varying degrees by the microbiota of the large intestine.

### Hemicelluloses

Hemicelluloses are a mixture of linear and highly branched polysaccharides containing various types of sugars (Scheller and Ulvskov 2010). D-Xylan is an extensively studied hemicellulose, whose main chain is primarily composed of D-xylopyranoses linked in β-1,4 bonds and which has 4-*O*-methyl-D-glucopyranosyl uronic acid units linked in α-1,2 bonds (Figure 2.11). Side chains may contain D-xylose, D-galactose, fucose, and other saccharides. The major sugar residues in hemicelluloses include β-D-xylopyranose, β-D-xylose, β-D-mannose, β-D-arabinose, β-D-glucose, β-D-galactose, and uronic acid (Scheller and Ulvskov 2010). Hemicelluloses are present on the cell walls of forage plants and are less resistant to chemical degradation than celluloses. For example, hemicelluloses can be hydrolyzed by a relatively mild acid, whereas cellulose hydrolysis requires a concentrated acid. Bacteria in the large intestine of nonruminants are able to ferment hemicelluloses more extensively than cellulose (McDonald et al. 2011). In ruminants, most hemicelluloses are digested in the rumen just like cellulose, and some escape the rumen to be further degraded in the lower intestinal tract.

### Inulins

Inulins are fructans in the roots and tubers of many plants and in some species of algae (Apolinário et al. 2014). These polysaccharides contain 20–30 D-fructofuranose units exclusively in β-2,1 glycosidic linkages. The C-2 position of their terminal D-fructofuranose units is linked with D-glucopyranose. Inulin is soluble in water and has a molecular weight of 3000–5000 Da. Inulins serve as the storage form of carbohydrates instead of starch in certain plants (Robyt 1998). Animal-source digestive enzymes do not degrade inulins.

### Mannans as Glucomannans, Galactomannans, or Galactoglucomannans

Besides the pure mannans noted previously, some mannans exist in plants as main β-1,4-D-mannose backbones with branches of other carbohydrates. When some C-6 carbons of the main mannose backbone are attached to β-D-glucose via a β-1,6- or α-1,6-glycosidic bond or to D-galactose via an α-1,6-glycosidic bond in side chains, the mannan-based heteropolysaccharides are called glucomannans or galactomannans, respectively (Moreira and Filho 2008). If the side-chain D-galactose residues are also linked with D-glucose residues, the mannan-based heteropolysaccharides are called galactoglucomannans. Glucomannan contains 8% β-D-glucose and is acetylated at the *O*-2 and/or *O*-3 positions. In contrast, galactomannans have variable amounts of α-D-galactose residues in their side chains. For example, the ratio of mannose to galactose is 3.5:1 for locust bean gum; 3:1 for tara (*Caesalpinia spinosa*) gum; and 1.5:1 for guar gum (Melton et al. 2009).

#### Mucilages

Mucilages are gelatinous substances of nearly all plants (including legumes or seaweeds) and some microorganisms, and are very similar to gums. They contain polysaccharides that are linked to protein via covalent bonding. The structures of mucilages are unknown and their hydrolysis generates pentoses and hexoses, including arabinose, galactose, glucose, mannose, rhamnose, and xylose (Hamman et al. 2015). The most common acids in mucilages are uronic acids (e.g., galacturonic acid), but other acids (e.g., sulfonic acids) are also present in the polysaccharides.

#### Pectins

Pectins are present primarily on the cell wall of all plants but also in the spaces between the cell wall and intracellular membranes. The structures of pectins are more uniform than those of hemicelluloses. All pectins are composed of D-galactopyranosyl uronic acid units linked with α-1,4 bonds, and some also contain araban (a short chain of D-arabinose) and rhamnose units (Atmodjo et al. 2013). The average molecular weight of pectin is 100,000 Da. Many of the carboxyl groups in the galacturonic acid units are esterified with methanol ($-CH_3OH$) or neutralized with calcium or magnesium. Some pectins also have 2-*O*-acetyl, 3-*O*-acetyl, and α-L-rhamnopyranosyl groups on the D-galactopyranosyl uronic acid units. Of note, in a pectin molecule, the C-1 hydroxyl group of the first monosaccharide above the plane of its ring reacts with the C-4 hydroxyl group of the second monosaccharide below the plane of its ring to form the glycosidic linkage (Robyt 1998). This cross-planar bond is not hydrolyzed by animal-source enzymes. However, pectins are hydrolyzed by microbial enzymes and thus are well utilized by ruminants. Pectins have water-holding capacity, and therefore pectins prepared from citrus peels are used to reduce diarrhea in calves. Of note, pectins can also form gels in the presence of $Mg^{2+}$ or $Ca^{2+}$ or at an acidic pH in the presence of high concentrations of sugar.

### Heteropolysaccharides in Animals

#### Definition

Heteropolysaccharides in animals usually contain amino, sulfate, or carboxyl groups. They are important structures in the extracellular matrix and cell membranes (Sinnott 2013). Examples of these substances are glycoaminoglycans, which consist of repeating disaccharide units of uronic acids and 2-acetamido-2-deoxy sugars (Figure 2.14). Such heteropolysaccharides (e.g., hyaluronic acid, chondroitin sulfates, dermatan sulfate, heparan sulfate, heparin sulfate, keratan sulfate, and chitin) are widely present in animals, and most of them are galactans. Those molecules fulfill such important biological functions as: (1) constituents of the organic matter of bones, connective tissue, or substances with blood group specificity; (2) anticoagulants; and (3) cell signaling. The heteropolysaccharides are degraded by exoglycosidases and endoglycosidases to release *N*-acetylglucosamine, which is subsequently converted into glucosamine-6-P, fructose-6-P, and pyruvate in animals (Wu 2013). Glycoaminoglycans are degraded by animal-source digestive enzymes.

#### Hyaluronic Acid

Hyaluronic acid (also called hyaluronan) is a nonsulfated heteropolysaccharide (Viola et al. 2015). It has a linear chain of the repeating disaccharide units of D-glucuronic acid and D-*N*-acetyl-glucosamine linked via alternating β-1,4 and β-1,3 glycosidic bonds. Hyaluronic acid can be 250–25,000 disaccharide repeats in length. Of note, it is a primary glycosaminoglycan that is synthesized by placental cells and present in the placental stroma. This substance plays an important role in: (1) embryonic survival, growth, and development; (2) lubrication of the joints; (3) angiogenesis (the formation of new blood vessels from existing ones); and (4) support of connective tissue in the skin, blood vessels, and bones.

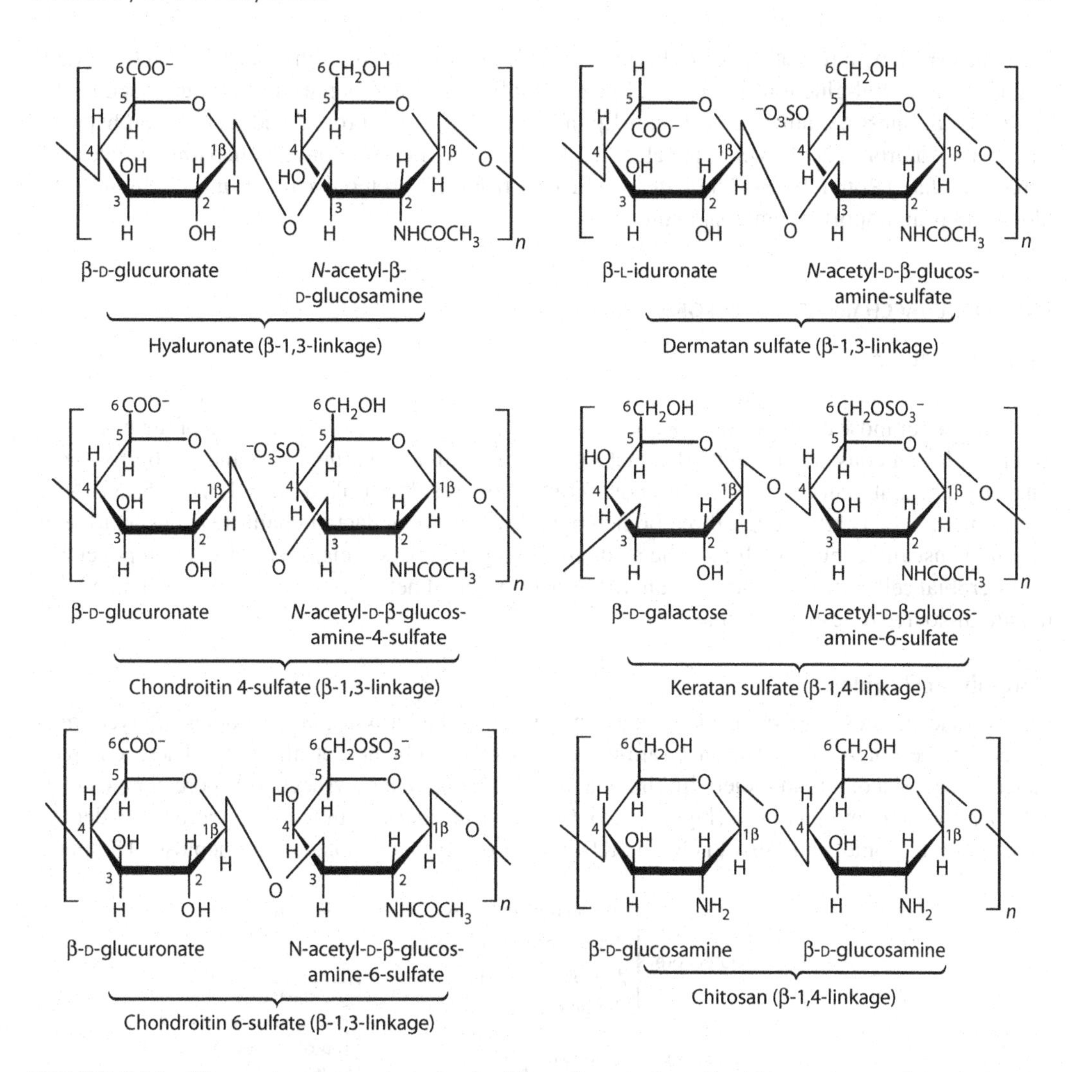


**FIGURE 2.14** Glycoaminoglycans in animals. These heteropolysaccharides are long unbranched polysaccharides consisting of a repeating disaccharide unit. They are widely present in mammals, birds, and fish. Except for keratan, the repeating unit contains an aminosugar (*N*-acetyl-glucosamine or *N*-acetyl-galactosamine) and a uronic sugar (glucuronic acid or iduronic acid) or galactose. Glucuronic acid or galactose is a derivative of D-glucose.

## Sulfated Heteropolysaccharides

Sulfated heteropolysaccharides are abundant components in connective tissue, including chondroitin sulfates, dermatan sulfate, keratan sulfate, and heparan sulfate (Mikami and Kitagawa 2013). Chondroitin sulfates have a repeating disaccharide unit of β-D-glucuronic acid and sulfated *N*-acetyl-galactosamine in β-1,3 and β-1,4 glycosidic linkages, and are major components in cartilage. Dermatan sulfate is a macromolecule with a repeating disaccharide unit of β-D-iduronic acid and sulfated *N*-acetyl-galactosamine in α-1,3 and β-1,4 glycosidic linkages, which is present mainly in the skin. Keratan sulfate is highly unique with the basic repeating disaccharide of β-D-galactose and sulfated *N*-acetyl-glucosamine in β-1,4 glycosidic linkages, and is found mainly in the erythrocytes, cornea, cartilage, and bone.

Heparan sulfate has the most common repeating disaccharide unit of glucuronic acid linked to sulfated *N*-acetyl-glucosamine via β-1,4 bonds in a linear chain, and is present in all animal tissues. It is the second most abundant glycosaminoglycan in placental tissue. In contrast, heparin sulfate is characterized by a repeating disaccharide unit of 2-*O*-sulfated L-iduronic acid and 6-*O*-sulfated, *N*-sulfated *N*-acetyl-glucosamine in α-1,4 glycosidic linkages, and is present in tissues such as the heart, blood, intestine, lungs, and skin. 5-Epimerization of D-glucuronic acid residues on heparan sulfate to L-iduronic acid, which is catalyzed by a C-5 epimerase, converts heparan sulfate into heparin sulfate (Robyt 1998). The latter is released from the proteoglycans of mast cells into the blood and is an important anticoagulant.

## Heteropolysaccharides in Microbes

### Arabinogalactan

In microorganisms, arabinogalactan is a heteropolysaccharide of arabinose and galactose residues solely in the furanose configuration (Knoch et al. 2014). The linear galactan portion of the microbial arabinogalactan consists of about 30 galactose residues with alternating β-1,5 and β-1,6 glycosidic linkages. The arabinan chain, which is about 30 arabinose residues linked via α-1,3, α-1,5, and β-1,2 glycosidic bonds, is attached at three branch points within the galactan chain (residues 8, 10, and 12) and is usually capped with mycolic acids. Arabinogalactan is a major structural component of the microbial cell wall. Arabinogalactan, like other microbial heteropolysaccharides, is indigestible to animal-source digestive enzymes.

### Lipopolysaccharides

Lipopolysaccharides (LPSs), also known as lipoglycans or endotoxins, are examples of glycolipids present in the outer membrane of Gram-negative bacteria (Gnauck et al. 2015). These complex molecules consist of a lipid moiety linking via the α-2,6 bond to a polysaccharide core composed of an inner core and an outer core (Figure 2.15). Common saccharides in the inner core are 3-deoxy-D-mannooctulosonic acid (also known as KDO, keto-deoxy-octulosonate) and heptose. The outer

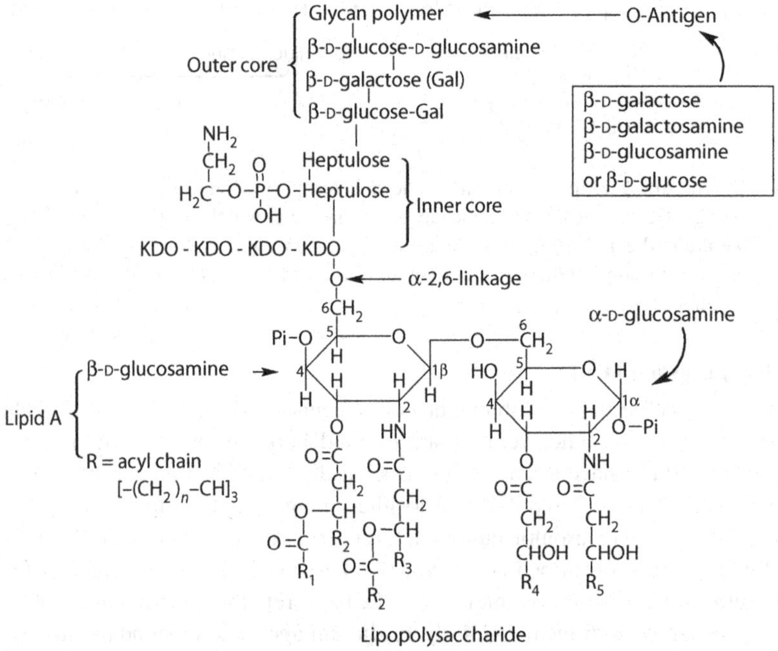

Outer core: Glycan polymer — β-D-glucose-D-glucosamine — β-D-galactose (Gal) — β-D-glucose-Gal
O-Antigen
β-D-galactose
β-D-galactosamine
β-D-glucosamine
or β-D-glucose
Inner core: Heptulose — Heptulose — KDO - KDO - KDO - KDO
α-2,6-linkage
α-D-glucosamine
Lipid A: β-D-glucosamine; R = acyl chain [-(CH2)n-CH]3
Lipopolysaccharide

**FIGURE 2.15** Structure of LPS in the outer membrane of Gram-negative bacteria. LPS (an endotoxin) is a complex carbohydrate that contains sugars, α-D-glucosamine, and lipids. The chemical structures and biological activities of LPS vary by bacterial species or strains.

core contains a repetitive glycan polymer (composed of β-D-Galactose, β-D-galactosamine, β-D-glucosamine, and β-D-glucose) as the *O*-antigen. In addition, α-D-glucosamine is attached to the lipid moiety by covalent bonding. Owing to these unique chemical structures, LPSs are strong stimuli of immune responses in animals.

### Murein

Murein is the major component of carbohydrates in the cell walls of microbes (Fiedler et al. 1973). It is a linear chain of alternating β-1,4-linked *N*-acetyl-glucosamine and *N*-acetyl-muramic acid residues. Murein is cross-linked to short peptides to form a water-insoluble peptidoglycan, which supports the shape and rigidity of bacteria.

### Xanthan

Xanthan is produced by Gram-negative bacteria. It is composed of a repeating pentasaccharide unit containing two D-glucose residues, two D-mannose residues, and one D-glucuronic acid residue (Becker et al. 1998). The two D-glucose residues are joined by the β-1,4-glycosidic bond. A trisaccharide is attached to every other D-glucose residue in the main chain via the α-1,3 bond. This results in a repeating unit of pentasaccharide. The trisaccharide is D-mannopyranosyl linked, via the β-1,4 bond, to D-glucopyranosyl uronic acid, which links to a D-mannopyranosyl residue via the β-1,2 bond. Xanthan is also highly soluble in water.

## Heteropolysaccharides in Algae and Seaweeds (Marine Plants)

Most of the heteropolysaccharides in algae and seaweeds consist of a galactan backbone linked with other sugars, such as D-glucuronic acid, uronic acid, D-manuronic acid, and L-guluronic acid. Thus, these substances are galactan-based heteropolysaccharides. Some of them are sulfated, and others may contain pyruvate and minerals (e.g., Na). Structural heteropolysaccharides in algae and seaweeds are not degraded by animal-source digestive enzymes.

### Agar (or Agar–Agar)

Agar is a mixture of two linear-chain polysaccharides (agaran and agaropectin). It is prepared from red-purple seaweeds (Mišurcová et al. 2012). The chemical structure of agaran is similar to that of κ-carrageenan and *l*-carrageenan, except that: (1) the first residue in the repeating disaccharide unit has no sulfated α-D-galactopyranose; (2) the second residue in the repeating disaccharide unit has the L-configuration instead of the D-configuration; and (3) approximately 20% of the α-D-galactopyranose residues have a 2-*O*-methyl group (Robyt 1998). Since the 3,6-anhydro-galactopyranose in agaran has the L-configuration, it is similar to the 3,6-anhydro-α-D-galactopyranose residue in κ- and *l*-carrageenans, as well as to the L-guluronic acid residue in alginic acid. Thus, agaran consists of repeating units of β-1,3-linked D-galactopyranose and α-1,4-linked 3,6-anhydro-L-galactopyranose. In contrast, agaropectin is a sulfated polysaccharide containing 3%–10% sulfate as ester sulfate, D-glucuronic acid, and small amounts of pyruvic acid (Robyt 1998). The proportion of agaran and agaropectin varies with the species of seaweed. Like other heteropolysaccharides in fungi, yeast, algae, or seaweeds, agar may have a beneficial role as a prebiotic in animal nutrition (Mišurcová et al. 2012; Rajapakse and Kim 2011).

### Algin (Alginic Acid)

Large amounts of algin are present in brown seaweeds, which amount to 20%–40% of their masses. Approximately 15%–20% of algin is localized in the cell wall, and 80%–85% of algin is present between cells. Algin is composed of uronic acid (Robyt 1998), which can exist both in the acid form (–COOH), which is not water soluble, and in the sodium form (–COONa) as sodium alginate, which is water soluble (Tavassoli-Kafrani et al. 2016). Algin is a linear polysaccharide chain consisting of β-D-mannopyranosyl uronic acid and α-L-gulopyranosyl uronic acid in β-1,4-linkages, as well as α-1,4-linkages, with the ratio of D-manuronic acid to L-guluronic acid being 2:1 for most algins (Robyt 1998).

### Carrageenans

Carrageenans are linear chains of D-galactans consisting of sulfated D-galactopyranose and its derivatives in β-1,4- and α-1,3-linkages (Tavassoli-Kafrani et al. 2016). They are the major polysaccharides of red seaweeds (types of algae). Carrageenans are composed of three linear D-galactans: κ-carrageenan, *l*-carrageenan, and λ-carrageenan. κ-Carrageenan has 4-*O*-sulfato-β-D-galactopyranose and 3,6-anhydro-α-D-galactopyranose as the main repeating disaccharide unit. The structure of *l*-carrageenan is similar to that of κ-carrageenan except that the 3,6-anhydro-α-D-galactopyranose molecule (the second residue in the repeating disaccharide unit) in κ-carrageenan is replaced by 3,6-anhydro-2-*O*-sulfato-α-D-galactopyranose in *l*-carrageenan. The structure of λ-carrageenan is similar to that of κ-carrageenan and *l*-carrageenan, except that the repeating disaccharide unit in λ-carrageenan consists of 2-*O*-sulfato-β-D-galactopyranose and 2,6-di-*O*-sulfato-α-D-galactopyranose (Robyt 1998).

## Phenolic Polymers in Plants

### Lignins

Lignins are cross-linked highly methoxylated (–$OCH_3$) phenolic polymers with a high molecular weight in plants (Boerjan et al. 2003). They are not soluble in water and are not carbohydrates. These substances are present in plants (forming tough woody fibers) and some algae, but are absent from animals. Owing to its association with cellulose and hemicellulose, lignin is usually discussed together with carbohydrates in nutrition. Lignin stiffens the cellulose fibers, providing strong structural support for the plant, and constitutes about 5%–10% of the DM of annual plants. Lignin's composition, such as the numbers of 3-phenylpropanol units and methyl groups, and nitrogen content, varies with plant species and maturity. For example, the methoxyl content (–$OCH_3$) of wood lignin is approximately 15%, that of grass lignin is approximately 8%, and that of legume lignin is approximately 5% (Mottiar et al. 2016; Robyt 1998). Lignin is very stable due to its condensed structure and is rarely attacked by microorganisms. Owing to its close association with cellulose and hemicellulose present in forages, lignin reduces their hydrolysis by microbes. However, the methoxyl content of lignin decreases progressively on passage through the ruminant gastrointestinal tract. The digestibility of low-quality forages and straw can be improved by treatment with alkali, which partially dissolves the lignin and breaks the bonds between lignin and cellulose or hemicellulose.

### Tannins

Tannins (also known as tannic acids) are phenolic polymers with numerous hydroxyl groups (–OH) in the plant and have a bitter taste (Sieniawska 2015). They are soluble in water and are not carbohydrates. Thus, there are major differences in the chemical structures and properties between tannins and lignins. Tannins can be classified as hydrolyzable tannins and condensed tannins (proanthocyanidins). The hydrolyzable tannins include taragallotannins (gallic acid and quinic acid) and caffetannins (e.g., caffeic acid and chlorogenic acid). Condensed tannins include cyanidin, delphinidin, malvidin, peonidin, perlargodinin, and petunidin. Tannins can bind protein, irons and other metal ions, carbohydrates, and alkaloids. Thus, a high content of tannins in the diet can decrease feed intake, growth rate, feed efficiency, and protein digestibility in nonruminants, but may protect high-quality dietary protein from rumen degradation in ruminants (Patra and Saxena 2011). Owing to their polyphenolic structures, tannins can scavenge oxygen-free radicals and ameliorate oxidative stress in animals.

### Non-Starch Polysaccharides in Plants, Algae, and Seaweeds

Non-starch polysaccharides (NSPs) include homo- and heteropolysaccharides other than starches in plants, as well as algae and seaweeds. As noted previously, they generally contain linear β-glucans and/or heteropolysaccharides in β-glucosidic linkages. NSPs are abundant in the cell walls of legumes, cereals, forages, and roughages, and are also present in marine plants. NSPs are classified as water soluble or water insoluble according to their solubility in water. Water-soluble NSPs include pectin, inulin,

**TABLE 2.10**
**The Content of Water-Soluble and Insoluble NSPs in Plant-Source Products**

| Feedstuff | Soluble NSPs (g/100 g) | Insoluble NSPs (g/100 g) | Total NSPs (g/100 g) |
|---|---|---|---|
| Apple fiber | 13.9 | 48.7 | 62.6 |
| Bamboo meal | <0.1 | 44.8 | 44.9 |
| Barley bran | 3.0 | 67 | 70 |
| Corn grain (wet weight) | 2.1 | 2.7 | 4.8 |
| Dried raw white beans | 4.3 | 13.4 | 17.7 |
| Kidney beans | 3.0 | 4.0 | 7.0 |
| Oat fiber | 1.5 | 73.6 | 75.1 |
| Oat hulls | 6.7 | 16.4 | 23.1 |
| Palm kernel expeller | 7.7 | 42.3 | 50 |
| Rice bran | 4.7 | 46.7 | 51.4 |
| Rice, brown | 0.8 | 6.0 | 6.8 |
| Rice, white | 0.0 | 0.7 | 0.7 |
| Soybean hulls | 8.4 | 48.3 | 56.7 |
| Tomato fiber | 8.3 | 57.6 | 65.9 |
| Wheat bran (for humans) | 4.6 | 49.6 | 54.2 |
| Wheat bran (for pigs) | 4.1 | 26.5 | 30.6 |

*Source:* Adapted from Chawla, R. and G.R. Patil. 2010. *Compr. Rev. Food Sci. Saf.* 9:178–196; Yu, C. et al. 2016. *Arch. Anim. Nutr.* 70:263–277.

xanthan gum, alginate (as sodium salt), and carrageenans (as sodium salt), whereas water-insoluble NSPs include cellulose, hemicellulose, resistant starch, chitin (marine plants), and lignin. In most plant-source products, insoluble NSPs are much more abundant than soluble NSPs (Table 2.10). Soluble and insoluble NSPs have different nutritional and physiological effects in animals (Grabitke and Slavin 2009). Although NSPs along with lignin are commonly called dietary fiber, this term is a misnomer because they are not all fibrous. Fermentable fiber is the fiber that is resistant to digestion and absorption in the small intestine but is broken down partially or completely by microbes in the large intestine (Gidenne 2015; Turner et al. 2013).

## CHEMICAL REACTIONS OF CARBOHYDRATES

Knowledge about chemical reactions of carbohydrates is useful for their analysis and therefore in conducting nutritional research. Some of these reactions may occur in animals and may provide a biochemical basis for adverse effects of excess carbohydrates in the body. Overall, chemical reactions of carbohydrates are dependent upon their functional groups such as ketones and aldehydes.

### Monosaccharides

#### Epimerization

In alkaline solutions, a monosaccharide is converted into a complex mixture of polyhydroxy aldehydes and polyhydroxy ketones. This reaction forms a pair of epimers at C-2 and therefore is called epimerization.

$$\text{D-Glucose} + {}^{-}\text{OH} \rightarrow \text{D-Mannose (epimerization at C-2)}$$

### Reduction

The carbonyl group of a monosaccharide can be reduced by $NaBH_4$ to form an alditol. For example, D-mannose is reduced to form D-mannitol, and D-fructose is reduced to yield both D-mannitol and D-sorbitol (also known as D-glucitol).

$$\text{D-Mannose} + NaBH_4 + H_3O^+ \rightarrow \text{D-Mannitol}$$

$$\text{D-Fructose} + NaBH_4 + H_3O^+ \rightarrow \text{D-Mannitol} + \text{D-Sorbitol}$$

### Oxidation

1. Oxidation by Tollens' reagent ($Ag^+$, $NH_3$, and $OH^-$). A ketose (–C=O) is converted to an aldose (–CHO) under alkaline conditions. An aldose sugar can be oxidized by Tollens' reagent to form a carboxylate ion. Thus, Tollens' reagent cannot be used to distinguish glucose from fructose.

$$\text{Ketose (e.g., Fructose)} + OH^- \rightarrow \text{Aldose (e.g., Glucose)}$$
$$+ \text{Tollens' reagent} \rightarrow \text{Carboxylate ion}$$

2. Oxidation by Benedict's reagent (sodium carbonate, sodium citrate, and copper (II) sulfate). Under alkaline conditions, an aldose sugar (e.g., glucose) is oxidized to an enediol (–CH=C–OH) by Benedict's reagent. The enediol then reduces the cupric ion ($Cu^{2+}$) to the cuprous ion ($Cu^+$), producing an insoluble brick-red copper (I) oxide ($Cu_2O$). Since a ketose (e.g., fructose) is converted into an aldose under alkaline conditions, Benedict's reagent can also be used to determine the presence of fructose.

$$\text{Ketose (e.g., Fructose)} + OH^- \rightarrow \text{Aldose (e.g., Glucose)}$$
$$+ \text{Benedict's reagent} \rightarrow Cu_2O \downarrow \text{(brick-red)}$$

3. Oxidation by $Br_2$. An aldehyde (e.g., glucose with –CHO) is oxidized by a $Br_2$ aqueous solution (red color) to gluconic acid (–COOH), with $Br_2$ being reduced to 2 $Br^-$ (colorless). A ketose (e.g., fructose) does not react with $Br_2$. Therefore, the red color of a $Br_2$ aqueous solution does not disappear in the presence of a ketose. This assay is useful to distinguish a ketose from an aldehyde.

$$\text{Aldose (e.g., Glucose)} + Br_2 \text{ solution (red color)} \rightarrow \text{Gluconic acid} + 2\ Br^- \text{(colorless)}$$

### Dehydration of Aldoses and Ketoses

A hexose can undergo dehydration under strong acidic conditions and at high temperature to form a hydroxymethyl-furfural. The furfural derivative condenses with two molecules of phenol (e.g., α-naphthol, resorcinol, or thymol) to generate a purple or cherry-red color product. Likewise, a pentose is dehydrated to yield furfural, which can react with anthrone to produce a blue–green color product.

$$\text{Hexose} + HCl \text{ (or } H_2SO_4) \rightarrow \text{Hydroxymethyl-furfural} + 3H_2O$$

$$\text{Pentose} + HCl \text{ (or } H_2SO_4) \rightarrow \text{Furfural} + 3H_2O$$

Dehydration of a ketose is a chemical basis for the determination of fructose in biological samples. Specifically, fructose is dehydrated in the presence of 18% HCl at 80°C to form 5-hydroxymethyl-furfural. The furfural derivative then reacts with resorcinol (a benzenediol) in the presence of alcohol (20% of a solution consisting of 0.5 g resorcinol in 500 mL of 95% ethyl alcohol) to generate a product with a cherry-red color. Under these conditions, no color develops when glucose is present in the assay mixture. This is a satisfactory method for fructose analysis in deproteinized plasma, urine, semen, and fetal fluid.

$$\text{Fructose} + \text{HCl} \rightarrow \text{5-Hydroxymethyl-furfural} + 3H_2O$$

## Formation of Glycosides

A hemiacetal (e.g., D-glucose) or hemiketal (e.g., D-fructose) reacts with an alcohol to form an acetal (e.g., β-D-glucoside and α-D-glucoside) or ketal (e.g., β-D-fructofuranoside and α-D-fructofuranoside). As noted previously, a hemiketal monosaccharide is a nonreducing sugar and cannot be oxidized by $Ag^+$ or $Br_2$. A glycoside of glucose, galactose, or fructose is called a glucoside, galactoside, or fructofuranoside, respectively. An example for the formation of a glycoside from glucose and alcohol is given as follows.

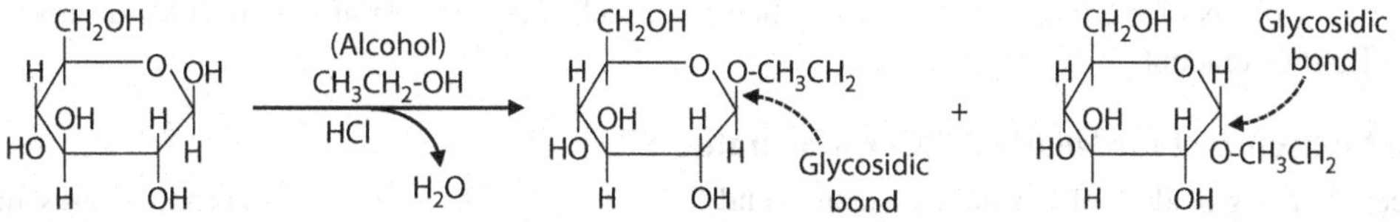

(Alcohol) $CH_3CH_2$-OH, HCl, $H_2O$; Glycosidic bond

β-D-glucose (β-D-glucopyranose) *a hemiacetal* → Ethyl-β-D-glucose (Ethyl-β-D-glucopyranose) *a glycoside and an acetal* + Ethyl-α-D-glucose (Ethyl-α-D-glucopyranose) *a glycoside and an acetal*

## Esterification

Esterification occurs chemically when an –OH group of a carbohydrate reacts with a –COOH group of a fatty acid in the presence of a catalyst (e.g., sulfuric acid) to form an ester. This reaction can be catalyzed by enzymes in cells. Glycerides, which are fatty acid esters of glycerol, are important esters in biology. Sulfate esters of galactose or glucosamine are present predominantly in proteoglycans of animals.

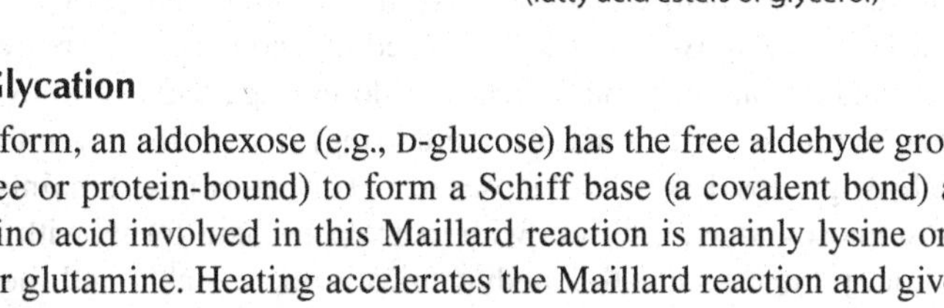

Glycerol ($CH_2OH$–$CH_2OH$–$CH_2OH$) + 3 R-$CH_2$-COOH (Fatty acid) → Glycerides (fatty acid esters of glycerol) ($CH_2O$-C(=O)-$CH_2$-R ×3) + 3 $H_2O$

## Nonenzymatic Glycation

In the open-chain form, an aldohexose (e.g., D-glucose) has the free aldehyde group that reacts with an amino acid (free or protein-bound) to form a Schiff base (a covalent bond) and then Amadori products. The amino acid involved in this Maillard reaction is mainly lysine or arginine, but can also be histidine or glutamine. Heating accelerates the Maillard reaction and gives rise to melanoidin polymers (brown color), which are not digestible by animals. Thus, nonenzymatic glycation has very important implications in feed pelleting and animal nutrition.

$$\text{D-Glucose } (-CHO, \text{open-chain}) + \varepsilon\text{-}NH_2 \text{ in Lysine}$$
$$\rightarrow \text{Schiff base } (-CH{=}N\text{-Lysine}) \rightarrow \text{Glycation}$$

### Disaccharides and Polysaccharides

#### Oxidation

Benedict's reagent can react with reducing disaccharides (e.g., lactose and maltose) as indicated previously, but not with nonreducing disaccharides (e.g., sucrose). However, sucrose can be hydrolyzed to D-glucose and D-fructose, if heated with dilute HCl. Subsequently, both glucose and fructose can be detected by Benedict's reagent. Starches and glycogen react very poorly with Benedict's reagent because they have only a limited number of reducing sugar moieties at the ends of their chains. Inositol (myoinositol) is another carbohydrate that cannot be detected by this assay.

#### Reacting with Iodine

Starch or glycogen reacts with Lugol's reagent (I-KI; iodine dissolved in an aqueous solution of potassium iodide) to give rise to a blue–black or brown–blue color, respectively. The intensity of the color decreases with increasing temperature and with the presence of water-miscible organic solvents (e.g., ethanol). The principle of this assay is that iodine binds to the helices of starch or glycogen to form a starch–iodine or glycogen–iodine complex, respectively. The helices of starch are longer than those of glycogen, therefore binding more iodine atoms and generating a more intense color, as compared with glycogen. This test should not be performed at very low pH due to the hydrolysis of starch and glycogen. Other polysaccharides and monosaccharides do not react with Lugol's reagent.

#### The Molisch Test for Nearly All Carbohydrates

Except for sugar alcohols, 2-deoxy sugars, and 2-amino-2-deoxy sugars, all carbohydrates in an aqueous solution are determined by the Molisch test (Robyt 1998). In this relatively broad assay with good specificity for carbohydrates, concentrated sulfuric acid hydrolyzes the glycosidic bonds in oligosaccharides or polysaccharides to monosaccharides. In the presence of the strong acid ($H_2SO_4$), monosaccharides are dehydrated to generate furfural derivatives, which condense with α-naphthol (a phenolic compound) to produce a characteristic purple color. The detection limit of the Molisch test for carbohydrates is 10 mg/L. 2-Deoxy sugars and 2-amino-2-deoxy sugars can be analyzed by high-performance liquid chromatography and mass spectrometry.

## SUMMARY

Carbohydrates are polyhydroxy aldehydes or ketones, as well as their amidated or sulfated derivatives (e.g., glucosamine, *N*-acetyl-glucosamine, and dermatan sulfate). They are important components of plants, animals, and microorganisms (Table 2.11). Carbohydrates can be classified into two types: simple or complex. Simple carbohydrates are monosaccharides (single sugars), which cannot be broken down by hydrolysis reactions. D-Glucose (an aldose), which is synthesized from $CO_2$ and $H_2O$ in green plants and from many glucogenic precursors in animals, is the most abundant single sugar in nature, followed by D-fructose (a ketose). All hexose monosaccharides (6-carbon sugars), either aldoses or ketoses, have an α- or β-isomer (called an anomer). A carbohydrate can spontaneously change its α- and β-configuration in water. Aldoses (e.g., D-glucose) exist predominantly as cyclic hemiacetals (pyranoses with a six-membered ring) in equilibrium with their open-chain forms with free aldehyde groups. Likewise, ketoses (e.g., D-fructose) exist mainly as cyclic hemiketals (pyranoses or furanoses) in equilibrium with their open-chain forms with ketone structures. In an aqueous solution, pyranoses are thermodynamically more stable and more abundant than furanoses.

Complex carbohydrates include disaccharides (e.g., lactose and sucrose), oligosaccharides (consisting of 3 or 10 monosaccharide units), and polysaccharides (e.g., starch, glycogen, cellulose, hemicellulose, and pectin). In main chains, monosaccharides are bonded primarily through α-1,4 and/or α-1,6 glycosidic linkages (starch and glycogen) or β-1,3 and β-1,4 glycosidic linkages (other complex

**TABLE 2.11**
**Glycosidic Linkages in Polysaccharides**

| Polysaccharide | Source | Monomer | Main Chain | Branch Linkages |
|---|---|---|---|---|
| **Homopolysaccharides** | | | | |
| Arabinan | Plants | D-Arabinose | α-1-3, α-1-5, β-1-2 | – |
| Amylose of starch | Green plants | D-Glucose | α-1,4 | – |
| Amylopectin of starch | Green plants | D-Glucose | α-1,4 | α-1,6 |
| Cellulose | Plants, others[a] | D-Glucose | β-1,4 | – |
| Chitin | Animals, others[b] | AGlcN | β-1,4 | – |
| Dextrans | Some bacteria | D-Glucose | α-1,6 | α-1,3 |
| Galactan | Plants | D-Galactose | β-1,4 | – |
| Galactan | Microbes | D-Galactose | | – |
| β-D-Glucans | Yeast, other fungi | D-Glucose | β-1,3 | β-1,6 |
| β-D-Glucans | Barley, oat | D-Glucose | β-1,3, β-1,4 | – |
| β-D-Glucans | Lichens | D-Glucose | β-1,3, β-1,6 | – |
| Glycogen | Animals, others[c] | D-Glucose | α-1,4 | α-1,6 |
| Mannans | Certain bacteria | D-Mannose | α-1,3 | α-1,2, β-1,6 |
| Mannans | Green algae | D-Mannose | β-1,4 | – |
| Mannans | Plants | D-Mannose | β-1,4 | – |
| Mannans | Yeast, other fungi | D-Mannose | α-1,6 | α-1,2, α-1,3 |
| Pullutan | Yeast, other fungi | D-Glucose | α-1,4, α-1,6 | – |
| **Heteropolysaccharides** | | Main sugars | | |
| Alginate | Seaweeds | MAN + GU | β-1,4 + α-1,4 | – |
| Agar | Red seaweeds | D-Galactose | β-1,4 + α-1,3 | – |
| Arabinogalactan | Plants | D-Arabinose +D-Galactose | α-1,5 α-1,4 or β-1,4 | β-1,3, β-1,6 |
| Arabinogalactan | Microbes | D-Arabinose +D-Galactose | α-1-3, α-1-5, β-1-2 β-1-5, β-1-6 | β-1,3, β-1,6 |
| Carageenan | Red seaweeds | G4S + G2S | β-1,4 + α-1,3 | – |
| Chondroitin sulfate | Animals | GlcN + AGN | β-1,3, β-1,4 | – |
| Dermatan sulfate | Animals | Idu + AGN | β-1,3, β-1,4 | – |
| Galactomannan | Plants | D-mannose (B) +D-galactose | β-1,4 | α-1,6 |
| Galactoglucomanann | Plants | D-Mannose (B) +D-galactose (S) +D-glucose (S) | β-1,4 | α-1,6 |
| Glucomannan | Plants | D-mannose (B) +D-glucose | β-1,4 | β-1,6, α-1,6 |
| Hemicellulose | Plants | Hexoses[d] | β-1,4, α-1,2 | – |
| Hyaluronan | Animals | GA + AGlcN | β-1,4, α-1-3 | – |
| Inulin | Plant tubers | D-Fructose | β-2,1 | – |
| Mannans | Plants | D-Mannose | β-1,4 | β-1,6, α-1,6 |
| Murein | Bacteria | AGlcN + AM | β-1,4 | – |
| Pectin | Green plants | GAU + others | β-1,4 + others | – |
| Xanthan | Bacteria | Hexoses[e] | β-1,4, α-1-3 | – |
| Xylans | Plants, others[f] | D-Xylose | β-1,3 | – |

[a] Some bacteria also contain cellulose.
[b] Fungi (including yeasts), green algae, as well as brown and red seaweeds (types of algae) also contain chitin.
[c] Bacteria, fungi (including yeasts), protozoa, and the blue–green algae also contain glycogen.
[d] Including β-D-xylopyranose, β-D-xylose, β-D-mannose, β-D-arabinose, β-D-glucose, β-D-galactose, and uronic acid.
[e] Including D-glucose, D-mannose, and V-glucuronic acid.
[f] Brown seaweeds also contain xylans.

AGlcN, *N*-acetyl-glucosamine; AGN, *N*-acetyl-D-galactosamine; AM, *N*-acetyl-D-muramic acid; B, backbone chain; GA, glucuronic acid; GlcN, D-glucosamine; GAU, D-galacturonate; GU, D-guluronate; G4S, D-galactose-4-sulfate; G2S, 3,6-anhydro-D-galactose-2-sulfate; Idu, α-L-iduronate; MAN, D-mannuronate; S, side chain.

carbohydrates). Starch and glycogen are the main homopolysaccharides in plants and animals, respectively. Other homopolysaccharides include cellulose, β-D-glucans, levans, mannans in plants, and chitin in animals. Heteropolysaccharides include: (1) exudate gums, hemicelluloses, inulins, mannans, mucilages, and pectins in plants; (2) hyaluronic acid, chondroitin sulfates, dermatan sulfate, heparan sulfate, heparin sulfate, keratan sulfate, and chitin in animals; (3) LPSs, murein, and xanthan in microbes; and (4) agar, algin (alginic acid), and carrageenans in algae and seaweeds. Except for lactose (with a galactosyl β-1,4-linkage) which is hydrolyzed by the small intestine-derived lactase, complex carbohydrates with D-glucosyl- or D-fructosyl β-1,4-linkages or dietary fibers are generally not broken down by animal-source enzymes but are fermented by microbes to varying degrees in the large intestine. NSPs are an important component of the diets for land-based animals to maintain their gut health. Although lignins and tannins are not carbohydrates, they are usually associated with polysaccharides in plants to affect their digestion in the gastrointestinal tract of animals.

Monosaccharides undergo chemical reactions, such as epimerization, reduction, oxidation, dehydration, formation of glycosides, esterification, and glycation, whereas starch or glycogen, but not other complex carbohydrates, can bind to and react with iodine to form a colored product. These reactions provide the bases for the determination of certain types of carbohydrates in feedstuffs and animals. Except for a few sugar alcohols, all carbohydrates in an aqueous solution can be analyzed by the Molisch test. Optimal animal feeding must be designed to ensure: (1) adequate supply of plant-source fibers and starch for post-weaning animals; (2) sufficient synthesis of glucose, glycogen, and heteropolysaccharides in all animals; and (3) maximum production of lactose in milk for mammals. Knowledge about the chemistry of carbohydrates provides a foundation for our understanding of their metabolism and nutrition in animals (Chapter 5).

## REFERENCES


Akhter, S., M.S. Ansari, B.A. Rakha, S.M.H. Andrabi, M. Qayyum, and N. Ullah. 2014. Effect of fructose in extender on fertility of buffalo semen. *Pakistan J. Zool.* 46:279–281.

Angyal, S.J. 1984. The composition of reducing sugars in solution. *Adv. Carbohydr. Chem. Biochem.* 42:15–68.

Apolinário, A.C., B.P. de Lima Damasceno, N.E. de Macêdo Beltrão, A. Pessoa, A. Converti, and J.A. da Silva. 2014. Inulin-type fructans: A review on different aspects of biochemical and pharmaceutical technology. *Carbohydr. Polym.* 101:368–378.

Arifkhodzhaev, A.O. 2000. Galactans and galactan-containing polysaccharides of higher plants. *Chem. Nat. Compd.* 36:229–244.

Aspinall, G.O. 1967. The exudate gums and their structural relationship to other groups of plant polysaccharides. *Pure Appl. Chem.* 14:43–55.

Atmodjo, M.A., Z. Hao, and D. Mohnen. 2013. Evolving views of pectin biosynthesis. *Annu. Rev. Plant Biol.* 64:747–779.

Bacon, J.S.D. and D.J. Bell. 1948. Fructose and glucose in the blood of the foetal sheep. *Biochem. J.* 42:397–405.

Bali, V., P.S. Panesar, M.B. Bera, and R. Panesar. 2015. Fructo-oligosaccharides: Production, purification and potential applications. *Crit. Rev. Food Sci. Nutr.* 55:1475–1490.

Barceló-Fimbres, M. and G.E. Seidel. 2008. Effects of embryo sex and glucose or fructose in culture media on bovine embryo development. *Reprod. Fertil. Dev.* 20:141–142.

Baronos, S. 1971. Seminal carbohydrates in boar and stallion. *J. Reprod. Fertil.* 24:303–305.

Bazer, F.W., T.E. Spencer, and W.W. Thatcher. 2012. Growth and development of the ovine conceptus. *J. Anim. Sci.* 90:159–170.

Bazer, F.W., W.W. Thatcher, F. Martinat-Botte, and M. Terqui. 1988. Conceptus development in large white and prolific Chinese Meishan pigs. *J. Reprod. Fertil.* 84:37–42.

Bearden, H.J. and J.W. Fuquay. 1980. *Applied Animal Reproduction.* Reston Publishing Company, Reston, Virginia.

Becker, A., F. Katzen, A. Pühler, and L. Ielpi. 1998. Xanthan gum biosynthesis and application: A biochemical/genetic perspective. *Appl. Microbiol. Biotechnol.* 50:145–152.

Benkeblia, N. 2013. Fructooligosaccharides and fructans analysis in plants and food crops. *J. Chromatogr. A.* 1313:54–61.

Bergman, E.N. 1983a. The pools of tissue constituents and products: Carbohydrates. In: *World Animal Science*. Edited by P.M. Riis, Elsevier, New York, Vol. 3, pp. 137–149.

Bergman, E.N. 1983b. The pool of cellular nutrients: Glucose. In: *World Animal Science*. Edited by P.M. Riis, Elsevier, New York, Vol. 3, pp. 173–196.

Boerjan, W., J. Ralph, and M. Baucher. 2003. Lignin biosynthesis. *Annu. Rev. Plant Biol.* 54:519–546.

Britton, H.G. 1962. Some non-reducing carbohydrates in animal tissues and fluids. *Biochem. J.* 85:402–407.

Brosnan, J.T. 2005. Metabolic design principles: Chemical and physical determinants of cell chemistry. *Adv. Enzyme Regul.* 45:27–36.

Bruice, P.Y. 2011. *Organic Chemistry*. Prentice Hall, New York, NY.

Cao, H., T. Chen, and Y. Shi. 2015. Glycation of human serum albumin in diabetes: Impacts on the structure and function. *Curr. Med. Chem.* 22:4–13.

Chandrasekaran, R. 1998. X-ray diffraction of food polysaccharides. *Adv. Food Nutr. Res.* 42:131–210.

Chawla, R. and G.R. Patil. 2010. Soluble dietary fiber. *Compr. Rev. Food Sci. Saf.* 9:178–196.

Cheng, K.C., A. Demirci, and J.M. Catchmark. 2011. Pullulan: Biosynthesis, production, and applications. *Appl. Microbiol. Biotechnol.* 92:29–44.

Demura, T. and Z.H. Ye. 2010. Regulation of plant biomass production. *Curr. Opin. Plant Biol.* 13:299–304.

Denzel, M.S. and A. Antebi. 2015. Hexosamine pathway and (ER) protein quality control. *Curr. Opin. Cell Biol.* 33:14–18.

Ege, S. 1984. *Organic Chemistry*. D.C. Heath and Company, Toronto, Canada.

Egusa, M., H. Matsui, T. Urakami, S. Okuda, S. Ifuku, H. Nakagami, and H. Kaminaka. 2015. Chitin nanofiber elucidates the elicitor activity of polymeric chitin in plants. *Front. Plant Sci.* 6:1098.

Farrokhi, N., R.A. Burton, L. Brownfield, M. Hrmova, S.M. Wilson, A. Bacic, and G.B. Fincher. 2006. Plant cell wall biosynthesis: Genetic, biochemical and functional genomics approaches to the identification of key genes. *Plant Biotechnol. J.* 4:145–167.

Fiedler, F., K. Schleifer, and O. Kandler. 1973. Amino acid sequence of the threonine-containing mureins of coryneform bacteria. *J. Bacteriol.* 113:8–17.

Fincher, G.B., W.H. Sawyer, and B.A. Stone. 1974. Properties of an arabinogalactan-peptide from wheat endosperm. *Biochem. J.* 139:535–545.

Frei, E and R.D. Preston. 1968. Non-cellulosic structural polysaccharides in algal cell walls. III. Mannan in siphoneous green algae. *Proc. R Soc. B.* 169:127–145.

Gaschen, F.P. and S.R. Merchant. 2011. Adverse food reactions in dogs and cats. *Vet. Clin. North Am. Small Anim. Pract.* 41:361–379.

Geraci, J.R. 1981. Dietary disorders in marine mammals: Synthesis and new findings. *J. Am. Vet. Med. Assoc.* 179:1183–1191.

Gidenne, T. 2015. Dietary fibres in the nutrition of the growing rabbit and recommendations to preserve digestive health: A review. *Animal* 9:227–242.

Gnauck, A., R.G. Lentle, and M.C. Kruger. 2015. The characteristics and function of bacterial lipopolysaccharides and their endotoxic potential in humans. *Int. Rev. Immunol.* 25:1–31.

Grabitke, H.A. and J.L. Slavin. 2009. Gastrointestinal effects of low-digestible carbohydrates. *Crit. Rev. Food Sci. Nutr.* 49:327–360.

Guo, S., W. Mao, Y. Han, X. Zhang, C. Yang, Y. Chen et al. 2010. Structural characteristics and antioxidant activities of the extracellular polysaccharides produced by marine bacterium *Edwardsiella tarda*. *Bioresour. Technol.* 101:4729–4732.

Hagely, K.B., D. Palmquist, and K.D. Bilyeu. 2013. Classification of distinct seed carbohydrate profiles in soybean. *J. Agric. Food Chem.* 61:1105–1111.

Hamman, H., J. Steenekamp, and J. Hamman. 2015. Use of natural gums and mucilages as pharmaceutical excipients. *Curr. Pharm. Des.* 21:4775–4797.

Heaney, R.P. 2013. Dairy intake, dietary adequacy, and lactose intolerance. *Adv. Nutr.* 4:151–156.

Henry, R.J. and H.S. Saini. 1989. Characterization of cereal sugars and oligosaccharides. *Cereal Chem.* 66:362–365.

Hinton, B.T., R.W. White, and B.P. Setchell. 1980. Concentrations of myo-inositol in the luminal fluid of the mammalian testis and epididymis. *J. Reprod. Fert.* 58:395–399.

Hitchcock, M.W.S. 1949. Fructose in the sheep fetus. *J. Physiol.* 108:117–126.

Keeling, P.L. and A.M. Myers. 2010. Biochemistry and genetics of starch synthesis. *Annu. Rev. Food Sci. Technol.* 1:271–303.

Kim, J.Y., G.W. Song, G. Wu, and F.W. Bazer. 2012. Functional roles of fructose. *Proc. Natl. Acad. Sci. USA* 109:E1619–E1628.

Knoch, E., A. Dilokpimol, and N. Geshi. 2014. Arabinogalactan proteins: Focus on carbohydrate active enzymes. *Front. Plant Sci.* 5:198.

Koehler, P. and H. Wieser. 2013. Chemistry of cereal grains. In: *Handbook of Sourdough Biotechnology*. Edited by M. Gobbetti and M. Gänzle. Springer, New York, pp. 11–45.

Li, N., D.N. Wells, A.J. Peterson, and R.S.F. Lee. 2005. Perturbations in the biochemical composition of fetal fluids are apparent in surviving bovine somatic cell nuclear transfer pregnancies in the first half of gestation. *Biol. Reprod.* 73:139–148.

Li, S., L. Lei, Y.G. Yingling, and Y. Gu. 2015. Microtubules and cellulose biosynthesis: The emergence of new players. *Curr. Opin. Plant Biol.* 28:76–82.

Lu, Y. and T.D. Sharkey. 2006. The importance of maltose in transitory starch breakdown. *Plant Cell Environ.* 29:353–366.

Lunn, J.E., I. Delorge, C.M. Figueroa, P. Van Dijck, and M. Stitt. 2014. Trehalose metabolism in plants. *Plant J.* 79:544–567.

McDonald, P., R.A. Edwards, J.F.D. Greenhalgh, J.F.D. Greenhalgh, C.A. Morgan, and L.A. Sinclair. 2011. *Animal Nutrition*, 7th ed. Prentice Hall, New York.

Melton, L.D., B.G. Smith, R. Ibrahim, and R. Schröder. 2009. Mannans in primary and secondary plant cell walls. *N. Z. J. Forestry Sci.* 39:153–160.

Messer, M., E. Trifonoff, W. Stern, and J.W. Bradbury. 1980. Structure of a marsupial milk trisaccharide. *Carbohydrate Res.* 83:327–334.

Mikami, T. and H. Kitagawa. 2013. Biosynthesis and function of chondroitin sulfate. *Biochim. Biophys. Acta.* 1830:4719–47133.

Mišurcová, L., S. Škrovánková, D. Samek, J. Ambrožová, and L. Machů. 2012. Health benefits of algal polysaccharides in human nutrition. *Adv. Food Nutr. Res.* 66:75–145.

Moreira, L.R. and E.X. Filho. 2008. An overview of mannan structure and mannan-degrading enzyme systems. *Appl. Microbiol. Biotechnol.* 79:165–178.

Mottiar, Y., R. Vanholme, W. Boerjan, J. Ralph, and S.D. Mansfield. 2016. Designer lignins: Harnessing the plasticity of lignification. *Curr. Opin. Biotechnol.* 37:190–200.

National Research Council. 2001. *Nutrient Requirements of Dairy Cattle*, 7th Revised ed. National Academy Press, Washington, DC.

National Research Council (NRC). 2012. *Nutrient Requirements of Swine*. National Academy Press, Washington, DC.

Patra, A.K. and J. Saxena. 2011. Exploitation of dietary tannins to improve rumen metabolism and ruminant nutrition. *J. Sci. Food Agric.* 91:24–37.

Peterbauer, T., J. Mucha, L. Mach, and A. Richter. 2002. Chain elongation of raffinose in pea seeds. Isolation, characterization, and molecular cloning of multifunctional enzyme catalyzing the synthesis of stachyose and verbascose. *J. Biol. Chem.* 277:194–200.

Pond, W.G., D.B. Church, K.R. Pond, and P.A. Schoknecht. 2005. *Basic Animal Nutrition and Feeding*, 5th ed. Wiley, New York.

Rajapakse, N. and S.K. Kim. 2011. Nutritional and digestive health benefits of seaweed. *Adv. Food Nutr. Res.* 64:17–28.

Rezaei, R., Z.L. Wu, Y.Q. Hou, F.W. Bazer, and G. Wu. 2016. Amino acids and mammary gland development: Nutritional implications for neonatal growth. *J. Anim. Sci. Biotechnol.* 7:20.

Roach, P.J., A.A. Depaoli-Roach, T.D. Hurley, and V.S. Tagliabracci. 2012. Glycogen and its metabolism: Some new developments and old themes. *Biochem. J.* 441:763–787.

Robyt, J.F. 1998. *Essentials of Carbohydrate Chemistry*. Springer, New York.

Römling, U. and M.Y. Galperin. 2015. Bacterial cellulose biosynthesis: Diversity of operons, subunits, products, and functions. *Trends Microbiol.* 23:545–557.

Ruan, Y.L. 2014. Sucrose metabolism: Gateway to diverse carbon use and sugar signaling. *Annu. Rev. Plant Biol.* 65:33–67.

Rumessen, J.J. 1992. Fructose and related food carbohydrates. Sources, intake, absorption, and clinical implications. *Scand. J. Gastroenterol.* 27:819–828.

Scheller, H.V. and P. Ulvskov. 2010. Hemicelluloses. *Annu. Rev. Plant Biol.* 61:263–289.

Schirren, C. 1963. Relation between fructose content of semen and fertility in man. *J. Reprod. Fertil.* 5:347–358.

Sengupta, S., S. Mukherjee, P. Basak, and A.L. Majumder. 2015. Significance of galactinol and raffinose family oligosaccharide synthesis in plants. *Front. Plant Sci.* 6:656.

Shelton, D.R. and W.J. Lee. 2000. Cereal carbohydrates. In: *Handbook of Cereal Science and Technology*. Edited by K. Kulp and J.G. Ponte, Jr. Marcell Dekker, New York, pp. 385–414.

Sieniawska, E. 2015. Activities of tannins: From *in vitro* studies to clinical trials. *Nat. Prod. Commun.* 10:1877–1884.

Sinnott, M. 2013. *Carbohydrate Chemistry and Biochemistry: Structure and Mechanism*, 2nd ed. Royal Society of Chemistry, London, UK.

Smith, A.M., S.C. Zeeman, and S.M. Smith. 2005. Starch degradation. *Annu. Rev. Plant Biol.* 56:73–98.

Srikanth, R., C.H. Reddy, G. Siddartha, M.J. Ramaiah, and K.B. Uppuluri. 2015. Review on production, characterization and applications of microbial levan. *Carbohydr. Polym.* 120:102–114.

Tavassoli-Kafrani, E., H. Shekarchizadeh, and M. Masoudpour-Behabadi. 2016. Development of edible films and coatings from alginates and carrageenans. *Carbohydr. Polym.* 137:360–374.

Trindade, C.E., R.C. Barreiros, C. Kurokawa, and G. Bossolan. 2011. Fructose in fetal cord blood and its relationship with maternal and 48-hour-newborn blood concentrations. *Early Hum. Dev.* 87:193–197.

Turner, N.D., L.E. Ritchie, R.S. Bresalier, and R.S. Chapkin. 2013. The microbiome and colorectal neoplasia—environmental modifiers of dysbiosis. *Curr. Gastroenterol. Rep.* 15(9):1–16.

van Arkel, J., R. Sévenier, J.C. Hakkert, H.J. Bouwmeester, A.J. Koops, and I.M. van der Meer. 2013. Tailor-made fructan synthesis in plants: A review. *Carbohydr. Polym.* 93:48–56.

Viola, M., D. Vigetti, E. Karousou, M.L. D'Angelo, I. Caon, P. Moretto, G. De Luca, and A. Passi. 2015. Biology and biotechnology of hyaluronan. *Glycoconj. J.* 32:93–103.

Wang, X.Q., G. Wu, and F.W. Bazer. 2016. mTOR: The master regulator of conceptus development in response to uterine histotroph during pregnancy in ungulates. In: *Molecules to Medicine with mTOR*. Edited by K. Maiese. Elsevier, New York, pp. 23–35.

Wang, Y., H. Yu, X. Shi, Z. Luo, D. Lin, and M. Huang. 2013. Structural mechanism of ring-opening reaction of glucose by human serum albumin. *J. Biol. Chem.* 288:15980–15987.

Wu, G. 2013. *Amino Acids: Biochemistry and Nutrition*. CRC Press, Boca Raton, Florida.

Yin, F., Z. Zhang, J. Huang, and Y.L. Yin. 2010. Digestion rate of dietary starch affects systemic circulation of amino acids in weaned pigs. *Br. J. Nutr.* 103:1404–1412.

Younes, I. and M. Rinaudo. 2015. Chitin and chitosan preparation from marine sources. Structure, properties and applications. *Mar. Drugs* 13:1133–1174.

Yu, C., S. Zhang, Q. Yang, Q. Peng, J. Zhu, X. Zeng, and S. Qiao. 2016. Effect of high fibre diets formulated with different fibrous ingredients on performance, nutrient digestibility and faecal microbiota of weaned piglets. *Arch. Anim. Nutr.* 70:263–277.

Zhang, G. and B.R. Hamaker. 2009. Slowly digestible starch: Concept, mechanism, and proposed extended glycemic index. *Crit. Rev. Food Sci. Nutr.* 49(10): 852–867.

# 3 Chemistry of Lipids

Lipids are defined as hydrocarbon compounds that are soluble in organic solvents (e.g., chloroform and ethanol) and, except for some small molecules, are generally insoluble in water (Gunstone 2012). These substances are highly reduced molecules, with the highest proportions of hydrogen atoms among all dietary macronutrients. Since lipids are classified solely on the basis of their hydrophobic properties, they have diverse chemical structures and biological functions. In nature, examples of lipids are fatty acids, triacylglycerols (TAGs), glycerolipids, glycerophospholipids, sphingolipids, cholesterol, cortisol, testosterone, progesterone, and vitamin A (Mead et al. 1986). Lipids account for 1%–50% of the body weights of animals, depending on their species, age, nutritional state, and disease (Cherian 2015; Pond et al. 2005). Plants and algae are excellent sources of fatty acids that are not synthesized by animals (NRC 2011, 2012). In proximate feedstuff analysis, lipids are determined together as the ether extract and are called crude fats.

Lipids are important structural and cellular components in plants, animals, and microorganisms. These substances are widely distributed in the cell membrane and the membranes of intracellular organelles to control the transport of gases, nutrients, ions, and metabolites into and out of cells (Ridgway and McLeod 2016). In animals, TAGs are the major form of energy storage, and fatty acids are the primary metabolic fuels for such key organs as the liver, skeletal muscle, and heart, while facilitating the digestion and absorption of fat-soluble vitamins (Conde-Aguilera et al. 2013; Smith and Smith 1995). In neonates, subcutaneous white adipose tissue insulates the body from the loss of heat. In many mammals, brown adipose tissue oxidizes fatty acids to produce large amounts of heat, thereby keeping the body warm during the neonatal period (Smith and Carstens 2005; Satterfield and Wu 2011). In all biological organisms, lipids serve as signaling molecules to regulate physiological processes. However, excessive fats also contribute to a variety of metabolic disorders and chronic diseases, including obesity, diabetes, and cardiovascular disease.

Our current knowledge of lipids has been built on the shoulders of the pioneers of the field (Block et al. 1946; Mead et al. 1986). The nineteenth century witnessed great discoveries of lipids in nature. In 1813, M.E. Chevreul reported the composition of animal fats and proposed the concept of fatty acids. Ten years later, this same author published a landmark book on the chemistry of lipids, in which he described several straight-chain fatty acids (margaric, oleic, stearic, butyric, and caproic acids) and a branched-chain fatty acid, isovaleric acid, which was isolated from the head oil of the dolphin and from porpoise oil. In 1884, Couerbe J-P introduced the method of using diethyl ether to extract lipids from animal tissues, which facilitated research in the field. G.O. Burr (1929) discovered linoleic acid, a long-chain fatty acid (LCFA), as a nutritionally essential fatty acid for the growth and health of young rats. Subsequently, Wesson and Burr (1931) reported that animals do not synthesize α-linolenic acid or linoleic acid. In the 1940s, K.E. Bloch discovered the synthesis of cholesterol from acetate in the liver. These ground-breaking findings ushered in a new era of lipid nutrition research in the twentieth century (Field et al. 2008; Kessler et al. 1970; Pedersen 2016; Spector and Kim 2015; Tso 1985; Wood and Harlow 1960). This chapter highlights the chemistry of lipids pertinent to animal nutrition.

## CLASSIFICATION AND STRUCTURES OF LIPIDS

Lipids are classified into four groups: fatty acids, simple lipids, compound lipids, and derived lipids (Figure 3.1). Fatty acids, also known as precursor lipids, include those fatty acids with various numbers of carbons and unsaturated double bonds. Some of them have *cis*, *trans*, or both types of the chemical configuration (Ma et al. 1999), whereas others may have a branched methyl group. Along

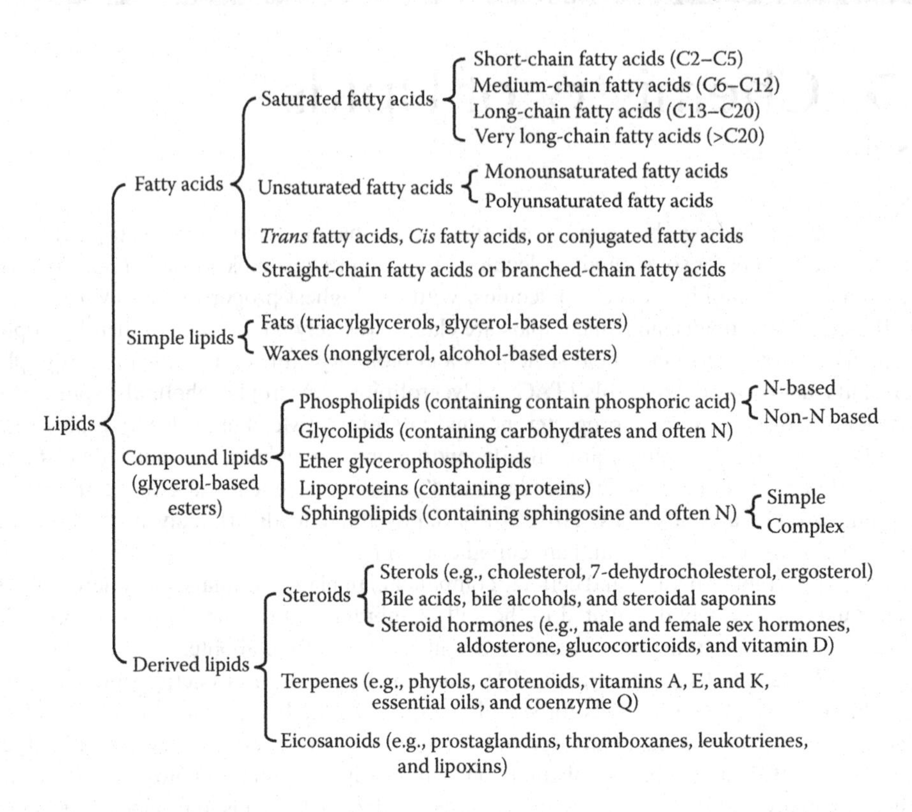


**FIGURE 3.1** Classification of lipids in animal nutrition. Lipids are composed of fatty acids (precursor lipids), as well as simple, compound, and derived lipids. Serine, choline, and ethanolamine are often components of phospholipids and sphingolipids. N, nitrogen.

with glycerol (1,2,3-propanetriol), alcohols, serine, sphingosine, choline, and ethanolamine, fatty acids are used to synthesize all other lipids in animals (Ridgway and McLeod 2016).

Simple lipids consist of fats and oils (esters of fatty acids [usually LCFAs] with glycerol) and waxes (esters of fatty acids [usually LCFAs] with fatty alcohols). Fats differ from waxes in both chemical and biochemical properties (Rijpstra et al. 2007; Schreiber 2010). Fats are also called TAGs or triglycerides because all three hydroxyl groups of glycerol are esterified to a glycerol backbone. In plants, oils are fats in the liquid state, with the fatty acids being primarily polyunsaturated fatty acids (PUFAs) (Mead et al. 1986).

$$\begin{array}{l} CH_2OH \\ | \\ CH_2OH \\ | \\ CH_2OH \\ \text{Glycerol} \end{array} + 3\,\underset{\text{Fatty acid}}{R\text{–}CH_2\text{–}COOH} \longrightarrow \begin{array}{l} CH_2O\text{–}C(=O)\text{–}CH_2\text{–}R \\ | \\ CH_2O\text{–}C(=O)\text{–}CH_2\text{–}R \\ | \\ CH_2O\text{–}C(=O)\text{–}CH_2\text{–}R \\ \text{Glycerides} \\ \text{(fatty acid esters of glycerol)} \end{array} + 3\,H_2O$$

Compound lipids are glycerol-based esters of fatty acids (e.g., usually LCFAs) that contain phosphoric acid (i.e., phospholipids and ether phospholipids), carbohydrates (i.e., glycolipids), sphingosine (i.e., simple and complex sphingolipids), and proteins (i.e., lipoproteins). Compound lipids often contain nitrogen in the form of choline, ethanolamine, or serine (Guidotti 1972; Ridgway and McLeod 2016). Like simple lipids, compound lipids are saponifiable in plants, bacteria, and animals.

Derived lipids include steroids, eicosanoids, and terpenes (carotenoids, coenzyme Q, vitamins A, E, and K, essential oils, and phytols). Except for steroidal saponins which are present in plants, other steroids such as sterols (e.g., cholesterol), steroid hormones (e.g., male and female reproductive hormones), bile acids, and bile alcohols are formed in animals (Pond et al. 2005). Terpenes (carotenoids, coenzyme Q, vitamins E and K, essential oils, and phytols) are produced by plants and frequently consumed by animals (Pichersky 2006). Vitamin A is formed from carotenoids in animals. In contrast, eicosanoids (prostaglandins [PGs], thromboxanes [TXs], leukotrienes [LTs], and lipoxins) are synthesized from LCFAs in nearly all cell types, particularly the endothelium, smooth muscle, and brain.

Lipids have structural, storage, regulatory, protective, secretory, and transport functions in animals. For example, excess energy is stored as fats in all animals (Bergen and Mersmann 2005). Insulation of the body by fats is crucial for keeping newborns warm and for protecting adult animals from the cold. In sperm whales, large amounts of lipids in the head may detect sound waves in the water. Fats are required for the digestion and absorption of lipid-soluble vitamins (Pond et al. 2005). Furthermore, phospholipids are signaling molecules that regulate nutrient metabolism, whereas lipoproteins play an important role in the interorgan transport of TAGs, cholesterol, and other lipids. Deficiencies of nutritionally essential fatty acids result in skin lesions, growth restriction, and diseases, but excess TAGs in white adipose tissue and excess cholesterol in plasma are the major causes of obesity and insulin resistance in animals (Fox et al. 2002; Hausman et al. 1982).

# Fatty Acids

## Definition of Fatty Acids

Fatty acids are hydrocarbon chains with 2 or more carbon atoms and a carboxyl group (Figure 3.2). The early isolation of these substances from animal fats led to the term "fatty acids." More than 300

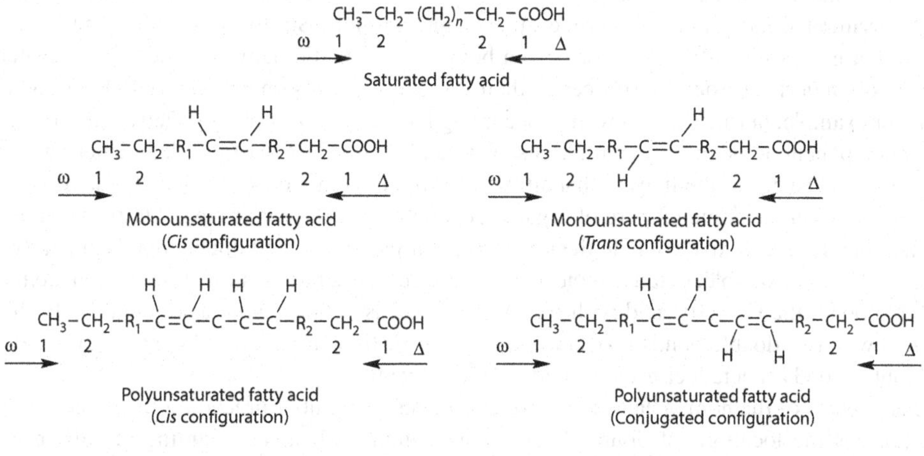

$CH_3{-}CH_2{-}(CH_2)_n{-}CH_2{-}COOH$

ω 1 2 → ... ← 2 1 Δ

Saturated fatty acid

$CH_3{-}CH_2{-}R_1{-}C(H){=}C(H){-}R_2{-}CH_2{-}COOH$

ω 1 2 → ... ← 2 1 Δ

Monounsaturated fatty acid
(*Cis* configuration)

$CH_3{-}CH_2{-}R_1{-}C(H){=}C(H){-}R_2{-}CH_2{-}COOH$

ω 1 2 → ... ← 2 1 Δ

Monounsaturated fatty acid
(*Trans* configuration)

$CH_3{-}CH_2{-}R_1{-}C(H){=}C(H){-}C{-}C(H){=}C(H){-}R_2{-}CH_2{-}COOH$

ω 1 2 → ... ← 2 1 Δ

Polyunsaturated fatty acid
(*Cis* configuration)

$CH_3{-}CH_2{-}R_1{-}C(H){=}C(H){-}C{-}C(H){=}C(H){-}R_2{-}CH_2{-}COOH$

ω 1 2 → ... ← 2 1 Δ

Polyunsaturated fatty acid
(Conjugated configuration)

**FIGURE 3.2** Nomenclature of fatty acids. Fatty acids are named according to delta (Δ), omega (ω), common (nonsystematic), and systematic (scientific) nomenclatures. In the Δ nomenclature, the carbon atom of the carboxyl group is counted as C-1. In the ω nomenclature, the carbon atom of the terminal methyl group is counted as C-1. Common names for fatty acids were often derived from the sources of their discoveries, whereas systematic names of fatty acids are given by following the nomenclature of organic chemistry. Saturated fatty acids have no double bond. Fatty acids with one or more double bonds are called mono- or poly-unsaturated fatty acids. Unsaturated fatty acids are grouped as: (1) *cis* fatty acids, with the hydrogen atoms being on the same side of the double bond; (2) *trans* fatty acids, with the hydrogen atoms being on the opposite side of the double bond; and (3) conjugated fatty acids, with at least one pair of double bonds being separated by only one carbon atom. Most naturally occurring fatty acids have the *cis* configuration, although the prefix "*cis*" is often omitted.

fatty acids have been isolated from plants and animals (Gunstone 2012). According to the length of the carbon chain, fatty acids are categorized as: (1) short-chain fatty acids (SCFAs) with 2–5 carbon atoms; (2) medium-chain fatty acids (MCFAs) with 6–12 carbon atoms; (3) LCFAs with 13–20 carbon atoms; and very LCFAs with more than 20 carbon atoms.

On the basis of the number of double bonds in the carbon chain, fatty acids are classified as: (1) saturated fatty acids without a double bond; (2) monounsaturated fatty acids with one double bond; and (3) PUFAs with two or more double bonds (Mead et al. 1986). Owing to the different structures of the double bonds, fatty acids are grouped as: (1) *cis* fatty acids, with the hydrogen atoms being on the same side of the double bond; (2) *trans* fatty acids, with the hydrogen atoms being on the opposite side of the double bond; and (3) conjugated fatty acids, with at least one pair of double bonds being separated by only one carbon atom (Barnes et al. 2012; Brandebourg and Hu 2005).

Most naturally occurring fatty acids have an even number of carbons because of their synthesis from acetyl-CoA (a 2-carbon compound), and are unbranched (Table 3.1). However, some fatty acids have an odd number of carbons or a branched chain. Additionally, most fatty acids contain *cis* double bonds, because fatty acid desaturases in plants and animals cannot produce *trans* double bonds. The solubility and acidity (ionization of the carboxyl group) of fatty acids in water decrease markedly with the length of the carbon chain (Table 3.2). The diversity of fatty acids fulfills their versatile nutritional and physiological functions in animals (Clandinin 1999; Swift et al. 1988).

### Nomenclature of Fatty Acids

There are four naming systems used for fatty acids: delta (Δ) nomenclature, omega (ω) nomenclature, common (nonsystematic) names, and systematic (scientific) names (Gunstone 2012). In the delta nomenclature, the carbon atom of the carboxyl group is counted as C-1, and the number of the carbon (e.g., C-9) in the first double bond is indicated by "Δ" plus the number of the carbon (e.g., Δ9) (Figure 3.3). In the omega nomenclature, the carbon atom of the terminal methyl group is accounted as C-1, and the number of the carbon (e.g., C-3) in the first double bond is indicated by "ω" or "n-" plus the number of the carbon (e.g., "ω3" or "n-3") (Figure 3.3). There are ω3, ω6, ω7, and ω9 unsaturated fatty acids in microbes, plants, and animals (Smith and Smith 1995).

Common names for fatty acids were given before a systematic naming system was developed, and were often derived from the sources of their discoveries (Ralston and Hoerr 1942; Mead et al. 1986). For example, lauric acid is a widely occurring fatty acid in *Lauraceae* seeds, palmitic acid is a major component of the oil from palm trees, oleic acid is abundant in olive oil, and melissic acid is abundant in the nectar of the flowers that attract bees (melissa in Greek). Systematic names of fatty acids are based on the nomenclature of organic chemistry. Greek prefixes (e.g., *di*, *tri*, *tetra*, *penta*, *hexa*, and *octa*) are used to designate the numbers of carbon atoms and double bonds in a fatty acid (Bruice 2011). For example, octadecanoic acid (stearic acid) is a fatty acid with 18 carbon atoms and no double bond, the $C_{18}$ fatty acid with one double bond is octadec*enoic* acid (oleic acid), the $C_{18}$ fatty acid with two double bonds is octadeca*dienoic* acid (linoleic acid), and the $C_{18}$ fatty acid with three double bonds is octadeca*trienoic* acid (linolenic acid).

Other aspects of the nomenclature deserve comments. A number preceding the name of a fatty acid indicates the locations of double bonds. For example, when the counting of carbon atoms begins from the carboxyl group, 9,12-octadeca*dienoic* acid is a fatty acid with 18 carbon atoms with two double bonds being located between carbons 9 and 10 and between carbons 12 and 13. In addition, the salt of a fatty acid (e.g., oleic acid) has a name ending with "-ate" (e.g., ole*ate*). The composition of fatty acids in common feedstuffs for animals is listed in Table 3.3.

### Short-Chain Fatty Acids

SCFAs are volatile organic substances, including acetic, propionic, butyric, isobutyric, valeric, and isovaleric acids. They are highly soluble in water and are present in the rumen and blood of ruminants as products of carbohydrate and amino acid fermentation (Rook 1964). Since silages (e.g., corn, sorghum, and other cereals) are fermented during long-term storage at high moisture,

**TABLE 3.1**
**Fatty Acids Commonly Present in Feedstuffs and Animals**

| Common Name | Systematic Name (Δ Nomenclature for Unsaturated Fatty Acids; Carboxyl Group = C-1) | Number of Carbons | Number of Double Bonds | Symbols of Fatty Acids |
|---|---|---|---|---|
| | **Saturated Fatty Acids** | | | |
| Acetic acid | Ethanoic acid | 2 | 0 | C2:0 |
| Propionic acid | Propanoic acid | 3 | 0 | C3:0 |
| Butyric acid | Butanoic acid | 4 | 0 | C4:0 |
| Isobutyric acid | 2-Methylpropanoic acid | 4 | 0 | C4:0[a] |
| Valeric acid | Pentanoic acid | 5 | 0 | C5:0 |
| Isovaleric acid | 3-Methylbutanoic acid | 5 | 0 | C5:0[b] |
| Caproic acid | Hexanoic acid | 6 | 0 | C6:0 |
| Caprylic acid | Octanoic acid | 8 | 0 | C8:0 |
| Capric acid | Decanoic acid | 10 | 0 | C10:0 |
| Lauric acid | Dodecanoic acid | 12 | 0 | C12:0 |
| Myristic acid | Tetradecanoic acid | 14 | 0 | C14:0 |
| Palmitic acid | Hexadecanoic acid | 16 | 0 | C16:0 |
| Stearic acid | Octadecanoic acid | 18 | 0 | C18:0 |
| Arachidic acid | Eicosanoic acid | 20 | 0 | C20:0 |
| Behenic acid | Docosanoic acid | 22 | 0 | C22:0 |
| Lignoceric acid | Tetracosanoic acid ($C_{23}H_{47}COOH$) | 24 | 0 | C24:0 |
| Melissic acid | Triacontanoic acid ($C_{29}H_{59}COOH$) | 30 | 0 | C30:0 |
| | **Unsaturated Fatty Acids (All Double Bonds Are *Cis*)** | | | |
| Palmitoleic acid | 9-Hexadecenoic acid | 16 | 1 | C16:1 (ω7) |
| Oleic acid | 9-Octadecenoic acid | 18 | 1 | C18:1 (ω9) |
| Linoleic acid | 9,12-Octadecadienoic acid | 18 | 2 | C18:2 (ω6) |
| α-Linolenic acid | 9,12,15-Octadecatrienoic acid | 18 | 3 | C18:3 (ω3) |
| γ-Linolenic acid | 6,9,12-Octadecatrienoic acid | 18 | 3 | C18:3 (ω6) |
| Arachidonic acid | 5,8,11,14-Eicosatetraenoic acid | 20 | 4 | C20:4 (ω6) |
| Timnodonic acid | EPA | 20 | 5 | C20:5 (ω3) |
| Cervonic acid | DHA | 22 | 6 | C22:6 (ω3) |
| Nervonic acid | 15-Tetracosenoic acid | 24 | 1 | C24:1 (ω9) |

[a] $(CH_3)_2$–CH–COOH.
[b] $(CH_3)_2$–CH–$CH_2$–COOH.
EPA, 5,8,11,14,17-Eicosapentaenoic acid.
DHA, 5,8,11,14,17,20-Docosahexaenoic acid.

they contain SCFAs. Valeric acid is also found naturally in the perennial flowering plant valerian. Production of SCFAs by ruminal bacteria is crucial for ruminant nutrition. Butyrate is a major metabolic fuel for colonocytes and also plays an important role in the health of the large intestine.

## Medium-Chain Fatty Acids

MCFAs account for approximately 58.7% and 56.4% of total fatty acids in coconut oil and palm kernel oil, respectively (Table 3.4). MCFAs with 6 carbons have a good solubility in water, whereas those with 8–12 carbons have a much lower solubility in water. At physiological temperatures and concentrations, MCFAs are soluble in water (Odle 1997). Approximately 10%–20% of the fatty

**TABLE 3.2**
**Melting Points of Fatty Acids and Their Solubility in Water**

| Fatty Acid | Molecular Weight (Daltons) | Melting Point (°C) | Solubility in Water (g/100 mL) | |
|---|---|---|---|---|
| | | | 20°C | 30°C |
| | **Saturated Fatty Acids** | | | |
| Acetic acid (C2:0) | 60.05 | 16.5 | Miscible | Miscible |
| Propionic acid (C3:0) | 74.08 | −20.5 | Miscible | Miscible |
| Butyric acid (C4:0) | 88.11 | −5.1 | Miscible | Miscible |
| Isobutyric acid (C4:0) | 88.11 | −47 | Miscible | Miscible |
| Valeric acid (C5:0) | 102.13 | −34.5 | 4.03 | 5.03 |
| Isovaleric acid (C5:0) | 102.13 | −29.3 | 4.07 | 5.27 |
| Caproic acid (C6:0) | 116.16 | −3.4 | 0.968 | 1.02 |
| Caprylic acid (C8:0) | 144.21 | 16.7 | 0.068 | 0.079 |
| Capric acid (C10:0) | 172.27 | 31.6 | 0.015 | 0.018 |
| Lauric acid (C12:0) | 200.32 | 44.2 | 0.0055 | 0.0063 |
| Myristic acid (C14:0) | 228.38 | 53.9 | 0.0020 | 0.0024 |
| Palmitic acid (C16:0) | 256.43 | 63.1 | 0.00072 | 0.00083 |
| Stearic acid (C18:0) | 284.48 | 69.6 | 0.00029 | 0.00034 |
| Arachidic acid (C20:0) | 312.54 | 75.5 | Insoluble | Insoluble |
| Behenic acid (C22:0) | 340.59 | 81.0 | Insoluble | Insoluble |
| Lignoceric acid (C24:0) | 368.63 | 86.0 | Insoluble | Insoluble |
| Melissic acid (C30:0) | 452.46 | 93.0 | Insoluble | Insoluble |
| | **Unsaturated Fatty Acids (All Double Bonds Are *Cis*)** | | | |
| Palmitoleic acid (C16:1, ω7) | 254.41 | −0.5 | Insoluble | Insoluble |
| Oleic acid (C18:1, ω9) | 282.47 | 13.4 | Insoluble | Insoluble |
| Linoleic acid (C18:2, ω6) | 280.45 | −5 | Insoluble | Insoluble |
| α-Linolenic acid (C18:3, ω3) | 278.44 | −11 | Insoluble | Insoluble |
| γ-Linolenic acid (C18:3, ω6) | 278.44 | −11 | Insoluble | Insoluble |
| Arachidonic acid (C20:4, ω6) | 304.47 | −49.5 | Insoluble | Insoluble |
| Timnodonic acid (EPA, C20:5, ω3) | 302.45 | −53.5 | Insoluble | Insoluble |
| Cervonic acid (DHA, C22:6, ω3) | 328.49 | −44.0 | Insoluble | Insoluble |
| Nervonic acid (C24:1, ω9) | 366.62 | 42.5 | Insoluble | Insoluble |

*Source:* Adapted from Bruice, P.Y. *Organic Chemistry*. Prentice Hall, Boston, 2011; Lehninger, A.L. et al. 1993. *Principles of Biochemistry*, Worth Publishers, New York, NY, 1993; Mead, J.F. et al. 1986. *Lipids: Chemistry, Biochemistry, and Nutrition*, Plenum Press, New York; Ralston, A.W. and C.W. Hoerr. 1942. *J. Org. Chem.* 7:546–555.

EPA, 5,8,11,14,17-Eicosapentaenoic acid.

DHA, 5,8,11,14,17,20-Docosahexaenoic acid.

acids in the milk of horses, cows, sheep, and goats are MCFAs (Breckenridge and Kuksis 1967; Park and Haenlein 2006). Owing to their solubility in water, these nutrients are absorbed from the small intestine into the portal vein.

### Long-Chain Fatty Acids

LCFAs are generally insoluble in water. They include saturated fatty acids (e.g., palmitic, stearic, and arachidic acids) and unsaturated fatty acids (e.g., palmitoleic, oleic, linoleic, α-linolenic, γ-linolenic, and arachidonic acids). In cells, myristic acid is covalently linked to some proteins, and

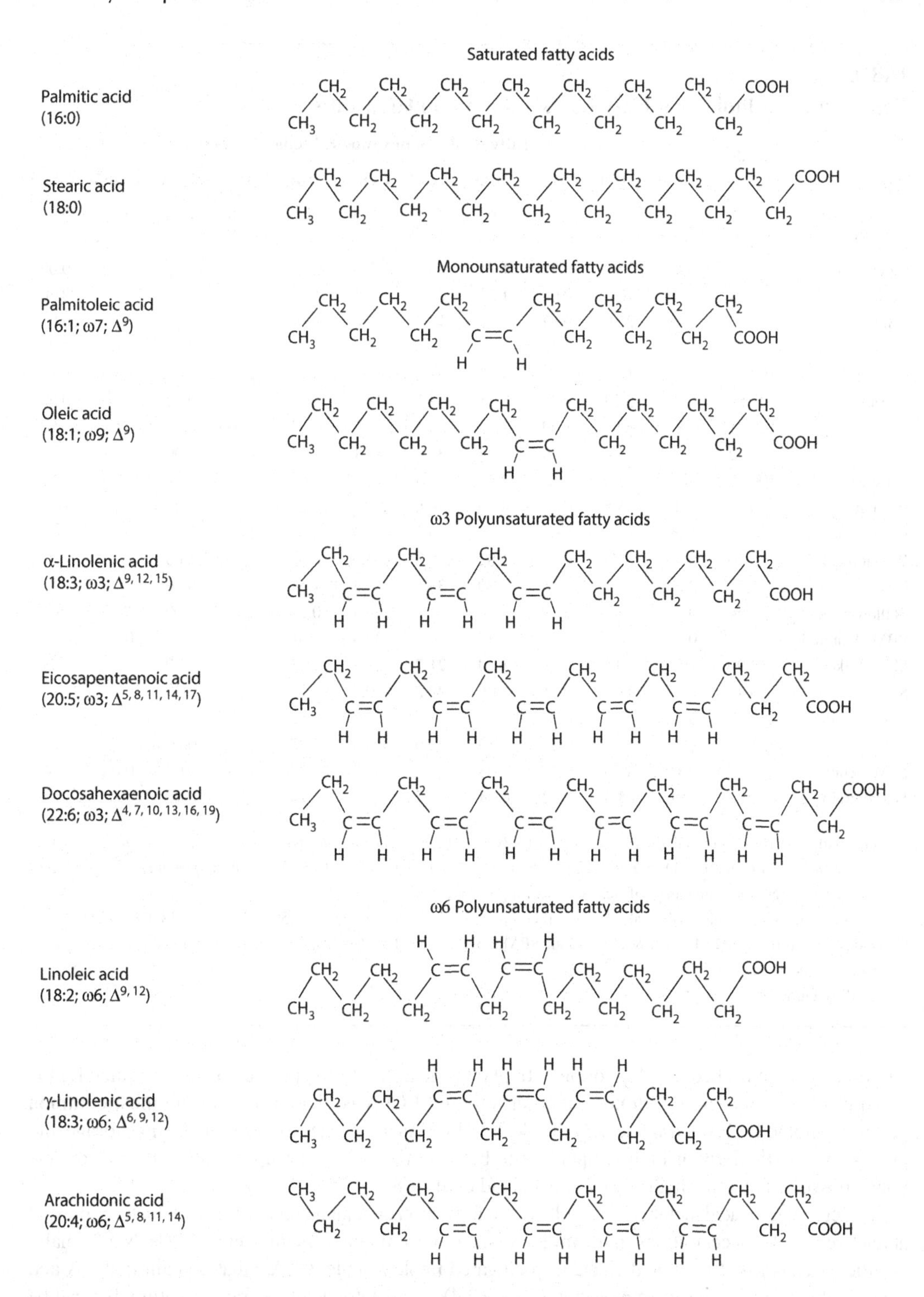


**FIGURE 3.3** Saturated, monounsaturated (ω7 or ω9), ω3 polyunsaturated, and ω6 polyunsaturated fatty acids. In most animals, a double bond can be formed in an LCFA between its Δ1 and Δ9 carbons but not beyond the Δ9 carbon. α-Linolenic acid (ω3) is the precursor of eicosapentaenoic acid and docosahexaenoic acid in animals, but is not synthesized by animals. Linoleic acid (ω6) is the precursor of γ-linolenic acid and arachidonic acid in animals, but is not synthesized by animals. Thus, α-linolenic acid and linoleic acid are nutritionally essential fatty acids in animals.

**TABLE 3.3**
**Composition of Individual Fatty Acids in Common Foodstuffs**

| Type | Crude Fat[a] (%) | Fatty Acids, % of Crude Fat (Ether Extract) | | | | | | | | | | |
|---|---|---|---|---|---|---|---|---|---|---|---|---|
| | | C14:0 | C16:0 | C16:1 | C18:0 | C18:1 | C18:2 | C18:3 | C18:4 | C20:0 | C20:5 | C22:6 |
| Alfalfa meal | 1.70 | 0.95 | 12.8 | 0.70 | 1.90 | 2.20 | 9.65 | 18.5 | 0.00 | 1.80 | 0.00 | 0.00 |
| Beef oil | 100 | 5[b] | 28 | – | 22.5 | 40 | 3 | – | – | – | – | – |
| Canola oil | 100 | 0.10 | 3.99 | 0.38 | 1.71 | 55.1 | 19.5 | 9.31 | 0.00 | 0.00 | 0.00 | 0.00 |
| Corn grain | 3.48 | 0.00 | 12.0 | 0.08 | 1.58 | 26.3 | 44.2 | 1.37 | – | – | – | 0.00 |
| CSM | 5.50 | 0.88 | 22.0 | 0.67 | 2.22 | 17.3 | 46.6 | 0.19 | – | 0.00 | 0.00 | 0.00 |
| Feather meal | 5.97 | 1.00 | 17.4 | 3.10 | 6.90 | 20.0 | 1.65 | 0.00 | 0.00 | 0.00 | 0.00 | 0.00 |
| Fish oil | 100 | 7.3 | 19.0 | 9.0 | 4.2 | 13.2 | 1.3 | 0.3 | 2.80 | – | 11.0 | 9.1 |
| Flaxseed | 33.8 | 0.02 | 5.14 | 0.06 | 3.15 | 17.5 | 14.0 | 54.1 | – | 0.12 | 0.00 | 0.00 |
| MBM | 9.21 | 1.89 | 19.3 | 2.59 | 13.4 | 28.5 | 2.52 | 0.63 | 0.00 | 1.05 | 0.00 | 0.00 |
| Oats | 5.42 | 0.22 | 15.0 | 0.19 | 0.94 | 31.4 | 35.1 | 1.61 | – | 0.00 | – | – |
| Olive oil | 100 | 0.0 | 11.0 | 0.8 | 2.2 | 72.5 | 7.9 | 0.6 | – | – | – | – |
| Palm oil | 100 | 1.0 | 43.5 | 0.3 | 4.3 | 36.6 | 9.1 | 0.2 | – | – | – | – |
| Palm kernel oil | 100 | 16.0 | 8.2 | 0.00 | 2.5 | 15.3 | 2.5 | 0.2 | 0.00 | | | |
| Peanut meal | 6.50 | 0.00 | 8.73 | 0.00 | 1.82 | 39.8 | 26.0 | 0.00 | – | 0.00 | – | – |
| Rice | 1.30 | 0.36 | 17.1 | 0.36 | 1.80 | 35.9 | 34.3 | 1.51 | – | 0.00 | – | – |
| Safflower meal | 2.24 | 0.08 | 6.03 | 0.08 | 2.18 | 11.3 | 65.9 | 0.25 | – | 0.00 | – | – |
| SBM, dehulled | 6.64 | 0.08 | 7.88 | 0.15 | 2.85 | 16.3 | 39.8 | 5.55 | 0.00 | 0.00 | 0.00 | 0.00 |
| Skim milk | 0.90 | 10.8 | 30.5 | 2.86 | 11.0 | 21.7 | 2.47 | 1.43 | – | 0.00 | – | – |
| Sorghum | 3.42 | 0.27 | 12.3 | 0.88 | 1.06 | 29.2 | 40.0 | 1.97 | – | 0.00 | – | – |
| Soybean oil | 100 | 0.1 | 10.3 | 0.2 | 3.8 | 22.8 | 51.0 | 6.8 | – | – | – | – |
| SPC | 1.05 | 0.22 | 8.26 | 0.22 | 2.83 | 17.0 | 38.5 | 5.22 | – | 0.00 | – | – |
| SFM, dehulled | 2.90 | 0.15 | 4.73 | 0.30 | 3.23 | 15.2 | 48.7 | 0.23 | 0.00 | 0.00 | 0.00 | 0.00 |
| Wheat grain | 1.82 | 0.06 | 15.2 | 0.52 | 0.84 | 12.5 | 39.0 | 1.75 | – | 0.00 | – | – |

*Source:* Adapted from National Research Council (NRC). 2012. *Nutrient Requirements of Swine, National Academy of Science*, Washington, DC; and National Research Council (NRC). 2011. *Nutrient Requirements of Fish and Shrimp*, National Academy of Science, Washington, DC.

[a] Expressed on a wet-weight basis. Palm kernel oil contains 0.3% C6:0, 3.6% C8:0, 3.5% C10:0, and 48.3% C12:0.

CSM, cottonseed meal; MBM, meat & bone meal; SBM, soybean meal (45% CP); SFM, sunflower meal (40% CP); SPC, soy protein concentrate (65% CP).

[b] Including lauric acid.

nervonic acid is enriched in sphingolipids. In plants and animals, the most common saturated LCFA is palmitic acid, the most common monounsaturated LCFA is oleic acid, and the most common polyunsaturated LCFA is linoleic acid (Table 3.3). PUFAs are prone to oxidation during storage and processing, particularly at high temperatures, because the $-CH_2-$ group between the two double bonds possesses reactive hydrogen atoms (Mead et al. 1986).

In bacteria, fatty acid metabolism results in the formation of conjugated fatty acids, which are present at relatively high concentrations in the milk and meat of ruminants (Bauman et al. 2011). Nutritionally significant conjugated fatty acids include conjugated linoleic acids (CLAs) that contain both *cis* and *trans* double bonds in the same molecule (Figure 3.4). *Trans* fatty acids are rare in nature, but can be produced during food processing and may have adverse effects on animal health. *Cis* fatty acids with 16–18 carbons comprise the bulk of the fatty acids in TAGs and compound lipids (Tan et al. 2011). Concentrations of *cis*- and *trans*-unsaturated fatty acids in cow's milk are shown in Table 3.5. Note that *trans*-unsaturated fatty acids are normally not found in the milk of nonruminants. Most naturally occurring fatty acids have the *cis* configuration, and the word "*cis*" is often omitted.

**TABLE 3.4**
**Types of Fatty Acids in Foodstuffs**

| Type of Fatty Acid | % Saturated | % Monounsaturated | % Polyunsaturated |
|---|---|---|---|
| | **Mostly Saturated** | | |
| Beef fat | 52 | 40 | 8 |
| Butter | 66 | 30 | 4 |
| Coconut oil[a] | 92 | 6 | 2 |
| Meat & bone meal | 51 | 44 | 5 |
| Palm oil | 52 | 37 | 11 |
| Palm kernel[b] | 83 | 15 | 2 |
| Skim milk powder | 66 | 29 | 5 |
| | **Mostly Monounsaturated** | | |
| Canola (rapeseed) oil | 7 | 62 | 31 |
| Chicken fat | 31 | 47 | 22 |
| Lard (pork fat) | 41 | 47 | 12 |
| Margarine, hard | 21 | 50 | 29 |
| Olive oil | 14 | 73 | 13 |
| Peanut oil | 18 | 46 | 36 |
| Rice | 21 | 40 | 39 |
| Sesame seed oil | 18 | 42 | 40 |
| Vegetable shortening (hydrogenated) | 27 | 50 | 33 |
| | **Mostly Polyunsaturated** | | |
| Alfalfa meal | 40 | 6 | 54 |
| Barley | 25 | 14 | 61 |
| Corn oil | 13 | 24 | 63 |
| Cottonseed oil | 27 | 18 | 55 |
| Fish oil, Menhaden | 33 | 25 | 42 |
| Flaxseed (linseed oil) | 9 | 19 | 72 |
| Margarine, soft | 13 | 26 | 61 |
| Margarine, tub | 19 | 35 | 46 |
| Oats | 19 | 37 | 44 |
| Safflower oil | 10 | 12 | 78 |
| Sorghum | 16 | 35 | 49 |
| Soybean oil | 15 | 23 | 62 |
| Soy protein concentrate | 16 | 24 | 60 |
| Sunflower oil | 11 | 20 | 69 |
| Wheat grain | 23 | 19 | 58 |

*Source:* Adapted from National Research Council (NRC). 2012. *Nutrient Requirements of Swine*, National Academy of Science, Washington DC; and National Research Council (NRC). 2011. *Nutrient Requirements of Fish and Shrimp*, National Academy of Science, Washington DC.

[a] Saturated fatty acids with $\leq$12 carbons account for 58.7% of total fatty acids.

[b] Saturated fatty acids with $\leq$12 carbons account for 56.4% of total fatty acids.

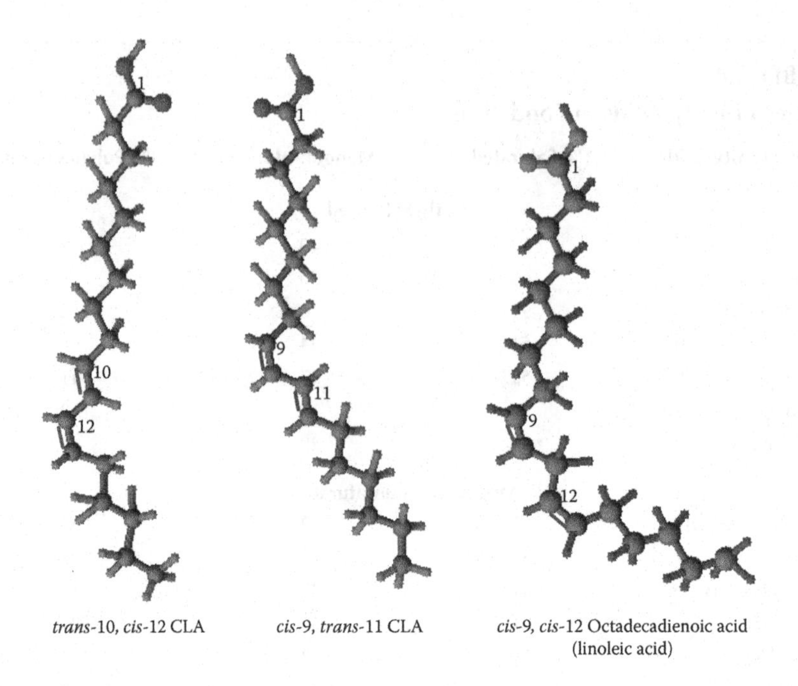


**FIGURE 3.4** Conjugated fatty acids. These fatty acids are formed by bacteria (e.g., ruminal bacteria) and are present at relatively high concentrations in ruminant milk and tissues. CLA, conjugated linoleic acid. *Cis*-linoleic acid is shown for comparison.

**TABLE 3.5**
**The Major Fatty Acids of Bovine and Sow's Milk**

| Fatty Acid | Bovine Milk | Sow's Milk |
|---|---|---|
| | Weight Percentage (%) of Total Fatty Acids | |
| 4:0 | 3.25 | – |
| 6:0 | 2.28 | – |
| 8:0 | 1.57 | – |
| 10:0 | 3.36 | – |
| 12:0 | 4.11 | 2 ($C_2$-$C_{12}$) |
| 14:0 | 13.13 | 2 |
| 14:1, *cis*-9 | 0.95 | – |
| 15:0 | 1.10 | – |
| 16:0 | 32.58 | 28 |
| 16:1, *cis*-9 | 1.83 | – |
| 18:0 | 10.74 | – |
| 18:1, *cis*-9 | 20.23 | 35 |
| 18:1, *trans*-11 | 7.07 | – |
| 18:2 | 2.70 | 14 |
| 18:3 | 1.28 | <1 |

*Sources:* Palmquist, D.L. 2006. In: *Advanced Dairy Chemistry*, Vol. 2: Lipids, 3rd ed. Edited by P.F. Fox and P.L.H. McSweeney, Springer, New York; Park, Y.W. and G.F.W. Haenlein. 2006. *Handbook of Milk of Non-Bovine Mammals*, Blackwell Publishing, Oxford, UK.

Vegetable oils usually contain more unsaturated LCFAs and ω6 PUFAs than animal-source fats (Table 3.4). Except for marine fish tissues, the content of ω3 PUFAs is much lower in animal than in plant products (Smith and Smith 1995). The composition of LCFAs in common feedstuffs is shown in Table 3.3. Linoleic acid ($C_{18:2}$, ω6) and α-linolenic acid ($C_{18:3}$, ω3) cannot be synthesized by animals and are nutritionally essential for them. Therefore, these two fatty acids must be provided to all animal diets (Spector and Kim 2015). In contrast, both linoleic acid and α-linolenic acid are synthesized by bacteria, marine algae, and plants. Safflower oil and corn oil are abundant sources of ω6 PUFAs, as are cod liver oil and salmon oil for ω3 PUFAs (Table 3.6). High amounts of both ω6 and ω3 PUFAs are available from certain plant products, such as canola oil and soybean oil (Adeola et al. 2013; Calder 2006). Most LCFAs are esterified with glycerol as TAGs in microbes, plants, and animals (Gunstone 2012).

## Simple Lipids

### Fats

Fats are the esters of saturated or unsaturated fatty acids with glycerol and make up the largest fraction (~98%) of lipids in most concentrate feedstuffs for animals (Ding et al. 2003; Pond et al. 2005). The first, second, and third carbons of the glycerol molecule are denoted as the *sn*-1, *sn*-2, and *sn*-3 positions, respectively. Among fats, TAGs are most predominant in nature for the storage and toxicity prevention of LCFAs. However, small amounts of mono- and di-acylglycerols are present in bacteria, yeast, plants, and animals (Ridgway and McLeod 2016; Zinser et al. 1991). Within the same TAG molecule, the type of three fatty acids may be either the same (e.g., tristearin and triolein), which is rare, or different (e.g., 1-palmitoleoyl-2-oleoyl-3-stearoyl-glycerol) (Figure 3.5). TAGs of saturated fatty acids containing ≥10 carbons are solid at 25°C, whereas those with <10 carbons are liquids. In plant oils, the percentage of unsaturated fatty acids greatly exceeds that of saturated fatty acids.

In animals, fats are either solid or soft, depending on the species or compositions of fatty acids (Ramsay et al. 2001; Smith et al. 1998; Whitney and Smith 2015). The fat content of the body is low at birth but increases with age (Table 3.7). As noted previously, TAG is the main form of energy storage in animals. Fats are hydrophobic and have protective functions in the skin and subcutaneous tissues. In marine mammals (e.g., whales whose heads represent 30% of the body weight), fats in their heads have an acoustic sensory role (Madsen and Surlykke. 2013). Excess white adipose tissue results in obesity, insulin resistance, and numerous health problems (Bergen and Brandebourg 2016; Jobgen et al. 2006). Thus, the amount of fats in animals must be precisely regulated.

### Waxes

Waxes are esters of fatty acids with aliphatic or alicyclic higher molecular weight monohydric alcohols. The fatty acids are usually LCFAs (≥C12), including stearic acid ($C_{18:0}$), lignoceric acid

**TABLE 3.6**
**Abundant Sources of ω6 and ω3 PUFAs for Animal Diets**

| Foodstuff | ω6 PUFAs | ω3 PUFAs |
|---|---|---|
| Safflower oil | 73% C18:2 | 0.4% C18:3 |
| Corn oil | 57% C18:2 | 0.7% C18:3 |
| Cod liver oil | 1.4% C18:2; 1.6% C20:4 | 11.2% C20:5; 12.6% C22:6 |
| Salmon oil | 1.2% C18:2; 0.9% C20:4 | 12.0% C20:5; 13.8% C22:6 |
| Canola oil | 22% C18:2 | 9.5% C18:3 |
| Soybean oil | 51% C18:2 | 7% C18:3 |

*Source:* National Research Council (NRC). 2011. *Nutrient Requirements of Fish and Shrimp*, National Academy of Science, Washington DC.

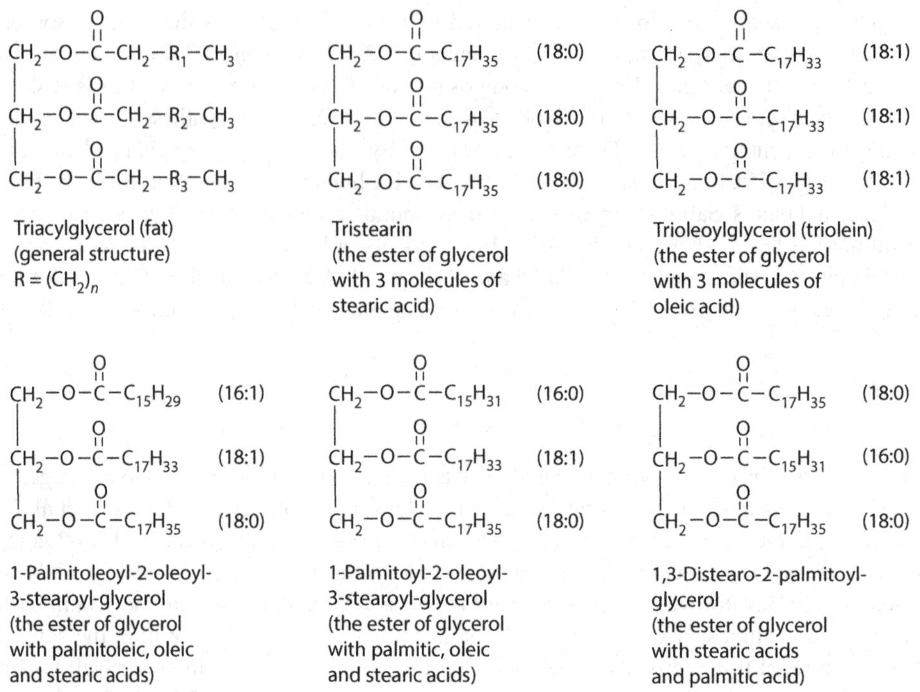

$CH_2{-}O{-}C(=O){-}CH_2{-}R_1{-}CH_3$
$CH_2{-}O{-}C(=O){-}CH_2{-}R_2{-}CH_3$
$CH_2{-}O{-}C(=O){-}CH_2{-}R_3{-}CH_3$

Triacylglycerol (fat)
(general structure)
$R = (CH_2)_n$

$CH_2{-}O{-}C(=O){-}C_{17}H_{35}$ (18:0)
$CH_2{-}O{-}C(=O){-}C_{17}H_{35}$ (18:0)
$CH_2{-}O{-}C(=O){-}C_{17}H_{35}$ (18:0)

Tristearin
(the ester of glycerol
with 3 molecules of
stearic acid)

$CH_2{-}O{-}C(=O){-}C_{17}H_{33}$ (18:1)
$CH_2{-}O{-}C(=O){-}C_{17}H_{33}$ (18:1)
$CH_2{-}O{-}C(=O){-}C_{17}H_{33}$ (18:1)

Trioleoylglycerol (triolein)
(the ester of glycerol
with 3 molecules of
oleic acid)

$CH_2{-}O{-}C(=O){-}C_{15}H_{29}$ (16:1)
$CH_2{-}O{-}C(=O){-}C_{17}H_{33}$ (18:1)
$CH_2{-}O{-}C(=O){-}C_{17}H_{35}$ (18:0)

1-Palmitoleoyl-2-oleoyl-
3-stearoyl-glycerol
(the ester of glycerol
with palmitoleic, oleic
and stearic acids)

$CH_2{-}O{-}C(=O){-}C_{15}H_{31}$ (16:0)
$CH_2{-}O{-}C(=O){-}C_{17}H_{33}$ (18:1)
$CH_2{-}O{-}C(=O){-}C_{17}H_{35}$ (18:0)

1-Palmitoyl-2-oleoyl-
3-stearoyl-glycerol
(the ester of glycerol
with palmitic, oleic
and stearic acids)

$CH_2{-}O{-}C(=O){-}C_{17}H_{35}$ (18:0)
$CH_2{-}O{-}C(=O){-}C_{15}H_{31}$ (16:0)
$CH_2{-}O{-}C(=O){-}C_{17}H_{35}$ (18:0)

1,3-Distearo-2-palmitoyl-
glycerol
(the ester of glycerol
with stearic acids
and palmitic acid)

**FIGURE 3.5** Triacylglycerols (triglycerides or fats) in plants, bacteria, and animals. Fats are the esters of saturated or unsaturated fatty acids with glycerol. Within the same fat molecule, the three fatty acids may be the same (e.g., tristearin and triolein) or different (e.g., 1-palmitoleoyl-2-oleoyl-3-stearoyl-glycerol). $R_1$, $R_2$, and $R_3$ represent alkyl groups $[-(CH_2)_n]$, with either the same or different numbers of carbons. The first, second, and third carbons of the glycerol molecule are denoted as the sn1, sn2, and sn3 positions, respectively.

## TABLE 3.7
## Fat Content in Animals at Birth and Older Ages[a]

| | Birth | | Older Ages | | |
|---|---|---|---|---|---|
| **Species** | **Body Weight (kg)** | **Fat Content (%, g/100 g)** | **Bogy Weight (kg)** | **Age (Days)** | **Fat Content (%, g/100 g)** |
| Broilers | 0.038 | 1.5 | 2.6 | 42 | 13 |
| Cat | 0.12 | 1.8 | 4.5 | 360 | 15 |
| Cattle | 35 | 3.0 | 545 | 540 | 31 |
| Guinea pig | 0.08 | 10.1 | 1.0 | 200 | 30 |
| Horse | 45 | 3.0 | 450 | 1800 | 18 |
| Human | 3.5 | 16.1 | 70 | 9125 | 13 |
| Mouse | 0.0016 | 2.1 | 0.03 | 60 | 15 |
| Pig | 1.4 | 1.1 | 110 | 180 | 36 |
| Rabbit | 0.054 | 2 | 2.3 | 63 | 8.0 |
| Rat | 0.0058 | 1.1 | 0.3 | 90 | 15 |
| Sheep | 4.0 | 3.0 | 52 | 180 | 20 |

*Source:* Cherian, G. 2015. *J. Anim. Sci. Biotechnol.* 6:28; Conde-Aguilera, J.A. et al. 2013. *Poult. Sci.* 92:1266–1275; Fox, J.G. et al. 2002. *Laboratory Animal Medicine*, 2nd ed. Academic Press, New York. Pond, W.G. et al. 1995. *Basic Animal Nutrition and Feeding.* 4th ed., John Wiley & Sons, New York.

[a] The values for body weight and fat content were reported in the literature, and may vary with breeds, feeding levels, and the ambient environment.

(also called carnaubic acid, $C_{24:0}$), and melissic acid ($C_{30:0}$), while fatty acids with < C12 are rare (Butovich et al. 2009). Waxes are widely present in plants and animals (e.g., animal skins and bird feathers) to provide protective function and a waterproof layer (Buschhaus and Jetter 2011; Chung and Carroll 2015).

The most common alcohols in natural waxes are oleoyl [$CH_3$–$(CH_2)_7$–CH = CH–$(CH_2)_8$–OH], cetyl [$CH_3$–$(CH_2)_{15}$–OH], carnaubyl [$CH_3$–$(CH_2)_{23}$–OH], and melissyl [$CH_3$–$(CH_2)_{29}$–OH]. Of note, the uropygial glands of birds produce unique waxes, which are esters of hydroxy acids (type I wax) or alkane-1,2-diols (type II wax) with medium- to long-chain fatty acids (Kolattukudy et al. 1987; Rijpstra et al. 2007). Carnauba wax is abundant in the leaves of the Carnauba palm, a plant native to the northeastern Brazilian states. Lanolin (also called wool wax or wool grease) is an animal wax secreted by the sebaceous glands of wool-bearing animals (e.g., sheep), whereas spermaceti is another type of animal wax produced by some marine animals (e.g., sperm whale) (Takagi and Itabashi 1977). Cetyl palmitate is a major component of beeswax. Waxes are water-insoluble due to the weakly polar nature of the ester group (Figure 3.6). Unlike fats, waxes cannot be digested or utilized as a nutrient by animals.

## Compound Lipids

### Glycolipids (Glycerol–Glycolipids)

Glycolipids are esters of glycerol. They are lipids with a carbohydrate (e.g., monosaccharide or oligosaccharide) joined together by a glycosidic bond (Figure 3.7), and are widely present in plants, bacteria, fungi, and animals (Mead et al. 1986). These substances are amphiphilic components of cell membranes, with a hydrophilic polar sugar backbone on the outer surface of all eukaryotic cell membranes and a hydrophobic nonpolar lipid moiety anchoring in the membrane.

Glycolipids are the major lipid component of forages (McDonald et al. 2011). In these compounds, two of the hydroxy groups of glycerol are esterified by fatty acids, mainly linoleic acid, and

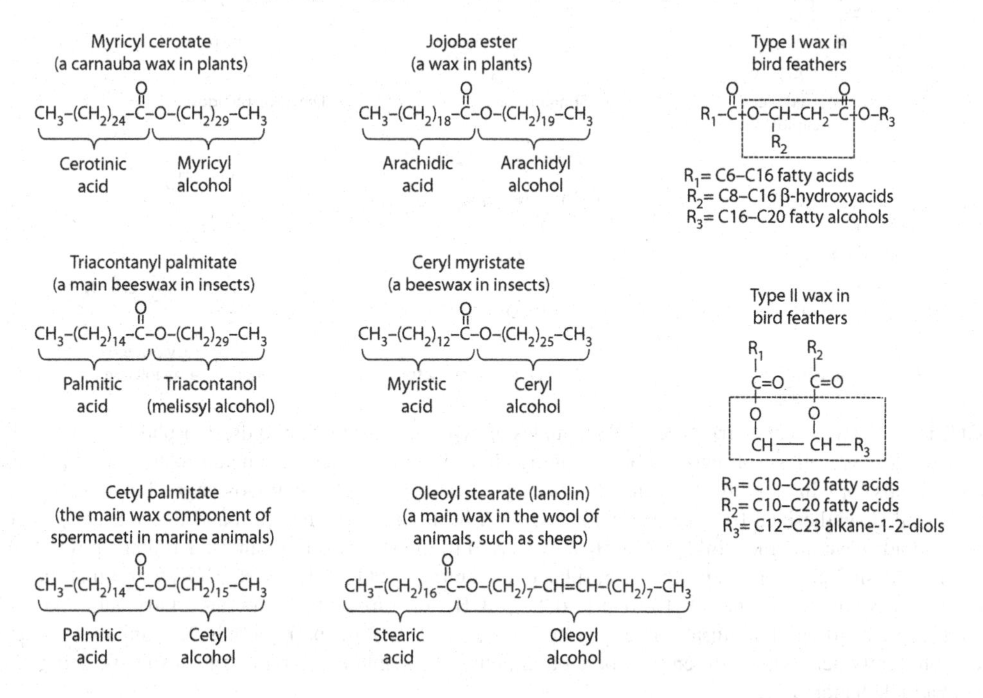


**FIGURE 3.6** Waxes in plants and animals. Waxes are the esters of fatty acids with aliphatic or alicyclic higher molecular-weight monohydric alcohols. This class of lipids provides plants and animals with a waterproof layer of protection. Unlike fats, waxes cannot be digested or utilized as a nutrient by animals.

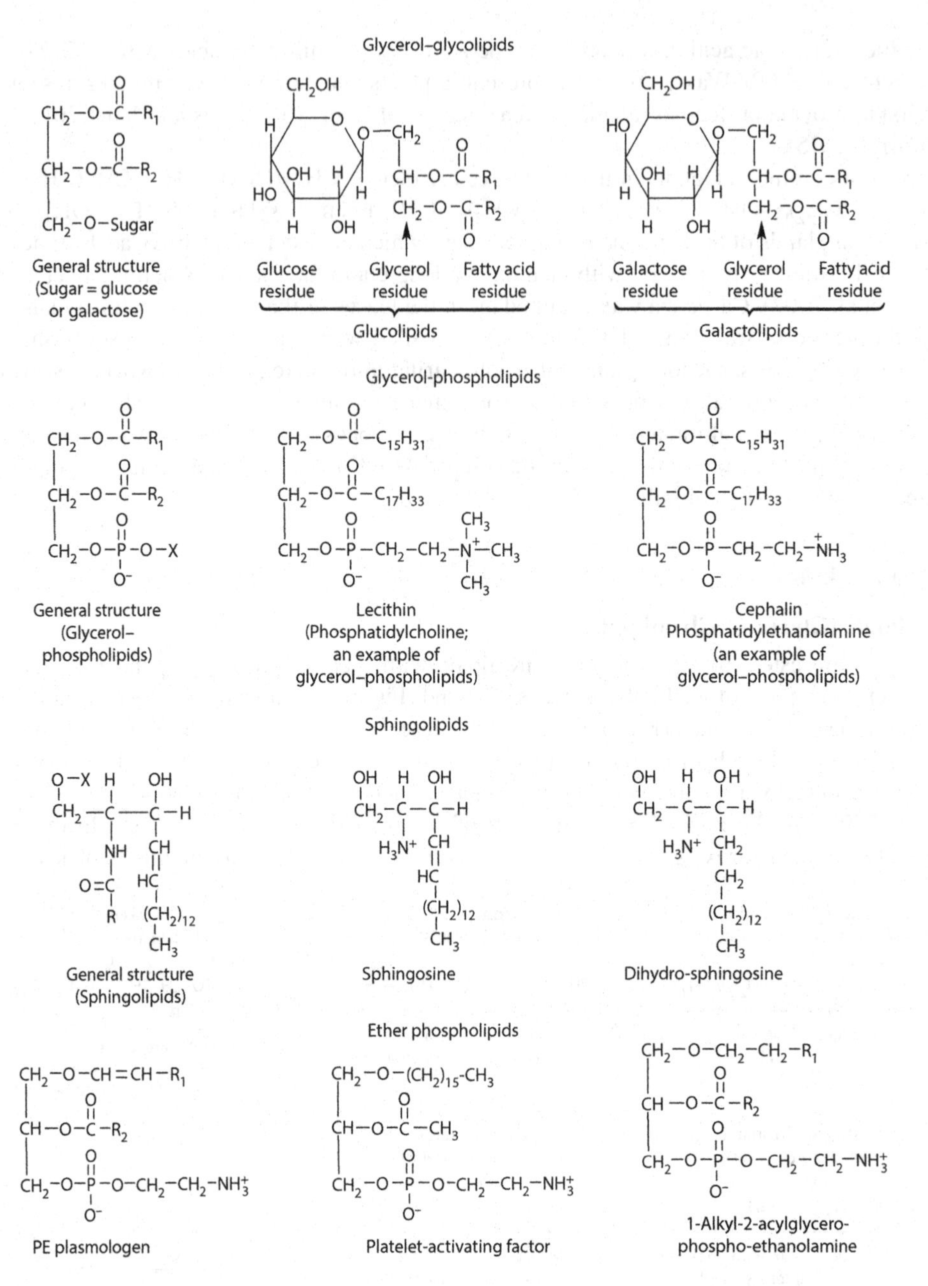


**FIGURE 3.7** The general structures and examples of glycerol-based glycolipids, phospholipids, and ether phospholipids, as well as sphingosine-based sphingolipids in plants, bacteria, and animals. Glycolipids and phospholipids contain carbohydrates and phosphate groups, respectively. Sphingosine is a long-chain amino alcohol and is synthesized from serine and acetyl-CoA in tissues (e.g., the brain and liver). Ether glycerophospholipids have an ether linkage ($-CH_2-O-CH_2-$) in the sn-1 position, an ester linkage ($-O-CO-CH_2-$) at the sn-2 position, and often a phosphoethanolamine ($-PO_3-CH_2-CH_2-NH_3^+$) group at the sn-3 position. $R_1$ is commonly the alkyl group [$-(CH_2)_n-CH_3$] of a long-chain saturated fatty acid and $R_2$ is often the hydrocarbon of an unsaturated fatty acid (e.g., oleic acid). In sphingolipids, R is an alkyl group of a saturated fatty acid with different numbers of carbons. The symbol "X" represents a specific group. PE, phosphatidylethanolamine.

one or two moles of a sugar (e.g., galactose) are added to the *sn*-3 position of the glycerol. In the leaf tissue, the lipid content (consisting of ~60% galactolipids) ranges from 3% to 10% of the dry matter. In myelin, which coats the axon of a neuron to confer protection and help speed nerve transmission, glycolipids are the most abundant compound lipids (Tanford 1980). In animals, glycolipids serve as markers for cell recognition and as an energy source.

### Phospholipids (Phosphatides)

Phospholipids are esters of glycerol, in which two of its hydroxyl groups are esterified by LCFAs and its *sn*-3 hydroxyl group is esterified to phosphoric acid (Figure 3.7). Thus, phosphatidic acid (the glycerol-based phospholipids with fatty acids being esterified at the *sn*-1 and *sn*-2 positions) is the common precursor for the synthesis of other phospholipids (Colbeau et al. 1971). In most cases, a saturated fatty acid is at the *sn*-1 position and an unsaturated fatty acid at the *sn*-2 position (Table 3.8). The *sn*-3 position contains a nitrogenous or non-nitrogenous compound (Gunstone 2012).

On the basis of its chemical structure, the phospholipid molecule generally has two "tails" of hydrophobic fatty acids and one "head" of hydrophilic phosphate moiety, joined together by a glycerol molecule (Vance 2014). The replacement of the "X" group in the general glycerol–phospholipid structure (Figure 3.7) by ethanolamine, choline, serine, myo-inositol, glycerol, or phosphatidylglycerol generates a corresponding phospholipid derivative (Figure 3.8). For example, phosphatidylcholine, which was the first phospholipid to be identified in the egg yolk of chickens in 1847, contains choline. Other common phospholipids are phosphatidylethanolamine (cephalins), phosphatidylserine, phosphatidylinositol, and diphosphatidylglycerol (cardiolipin). Phosphatidylcholine is the most abundant phospholipid in animal tissues, and is also predominant in the membranes of animal cells and yeast (Table 3.9). In nutrition, soybean lecithin (98% acetone insolubles) is often used as a rich source of phosphatidylcholine, phosphatidylethanolamine, and phosphatidylinositol. Other good sources of phospholipids are rapeseed, sunflower, chicken eggs, bovine milk, brain, liver, and fish. Phospholipids are: (1) a major component of all cell membranes; (2) second messengers in cell signaling; (3) sources of choline, inositol, and physiologically important fatty acids; and (4) mediators of the metabolism of nutrients (including lipids, amino acids, and glucose), intestinal absorption of lipids; and interorgan transport of cholesterol and lipoproteins (Jacobs et al. 2005).

### Sphingolipids

This class of lipids is based on sphingosine (a C18 amino alcohol), instead of glycerol (Figure 3.7). They were discovered in brain extracts in the 1870s, and are now known to be synthesized from serine plus acetyl-CoA (Morell and Braun 1972). The replacement of the "X" group in the general sphingolipid structure (Figure 3.7) by phosphocholine, glucose, galactose, lactose, and complex oligosaccharides yields a corresponding new sphingolipid derivative (Figure 3.9). Typically, the sphingosine backbone is linked to: (1) an acyl group (e.g., a fatty acid) via the amide linkage to form

**TABLE 3.8**
**Positional Distribution of Fatty Acids in Liver and Brain Phosphatidylserine**

| | | Fatty Acid | | | | | |
|---|---|---|---|---|---|---|---|
| **Tissue** | **Position** | **16:0** | **18:0** | **18:1** | **18:2** | **20:4** | **22:6** |
| Rat liver | *sn*-1 | 5 | 93 | 1 | 0 | 0 | 0 |
| | *sn*-2 | 6 | 29 | 8 | 4 | 32 | 19 |
| Bovine brain | *sn*-1 | 3 | 81 | 13 | 0 | 0 | 0 |
| | *sn*-2 | 2 | 1 | 25 | Trace | 1 | 60 |

*Source:* Wood, R. and R.D. Harlow. 1960. *Arch. Biochem. Biophys.* 135:272–281; Yabuuchi, H. and J.S. O'Brien. 1968. *J. Lipid Res.* 9:65–67.

| Name of X | Formula of X | Name of Phospholipid |
|---|---|---|
| - | $-H$ | Phosphatidic acid |
| Ethanolamine | $-CH_2CH_2\overset{+}{N}H_3$ | Phosphatidylethanol-amine (cephalin) |
| Choline | $-CH_2CH_2\overset{+}{N}(CH_3)_3$ | Phosphatidylcholine (lecithin) |
| Serine | $-CH_2CH(\overset{+}{N}H_3)COO^-$ | Phosphatidylserine |
| myo-Inositol | 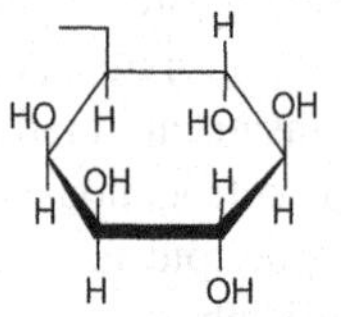 H; HO, H, HO, OH; OH, H; H, H; H, OH | Phosphatidylinositol |
| Glycerol | $-CH_2CH(OH)CH_2OH$ | Phosphatidylglycerol |
| Phosphatidylglycerol | 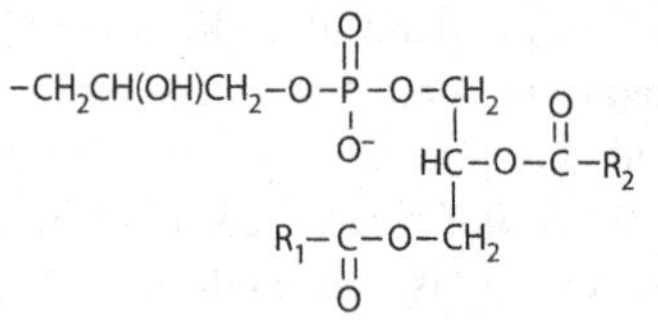 $-CH_2CH(OH)CH_2-O-P(=O)(O^-)-O-CH_2-CH(-O-C(=O)-R_2)-CH_2-O-C(=O)-R_1$ | Diphosphatidylglycerol (cardiolipin) |

**FIGURE 3.8** The structures of abundant phospholipids in plants, bacteria, and animals. The symbol "X" in the general structure of phospholipids (Figure 3.7) is replaced by various groups (e.g., ethanolamine, choline, serine, or myo-inositol) to form different phospholipids (e.g., phosphatidylethanolamine, phosphatidylcholine, phosphatidylserine, or phosphatidylinositol). These compounds are all glycerol-based lipids.

a ceramide; (2) a nitrogenous charged head group (e.g., ethanolamine, serine, or choline) to yield a sphingomyelin; or (3) various sugar monomers or dimers to generate glycosphingolipids (e.g., cerebrosides) (Ridgway and McLeod 2016). Like phosphatidylcholine and cephalins, sphingomyelins are surface active and serve as important components of cell membranes in animal cells (Daum 1985). Of note, *E. coli* and yeasts do not have sphingomyelin (major phosphosphingolipids in mammals). Instead, yeasts have inositol phosphosphingolipids, which may function like the mammalian sphingomyelin (Horvath and Daum 2013).

Sphingolipids have a common structural feature: a backbone of sphingoid bases (aliphatic amino alcohols), including sphingosine. On the basis of their structures, sphingolipids are classified as simple or complex. Simple sphingolipids include sphingoid bases (the fundamental building blocks of all sphingolipids) and ceramides, whereas complex sphingolipids are sphingomyelins, glycosphingolipids, cerebrosides (including sulfated cerebrosides), gangliosides (having at least three sugars, with one being sialic acid), and inositol-containing ceramides (Figure 3.10). Sphingolipids are particularly abundant in tissues (e.g., the brain) of the nervous system, constituting, for example, up to 25% of the total lipids in the myelin sheaths of nerve cells (Maceyka and Spiegel 2014). In addition, sphingolipids serve as adhesion sites for extracellular proteins and play important roles in cell signal transmission and cell recognition. Meat, dairy products, eggs, and soybeans are good dietary sources of ceramides, sphingomyelins, cerebrosides, gangliosides, and sulfatides as sphingolipids.

## Ether Glycerophospholipids

Ether glycerophospholipids are derivatives of glycerol, fatty acids, phosphorus, and ethanolamine. This class of lipids possesses an ether linkage ($-CH_2-O-CH_2-$) in the *sn*-1 position, an ester linkage ($-O-CO-CH_2-$) at the *sn*-2 position, and a phosphoryl nitrogenous head group up at the *sn*-3

**TABLE 3.9**
**Composition of Lipids, Protein, and Carbohydrates in Some Biological Membranes**

| | Cell Membrane | | | | Outer MM | | Inner MM | | Bovine | | |
|---|---|---|---|---|---|---|---|---|---|---|---|
| **Variable** | **Human RBCs** | **Rat Liver[a]** | ***E. Coli*** | **Yeast[b]** | **Rat Liver** | **Yeast** | **Rat Liver** | **Yeast** | **Heart Mit** | **ER** | **Human Myelin** |
| Protein, % (g/100 g) | 49 | 52 | 68 | 53 | 52 | 52 | 76 | 84 | 74 | 55 | 18 |
| Carbohydrates, % (g/100 g) | 8 | 8 | – | – | 2–4 | – | 1–2 | – | – | – | 3 |
| Lipids, % (g/100 g) | 43 | 40 | 32 | 47 | 48 | 48 | 24 | 16 | 24 | 45 | 79 |
| Phosphatidic acid[c] | 1.5 | 2.4 | 0 | 1 | 1 | 4 | 1 | 1.7 | 0 | 1 | 0.5 |
| Phosphatidylcholine[c] | 19 | 20 | 0 | 4.4 | 42 | 46 | 40 | 32 | 39 | 60 | 10 |
| Phosphatidylethanolamine[c] | 18 | 11 | 65 | 5.1 | 27 | 33 | 34 | 20 | 27 | 23 | 20 |
| Phosphatidylglycerol[c] | 0 | 2.7 | 18 | 1.8 | – | – | – | – | 0 | – | 0 |
| Phosphatidylinositol[c] | 1 | 4.0 | 2 | 4.7 | 11 | 10 | 2 | 13 | 7 | 10 | 1 |
| Phosphatidylserine[c] | 8.5 | 5.0 | 2 | 8.7 | 2 | 1 | 3 | 3.3 | 0.5 | 2 | 8.5 |
| Cardiolipin[c] | 0 | 0.3 | 12 | 0.3 | 5 | 6 | 18 | 13 | 22.5 | 1 | 0 |
| Sphingomyelin[c] | 17.5 | 10 | 0 | 0 | 2 | 0 | 2 | 0 | 0 | 3 | 8.5 |
| Glycolipids[c] | 10 | 5.6 | 0 | – | 0 | 0 | 0 | 0 | 0 | – | 26 |
| Cholesterol[c] | 25 | 20.4 | 0 | 0[d] | 10 | 0 | 1.5 | 0 | 3 | – | 26 |

*Source:* Colbeau, A. et al. 1971. *Biochim. Biophys. Acta.* 249:462–492; Daum, G. 1985. *Biochim. Biophys. Acta.* 882:1–42; Guidotti, G. 1972. *Annu. Rev. Biochem.* 41:731–752; Horvath, S.E. and G. Daum. 2013. *Prog. Lipid Res.* 52:590–614; Ray, T.K., et al. 1969. *J. Biol. Chem.* 244:5528–5536; Tanford, C. 1980. *The Hydrophobic Effect: Formation of Micelles and Biological Membranes*, Wiley, New York; Zinser, E. et al. 1991. *J. Bacteriol.* 173:2026–2034.

[a] In the liver cell membrane, phospholipids, glycolipids, and neutral lipids account for 55.4%, 5.6%, and 39% of the total lipids by weight. Neutral lipids (% of the total lipids) consist of the following: triacylglycerols, 3.9; diacylglycerols, 1.6; monoacylglycerols, 1.8; free cholesterol, 18.1; esterified cholesterol, 0.9; cholesterol esters, 1.4; free fatty acids, 7.9; hydrocarbons, 2.5; unidentified lipids, 0.9 (Ray et al. 1969).

[b] Yeast *Saccharomyces cerevisiae*.

[c] Expressed as % of total lipids by weight.

[d] Yeast *Saccharomyces cerevisiae* contains no sterol or sphingomyelin, but its cell membrane has ergosterol and sphingolipids instead. The content of phospholipids, ergosterol, and sphingolipids in the yeast cell membrane (mg/mg protein) is 0.23, 0.4, and 0.27, respectively.

MM, mitochondrial membrane; RBCs, red blood cells.

position (Lehninger et al. 1993). Examples of ether glycerophospholipids are plasmalogens and the platelet-activating factor (Figure 3.10).

Plasmalogens, which were first reported in 1924, are a major group of ether phospholipid. In these compounds, the *sn*-1 position is usually derived from a $C_{16:0}$, $C_{18:0}$, or $C_{18:1}$ fatty alcohol, the *sn*-2 position is most commonly linked to a PUFA, and the head group at the *sn*-3 position contains choline, ethanolamine, or serine. In mammals and birds, the most common head groups present in plasmalogens are phosphoethanolamine [$-PO_3-CH_2-CH_2-NH_3^+$] or phosphocholine (Lehninger et al. 1993). Plasmalogens are abundant in many tissues, particularly those of the nervous, immune, and cardiovascular systems. Notably, in the heart, plasmalogens represent 30%–40% of choline glycerophospholipids, 30% of the glycerophospholipids in the brain, and up to 70% of myelin sheath ethanolamine glycerophospholipids (Ridgway and McLeod 2016).

The platelet-activating factor (acetyl-glyceryl-ether-phosphorylcholine) was discovered in the 1970s, and was the first phospholipid known to have intracellular messenger functions. Its *sn*-1 position is linked via an ether linkage to a saturated fatty acid (palmitate), its *sn*-2 position is connected to an acetate unit via an ester linkage (for increasing solubility in water), and its *sn*-3 position is occupied by phosphocholine (Gunstone 2012). The platelet-activating factor plays an important role

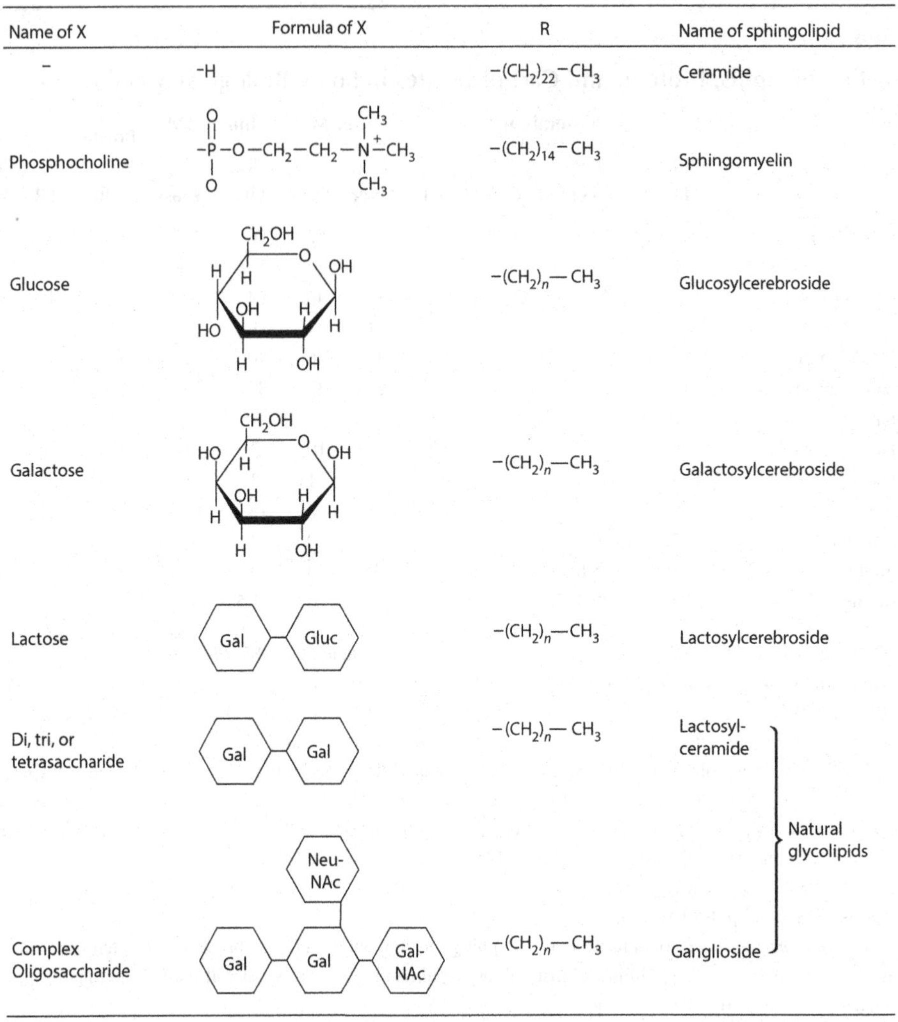

| Name of X | Formula of X | R | Name of sphingolipid |
|---|---|---|---|
| - | -H | $-(CH_2)_{22}-CH_3$ | Ceramide |
| Phosphocholine | $-P(=O)(O)-O-CH_2-CH_2-N^{+}(CH_3)_3$ | $-(CH_2)_{14}-CH_3$ | Sphingomyelin |
| Glucose | $CH_2OH$, O, OH, H, H, OH, H, HO, H, H, OH (glucose ring) | $-(CH_2)_n-CH_3$ | Glucosylcerebroside |
| Galactose | $CH_2OH$, O, HO, H, OH, OH, H, H, H, H, OH (galactose ring) | $-(CH_2)_n-CH_3$ | Galactosylcerebroside |
| Lactose | Gal–Gluc | $-(CH_2)_n-CH_3$ | Lactosylcerebroside |
| Di, tri, or tetrasaccharide | Gal–Gal | $-(CH_2)_n-CH_3$ | Lactosyl-ceramide (Natural glycolipids) |
| Complex Oligosaccharide | Gal–Gal(–Neu-NAc)–Gal-NAc | $-(CH_2)_n-CH_3$ | Ganglioside (Natural glycolipids) |

**FIGURE 3.9** The structures of abundant sphingolipids in plants, bacteria, and animals. The symbols "X" and "R" in the general structure of sphingolipids (Figure 3.7) are replaced by various groups to form different sphingolipids. For example, when X = "H" and R = "$-(CH_2)_{22}-CH_3$)," the sphingolipid is called ceramide; when X = "phosphocholine" and R = "$-(CH_2)_{14}-CH_3$)," the sphingolipid is called sphingomyelin.

in mediating the chemotaxis and functions of leukocytes, platelet aggregation and degranulation, inflammation, anaphylaxis, vascular permeability, and the oxidative burst in animals.

## Lipoproteins

Lipoproteins are lipids associated noncovalently with specific proteins, and are synthesized and released by the small intestine and liver (Ridgway and McLeod 2016). The protein moiety serves to emulsify the lipid molecules. Examples of lipoproteins are high-, intermediate-, low-, and very low-density lipoproteins, as well as chylomicrons (Table 3.10). They have different proportions of protein, cholesterol, cholesteryl ester, phospholipids, and TAGs and therefore different density values. In essence, high-density lipoproteins and chylomicrons (the major small-intestinal lipoprotein) contain the highest proportions of protein and TAGs, respectively (Besnard et al. 1996).

Lipoproteins are present in the blood, transmembrane proteins, and intracellular fatty acid-binding proteins, as well as some antigens, adhesins, and toxins. Apolipoproteins function to (1) guide the formation of lipoproteins; (2) transport LCFAs, TAGs, and cholesterol from the small intestine

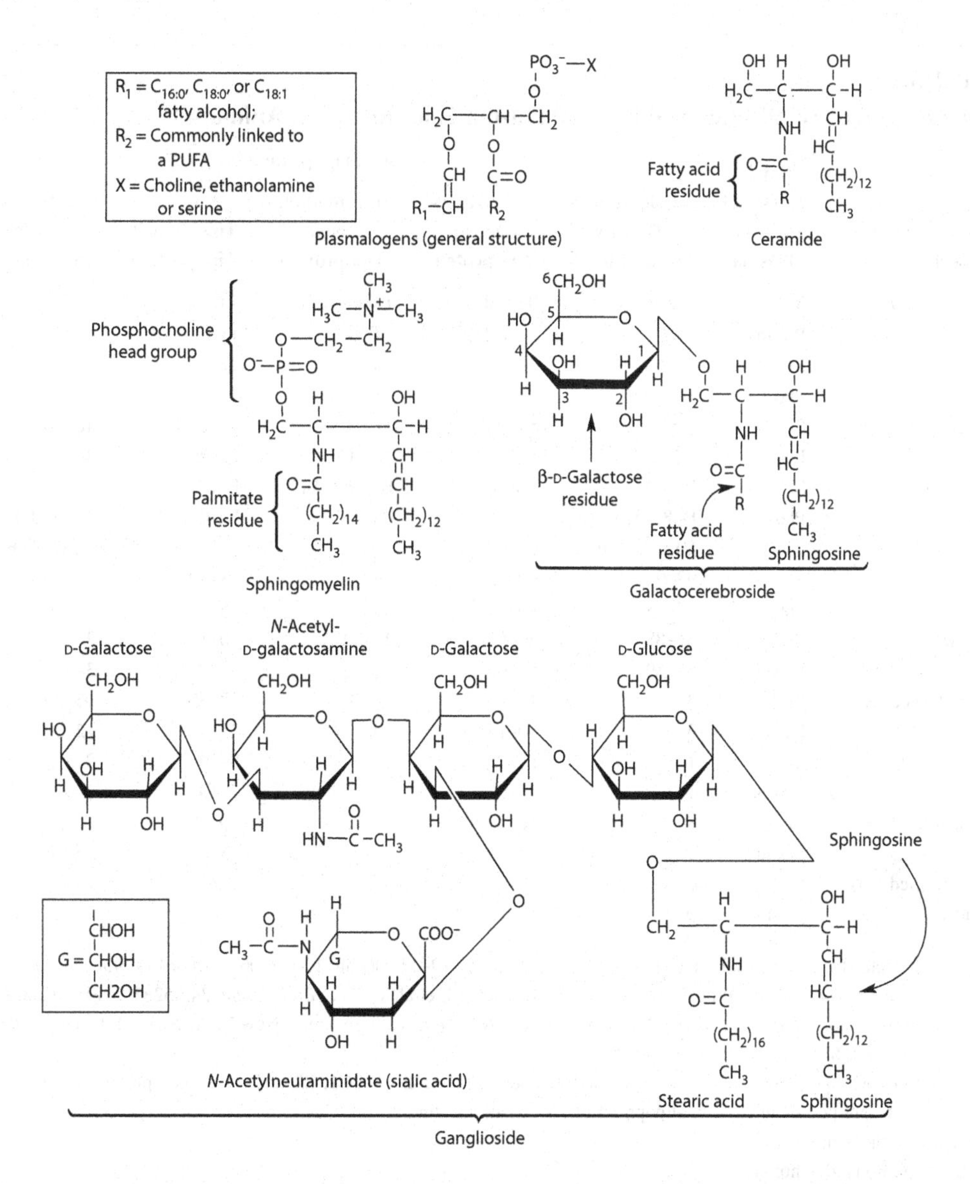


**FIGURE 3.10** The general structure of plasmalogens, as well as specific structures of ceramide, phosphocholine sphingomyelin, galactocerebroside, and ganglioside. The sphingosine backbone is linked to: (1) an acyl group (e.g., a fatty acid) via the amide linkage to form a ceramide; (2) a nitrogenous charged head group (e.g., ethanolamine, serine, or choline) to yield a sphingomyelin; or (3) various sugar monomers or dimers to generate glycosphingolipids (e.g., cerebrosides).

to lymph vessels (lacteals), from the liver to peripheral tissues, and in the circulation; (3) act as ligands for lipoprotein receptors; and (4) regulate the metabolism of lipoproteins (Gunstone 2012; Ridgway and McLeod 2016). Chylomicron remnants, VLDLs, IDLs, and LDLs (bad cholesterol) are pro-atherogenic, whereas HDL is antiatherogenic and anti-oxidative (good cholesterol).

## Derived Lipids

### Definition

Derived lipids are lipids that are formed from cholesterol or isoprene compounds (Gunstone 2012). Their structures are complex and can be classified as steroids, eicosanoids, and terpenes. Both

**TABLE 3.10**
**Composition of Small-Intestinal (SI) and Plasma Lipoproteins in Animals**

| Physicochemical Property | Small-Intestinal Source or Plasma | Class of Lipoprotein | | | | |
|---|---|---|---|---|---|---|
| | | Chylomicrons Density Lipoproteins | Very-Low-Density Lipoproteins | Intermediate-Density Lipoproteins | Low-Density Lipoproteins | High-Density Lipoproteins |
| Density, g/mL | SI | <0.95 | 0.95–1.006 | 1.006–1.040 | 1.04 | 1.12 |
| | Plasma | 0.94 | 0.94–1.006 | 1.006–1.019 | 1.019–1.063 | 1.063–1.21 |
| Size, nm | SI | 70–600 | 28–70 | 40 | 22–26 | 5–15 |
| | Plasma | 80–500 | 30–80 | 25–30 | 16–25 | 7–13 |
| Protein, % | SI | 1.5–2 | 5–10 | 11 | 20–22 | 40–50 |
| | Plasma | 1.5–2.5 | 5–10 | 15–20 | 20–25 | 40–55 |
| Major apoproteins | SI | B48,A1,A4 | B48,A1,A4 | B48,A1,A4 | B48 | A1 |
| (Apo) | Plasma | B48,A1,A2 C1,C2,C3,E | B100,C1,C2 C3,E | B100,C3,E | B100 | A1,A2,C1 C2,C3,D,E |
| Total lipids, % | SI | 98–98.5 | 90–95 | 89 | 78–80 | 50–60 |
| | Plasma | 97–98.5 | 90–95 | 80–85 | 75–80 | 45–60 |
| Triacylglycerols, % | SI | 85–88 | 50–55 | 24–30 | 10–15 | 3–5 |
| | Plasma | 84–89 | 50–65 | 22 | 7–10 | 3–5 |
| Cholesteryl ester, % | SI | 3 | 12–15 | 25–30 | 37–45 | 15–20 |
| | Plasma | 3–5 | 10–15 | 30 | 35–42 | 12–20 |
| Free cholesterol[a], % | SI | 1 | 8–10 | 8–10 | 8–10 | 2–5 |
| | Plasma | 1–3 | 5–10 | 8 | 7–10 | 3–5 |
| Phospholipids, % | SI | 8 | 18–20 | 25–27 | 20–28 | 26–30 |
| | Plasma[b] | 7–9 | 15–20 | 22 | 15–22 | 25–30 |
| Nonesterified fatty | SI | 0 | 1 | 1 | 1 | 2 |
| acids, % | Plasma[b] | 0 | 1 | 1 | 1 | 2 |

*Source:* Adapted from Besnard, P. et al. 1996. *Proc. Nutr. Soc.* 55:19–37; Devlin, T.M. 2006. *Textbook of Biochemistry with Clinical Correlations*, Wiley-Liss, New York; Kessler, J.I. et al. 1970. *J. Biol. Chem.* 245:5281–5288; Mead, J.F. et al. 1986. *Lipids: Chemistry, Biochemistry, and Nutrition*, Plenum Press, New York; Swift, L.L. et al. 1988. *Biochim. Biophys. Acta.* 962:186–195.

*Note:* A1 and A2, apolipoproteins A-1 and A-2; B100, apolipoprotein B-100; C1, C2, and C3, apolipoproteins C1, C2, and C3; D, apolipoprotein D; E, apolipoprotein E; SI, small intestine.

[a] Surface components.

[b] Mainly phosphatidylcholine.

steroids and terpenes are nonsaponifiable. Steroids have the cyclopentanophenanthrene ring (Figure 3.11) and include sterols, steroid hormones, bile acids, and bile alcohols. Eicosanoids are products of ω3 and ω6 PUFAs. Terpenes are a diverse group of organic compounds that contain isoprene units (Zerbe and Bohlmann 2015). The name "terpene" is derived from the Greek word "turpentine," meaning a species of the terebinth tree. Terpenes are produced by a variety of plants, green algae, and some insects (e.g., termites and swallowtail butterflies). The difference between terpenes and terpenoids is that terpenoids contain additional functional groups beyond the terpene hydrocarbon chain.

## Steroids

1. *Sterols.* Sterols are steroid alcohols, such as phytosterols of plant origin, mycosterols of fungal origin, and zoosterols of animal origin. Zoosterols include cholesterol, 7-dehydrocholesterol, and the sulfated conjugate of cholesterol, all of which are a component of

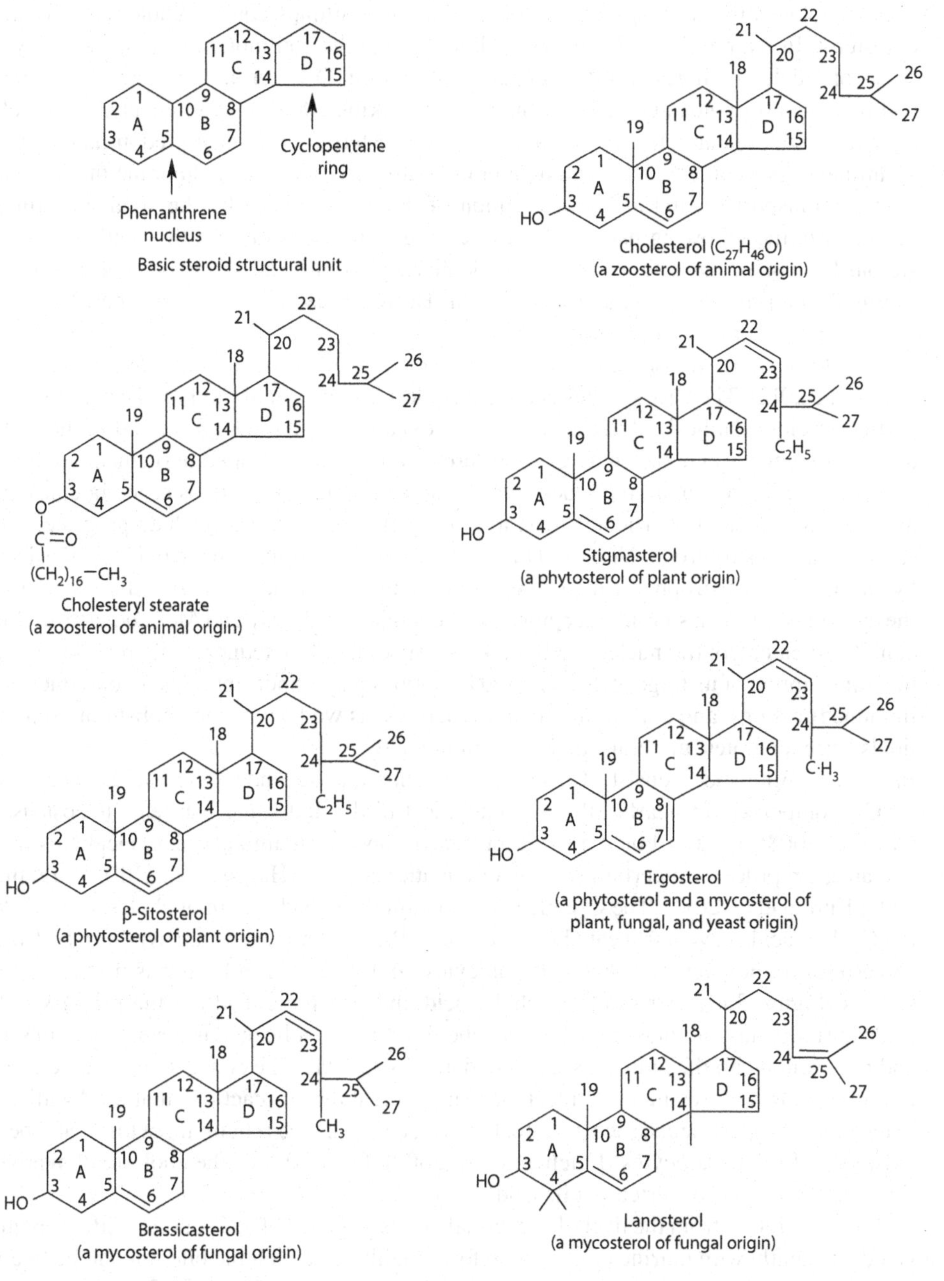

Phenanthrene nucleus

Cyclopentane ring

Basic steroid structural unit

Cholesterol ($C_{27}H_{46}O$)
(a zoosterol of animal origin)

Cholesteryl stearate
(a zoosterol of animal origin)

Stigmasterol
(a phytosterol of plant origin)

β-Sitosterol
(a phytosterol of plant origin)

Ergosterol
(a phytosterol and a mycosterol of plant, fungal, and yeast origin)

Brassicasterol
(a mycosterol of fungal origin)

Lanosterol
(a mycosterol of fungal origin)

**FIGURE 3.11** Structures of sterols in plants and animals. Sterols are steroid alcohols, including zoosterols of animal origin (e.g., cholesterol and cholesteryl stearate), phytosterols of plant origin (e.g., stigmasterol and β-sitosterol), mycosterols of fungal origin (e.g., brassicasterol and lanosterol). Ergosterol is present in plants, fungi, and yeasts.

skin lipids (Gunstone 2012). The term cholesterol was originally coined from the Greek *chole-* (bile) and *stereos* (solid), followed by the chemical suffix *-ol* meaning an alcohol. Zoosterols, but not the phytosterols or mycosterols, are absorbed by the small intestine of animals (Ridgway and McLeod 2016). However, ergosterol is a sterol widely distributed in brown algae, bacteria, yeast, and higher plants, and these organisms contain little or no cholesterol. Ergosterol is converted by sunlight into ergocalciferol (vitamin $D_2$), which is then biologically available to animals. In contrast, animals contain cholesterol but not ergosterol. In mammals, birds, and fish, cholesterol is the common precursor for the synthesis of 7-dehydrocholesterol (the precursor of vitamin $D_3$), steroid hormones, bile acids, and bile alcohols (Mead et al. 1986; Stamp and Jenkins 2008). Quantitatively, the sterols are the most abundant steroids in nature, and cholesterol is the most predominant sterol in animals. As a component of cell membranes, cholesterol affects membrane fluidity and nutrient transport (including the absorption of dietary nutrients by the small intestine). As noted in the following paragraphs, by serving as the substrate for the synthesis of all steroid hormones and bile acids or bile alcohols, physiological levels of cholesterol are essential to animal nutrition and metabolism. However, excess cholesterol increases risk for cardiovascular disease in animals.

2. *Steroid hormones.* Steroid hormones are steroids with hormone functions in biology (Gunstone 2012). They are synthesized from cholesterol in animals and can be classified as corticosteroids (synthesized in the adrenal cortex) and sex steroids (generated in the male and female gonads and placenta). Corticosteroids are further grouped into glucocorticoids (e.g., cortisol in most mammals such as pigs and ruminants, or corticosterone in chickens and rats), and mineralocorticoids (e.g., aldosterone). Sex hormones include progesterone, estrogen, and testosterone. Vitamin D is another steroid hormone that can be synthesized by animals. As a hydrophobic molecule, a steroid hormone binds to its specific receptor in the cytosol, forming a steroid–receptor ligand complex (Ridgway and McLeod 2016). This complex then enters the nucleus to bind with a specific DNA sequence, thereby inducing the transcription of its target genes. Steroid hormones play important roles in reproduction, immune functions, and anti-inflammatory reactions, as well as the metabolism of protein, lipids, carbohydrates, minerals, and water in the body.
3. *Bile acids.* Bile acids consist of primary bile acids and secondary bile acids. They are all $C_{24}$ compounds in nearly all mammals, most birds, and some fish (e.g., teleost fish) (Agellon 2008), but $C_{27}$ bile acids are present in ancient mammals (e.g., elephants and manatees), reptiles, and certain species of aquatic animals (Hagey et al. 2010; Hofmann 1999; Kurogi et al. 2011). The $C_{27}$ bile acids contain the $C_8$ side chain of cholesterol, while the $C_{24}$ bile acids have a truncated $C_5$ side chain. Primary bile acids are synthesized from cholesterol in the liver (perivenous hepatocytes) and their molecular forms differ among species (Figure 3.12). For example, cholic acid and hyocholic acid are the primary bile acids in ruminants and pigs, respectively, whereas β-muricholic acid is formed only in rats and mice among all the animals studied to date (Table 3.11). The conversion of cholesterol into bile acids requires many intracellular enzyme-catalyzed reactions that are localized in different compartments, such as mitochondria, endoplasmic reticulum, cytosol, and peroxisomes of the hepatocytes (Lefebvre et al. 2009). Over 50% of the cholesterol synthesized in the liver is converted to bile acids.

   Before secretion from the liver, the terminal carboxyl group of 98% of bile acids is conjugated covalently with taurine or glycine to form highly water-soluble bile salts in the livers of mammals and birds (Stamp and Jenkins 2008). The bile salts in teleost fish are the same as those in mammals. Of note, the amounts of taurine and glycine in the bile salts vary with animal species (Washizu et al. 1991). There are reports that bile acids are conjugated mainly with taurine in carnivores, with glycine in herbivores, and with both taurine or glycine in omnivores (Agellon 2008). Examples are taurocholic acid (the derivative of cholic acid and taurine) and glycocholic acid (the derivative of cholic acid and glycine). However, it should be borne in mind that both taurine- and glycine-conjugated forms of bile acids can be present in the same animal, but their concentrations may be markedly different as noted previously. The liver releases bile acids into the gall bladder for storage. Of interest, the concentrations of bile acids in the gallbladder are extremely high (>300 mM) because of a constant removal of water and electrolytes (Stamp and Jenkins 2008). In response to

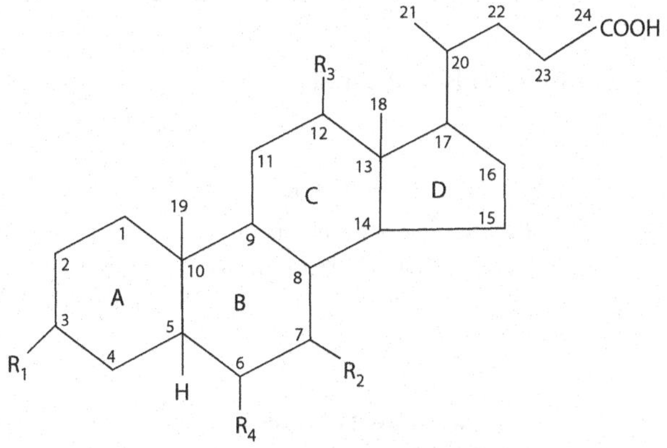

Structures of bile acids in animals

| Bile acid | $R_1$ | $R_2$ | $R_3$ | $R_4$ |
|---|---|---|---|---|
| Lithocholic acid | αOH | H | H | H |
| Deoxycholic acid | αOH | H | αOH | H |
| Chenodeoxycholic acid | αOH | αOH | H | H |
| Ursodeoxycholic acid | αOH | βOH | H | H |
| Cholic acid | αOH | αOH | αOH | H |
| Ursocholic acid | αOH | βOH | αOH | H |
| Hyocholic acid | αOH | αOH | H | αOH |
| β-Muricholic acid | αOH | βOH | H | βOH |
| Hyodeoxycholic acid | αOH | H | H | αOH |

**FIGURE 3.12** Structures of primary and secondary bile acids in animals. The carboxyl group of bile acids can conjugate with taurine or glycine. Dehydroxylation of a primary bile acid at the C-6 position by liver and intestinal bacteria generates a secondary bile acid. The major forms of bile acid differ among animals. When the C6-position of chenodeoxycholic acid contains an α-hydroxyl group, the modified molecule is called hyocholic acid (the major bile acid synthesized by the liver of pigs). When the C6-position of ursodeoxycholic acid contains a β-hydroxyl group, the modified molecule is called β-muricholic acid (a bile acid synthesized by the liver of mice and rats).

feeding, the gall bladder secretes the bile acids, via the bile duct, into the duodenum of the small intestine (Tso 1985).

The bile salts are actively secreted as bile into the lumen of the duodenum where their concentrations range from 0.2% to 2% (g/100 mL fluid) (Agellon 2008). The typical mammalian bile (a yellow-green aqueous solution) comprises 82% water, 12% bile salts, 4% phospholipids (mostly phosphatidylcholines), 1% unesterified cholesterol, and 1% other compounds (including proteins and pigments [biliverdin and bilirubin conjugated with the water-soluble glucuronides]) (Ridgway and McLeod 2016). In the small intestine, bile acids facilitate the digestion and absorption of lipids by forming micelles, while activating the farnesoid X receptor (FXR; a member of the superfamily of ligand-activated nuclear receptor transcription factors).

At the terminal ileum, 95% of bile salts return to the liver via the portal vein through enterohepatic circulation, and the remaining 5% enters the large intestine where they undergo modifications by bacterial enzymes (Devlin 2006). The biochemical reactions mainly involve the removal of one hydroxyl group from the primary bile acids and their deconjugation (e.g., removal of the taurine or glycine). Examples for dehydroxylation are the conversion of cholic acid into deoxycholic acid, chenodeoxycholic acid into lithocholic acid, hyocholic acid or β-muricholic acid into hyodeoxycholic acid, and ursocholic acid into ursodeoxycholic acid. The resultant products are called secondary bile acids. In feces,

**TABLE 3.11**
**Primary and Secondary Bile Acids in Animals**

| Bile Acid | Animals |
|---|---|
| | **Primary Bile Acids** |
| Chenodeoxycholic acid[a,b] | Bear, hamster, horse, human, pig |
| Cholic acid[a,c] | Bear, cat, cattle, chicken, dog, hamster, human, mouse, rabbit, rat, sheep |
| Ursocholic acid[d] | Bear |
| Hyocholic acid[e] | Pig |
| β-Muricholic acid[f] | Mouse, rat |
| | **Secondary Bile Acids** |
| Lithocholic acid | Bear, hamster, human, pig |
| Deoxycholic acid | Bear, cat, cattle, chicken, dog, hamster, human, mouse, rabbit, rat, sheep |
| Ursodeoxycholic acid[d] | Bear |
| Hyodeoxycholic acid | Pig |

*Note:* Dehydroxylation of a primary bile acid at the C6 position results in the formation of the corresponding secondary bile acid.

[a] Principal primary bile acid in hamsters and humans.
[b] Principal primary bile acid in horses.
[c] Principal primary bile acid in cats, cattle, chickens, dogs, hamsters, mice, rabbits, rats, and sheep.
[d] Principal bile acid in bears.
[e] Principal primary bile acid in pigs.
[f] Another principal primary bile acid in mice and rats.

98% of bile acids are not conjugated with taurine or glycine, such that these two AAs can be conserved.

4. *Bile alcohols.* Bile alcohols are usually $C_{27}$ compounds synthesized from cholesterol in the liver of fish and reptiles, with the terminal –OH group at the $C_{27}$ position (Figure 3.13). In mammals, impaired mitochondrial 26-hydroxylation of intermediates in the pathway for the conversion of cholesterol into bile acids generates bile alcohols. Like the $C_{27}$ bile acids, the $C_{27}$ bile alcohols contain the $C_8$ side chain of cholesterol. Thus, the conversion of cholesterol into bile alcohols does not involve the removal of any carbons.

   The molecular forms of bile alcohols differ among fish and reptile species. Typically, bile alcohols are secreted from the liver of these animals as sulfate conjugates, which usually form salts with minerals, such as sodium (Kurogi et al. 2011). For example, zebrafish produce cyprinol and cyprinol sulfate, but no bile acids. In contrast, myxinol and myxinol sulfate are synthesized by hagfish, and scymnol and scymnol sulfate by marine elasmobranch vertebrates (Figure 3.13). Concentrations of bile alcohol sulfate salts in the lumen of the fish intestine are comparable to those of bile salts in mammals and birds (Lefebvre et al. 2009).

5. *Steroidal saponins.* Steroidal saponins are plant metabolites. They are abundant (up to 10% of dry matter) in Yucca trees native to North America (e.g., Mexico, California, and Arizona). The name yucca applies to as many as 40 species of trees and shrubs, including *Yucca aloifolia, Yucca whipplei, and Yucca schidigera.* Steroidal saponins contain an ether linkage (C–O–C) and one or more monosaccharides joined via β-1,2 or β-1,3 bonds. Oleszek et al. (2001) reported the structures of 8 steroidal saponins in *Yucca schidigera* Roezl (Figure 3.14). They are similar in structure to glucocorticoids in animals.

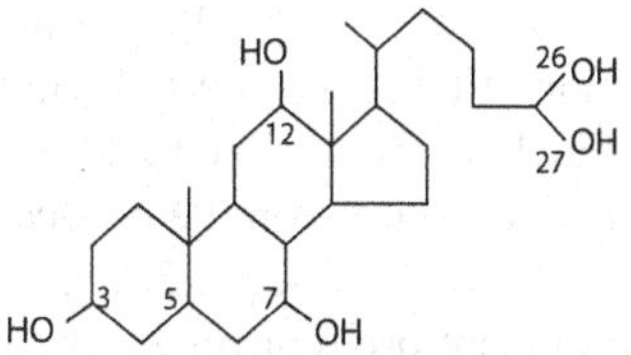

5α-Cyprinol
(a bile alcohol; e.g., zebrafish)

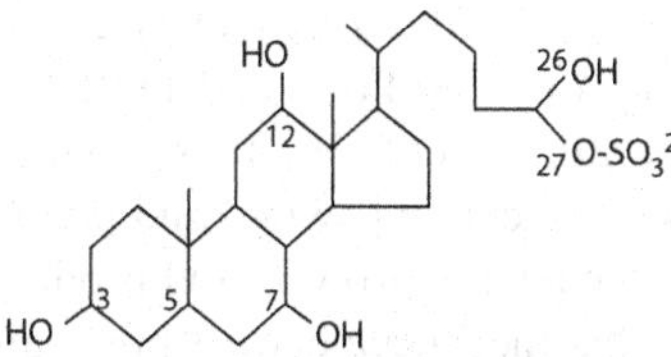

5α-Cyprinol-27-sulfate
(a bile alcohol; e.g., zebrafish)

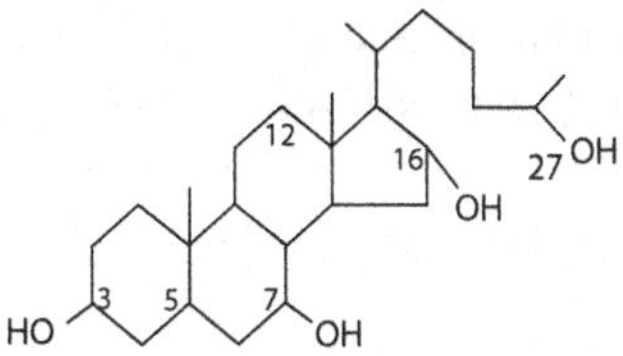

5α-Myxinol
(a bile alcohol; e.g., hagfish)

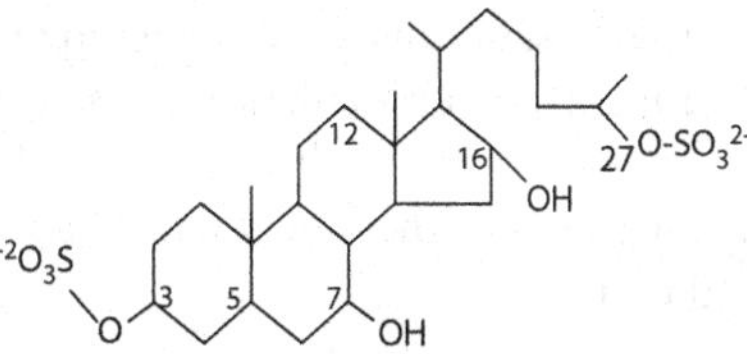

5α-Myxinol-3β,27-disulfate
(a bile alcohol; e.g., hagfish)

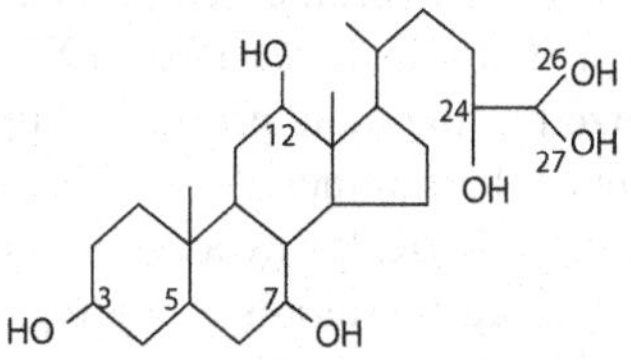

5β-Scymnol
(a bile alcohol; e.g., elasmobranch fish)

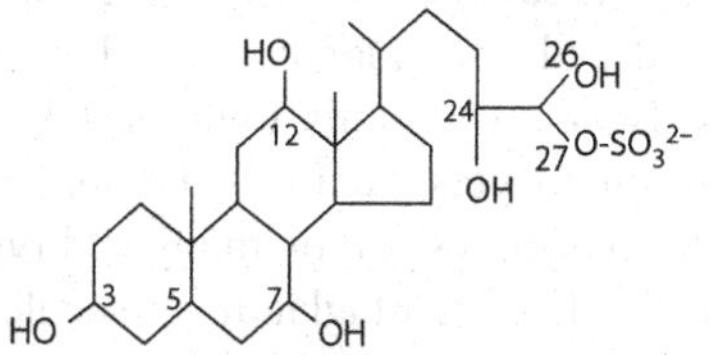

5β-Scymnol-27-sulfate
(a bile alcohol; e.g., elasmobranch fish)

**FIGURE 3.13** Structures of bile alcohols in fish. They are usually $C_{27}$ compounds synthesized from cholesterol in the liver of aquatic animals and reptiles, with the terminal –OH group at the $C_{27}$ position. The sulfate group forms a salt with sodium in the body.

Steroidal saponins in Yucca extracts
Compound 1: R = Glc (1-2) [Xyl (1-3)] Glc
Compound 2: R = Glc (1-2) [Glc (1-3)] Glc

Steroidal saponins in Yucca extracts
Compound 3: R = Glc (1-2) Xyl; $R_1$ = H
Compound 4: R = Glc (1-2) [Xyl (1-3)] Glc; $R_1$ = H
Compound 5: R = Glc (1-2) Gal; $R_1$ = OH

Steroidal saponins in Yucca extracts
Compound 6: R = Glc (1-2) Glc
Compound 7: R = Glc (1-2) [Xyl (1-3)] Glc

Steroidal saponins in Yucca extracts
Compound 8: R = Glc (1-2) [Xyl (1-3)] Glc

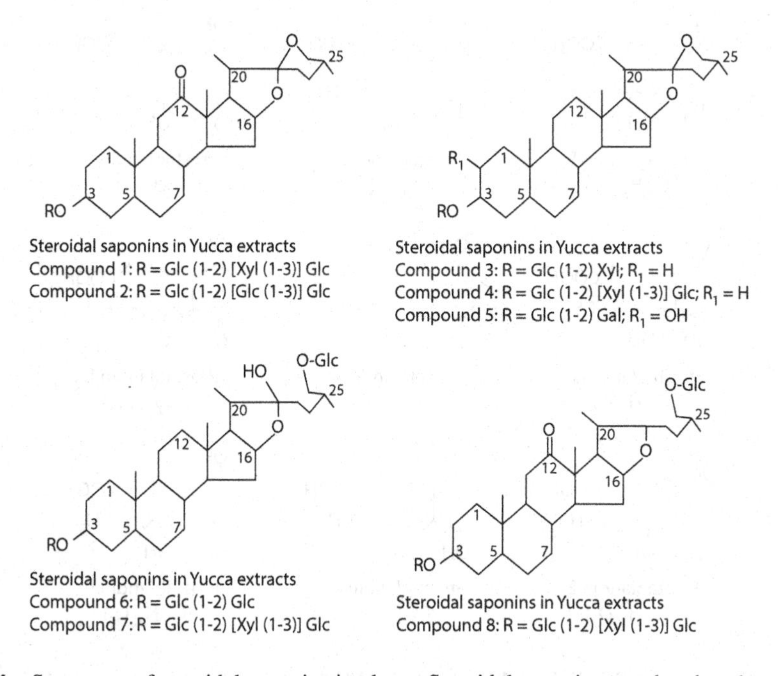

**FIGURE 3.14** Structures of steroidal saponins in plants. Steroidal saponins are abundant (up to 10% of dry matter) in Yucca trees native to North America. These substances contain an ether linkage (C–O–C) and one or more monosaccharides joined via β-1,2 or β-1,3 bonds. The structures of 8 steroidal saponins present in the *Yucca schidigera* plants are illustrated to show their similarities and differences. Glc, glucose; Xyl, xylose.

The *Yucca schidigera* extract is generally recognized as a safe (GRAS) product and approved by the U.S. Food and Drug Administration (FDA) as a natural food adjuvant under Title 21CFR 172.510. This product is also widely used as a feed additive for livestock species (including swine) and poultry to improve air quality in the production barns as well as the health, growth, and productivity of the animals (Cheeke 2000). It has been suggested that the Yucca extract binds ammonia and therefore reduces its emission from animals (Colina et al. 2001). As steroidal derivatives, Yucca saponins may also have potent anabolic and anti-oxidative effects on animals. For example, under high-temperature conditions, steroidal saponins may antagonize the action of glucocorticoids and oxidative stress in animals, thereby enhancing feed efficiency and production performance. This view represents a paradigm shift in our understanding of the mechanisms responsible for the beneficial effects of the *Yucca schidigera* extracts on the growth and health of livestock species and poultry.

## Eicosanoids

1. *Precursors.* Eicosanoids are derivatives of ω3 PUFAs (α-linolenic acid) and ω6 PUFAs (linoleic acid and arachidonic acid). This group of lipids includes PGs, TXs, LTs, and lipoxins. PGs were originally found to be synthesized in the male prostate gland, TXs in platelets (thrombocytes), and LTs in leukocytes, hence their names. Now, it is known that eicosanoids are synthesized by many cell types in animals (Ridgway and McLeod 2016).
2. *Prostaglandins.* Each prostaglandin molecule contains 20 carbon atoms, including a 5-carbon ring (Figure 3.15). They act like hormones but differ from endocrine hormones because these eicosanoids are not produced at a specific site, but in many cell types throughout the body (Gunstone 2012). There are 3 series of PGs. Series 1 and 2 PGs (with 1 and 2 double bonds, respectively) are derived from linoleic acid and arachidonic acid (ω6 PUFAs),

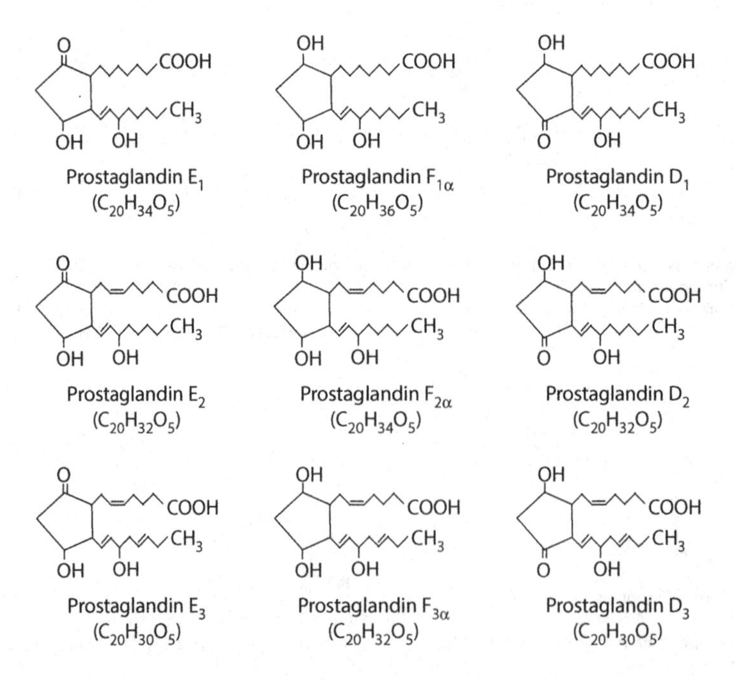


**FIGURE 3.15** Structures of PGs E, F, and D in animals. PGs contain 20 carbon atoms, including a 5-carbon ring. There are 3 series of PGs. Series 1 and 2 of PGs (with 1 and 2 double bonds, respectively) are derived from linoleic acid and arachidonic acid, respectively. Series 3 of PGs (with 3 double bonds) is derived from α-linolenic acid.

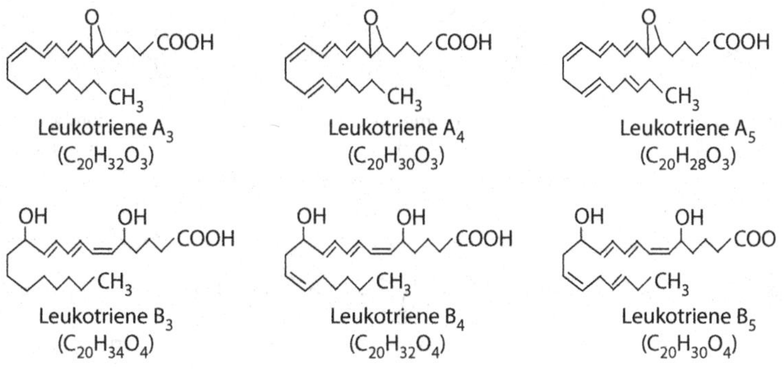

Leukotriene $A_3$ ($C_{20}H_{32}O_3$) | Leukotriene $A_4$ ($C_{20}H_{30}O_3$) | Leukotriene $A_5$ ($C_{20}H_{28}O_3$)

Leukotriene $B_3$ ($C_{20}H_{34}O_4$) | Leukotriene $B_4$ ($C_{20}H_{32}O_4$) | Leukotriene $B_5$ ($C_{20}H_{30}O_4$)

**FIGURE 3.16** Structures of LTs in animals. LTs are derivatives of unsaturated LCFAs and contain three conjugated double bonds. LTA is an epoxide, whereas LTB has two –OH groups. Series 3, 4, and 5 LTs (LTA3 and LTB3) are synthesized from eicosatrienoic acid (20:3, ω9), arachidonic acid (20:4, ω6), and eicosapentaenoic acid (C20:5, ω3), respectively.

respectively. Series 1 PGs are $PGH_1$, $PGE_1$, $PGF_{1\alpha}$, $PGI_1$, and $PGD_1$, whereas series 2 PGs are $PGH_2$, $PGE_2$, $PGF_{2\alpha}$, $PGI_2$, and $PGD_2$. Series 3 PGs (with 3 double bonds) are derived from α-linolenic acid (ω3 PUFA), and include $PGH_3$, $PGE_3$, $PGF_{3\alpha}$, $PGI_3$, and $PGD_3$. Series 2 PGs are proinflammatory mediators, but series 1 and 3 PGs are anti-inflammatory (Folco and Murphy 2006).

3. *Leukotrienes*. LTs are derivatives of unsaturated LCFAs and contain three conjugated double bonds. LTA is an epoxide, whereas LTB has two –OH groups (Figure 3.16). Series 3 LTs ($LTA_3$ and $LTB_3$) are synthesized from eicosatrienoic acid ($C_{20:3}$ ω9, Mead's acid) and have three conjugated double bonds (Devlin 2006). $LTC_3$ (5-hydroxy-6-S-glutathionyl-7,9,1l-eicosatrienoic acid) is the conjugate of a hydroxylated $LTA_3$ intermediate with glutathione (Glu–Cys–Gly), $LTD_3$ is the conjugate of a hydroxylated $LTA_3$ intermediate with cysteine–glycine, and $LTE_3$ is the conjugate of a hydroxylated $LTA_3$ intermediate with one cysteine molecule.

   Series 4 LTs have four double bonds (including three conjugated double bonds) and were the first LTs discovered. They are synthesized from arachidonic acid, including $LTA_4$ and $LTB_4$, as well as $LTC_4$, $LTD_4$, $LTE_4$, and $LTF_4$. $LTC_4$, $LTD_4$, $LTE_4$, and $LTF_4$ are derivatives of $LTA_4$, and they all contain a cysteine moiety. Specifically, $LTC_4$ is the conjugate of a hydroxylated $LTA_4$ intermediate with glutathione, $LTD_4$ is the conjugate of a hydroxylated $LTA_4$ intermediate with cysteine–glycine, $LTE_4$ is the conjugate of a hydroxylated $LTA_4$ intermediate with one cysteine molecule, and $LTF_4$ is the conjugate of a hydroxylated $LTA_4$ intermediate with cysteine and glutamate. Thus, $LTC_4$, $LTD_4$, $LTE_4$, and $LTF_4$ are called cysteinyl LTs. Production of series 4 LTs is enhanced in response to inflammatory mediators, thereby inducing the adhesion and activation of leukocytes on the endothelium of blood vessels (Folco and Murphy 2006).

   Series 5 LTs (e.g., $LTA_5$, $LTB_5$, $LTC_5$, $LTD_5$, and $LTE_5$) have five double bonds, including three conjugated double bonds. They are synthesized from eicosapentaenoic acid, which is abundant in marine fish oil. $LTC_5$ (5-hydroxy-6-S-glutathionyl-7,9,11,14,17-eicosapentaenoic acid) is the conjugate of a hydroxylated $LTA_5$ intermediate with glutathione, $LTD_5$ is the conjugate of a hydroxylated $LTA_5$ intermediate with cysteine–glycine, and $LTE_5$ is the conjugate of a hydroxylated $LTA_5$ intermediate with one cysteine molecule. Series 5 LTs inhibit the synthesis of series 4 LTs and exert anti-inflammatory effects in blood vessels.

4. *Thromboxanes*. TX is named for its role in constricting blood vessels and promoting clot formation (thrombosis). This class of lipids contains a 6-membered ether-containing ring.

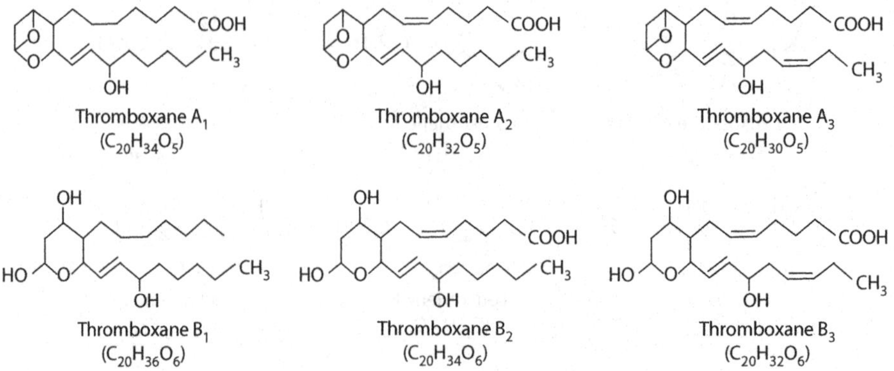

Thromboxane $A_1$ ($C_{20}H_{34}O_5$) Thromboxane $A_2$ ($C_{20}H_{32}O_5$) Thromboxane $A_3$ ($C_{20}H_{30}O_5$)

Thromboxane $B_1$ ($C_{20}H_{36}O_6$) Thromboxane $B_2$ ($C_{20}H_{34}O_6$) Thromboxane $B_3$ ($C_{20}H_{32}O_6$)

**FIGURE 3.17** Structures of TXs in animals. TXs are derivatives of unsaturated LCFAs and have a 6-membered ether-containing ring. TXA is an epoxide, whereas TXB has two –OH groups. There are 3 series of TXs. Series 1 ($TXA_1$ and $TXB_1$ with one double bond), 2 ($TXA_2$ and $TXB_2$ with two double bonds), and 3 TXs ($TXA_3$ and $TXB_3$ with three double bonds) are formed from dihomo-γ-linolenic acid (ω6 PUFA), arachidonic acid, and eicosapentaenoic acid, respectively.

Three series of TXs have been identified (Figure 3.17). Series 1 ($TXA_1$ and $TXB_1$ with one double bond), 2 ($TXA_2$ and $TXB_2$ with two double bonds), and 3 TXs ($TXA_3$ and $TXB_3$ with three double bonds) are formed from dihomo-γ-linolenic acid (ω6 PUFA), arachidonic acid, and eicosapentaenoic acid, respectively (Folco and Murphy 2006). $TXA_2$ and $TXB_2$ are quantitatively two major TXs identified to date. All three series of TXs act on specific receptors on the plasma membrane of platelets, thereby modulating the functions of these cells. $PGI_2$, a product of arachidonic acid in vascular endothelial cells, inhibits platelet aggregation and relaxes the smooth muscle cells of blood vessels.

5. *Lipoxins*. Lipoxins were first described in 1984 and are the newest type of eicosanoids to be discovered. They have four conjugated double bonds and three –OH groups (Figure 3.18). This class of lipids is synthesized from arachidonic acid via the formation of 15-hydroxyicosatetraenoic acid (15(*S*)-HETE) and its 15-hydroperoxy precursor. At present, four lipoxins have been identified in animal tissues: lipoxins $A_4$, $A_5$, $B_4$, and $B_5$. Lipoxins $A_4$ and $B_4$ have the same molecular weight. Lipoxins $A_5$ and $B_5$ also have the same molecular

Lipoxin $A_4$ ($C_{20}H_{32}O_5$) Lipoxin $A_5$ ($C_{20}H_{30}O_5$)

Lipoxin $B_4$ ($C_{20}H_{32}O_5$) Lipoxin $B_5$ ($C_{20}H_{30}O_5$)

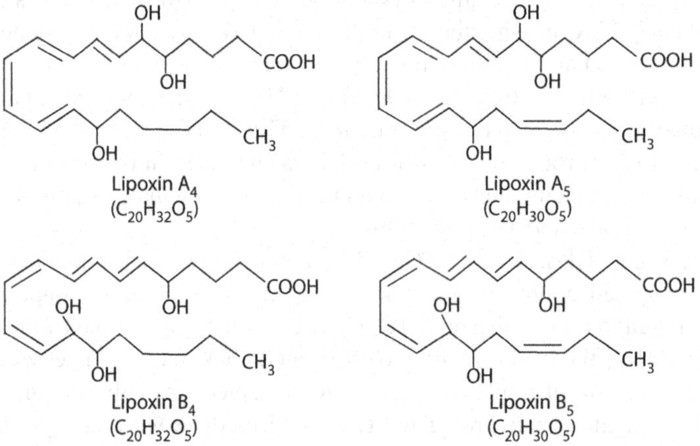

**FIGURE 3.18** Structures of lipoxins in animals. Lipoxins contain four conjugated double bonds and three –OH groups. Thus, this class of lipids has a conjugated trihydroxytetraene structure. At present, lipoxins A4, A5, B4, and B4 are known to be synthesized from arachidonic acid.

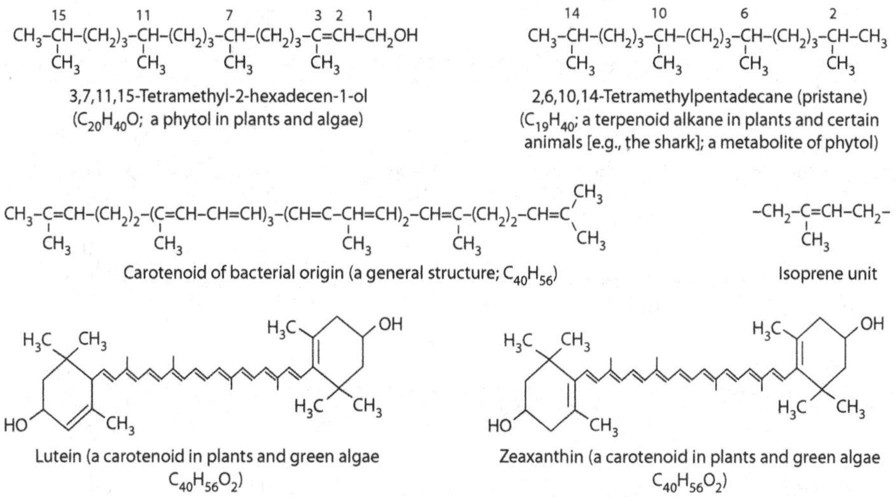

3,7,11,15-Tetramethyl-2-hexadecen-1-ol ($C_{20}H_{40}O$; a phytol in plants and algae)

2,6,10,14-Tetramethylpentadecane (pristane) ($C_{19}H_{40}$; a terpenoid alkane in plants and certain animals [e.g., the shark]; a metabolite of phytol)

Carotenoid of bacterial origin (a general structure; $C_{40}H_{56}$)

Isoprene unit

Lutein (a carotenoid in plants and green algae $C_{40}H_{56}O_2$)

Zeaxanthin (a carotenoid in plants and green algae $C_{40}H_{56}O_2$)

**FIGURE 3.19** Structures of phytols and carotenoids. Phytols and carotenoids are classified as terpenes that have an isoprene structure. Phytol is an acyclic diterpene alcohol present in plants, algae, and bacteria. Carotenoids consist of isoprenoid units with conjugated double bonds, and are derived from the acyclic $C_{40}H_{56}$ structure. More than 600 different types of carotenoids exist in nature, yielding pigments responsible for bright red, yellow, and orange colors in plants and certain organisms.

weight. These lipoxins stimulate superoxide anion generation and degranulation, as does $LTB_4$. Like LTs, lipoxins conjugate with cysteine to form cysteinyl-lipoxins. Emerging evidence shows that lipoxins have anti-inflammatory effects in animals (Romano et al. 2015).

## Terpenes

1. *Phytols*. Phytol is an acyclic diterpene alcohol. It is freely present in plants and algae as a constituent of chlorophyll, and is also produced by bacteria (including those in the gastrointestinal tract of animals). An example of a phytol of plant and algae origin is 3,7,11,15-tetramethyl-2-hexadecen-1-ol ($C_{20}H_{40}O$) (Figure 3.19). Plants, algae, and bacteria can convert phytol into vitamin E and vitamin $K_1$, as well as phytanic acid and pristine (a saturated terpenoid alkane). Thus, these substances are found in common fruits, vegetables, and algae products (Chung et al. 1989). Likewise, the liver of certain animals (e.g., the shark) can metabolize phytol into pristane, which was originally coined from the Latin *pristis* "shark." As compounds with fragrant properties, phytols are used by plants to protect against predation. Similarly, some insects (e.g., the sumac flea beetle) depend on plant phytols for defense.
2. *Carotenoids*. Carotenoids are lipids consisting of isoprenoid units with conjugated double bonds and thus are called isoprenoids (Mead et al. 1986). They are derived from the acyclic $C_{40}H_{56}$ structure (Figure 3.19) and are plant or algae pigments responsible for bright red, yellow, and orange colors in fruits, vegetables, and other foods (e.g., sweet potatoes and papaya). There are more than 600 different types of carotenoids in nature, which can be classified as carotenes (e.g., α-carotene, β-carotene, γ-carotene, and lycopene) and xanthophylls (e.g., lutein, zeaxanthin, antheraxanthin, and β-cryptoxanthin). Both groups are hydrocarbons by definition, but differ in structure. Specifically, xanthophylls contain oxygen, whereas carotenes do not. Animals do not synthesize carotenoids (Pond et al. 2005). However, these substances are important antioxidants in the diets of animals.

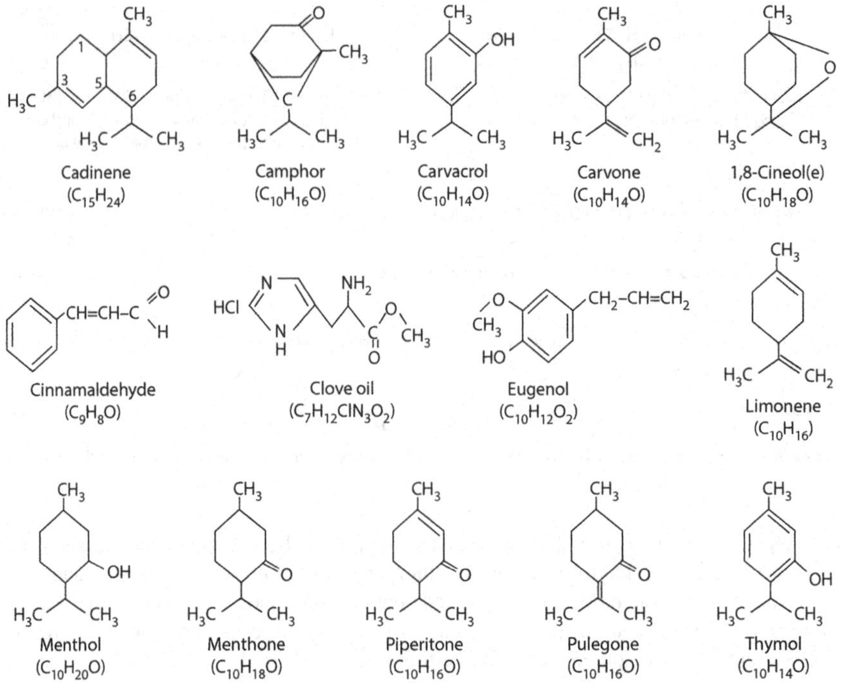

Cadinene ($C_{15}H_{24}$) Camphor ($C_{10}H_{16}O$) Carvacrol ($C_{10}H_{14}O$) Carvone ($C_{10}H_{14}O$) 1,8-Cineol(e) ($C_{10}H_{18}O$)

Cinnamaldehyde ($C_9H_8O$) Clove oil ($C_7H_{12}ClN_3O_2$) Eugenol ($C_{10}H_{12}O_2$) Limonene ($C_{10}H_{16}$)

Menthol ($C_{10}H_{20}O$) Menthone ($C_{10}H_{18}O$) Piperitone ($C_{10}H_{16}O$) Pulegone ($C_{10}H_{16}O$) Thymol ($C_{10}H_{14}O$)

**FIGURE 3.20** Structures of essential oils in plants. Essential oils are concentrated hydrophobic liquids containing a phenolic ring. They are present in certain plants as volatile aromatic compounds with characteristic fragrances and flavors. Many of them have the same molecular weight but different structures, whereas some are isomeric (e.g., thymol and carvacrol).

3. *Lipid-soluble vitamins.* Terpenes are lipid-soluble vitamins, including vitamins A, E, and K. Plants or algae contain vitamin-A precursors but not vitamin A. In animals, the small intestine converts β-carotene into vitamin A. In contrast, plants, algae, and bacteria synthesize vitamins E and K from shikimate (Bentley and Meganathan 1983; DellaPenna 2005), but these two vitamins are not made by animals (Pond et al. 2005).
4. *Essential oils.* An essential oil is a concentrated hydrophobic liquid containing a phenolic ring. It is not an "oil" in the same way as the liquid state of the ester of an LCFA with glycerol. Steam distillation is the usual method for extracting essential oils from certain plants (Tongnuanchan and Benjakul 2014). The term "essential" does not imply that these substances are nutritionally essential for animals. Rather, the name was used because the *essence* of the plant has been extracted. The structures of various components of some essential oils are shown in Figure 3.20. Many of them have the same molecular weight but different structures, whereas some are isomeric (e.g., thymol and carvacrol). Note that essential oils are volatile aromatic compounds with characteristic fragrances and flavors.

   Essential oils are unique to certain plants. For example, cinnamaldehyde is a pale yellow, viscous liquid present in the bark of cinnamon trees and other species of the genus *Cinnamomum.* Eugenol is an allyl chain-substituted guaiacol, which is a member of the phenylpropanoids class of phytochemicals (Figure 3.20). It is a pale yellow to colorless liquid extracted from certain plants, such as cloves, nutmeg, cinnamon, basil, and bay leaves. Thymol (also known as 2-isopropyl-5-methylphenol) is a natural monoterpene phenol derivative of cymene and is isolated from *Thymus vulgaris* (common thyme) and various other kinds of plants. Thymol is a white crystalline substance with a pleasant aromatic odor.

Essential oils have antimicrobial, antiparasitic, anti-inflammatory, anti-oxidative, and immunomodulatory functions (Benchaar et al. 2008; Zeng et al. 2015). They can be added to a diet as a single substance or a mixture of two or more compounds. For example, supplementing cinnamaldehyde to the diet of weanling piglets reduces the intestinal expression of inflammatory cytokines in response to LPS challenge genes (Wang et al. 2015). In addition, supplementing cinnamaldehyde plus thymol to the diet of chickens can beneficially enhance feed intake, modulate the gut microbiota, and improve body weight gain (Zeng et al. 2015). However, it should be borne in mind that, owing to their lipid-soluble properties and involvement in chemical reactions, excessive amounts of essential oils are toxic to animals.

5. *Coenzyme Q.* Coenzyme Q (CoQ), which was discovered in 1957, is chemically known as 2,3-dimethoxy-5-methyl-6-multiprenyl-1,4-benzoquinone. It is a hydrophobic compound present in the organelles (particularly the mitochondria) of all animals. The various forms of CoQ are distinguished by the number (usually between 6 and 10) of isoprenoid repeats in their side chains. In mammals and birds, the most common CoQ is either $CoQ_{10}$ or $CoQ_9$, where the number refers to the number of isoprene repeats in the molecule (Turunen et al. 2004). For example, ~90% of ubiquinone is $CoQ_9$ in mice and rats. In contrast, in chickens, cows, goats, guinea pigs, horses, humans, rabbits, and pigs, ≥96% of ubiquinone is $CoQ_{10}$, with ≤4% of ubiquinone being $CoQ_9$ (Lass et al. 1997). Fish is also an excellent source of $CoQ_{10}$. CoQ plays an essential role in mitochondrial electron transport and ATP synthesis, and also acts as an antioxidant in cell membranes, lipoproteins, and mitochondria.

   All animals can synthesize CoQ and do not require this fat-soluble ubiquinone from diets. This synthetic pathway occurs in many tissues, including the liver and brain. The biosynthesis of coenzyme $Q_{10}$ involves three major steps: (1) the synthesis of the benzoquinone structure from tyrosine, with the first step being the vitamin $B_6$-dependent conversion of tyrosine to 4-hydroxyphenylpyruvic acid; (2) the synthesis of the isoprene side chain from acetyl-CoA via the mevalonate (cholesterol-synthetic) pathway; and (3) the condensation of the benzoquinone and mevalonate structures (Turunen et al. 2004). Hydroxymethylglutaryl (HMG)-CoA reductase plays a critical role in regulating the synthesis of both cholesterol and CoQ.

## CHEMICAL REACTIONS

### Hydrolysis of TAG and Saponification of Fatty Acids

TAG can be hydrolyzed by boiling in the presence of an alkali compound (e.g., NaOH) to form glycerol and fatty acids. The fatty acids then react with the base to produce soaps (i.e., alkali salts of fatty acids) (Ridgway and McLeod 2016). This reaction of salt formation is called saponification, a process of manufacturing soaps in the chemical industry. Similarly, a fatty acid reacts with calcium hydroxide to form a salt. Such a reaction has been used to manufacture a rumen-protected fatty acid calcium salt from fatty acids plus calcium oxide.

$$\text{Triacylglycerols} + 3\,H_2O \xrightarrow{\text{Boiling with alkali}} 3\,\text{R-COOH} + \text{Glycerol}$$

$$\text{R-COOH} + \text{NaOH} \longrightarrow \text{R-COONa} + H_2O$$

$$2\,\text{R-COOH} + Ca(OH)_2 \longrightarrow (\text{R-COO})_2Ca + 2\,H_2O$$

$$2\,\text{R-COOH} + CaO + H_2O \longrightarrow (\text{R-COO})_2Ca + 2\,H_2O$$

In animals, fat hydrolysis, which takes place in the lumen of the small intestine, is catalyzed by lipases in the presence of bile salts to yield *sn*-2-mono- or di-acylglycerols, fatty acids, and/or glycerol (Lefebvre et al. 2009). These digestion products, together with the bile salts, form water-miscible micelles, with the hydrophilic "head" regions in contact with the surrounding water and the hydrophobic single-tail regions being sequestered in the micelle center.

Feed analysis of lipids often calls for the determination of "the acid value" of fatty acids, namely the quantity of KOH that is required to neutralize the free organic acids in a gram of fat. The acid value is a measure of the amount of free fatty acids present in the sample. This method provides a very rapid way to quantify fatty acids, but its accuracy should be verified by HPLC or gas chromatography.

### Esterification with Alcohols

A fatty acid forms an ester with glycerol (a sugar alcohol with three –OH groups) as noted previously. This condensation reaction is important for fat storage in the animal body (Tso 1985; Yabuuchi and O'Brien 1968). For comparison, phosphoric acid reacts with a hydroxyl group in glycerol to yield a phosphate ester (e.g., phospholipids). Furthermore, a fatty acid forms an ester with a straight-chain alcohol (e.g., ethanol) (Gunstone 2012), as shown in the following reaction, which is the chemical basis for the industrial production of polyesters. Of note, ethyl acetate is the most common ester in wine that is formed enzymatically from acetic acid and ethanol during the fermentation process.

$$\underset{\text{Acetic acid}}{CH_3\text{-}\overset{\overset{O}{\|}}{C}\text{-}OH} + \underset{\text{Ethanol}}{CH_3CH_2\text{-}OH} \xrightarrow{H_2SO_4} \underset{\text{Ethyl acetate}}{CH_3\text{-}\overset{\overset{O}{\|}}{C}\text{-}O\text{-}CH_2CH_3} + H_2O$$

### Substitution of the Hydroxyl Hydrogen

An electrophile (an electron-seeking reagent) extracts the hydrogen atom from the hydroxyl group of an LCFA (Gunstone 2012). Electrophiles have vacant orbitals attracted to an electron-rich center and participate in chemical reactions by accepting a pair of electrons. Examples of this class of substances are alkyl halides, acyl halides, carbonyl compounds, hydrogen sulfide anion, alcohols and hydrogen, and oxidizing agents. Substitution of the hydroxyl hydrogen in fatty acids renders both saturated and unsaturated fatty acids prone to oxidation, leading to reductions in their chemical stability and biological activity.

$$R\text{-}COOH + E^+ \rightarrow R\text{-}COO\text{-}E + H^+, \text{ Where } E^+ \text{ is an electrophile}$$

### Hydrogenation of Unsaturated Fatty Acids

An unsaturated fatty acid, which is liquid at 37°C, can be converted into a saturated fatty acid by the hydrogenation of its double bonds (Mead et al. 1986). This process is used to convert oil into solid margarine. Rumen microorganisms enzymatically hydrogenate unsaturated fatty acids, which is called biohydrogenation. This explains why the percentage of saturated fatty acids among total lipids in white adipose tissue and skeletal muscle is higher in ruminants than in nonruminants (Smith and Smith 1995; Tan et al. 2011) and why the body fat is "harder" in ruminants than in nonruminants.

$$\underset{\text{Unsaturated fatty acid}}{R\text{-}CH_2\text{-}CH{=}CH\text{-}CH_2\text{-}\overset{\overset{O}{\|}}{C}\text{-}OH} + 2H \longrightarrow \underset{\text{Saturated fatty acid}}{R\text{-}CH_2\text{-}CH_2\text{-}CH_2\text{-}CH_2\text{-}\overset{\overset{O}{\|}}{C}\text{-}OH}$$

### IODINATION AND BROMINATION OF THE DOUBLE BONDS OF UNSATURATED FATTY ACIDS

A double bond in an unsaturated fatty acid is highly reactive with iodine ($I_2$), forming an iodinated fatty acid. This reaction has been widely used as a measure of the degree of unsaturation of a lipid (e.g., an oil, fat, or wax), and quantified as an iodine value (or iodine number), which is defined as the amount of iodine (in g) that is taken up by 100 g of a lipid. Saturated oils, fats, and waxes do not react with iodine and therefore have an iodine value of zero. The more double bonds a fatty acid has, the higher its iodine value will be. This test is often performed with a known excess of iodine, usually in the form of iodine monochloride (ICl), and the amount of iodine remaining unreacted is then determined by titration. Note that a double bond in an unsaturated fatty acid also reacts with bromine ($Br_2$) to yield a brominated fatty acid.

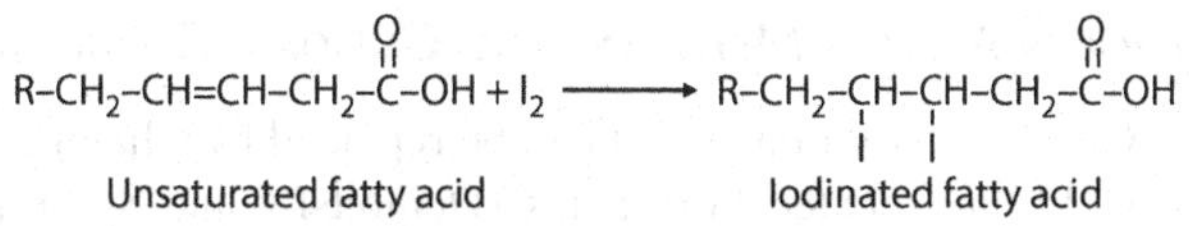

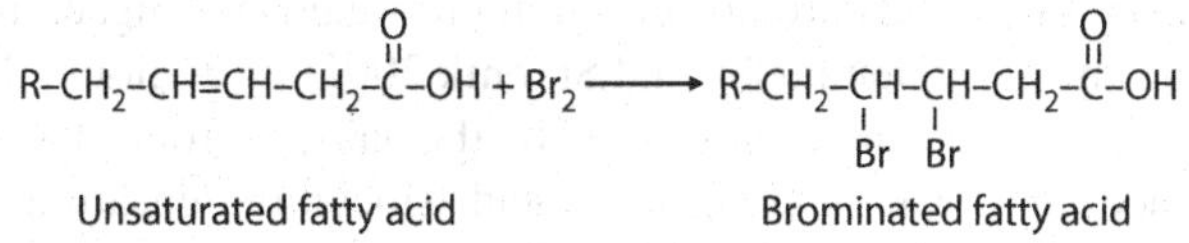

$$\underset{\text{Unsaturated fatty acid}}{R\text{-}CH_2\text{-}CH{=}CH\text{-}CH_2\text{-}\overset{O}{\overset{\|}{C}}\text{-}OH} + I_2 \longrightarrow \underset{\text{Iodinated fatty acid}}{R\text{-}CH_2\text{-}\underset{I}{CH}\text{-}\underset{I}{CH}\text{-}CH_2\text{-}\overset{O}{\overset{\|}{C}}\text{-}OH}$$

$$\underset{\text{Unsaturated fatty acid}}{R\text{-}CH_2\text{-}CH{=}CH\text{-}CH_2\text{-}\overset{O}{\overset{\|}{C}}\text{-}OH} + Br_2 \longrightarrow \underset{\text{Brominated fatty acid}}{R\text{-}CH_2\text{-}\underset{Br}{CH}\text{-}\underset{Br}{CH}\text{-}CH_2\text{-}\overset{O}{\overset{\|}{C}}\text{-}OH}$$

### PEROXIDATION OF UNSATURATED FATTY ACIDS

The double bonds in unsaturated fatty acids are chemically reactive (Mead et al. 1986). Thus, unsaturated fatty acids, particularly PUFAs, undergo peroxidation by reactive oxygen species (ROS, such as, OH and HOO·) to form lipid peroxides or lipid oxidation products. This reaction occurs *in vitro* and *in vivo*, and is accelerated at high ambient temperatures and increased oxygen exposure (Rosero et al. 2015). Lipid peroxidation involves three major steps: initiation, propagation, and termination (Figure 3.21). During initiation, a free radical extracts a proton and an electron from the carbon adjacent to the double bond, yielding an unstable fatty acid radical. The fatty acid radical then reacts with molecular oxygen to produce an unstable peroxyl-fatty acid radical, which reacts with another molecule of unsaturated fatty acid to form a new fatty acid radical and a lipid peroxide (Gunstone 2012). This ROS-initiated chain reaction results in the propagation of fatty acid radicals.

A radical reaction stops after two radicals react to produce a non-radical species. In animals, termination of the free radical reaction can be facilitated by antioxidants (e.g., vitamins E and C,

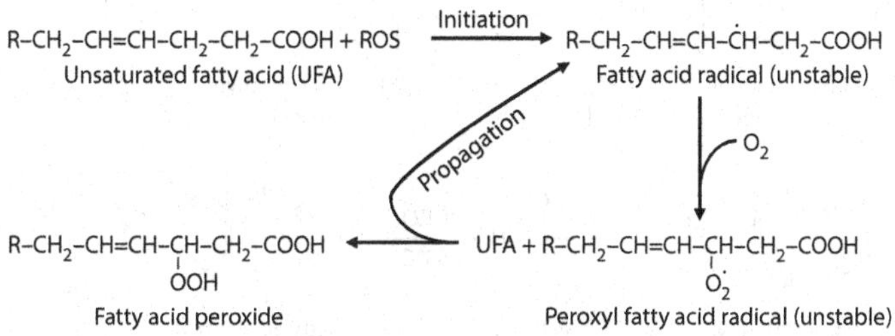

$$\underset{\text{Unsaturated fatty acid (UFA)}}{R\text{-}CH_2\text{-}CH{=}CH\text{-}CH_2\text{-}CH_2\text{-}COOH} + ROS \xrightarrow{\text{Initiation}} \underset{\text{Fatty acid radical (unstable)}}{R\text{-}CH_2\text{-}CH{=}CH\text{-}\dot{C}H\text{-}CH_2\text{-}COOH}$$

$$\xrightarrow{O_2} UFA + \underset{\text{Peroxyl fatty acid radical (unstable)}}{R\text{-}CH_2\text{-}CH{=}CH\text{-}\underset{O_2^{\cdot}}{CH}\text{-}CH_2\text{-}COOH} \longrightarrow \underset{\text{Fatty acid peroxide}}{R\text{-}CH_2\text{-}CH{=}CH\text{-}\underset{OOH}{CH}\text{-}CH_2\text{-}COOH}$$

Propagation

**FIGURE 3.21** Peroxidation of unsaturated fatty acids. The double bonds in unsaturated fatty acids undergo peroxidation by ROS to form lipid peroxides or lipid oxidation products. Lipid peroxidation involves three major steps: initiation, propagation, and termination. An unstable fatty acid radical is formed during the initiation phase, followed by the propagation of fatty acid radicals. The radical reaction stops when two radicals react and produce a non-radical species.

and phenolic compounds) and antioxidant enzymes (e.g., superoxide dismutase, catalase, and peroxidase) (Fang et al. 2002). The antioxidants react with fatty acid radicals to form nonreactive products, thereby breaking the propagation chain of the peroxidation reaction (Mao et al. 2010). In fact, these compounds are able to donate a hydrogen atom to the fatty acid radical formed during the propagation phase of lipid acid oxidation.

The knowledge of fatty acid peroxidation is useful for the storage (shelf life) and analysis of unsaturated fatty acids and for protecting animals from oxidative damage, a contributor to chronic diseases in mammals and birds. The Rancimat method for detecting peroxides provides useful information about the oxidative stability of fats and oils, as well as fatty acids in feedstuffs (Aparicio et al. 1999).

### Reaction of the Hydrogen Atom in Methylene and Carboxyl Groups with Halogens

A hydrogen atom in a $-CH_2$ group of a fatty acid can be replaced by a halogen (fluorine, chlorine, bromine, or iodine) to yield halogenated fatty acids (Dembitsky and Srebnik 2002). More than 200 different halogenated fatty acids are present in microorganisms, algae, marine invertebrates, higher plants, and some animals (Dembitsky and Srebnik 2002). In addition, the hydrogen atom of the carboxyl group in a fatty acid can be substituted by the halogen from a halogenated compound. For example, short-, medium-, or long-chain fatty acids (including unsaturated fatty acids) react with 9-chloromethyl-anthracene (Xie et al. 2012) or 2-bromomethyl-anthraquinone (Tapia 2014) in the presence of a base (e.g., $K_2CO_3$) to yield fluorescent, stable fatty acyl derivatives (Figure 3.22). The derivatives are separated on a reversed-phase HPLC column and detected by fluorescence. These chemical reactions provide a useful tool for sensitive analysis of fatty acids in biological samples.

## SUMMARY

Lipids are a diverse group of hydrocarbons that are defined on the basis of their common hydrophobic property. This class of organic substances consists of fatty acids, as well as simple, compound, and derived lipids, with essential nutritional and physiological functions. Fatty acids have 2–30 carbon atoms and a carboxyl group, including short ($C_{2-5}$)-, medium ($C_{6-12}$)-, long ($C_{13-20}$)-, and very long ($>C_{20}$)-chain fatty acids. LCFAs are much more abundant than SCFAs and MCFAs in the tissues of animals, and possess 0–6 double bonds. In unsaturated fatty acids, the hydrogen atoms are

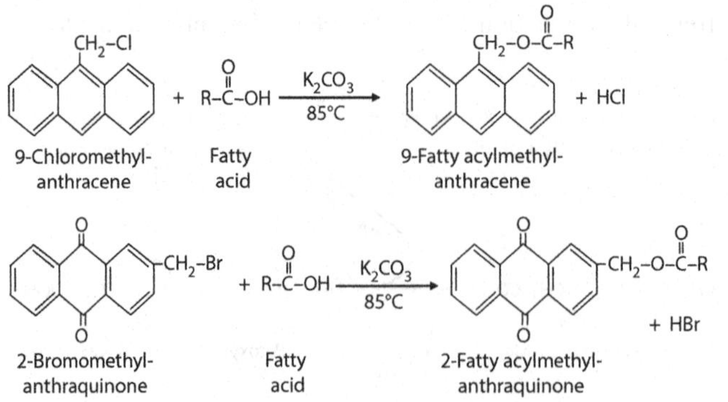

9-Chloromethyl-anthracene + Fatty acid (R-C(=O)-OH) $\xrightarrow[85°C]{K_2CO_3}$ 9-Fatty acylmethyl-anthracene + HCl

2-Bromomethyl-anthraquinone + Fatty acid (R-C(=O)-OH) $\xrightarrow[85°C]{K_2CO_3}$ 2-Fatty acylmethyl-anthraquinone + HBr

**FIGURE 3.22** Reaction of fatty acids with halogens. The hydrogen atom of the carboxyl group in a fatty acid can be substituted by the halogen of a halogenated compound, such as 9-chloromethyl-anthracene or 2-bromomethyl-anthraquinone in the presence of a base (e.g., $K_2CO_3$), to yield a fluorescent, stable fatty acyl derivative. These reactions provide a basis for the analysis of fatty acids by chromatographic methods, such as high-performance liquid chromatography.

usually on the same (*cis*) side of the double bond, but may also be on its opposite (*trans*) side. Most of the naturally occurring fatty acids have an even number of carbons, but some have an odd number of carbons or a branched chain. Since elevated concentrations of LCFAs are toxic to cells, they are stored in animals primarily as glycerol-based esters (fats or TAGs) and, to a much lesser extent, as alcohol-based waxes. Oils are fats in the liquid state, which contain mainly PUFAs. Fats and waxes are collectively known as simple lipids, but differ in compositions and functions. For example, fats are digestible as the major source of energy, whereas waxes are indigestible and provide a waterproof layer of protection.

Compound lipids are composed of (a) glycolipids containing a carbohydrate moiety; (b) phospholipids containing a phosphate group and an ethanolamine, choline, serine, myo-inositol, glycerol, or phosphatidylglycerol group; (c) sphingosine-based sphingolipids containing an acyl group to form a ceramide, a nitrogenous group (e.g., ethanolamine, serine, or choline) to yield a sphingomyelin, or sugars to generate glycosphingolipids; (d) ether glycerophospholipids containing an ether linkage ($-CH_2-O-CH_2-$) in the phospholipids (e.g., PAF and plasmalogens); and (e) lipoproteins formed and released by the small intestine and liver, with the protein moiety transporting LCFAs and cholesterol. Phosphatidylcholine, cephalins, and sphingomyelins are important components of cell membranes (Table 3.10) and highly abundant in the nervous system. Plasma chylomicrons and HDLs have the highest content of TAGs and proteins, respectively. The proportions of cholesterols in lipoproteins have important implications for cardiovascular health.

Derived lipids include steroids, eicosanoids, and terpenes. Steroids include sterols (e.g., cholesterol) and their derivatives, such as steroid hormones (e.g., male and female reproductive hormones), bile acids, and bile alcohols that are synthesized in animals, as well as steroidal saponins that are present in plants. Eicosanoids are composed of series 1, 2, and 3 PGs and TXs with 1, 2, or 3 double bonds, as well as series 4 and 5 LTs and lipoxins with 4 or 5 double bonds. Terpenes, which have one or more isoprene units, include carotenoids, coenzyme Q, vitamins A, E, and K, essential oils, and phytols.

Lipids undergo many reactions, such as the hydrolysis of TAGs, the saponification of fatty acids, esterification with alcohols, substitution of the hydroxyl hydrogen, hydrogenation of unsaturated fatty acids, peroxidation of unsaturated fatty acids, particularly at high temperatures, and reaction with chlorine or bromine. Although the diverse structures of lipids present challenges in their laboratory analysis, recent advances in chemistry have laid down a solid foundation for nutritional research on precursor fatty acids and their metabolites. Knowledge about the chemistry of lipids provides a foundation for our understanding of their metabolism and nutrition in animals (chapter 6).

## REFERENCES

Adeola, O., D.C. Mahan, M.J. Azain, S.K. Baidoo, G.L. Cromwell, G.M. Hill, J.E. Pettigrew, C.V. Maxwell, and M.C. Shannon. 2013. Dietary lipid sources and levels for weanling pigs. *J. Anim. Sci.* 91:4216–4225.

Agellon, J.B. 2008. Metabolism and function of bile acids. In: *Biochemistry of Lipids, Lipoproteins and Membranes (Fifth Edition)*. Edited by D.E. Vance and J.E. Vance, Elsevier, New York, pp. 423–440.

Aparicio, R., L. Roda, M.A. Albi, and F. Gutiérrez. 1999. Effect of various compounds on virgin olive oil stability measured by Rancimat. *J. Agric. Food Chem.* 47:4150–4155.

Bauman, D.E., K.J. Harvatine, and A.L. Lock. 2011. Nutrigenomics, rumen-derived bioactive fatty acids, and the regulation of milk fat synthesis. *Annu. Rev. Nutr.* 31:299–319.

Benchaar, C., S. Calsamiglia, A.V. Chaves, G.R. Fraser, D. Colombatto, T.A. McAllister, and K.A. Beauchemin. 2008. A review of plant-derived essential oils in ruminant nutrition and production. *Anim. Feed Sci. Technol.* 145:209–228.

Bentley, R. and R. Meganathan. 1983. Vitamin K biosynthesis in bacteria: Precursors, intermediates, enzymes, and genes. *J. Nat. Prod.* 46:44–59.

Bergen, W.G. and T.D. Brandebourg. 2016. Regulation of lipid deposition in farm animals: Parallels between agriculture and human physiology. *Exp. Biol. Med.* 241:1272–1280.

Bergen, W.G. and H.J. Mersmann. 2005. Comparative aspects of lipid metabolism: Impact on contemporary research and use of animal models. *J. Nutr.* 135:2499–2502.

Besnard, P., Niot, I., Bernard, A., and Carlier, H. 1996. Cellular and molecular aspects of fat metabolism in the small intestine. *Proc. Nutr. Soc.* 55:19–37.

Block, K., E. Borek, and D. Rittenberg. 1946. Synthesis of cholesterol in living liver. *J. Biol. Chem.* 162:441–449.

Brandebourg, T.D. and C.Y. Hu. 2005. Isomer-specific regulation of differentiating pig preadipocytes by conjugated linoleic acids. *J. Anim. Sci.* 83:2096–2105.

Breckenridge, W.C. and A. Kuksis. 1967. Molecular weight distributions of milk fat triglycerides from seven species. *J. Lipid Res.* 8:473–478.

Burr, G.O. and M.M. Burr. 1929. A new deficiency disease produced by the rigid exclusion of fat from the diet. *J. Biol. Chem.* 82:345–367.

Buschhaus, C. and R. Jetter. 2011. Composition differences between epicuticular and intracuticular wax substructures: How do plants seal their epidermal surfaces? *J. Exp. Bot.* 62:841–853.

Butovich, I.A., J.C. Wojtowicz, and M. Molai. 2009. Human tear film and meibum. Very long chain wax esters and (O-acyl)-omega-hydroxy fatty acids of meibum. *J. Lipid Res.* 50:2471–2485.

Calder, P.C. 2006. n-3 polyunsaturated fatty acids, inflammation, and inflammatory diseases. *Am. J. Clin. Nutr.* 83:1505S–1519S.

Cheeke, P.R. 2000. Actual and potential applications of *Yucca schidigera* and *Quillaja saponaria* saponins in human and animal nutrition. *Proc. Phytochem. Soc. Eur.* 45:241–254.

Cherian, G. 2015. Nutrition and metabolism in poultry: Role of lipids in early diet. *J. Anim. Sci. Biotechnol.* 6:28.

Clandinin, M.T. 1999. Brain development and assessing the supply of polyunsaturated fatty acid. *Lipids* 34:131–137.

Colbeau, A., J. Nachbaur, and P.M. Vignais. 1971. Enzymic characterization and lipid composition of rat liver subcellular membranes. *Biochim. Biophys. Acta.* 249:462–492.

Colina, J.J., A.J. Lewis, P.S. Miller, and R.L. Fischer. 2001. Dietary manipulation to reduce aerial ammonia concentrations in nursery pig facilities. *J. Anim. Sci.* 79:3096–3103.

Conde-Aguilera, J.A., C. Cobo-Ortega, S. Tesseraud, M. Lessire, Y. Mercier, and J. van Milgen. 2013. Changes in body composition in broilers by a sulfur amino acid deficiency during growth. *Poult. Sci.* 92:1266–1275.

Chung, H. and S.B. Carroll. 2015. Wax, sex and the origin of species: Dual roles of insect cuticular hydrocarbons in adaptation and mating. *Bioessays* 37:822–830.

Chung, J.G., L.R. Garrett, P.E. Byers, and M.A. Cuchens. 1989. A survey of the amount of pristane in common fruits and vegetables. *J. Food Comp. Anal.* 2(22):22.

Daum, G. 1985. Lipids of mitochondria. *Biochim. Biophys. Acta* 882:1–42.

DellaPenna, D. 2005. A decade of progress in understanding vitamin E synthesis in plants. *J. Plant Physiol.* 162:729–737.

Dembitsky, V.M. and M. Srebnik. 2002. Natural halogenated fatty acids: Their analogues and derivatives. *Prog. Lipid Res.* 41:315–67.

Devlin, T.M. 2006. *Textbook of Biohemistry with Clinical Correlations*. Wiley-Liss, New York, NY.

Ding, S.T., A. Lapillonne, W.C. Heird, and H.J. Mersmann. 2003. Dietary fat has minimal effects on fatty acid metabolism transcript concentrations in pigs. *J. Anim. Sci.* 81:423–431.

Fang, Y.Z., S. Yang, and G. Wu. 2002. Free radicals, antioxidants, and nutrition. *Nutrition* 18:872–879.

Field, C.J., J.E. Van Aerde, L.E. Robinson, and M.T. Clandinin. 2008. Effect of providing a formula supplemented with long-chain polyunsaturated fatty acids on immunity in full-term neonates. *Br. J. Nutr.* 99:91–99.

Folco, G. and R.C. Murphy. 2006. Eicosanoid transcellular biosynthesis: From cell-cell interactions to *in vivo* tissue responses. *Pharmacol. Rev.* 58:375–388.

Fox, J.G., L.C. Anderson, F.M. Loew, and F.W. Quimby. 2002. *Laboratory Animal Medicine*, 2nd ed. Academic Press, New York.

Guidotti, G. 1972. Membrane proteins. *Annu. Rev. Biochem.* 41:731–752.

Gunstone, F.D. 2012. *Fatty Acid and Lipid Chemistry*, Springer, New York.

Hagey, L.R., P.R. Møller, A.F. Hofmann, and M.D. Krasowski. 2010. Diversity of bile salts in fish and amphibians: Evolution of a complex biochemical pathway. *Physiol. Biochem. Zool.* 83:308–321.

Hausman, G.J., T.R. Kasser, and R.J. Martin. 1982. The effect of maternal diabetes and fasting on fetal adipose tissue histochemistry in the pig. *J. Anim. Sci.* 55:1343–1350.

Hofmann, A.F. 1999. Bile acids: The good, the bad, and the ugly. *Physiology* 14:24–29.

Horvath, S.E. and G. Daum. 2013. Lipids of mitochondria. *Prog. Lipid Res.* 52:590–614.

Jacobs, R.L., L.M. Stead, C. Devlin, I. Tabas, M.E. Brosnan, J.T. Brosnan, and D.E. Vance. 2005. Physiological regulation of phospholipid methylation alters plasma homocysteine in mice. *J. Biol. Chem.* 280:28299–28305.

Jobgen, W.S., S.K. Fried, W.J. Fu, C.J. Meininger, and G. Wu. 2006. Regulatory role for the arginine-nitric oxide pathway in metabolism of energy substrates. *J. Nutr. Biochem.* 17:571–588.

Kessler, J.I., J. Stein, D. Dannacker, and P. Narcessian. 1970. Intestinal mucosa biosynthesis of low density lipoprotein by cell-free preparations of rat. *J. Biol. Chem.* 245:5281–5288.

Kolattukudy, P.E., S. Bohnet, and L. Rogers. 1987. Diesters of 3-hydroxy fatty acids produced by the uropygial glands of female mallards uniquely during the mating season. *J. Lipid Res.* 28:582–588.

Kurogi, K., M.D. Krasowski, E. Injeti, M.Y. Liu, F.E. Williams, Y. Sakakibara, M. Suiko, and M.C. Liu. 2011. A comparative study of the sulfation of bile acids and a bile alcohol by the *Zebra danio (Danio rerio)* and human cytosolic sulfotransferases (SULTs). *J. Steroid. Biochem. Mol. Biol.* 127:307–314.

Lass, A., S. Agarwal, and R.S. Sohal. 1997. Mitochondrial ubiquinone homologues, superoxide radical generation, and longevity in different mammalian species. *J. Biol. Chem.* 272:19199–19204.

Lefebvre, P., B. Cariou, F. Lien, F. Kuipers, and B. Staels. 2009. Role of bile acids and bile acid receptors in metabolic regulation. *Physiol. Rev.* 89:147–191.

Lehninger, A.L., D.L. Nelson, and M.M. Cox. 1993. *Principles of Biochemistry*, Worth Publishers, New York, NY.

Ma, D.W., A.A. Wierzbicki, C.J. Field, and M.T. Clandinin. 1999. Conjugated linoleic acid in Canadian dairy and beef products. *J. Agric. Food Chem.* 47:1956–1960.

Maceyka, M. and S. Spiegel. 2014. Sphingolipid metabolites in inflammatory disease. *Nature* 510:58–67.

Madsen, P.T. and A. Surlykke. 2013. Functional convergence in bat and toothed whale biosonars. *Physiology (Bethesda)* 28:276–283.

Mao, G., G.A. Kraus, I. Kim, M.E. Spurlock, T.B. Bailey, Q. Zhang, and Beitz DC. 2010. A mitochondria-targeted vitamin E derivative decreases hepatic oxidative stress and inhibits fat deposition in mice. *J. Nutr.* 140:1425–1431.

McDonald, P., R.A. Edwards, J.F.D. Greenhalgh, J.F.D. Greenhalgh, C.A. Morgan, and L.A. Sinclair. 2011. *Animal Nutrition*, 7th ed. Prentice Hall, New York.

Mead, J.F., E.B. Alfin-Slater, D.R. Howton, and G. Popják. 1986. *Lipids: Chemistry, Biochemistry, and Nutrition.* Plenum Press, New York.

Morell, P. and P. Braun. 1972. Biosynthesis and metabolic degradation of sphingolipids not containing sialic acid. *J. Lipid Res.* 13:293–310.

National Research Council (NRC). 2011. *Nutrient Requirements of Fish and Shrimp*, National Academy of Science, Washington, DC.

National Research Council (NRC). 2012. *Nutrient Requirements of Swine*, National Academy of Science, Washington, DC.

Odle, J. 1997. New insights into the utilization of medium-chain triglycerides by the neonate: Observations from a piglet model. *J. Nutr.* 127:1061–1067.

Oleszek, W., M. Sitek, A. Stochmal, S. Piacente, C. Pizza, and P. Cheeke. 2001. Steroidal saponins of *Yucca schidigera* Roezl. *J. Agric. Food Chem.* 49:4392–4396.

Palmquist, D.L. 2006. Milk fat: Origin of fatty acids and influence of nutritional factors thereon. In: *Advanced Dairy Chemistry*, Volume 2: Lipids, 3rd edition. Edited by P.F. Fox and P.L.H. McSweeney, Springer, New York, NY.

Park, Y.W. and G.F.W. Haenlein. 2006. *Handbook of Milk of Non-Bovine Mammals*, Blackwell Publishing, Oxford, UK, 2006.

Pedersen, T.R. 2016. The success story of LDL cholesterol lowering. *Circ. Res.* 118:721–731.

Pichersky, E. 2006. Biosynthesis of plant volatiles: Nature's diversity and ingenuity. *Science* 311: 808–811.

Pond, W.G., D.C. Church, and K.R. Pond. 2005. *Basic Animal Nutrition and Feeding.* 4th ed., John Wiley & Sons, New York.

Ralston, A.W. and C.W. Hoerr. 1942. The solubilities of the normal saturated fatty acids. *J. Org. Chem.* 7:546–555.

Ramsay, T.G., C.M. Evock-Clover, N.C. Steele, and M.J. Azain. 2001. Dietary conjugated linoleic acid alters fatty acid composition of pig skeletal muscle and fat. *J. Anim. Sci.* 79:2152–2161.

Ray, T.K., V.P. Skipski, M. Barclay, E. Essner, and F.M. Archibald. 1969. Lipid composition of rat liver plasma membranes. *J. Biol. Chem.* 244:5528–5536.

Ridgway, N.D. and R.S. McLeod. 2016. *Biochemistry of Lipids, Lipoproteins and Membranes*, Elsevier, New York.

Rijpstra, W.I., J. Reneerkens, T. Piersma, and J.S. Damsté. 2007. Structural identification of the beta-hydroxy fatty acid-based diester preen gland waxes of shorebirds. *J. Nat. Prod.* 70:1804–1807.

Romano, M., E. Cianci, F. Simiele, and A. Recchiuti. 2015. Lipoxins and aspirin-triggered lipoxins in resolution of inflammation. *Eur. J. Pharmacol.* 760:49–63.

Rook, J.A.F. 1964. Ruminal volatile fatty acid production in relation to animal production from grass. *Proc. Nutr. Soc.* 23:71–80.

Rosero, D.S., J. Odle, A.J. Moeser, R.D. Boyd, and E. van Heugten. 2015. Peroxidised dietary lipids impair intestinal function and morphology of the small intestine villi of nursery pigs in a dose-dependent manner. *Br. J. Nutr.* 114:1985–1992.

Satterfield, M.C. and G. Wu. 2011. Growth and development of brown adipose tissue: Significance and nutritional regulation. *Front. Biosci.* 16:1589–1608.

Schreiber, L. 2010. Transport barriers made of cutin, suberin and associated waxes. *Trends Plant Sci.* 15:546–553.

Smith, S.B. and G.E. Carstens. 2005. Ontogeny and metabolism of brown adipose tissue in livestock species. In: *Biology of Metabolism in Growing Animals*. Edited by D.G. Burren and H.J. Mersmann. Elsevier Science Publishers, Oxford.

Smith, S.B. and D.R. Smith. 1995. *The Biology of Fat in Meat Animals: Current Advances*. Am. Soc. Anim. Sci., Champaign, IL.

Smith, S.B., A. Yang, T.W. Larsen, and R.K. Tume. 1998. Positional analysis of triacylglycerols from bovine adipose tissue lipids varying in degree of unsaturation. *Lipids* 33:197–207.

Spector, A.A. and H.Y. Kim. 2015. Discovery of essential fatty acids. *J. Lipid Res.* 56:11–21.

Stamp, D. and G. Jenkins 2008. An overview of bile-acid synthesis, chemistry and function. In: *Bile Acids: Toxicology and Bioactivity*. Edited by G. Jenkins and L.J. Hardie. Royal Society of Chemistry, pp. 1–13.

Swift, L.L., M.E. Gray, and V.S. LeQuire. 1988. Intestinal lipoprotein synthesis in control and hypercholesterolemic rats. *Biochim. Biophys. Acta.* 962:186–195.

Takagi, T. and Y. Itabashi. 1977. Random combinations of acyl and alcoholic groups through overall wax esters of sperm whale head oils. *Comp. Biochem. Physiol. B.* 57:37–39.

Tan, B.E., Y.L. Yin, Z.Q. Liu, W.J. Tang, H.J. Xu, X.F. Kong, X.G. Li et al. 2011. Dietary L-arginine supplementation differentially regulates expression of lipid-metabolic genes in porcine adipose tissue and skeletal muscle. *J. Nutr. Biochem.* 22:441–445.

Tanford, C. 1980. *The Hydrophobic Effect: Formation of Micelles and Biological Membranes*. Wiley, New York.

Tapia, J.B. 2014. Chromatographic analysis of fatty acids using 9-chloromethyl-anthracene and 2-bromomethylanthraquinone. Thesis. University of Northern Colorado, Greeley, CO.

Tongnuanchan, P. and S. Benjakul. 2014. Essential oils: Extraction, bioactivities, and their uses for food preservation. *J. Food Sci.* 79:R1231–R1249.

Tso, P. 1985. Gastrointestinal digestion and absorption of lipid. *Adv. Lipid Res.* 21:143–186.

Turunen, M., J. Olsson, and G. Dallner. 2004. Metabolism and function of coenzyme Q. *Biochim. Biophys. Acta* 1660:171–199.

Vance, D.E. 2014. Phospholipid methylation in mammals: From biochemistry to physiological function. *Biochim. Biophys. Acta.* 1838:1477–1487.

Wang, L., Y.Q. Hou, D. Yi, B.Y. Ding, D. Zhao, Z.X. Wang, H.L. Zhu et al. 2015. Dietary oleum cinnamomi alleviates intestinal injury. *Front. Biosci.* 20:814–828.

Washizu, T., I. Tomoda, and J.J. Kaneko. 1991. Serum bile acid composition of the dog, cow, horse and human. *J. Vet. Med. Sci.* 53:81–86.

Wesson, L.G. and G.O. Burr. 1931. The metabolic rate and respiratory quotients of rats on a fat-deficient diet. *J. Biol. Chem.* 91:525–539.

Whitney, T.R. and S.B. Smith. 2015. Substituting redberry juniper for oat hay in lamb feedlot diets: Carcass characteristics, adipose tissue fatty acid composition, and sensory panel traits. *Meat Sci.* 104:1–7.

Wood, R. and R.D. Harlow. 1960. Structural analyses of rat liver phosphoglycerides. *Arch. Biochem. Biophys.* 135:272–281.

Xie, Z., L. Yu, and Q. Deng. 2012. Application of a fluorescent derivatization reagent 9-chloromethyl anthracene on determination of carboxylic acids by HPLC. *J. Chromatogr. Sci.* 50:464–468.

Yabuuchi, H. and J.S. O'Brien. 1968. Positional distribution of fatty acids in glycerophosphatides of bovine gray matter. *J. Lipid Res.* 9:65–67.

Zeng, Z., S. Zhang, H. Wang, and X. Piao. 2015. Essential oil and aromatic plants as feed additives in non-ruminant nutrition: A review. *J. Anim. Sci. Biotechnol.* 6(1):7–8.

Zerbe, P. and J. Bohlmann. 2015. Plant diterpene synthases: Exploring modularity and metabolic diversity for bioengineering. *Trends Biotechnol.* 33:419–428.

Zinser, E., C.D. Sperka-Gottlieb, E.V. Fasch, S.D. Kohlwein, F. Paltauf, and G. Daum. 1991. Phospholipid synthesis and lipid composition of subcellular membranes in the unicellular eukaryote *Saccharomyces cerevisiae*. *J. Bacteriol.* 173:2026–2034.

# 4 Chemistry of Protein and Amino Acids

The word "protein" originated from the Greek word "*proteios*," meaning prime or primary (Meister 1965). A protein is a large polymer of amino acids (AAs) linked via the peptide bond (–CO–NH–). Different proteins have different chemical properties (e.g., AA sequences, molecular weights, ionic charges, three-dimensional (3D) structures, hydrophobicity, and function). The general structure of an AA is shown in Figure 4.1. There may be one or more polypeptide chains in a protein, which contains its constituents (nitrogen, carbon, oxygen, hydrogen, and sulfur atoms). A protein may be covalently bonded to other atoms and molecules (e.g., phosphates) and non-covalently attached with minerals (e.g., calcium, iron, copper, zinc, magnesium, and manganese), certain vitamins (e.g., vitamin $B_6$, vitamin $B_{12}$, and lipid-soluble vitamins), and/or lipids. Protein is the major nitrogenous macronutrient in foods and the fundamental component of animal tissues (Wu 2016). It has structural, signaling, and physiological functions in animals (Table 4.1).

AAs are classified according to their molecular weights (small vs. large), chemical properties (hydrophobic or hydrophilic; net ionic charges [neutral, acidic, or basic]; straight- or branched-chain; structure [primary amino vs. imino group]; and the composition of nitrogen [one to four N atoms] and sulfur [zero to two S atoms]), and physiological functions (e.g., proteinogenic vs. nonproteinogenic). The 20 AAs which are the precursors for protein synthesis are called proteinogenic AAs (Figure 4.2), whereas the AAs which are not substrates for protein synthesis are referred to as nonproteinogenic AAs (Wu et al. 2016). Examples of nonproteinogenic AAs with important physiological functions in animals are shown in Figure 4.3. Both proteinogenic and nonproteinogenic AAs have diverse roles in animals, and all of them are needed to maintain the homeostasis of organisms (Wu 2013). Animal- and plant-source proteins in feed ingredients have different compositions of AAs (Li et al. 2011), as do various proteins in the body.

There is a rich history of AA chemistry (Greenstein and Winitz 1961; Vickery and Schmidt 1931). Research on natural and synthetic AAs was pioneered in Europe and has spanned over 200 years. In 1806, asparagine was the first AA to be discovered in nature by French chemists L.N. Vauquelin and P.J. Robiquet. This was followed by the first isolation of glycine from a protein (i.e., gelatin) in 1820 by another French chemist H. Braconnot. In 1925, threonine was discovered in oat protein and teozein, and was the last addition to the long list of 20 proteinogenic AAs in organisms. Ten years later, W.C. Rose identified the presence of threonine in casein. This work led to the formulation of purified diets with which to determine the dietary requirements of individual AAs by animals. The analysis of peptide-bound AAs in feedstuff and animal proteins is now feasible based on their acid, alkaline, and enzymatic hydrolysis (Dai et al. 2014; Li et al. 2011). Protein ingredients (the primary sources of dietary AAs) are the most expensive components of animal diets. Thus, maximum economic returns and sustainability of animal production require an adequate knowledge of protein and AA chemistry (Wu et al. 2014a,b). This essential aspect of animal nutrition is highlighted in Chapter 4.

## DEFINITION, CHEMICAL CLASSIFICATION, AND PROPERTIES OF AAS

### Definition of AAs

#### α-, ß-, γ-, δ-, or ε-AAs

An AA is defined as an organic substance that contains both amino and acid groups. The acid group is the carboxyl group (–COOH) in proteinogenic AAs but can be a sulfonic acid group

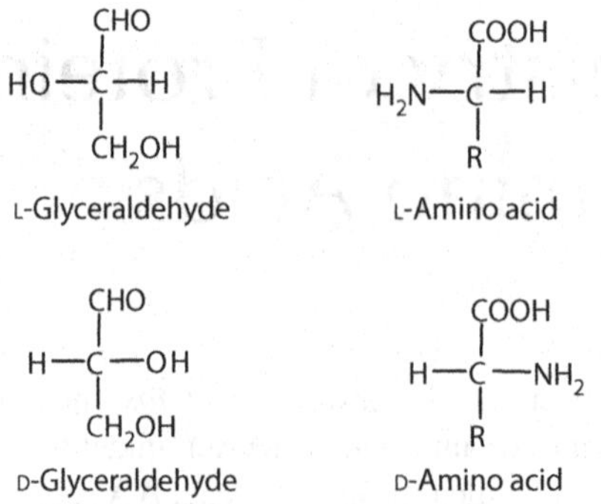

CHO
HO—C—H
$CH_2OH$
L-Glyceraldehyde

COOH
$H_2N$—C—H
R
L-Amino acid

CHO
H—C—OH
$CH_2OH$
D-Glyceraldehyde

COOH
H—C—$NH_2$
R
D-Amino acid

**FIGURE 4.1** Fisher projections for configurations of AAs relative to L- and D-glyceraldehydes. The general structure of an AA in the non-ionized form is shown. For AAs, L- or D-isomers refer only to the chemical configuration of their α-carbon.

($-SO_2-OH$; its ionized form being called sulfonate) in nonproteinogenic AAs (Wu 2013). The number of carbons in an AA is ≥2, with the carbon adjacent to the primary acid group being called the α-carbon. The other carbon atoms of the AA beyond the α-carbon are named in sequence according to the Greek alphabet, that is, ß-, γ-, δ-, or ε-carbon. If the amino group ($-NH_2$) is linked to the α-carbon, the AA is called an α-AA. Likewise, if the amino group is linked to the ß-, γ-, δ-, or ε-carbon, the AA is known as a ß-, γ-, δ-, or ε-AA, respectively. All of these types of AAs occur in nature.

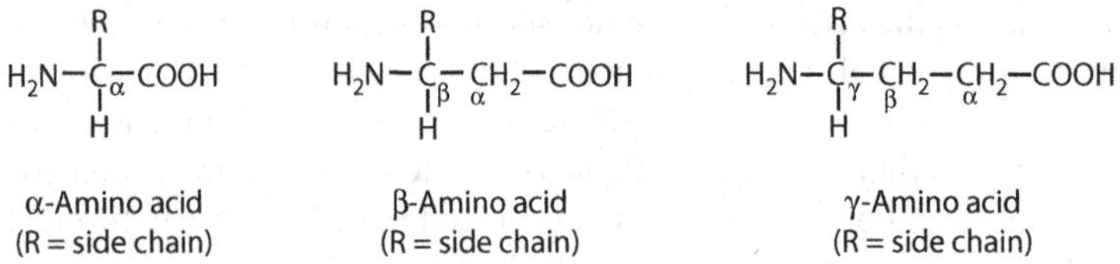

R
$H_2N-C_{\alpha}-COOH$
H
α-Amino acid
(R = side chain)

R
$H_2N-C_{\beta}-CH_2{}_{\alpha}-COOH$
H
β-Amino acid
(R = side chain)

R
$H_2N-C_{\gamma}-CH_2{}_{\beta}-CH_2{}_{\alpha}-COOH$
H
γ-Amino acid
(R = side chain)

**TABLE 4.1**
**Structural and Physiological Roles of Proteins in Animals**

| Roles | Examples of Proteins |
|---|---|
| Buffering | Hemoglobin and myoglobin |
| Cell and tissue structures | Collagen, elastin, keratin, mucins, proteoglycans, vimentin |
| Colloidal properties | Proteins in plasma (albumin and globulins) and gelatin |
| Enzyme-catalyzed reactions | Decarboxylase, dehydrogenase, kinase, lipases, proteases |
| Gene expression | DNA-binding proteins, histones, repressor proteins |
| Hormone-mediated effects | FSH, insulin, LH, placental lactogen, somatotropin, TSH |
| Muscle contraction | Actin, myosin, tropomyosin, troponin, tubulin |
| Protection | Blood clotting factors, immunoglobulins, interferon |
| Regulation of cell signaling | Calmodulin, GPCRs, leptin, MTOR, AMPK, osteopontin |
| Storage of nutrients and $O_2$ | FABs, ferritin, metallothionein, myoglobin, perilipins |
| Transport of nutrients and $O_2$ | Albumin, hemoglobin, plasma lipoproteins, transporters |

*Note:* AMPK, AMP-activated protein kinase; FABs, fatty acid-binding proteins; FSH, follicle-stimulating hormone; GPCRs, G-protein-coupled receptors; LH, luteinizing hormone; MTOR, mechanistic target of rapamycin; TSH, thyroid-stimulating hormone.

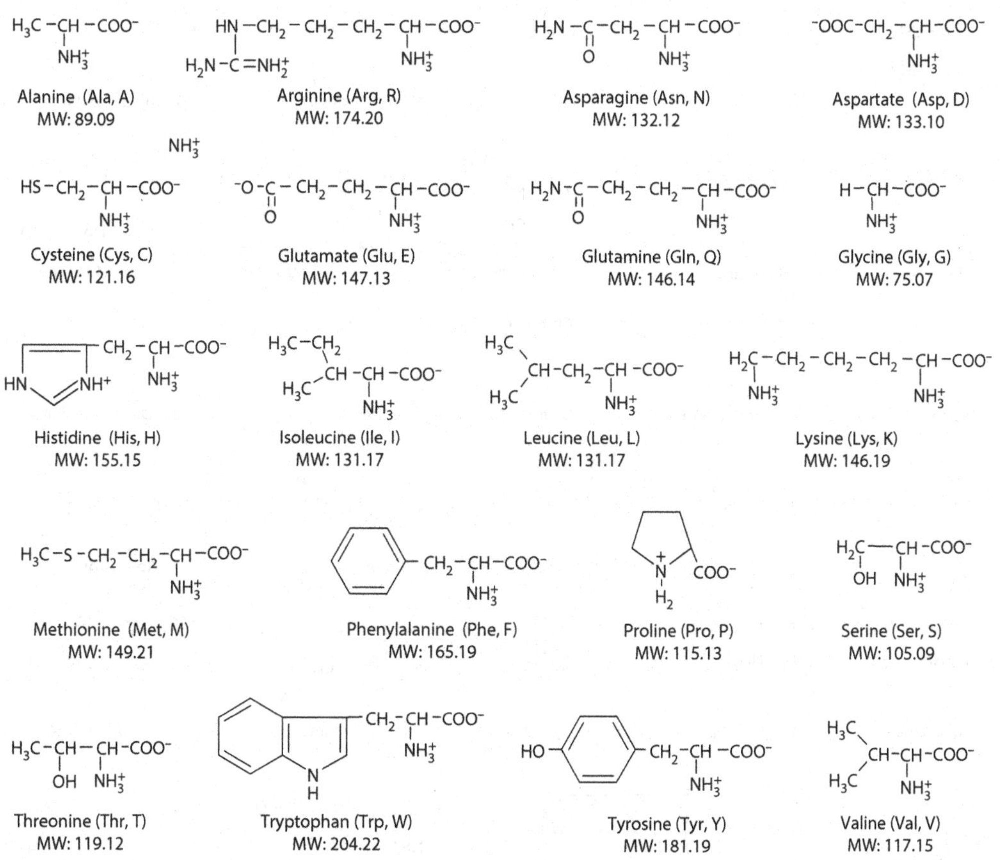

Alanine (Ala, A) MW: 89.09
Arginine (Arg, R) MW: 174.20
Asparagine (Asn, N) MW: 132.12
Aspartate (Asp, D) MW: 133.10
Cysteine (Cys, C) MW: 121.16
Glutamate (Glu, E) MW: 147.13
Glutamine (Gln, Q) MW: 146.14
Glycine (Gly, G) MW: 75.07
Histidine (His, H) MW: 155.15
Isoleucine (Ile, I) MW: 131.17
Leucine (Leu, L) MW: 131.17
Lysine (Lys, K) MW: 146.19
Methionine (Met, M) MW: 149.21
Phenylalanine (Phe, F) MW: 165.19
Proline (Pro, P) MW: 115.13
Serine (Ser, S) MW: 105.09
Threonine (Thr, T) MW: 119.12
Tryptophan (Trp, W) MW: 204.22
Tyrosine (Tyr, Y) MW: 181.19
Valine (Val, V) MW: 117.15

**FIGURE 4.2** Chemical structures of AAs that are substrates for the synthesis of proteins in animals at a neutral pH. These proteinogenic AAs also occur in microorganisms and plants.

## Imino Acids

Proline and hydroxyproline are special nitrogenous compounds with a pyrrolidine ring. They contain a secondary α-amino (α-imino; –NH) group and therefore are α-imino acids (Phang et al. 2008). The chemical reactivity of the imino group differs remarkably from that of the amino group. Since proline is a common substrate for protein synthesis like α-AAs and hydroxyproline is the posttranslational derivative of proline, both proline and hydroxyproline are loosely referred to as α-AAs in biochemistry and nutrition. Hydroxyproline occurs as both 4-hydroxyproline (the major form) and 3-hydroxyproline (the minor form) in animals, but is rare in plants and microbes.

## Differences in the Structures of AAs

The numbers of amino and acid groups, as well as side-chain groups, vary with AAs (Greenstein and Winitz 1961). For example, glutamate and aspartate have two carboxyl groups and one α-amino group, whereas lysine and ornithine have two amino groups and one carboxyl group. Both arginine and some of its metabolites (e.g., methylarginines and homoarginine) possess a guanidino group, while other members of the arginine family of AAs, citrulline and homocitrulline, contain a ureido group. Although most AAs have a straight carbon chain (e.g., alanine, glutamine, and glycine), some AAs (e.g., leucine, isoleucine, and valine) are branched in structure. The differences in the side chains of AAs greatly affect their chemical properties.

All AAs are composed of nitrogen (N), carbon (C), oxygen (O), and hydrogen (H) atoms. The abundance of the N atom in AAs can be very different. For example, the number of N atoms per

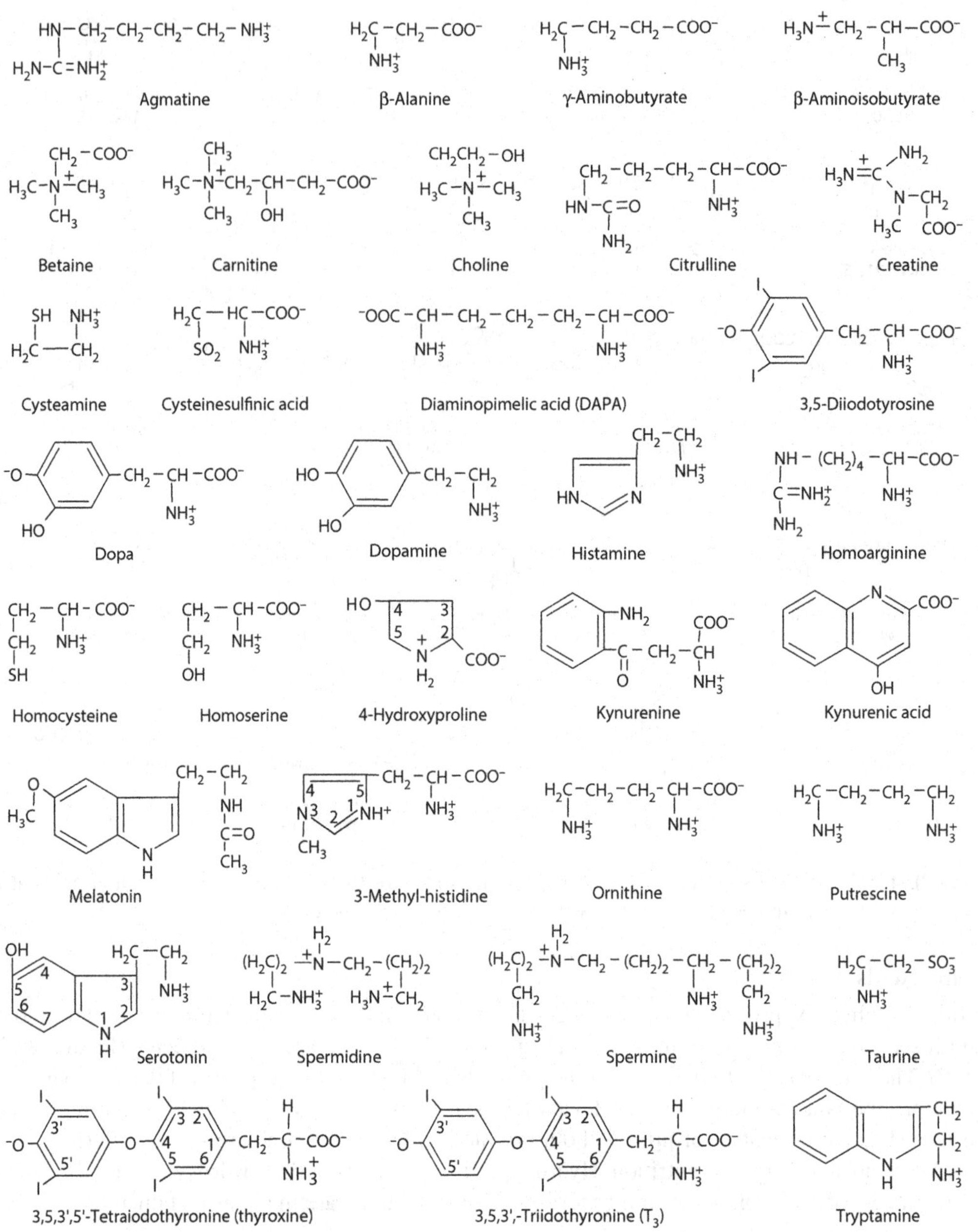

Agmatine β-Alanine γ-Aminobutyrate β-Aminoisobutyrate

Betaine Carnitine Choline Citrulline Creatine

Cysteamine Cysteinesulfinic acid Diaminopimelic acid (DAPA) 3,5-Diiodotyrosine

Dopa Dopamine Histamine Homoarginine

Homocysteine Homoserine 4-Hydroxyproline Kynurenine Kynurenic acid

Melatonin 3-Methyl-histidine Ornithine Putrescine

Serotonin Spermidine Spermine Taurine

3,5,3',5'-Tetraiodothyronine (thyroxine) 3,5,3',-Triidothyronine ($T_3$) Tryptamine

**FIGURE 4.3** Chemical structures of nonprotein AAs in animals at a neutral pH. These substances occur in physiological fluids of animals, and some of them are also present in microorganisms and plants. Taurine is present only in animals as a free AA.

molecule is 4 in arginine, homoarginine, and argininosuccinate; 3 in citrulline and histidine; 2 in glutamine, lysine, ornithine, tryptophan, and cystine; and 1 in alanine, glutamate, glycine, and leucine. The mean content of N in skeletal muscle and most other tissues is 16%.

Some AAs (e.g., methionine, cysteine, homocysteine, taurine, and selenocysteine) also contain one S atom, while there are two S atoms in cysteine and djenkolic acid. They are all called sulfur-containing AAs. Selenocysteine is a rare AA only present in selenoproteins (Stadtman 1996), and is derived, at the translation step, from serine and selenium (in the form of selenophosphate synthesized from selenide and ATP by selenophosphate synthetase 2) (Leibundgut et al. 2005). Free selenocysteine is not a substrate for protein synthesis. The presence of the S atom greatly influences the reactivity of the α-amino group in the sulfur-containing AAs and proteins.

### Naming and Chemical Expression of AAs

The common or trivial names of AAs were derived from: (1) the history of their discoveries, (2) their characteristics, including appearance (e.g., arginine and leucine), taste (e.g., glycine), and chemical structure (hydroxyproline, isoleucine, lysine, methionine, proline, and threonine), (3) their sources of isolation (e.g., asparagine, citrulline, cysteine, glutamate, serine, tryptophan, tyrosine, and valine), or (4) the precursors of their chemical syntheses (e.g., alanine and phenylalanine). Owing to variations in their side chains, AAs have remarkably different chemical properties and physiological functions (Greenstein and Winitz 1961).

According to the International Union of Biochemistry and Molecular Biology, a three-letter abbreviation can be used to designate a protein AA, with one capital letter followed by two lowercase letters (e.g., Gln for glutamine). A one-letter abbreviation is used to represent an AA in protein or polypeptide sequences (e.g., E, Q, and R for glutamate, glutamine, and arginine, respectively). This annotation is very useful to indicate the primary structure of a protein.

## The Zwitterionic (Ionized) Form of AAs

The amino (or imino) and acid groups have opposite electrical charges. Therefore, an AA can act as a base or an acid by accepting or donating a hydrogen ion ($H^+$, also called proton), respectively. All AAs form intramolecular salts both in the crystalline state and in an aqueous solution. This structure, in which a molecule has both positive and negative electrical charges, is known as a zwitterion. All AAs are ionized in physiological fluid and cellular protein. The dissociation constants for the acid, amino, and side-chain groups are termed $pK_1$, $pK_2$, and $pK_3$, respectively (Table 4.2).

$$H_3\overset{+}{N}-\underset{H}{\overset{R}{|}}C_\alpha-COO^-$$

The pH of an aqueous solution at which an AA has no net electrical charge is called the isoelectric point (pI). When an AA is dissolved in pure water until the solution is saturated, the pH of this solution will approach the pI value of the AA. For an AA without an ionizable side chain (e.g., glutamine and glycine), pI = $(pKa_1 + pKa_2)/2$.

Examples: for glutamine, pI = (2.17 + 9.13)/2 = 5.65; for glycine, pI = (2.35 + 9.78)/2 = 6.07.

For an AA with an ionizable side chain (e.g., glutamate and arginine), pI = average of the pKa values of the two most similar acid groups.

Examples: for glutamate, pI = (2.19 + 4.25)/2 = 3.22; for arginine, pI = (9.04 + 12.48)/2 = 10.76.

Since the pKa values of the α-carboxylic acid groups of α-AA are approximately 2.0–2.4 (Table 4.2), these groups are almost entirely in their carboxylate forms at pH > 3.5. Similarly, since the pKa values of the α-amino groups of α-AAs are approximately 9.0–10.0, these groups are almost entirely in their ammonium ion forms at pH < 8.0. Thus, at a physiological pH (e.g., pH 7.4 in the blood and pH 7.0 in the cytoplasm), the α-carboxylic acid and α-amino groups of α-AAs are completely ionized to take the zwitterion form. In their ionized form, glutamic acid and aspartic acid are called glutamate and aspartate, respectively.

Based on their net charges at a neutral pH, AAs are classified as neutral (net charge = 0), basic (net charge ≥ +1), or acidic (net charge ≤ −1). Thus, the addition of an acidic or basic AA to a

**TABLE 4.2**
**Molecular Weights and Chemical Properties of AAs**

| AA | MW | MP (°C) | Solubility[a] | $pK_1$[b] | $pK_2$[c] | $pK_3$[d] | pI |
|---|---|---|---|---|---|---|---|
| **1. Neutral** | | | | | | | |
| L-Alanine | 89.09 | 297 | 16.5 | 2.35 | 9.87 | | 6.11 |
| β-Alanine | 89.09 | 197 | 82.8 | 3.55 | 10.24 | | 6.90 |
| γ-Aminobutyrate | 103.12 | 202 | 107.3 | 4.03 | 10.56 | | 7.30 |
| L-Asparagine | 132.12 | 236 | 2.20 | 2.02 | 8.80 | | 5.41 |
| L-Citrulline | 175.19 | 222 | 15.2 | 2.43 | 9.41 | | 5.92 |
| L-Cysteine | 121.16 | 178 | 17.4 | 1.96[e] | 8.18[e] | 10.28[e] | 5.07[e] |
| L-Cystine | 240.30 | 261 | 0.011 | 1.04[f] | 8.02[f] | | 5.06[f] |
| | | | | 2.10[f] | 8.71[f] | | |
| L-Glutamine | 146.14 | 185 | 4.81[e] | 2.17 | 9.13 | | 5.65 |
| Glycine | 75.07 | 290 | 25.0 | 2.35 | 9.78 | | 6.07 |
| L-Hydroxyproline | 131.13 | 270 | 36.1 | 1.92 | 9.73 | | 5.83 |
| L-Isoleucine | 131.17 | 284 | 4.12 | 2.36 | 9.68 | | 6.02 |
| L-Leucine | 131.17 | 337 | 2.19 | 2.33 | 9.75 | | 6.04 |
| L-Methionine | 149.21 | 283 | 5.06 | 2.28 | 9.21 | | 5.74 |
| L-Phenylalanine | 165.19 | 284 | 2.96 | 2.20 | 9.31 | | 5.76 |
| L-Proline | 115.13 | 222 | 162.3 | 1.99 | 10.6 | | 6.30 |
| L-Serine | 105.09 | 228 | 41.3 | 2.21 | 9.15 | | 5.68 |
| Taurine | 125.15 | 328 | 10.5 | 1.50 | 8.74 | | 5.12 |
| L-Threonine | 119.12 | 253 | 9.54 | 2.15 | 9.12 | | 5.64 |
| L-Tryptophan | 204.22 | 282 | 1.14 | 2.38 | 9.39 | | 5.89 |
| L-Tyrosine | 181.19 | 344 | 0.045 | 2.20 | 9.11 | 10.07 | 5.66 |
| L-Valine | 117.15 | 315 | 5.82 | 2.29 | 9.72 | | 6.01 |
| **2. Basic** | | | | | | | |
| L-Arginine | 174.20 | 238 | 18.6 | 2.17 | 9.04 | 12.48 | 10.76 |
| L-Histidine | 155.15 | 277 | 4.19 | 1.80 | 9.33 | 6.04 | 7.69 |
| L-Lysine | 146.19 | 224 | 78.2[g] | 2.18 | 8.95 | 10.53 | 9.74 |
| L-Ornithine | 132.16 | 231[h] | 54.5[h] | 1.94 | 8.65 | 10.76 | 9.71 |
| **3. Acidic** | | | | | | | |
| L-Aspartic acid | 133.10 | 270 | 0.45 | 1.88 | 9.60 | 3.65 | 2.77 |
| L-Glutamic acid | 147.13 | 249 | 0.86 | 2.19 | 9.67 | 4.25 | 3.22 |

*Source:* Wu, G. 2013. *Biochemistry and Nutrition of Amino Acids*. CRC Press, Boca Raton, Florida.

[a] Solubility in water (g/100 mL at 25°C unless otherwise indicated).

[b] pK for α-COOH ($SO_3H$ for taurine) at 25°C unless otherwise indicated.

[c] pK for α-$NH_3^+$ at 25°C unless otherwise indicated.

[d] pK for the ionized group in the side chain at 25°C unless otherwise indicated.

[e] Determined at 30°C.

[f] Determined at 35°C.

[g] L-Lysine-$H_2O$.

[h] L-Ornithine-HCl.

MP = melting point; MW = molecular weight.

solution with a weak buffering capacity will substantially decrease or increase its pH, respectively. Similarly, intravenous infusion of large amounts of an acidic AA (e.g., aspartic acid) or basic AA (e.g., arginine) into animals and humans will adversely disturb the acid–base balance of the body. Thus, acidic or basic AAs should be neutralized (e.g., in the form of the aspartate-sodium salt or the arginine-HCl salt) before their use for intravenous administration. Interestingly, supplementing an appropriate amount of an acidic AA (e.g., 1% glutamic acid) or basic AA (e.g., 1% arginine) to a corn- and soybean meal (SBM)-based diet does not affect the pH in the lumen of the swine gastrointestinal tract. This is likely due to the highly acidic environment of the stomach (pH 2–2.5) and bicarbonate-containing pancreatic secretions in the lumen of the small intestine.

## D- OR L-CONFIGURATIONS OF AAs

### Definition of L- and D-AAs

The absolute configuration of AAs (L- or D-isomers as introduced by Emil Fischer in 1908) was arbitrarily defined with reference to glyceraldehyde (Figure 4.1), and is now mostly used in AA chemistry and nutrition. For AAs, L- or D-isomers refer only to the chemical configuration of their α-carbon. An asymmetric carbon is also called a chirality center. Since each asymmetric carbon can have two possible configurations, an AA with *n* asymmetric carbons has $2^n$ different possible stereoisomers. Except for glycine (the simplest AA in nature) which has no chirality center and therefore no L- or D-configuration, all proteinogenic AAs (Figure 4.2) exist only as L-AAs in animal cells. Most nonproteinogenic AAs can exist as L- or D-AAs or both, but some nonproteinogenic AAs (e.g., taurine, β-alanine, and γ-aminobutyric acid) do not have a chirality center and therefore have no D- or L-isomers. Chemical synthesis may yield both D- and L-isoforms of the AA.

### Optical Activity of L- and D-AAs

An optical isomer (e.g., L- or D-AA) exhibits optical activity or rotatory polarization. That is, when a beam of plane-polarized light is passed through a solution of the optical isomer, the light will be rotated either to the right or to the left. Optical rotations of AAs can be determined with a photoelectric polarimeter at 20°C–28°C and their concentrations of 0.5%–2% (Greenstein and Winitz 1961). When equal amounts of D- and L-AA (e.g., synthetic DL-methionine) are present in a solution, the resulting mixture has no optical activity.

Optical isomerism of organic molecules has traditionally been described as dextrorotatory (right, "+," or *d*) or levorotatory (left, "−," or *l*), depending on the direction of optical rotation. Since measurement conditions can affect the angle of optical rotation, the terms "dextrorotatory" and "levorotatory" have been abandoned. It should be noted that the D- and L-configurations for an organic substance may not necessarily determine the rotation of plane-polarized light. For example, the naturally occurring form of fructose is the D(−) isomer (D-configuration) with a levorotatory optical activity.

### L- and D-AAs in Nature

Approximately 700 natural L- and D-AAs had been reported to be present in animals, plants, and microorganisms by the 1980s (Wagner and Musso 1983). Interestingly, only 20 of them are the building blocks of cellular proteins. Thus, >97% of the naturally occurring AAs are nonproteinogenic. Some of them are present in animals (Figure 4.4), as well as feedstuffs, microbes, and plants

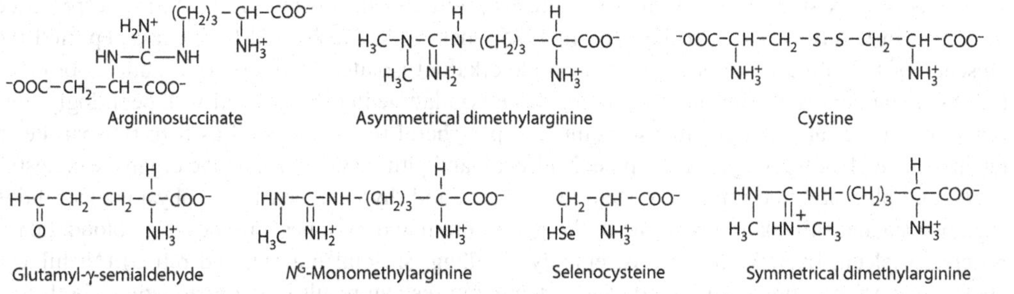

Argininosuccinate

Asymmetrical dimethylarginine

Cystine

Glutamyl-γ-semialdehyde

$N^G$-Monomethylarginine

Selenocysteine

Symmetrical dimethylarginine

**FIGURE 4.4** Chemical structures of methylarginines and some special AAs in animals at a neutral pH. These substances also occur in microorganisms and plants.

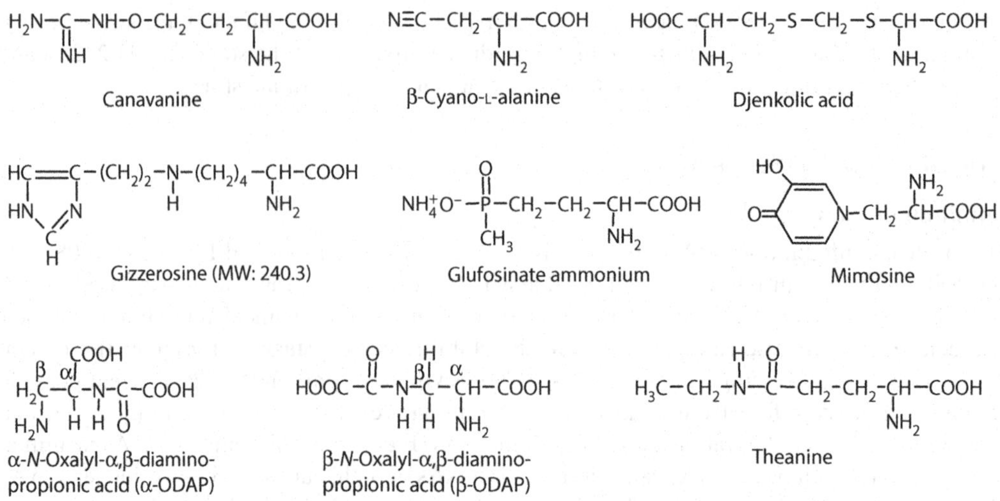

Canavanine

β-Cyano-L-alanine

Djenkolic acid

Gizzerosine (MW: 240.3)

Glufosinate ammonium

Mimosine

α-*N*-Oxalyl-α,β-diamino-propionic acid (α-ODAP)

β-*N*-Oxalyl-α,β-diamino-propionic acid (β-ODAP)

Theanine

**FIGURE 4.5** Chemical structures of gizzerosine, glufosinate ammonium, and some plant AAs in the non-ionized form. Gizzerosine may be formed from histamine and lysine in fish meal during processing and storage. Glufosinate ammonium and β-cyano-L-alanine are produced by microbes. All the other AAs presented in this figure occur in plants. Canavanine is structurally similar to arginine, djenkolic acid to cystine, mimosine to tyrosine, and theanine to glutamine. Except for theanine, all the AAs shown herein are highly toxic to animals.

(Figure 4.5). Besides proteinogenic AAs, many nonproteinogenic AAs are commonly present in all living organisms. However, some nonproteinogenic AAs are specific to only certain kingdoms of organisms. For example, taurine is synthesized only by the liver of animals and is not formed in either plants or microbes (Wu 2013). In contrast, theanine (*N*-ethyl-L-glutamine) is found only in plants and is not produced in either animals or microbes.

Some nonproteinogenic AAs in plants (e.g., L-theanine in teas and citrulline in watermelon) are beneficial for animal health, whereas others (e.g., β-cyanoalanine, djenkolic acid [two cysteine radicals connected by a methylene group], mimosine [chemically similar to tyrosine], gizzerosine, and glufosinate ammonium) can be highly toxic to animals (Nunn et al. 2010). Gizzerosine, which is formed from histamine and lysine in fish meal at a high temperature (e.g., >140°C), causes severe gizzard erosion (known as black vomit) in chickens even at a very low dose of 0.2 ppm in the diet (Sugahara 1995). It is L-gizzerosine, but not D-gizzerosine, that exerts the toxic effect in animals. Some naturally occurring AA derivatives exhibit activities against weeds, fungi, and insects (Lamberth 2016). For example, glufosinate ammonium, a naturally occurring broad-spectrum systemic herbicide from several species of *Streptomyces* (soil bacteria), can inhibit glutamine synthesis in animals (Hack et al. 1994).

D-AAs also exist naturally in microorganisms, animals, and plants (Table 4.3). The presence of D-AAs in nature was first recognized in 1935 when W.A. Jacobs and L.C. Craig reported the presence of D-proline in ergotinine (a tripeptide alkaloid isolated from ergot). Examples of other D-AAs are numerous: D-aspartate, D-glutamate, and D-alanine in bacterial cell-wall peptidoglycans; D-alanine in the rat pancreas, mouse brain, and peripheral tissues, as well as fish; D-aspartate in rat endocrine glands (e.g., pancreas, pineal, adrenal, and pituitary), reproductive organs (e.g., testis, ovary, and placenta), the immune system (e.g., spleen and thymus), heart, and physiological fluids (e.g., plasma and saliva); and D-serine in the mouse brain and peripheral tissues (e.g., blood, heart, pancreas, spleen, liver, kidney, testis, epididymis, lung, skeletal muscle, and retina) (Nishikawa 2011). Furthermore, processing food at high temperatures can result in the formation of both free and peptide-bound D-AAs in a time and pH-dependent manner (0.2%–2%). Rates of racemization of different L-AA residues to their respective D-isomers in a food protein vary, but the relative rates

**TABLE 4.3**
**Presence of Naturally Occurring Peptides Containing D-AAs**

| Common Name | Structure and Origin |
|---|---|
| Ergotinine (ergocristinine) | Phe-D-Pro–Val–Lysergic acid (a tripeptide, with the $NH_2$ of Val linking to lysergic acid)<br>Produced by ergot (fungus) |
| Tyrocidine A[a] | D-Phe-Pro–Phe-D-Phe–Asn–Gln–Tyr–Val–Orn–Leu (a cyclic decapeptide)<br>Produced by Gram-positive bacteria *Bacillus brevis* found in soil |
| Gramicidin[a] | Formyl–Val–Gly–Ala-D-Leu-Ala-D-Val-Val-D-Val-Trp-D-Leu-Trp-D-Leu-Trp-D-Leu-Trp-Ethanolamine (a cyclodecapeptide)<br>Produced by Gram-positive bacteria *B. brevis* found in soil |
| Lactocin S[a] | A peptide containing 37 AA residues, including Lanthionine and D-Ala |
| Enkephalins | Tyr–Gly–Gly–Phe–Met and Tyr–Gly–Gly–Phe–Leu (pentapeptides)<br>Produced by the brain (pentapeptide); bind opioid receptors |
| Dermorphin[b] | Tyr-D-Ala-Phe–Gly–Tyr–Pro–Ser–$NH_2$; Tyr-D-Ala–Phe–Gly–Tyr–Pro–Lys–$NH_2$<br>Tyr-D-Ala-Phe–Trp–Tyr–Pro–Asn–$NH_2$ (a hepta-peptide)<br>Produced by South American frogs *Phyllomedusa*, bacteria, amphibians, and molluscs |
| Deltorphins | Tyr-D-Met–Phe–His–Leu–Met–Asp–$NH_2$; Tyr-D-Ala–Phe–Asp–Val–Val–Gly–$NH_2$;<br>Tyr-D-Ala–Phe–Glu–Val–Val–Gly–$NH_2$<br>Produced by opioid peptides from the amphibian skin |
| Achatin I[c] | Gly-D-Phe–Ala–Asp–$NH_2$ (a tetrapeptide)<br>Produced by the ganglia and atrium of the African snail *Achatina fulica* |
| Fulicin | Phe-D-Asn–Glu–Phe–$NH_2$ (a tetrapeptide)<br>Produced by the ganglia of the African snail *A. fulica* |
| ω-Agatoxins | A peptide containing 48 AA residues, including Lanthionine and D-Ser<br>Produced by the funnel web spider *Agelenopsis aperta* and present in its venom |
| Petidoglycans | Polypeptides containing D-Ala, D-Asp, and D-Glu<br>Produced by bacteria and present on the bacterial cell walls |

*Source:* Kreil, G. 1997. *Annu. Rev. Biochem.* 66:337–345; Li, H. et al. 2016. *Int. J. Mol. Sci.* 17. pii: E1023.

[a] Antibiotic.

[b] Acts through binding to opiate receptors. Dermorphin is more potent than morphine in inducing deep long-lasting analgesia. This peptide has no biological activity if D-Ala is replaced by L-Ala.

[c] Acts as a neuropeptide for the control of muscle contraction. This peptide has no excitatory activity on the heart or other muscles of the snail if D-Phe is replaced by L-Phe.

Except for Gly, AAs not indicated as the D-isoform is present in the L-isoform.

for the same D-AA in different proteins are similar under the same conditions. Compared to L-AAs, D-AAs are quantitatively the minor isomers of AAs in nature (Li et al. 2016; Wu 2013). The ratio of total L-AAs to total D-AAs is likely greater than 100:0.02 in organisms. The physiological functions of D-AAs in animals remain to be defined (Brosnan 2001).

The configuration of L- or D-AAs in water or buffered solutions is not changed at room temperature (e.g., 25°C). Standard conditions for hydrolysis under acid (6 M HCl at 110°C for 24 h under nitrogen gas), base (4.2 N NaOH plus 1% thiodiglycol, antioxidant, at 110°C for 20 h), or enzymes does not affect the preexisting isomer of an AA in peptides. However, L- or D-AAs may lose their optical activity (known as racemization) in higher concentrations of acid or alkaline solutions at high temperatures (e.g., >105°C). Heating of feed protein above 105°C may generate a small amount of D-AAs (Friedman 1999). To date, D-AAs are often analyzed by high-performance liquid chromatography (HPLC) on a chiral or ligand column, or involving pre-column derivatization with reagents that convert the enantiomers to diastereomers to improve chromatographic resolution.

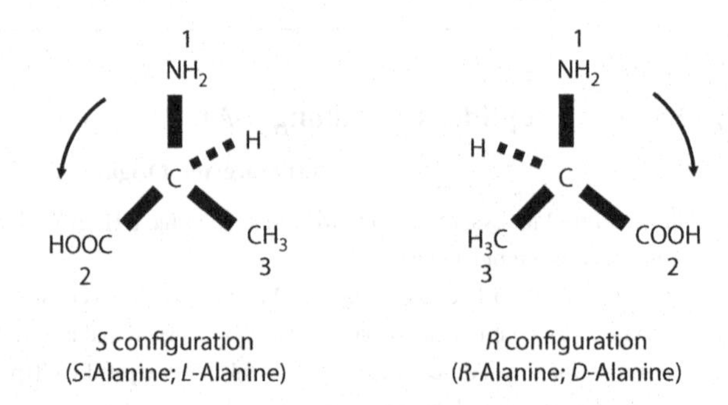


**FIGURE 4.6** *R* and *S* configurations of organic substances. This nomenclature system does not involve a reference molecule such as glyceraldehyde. 1 = the group with the highest atomic number; 2 = the group with the second highest atomic number; 3 = the group with the third highest atomic number; and 4 = the group with the lowest atomic number. To determine whether the chirality center is *R* or *S* configuration, one needs to first prioritize all four of the groups connected to the chirality center based on their atomic numbers (i.e., a higher atomic number takes precedence over a lower atomic number). Then rotate the molecule so that the fourth (the lowest) priority group points away from you (a dash line). If the sequence for the first three priority groups 1–2–3 is clockwise, the designation is *R*. If the sequence for the first three priority groups 1–2–3 is counterclockwise, the designation is *S*.

## *R/S* Configurations of AAs

To better distinguish some naturally occurring and synthetic AAs (e.g., threonine, isoleucine, and hydroxyproline) with more than one chirality center, the *R/S* nomenclature is used to name their absolute configurations, where *R* is *rectus* (right) and *S* is *sinister* (left) in Latin (Figure 4.6). This nomenclature system does not involve a reference molecule such as glyceraldehyde, but is based on the prioritized spatial arrangement of the four different groups which are attached to the chirality center. The *R/S* system has no fixed relation to the (+; dextrorotatory form)/(−; levorotary form) system. An *R* isomer can be either dextrorotatory or levorotatory, depending on its exact substituents. In the *R/S* system, naturally occurring AAs are mostly in the *S* configuration for the first chiral center just like carbohydrates. The *R/S* configurations of L-threonine, D-threonine, L-isoleucine, and D-isoleucine are shown in Figure 4.7.

The collagen and plasma of animals contain 4-hydroxy-L-proline (4-hydroxy-L-pyrrolidine-2-carboxylic acid) and 3-hydroxy-L-proline (3-hydroxy-L-pyrrolidine-2-carboxylic acid), with their ratio being approximately 100:1. According to the *R/S* nomenclature system, the physiological isoform of 4-hydroxy-L-proline in collagen and its enzymatic hydrolysates is (2*S*,4*R*)-4-hydroxy-proline (Figure 4.8), and that of 3-hydroxy-L-proline is (2*S*,3*S*)-3-hydroxyproline; both L-4-hydroxyproline and L-3-hydroxyproline are present only in the *trans* isoform. However, the acid hydrolysis of collagen at high temperatures (e.g., 110°C) yields a small amount of 4-hydroxyproline and 3-hydroxyproline in the *cis* isoform. *cis*-4-Hydroxy-L-proline (*cis*-(2*S*,4*S*)-4-hydroxyproline), a diastereomer of L-4-hydroxyproline, is present in the toxic cyclic peptides from *Amanita* mushrooms. Also, marine sponges and cyclopeptide antibiotics (e.g., telomycin) have both (2*S*, 3*S*) and (2*S*, 3*R*) 3-hydroxyproline.

## Allo-Forms of AAs

The nomenclature of an AA with more than one asymmetric carbon includes an allo-form. Specifically, if two diastereomers have a different configuration in the β- or γ-carbon, they are designated with the prefix “allo.” For example, a synthetic L-threonine (2*S*, 3*S*) whose β-carbon has a configuration opposite to that of its naturally occurring diastereomer (L-(2*S*, 3*R*) threonine) is called L-allo-threonine (Figure 4.7). L-Threonine and L-allo-threonine are called diastereomers, and the relationship between the two AAs is known as diastereomerism. This also applies to D-threonine and D-allo-threonine. The allo-forms of isoleucine are illustrated in Figure 4.7.

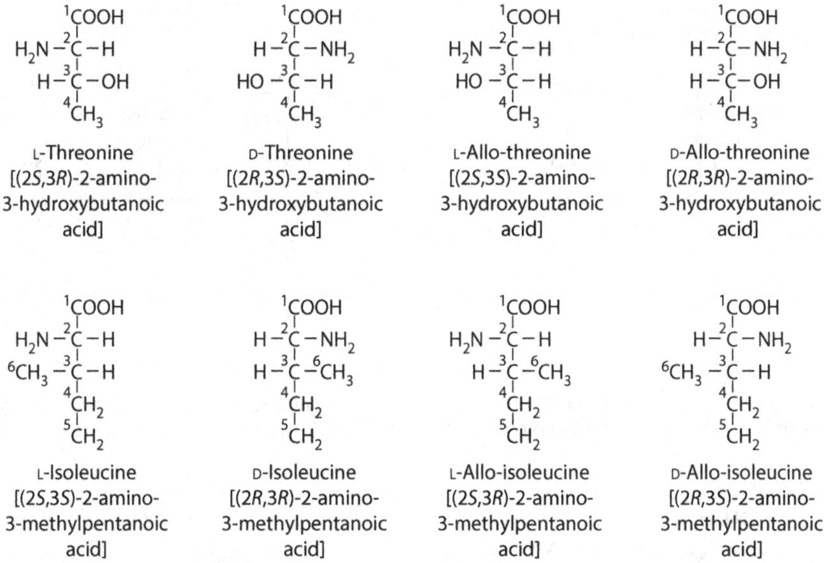

L-Threonine [(2*S*,3*R*)-2-amino-3-hydroxybutanoic acid]
D-Threonine [(2*R*,3*S*)-2-amino-3-hydroxybutanoic acid]
L-Allo-threonine [(2*S*,3*S*)-2-amino-3-hydroxybutanoic acid]
D-Allo-threonine [(2*R*,3*R*)-2-amino-3-hydroxybutanoic acid]

L-Isoleucine [(2*S*,3*S*)-2-amino-3-methylpentanoic acid]
D-Isoleucine [(2*R*,3*R*)-2-amino-3-methylpentanoic acid]
L-Allo-isoleucine [(2*S*,3*R*)-2-amino-3-methylpentanoic acid]
D-Allo-isoleucine [(2*R*,3*S*)-2-amino-3-methylpentanoic acid]

**FIGURE 4.7** The *R/S* configurations of L-threonine, D-threonine, L-isoleucine, and D-isoleucine. Specifically, if two diastereomers have a different configuration in the β- or γ-carbon, they are designated with the prefix "allo." Note that diastereomers are stereoisomers with two or more stereocenters that are not mirror images of one another and are non-superimposable on one another.

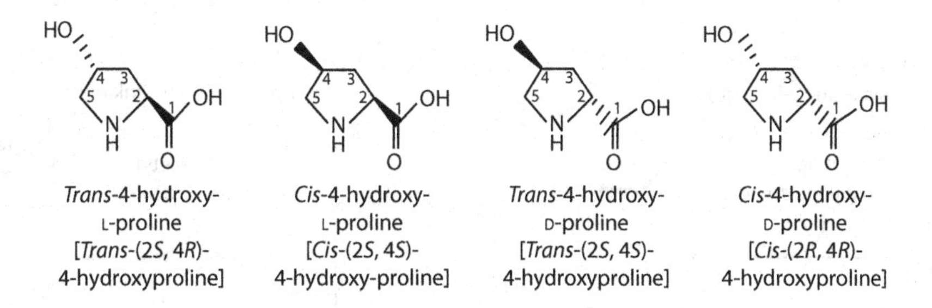


**FIGURE 4.8** The *R/S* configurations of 4-hydroxy-L-proline and 4-hydroxy-D-proline in *trans* and *cis* forms. Proline is also known as pyrrolidine-2-carboxylic acid. The physiological isoform of 4-hydroxyproline in animal collagen and its enzymatic hydrolysates is *trans* 4-hydroxy-L-proline. In general, when an organic compound contains double bonds that cannot rotate, or when an organic compound (e.g., proline) has a ring structure where the rotation of bonds is restricted, *cis* and *trans* isomers occur. When two functional groups of a diastereomer are oriented in the same direction, the diastereomer (also called diastereoisomer) is referred to as *cis*. In contrast, when two functional groups of a diastereomer are oriented in opposite directions, the diastereomer is referred to as *trans*. Note that the *cis*/*trans* nomenclature is not the same as the *R*/*S* nomenclature.

## Modified AA Residues in Proteins or Polypeptides

Certain AA residues in proteins undergo modifications, such as phosphorylation (Bischoff and Schlüter 2012), as well as acetylation, methylation, nitrosylation, hydroxylation, and glycosylation (*N*- or *O*-linkage) (Figure 4.9). The posttranslational phosphorylation of proteins results in the covalent linkage of an AA to the phosphate group, yielding phospho-serine, phospho-tyrosine, and phospho-threonine. Certain free naturally occurring AAs are phosphorylated to generate new derivatives (e.g., phospho-arginine in various invertebrates [such as crustaceans] and phospho-glutamate in certain plants). The methylation of AA residues in proteins yields methylated AAs (e.g., 1-methylhistidine

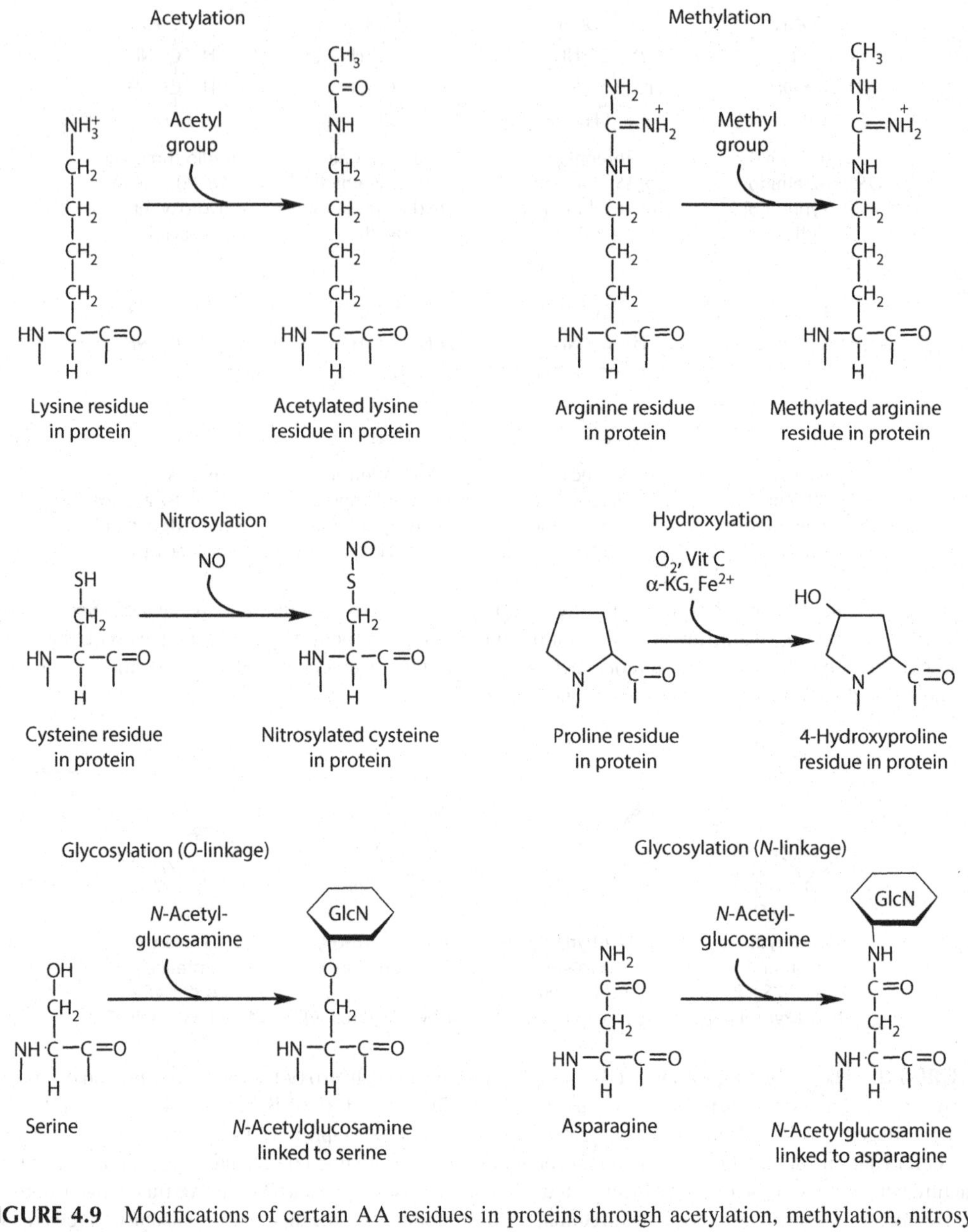

**FIGURE 4.9** Modifications of certain AA residues in proteins through acetylation, methylation, nitrosylation, hydroxylation, and glycosylation. These reactions occur in animals, microorganisms, and plants.

and 3-methylhistidine from histidine; asymmetric dimethylarginine, symmetric dimethylarginine, and $N^G$-monomethyl-arginine from arginine) (Wu and Morris 1998). Furthermore, the hydroxylation of AA residues in proteins yields hydroxylated AAs (e.g., 4-hydroxyproline and 3-hydroxyproline from proline; hydroxyserine from serine; hydroxythreonine from threonine; and hydroxytyrosine from tyrosine). Other examples of the formation of new AA residues in polypeptides due to post-translational modifications include citrulline from arginine; nitrosylated tyrosine from tyrosine; and acetylated lysine, hydroxylysine, methylated lysine, and hypusine from lysine. Of note, hypusine is present in eukaryotic translation initiation factor 5A (eIF5A) and is formed by (1) deoxyhypusine synthase, which catalyzes the cleavage of the polyamine spermidine and the transfer of its 4-aminobutyl moiety to the ε-amino group of one specific lysine residue of the eIF-5A precursor to form deoxyhypusine and 1,3-diaminopropane; and (2) deoxyhypusine hydroxylase, which mediates the formation of hypusine through the addition of a hydroxyl group to the deoxyhypusine residue. Finally, glutamine residues in certain proteins (e.g., blood coagulation protein factor XIII, as well as skin and hair proteins) can be modified by primary amines or protein-bound lysine through transglutaminases 1 and 2 to incorporate amines into proteins or cross-linked proteins, respectively. Bonds formed by transglutaminases exhibit high resistance to proteolytic degradation. Transglutaminases also catalyze the removal of the $-NH_2$ group in the side chain of glutamine residues in proteins (deamidation). Examples of these reactions are provided below:

Protein–Gln–$NH_2$ + Primary amine ($H_2N$–R) = Protein–Gln–NH–R + $NH_3$ (Transglutaminases 1)
Protein–Gln–$NH_2$ + $H_2N$–$CH_2$–Lys–Protein = Protein–Gln–NH–$CH_2$–Lys–Protein + $NH_3$ (Transglutaminases 2)
Protein–Gln–$NH_2$ + $H_2O$ = Protein–Glu + $NH_3$ (Deamidation)

## Free AAs and Peptide (Protein)-Bound AAs

Free AAs are defined as those AAs which are not covalently bound in peptides or proteins. All nonproteinogenic AAs are free AAs. Peptide (protein)-bound AAs are those AAs which are present in peptides or proteins. Except for selenocysteine, all proteinogenic AAs are present in the free pool. The total amount of a proteinogenic AA in the cell is its sum in the peptide-bound and free-AA pools. The concentrations of individual free AAs can differ markedly among cells, tissues, and species. For example, concentrations of free glutamine are 0.5 and 1 mM in the plasma of healthy humans and chickens, respectively, and are 20–25 and 1.5–15 mM in the skeletal muscle of the same species, respectively, depending on muscle type (Hou et al. 2016; Watford and Wu 2005). Also, the concentrations of free glycine are 0.25 and 1 mM in the plasma of healthy humans and pigs, respectively (Table 4.4). Interestingly, glycine, rather than glutamine, is the most abundant free AA in the plasma of postnatal pigs (Flynn et al. 2000). Furthermore, the concentrations of arginine, glutamine, citrulline, and serine can be as high as 1, 25, 10, and 20 mM, respectively, in ovine allantoic fluid during gestation, whereas values for the corresponding AAs in porcine allantoic fluid are 6, 2.5, 0.1, and 0.2 mM, respectively (Kwon et al. 2003; Wu et al. 1996). These differences in concentrations of free AAs reflect tissue- and species-differences in AA metabolism.

The composition of peptide-bound AAs in animal products or tissues can vary greatly among different proteins (Davis et al. 1994; Wu et al. 2016). For example, sow's milk protein contains approximately 10% glutamate and 10% glutamine (Table 4.5), but muscle protein contains approximately 5% glutamate and 5% glutamine. The overall composition of AAs in whole body proteins is largely similar among different species, such as chickens, fish, humans, cattle, rats, pigs, and sheep. The ratio of total free AAs to total peptide-bound AAs in the whole body and most tissues (e.g., skeletal muscle, liver, and small intestine) is approximately 1:30 (g:g), meaning that total free AAs represent approximately 3% of total AAs (free plus peptide-bound) in humans and other animals. However, a ratio of some individual free AAs to the same peptide-bound AAs can be greater than 1:10 or lower than 0.1:100 (g:g). For example, in human skeletal muscle, the ratio of free glutamine to peptide-bound glutamine is approximately 2:10 (g:g), whereas the ratio of free tryptophan to peptide-bound tryptophan is only 0.06:100 (g:g). Depending on age and nutritional status, protein content in animals ranges from 12% to 16%. Selenocysteine is rare in proteins as noted previously, but there is virtually no free selenocysteine in animal cells or plasma.

In most food ingredients of plant and animal origin, more than 98% of total AAs are present in proteins and polypeptides, whereas only small amounts (<2% of total AAs) occur in a free form (Li et al. 2011). However, some free AAs represent significant amounts of total AAs in certain animal products. Notably, free glutamate and glutamine (1 and 4 mM, respectively) account for approximately 2.5% and 10% of total glutamate and glutamine (free plus peptide-bound), respectively,

## TABLE 4.4
## Concentrations of AAs in the Plasma of Animals (μmol/L)

| AA | Cats[a] | Cattle[b] | Chickens[c] | Dogs[d] | Fish[e] | Goats[f] | Horses[g] | Mice[h] | Pigs[i] | Rats[j] | Sheep[k] |
|---|---|---|---|---|---|---|---|---|---|---|---|
| Ala | 570 | 192 | 665 | 312 | 865 | 186 | 121 | 673 | 763 | 492 | 270 |
| Arg | 111 | 55 | 297 | 187 | 144 | 145 | 70 | 235 | 126 | 279 | 191 |
| Asn | 96 | 25 | 121 | 26 | 145 | 67 | 28 | 50 | 101 | 120 | 38 |
| Asp | 8 | 10 | 87 | 5.7 | 8 | 21 | 9.7 | 39 | 16 | 46 | 17 |
| Cit | 19 | 47 | 1.0 | 39 | 20 | 111 | 61 | 70 | 65 | 70 | 181 |
| Cys* | 14 | 156 | 162 | 33 | 9 | 92 | 147 | 124 | 158 | 157 | 188 |
| Gln | 816 | 200 | 912 | 967 | 281 | 256 | 323 | 754 | 521 | 559 | 248 |
| Glu | 43 | 56 | 290 | 48 | 35 | 131 | 22 | 308 | 151 | 137 | 137 |
| Gly | 299 | 243 | 391 | 257 | 505 | 912 | 405 | 234 | 912 | 384 | 566 |
| His | 141 | 45 | 89 | 73 | 107 | 67 | 59 | 75 | 103 | 120 | 70 |
| Ile | 84 | 62 | 96 | 65 | 225 | 136 | 39 | 149 | 119 | 144 | 66 |
| Leu | 157 | 131 | 219 | 179 | 419 | 158 | 64 | 279 | 180 | 216 | 111 |
| Lys | 124 | 57 | 162 | 234 | 437 | 146 | 100 | 246 | 237 | 259 | 119 |
| Met | 54 | 27 | 70 | 62 | 96 | 18 | 19 | 120 | 80 | 107 | 22 |
| Orn | 16 | 72 | 19 | 19 | 57 | 84 | 32 | 54 | 75 | 68 | 98 |
| Phe | 89 | 47 | 137 | 59 | 95 | 42 | 42 | 67 | 95 | 106 | 33 |
| Pro | 149 | 102 | 315 | 160 | 115 | 225 | 128 | 195 | 580 | 286 | 115 |
| Ser | 138 | 72 | 446 | 145 | 160 | 134 | 210 | 472 | 252 | 353 | 80 |
| Tau | 136 | 31 | 170 | 69 | 417 | 52 | 23 | 632 | 127 | 670 | 54 |
| Thr | 156 | 41 | 220 | 207 | 278 | 81 | 61 | 195 | 254 | 381 | 98 |
| Trp | 68 | 44 | 58 | 83 | 21 | 38 | 62 | 45 | 43 | 115 | 30 |
| Tyr | 65 | 48 | 158 | 55 | 87 | 52 | 45 | 126 | 164 | 125 | 43 |
| Val | 210 | 54 | 156 | 250 | 468 | 238 | 115 | 485 | 294 | 249 | 171 |

[a] The plasma was prepared from blood samples of adult cats in the fed state (Sabatino et al. 2013).

[b] Growing Angus steers fed a ground corn-, ground milo-, and cottonseed hulls-based diet (Choi et al. 2014).

[c] Forty two-day-old broilers fed a corn- and SBM-based diet containing 18.4% CP; plasma was prepared from the wing vein blood at 2 h after the feeding. AAs were analyzed as described by Watford and Wu (2005).

[d] The plasma was prepared from blood samples of adult dogs at 3 h after feeding for the analysis of most AAs, except for Asn, Cit, Gln, and Orn (Ikada et al. 2002). The values for these four AAs were reported by Outerbridge et al. (2002).

[e] Rainbow trout with a body weight of 695–1483 g. The plasma was prepared from arterial blood samples at 3 h after the last feeding (Karlsson et al. 2006).

[f] Lactating goats; the plasma was prepared from the arterial blood samples for the analysis of most AAs, except for Cys, Taurine, and Trp (Mepham and Linzell 1966). Values of these three AAs were obtained by G. Wu (unpublished data).

[g] Twelve-month-old horse housed on pasture with free access to grass and hay and received twice daily supplementation with a pellet diet containing 15% CP; the plasma was prepared from blood samples at 14 h after the last feeding (Manso Filho et al. 2009).

[h] The plasma was prepared from the blood samples of adult mice in the fed state (Nagasawa et al. 2012; G. Wu, unpublished work).

[i] Twenty one-day-old piglets nursed by lactating sows; the plasma was prepared from blood samples at 1.5 h after suckling (Flynn et al. 2000).

[j] Thirteen-week-old male rats fed a semi-purified diet containing 20% casein; the plasma was prepared from blood samples at 5 h after feeding (Assaad et al. 2014).

[k] Sheep on Day 30 of gestation fed an alfalfa-based diet containing 15.8% CP; the plasma was prepared from blood samples at 24 h after feeding (Kwon et al. 2003).

* Total cysteine (1/2 cystine + free cysteine). In the pig plasma, cystine = 77 μmol/L and free cysteine = 4.2 μmol/L.

Cit = citrulline; Orn = ornithine; Tau = taurine.

**TABLE 4.5**
**Composition of Free, Peptide-Bound, and Total AAs in Sow's Colostrum and Milk**

| | Day 2 of Lactation | | | Day 14 of Lactation | | | Day 28 of Lactation | | |
|---|---|---|---|---|---|---|---|---|---|
| AA | Total AA | Free AA | Peptide-Bound AA | Total AA | Free AA | Peptide-Bound AA | Total AA | Free AA | Peptide-Bound AA |
| | | | | g/L of Whole Milk | | | | | |
| Ala | 3.74 | 0.025 | 3.72 | 1.99 | 0.056 | 1.93 | 1.84 | 0.058 | 1.78 |
| Arg | 2.89 | 0.008 | 2.89 | 1.43 | 0.010 | 1.42 | 1.35 | 0.011 | 1.34 |
| Asn | 4.31 | 0.004 | 4.31 | 2.51 | 0.017 | 2.49 | 2.17 | 0.032 | 2.14 |
| Asp | 4.58 | 0.027 | 4.55 | 2.77 | 0.060 | 2.71 | 2.35 | 0.066 | 2.28 |
| Cys[a] | 1.72 | 0.028 | 1.69 | 0.72 | 0.048 | 0.67 | 0.75 | 0.095 | 0.65 |
| Glu | 7.72 | 0.062 | 7.59 | 4.97 | 0.187 | 4.78 | 4.40 | 0.176 | 4.22 |
| Gln | 7.65 | 0.054 | 7.41 | 4.85 | 0.226 | 4.62 | 4.71 | 0.546 | 4.16 |
| Gly | 2.20 | 0.024 | 2.18 | 1.12 | 0.068 | 1.05 | 1.03 | 0.104 | 0.93 |
| His | 1.54 | 0.136 | 1.40 | 0.94 | 0.116 | 0.82 | 0.83 | 0.079 | 0.75 |
| Ile | 3.89 | 0.001 | 3.89 | 2.29 | 0.002 | 2.29 | 2.11 | 0.003 | 2.11 |
| Leu | 8.04 | 0.003 | 8.04 | 4.58 | 0.005 | 4.57 | 4.23 | 0.006 | 4.22 |
| Lys | 4.23 | 0.005 | 4.22 | 4.18 | 0.008 | 4.17 | 3.77 | 0.009 | 3.76 |
| Met | 1.81 | 0.001 | 1.81 | 1.05 | 0.003 | 1.05 | 0.93 | 0.003 | 0.93 |
| Phe | 3.35 | 0.003 | 3.35 | 2.03 | 0.006 | 2.02 | 1.90 | 0.006 | 1.89 |
| Pro | 7.49 | 0.004 | 7.49 | 5.61 | 0.009 | 5.60 | 5.28 | 0.014 | 5.27 |
| OH-Pro | 1.37 | 0.015 | 1.35[b] | 1.04 | 0.009 | 1.03[b] | 0.69 | 0.007 | 0.68[b] |
| Ser | 4.48 | 0.005 | 4.47 | 2.35 | 0.031 | 2.32 | 2.20 | 0.048 | 2.15 |
| Thr | 4.36 | 0.013 | 4.35 | 2.28 | 0.019 | 2.26 | 2.07 | 0.054 | 2.02 |
| Trp | 1.28 | 0.001 | 1.28 | 0.66 | 0.003 | 0.66 | 0.62 | 0.004 | 0.62 |
| Val | 4.70 | 0.006 | 4.69 | 2.53 | 0.013 | 2.52 | 2.26 | 0.017 | 2.24 |
| β-Ala | 0.001 | 0.001 | 0.000 | 0.003 | 0.003 | 0.000 | 0.004 | 0.004 | 0.000 |
| Cit | 0.001 | 0.001 | 0.000 | 0.007 | 0.007 | 0.000 | 0.009 | 0.009 | 0.000 |
| Orn | 0.005 | 0.005 | 0.000 | 0.008 | 0.008 | 0.000 | 0.008 | 0.008 | 0.000 |
| Taurine | 0.134 | 0.134 | 0.000 | 0.176 | 0.176 | 0.000 | 0.186 | 0.186 | 0.000 |
| All AAs | 81.2 | 0.57 | 80.7 | 50.1 | 1.09 | 49.0 | 45.7 | 1.55 | 44.1 |

[a] Total cysteine (1/2 cystine + free cysteine).
[b] Present in small peptides.

*Note:* Milk samples were obtained from lactating sows fed an 18.5% CP (Mateo et al. 2008) and analyzed for free and peptide-bound AAs (Wu et al. 2016). Values are the means for 10 sows. Day 0 of lactation is defined as the day of farrowing. The molecular weights of intact AAs were used for the calculation of concentrations of peptide-bound AAs in the milk.

in sow's milk on Day 28 of lactation (Table 4.5). Similar results have been reported for human milk. Also, the concentration of free taurine in human and porcine milk can be as high as 1 mM. These AAs play an important role in the growth and development of the neonatal small intestine.

## Physical Appearance, Melting Points, and Tastes of AAs

The crystals of AAs are generally white (Ajinomoto 2003). All crystalline α-AAs, except for glutamine and cysteine, have a high melting point of over 200°C. Glutamine and cysteine have melting points of 185°C and 178°C, respectively. At or above their melting points, AAs decompose spontaneously. The hydrochlorides of L-arginine (L-arginine-HCl), L-lysine (L-lysine-HCl), and L-ornithine (L-ornithine-HCl) have melting points of 235°C, 236°C, and 231°C, respectively (Table 4.2). Interestingly, the melting points of L-arginine and L-arginine-HCl are nearly identical.

The taste of AAs results from their interactions with specific receptors (guanine nucleotide-binding protein [G protein]-coupled receptors) on the tongue (Fernstrom et al. 2012). L-Glutamate has a "meaty" taste. L-Alanine and glycine have a sweet taste, L-serine and L-threonine have a faintly sweet taste, and L-citrulline has a slightly sweet taste. The L-arginine base has a bitter and unpleasant taste by itself, but in a mixture with citric acid in drinking water, it is palatable. L-Isoleucine has a bitter taste, whereas L-lysine, L-aspartate, and L-phenylalanine have a slightly bitter taste. L-Glutamine, β-alanine, and taurine are flat (lacking tastiness). L-Asparagine, L-cysteine, L-cystine, L-methionine, L-tryptophan, L-proline, L-ornithine, L-histidine, L-leucine, L-tyrosine, and L-valine have a flat-to-bitter taste. D-Glutamate is almost tasteless, whereas D-aspartate is flat. D-Alanine, D-leucine, D-serine, D-tryptophan, and D-valine are very sweet, whereas D-glutamine, D-histidine, D-isoleucine, D-methionine, D-phenylalanine, D-threonine, and D-tyrosine are sweet (Kawai et al. 2012). The taste of a basic AA is altered by its hydrochloride salt (San Gabriel et al. 2009).

## Solubility of AAs in Water and Solutions

All AAs are soluble in water at room temperature. Leucine, isoleucine, valine, phenylalanine, tryptophan, methionine, tyrosine, and cysteine are among the most hydrophobic AAs. All AAs (except for cystine) are soluble in Krebs bicarbonate buffer (pH 7.4 at 25°C) at concentrations that are at least 10 times greater than those in animal plasma. The solubility of α-AAs in water varies with their side chains, with proline and cystine being the most and least soluble, respectively (Table 4.2). The solubility of β-alanine and γ-aminobutyrate in water is higher than that of lysine. Salts affect the solubility of AAs in water, and such an effect depends on their structures (Wu 2013). The hydrochlorides of AAs (both neutral and basic), such as cystine, arginine, histidine, and lysine, are generally more soluble in water than the corresponding free AAs. Most of the AA hydrochloride salts are highly soluble in absolute ethanol. The hydrochloride salts of basic AAs (e.g., arginine and lysine) are often used for their neutralization in water and in physiological solutions. The sodium salts of most AAs dissolve more readily in water and are more ethanol soluble than the corresponding free AAs.

The solubility of AAs generally increases in acidic or alkaline solutions and with elevated temperatures. With the exception of proline and hydroxyproline, AAs are generally insoluble in organic solvents (e.g., absolute ethanol). Owing to their pyrrole ring structures, proline and hydroxyproline are fairly soluble in absolute ethanol (~1.6 g/100 mL at 20°C). Thus, proteins with a high content of proline are soluble in 70%–80% ethanol.

## Chemical Stability of AAs

### Stability of Crystalline AAs

The crystalline forms of all AAs are stable at room temperature (i.e., 25°C) for at least 25 years without any detectable loss. This applies to L- and D-AAs, as well as proteinogenic and nonproteinogenic AAs. However, like all substances, AAs should be protected from light and should not be exposed to a high humidity environment during storage (Ajinomoto 2003).

### Stability of AAs in Water and Buffers

Except for cysteine, all AAs in water, in buffered solutions (e.g., Krebs bicarbonate buffer), or in deproteinized and neutralized biological samples, are stable at −80°C for 6 months without any detectable loss. Likewise, AAs are generally stable in an aqueous solution at a physiological pH and 37°C –40°C, except for (1) cysteine, which undergoes rapid oxidation to cystine, particularly in the presence of metal ions and the absence of reducing agents; and (2) glutamine, whose side-chain amide group and the α-amino group spontaneously and slowly interact to form the cyclic product, the ammonium salt of pyrrolidone carboxylate (pyroglutamate, a potential neurotoxin). This reaction occurs at a rate of <1%/day for 1 mM glutamine at 37°C.

The ratio of cystine to cysteine is approximately 10:1 in the plasma or serum of healthy subjects. Cystine is readily converted to cysteine inside the cell under physiological reducing conditions. *N*-Acetylcysteine (a water-soluble synthetic substance) is a stable precursor of cysteine for cultured cells and for intravenous or oral administration into humans and other animals (Hou et al. 2015b). In chemical analysis, the thiol (–SH) group of cysteine can be protected by iodoacetic acid, whereas cystine can be readily reduced to cysteine by 2-mercaptoethanol. In contrast to cysteine, few means are available to protect glutamine from spontaneous cyclization in an aqueous solution.

### Stability of AAs in Acid and Alkaline Solutions

At concentrations between 0.01 and 5 mM, all AAs, except for cysteine and glutamine, are stable in a 5% trichloroacetic acid (TCA) or 0.75 M $HClO_4$ solution, or an alkaline solution (pH 8.4), at room temperature (e.g., 25°C) for at least 12 h or at −80°C for 2 months, without any detectable loss. However, under the standard conditions of acid hydrolysis at high temperatures (i.e., 6 M HCl, 110°C, and 24 h under N gas), changes in the following AAs occur: (1) all glutamine and asparagine are converted to glutamate and aspartate, respectively; (2) tryptophan is completely destroyed; and (3) 20% of methionine undergoes oxidation to generate methionine sulfoxide. Notably, under these conditions, other AAs are either completely stable (i.e., no detectable loss for alanine, arginine, cystine, glutamate, glycine, histidine, leucine, lysine, phenylalanine, and valine) or relatively stable (3% loss for aspartate and threonine; 5% loss for tyrosine and proline; and 10% loss for serine). Most AAs (including glycine, histidine, serine, and threonine) are almost completely destroyed, many AAs (e.g., cysteine and methionine) undergo degradation to a great extent, and some AAs are hydrolyzed (e.g., glutamine to glutamate, asparagine to aspartate, and arginine to ornithine), under the conditions of alkaline hydrolysis at a high temperature (e.g., 4.2 M NaOH and 105°C). In contrast, tryptophan is stable (100% recovery) in alkaline solution for 20 h even at 105°C. Thus, the analysis of tryptophan in protein can be successfully accomplished by alkaline hydrolysis in the presence of 4.2 M NaOH and 1% thiodiglycol (an antioxidant) at 110°C for 20 h.

With three exceptions, free AAs in water or a neutral solution are stable under high pressure and high temperature conditions (e.g., in an autoclave); glutamine and asparagine are almost completely destroyed, while cysteine is oxidized to cystine. Cystine, however, is stable under these same conditions. In a dipeptide form (e.g., L-alanyl-glutamine and glycyl-glutamine, as well as L-leucyl-asparagine and glycyl-asparagine), glutamine and asparagine are stable under these conditions. To prevent the loss of glutamine and asparagine under autoclaving conditions, a solution containing free glutamine and asparagine can be sterilized through a 0.2 μm filter before use for cell or tissue culture. Note that, under autoclaving conditions, cysteine (2%, w/v) in deoxygenated water is stable at pH 4.9 but undergoes 8% and 17% losses at pH 7 and 8, respectively.

## DEFINITION, CHEMICAL CLASSIFICATIONS, AND PROPERTIES OF PEPTIDES AND PROTEIN

### Definitions of Peptides and Proteins

A peptide is defined as an organic molecule consisting of 2 or more AA residues linked by peptide bonds. In most peptides, the typical peptide bonds are formed from the α-amino and α-carboxyl groups of adjacent AAs. Peptides can be chemically and biochemically synthesized from AAs (Fridkin and Patchornik 1974). The formation of one peptide bond results in the removal of one water molecule (Figure 4.10). Peptides can be classified according to the number of their AA

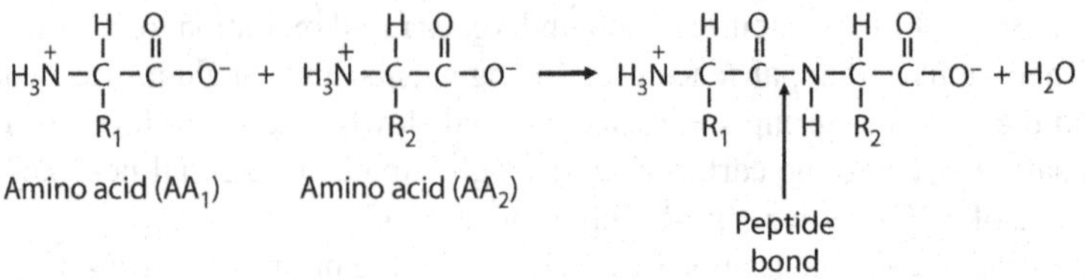

$$H_3\overset{+}{N}-\underset{R_1}{\overset{H}{C}}-\overset{O}{\overset{\|}{C}}-O^- + H_3\overset{+}{N}-\underset{R_2}{\overset{H}{C}}-\overset{O}{\overset{\|}{C}}-O^- \longrightarrow H_3\overset{+}{N}-\underset{R_1}{\overset{H}{C}}-\overset{O}{\overset{\|}{C}}-\underset{H}{N}-\underset{R_2}{\overset{H}{C}}-\overset{O}{\overset{\|}{C}}-O^- + H_2O$$

Amino acid ($AA_1$) Amino acid ($AA_2$) Peptide bond

**FIGURE 4.10** Synthesis of a dipeptide from two AAs. $R_1$ and $R_2$ represent the side chains of the two AAs. With the loss of one $H_2O$ molecule, a peptide bond (–CONH–) is formed.

residues. An oligopeptide comprises 2–20 AA residues (Hughes 2012). An oligopeptide containing ≤10 AA residues is called a small oligopeptide (or small peptide); an example is oxytocin with 9 AA residues, which stimulates lactation. An oligopeptide containing 11–20 AA residues is called a large oligopeptide (or large peptide); an example is somatostatin with 14 AA residues, which is an inhibitor of growth hormone release. A peptide that contains ≥21 AA residues and does not have a 3D structure is termed a polypeptide; an example is endothelin with 21 AA residues, which is a potent vasoconstrictor. A protein consists of one or more polypeptides and has a well-defined 3D structure; an example is mature bovine serum albumin with a molecular weight of 66,463 Daltons (583 AA residues). All peptides and proteins are polymers, and are abundant in blood (Gilbert et al. 2008).

The dividing line between proteins and polypeptides is usually their molecular weights and the number of their AA residues (Kyte 2006). Generally speaking, a protein has a molecular weight of ≥8000 Daltons (i.e., ≥72 AA residues), because such a molecule will have a well-defined 3D structure. For example, growth hormone, which has 191 AAs with a molecular weight of approximately 22,000 Daltons, is a protein. Ubiquitin (a single chain of 72 AA residues) and casein α-S1 (200 AA residues) are proteins as well. Polypeptides with a molecular weight less than 8000 Daltons and 72 AA residues are generally not considered to be proteins, unless they have a well-defined 3D structure. For example, glucagon (29 AA residues with a molecular weight of ~3500 Daltons) is a polypeptide. Likewise, PEC-60 (a single chain of 60 AA residues; Agerberth et al. 1989) and dopuin (a single chain of 62 AA residues; Chen et al. 1997), which are isolated from the pig small-intestinal mucosae, are called polypeptides. However, the classification of proteins or polypeptides simply on the basis of their molecular weights or their number of AA residues is certainly not absolute. For example, insulin (51 AA residues [20 in chain A and 31 in chain B]) is well recognized as a protein, because it has the defined 3D structure exhibited by proteins. To date, the number of different proteins with various AA compositions has been estimated to be approximately 100,000 in domestic animals and up to 50,000 in plants (Sterck et al. 2007).

Some substances with nontypical peptide bonds (e.g., glutathione [GSH] and *N*-pteroyl-L-glutamate [folate]) are beneficial for nutrition and physiology, whereas others (e.g., ergovaline [present in endophyte-infected Tall fescue, a cool season grass] and phalloidine) are toxic to animals, including humans. GSH, which consists of L-glutamate, L-cysteine, and glycine, is the most abundant low-molecular-weight antioxidant tripeptide in animal cells and fluids (up to 10 mM). GSH is a very special small peptide, as it is the γ-carboxyl group (Figure 4.11), rather than the α-carboxyl group, of the L-glutamate molecule that reacts with the α-amino group of L-cysteine to form a peptidic γ-linkage, which protects GSH from hydrolysis by extracellular or intracellular peptidases.

## Major Proteins in Animals

### Actin and Myosin

Actin and myosin are major intracellular proteins in most animal cells (e.g., muscles). For example, actin and myosin comprise 65% and 2%–10% of total cellular protein in skeletal muscle and non-muscle cells, respectively (Rennie and Tipton 2000). Actin has three α-isoforms (e.g., in skeletal, cardiac, and smooth muscles), as well as β- and γ-isoforms (e.g., in both muscle and non-muscle

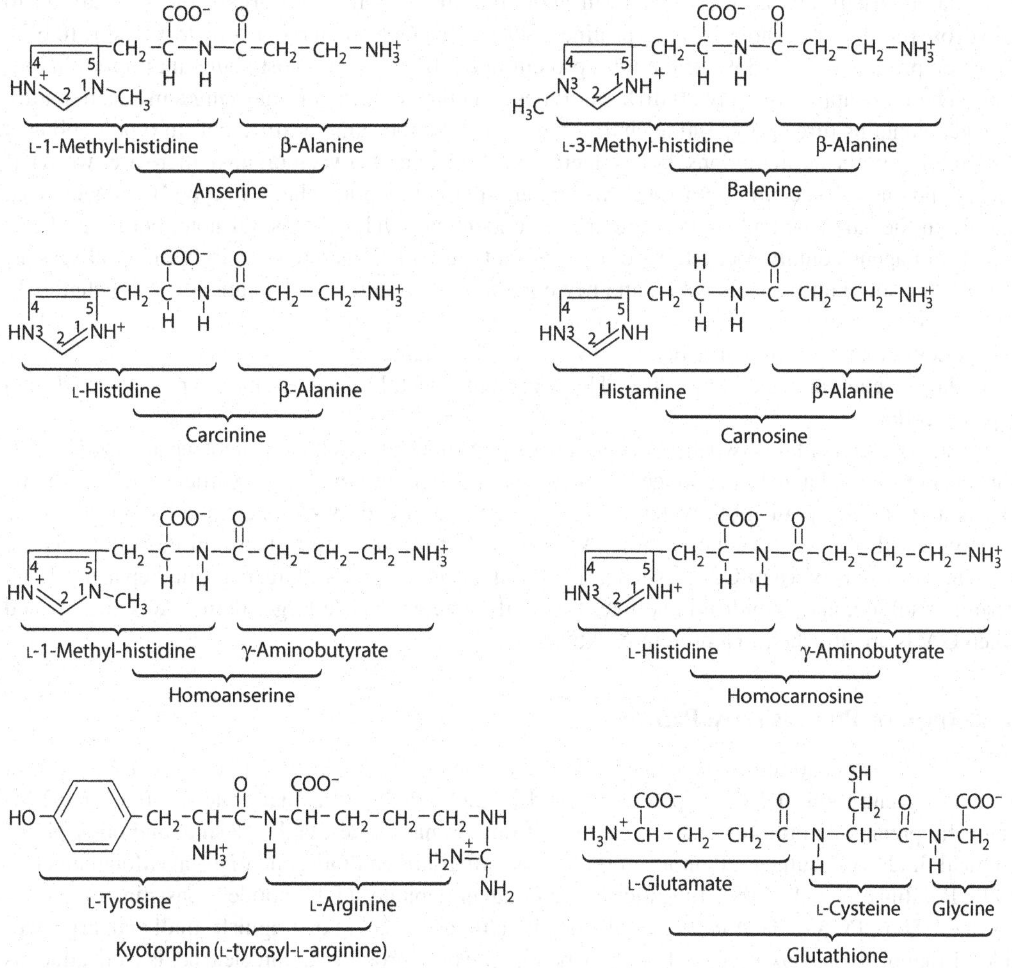

L-1-Methyl-histidine β-Alanine

Anserine

L-3-Methyl-histidine β-Alanine

Balenine

L-Histidine β-Alanine

Carcinine

Histamine β-Alanine

Carnosine

L-1-Methyl-histidine γ-Aminobutyrate

Homoanserine

L-Histidine γ-Aminobutyrate

Homocarnosine

L-Tyrosine L-Arginine

Kyotorphin (L-tyrosyl-L-arginine)

L-Glutamate L-Cysteine Glycine

Glutathione

**FIGURE 4.11** Physiologically important dipeptides and glutathione in animal tissues.

cells) (Dominguez and Holmes 2011). The actin isoforms differ by only a few AA residues, and undergo posttranslational modifications (e.g., the methylation of His-73 of skeletal muscle α-actin to form 3-methyl-histidine). Of interest, actin can exist in monomeric globular (G-actin) and filamentous (F-actin) states. Myosin consists of six polypeptides: two heavy chains, as well as two pairs of different light chains (essential light chains and regulatory light chains) (Sweeney and Houdusse 2010). Both myosin and F-actin possess ATPase activity. In the resting state, actin and myosin filaments partially overlap each other in an interdigitating manner. When muscle contracts, the actin and the myosin slide past each other, with the required energy being provided through ATP hydrolysis by the myosin globular head. Besides contraction, actin and myosin also have other biological activities, such as cell motility, division, signaling, and organelle movement, as well as the maintenance of cell cytoskeleton and shape.

### Proteins in Connective Tissues

The four major types of proteins in connective tissue (e.g., the skin) are collagen, elastin, glycosoaminoglycans (GAGs), and proteoglycans. They are extracellular proteins, which are synthesized and released by fibroblasts. Collagen, which is unusually rich in proline, hydroxyproline, and glycine in the repeated form of tripeptides (Gly-Pro-Y and Gly-X-Hyp, where X and Y can be any

AA), has a structural role to confer form and strength to tissues and organisms. In addition to 4-hydroxyproline (9%) and 3-hydroxyproline (0.1%), collagen also contains 5-hydroxylysine (0.6%). Collagen protein (~30%–33% of the total protein in the body) is the most abundant protein in animals. There are approximately 20 different types of collagen in the animal kingdom. Each mature collagen contains three polypeptide chains, which may be the same or different. In type I collagen (e.g., mainly in the skin, tendons, bones, teeth, ligaments, and between organs), there are two α1(I) chains and one α2(I) chain, with 1000 AA residues per polypeptide chain. In type II collagen (e.g., mainly in the cartilage and eyes), there are three identical α1(II) chains. Of note, both type I and type II collagens contain no cysteine or cystine. In type III collagen (e.g., mainly in blood vessels, muscle, intestinal and uterine walls, and newborn skin), there are three identical α1(III) chains. In type IV collagen (mainly in the basement membrane, eye lens, and the capillaries and glomeruli of the kidneys), there are three identical α1(IV) or α2(IV) chains. Interestingly, both type III and type IV collagens contain cysteine residues. The heart and skeletal muscle contain type I, type III, and type IV collagens.

Elastin, which contains two special derivatives of lysine residues (i.e., desmosine and isodesmonsine), is more stretchable than collagen, thereby helping to maintain a tissue resilience and elasticity. GAGs and proteoglycans hold water within a tissue and also provide mechanical support. GAGs are composed of *N*-acetyl glucosamine, *N*-acetyl galactosamine, and glucosamine sulfate. These units form various types of GAGs, such as hyaluronic acid, keratin sulfate, heparin, heparin sulfate, dermatin sulfate, and chondroitin sulfate. Proteoglycans, which are larger than GAGs, are formed when GAGs are attached to a protein backbone.

### Separation of Peptides from Proteins

Proteins can be denatured by heat, acids, bases, alcohols, urea, and salts of heavy metals. TCA (at a final concentration of 5%) or perchloric acid ($HClO_4$, PCA; at a final concentration of 0.2 M) can fully precipitate proteins, but not peptides, from animal tissues, cells, plasma, and other physiological fluids (e.g., rumen, allantoic, amniotic, intestinal-lumen fluids, and digesta) (Moughan et al. 1990; Rajalingam et al. 2009). Tungstic acid (1%) can precipitate small peptides consisting of ≥4 AA residues. Thus, PCA or TCA can be used along with tungstic acid to distinguish small and large peptides. Ethanol (80%, vol/vol) can effectively precipitate both proteins and nucleic acids from aqueous solutions (Wilcockson 1975). This method may be useful to remove water-soluble inorganic compounds (e.g., aluminum) from protein hydrolysates. Note that certain plant proteins with high proline content (e.g., zein, glidin, and hordein) are soluble in 70%–80% ethanol but insoluble in water or 100% ethanol; these proteins are called prolamines. Finally, ammonium sulfate (e.g., at a final concentration of 35%) can precipitate proteins from a solution without altering their biological structure.

### Protein Structures

Proteins are the most abundant macromolecules in cells. They have four orders of structures: (1) a primary structure (the sequence of AAs along the polypeptide chain); (2) a secondary structure (the conformation of the polypeptide backbone); (3) a tertiary structure (the 3D arrangement of the protein molecule); and (4) a quaternary structure (the spatial arrangement of polypeptide subunits) (Figure 4.12). The primary sequence of AAs in protein determines its secondary, tertiary, and quaternary structures, as well as its biological functions. The forces stabilizing polypeptide aggregates are hydrogen and electrostatic bonds between AA residues. Peptides and proteins are usually stable in a sterile aqueous solution at room temperature (Lubec and Rosenthal 1990).

The secondary structure of protein consists of several repeating patterns (Jones 2012). The most commonly observed types of secondary structure are the α-helix and the β-pleated sheet. The α-helix is a rigid, rodlike structure that arises when a polypeptide chain twists into a right-handed helical conformation, where hydrogen bonds form between the NH group of each AA and the carbonyl group

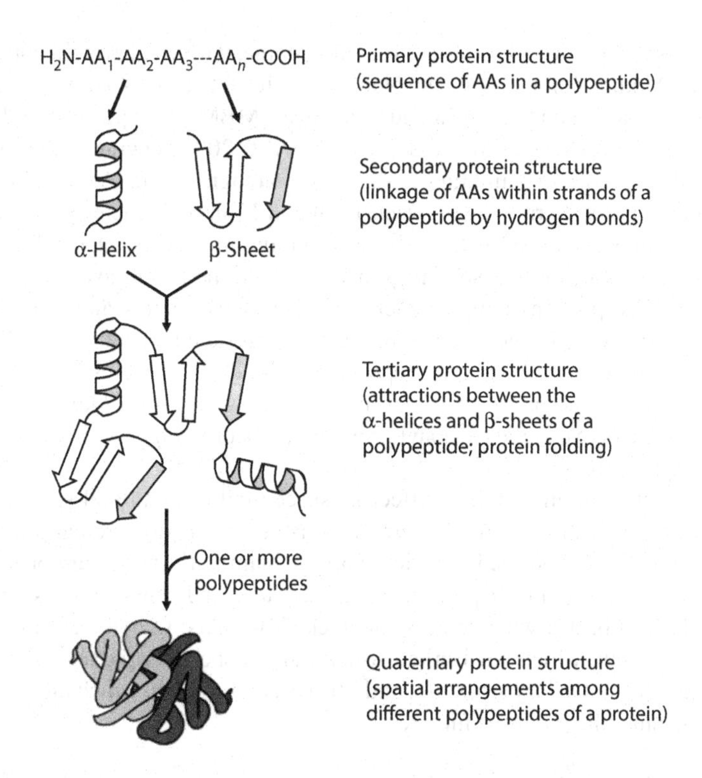


**FIGURE 4.12** The four orders of protein structures. A protein has: (1) a primary structure (the sequence of AAs along the polypeptide chain); (2) a secondary structure (the conformation of the polypeptide backbone); (3) a tertiary structure (the 3D arrangement of protein); and (4) a quaternary structure (the spatial arrangement of polypeptide subunits). The primary sequence of AAs in protein determines its secondary, tertiary, and quaternary structures, as well as its biological functions. (Courtesy of Hou, Y.Q. et al. 2017. *J. Anim. Sci. Biotechnol.* 8:24.)

of the AA four residues away. Some AAs foster or inhibit the formation of specific secondary structures. For example, glycine's R group (a hydrogen atom) is so small that the polypeptide chain may be too flexible, while proline contains a rigid ring that prevents the N–C bond from rotating. In addition, proline has no NH group available to form the intra-chain hydrogen bonds that are crucial in an α-helix structure. Likewise, AA sequences with large numbers of charged AAs (e.g., glutamate and aspartate) and bulky R groups (e.g., tryptophan) are also incompatible with α-helix structures. On the other hand, β-pleated sheets form when two or more polypeptide chain segments line up side by side, with each individual segment being called a β-strand. Instead of being coiled, each β-strand is fully extended. The β-pleated sheets are either parallel or antiparallel. In the parallel β-pleated sheet structures, the hydrogen bonds in the polypeptide chains are arranged in the same direction; in the antiparallel chains, these bonds are arranged in opposite directions. In the secondary structure, both α-helix and β-pleated sheet patterns are stabilized by localized hydrogen bonding between the carbonyl and NH groups in the protein's backbone. Proline plays a key role in forming the β-turns of β-sheets.

Proteins can be classified according to their overall shape (globular or fibrous), solubility in water (hydrophobic or hydrophilic), 3D structure, or biological functions (Table 4.1). On the basis of the combined chemical properties, proteins can be classified as simple proteins, scleroproteins, and complex proteins (e.g., flavoproteins, glycoproteins, hemoproteins, lipoproteins, metalloproteins, mucoproteins, nucleoproteins, and phosphoproteins). Albumin and hemoglobin are globular proteins, which are common to all feedstuffs of plant origin. Fibrous proteins include actin, myosin, collagens, elastin, α-keratins, and β-keratins, which are limited to the feedstuffs of animal and marine origin. Collagens are rich in proline and glycine (~1/3 each), and constitute approximately

30% of total proteins in animals. Keratins are rich in cysteine, with wool protein containing approximately 4% sulfur. Mature collagens are insoluble in water. Feedstuffs with high percentages of water-insoluble protein are fish meal, meat and bone meal (MBM), beet pulp, dried brewers grains, dried distillers grains, forages, sorghum, and soy hulls (NRC 2001). Owing to their large size, proteins have colloidal properties to maintain stability in physiological fluid. A colloid is a solution that has evenly distributed particles ranging between 1 nm and 1 μm in diameter.

Proteins interact among themselves and the surrounding molecules. Depending on concentration and type, proteins differ in their solubility in water, with the membrane-bound proteins being hydrophobic. Like AAs, proteins have characteristic isoelectric points and buffering capacities. All proteins can be denatured or modified from their natural state by heat, acids, alkalis, alcohols, urea, and the salts of heavy metals. The susceptibility of foodstuff proteins to heat damage during processing is increased in the presence of carbohydrates, owing to the Maillard reaction, which involves a condensation between the carbonyl group of a reducing sugar with the free amino group of an AA residue (e.g., lysine).

The structures of the proteins in diets affect its susceptibility to animal-source proteases. For example, digestive proteases of mammals, birds and fish do not hydrolyze natural α-keratins (the major proteins of hair, wool, hooves, horns, and nails in mammals), which are primarily α-helical in structure, or β-keratins (the major proteins of nails, scales and claws in birds and reptiles, and of beaks and feathers in birds), which consist of stacked β-sheets. In contrast, digestive proteases readily degrade: (1) casein, which has limited α-helix and β-sheet secondary structure, as well as no disulfide bridges and no tertiary structure; and (2) actin and myosin, which are the main globular proteins in skeletal, smooth, and heart muscles.

## The Concept of Crude Protein and True Protein

The content of mixed proteins in a feed or biological sample is often obtained by multiplying their nitrogen content by a factor of 6.25, on the basis of the average nitrogen content (16%) in protein. The value obtained from the analysis is referred to as crude protein (CP) content. Such calculation, however, is not very precise for determining true protein content, because (1) some proteins contain more or less nitrogen due to their AA composition; and (2) different feedstuffs contain various percentages of nonprotein nitrogen (NPN) (e.g., peptides, AAs, ammonia, urea, amides, amines, choline, betaine, purines, pyrimidines, nitrite, and nitrate). The NPN substances are abundant in grasses and legume forages (NRC 2001). NPN content is generally higher in hays and silages than the same feedstuffs when fresh, because proteolysis occurs during wilting or fermentation. Some nitrogen-rich substances (e.g., melamine, which contains 66% nitrogen) lead to high CP content and are highly toxic to animals. With the availability of advanced analytical methods, the composition of AAs in dietary or tissue proteins can be precisely determined and used to calculate the content of true protein on the basis of the molecular weights (Daltons) of constituent AA residues (i.e., the molecular weight of an intact AA-18) (Dai et al. 2014).

Animal-source ingredients (casein, gelatin, blood meal, hydrolyzed feather meal, MBM, poultry by-product meal [PBM], and Menhaden fish meal) generally contain a higher content of CP and true protein than plant-source ingredients (cookie meal, SBM, dehulled SBM, cottonseed meal, peanut meal, corn grain, and sorghum grain) (Table 4.6). The percentages of CP in these ingredients vary from 9% to 100%, depending on type, and are greater than those in forages and roughages (as low as 3% CP on the fed-basis) for ruminants (Table 4.7). The content of true protein is approximately 80%–100% of CP in ingredients, depending on type. Differences between CP and true protein are smaller for blood meal, casein, feather meal, fish meal, gelatin, MBM, PBM, and SBM, compared with cookie meal, cottonseed meal, peanut meal, and dehulled SBM (Li et al. 2011). In all these ingredients, the total content of the AAs that are not synthesizable in animal cells is lower than that of the AAs which are synthesizable in animal cells.

**TABLE 4.6**
**Composition of AAs in Feed Ingredients**

| AA | Blood Meal | Casein | Cookie Meal | Corn Grain | CSM | Feather Meal | Fish Meal | Gelatin | MBM | Peanut Meal | PBM | SBM | SBM (P) | SGH Grain |
|---|---|---|---|---|---|---|---|---|---|---|---|---|---|---|
| | | | | | **General Nutrients (% of Foodstuff, As-Fed Basis)** | | | | | | | | | |
| DM | 91.8 | 91.7 | 90.8 | 89.0 | 90.0 | 95.1 | 91.8 | 88.9 | 96.1 | 91.8 | 96.5 | 89.0 | 96.4 | 89.1 |
| CP | 89.6 | 88.0 | 12.3 | 9.3 | 40.3 | 82.1 | 63.4 | 100.1 | 52.0 | 43.9 | 64.3 | 43.6 | 51.8 | 10.1 |
| TP | 88.0 | 86.2 | 10.5 | 8.2 | 32.3 | 81.0 | 63.7 | 97.4 | 50.7 | 35.1 | 60.4 | 38.2 | 41.6 | 8.8 |
| EA | 41.9 | 37.2 | 3.3 | 3.0 | 10.7 | 24.9 | 24.9 | 14.4 | 15.4 | 10.7 | 18.4 | 14.5 | 15.5 | 3.2 |
| SA | 46.1 | 49.0 | 7.2 | 5.2 | 21.6 | 56.1 | 38.8 | 83.0 | 35.3 | 24.3 | 42.0 | 23.7 | 26.1 | 5.6 |
| | | | | | **Individual AA (% of Foodstuff, As-Fed Basis)** | | | | | | | | | |
| Ala | 7.82 | 2.77 | 0.52 | 0.71 | 1.42 | 4.18 | 5.07 | 9.01 | 4.78 | 1.86 | 4.91 | 1.95 | 2.08 | 0.96 |
| Arg | 4.91 | 3.40 | 0.58 | 0.38 | 4.32 | 5.74 | 4.85 | 7.68 | 3.67 | 5.68 | 4.63 | 3.18 | 3.12 | 0.41 |
| Asn | 4.67 | 2.56 | 0.40 | 0.35 | 1.57 | 1.67 | 2.92 | 1.42 | 2.21 | 1.80 | 2.73 | 2.10 | 2.41 | 0.31 |
| Asp | 6.20 | 3.88 | 0.45 | 0.43 | 1.94 | 2.92 | 4.34 | 2.86 | 3.08 | 2.52 | 4.10 | 3.14 | 3.40 | 0.36 |
| Cys | 1.92 | 0.43 | 0.18 | 0.20 | 0.70 | 4.16 | 0.67 | 0.05 | 0.49 | 0.65 | 1.05 | 0.70 | 0.69 | 0.19 |
| Gln | 4.32 | 11.2 | 1.44 | 1.02 | 3.60 | 2.86 | 3.94 | 3.03 | 2.81 | 2.66 | 3.54 | 3.80 | 4.11 | 0.85 |
| Glu | 6.38 | 9.38 | 1.92 | 0.64 | 4.59 | 4.81 | 6.01 | 5.26 | 4.05 | 4.18 | 4.89 | 4.17 | 4.53 | 1.18 |
| Gly | 3.86 | 1.86 | 0.78 | 0.40 | 2.12 | 8.95 | 6.58 | 33.6 | 8.67 | 3.17 | 9.42 | 2.30 | 2.72 | 0.39 |
| His | 5.57 | 2.78 | 0.22 | 0.23 | 1.08 | 0.88 | 1.51 | 0.74 | 1.19 | 0.95 | 1.30 | 1.13 | 1.15 | 0.23 |
| Hyp | 0.20 | 0.14 | 0.00 | 0.00 | 0.05 | 4.95 | 1.86 | 12.8 | 2.88 | 0.07 | 3.31 | 0.09 | 0.07 | 0.00 |
| Ile | 2.54 | 4.91 | 0.51 | 0.34 | 1.19 | 3.79 | 3.26 | 1.17 | 1.92 | 1.41 | 2.32 | 2.03 | 2.10 | 0.38 |
| Leu | 11.4 | 8.82 | 0.88 | 1.13 | 2.26 | 6.75 | 5.24 | 2.61 | 3.56 | 2.48 | 4.21 | 3.44 | 3.70 | 1.21 |
| Lys | 8.25 | 7.49 | 0.41 | 0.25 | 1.66 | 2.16 | 5.29 | 3.75 | 3.13 | 1.37 | 3.44 | 2.80 | 2.87 | 0.21 |
| Met | 1.16 | 2.64 | 0.19 | 0.21 | 0.66 | 0.75 | 2.02 | 1.03 | 1.10 | 0.47 | 1.39 | 0.60 | 0.64 | 0.20 |
| Phe | 5.83 | 4.87 | 0.50 | 0.46 | 2.02 | 3.95 | 2.76 | 1.67 | 1.85 | 1.93 | 2.36 | 2.21 | 2.44 | 0.51 |
| Pro | 6.29 | 10.8 | 0.98 | 1.06 | 1.89 | 11.7 | 4.25 | 20.6 | 5.86 | 2.29 | 6.72 | 2.40 | 3.18 | 0.96 |
| Ser | 4.49 | 5.08 | 0.56 | 0.45 | 1.72 | 8.80 | 2.80 | 3.44 | 2.08 | 2.03 | 2.67 | 2.12 | 2.35 | 0.46 |
| Trp | 1.30 | 1.19 | 0.15 | 0.07 | 0.44 | 0.79 | 0.70 | 0.22 | 0.39 | 0.38 | 0.49 | 0.62 | 0.63 | 0.10 |
| Thr | 3.95 | 4.10 | 0.42 | 0.31 | 1.25 | 3.97 | 4.11 | 3.45 | 2.42 | 1.67 | 2.85 | 1.76 | 2.03 | 0.32 |
| Tyr | 2.86 | 5.06 | 0.55 | 0.43 | 1.10 | 2.04 | 2.36 | 0.93 | 1.45 | 1.39 | 1.84 | 1.66 | 1.72 | 0.45 |
| Val | 8.21 | 6.03 | 0.53 | 0.44 | 1.69 | 5.76 | 3.80 | 1.96 | 2.23 | 1.69 | 2.89 | 2.09 | 2.25 | 0.50 |

*Source:* Li, X.L. et al. 2011. *Amino Acids.* 40:1159–1168.
Molecular weights of intact AA were used to calculate the content of peptide-bound AA in feed ingredients.
CP = Crude protein (N% × 6.25).
CSM = Cottonseed meal.
DM = Dry matter.
EA = Total amounts of AAs which are not synthesized in animal cells.
MBM = Meat and bone meal.
(P) = (Processed).
PBM = Poultry byproduct meal.
SA = Total amounts of AAs which are synthesizable in animal cells.
SBM = Soybean meal.
SGH = Sorghum.
TP = True protein, which was calculated on the basis of molecular weights of AA residues in protein.

**TABLE 4.7**
**The Content of CP in Forages and Roughages for Ruminant Diets**

| Feedstuff | DM (%) | CP (%) |
|---|---|---|
| Bermudagrass hay | 87.1 | 10.4 |
| **Corn (yellow)** | | |
| Cobs | 90.8 | 3.0 |
| Silage (immature) | 23.5 | 9.7 |
| Silage (normal) | 35.1 | 8.8 |
| Silage (mature) | 44.2 | 8.5 |
| Hulls | 89.0 | 6.2 |
| **Grasses** | | |
| Pasture (intensively managed) | 20.1 | 5.3 |
| Hay (immature) | 84.0 | 18.0 |
| Hay (mid-mature) | 83.8 | 13.3 |
| Hay (mature) | 84.4 | 10.8 |
| Silage (immature) | 36.2 | 16.8 |
| Silage (mid-mature) | 42.0 | 16.8 |
| Silage (mature) | 38.7 | 12.7 |
| **Legumes, forage** | | |
| Pasture (intensively managed) | 21.4 | 5.7 |
| Hay (immature) | 84.2 | 22.8 |
| Hay (mid-mature) | 83.9 | 20.8 |
| Hay (mature) | 83.8 | 17.8 |
| Silage (immature) | 41.2 | 23.2 |
| Silage (mid-mature) | 42.9 | 21.9 |
| Silage (mature) | 42.6 | 20.3 |
| **Soybean hulls** | 90.9 | 13.9 |
| **Wheat** | | |
| Bran | 89.1 | 17.3 |
| Hay, headed | 86.8 | 9.4 |
| Middlings | 89.5 | 18.5 |
| Straw | 92.7 | 4.8 |

*Source:* National Research Council. 2001. *Nutrient Requirements of Dairy Cattle*. National Academies Press, Washington, DC.

## CRYSTALLINE AAS, PROTEIN INGREDIENTS, AND PEPTIDE ADDITIVES FOR ANIMAL DIETS

### Crystalline AAs

A dietary supplement is a substance taken by mouth to provide a nutrient that animals may not obtain adequately from their regular diet relative to their optimal growth, development, and health. In the United States, most of the proteinogenic AAs are permitted as feed additives for animals. Over the past 60 years, animal production has greatly benefited from dietary supplementation with some AAs. Farm animals (e.g., chickens, pigs, cows, and sheep) are usually fed plant-based diets that generally contain low levels of lysine, methionine, threonine, and tryptophan. Deficiencies of these AAs limit the maximum growth and production performance of these animals, while impairing their immunity (Li et al. 2007). To partially correct this problem, DL-methionine was first used in the late 1950s as a supplement in feeds for broiler chickens. In the 1960s, L-lysine-HCl became commercially available for piglet diets. The 1980s witnessed the beginning of the use of L-threonine and L-tryptophan as supplements for swine and poultry feeds to enhance growth, improve immune function, and reduce glucocorticoid-induced stress. In the 1990s and 2000s, there was interest in the use of isoleucine and valine to improve milk production by lactating sows, but inconsistent results were reported in the literature, likely due to different experimental conditions (Wu et al. 2014b). In the past decade, rumen-protected lysine came into use for ruminants (e.g., cows and beef cattle) to increase milk production of lactating cows and growth performance of postweaning calves.

Although traditional research logically focused on dietary supplementation with AAs which are not synthesized in animal cells, recent advances in the physiological roles of synthesizable AAs have resulted in their use in swine and poultry production. For example, in 2005, a mixture of glutamate and glutamine was first produced for feeding postweaning pigs and chickens in some countries (including Brazil and Mexico) to prevent intestinal atrophy and improve feed efficiency. The nutrition of glutamate and glutamine in animals had long been ignored because of historic reasons including: (1) the absence of data on glutamine content in feedstuffs due to analytical problems; (2) the complete lack of glutamine research in livestock production prior to the 1990s; and (3) the failure to describe glutamine as a component of proteins in classic animal nutrition textbooks. To date, many states in the United States have approved the use of these two AAs as supplements for animal feeds. Finally, based on discoveries driven by basic research, arginine (Progenos™) was first marketed in 2006 to enhance embryonic survival and litter size in gilts and sows. Feed-grade arginine is now available from Ajinomoto Inc. (Tokyo, Japan) as a feed additive for swine, poultry, and fish. Aside from its use to promote lean tissue growth, arginine can also reduce whole-body white fat and enhance immunity in livestock and avian species.

Crystalline AAs in the diet are directly available for absorption by the small intestine. Therefore, they are absorbed into enterocytes and appear in the portal vein more rapidly than peptide-bound AAs released from protein digestion (Yen et al. 2004). This may result in a transient imbalance among AAs in the systemic circulation, the extent of which likely depends on both the quality and quantity of dietary protein. Such a phenomenon raises a question about the bioequivalence of supplemental AAs relative to AAs in dietary proteins and peptides. However, experimental evidence from studies with humans, pigs, chickens, and rats consistently indicates that crystalline AAs have high-nutritional values when they are added to a diet deficient in those AAs. Advantages of dietary AA supplementation include: (1) balancing AA composition in the diet; (2) reducing total protein content in the diet without compromising maximal growth or production performance; (3) minimizing the impact of animal production on environmental pollution; (4) improving health status and reducing infectious diseases and the associated costs of treatment; (5) enhancing feed efficiency and economic returns; and (6) mitigating the global shortage of protein resources. Extensive research has also shown that supplementing appropriate amounts of an AA (usually 0.2%–2.5% of the diet on a dry matter basis depending on individual AAs, age, and species) is generally safe for animals. For example, supplementing up to 2% alanine, 1% arginine, 0.2% cysteine, 4% glutamate, 1% glutamine, 1% isoleucine, 2% leucine, 2% glycine, 0.2% methionine, 2% proline, 0.5% threonine, 0.2% tryptophan, or 1% valine in diets (on an as-fed basis) is safe for lactating sows and postweaning pigs fed a corn- and SBM-based diet containing 16%–20% CP. Pregnant gilts and sows fed a corn- and SBM-based diet containing 12% CP can also tolerate dietary supplementation with: (1) 1% arginine between Days 14 and 25 or between Days 14 and 114 of gestation; or (2) 1% glutamine between Days 90 and 114 of gestation, as can lactating sows between Days 1 and 21 postpartum. However, dietary supplementation with 0.83% arginine immediately after breeding until Day 25 of gestation (i.e., between Days 0 and 25 of gestation) reduces progesterone production and embryonic survival in gilts.

### Protein Ingredients

Both plant- and animal-source ingredients are the regular sources of protein in animal diets. Different proteins in feedstuffs and animal tissues have different compositions of AAs. On a dry-matter basis, plant-source feedstuffs generally contain a lower content of protein and AAs than animal-source feedstuffs (Table 4.6). For example, while corn grain and sorghum are excellent sources of energy for swine and poultry, they contain only 9%–10% CP, 0.21%–0.25% lysine, and 0.07%–0.1% tryptophan, as well as imbalanced proportions of AAs. For comparison, fish meal contains 63.4% CP, 5.28% lysine, and 0.7% tryptophan (Li et al. 2011). Also, PBM contains 64.3% CP, 3.44% lysine, and 0.49% tryptophan.

The quality of a protein feedstuff depends upon many factors, including: (a) its ability to supply sufficient amounts of all proteinogenic AAs; (b) its protein digestibility; and (c) the presence of anti-nutritional or toxic substances. Globally, SBM, which contains 40%–48% CP depending on the processing method (e.g., the removal of hulls and oil extraction), is the preferred protein source for nonruminant feeds because of its wide availability, high protein digestibility, well-balanced AA profile, and reasonably low cost. Various processed soybean products that have been used in animal (including fish) feeding include soybean protein concentrates (SPC), soybean protein isolates (SPI), extruded SBMs, and protein hydrolysates (McCalla et al. 2010). Other commonly used plant protein sources include wheat, canola meal, cottonseed meal, peanut meal, sunflower meal, peas, dried brewers grains, and dried distillers grains. Of note, these products contain many anti-nutritional factors (e.g., gossypol, oxalates, goitrogens, tannins, cyanogenic glycosides, chlorogenic acids, and toxic AAs), in addition to those found in the SBM. The plant-source anti-nutritional factors can be divided into heat-labile (e.g., trypsin inhibitors, hemagglutinins, phytate, goitrogens, and antivitamin factors) and heat-stable (e.g., saponins, oestrogens, flatulence factors, and lysinoalanine) factors.

Distiller's dried grains with solubles (DDGS) as new sources of feed protein deserve much attention from animal nutritionists. With the rapid growth of the ethanol industry, amounts of low-cost DDGS for ruminant and nonruminant rations are increasing worldwide. Corn- and wheat-source DDGS contain 26%–30% and 40%–45% CP (DM basis), respectively (Cromwell et al. 2011; Widyaratne and Zijlstra 2007). DDGS contains a higher content of CP than its parent grain because of microbial fermentation (carbohydrate catabolism and protein/AA synthesis) during ethanol production. DDGS is an excellent source of fiber and phosphorus for animals. A concern over the use of DDGS to feed animals is its high and variable levels of sulfur (0.4–1.5% of DM). This is primarily because: (1) various amounts of sulfuric acid are employed to maintain fermenter pH levels in the biofuels industry with rapidly changing technologies; and (2) grains and possibly water also contain some sulfur. Inclusion rates of DDGS in rations depend on animal species and production phases, such as 15%, 20%, 30%, and 40% for pigs during grower, finisher, lactation, and gestation periods, respectively (Cromwell et al. 2011; Song et al. 2010), as well as 10%, 20%, and 40% for poultry, dairy cattle, and beef cattle, respectively (Shurson 2017).

As noted previously, plant protein ingredients (including SBM) contain a lower content of many AAs (e.g., cysteine, glycine, lysine, methionine, tryptophan, and threonine) than animal-source proteins, and there is a limitation to the inclusion of plant ingredients in the diet (particularly for young animals) due to their content of anti-nutritional factors. Thus, animal nutritionists have used animal-source proteins to formulate AA-balanced diets. To date, animal protein supplements are manufactured from poultry, pork, beef, and fish by-products at poultry, meat, rendering operation, fish, and dairy processing plants. Bone meal, MBM, poultry meal, hydrolyzed feather meal, intestine-mucosa product, and blood meal are cost-effective feedstuffs for livestock, poultry, and fish. In addition to their high content of AAs, animal-source feeds provide high levels of available phosphorus, calcium, and other minerals, as well as moderate levels of energy. Importantly, animal-source ingredients contain little or no anti-nutritional factors. While all animal protein products have a high content of AAs, blood meal (a by-product of slaughterhouses after protein coagulation by heating) has low levels of isoleucine (only 2.54%) and glycine (3.86%) in comparison with other branched-chain AAs and synthesizable AAs, respectively (Li et al. 2011). Of note, dried blood products (e.g., spray-dried plasma protein and spray-dried blood cells obtained by the separation of whole blood into plasma and cell fractions) have been used in the feed industry as high-quality protein sources. The quality of these products, which contain immunoglobulins, growth factors, polyamines, and bioactive peptides, is greatly influenced by the method of drying (e.g., heating vs. spray-drying).

## Peptides Used as Feed Additives

Industrially produced peptides are now widely used as feed supplements in animal nutrition (McCalla et al. 2010). Chemical, enzymatic, or microbial hydrolysis of proteins in animal by-products or plant-source feedstuffs before feeding is an attractive means of generating high-quality small or large peptides that have both nutritional and physiological or regulatory functions in live-stock, poultry, and fish (Zhang et al. 2015). Antioxidative peptides generated from the hydrolysis of animal proteins are shown in Table 4.8.

**TABLE 4.8**
**Antioxidative Peptides Generated from the Hydrolysis of Animal Proteins**

| Source | Protease(s) | AA Sequence |
|---|---|---|
| Pig muscle actin | Papain + Actinase E | Asp–Ser–Gly–Val–Thr |
| Pig muscle | Papain + Actinase E | Ile–Glu–Ala–Glu–Gly–Glu |
| Pig muscle tropomyosin | Papain + Actinase E | Asp–Ala–Gln–Glu–Lys–Leu–Glu |
| Pig muscle tropomyosin | Papain + Actinase E | Glu–Glu–Leu–Asp–Asn–Ala–Leu–Asn |
| Pig muscle myosin | Papain + Actinase E | Val–Pro–Ser–Ile–Asp–Asp–Gln–Glu–Glu–Leu–Met |
| Pig collagen | Pepsin + Papain + others[a] | Gln–Gly–Ala–Arg |
| Pig blood plasma | Alcalase | His–Asn–Gly–Asn |
| Chicken muscle | – | His–Val–Thr–Glu–Glu |
| Chicken muscle | – | Pro–Val–Pro–Val–Glu–Gly–Val |
| Deer muscle | Papain | Met–Gln–Ile–Phe–Val–Lys–Thr–Leu–Thr–Gly |
| Deer muscle | Papain | Asp–Leu–Ser–Asp–Gly–Glu–Gln–Gly–Val–Leu |
| Bovine milk casein | Pepsin, pH 2, 24 h | Tyr–Phe–Tyr–Pro–Glu–Leu |
| Bovine milk casein | Pepsin, pH 2, 24 h | Phe–Tyr–Pro–Glu–Leu |
| Bovine milk casein | Pepsin, pH 2, 24 h | Tyr–Pro–Glu–Leu |
| Bovine milk casein | Pepsin, pH 2, 24 h | Pro–Glu–Leu |
| Bovine milk casein | Pepsin, pH 2, 24 h | Glu–Leu |
| Bovine milk casein | Trypsin, pH 7.8, 24–28 h | Val–Lys–Glu–Ala–Met–Pro–Lys |
| Bovine milk casein | Trypsin, pH 7.8, 24–28 h | Ala–Val–Pro–Tyr–Pro–Gln–Arg |
| Bovine milk casein | Trypsin, pH 7.8, 24–28 h | Lys–Val–Leu–Pro–Val–Pro–Glu–Lys |
| Bovine milk casein | Trypsin, pH 7.8, 24–28 h | Val–Leu–Pro–Val–Pro–Glu–Lys |
| Bovine whey protein | Thermolysin, 80°C, 8 h | Leu–Gln–Lys–Trp |
| Bovine whey protein | Thermolysin, 80°C, 8 h | Leu–Asp–Thr–Asp–Tyr–Lys–Lys |
| Bovine β-Lactoglobulin | Corolase PP, 37°C, 24 h | Trp–Tyr–Ser–Leu–Ala–Met–Ala–Ala–Ser–Asp–Ile |
| Bovine β-Lactoglobulin | Corolase PP, 37°C, 24 h | Met–His–Ile–Arg–Leu |
| Bovine β-Lactoglobulin | Corolase PP, 37°C, 24 h | Try–Val–Glu–Glu–Leu |
| Egg yolk | Pepsin | Tyr–Ile–Glu–Ala–Val–Asn–Lys–Val–Ser–Pro–Arg–Ala–Gly–Gln–Phe |
| Egg yolk | Pepsin | Tyr–Ile–Asn–Gln–Met–Pro–Gln–Lys–Ser–Arg–Glu |

*Source:* Hou, Y.Q. et al. 2017. *J. Anim. Sci. Biotechnol.* 8:24.

[a] Bovine pancreatic proteases plus bacterial proteases from *Streptomyces bacillus*.

Acid hydrolysis of a protein (gelatin) at a high temperature was first reported by the French chemist H. Braconnot in 1920. A much shorter period of time (e.g., 2–6 h) is now used to produce peptides as flavor enhancers in animal diets (e.g., hydrolyzed vegetable protein) (Pasupuleki and Braun 2010). Acid hydrolysis of a protein offers the advantage of low cost, but results in the complete destruction of tryptophan, a partial loss of methionine, and the conversion of glutamine into glutamate and of asparagine into aspartate. Alkaline hydrolysis of protein (such as 1 M NaOH) is usually performed at 27°C–55°C for 4–8 h (Pasupuleki et al. 2010) for the production of foaming agents (e.g., substitutes for egg proteins). This method results in the complete destruction of most AAs and the partial loss of many AAs.

Most enzymes for producing peptides are obtained from animal, plant, and microbial sources, such as pancreatin, trypsin, pepsin, carboxypeptidases, and aminopeptidases from pigs, papain, and bromelain from plants, and proteases of bacterial and fungal sources with a broad spectrum of optimal temperatures, pHs, and ion concentrations. Either a single enzyme (e.g., trypsin) or multiple enzymes (e.g., a mixture of proteases known as pronase, pepsin, and prolidase) can be used for protein hydrolysis, depending on raw materials and the desired degree of hydrolysis. Hydrophobic peptides and AAs with bitterness can be degraded by treatment with porcine kidney cortex homogenate or activated carbon (Pasupuleki and Braun 2010). The enzymatic hydrolysis of proteins offers the following advantages: (a) the hydrolysis conditions (e.g., like temperature and pH) are mild and do not result in any loss of AAs; (b) proteases are more specific and precise to control the degree of peptide-bond hydrolysis; (c) the small amounts of enzymes can be easily deactivated after the hydrolysis (e.g., 85°C for 3 min); and (d) the resulting products have anti-oxidative (Table 4.8) and antimicrobial activities (Table 4.9).

**TABLE 4.9**
**Antimicrobial Peptides Generated from the Hydrolysis of Animal Proteins**

| Source | AA Sequence | Against Gram-Positive Bacteria | Against Gram-Negative Bacteria |
|---|---|---|---|
| Bovine meat | Gly–Leu–Ser–Asp–Gly–Glu–Trp–Gln | *Bacillus cereus*<br>*Listeria monocytogenes* | *Salmonella typhimurium*<br>*Escherichia coli* |
| | Gly–Phe–His–Ile | No effect | *Pseudomonas aeruginosa* |
| | Phe–His–Gly | No effect | *Pseudomonas aeruginosa* |
| Bovine collagen | Peptides <2 kDa (by collagenase)[a] | *Staphylococcus aureus* | *Escherichia coli* |
| Goat whey | GWH (730 Da) and SEC-F3 (1183 Da) (hydrolysis by Alcalase) | *Bacillus cereus*<br>*Staphylococcus aureus* | *Salmonella typhimurium*<br>*Escherichia coli* |
| Red blood cells | Various peptides (24-h hydrolysis by fungal proteases) | *Staphylococcus aureus* | *Escherichia coli*<br>*Pseudomonas aeruginosa* |
| Hen egg white lysozyme | Asn–Thr–Asp–Gly–Ser–Thr–Asp–Tyr–Gly–Ile–Leu–Gln–Ile–Asn–Ser–Arg (hydrolysis by papain and trypsin)[b] | *Leuconostoc-mesenteroides* | *Escherichia coli* |
| Trout by-products | Various peptides (20%–30% of hydrolysis) (hydrolysis by trout pepsin) | *Renibacterium-salmoninarum* | *Flavobacterium psychrophilum* |
| Small intestine (Paneth cells) | α-Defensins, lysozyme C, angiogenin-4, and cryptdin-related sequence peptides | Gram-positive bacteria (broad-spectrum) | Gram-negative bacteria (broad-spectrum) |
| | Phospholipid-*sn*-2 esterase and C-type lectin | Gram-positive bacteria (broad-spectrum) | No effect |

*Source:* Hou, Y.Q. et al. 2017. *J. Anim. Sci. Biotechnol.* 8:24.
[a] Minimal inhibition concentrations = 0.6–5 mg/mL.
[b] Minimal inhibition concentrations = 0.36–0.44 μg/mL.

Microbial hydrolysis of protein generates large and small peptides using liquid (high-moisture conditions) or solid (high-moisture conditions)-state fermentation. The suitable microbes may be *Aspergillus oryzae, Aspergillus sojae*, and *Aspergillus tamari* (fungi); *S. cerevisiae* (yeasts); and bacteria, such as *Bacillus* and *Lactobacillus* species. Compared with the conventional SBM, fermented hydrolyzed soy products contain much lower levels of hyper-allergenic or anti-nutritional factors (e.g., protease [e.g. trypsin] inhibitors, amylase inhibitors, glycinin, β-conglycinin, phytate, lectins, oligosaccharides [raffinose and stachyose], and saponins in soybeans), and can be included in diets at higher levels (McCalla et al. 2010).

## CHEMICAL REACTIONS OF FREE AAs

Knowledge about the chemical reactions of free AAs is useful for their analysis and metabolism and therefore in conducting AA nutrition research. Some of these reactions may occur in animals and may be of biochemical importance for understanding the safety of AAs in animals. Many AA metabolites (including newly derived AAs) are commonly present in animals, plants, and microorganisms (Wu 2013). Of particular interest are the biologically active amines, which are a class of compounds synthesized in living organisms, including polyamines and other amines (agmatine, serotonin, tyramine, histamine, phenylethylamine, tryptamine, and catecholamines). Overall, chemical reactions of AAs are dependent upon the amino group, the carboxyl group, the side chain, and the intact molecule.

### CHEMICAL REACTIONS OF THE AMINO GROUP IN α-AAs

The amino group of α-AAs is chemically active and participates in reactions with a variety of substances. These chemical reactions include: acetylation, benzoylation, carbobenzoxylation, condensation, deamination, dinitrophenylation, group protection, methylation, oxymethylation, and transamination (Wu 2013). Four of these reactions, conjugation, deamination, transamination, and oxymethylation, are briefly discussed here because of their biological relevance and use in the analysis of AAs and their metabolites.

#### Reaction of the α-Amino Group of AAs with a Strong Acid

Basic AAs, such as arginine and lysine, are often prepared as their hydrochloride salts for intravenous infusion or dietary additives. This involves the reaction of the α-amino group of the AA with HCl at room temperature (e.g., 25°C). The resulting products have no bitter or unpleasant tastes.

$$\underset{\text{Amino acid}}{R{-}\overset{\displaystyle H}{\underset{\displaystyle NH_2}{C}}{-}COOH} + HCl \longrightarrow \underset{\text{Aminoacid-HCl}}{R{-}\overset{\displaystyle H}{\underset{\displaystyle NH_3^+Cl^-}{C}}{-}COOH}$$

#### Acetylation of the α-Amino Group of AAs

The amino group of AAs readily undergoes acetylation (addition of $-COCH_3$ to an AA) by acetylating reagents such as acetyl chloride and acetic anhydride. In cells, the acetylation of AA residues in protein plays an important role in its biological activity. In the chemical synthesis of peptides, acetylation of the amino group by agents, such as benzyloxycarbonyl chloride and tert-butoxycarbonyl chloride, is required to generate a desired sequence of AAs.

$$\underset{\text{Amino acid (AA)}}{R{-}\overset{\displaystyle H}{\underset{\displaystyle NH_2}{C}}{-}COOH} + \underset{\text{Acetyl chloride}}{CH_3COCl} \longrightarrow \underset{\text{Acetylated AA}}{R{-}\overset{\displaystyle H}{\underset{\displaystyle NHCOCH_3}{C}}{-}COOH} + HCl$$

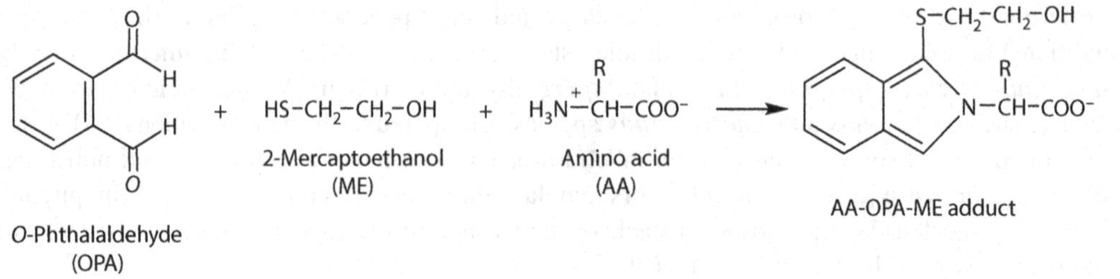

$$O\text{-Phthalaldehyde (OPA)} + HS{-}CH_2{-}CH_2{-}OH \text{ (2-Mercaptoethanol, ME)} + H_3\overset{+}{N}{-}CH(R){-}COO^- \text{ (Amino acid, AA)} \longrightarrow \text{AA-OPA-ME adduct}$$

**FIGURE 4.13** Analysis of primary AAs as their OPA derivatives. The concentration of each AA standard used for the reaction with OPA is 10 μM. The resultant products are separated by HPLC, followed by detection at an excitation wavelength of 340 nm and an emission wavelength of 455 nm.

## Conjugation of the α-Amino Group in AAs with a Reagent

*o*-Phthaldialdehyde (OPA, a nonfluorescent substance) is a reagent that reacts with primary AAs, β-AAs, and γ-AAs, as well as small peptides (e.g., alanyl-glutamine and glutathione) (Wu and Meininger 2008). OPA was first chemically synthesized from α, α, α′,α′-tetrachloro-ortho-xylene by A. Colson and H. Gautier in 1887. OPA reacts rapidly with a molecule containing a primary amino group at room temperature in the presence of 2-mercaptoethanol or 3-mercaptopropionic acid to form a highly fluorescent adduct (Figure 4.13). Proline does not react with OPA (Wu 1993), and the reaction of cysteine or cystine with OPA is very limited (Dai et al. 2014). However, OPA also readily reacts with (1) 4-amino-1-butanol, which is produced from the oxidation of proline in the presence of chloramine-T and sodium borohydride at 60°C; and (2) S-carboxymethyl-cysteine, which is formed from cysteine in the presence of iodoacetic acid.

The OPA method is most widely used for AA analysis by HPLC because of the following advantages: simple procedures for the preparation of samples, reagents, and mobile phase solutions; rapid formation of OPA derivatives and their efficient separation at room temperature; high sensitivity of detection at picomole levels; easy automation of the instrument; few interfering side reactions; a stable chromatography baseline and accurate integration of peak areas; and rapid regeneration of guard and analytical columns. This method is suitable for the analysis of AAs and related metabolites in both tissues and protein hydrolysates (Dai et al. 2014; Hou et al. 2015a).

## Deamination of AAs

Removal of the α-amino group from an AA after treatment with nitrous acid to yield the corresponding hydroxy acid and nitrogen gas was recognized in the early 1910s. This reaction, known as the Van Slyke assay, was first used in 1911 by D.D. Van Slyke to determine AAs. The nitrogen gas is measured by volumetric or manometric methods and its production is directly proportional to the amount of the AA. Note that secondary AAs (e.g., proline and hydroxyproline) do not react with nitrous acid.

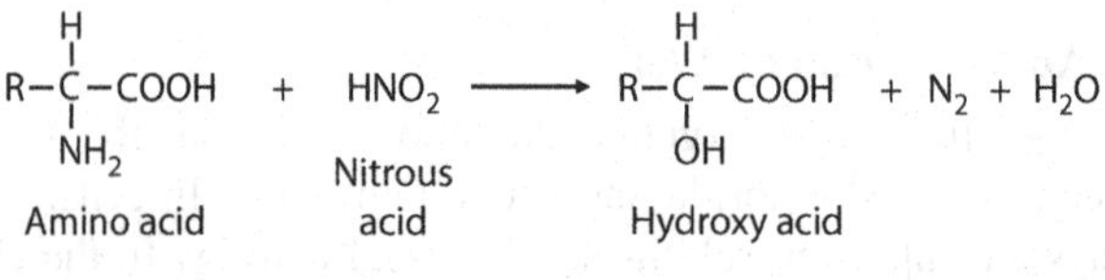

$$\underset{\text{Amino acid}}{R{-}CH(NH_2){-}COOH} + \underset{\text{Nitrous acid}}{HNO_2} \longrightarrow \underset{\text{Hydroxy acid}}{R{-}CH(OH){-}COOH} + N_2 + H_2O$$

An AA can undergo deamination to yield ammonia and the corresponding α-ketoacid in the presence of reactive carbonyls (e.g., alloxan, isatin, and quinones) or α-dicarbonyls (e.g., methylglyoxal and phenylglyoxal). In biology, deamination is catalyzed by D-AA deaminase (oxidase) and L-AA deaminase (oxidase). In 1909, O. Neubauer reported the deamination of α-AAs in the mammalian body. Enzyme-catalyzed deamination of AAs in animal tissues was discovered by H.A. Krebs in 1935. This biochemical reaction has important functions in both neurological and immunological systems.

### Transamination of AAs with α-Ketoacids

The nonenzymatic transamination of AAs with an α-ketoacid occurs in response to heating. For example, α-aminophenyl-acetic acid [$C_6H_5CH(NH_2)COOH$] reacts with pyruvic acid in an aqueous solution to yield alanine, benzaldehyde ($C_6H_5CHO$), and $CO_2$. This chemical reaction was discovered in 1934 by R.M. Herbst and L.L. Engel, and is used to synthesize dipeptides, such as alanyl-alanine. The enzyme-catalyzed transamination of AAs is widespread in animals, plants, and microorganisms, and plays an essential role in the synthesis and catabolism of many AAs (Brosnan 2001).

$$R_1\text{-CH(NH}_2\text{)-COOH} + R_2\text{-C(=O)-COOH} \longrightarrow R_2\text{-CH(NH}_2\text{)-COOH} + R_1\text{-C(=O)-COOH}$$

Amino acid$_1$ α-Ketoacid$_1$ Amino acid$_2$ α-Ketoacid$_2$

### Oxymethylation of AAs

In oxymethylation, the α-amino group of an AA reacts with formaldehyde to form an *N*-hydroxymethyl AA. This reaction was proposed by H. Schiff in 1899 and developed in 1907 by S.P.L. Sörensen for AA analysis. In this method, excess formaldehyde is added to an AA solution, followed by titration with standard alkali to a strong red color with phenolphthalein as the indicator. It should be noted that: (1) the AA must be dissolved in a colorless solution to prevent any interference of the assay; (2) cysteine, but not cystine, reacts with formaldehyde or 1,2-naphthoquinone-4-sodium sulfonate; and (3) many nitrogenous substances, including ammonia, peptides, primary amines (substances in which one hydrogen atom in ammonia is replaced by an alkyl group), nitrite, and nitrate also react with formaldehyde. Thus, this method greatly overestimates concentrations of free AAs in animal products or tissue enzymatic hydrolysates.

$$R\text{-CH(NH}_2\text{)-COOH} + H\text{-CHO} \longrightarrow R\text{-CH(NH-CH}_2\text{-OH)-COOH}$$

Amino acid (AA) Formaldehyde N-Hydroxymethyl AA

## Chemical Reactions of the Carboxyl Group in α-AAs

### Reaction of the Carboxyl Group of AAs with an Alkaline

The carboxyl group of most AAs reacts with strong bases (e.g., NaOH; pH > 12) to form sodium carboxylate salts at room temperature (e.g., 25°C). This explains the instability of these AAs under strong alkaline conditions. An exception is tryptophan, which is very stable in strong bases (e.g., 4.2 M NaOH) for at least 20 h even at 105°C.

$$R\text{-CH(NH}_2\text{)-COOH} + NaOH \longrightarrow R\text{-CH(NH}_2\text{)-C(=O)O}^-Na^+ + H_2O$$

Amino acid (AA) Sodium salt of AA

### Decarboxylation of AAs

The α-carboxyl group of AAs is involved in several chemical reactions. These reactions include the following: decarboxylation, esterification, and reduction (Wu 2013). Examples of the decarboxylation of AAs are the conversion of histidine into histamine and of glutamate into γ-aminobutyrate. These two reactions are catalyzed by enzymes in animal cells.

Glutamate → γ-Aminobutyrate + $CO_2$ (glutamate decarboxylase)
Histidine → Histamine + $CO_2$ (histidine decarboxylase)

AAs can be esterified by a strong base (e.g., NaOH). In addition, methyl, ethyl, and benzyl esters of many AAs can be chemically prepared using 2,2-dimethoxypropane, absolute ethanol, and *p*-toluenesulfonic acid plus benzyl alcohol, respectively. Esterification of AAs serves to block its α-carboxyl group. Finally, α-AAs can be chemically converted into 1,2-amino alcohols. In these methods, the modification of unprotected or *N*-protected α-AAs to the corresponding amino alcohols involves the activation of the acid group to become an anhydride, acid fluoride, or active ester, followed by reduction with sodium borohydride. Alternatively, AAs can be reduced to form the corresponding alcohols directly using sodium borohydride and iodine in tetrahydrofuran.

## Chemical Reactions of the Side Chains in α-AAs

The amino or carboxyl group of the side chain of α-AAs can take part in certain chemical reactions. For example, the ε-amino group of lysine and the guanidino amino group of arginine can participate in hydrogen bonding, methylation, and reactions involving carbohydrates. In addition, the guanidino group of arginine, not its amino group, can react specifically with diketones (Dinsmore and Beshore 2002). This reaction is used to determine a putative role of arginine residues in the stabilization of the tertiary and quaternary structures of proteins and in the allosteric and active sites of enzymes. Furthermore, the γ-amino group of asparagine can react with reducing carbohydrates, thereby providing key sites for *N*-linked glycosylation of proteins. Asparagine can also react with reactive carbonyls, that is, carbohydrates, at high temperatures to generate acrylamide (a potential carcinogen), which is present in baked foods.

### Amidation

An example of the amidation of an AA is the formation of glutamine from glutamate and $NH_4^+$. Another example is the synthesis of asparagine from aspartate and $NH_4^+$. These are important reactions in animals, plants, and microbes.

Glutamate + $NH_4^+$ → Glutamine (glutamine synthetase)
Aspartate + $NH_4^+$ → Asparagine (asparagine synthetase in microbes)

### Deamidination

As noted previously, glutamine and asparagine undergo deamidination in the presence of a strong acid (e.g., 6 M HCl) at a relatively high temperature (i.e., 110°C) to produce glutamate and aspartate, respectively. These reactions also yield $NH_4^+$. Hydrolysis of glutamine or asparagine is not detectable in the presence of 0.75 M $HClO_4$ or 5% TCA at room temperature (e.g., 25°C).

### Iodination of the Phenol Ring in Tyrosine

The phenol ring of tyrosine is iodinated under alkaline conditions. The synthesis of thyroid hormones from tyrosine in animals also involves tyrosine iodination, which includes a series of $H_2O_2$-dependent peroxidative reactions, such as peroxidase-catalyzed oxidation of iodide, the iodination of tyrosyl residues, and the coupling of iodotyrosyl in thyroglobulin.

$$H_2N{-}\underset{COOH}{\overset{H}{C}}{-}CH_2{-}C_6H_4{-}OH + I_2 \longrightarrow H_2N{-}\underset{COOH}{\overset{H}{C}}{-}CH_2{-}C_6H_2I_2{-}OH$$

Tyrosine → Iodinatedtyrosine

## Chemical Reactions Involving the ε-$NH_2$ Group of Lysine

A guanidination reaction of either free lysine or lysine residue in feed protein with methylisourea generates homoarginine. Specifically, a test material (containing 200 g of CP) is thoroughly mixed with 1 L of 0.5 M methylisourea (adjusted to pH 10.5 using 1 M NaOH), and the mixture is then

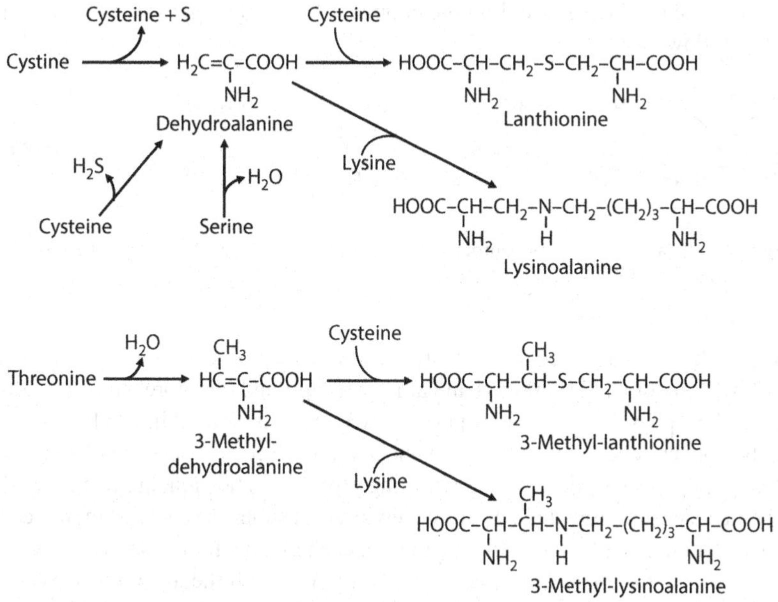

Cystine → (Cysteine + S) → $H_2C{=}C(NH_2){-}COOH$ (Dehydroalanine) → (Cysteine) → $HOOC{-}CH(NH_2){-}CH_2{-}S{-}CH_2{-}CH(NH_2){-}COOH$ (Lanthionine)

Cysteine → ($H_2S$) → Dehydroalanine; Serine → ($H_2O$) → Dehydroalanine

Dehydroalanine → (Lysine) → $HOOC{-}CH(NH_2){-}CH_2{-}N(H){-}CH_2{-}(CH_2)_3{-}CH(NH_2){-}COOH$ (Lysinoalanine)

Threonine → ($H_2O$) → $HC(CH_3){=}C(NH_2){-}COOH$ (3-Methyl-dehydroalanine) → (Cysteine) → $HOOC{-}CH(NH_2){-}CH(CH_3){-}S{-}CH_2{-}CH(NH_2){-}COOH$ (3-Methyl-lanthionine)

3-Methyl-dehydroalanine → (Lysine) → $HOOC{-}CH(NH_2){-}CH(CH_3){-}N(H){-}CH_2{-}(CH_2)_3{-}CH(NH_2){-}COOH$ (3-Methyl-lysinoalanine)

**FIGURE 4.14** Formation of lanthionine, lysinoalanine, 3-methyl-lanthionine, 3-methyl-lysinoalanine after heating of free AAs. These reactions can also occur in peptide-bound AAs.

incubated at 4°C for 4–6 days. The protein with homoarginine residues is fed to animals (e.g., pigs and poultry) to determine the true digestibility of AAs (Yin et al. 2015). This method was based on the assumption that homoarginine was not synthesized by the test animals. This assumption is now known to be invalid because many tissues of animals (e.g., pigs and rats) can synthesize homoarginine from arginine and glycine (Hou et al. 2016).

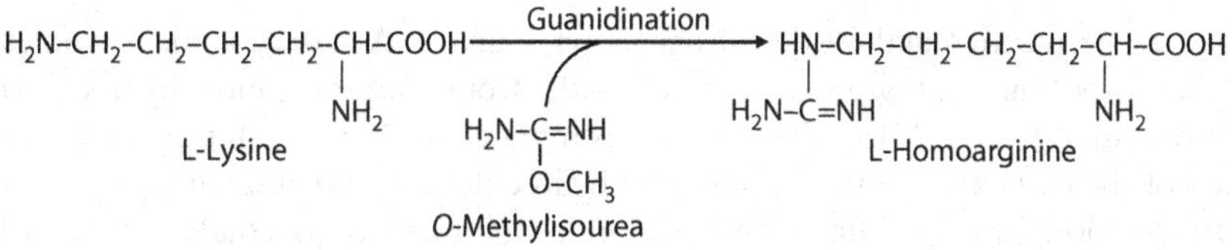

$H_2N{-}CH_2{-}CH_2{-}CH_2{-}CH_2{-}CH(NH_2){-}COOH$ (L-Lysine) → Guanidination, with $H_2N{-}C(=NH){-}O{-}CH_3$ (*O*-Methylisourea) → $(H_2N{-}C{=}NH){-}HN{-}CH_2{-}CH_2{-}CH_2{-}CH_2{-}CH(NH_2){-}COOH$ (L-Homoarginine)

### Condensation of Two AAs

At high temperature (e.g., feed heating), two AAs can be condensed to form a new AA through chemical reactions of their side chains. Such condensation does not involve the formation of a peptide bond. Examples are the generation of lanthionine and lysinoalanine from cystine plus cysteine and cysteine (or serine) plus lysine, respectively; as well as the formation of 3-methyl-lanthionine and 3-methyl-lysinoalanine from threonine plus cysteine and threonine plus lysine, respectively (Figure 4.14). Such reactions, which also occur in peptide-bound lysine, threonine, serine, and cysteine, can reduce protein quality, because these AA derivatives are not hydrolyzed by any enzymes and have no nutritional value to animals.

## Chemical Reactions Involving Both the Amino and Carboxyl Groups of the Same α-AA

Since α-AAs contain both amino and carboxyl groups that are chemically active, they participate in some unique reactions, including chelation, cyclization, racemization, formation of *N*-carboxy anhydride, and oxidative deamination (decarboxylation) (Wu 2013). These reactions yield AA chelates, azlactone, diketopiperazine, *N*-carboxy AA anhydride (NCA), peptide bonds, and aldehyde.

The structures of some products (including the copper-AA complex) generated from these reactions are illustrated as follows:

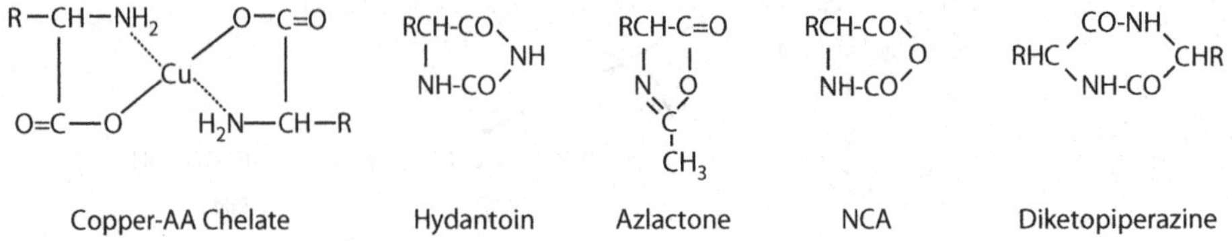

R—CH—NH$_2$ O—C=O / Cu / O=C—O H$_2$N—CH—R | RCH-CO, NH, NH-CO | RCH-C=O, N O, C, CH$_3$ | RCH-CO, O, NH-CO | CO-NH, RHC CHR, NH-CO

Copper-AA Chelate | Hydantoin | Azlactone | NCA | Diketopiperazine

## Chelation of AAs with Metals

Chelates of AAs with metals are used to efficiently supply an inorganic nutrient (e.g., Zn, Cu, and Fe) to animals. AAs have both ionizable carboxyl and amino groups, and therefore have the capacity to form metal complexes. This physicochemical property of AAs was discovered in 1854 when A. Gössmann first prepared the copper–leucine chelate. Subsequently, the copper complex of glycine in the ratio of 1:2 [$(NH_2CH_2COO)_2Cu$] was made in 1904 by mixing glycine in a hot aqueous solution with an excess of copper carbonate. AA-mineral chelates are widely used as supplements in animal feeds.

In the copper-glycine complex, a hydrogen atom in each glycine molecule is displaced by a single copper atom, and the metal forms coordinate covalent bonds with the amino groups of two glycine molecules (Yamauchi et al. 2002). In contrast to the salts of the alkaline metals with glycine, aqueous solutions of the copper-glycine complex have virtually no conductivity. It is now known that only α- and β-AAs, but not γ- or δ-AAs, may form stable copper complexes, and that their stability depends on the dissociation constant of the complexing nitrogen atom rather than simply the nature of the side chain. In addition to copper, α- and β-AAs can also form chelates with $Ni^{2+}$, $Zn^{2+}$, $Co^{2+}$, $Fe^{2+}$, $Mn^{2+}$, $Mg^{2+}$, and $Ca^{2+}$. Examples include Zn–Met, Cu–Lys, and Mn–Gly, which are now commercially available as feed additives for farm animals. For serine, threonine, and tyrosine, $Ca^{2+}$ can form covalent bonds with all their functional groups (i.e., carboxyl, amino, and hydroxyl groups).

## Esterification and $N^{\alpha}$-Dehydrogenation of α-AAs

An example for esterification and $N^{\alpha}$-dehydrogenation of an α-AA is the chemical synthesis of lauric arginate (ethyl-$N^{\alpha}$-lauroyl-L-arginate hydrochloride) from L-arginine monohydrochloride, ethanol, and lauroyl chloride (Wu 2013). This reaction is initiated by thionyl chloride ($SOCl_2$)-catalyzed esterification of the carboxyl group of L-arginine hydrochloride with ethanol in the presence of a base (NaOH) to form ethyl arginine dihydrochloride, followed by its condensation with lauroyl chloride to finally yield lauric arginate. This substance is a novel cationic surfactant that has a potent antimicrobial effect. Thus, lauric arginate (e.g., 200 ppm) is now used as a safe preservative in food and beverage industries. It may also be a useful feed additive to diets for animals (e.g., weanling pigs) to improve intestinal health and the efficiency of nutrient utilization.

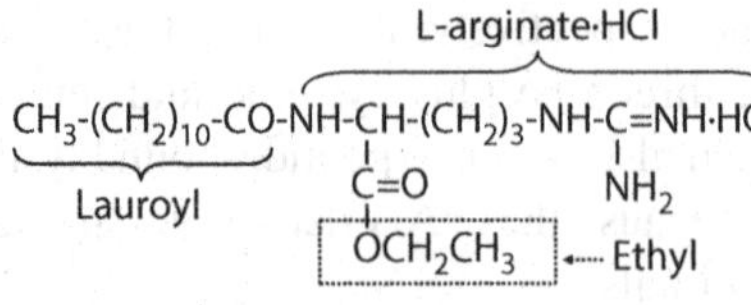

L-arginate·HCl

$CH_3$-$(CH_2)_{10}$-CO-NH-CH-$(CH_2)_3$-NH-C=NH·HCl

Lauroyl | C=O | $NH_2$

$OCH_2CH_3$ ← Ethyl

Ethyl-$N^{\alpha}$-lauroyl-L-arginate hydrochloride

## Oxidative Deamination (Decarboxylation) of AAs

Oxidative deamination (decarboxylation) of an AA to form ammonia, $CO_2$, and aldehyde in response to a mixture of lead dioxide and dilute sulfuric acid was first recognized by J. von Liebig in 1849. Such a reaction also occurs when AAs are treated with sodium hypochlorite or chloramine-T. The formation of the aldehyde is specific to the AA under consideration, whereas ammonia and

$CO_2$ are generated nonspecifically from all AAs. Another well-utilized oxidative deamination (decarboxylation) of an AA is its reaction with ninhydrin to yield colored products. This chemical reaction was discovered by S. Ruhemann in 1911 and its chemistry is very complex. First, an AA reacts with ninhydrin to form an intermediate amine, the corresponding aldehyde, carbon dioxide, and ammonia. Interestingly, the initial products vary with individual AAs. For example, aspartate and cystine yield 2 moles of $CO_2$, whereas proline and hydroxyproline do not generate ammonia. Second, the intermediate amine reacts with ninhydrin to yield indandione-2-*N*-2′-indanone enolate (Ruhemann's purple), hydrindantin (which can be detected by UV absorption), and ammonia. Third, hydrindantin reacts with ammonia to form Ruhemann's purple (blue–violet color with maximum absorption at 570 nm). In addition, ammonia reacts with ninhydrin and the reduced ninhydrin to also yield Ruhemann's purple. Overall, the nitrogen atom of this enolate pigment arises from α-AAs. On paper chromatography, the reaction of proline or hydroxyproline with ninhydrin gives a yellow color product (maximum absorption at 440 nm), whereas purple–blue color is formed for other AAs. In addition to AAs and ammonia, peptides can also react with ninhydrin to yield color products. To date, ninhydrin is often used to analyze AAs.

$$\text{Ninhydrin} + \text{Amino acid} \rightarrow \text{RCHO (Aldehyde)} + CO_2 + H_2O + \text{Ruhemann's purple}$$

### Intramolecular Cyclization Reactions Involving the Side Chain Group and the α-Amino Group of α-AAs

As noted previously, glutamine in an aqueous solution at room temperature undergoes very slow spontaneous cyclization between the amide group and the α-amino group to yield pyroglutamate, with the associated release of ammonia. At 180°C, within the glutamate molecule, the side-chain carboxyl group cyclizes with the α-amino group to also form pyroglutamate, with the associated release of $H_2O$. These reactions are shown below.

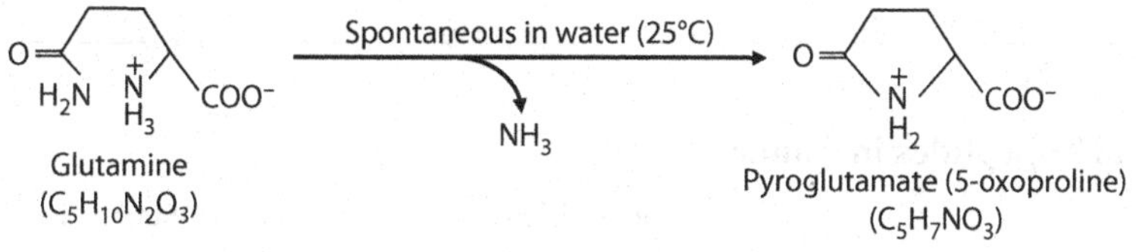

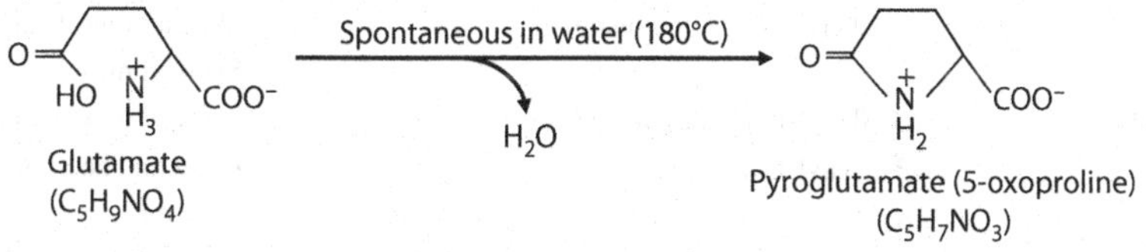

Glutamine ($C_5H_{10}N_2O_3$) —Spontaneous in water (25°C), − $NH_3$ → Pyroglutamate (5-oxoproline) ($C_5H_7NO_3$)

Glutamate ($C_5H_9NO_4$) —Spontaneous in water (180°C), − $H_2O$ → Pyroglutamate (5-oxoproline) ($C_5H_7NO_3$)

### Peptide Synthesis

A carboxyl group of one AA and the amino group of another AA can form a peptide bond (–CONH–) with the loss of one molecule of $H_2O$, which has the molecular weight of 18 Dalton (Figure 4.10). *N*-carboxy AA anhydride is an important activated derivative of an AA for the chemical synthesis of small peptides and proteins. Liquid-phase peptide synthesis is a classical method for peptide formation and is useful for large-scale production of peptides for industrial purposes. Solid-phase peptide synthesis, pioneered by R.B. Merrifield in 1963, is now widely used to synthesize peptides and proteins in the laboratory (Marglin and Merrifield 1970). Unlike ribosomal protein synthesis, the chemical synthesis of peptides proceeds in a C-terminal to N-terminal manner, with the N-terminus being protected by either t-butyloxy carbamate (t-BOC) or 9-fluorenylmethyl chloroformate (FMOC).

In animal cells, polypeptide synthesis requires mRNA templates, tRNAs, rRNAs, many enzymes, translation initiation factors, elongation factors, and biological energy (ATP and GTP). Of note, the formation of some special antioxidant dipeptides (e.g., anserine, balenine, carcinine, carnosine, homoanserine, and homocarnosine) is catalyzed by specific enzymes and does not require mRNAs, tRNAs, or rRNAs (Figure 4.15). Likewise, a neuroactive dipeptide (kyotorphin) is synthesized from L-tyrosine and L-arginine by ATP-dependent kyotorphin synthetase in the brain. The distribution of these dipeptides varies with tissues (Table 4.10). For example, carnosine and anserine are the

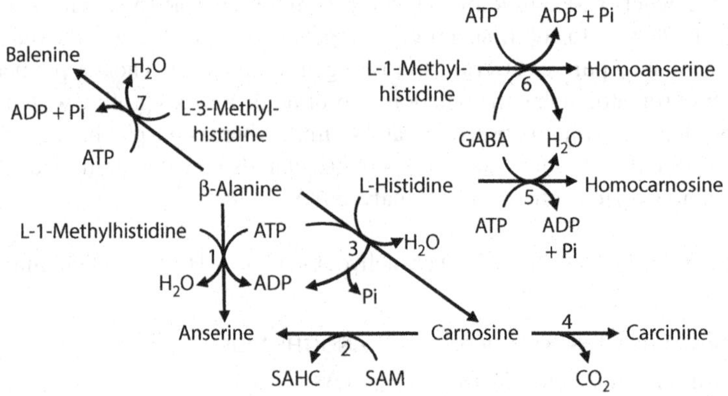

**FIGURE 4.15** Synthesis of special antioxidants in animal tissue. The enzymes that catalyze the indicated reactions are: (1) anserine synthetase; (2) carnosine-*N*-methyltransferase; (3) carnosine synthetase; (4) carnosine decarboxylase; (5) homocarnosine synthetase; (6) homoserine synthetase; and (7) balenine synthetase. Expression of these enzymes is species- and tissue-specific. GABA, γ-aminobutyrate. (Reproduced from Wu G. 2013. *Amino Acids: Biochemistry and Nutrition.* Copyright 2013, with permission from CRC Press.)

## TABLE 4.10
## Dipeptides and Tripeptides in Animals[a]

| Common Name | Composition | Storage in Major Tissue |
|---|---|---|
| **1. Dipeptides** | | |
| Anserine[b] | β-Alanyl-L-1-Methylhistidine | Skeletal muscle and brain in birds; Skeletal muscle in mammals |
| Balenine (Ophidine) | β-Alanyl-L-3-Methylhistidine | Skeletal muscle and brain |
| Carcinine | β-Alanyl-Histamine | Brain and heart of vertebrates; Crab muscle |
| Carnosine[c] | β-Alanyl-L-Histidine | Skeletal muscle and brain |
| Homocarnosine | γ-Aminobutyryl-L-Histidine | Brain of vertebrates |
| Homoanserine | γ-Aminobutyryl-L-1-Methylhistidine | Brain of vertebrates |
| Kyotorphin | L-Tyrosyl-L-Arginine | Mammalian brain |
| **2. Tripeptides** | | |
| Glutathione | γ-Glu-Cys-Gly | Cells, bile acid, pancreatic juice, and uterine fluid |
| Collagen peptide | Gly-Pro-Hydroxyproline | Milk and plasma |

[a] Present in both mammals and birds, unless indicated otherwise.
[b] Also known as methyl carnosine, not found in mammalian muscle or brain.
[c] Absent from birds.

most abundant dipeptides in skeletal muscles of mammals (Wu et al. 2016) and birds, respectively. Balenine is also present in pig skeletal muscle, and anserine in the retina of birds. In the mammalian brain, homocarnosine and homoanserine are more abundant than carnosine. Finally, carcinine is abundant in crab muscle, as well as in the nervous tissue and heart of vertebrates.

## CHEMICAL REACTIONS OF PROTEINS AND POLYPEPTIDES

### Hydrolysis of the Peptide Bond in Protein and Polypeptides

The peptide bond in a protein can be broken down in the presence of strong acids (e.g., 6 M HCl) or bases (e.g., 4 M NaOH) and high temperature (e.g., 105°C–110°C). The degree of hydrolysis is time dependent. Acid hydrolysis is the standard method for the determination of most AAs in protein, whereas alkaline hydrolysis is the standard method for the determination of tryptophan in protein. In animals, proteins are hydrolyzed by proteases in the gastrointestinal tract (extracellular proteolysis) and within all cell types (intracellular proteolysis).

Protein + $H_2O$ → AAs (6 M HCl, 110°C, 24 h)
Protein + $H_2O$ → Tryptophan (4 M NaOH, 105°C, 20 h)

The molecular weight of an intact AA (e.g., aspartate, 133.10 Dalton) is greater by 18 Dalton than that of its residue in protein (e.g., aspartate residue, 115.10 Dalton). Thus, care should be taken when true protein content in feedstuffs or animal tissues is calculated after their acid or alkaline hydrolysis. In the animal body (e.g., the pig), the average molecular weight of protein (the sum of the molecular weight of its constituent AA residues) is 100 Dalton (Table 4.11), which corresponds to the chemical formula of $C_{4.3}H_7O_{1.4}N_{1.2}S_{0.069}$. A total of 118 g of AAs is generally required to produce 100 g protein in animals (Table 4.11). If the molecular weights of intact AAs were used to calculate the amount of protein, the value would have been 118 g. This would have overestimated the true quantity of protein by 18%.

### Dye-Binding of Protein and Polypeptides

Protein can bind the Coomassie dye under acidic conditions. The binding of protein to the dye results in a spectral shift, so that the color of the Coomassie solution changes from brown (absorbance maximum 465 nm) to blue (absorbance maximum 610 nm). The change in color density is read at 595 nm and is proportional to the protein concentration in the solution. This method is very useful in protein identification and quantification (e.g., proteomics).

### Biuret Assay of Protein and Peptides

Under alkaline conditions, substances containing two or more peptide bonds form a purple complex with cupric ions ($Cu^{2+}$) in the reagent (9 g sodium potassium tartrate, 3 g copper sulfate · 5 $H_2O$, and 5 g potassium iodide, all dissolved in order in 400 mL of 0.2 M NaOH, followed by the addition of water to a final volume of 1 L). The underlying principle is that $Cu^{2+}$ ions chelate with the peptide bonds. The absorbance of the solution at 545 nm is measured. The intensity of the color produced is proportional to protein and peptide concentration in the solution. Note that this assay reagent does not actually contain biuret (a chemical compound with the chemical formula $C_2H_5N_3O_2$, also known as carbamylurea). The Biuret test is so named because both biuret and protein (or peptides) have the same response to the alkaline copper reagent.

### Lowry Assay of Protein and Peptides

Under alkaline conditions, cupric ions ($Cu^{2+}$) chelate with the peptide bonds, resulting in the reduction of cupric ions ($Cu^{2+}$) to cuprous ions ($Cu^+$). The cuprous ions react with Folin Ciocalteu Reagent

**TABLE 4.11**
**Composition of AAs in Proteins of the Pig Body**

| AA | Molecular Weight of Intact AA (Dalton) | Molecular Weight of AA Residue (Dalton) | g of AA Residue in 100 g Protein | mmol of AA Residue in 100 g Protein | g of AA Needed to Produce 100 g Protein | Energy of Intact AA (kJ/mol) | Energy (kJ) of Intact AA Needed to Produce 100 g Protein |
|---|---|---|---|---|---|---|---|
| | A | B = (A − 18) | C | D = C × 1000/B | E = A × D/1000 | F | G = D × F/1000 |
| Ala | 89.09 | 71.09 | 6.16 | 86.7 | 7.72 | 1577 | 136.6 |
| Arg | 174.2 | 156.2 | 7.14 | 45.7 | 7.96 | 3739 | 170.9 |
| Asn | 132.12 | 114.12 | 3.65 | 32.0 | 4.23 | 1928 | 61.7 |
| Asp | 133.1 | 115.1 | 4.36 | 37.9 | 5.04 | 1601 | 60.6 |
| Cys | 121.16 | 103.16 | 1.32 | 12.8 | 1.55 | 2249 | 28.8 |
| Gln | 146.14 | 128.14 | 5.28 | 41.2 | 6.02 | 2570 | 105.9 |
| Glu | 147.13 | 129.13 | 8.7 | 67.4 | 9.91 | 2244 | 151.2 |
| Gly | 75.07 | 57.07 | 10.5 | 184.0 | 13.81 | 973 | 179.0 |
| His | 155.15 | 137.15 | 2.16 | 15.7 | 2.44 | 3213 | 50.6 |
| OH-Pro | 131.13 | 113.13 | 3.85 | 34.0 | 4.46 | 2593 | 88.2 |
| Ile | 131.17 | 113.17 | 3.59 | 31.7 | 4.16 | 3581 | 113.6 |
| Leu | 131.17 | 113.17 | 6.93 | 61.2 | 8.03 | 3582 | 219.3 |
| Lys | 146.19 | 128.19 | 6.22 | 48.5 | 7.09 | 3683 | 178.7 |
| Met | 149.21 | 131.21 | 1.93 | 14.7 | 2.19 | 3245 | 47.7 |
| Phe | 165.19 | 147.19 | 3.59 | 24.4 | 4.03 | 4647 | 113.3 |
| Pro | 115.13 | 97.13 | 8.53 | 87.8 | 10.11 | 2730 | 239.7 |
| Ser | 105.09 | 87.09 | 4.31 | 49.5 | 5.20 | 1444 | 71.5 |
| Thr | 119.12 | 101.12 | 3.5 | 34.6 | 4.12 | 2053 | 71.1 |
| Trp | 204.22 | 186.22 | 1.19 | 6.4 | 1.31 | 5628 | 36.0 |
| Tyr | 181.19 | 163.19 | 2.86 | 17.5 | 3.18 | 4429 | 77.6 |
| Val | 117.15 | 99.15 | 4.2 | 42.4 | 4.96 | 2933 | 124.2 |
| Mean | 136.6 | 118.6 | – | – | – | – | – |
| Total | – | – | 100 | – | 118 | – | 2326 |

*Source:* Adapted from Wu, G. 2013. *Amino Acids: Biochemistry and Nutrition*. CRC Press, Boca Raton, Florida.

(phosphomolybdic/phosphotungstic acid) to produce a blue color, which can be read at 650–750 nm. The blue color of the solution is intensified by the oxidation of aromatic AA residues in protein and peptides. The intensity of the color produced is proportional to the amount of peptide bonds. This method is commonly known as the Lowry method for protein or peptide quantification.

## Maillard Reaction of Protein and Peptides

The susceptibility of proteins or free AAs to heat damage is increased in the presence of carbohydrates, owing to the Maillard reaction. This reaction occurs between the free amino groups of certain AAs (particularly the ε-amino groups [$-NH_2$] of lysine residues in protein) and carbonyl compounds ($-HC=O$), notably reducing sugars (e.g., glucose, fructose, or ribose) (Figure 4.16). The guanidino group of arginine residues or the side chain $-CH_2$ group of glutamine residues in protein can also react with the carbonyl compounds. Free lysine, arginine, and glutamine can also participate in the Maillard reaction.

The initial step is the formation of a Schiff's base, followed by Amadori rearrangement of Schiff's base to generate an Amadori compound. The formation of Schiff's base is reversible. However,

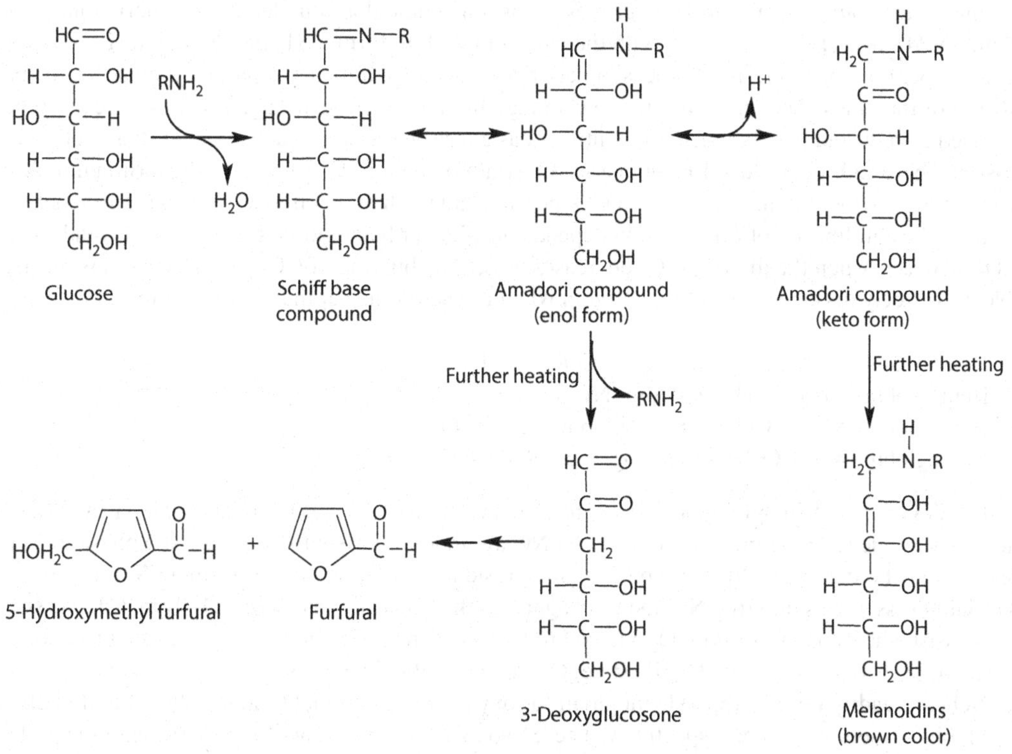

**FIGURE 4.16** The Maillard reaction between amino acids and carbohydrates. (Reproduced from Wu G. 2013. *Amino Acids: Biochemistry and Nutrition*. Copyright 2013, with permission from CRC Press).

further heating results in the production of melanoidin polymers that give a brown color. The dark coloration of overheated hays and silages is symptomatic of the Maillard reaction. The modified lysine in the form of melanoidin polymers is nutritionally unavailable to animals. Therefore, excess heating of feed proteins poses a problem. If the heated proteins escape breakdown by proteases in the rumen, these proteins may also escape breakdown by proteases in the abomasum and the small intestine. The Maillard reaction, which can occur in animals at a low rate under hyperglycemic conditions, also has important implications for their nutrition and health.

## Buffering Reactions of Proteins

Proteins contain AA residues (e.g., histidine, arginine, lysine, and glycine) with ionizable groups, with each having different pKa values. Owing to their high concentrations in blood and cells, proteins provide important buffering capacities to cells and organisms. A good example of intracellular buffering by a protein is hemoglobin, which is rich in histidine and abundant within red blood cells. Owing to the permeability of the erythrocyte membrane to $H^+$, this buffering action also affects the pH of blood.

$$\text{H} \cdot \text{Protein} \leftrightarrow \text{H}^+ + \text{Protein}$$

## Binding of Hemoglobin to $O_2$, $CO_2$, CO, and NO

Deoxygenated hemoglobin is the form of hemoglobin without the bound oxygen. Hemoglobin inside red blood cells carries oxygen to cells and $CO_2$ to the lungs. This protein is made up of four symmetrical subunits and four heme groups. Thus, one hemoglobin molecule transports four molecules of $O_2$. Iron ($Fe^{2+}$) associated with the heme binds $O_2$ to form oxyhemoglobin [Hb(Fe(II)-$O_2$)] in a cooperative manner. This process takes place in the pulmonary capillaries adjacent to the alveoli of the lungs. The oxygen in the oxyhemoglobin then travels through the bloodstream to be released at cells and tissues where $O_2$ is utilized as a terminal electron acceptor. At those cells and tissues where $CO_2$ is produced from energy-substrate oxidation, $CO_2$ binds to the terminal amino group of hemoglobin (four molecules of $CO_2$ per molecule of hemoglobin) to form carbaminohemoglobin. The equilibrium of this reaction depends on whether hemoglobin binds to $O_2$, as binding to $CO_2$ increases when the dissolved $O_2$ decreases. Since the binding of $CO_2$ to hemoglobin is reversible, $CO_2$ freely dissociates from this protein when it reaches the capillaries in the lungs.

$$\text{Protein–NH}_2 + \text{CO}_2 \leftrightarrow \text{Protein–NH–COO}^- + \text{H}^+$$
$$\text{Hemoglobin–NH}_3^+ \leftrightarrow \text{Hemoglobin–NH}_2 + \text{H}^+$$
$$\text{Hemoglobin–NH}_2 + \text{CO}_2 \leftrightarrow \text{Hemoglobin–NH–COOH}$$
$$\text{Hemoglobin–NH–COOH} \leftrightarrow \text{Hemoglobin–NH–COO}^- + \text{H}^+$$

Besides oxygen, hemoglobin also binds to competitive inhibitors, such as carbon monoxide (CO) and nitric oxide (NO). High levels of CO and NO are therefore toxic to animals. At a physiological level, NO is bound to the thiol group of cysteine residues in hemoglobin to form an S-nitrosothiol. The latter dissociates into free NO and thiol again, as the hemoglobin releases $O_2$ from its heme site. This assists the transport of both $O_2$ and NO to tissues in the body. In the presence of CO, or when the heme Fe is oxidized to the Fe(III) state, $O_2$ cannot bind to hemoglobin.

NO can readily react with oxyhemoglobin or oxymyoglobin to yield nitrate ($NO_3^-$) and methemoglobin or metmyoglobin, respectively. These two met forms of hemoglobin or myoglobin are the oxidized hemoproteins, and cannot bind $O_2$. In addition, NO can react with the met and deoxy forms of hemoglobin or myoglobin to yield nitrite ($NO_2^-$) and the Hb(Fe(II)-NO complex. These reactions are summarized as follows.

$$\text{Hb(Fe(II)–O}_2) + \text{NO} \rightarrow \text{metHb[Fe(III)]} + \text{NO}_3^-$$
$$\text{metHb[Fe(III)]} + \text{NO} \rightarrow \text{deoxyHb[Fe(II)]} + \text{NO}_2^- + 2\text{H}^+$$
$$\text{deoxyHb[Fe(II)]} + \text{NO} \rightarrow \text{Hb[Fe(II)]–NO}$$

### Protein Solubility in Water

Most proteins in an animal are soluble in water, but some (e.g., transmembrane proteins, mature collagens with covalent intermolecular cross-linkages, as well as α- and β-keratins) are not. Mature collagens can be isolated from connective tissue through their solubilization in 1% acetic acid, followed by dialysis against distilled water (Veis and Anesey 1965). Keratins can be dissolved in 0.5 M sodium sulfide at pH 10-13 to break their disulfide linkages, precipitated by 35% ammonium sulfate, and re-solubilized, like any other proteins, in 1 M NaOH (Gupta et al. 2012). This method is useful for isolating proteins from bird feathers, mammalian horns, and reptile scales.

## SUMMARY

Proteins are macromolecules consisting of one or more polypeptide chains, with each chain composed of approximately 40 to over 1000 α-AAs linked by peptide bonds. They are the most abundant dry matter in cells other than adipocytes. Proteins have four orders of structures: (1) a primary structure (the sequence of AAs along the polypeptide chain); (2) a secondary structure (the conformation of the polypeptide backbone); (3) a tertiary structure (the 3D arrangement of protein); and (4) a quaternary structure (the spatial arrangement of polypeptide subunits). The primary sequence of AAs in protein determines its other structures and biological functions. The forces stabilizing polypeptide aggregates are hydrogen and electrostatic bonds between AA residues. Proteins are stable in aqueous solutions at a physiological pH (7–7.4) and temperatures (37°C in mammals and 40°C in birds). Unlike carbohydrates and fats, protein is the only macronutrient which provides nitrogen, carbon, and sulfur to animals. As the most fundamental components of animal tissues, proteins play important roles in the body, including their roles in cell and tissue structure, enzyme-catalyzed reactions, muscle contraction, hormone-mediated effects, immune response, oxygen storage and transport, nutrition, metabolic regulation, buffering, and gene expression. Animal-source ingredients usually contain more proteins and more balanced ratios of AAs relative to their composition in animals and therefore have higher nutritional values than plant-source ingredients. The digestion of dietary protein generates large peptides, which are further hydrolyzed to small peptides and free AAs for absorption into enterocytes of the small intestine. Thus, animals have dietary requirements of AAs but not protein.

Except for glycine, taurine, β-alanine, and γ-aminobutyric acid, AAs can exist in an L- and D-configuration. In animals, L-AAs and glycine are substrates for protein synthesis, but some D-AAs are also present in physiological fluids. The diversity of AAs is also expressed by different side chains. Quantitatively, L-AAs likely account for >99.98% of total AAs (L-AAs + D-AAs) in animal organisms. All AAs are generally stable in the crystalline form at room temperature (e.g., 25°C). Except for cysteine (which is readily oxidized to cystine in an oxygenated solution) and glutamine (which spontaneously cyclizes to form pyroglutamate at a very slow rate), all AAs are stable in water and physiological solutions at 25°C–40°C. All AAs, except for cysteine and glutamine, are stable in a 5% TCA or 0.75 M $HClO_4$ solution, or an alkaline solution (pH 8.4), at room temperature (e.g., 25°C) for at least 12 h or at −80°C for 2 months. Under the standard conditions of acid hydrolysis at high temperature (i.e., 6 M HCl, 110°C, and 24 h), all AAs, except for glutamine, asparagine, tryptophan, and methionine, are highly stable. In contrast, most AAs (including arginine, asparagine, cysteine, cystine, glutamine, and serine) are destroyed by alkaline hydrolysis at high temperature (e.g., 105°C), but tryptophan is stable in alkaline solution without any detectable loss.

Free AAs and peptide-bound AAs participate in various reactions. They include: (1) the reaction of the α-amino group of AAs with a strong acid or reaction of the carboxyl group of AAs with an alkaline; (2) the acetylation of the α-amino group of AAs; (3) the conjugation of the α-amino group of the AA with a reagent; (4) the deamination, oxidative deamination, transamination, decarboxylation, oxymethylation, condensation, esterification, and intramolecular cyclization of AAs; (5) chelation with metals; (6) dye binding; and (7) peptide synthesis (Wu 2013). Specific AAs are also involved in certain reactions, such as the iodination of the phenol ring in tyrosine, the guanidination of the ε-$NH_2$ group of lysine, and the Maillard reaction. The peptide bonds in protein and peptides can: (1) be hydrolyzed by strong acids and bases, as well as proteases and peptidases; (2) stabilize AAs; and (3) react with cupric ions ($Cu^{2+}$) to form colored products as the basis of protein/peptide analysis (Biuret and Lowry assays). Furthermore, hemoglobin binds to $O_2$, $CO_2$, and NO, thereby playing an important role in oxygenation and gas exchange. Collectively, protein is the most fundamental component of animals and exhibits versatile chemical reactions with enormous biological importance.

## REFERENCES


Agerberth, B., J. Söderling-Barros, H. Jörnvall, Z.W. Chen, C.G. Ostenson, S. Efendić, and V. Mutt. 1989. Isolation and characterization of a 60-residue intestinal peptide structurally related to the pancreatic secretory type of trypsin inhibitor: Influence on insulin secretion. *Proc. Natl. Acad. Sci. USA.* 86:8590–8594.

Ajinomoto. 2003. *Ajinomoto's Amino Acid Handbook.* Ajinomoto Inc., Tokyo, Japan.

Assaad, H., L. Zhou, R.J. Carroll, and G. Wu. 2014. Rapid publication-ready MS-Word tables for one-way ANOVA. *SpringerPlus.* 3:474.

Bischoff, R. and H. Schlüter. 2012. Amino acids: Chemistry, functionality and selected non-enzymatic post-translational modifications. *J. Proteomics.* 75:2275–2296.

Brosnan, J.T. 2001. Amino acids, then and now—A reflection on Sir Hans Krebs' contribution to nitrogen metabolism. *IUBMB Life*. 52:265–270.

Chen, Z.W., T. Bergman, C.G. Ostenson, S. Efendic, V. Mutt, and H. Jörnvall. 1997. Characterization of dopuin, a polypeptide with special residue distributions. *Eur. J. Biochem.* 249:518–522.

Choi, S.H., T.A. Wickersham, G. Wu, L.A. Gilmore, H.D. Edwards, S.K. Park, K.H. Kim, and S.B. Smith. 2014. Abomasal infusion of arginine stimulates *SCD* and *C/EBPβ* gene expression, and decreases *CPT1β* gene expression in bovine adipose tissue independent of conjugated linoleic acid. *Amino Acids.* 46:353–366.

Cromwell, C.L., M.J. Azain, O. Adeola, S.K. Baidoo, S.D. Carter, T.D. Crenshaw, S.W. Kim, D.C. Mahan, P.S. Miller, and M.C. Shannon. 2011. Corn distillers dried grains with solubles in diets for growing-finishing pigs: A cooperative study. *J. Anim. Sci.* 89:2801–2811.

Dai, Z.L., Z.L. Wu, S.C. Jia, and G. Wu. 2014. Analysis of amino acid composition in proteins of animal tissues and foods as pre-column *o*-phthaldialdehyde derivatives by HPLC with fluorescence detection. *J. Chromatogr. B.* 964:116–127.

Davis, T.A., H.V. Nguyen, R. Garciaa-Bravo, M.L. Fiorotto, E.M. Jackson, D.S. Lewis, D.R. Lee, and P.J. Reeds. 1994. Amino acid composition of human milk is not unique. *J. Nutr.* 124:1126–1132.

Dinsmore, C.J. and D.C. Beshore. 2002. Recent advances in the synthesis of diketopiperazines. *Tetrahedron* 58:3297–3312.

Dominguez, R. and K.C. Holmes. 2011. Actin structure and function. *Annu. Rev. Biophys.* 40:169–186.

Fernstrom, J.D., S.D. Munger, A. Sclafani, I.E. de Araujo, A. Roberts, and S. Molinary. 2012. Mechanisms for sweetness. *J. Nutr.* 142:1134S–1141S.

Flynn, N.E., D.A. Knabe, B.K. Mallick, and G. Wu. 2000. Postnatal changes of plasma amino acids in suckling pigs. *J. Anim. Sci.* 78:2369–2375.

Fridkin, M. and A. Patchornik. 1974. Peptide synthesis. *Annu. Rev. Biochem.* 43:419–443.

Friedman, M. 1999. Chemistry, nutrition, and microbiology of D-amino acids. *J. Agric. Food Chem.* 47:3457–3479.

Gilbert, E.R., E.A. Wong, and K.E. Webb, Jr. 2008. Board-invited review: Peptide absorption and utilization: Implications for animal nutrition and health. *J. Anim. Sci.* 86:2135–2155.

Greenstein, J.P. and M. Winitz. 1961. *Chemistry of Amino Acids.* John Wiley, New York.

Gupta, A, N.B. Kamarudin, C.Y.G. Kee, and R.B.M. Yunus. 2012. Extraction of keratin protein from chicken feather. *J. Chem. Chem. Eng.* 6:732–737.

Hack, R., E. Ebert, G. Ehling, and K.-H. Leist. 1994. Glufosinate ammonium—Some aspects of its mode of action in mammals. *Food Chem. Toxic.* 32:461–470.

Hou, Y.Q., S.D. Hu, S.C. Jia, G. Nawaratna, D.S. Che, F.L. Wang, F.W. Bazer, and G. Wu. 2016. Whole-body synthesis of L-homoarginine in pigs and rats supplemented with L-arginine. *Amino Acids.* 48:993–1001.

Hou, Y.Q., S.C. Jia, G. Nawaratna, S.D. Hu, S. Dahanayaka, F.W. Bazer, and G. Wu. 2015a. Analysis of L-homoarginine in biological samples by HPLC involving pre-column derivatization with *o*-phthalaldehyde and *N*-acetyl-L-cysteine. *Amino Acids.* 47:2005–2014.

Hou, Y.Q., L. Wang, D. Yi, and G. Wu. 2015b. N-acetylcysteine and intestinal health: A focus on mechanisms of its actions. *Front. Biosci.* 20:872–891.

Hou, Y.Q., Z.L. Wu, Z.L. Dai, G.H. Wang, and G. Wu. 2017. Protein hydrolysates in animal nutrition: Industrial production, bioactive peptides, and functional significance. *J. Anim. Sci. Biotechnol.* 8:24.

Hughes, A.B. 2012. *Amino Acids, Peptides and Proteins in Organic Chemistry.* Wiley-VCH Verlag Gmbh, Weinheim, Germany.

Ikada, K., M. Takeishi, N. Ishikawa, H. Hori, F. Sakurai, and T. Ishibashi. 2002. Relationship between dietary protein levels and concentration of plasma free amino acids in adult dogs. *J. Pet. Anim. Nutr.* 5:120–127.

Jones S. 2012. Computational and structural characterisation of protein associations. *Adv. Exp. Med. Biol.* 747:42–54.

Karlsson, A., E.J. Eliason, L.T. Mydland, A.P. Farrell, and A. Kiessling. 2006. Postprandial changes in plasma free amino acid levels obtained simultaneously from the hepatic portal vein and the dorsal aorta in rainbow trout (*Oncorhynchus mykiss*). *J. Exp. Biol.* 209:4885–4894.

Kawai, M., Y. Sekine-Hayakawa, A. Okiyama, and Y. Ninomiya. 2012. Gustatory sensation of L- and D-amino acids in humans. *Amino Acids.* 43:2349–2358.

Kreil, G. 1997. D-amino acids in animal peptides. *Annu. Rev. Biochem.* 66:337–345.

Kwon, H., T.E. Spencer, F.W. Bazer, and G. Wu. 2003. Developmental changes of amino acids in ovine fetal fluids. *Biol. Reprod.* 68:1813–1820.

Kyte, J. 2006. *Structure in Protein Chemistry*, 2nd ed. Garland Science, New York, p. 832.

Lamberth, C. 2016. Naturally occurring amino acid derivatives with herbicidal, fungicidal or insecticidal activity. *Amino Acids.* 48:929–940.
Leibundgut, M., C. Frick, M. Thanbichler, A. Böck, and N. Ban. 2005. Selenocysteine tRNA-specific elongation factor SelB is a structural chimaera of elongation and initiation factors. *EMBO J.* 24:11–22.
Li, H., N. Anuwongcharoen, A.A. Malik, V. Prachayasittikul, J.E. Wikberg, and C. Nantasenamat. 2016. Roles of d-amino acids on the bioactivity of host defense peptides. *Int. J. Mol. Sci.* 17:pii: E1023.
Li, P., Y.L. Yin, D.F. Li, S.W. Kim, and G. Wu. 2007. Amino acids and immune function. *Br. J. Nutr.* 98:237–252.
Li, X.L., R. Rezaei, P. Li, and G. Wu. 2011. Composition of amino acids in feed ingredients for animal diets. *Amino Acids.* 40:1159–1168.
Lubec, G. and G.A. Rosenthal (eds.) 1990. *Amino Acids: Chemistry, Biology and Medicine.* ESCOM Science Publisher B.V., Leiden, The Netherlands.
Manso Filho, H.C., K.H. McKeever, M.E. Gordon, H.E. Manso, W.S. Lagakos, G. Wu, and M. Watford. 2009. Developmental changes in the concentrations of glutamine and other amino acids in plasma and skeletal muscle of the Standardbred foal. *J. Anim. Sci.* 87:2528–2535.
Marglin, A. and R.B. Merrifield. 1970. Chemical synthesis of peptides and proteins. *Annu. Rev. Biochem.* 39:841–866.
Mateo, R.D., G. Wu, H.K. Moon, J.A. Carroll, and S.W. Kim. 2008. Effects of dietary arginine supplementation during gestation and lactation on the performance of lactating primiparous sows and nursing piglets. *J. Anim. Sci.* 86:827–835.
McCalla, J., T. Waugh, and E. Lohry. 2010. Protein hydrolysates/peptides in animal nutrition. In: *Protein Hydrolysates in Biotechnology.* Edited by V.K. Pasupuleki and A.L. Demain. Springer Science, New York, pp. 179–190.
Meister, A. 1965. *Biochemistry of Amino Acids.* Academic Press, New York.
Mepham, T.B. and J.L. Linzell. 1966. A quantitative assessment of the contribution of individual plasma amino acids to the synthesis of milk proteins by the goat mammary gland. *Biochem. J.* 101:76–83.
Moughan, P.J., A.J. Darragh, W.C. Smith, and C.A. Butts. 1990. Perchloric and trichloroacetic acids as precipitants of protein in endogenous ileal digesta from the rat. *J. Sci. Food Agric.* 52:13–21.
Nagasawa, M., T. Murakami, S. Tomonaga, and M. Furuse, 2012. The impact of chronic imipramine treatment on amino acid concentrations in the hippocampus of mice. *Nutr. Neurosci.* 15:26–33.
National Research Council (NRC). 2001. *Nutrient Requirements of Dairy Cattle.* National Academies Press, Washington, DC.
Nishikawa, T. 2011. Analysis of free D-serine in mammals and its biological relevance. *J. Chromatogr. B.* 879:3169–3183.
Nunn, P.B., E.A. Bell, A.A. Watson, and R.J. Nash. 2010. Toxicity of non-protein amino acids to humans and domestic animals. *Nat. Prod. Commun.* 5:485–504.
Outerbridge, C.A., S.L. Marks, and Q.R. Rogers. 2002. Plasma amino acid concentrations in 36 dogs with histologically confirmed superficial necrolytic dermatitis. *Vet. Dermatol.* 13:177–186.
Pasupuleki, V.K. and S. Braun. 2010. State of the art manufacturing of protein hydrolysates. In: *Protein Hydrolysates in Biotechnology.* Edited by V.K. Pasupuleki and A.L. Demain. Springer Science, New York, pp. 11–32.
Pasupuleki, V.K., C. Holmes, and A.L. Demain. 2010. Applications of protein hydrolysates in biotechnology. In: *Protein Hydrolysates in Biotechnology.* Edited by V.K. Pasupuleki and A.L. Demain. Springer Science, New York, pp. 1–9.
Phang, J.M., S.P. Donald, J. Pandhare, and Y. Liu. 2008. The metabolism of proline, a stress substrate, modulates carcinogenic pathways. *Amino Acids.* 35:681–690.
Rajalingam, D., C. Loftis, J.J. Xu, and T.K.S. Kumar. 2009. Trichloroacetic acid-induced protein precipitation involves the reversible association of a stable partially structured intermediate. *Protein Sci.* 18:980–993.
Rennie, M.J. and K.D. Tipton. 2000. Protein and amino acid metabolism during and after exercise and the effects of nutrition. *Annu. Rev. Nutr.* 20:457–483.
Sabatino, B.R., B.W. Rohrbach, P.J. Armstrong, and C.A. Kirk. 2013. Amino acid, iodine, selenium, and coat color status among hyperthyroid, siamese, and age-matched control cats. *J. Vet. Intern. Med.* 27:1049–1055.
San Gabriel, A., E. Nakamura, H. Uneyama, and K. Torii. 2009. Taste, visceral information and exocrine reflexes with glutamate through umami receptors. *J. Med. Invest.* 56(Suppl.):209–217.
Shurson, G.C. 2017. The Role of biofuels coproducts in feeding the world sustainably. *Annu. Rev. Anim. Biosci.* 5:229–254.

Song, M., S.K. Baidoo, G.C. Shurson, M.H. Whitney, L.J. Johnston, and D.D. Gallaher. 2010. Dietary effects of distillers dried grains with solubles on performance and milk composition of lactating sows. *J. Anim. Sci.* 88:3313–3319.

Stadtman, T.C. 1996. Selenocysteine. *Annu. Rev. Biochem.* 65:83–100.

Sterck, L., S. Rombauts, K. Vandepoele, P. Rouzé, and Y. Van de Peer. 2007. How many genes are there in plants (… and why are they there)? *Curr. Opin. Plant Biol.* 10:199–203.

Sugahara, M. 1995. Black vomit, gizzard erosion and gizzerosine. *Worlds Poult. Sci. J.* 51:293–306.

Sweeney, H.L. and A. Houdusse. 2010. Structural and functional insights into the myosin motor mechanism. *Annu. Rev. Biophys.* 39:539–557.

Veis, A. and J. Anesey. 1965. Modes of intermolecular cross-linking in mature insoluble collagen. *J. Biol. Chem.* 240:3899–3908.

Vickery, H.B. and C.A. Schmidt. 1931. The history of the discovery of the amino acids. *Chem. Rev.* 9:169–318.

Wagner, I. and H. Musso. 1983. New naturally occurring amino acids. *Angew. Chem. Int. Ed. Engl.* 22:816–828.

Watford, M. and G. Wu. 2005. Glutamine metabolism in uricotelic species: Variation in skeletal muscle glutamine synthetase, glutaminase, glutamine levels and rates of protein synthesis. *Comp. Biochem. Physiol. B.* 140:607–614.

Widyaratne, G.P. and R.T. Zijlstra. 2007. Nutritional value of wheat and corn distiller's dried grain with solubles: Digestibility and digestible contents of energy, amino acids and phosphorus, nutrient excretion and growth performance of grower-finisher pigs. *Can. J. Anim. Sci.* 87: 103–114.

Wilcockson, J. 1975. The differential precipitation of nucleic acids and proteins from aqueous solutions by ethanol. *Anal. Biochem.* 66:64–68.

Wu, G. 1993. Determination of proline by reversed-phase high performance liquid chromatography with automated pre-column *o*-phthaldialdehyde derivatization. *J. Chromatogr.* 641:168–175.

Wu, G. 2013. *Amino Acids: Biochemistry and Nutrition*. CRC Press, Boca Raton, Florida.

Wu, G. 2016. Dietary protein intake and human health. *Food Funct.* 7:1251–1265.

Wu, G., F.W. Bazer, and H.R. Cross. 2014a. Land-based production of animal protein: Impacts, efficiency, and sustainability. *Ann. N.Y. Acad. Sci.* 1328:18–28.

Wu, G., F.W. Bazer, Z.L. Dai, D.F. Li, J.J. Wang, and Z.L. Wu. 2014b. Amino acid nutrition in animals: Protein synthesis and beyond. *Annu. Rev. Anim. Biosci.* 2:387-417.

Wu, G., F.W. Bazer, W. Tuo, and S.P. Flynn. 1996. Unusual abundance of arginine and ornithine in porcine allantoic fluid. *Biol. Reprod.* 54:1261–1265.

Wu, G., H.R. Cross, K.B. Gehring, J.W. Savell, A.N. Arnold, and S.H. McNeill. 2016. Composition of free and peptide-bound amino acids in beef chuck, loin, and round cuts. *J. Anim. Sci.* 94:2603–2613.

Wu, G. and C.J. Meininger. 2008. Analysis of citrulline, arginine, and methylarginines using high-performance liquid chromatography. *Methods Enzymol.* 440:177–189.

Wu, G. and S.M. Morris, Jr. 1998. Arginine metabolism: Nitric oxide and beyond. *Biochem. J.* 336:1–17.

Yamauchi, O., A. Odani, and M. Takani. 2002. Metal-amino acid chemistry. Weak interactions and related functions of side chain groups. *J. Chem. Soc., Dalton Trans.* 2002:3411–3421.

Yen, J.T., B.J. Kerr, R.A. Easter, and A.M. Parkhurst. 2004. Difference in rates of net portal absorption between crystalline and protein-bound lysine and threonine in growing pigs fed once daily. *J. Anim. Sci.* 82:1079–1090.

Yin, J., W.K. Ren, Y.Q. Hou, M.M. Wu, H. Xiao, J.L. Duan, Y.R. Zhao, T.J. Li, Y.L. Yin, G. Wu, and C.M. Nyachoti. 2015. Use of homoarginine for measuring true ileal digestibility of amino acids in food protein. *Amino Acids.* 47:1795–1803.

Zhang, H., C.A. Hu, J. Kovacs-Nolan, and Y. Mine. 2015. Bioactive dietary peptides and amino acids in inflammatory bowel disease. *Amino Acids.* 47:2127–2141.

# 5 Nutrition and Metabolism of Carbohydrates

Carbohydrates are the most abundant nutrients in the feedstuffs of land herbivores and omnivores, and are ultimately the most abundant metabolic fuels for these animals. In contrast, the diets for fish contain much less carbohydrates than those for most terrestrial animals, and the foods of strict carnivores provide only a limited amount of carbohydrates. The digestion of polysaccharides differs markedly among species and, within a given species, the various parts of the digestive tract (McDonald et al. 2011). In nonruminants, starch and glycogen are the only complex carbohydrates that are digestible in the small intestine to yield free glucose, whereas dietary fibers are fermented by microbes in the large intestine to short-chain fatty acids (SCFAs), with the extent of fermentation varying tremendously among different species (Stevens and Hume 1998). In contrast, in ruminants, starch, glycogen, and dietary fibers are extensively fermented in the rumen to produce SCFAs and methane, and dietary fibers that escape the forestomach are further fermented in the large intestine. Consequently, in ruminants, there is little or no absorption of glucose from the small or large intestine into the blood circulation, but very active conversion of propionate into glucose in the liver (Thompson et al. 1975). Likewise, conversion of glucose into fructose in the seminal vesicles and conceptus is vital for successful reproduction in ungulates (Kim et al. 2012). Thus, the diversity of carbohydrate metabolism is a strategy for animals to adapt to their environments, survive, and evolve.

Glucose and SCFAs are important for both ruminants and nonruminants. Specifically, glucose is almost the exclusive metabolic fuel for the brain in the fed or postabsorptive state when the concentrations of ketone bodies in plasma are low (e.g., <0.1 mM; Brosnan 1999). Under all physiological conditions, glucose is also the exclusive source of energy for red blood cells, and is a metabolic fuel in the cells of the immune system, retina, and renal medulla (Swenson and Reece 1984). In all cell types, glucose is the major source of NADPH that is required by many enzymes, including nitric oxide synthase (Devlin 2011) and antioxidative enzymes (Fang et al. 2002; Krebs 1964). Thus, the maintenance of glucose homeostasis in the blood, which is achieved through the digestion of dietary carbohydrates as well as the endogenous synthesis and catabolism of glucose, is essential to the survival, growth, and development of mammals, birds, and fish. On the other hand, butyrate (an SCFA) is the major metabolic fuel for epithelial cells of the large intestine, and therefore dietary fiber plays an important role in gut health (Turner and Lupton 2011).

Dietary carbohydrates, particularly fiber, affect the digestion, absorption, and metabolism of nutrients in both ruminants and nonruminants (Bondi 1987; Pond et al. 1995). For example, high intake of starch impairs the utilization of dietary protein by ruminal bacteria in ruminants (Bondi 1987), whereas excess consumption of dietary fibers reduces the digestion of protein, soluble carbohydrates, and total dry matter (DM) by the small intestine in nonruminants (Zhang et al. 2013). This is a conundrum in animal nutrition, namely, how to take advantage of the benefits of non-starch and nonglycogen complex carbohydrates on improving intestinal health, while alleviating their negative impacts on nutrient digestion and absorption in the small intestine. Toward a better understanding of such a nutritional dilemma, Chapter 5 highlights the digestion and absorption of carbohydrates in nonruminants, ruminants, and fish, as well as glucose metabolism through glycolysis, the Krebs cycle, the pentose cycle, uronic acid pathway, gluconeogenesis, glycogenesis, glycogenolysis, and other related pathways.

## DIGESTION AND ABSORPTION OF CARBOHYDRATES IN NONRUMINANTS

### Digestion of Starch and Glycogen in Nonruminants

#### Roles of α-Amylase in the Mouth and Stomach

Starch content in typical diets for postweaning nonruminants is 46%–52%. These animals may ingest a small amount of glycogen from animal-source products. Starch and glycogen are the only polysaccharides which are digestible by animal-source enzymes in the oral cavity and small intestine of these animals. Digestion of homopolysaccharides begins in the mouth with the mechanical action of chewing and the chemical hydrolysis of salivary α-amylase (α-1,4 endo-glucosidase). This enzyme is secreted from the salivary gland. The time and extent of the hydrolysis of starch or glycogen in the mouth are limited. The enzymatic action of the salivary α-amylase continues in the esophageal region of the stomach and ends in its fundus region (fluid pH < 3.6), but the gastric digestion of carbohydrates is limited (Yen 2001). The products of the salivary α-amylase in the mouth and stomach are dextrins, α-limit dextrins, maltose, maltotriose, and isomaltose (Figure 5.1). Dextrins are low-molecular-weight polymers of α-D-glucose units linked by α-1,4 or α-1,6 glycosidic bonds, whereas α-limit dextrins are short-chained, branched glucose polymer remnants of amylopectin or glycogen. Note that the α-amylase cannot hydrolyze the α-1,6 glycosidic bond.

#### Roles of Pancreatic α-Amylase and Apical Membrane Disaccharidases in the Small Intestine

Starch and glycogen, as well as their partial digestion products, move from the mouth into the upper part of the small intestine. The small intestine contains: (a) the α-amylase released from the pancreas; and (b) sucrase-isomaltase (a bifunctional protein) and maltase-glucoamylase (amylo exoglucanase), which are secreted from the small intestine and bound to the apical (brush border)

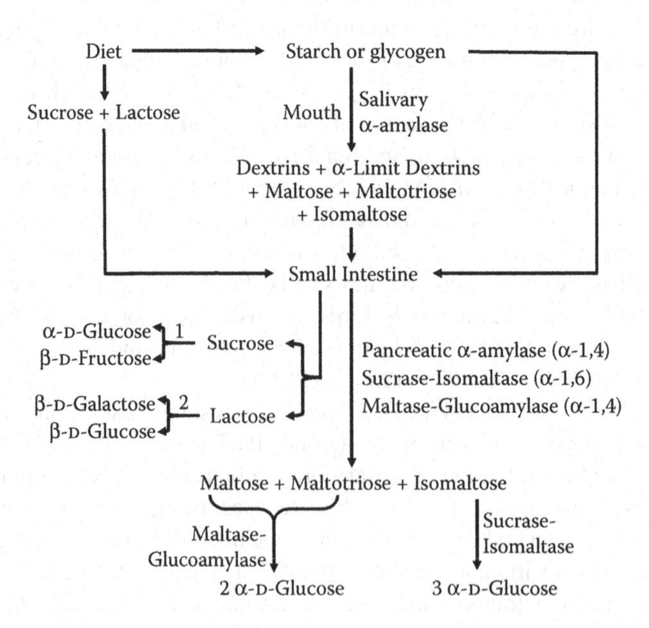


**FIGURE 5.1** Digestion of starch, glycogen, disaccharides, and oligosaccharides in the digestive tract of nonruminants. Except for the action of saliva-derived α-amylase in the mouth, other reactions (e.g., those catalyzed by pancreas-derived α-amylase) take place in the small intestine. Hydrolysis of maltose, maltotriose, and isomaltose to α-D-glucose is catalyzed, respectively, by maltase, α-1,4-glucosidase, and oligo-1,6-glucosidase, which are all located on the outer brush border of the apical membrane of the enterocyte. Isomaltase is also known as oligo-1,6-glucosidase. Both salivary α-amylase and pancreatic α-amylase require $Ca^{2+}$ for enzymatic activity. The enzymes that catalyze the indicated reactions are: (1) sucrase and (2) lactase.

membrane of the enterocyte. Like the salivary α-amylase, the pancreatic α-amylase has α-1,4 endo-glucosidase activity. The pancreatic α-amylase splits α-1,4 linkages in: (a) the amyloses (linear chains) of starch and glycogen to produce maltotriose and maltose; (b) the amylopectins (highly branched molecules) of starch and glycogen to yield not only maltotriose and maltose but also α-limit dextrins. At the same time, the amylo-1,6-glucosidase activity of sucrase-isomaltase breaks down α-1,6 branching points to expose the linear chains of starch and glycogen and facilitates the action of α-amylase. Collectively, these enzymatic reactions generate linear and branched glucose oligomers, such as maltose, maltotriose, and α-limit dextrins. The α-limit dextrins are broken down into maltose, maltotriose, and isomaltose by maltase-glucoamylase. Maltose and maltotriose are hydrolyzed by maltase-glucoamylase, and isomaltose by sucrase-isomaltase, to form α-D-glucose. Thus, in postweaning nonruminants, the digestion of starch and glycogen starts in the mouth and is completed in the small intestine, resulting in high concentrations of D-glucose in the intestinal lumen (Table 5.1). It should be borne in mind that in either fetuses or postnatal animals, the enterocytes of the small intestine do not express transporters for di-, tri-, or oligosaccharides (Drozdowski and Thomson 2006). To fulfill their nutritional roles, these carbohydrates must be degraded by the apical membrane sucrase-isomaltase and maltase-glucoamylase to monosaccharides for absorption into the enterocytes as described previously.

### Effects of the Structure of Starches on Their Digestion in the Small Intestine

The major site of the digestion of starches in the small intestine is dependent on their types. For example, in growing pigs, 82% of sticky rice starch, 47% of corn starch, and 30% of resistant starch are hydrolyzed in the anterior jejunum (Yin et al. 2010). In these animals, nearly 100% of sticky rice starch (23.6% amylose and 76.4% amylopectin), 93% of waxy corn starch (100% amylopectin and 0% amylose), and 67% of resistant starch (96.5% amylose and 3.5% amylopectin) are digested along the length of the entire small intestine, as determined through the collection of digesta from the terminal ileum. Rapidly digestible starch yields a rapid increase in the concentrations of plasma glucose and insulin, and the opposite is true for slowly digestible starch. Thus, owing to moderate glycemic and insulinemic responses, resistant starch may be beneficial for the nutritional control of glucose homeostasis in obese and diabetic animals.

The digestibilities of dietary starches are affected by their ratios of amylose to amylopectin, the length of their α-1,4 chains, and the frequency of their α-1,6 branching, all of which vary among different plant species or varieties. The true digestibilities (%) of starch in most cereal grains and in

**TABLE 5.1**
**Glucose Concentrations in the Lumen of the Small Intestine and in the Tissues of Animals[a]**

| Animals | Lumen of the SI | Plasma | Liver | Brain | Kidney | Skeletal Muscle | Heart | Adipose Tissue |
|---|---|---|---|---|---|---|---|---|
| Rat[b] | 42.8 ± 1.3 | 6.0 ± 0.2 | 7.4 ± 0.3 | 1.6 ± 0.1 | 3.3 ± 0.2 | 2.1 ± 0.1 | 0.65 ± 0.04 | 0.45 ± 0.02 |
| Pig[c] | 36.4 ± 1.0 | 5.9 ± 0.2 | 7.2 ± 0.4 | 1.7 ± 0.1 | 3.2 ± 0.2 | 2.0 ± 0.1 | 0.70 ± 0.05 | 0.48 ± 0.02 |
| Chicken[d] | 39.2 ± 1.6 | 12.4 ± 0.5 | 7.6 ± 0.4 | 1.9 ± 0.1 | 3.5 ± 0.3 | 1.6 ± 0.1 | 0.73 ± 0.05 | 0.51 ± 0.03 |
| Sheep[e] | 0.15 ± 0.01 | 3.4 ± 0.1 | 3.8 ± 0.2 | 1.0 ± 0.1 | 1.9 ± 0.1 | 1.2 ± 0.1 | 0.54 ± 0.03 | 0.37 ± 0.02 |

[a] Values, expressed as mM, are means ± SEM, $n = 6$. All animals were fed their conventional diets. All tissue samples and the digesta in the lumen of the proximal part of the jejunum were obtained from animals at 1 h after feeding. Glucose was measured using an enzymatic method (Wu et al. 1991).
[b] Three-month-old male rats.
[c] Thirty-five-day-old barrows.
[d] Thirty-five-day-old male broilers.
[e] Nine-month-old female sheep (nonpregnant and non-lactating).

field peas for postweaning swine are >95% and approximately 90%, respectively (Bach Knudsen 2001). Compared with cereal grains, some of the pea starch is entrapped within the cell wall and is not accessible to digestive enzymes, and the pea starch contains a higher ratio of amylose to amylopectin. In chickens, the true digestibilities (%) of starch in most cereal grains range from 82% to 89% between 4 and 21 days of age (Noy and Sklan 1995) and reach ≥95% after 3-weeks of age (Svihus 2014). In horses, whose diets typically contain only 6%–8% starch on a DM basis, the digestibility of starch in cereals is affected by feed processing methods: 20%–30%, 45%–80%, and 50%–70%, respectively, in whole, ground, and pelleted corn; 25%, 80%, and 95%, respectively, in rolled, ground, and pelleted barley; and 55%–85%, 50%–90%, and 85%–95%, respectively, in whole, rolled, and ground oat (Julliand et al. 2006).

### Digestion of Milk- and Plant-Source Di- and Oligosaccharides in Nonruminants

Milk- and plant-source disaccharides are hydrolyzed by disaccharidases in the small intestine into their constituent monosaccharides. These enzymes are synthesized by enterocytes and bound to their apical membrane. For example, lactose is hydrolyzed by lactase (a β-galactosidase, also known as lactase-phlorizin hydrolase) into β-D-galactose and β-D-glucose, whereas sucrose is hydrolyzed by the apical membrane-bound sucrose-isomaltase into α-D-glucose and β-D-fructose. In *E. coli* (e.g., intestinal bacteria), the β-galactosidase gene (*lacZ* gene) is expressed as part of the inducible system *lac* operon, which is activated by lactose when glucose concentration is low. Oligosaccharides in α-1,4- and α-1,6-glycosidic linkages are hydrolyzed by α-1,4-glucosidase and oligo-1,6-glucosidase, respectively, to produce their constituent monosaccharides. The digestibility of dietary lactose by neonates (e.g., piglets) is nearly 100% (Manners 1976).

### Substrate Specificity of Carbohydrases in Nonruminants

Except for trehalase and lactase, the saccharidases secreted by the small-intestinal mucosa are not specific for one substrate, but rather they have a broad specificity for a group of substrates with a similar chemical structure. Trehalase, which is bound to the apical membrane of the enterocyte, specifically hydrolyzes one molecule of trehalose into two molecules of glucose, and does not act on other substrates. As alluded to previously, lactase only hydrolyzes lactose and does not use other substances as substrates. In contrast, sucrose-isomaltase can hydrolyze starch, glycogen, and isomaltose, whereas maltase-glucoamylase can hydrolyze maltose, maltotriose, and low-molecular-weight glucose oligomers (e.g., α-limit dextrins), as noted previously.

### Developmental Changes of Carbohydrases in Nonruminants

#### Nonruminant Mammals

Developmental changes of carbohydrases result from changes in: (1) transport activity per cell or unit of mucosal mass; and (2) the total number of cells or intestinal mass. The specific activity of substrate transport refers to the amount of transported substance per cell or unit of mucosal mass, whereas the total activity of substrate transport is defined as the amount of transported substance per animal or the small intestine. In mammals, except for lactase (β-galactosidase), specific (μmol product/g tissue), and total (μmol product/total tissue) activities of α-amylase, sucrase-isomaltase and maltase-glucoamylase are very low or absent at birth and then increase with advancing age until the small intestine becomes mature (Manners 1976). For example, in pigs, specific and total activities of maltase are minimal at birth, increase from birth to 56 days of age, and then decline moderately, whereas both sucrase-isomaltase and trehalase are completely absent from the small-intestinal mucosa at birth, and are expressed after 7 days of age; specific and total activities of these two enzymes increase markedly until 56 days of age. Thus, feeding large amounts of sucrose to young mammals results in diarrhea because of an insufficiency of sucrase to hydrolyze sucrose. Two-week-old piglets can digest a small amount of dietary sucrose. In contrast, specific and total lactase activities in the mammalian small-intestinal mucosa peak at birth, remain high until weaning, and decline markedly thereafter. These changes in intestinal enzymes prepare mammals for transition from the milk containing lactose to the solid foods containing starch or glycogen. Glucocorticoids play an important role in regulating the expression of these digestive enzymes.

In mammals exhibiting sucrose or lactose intolerance, the osmotic effect of undigested disaccharides attracts water from the small-intestinal mucosa and the blood into the lumen of the small intestine, leading to the formation of the watery digesta. Similarly, humans with a low activity of lactase in their small intestines have a reduced capacity for utilizing dietary lactose, and the affected individuals cannot tolerate a large amount of milk. Many cheeses are well tolerated by these individuals because the bacteria used in cheese production have degraded the majority of the lactose that was originally present in the milk.

#### Avian Species

Birds exhibit a different pattern of developmental changes in gastrointestinal carbohydrases than mammals (Chotinsky et al. 2001). Significant activities of α-amylase and sucrase-isomaltase are present on the apical membrane of the enterocyte in newly hatched broiler chickens. This, along with the grinding function of the gizzard, provides the basis for poultry to utilize a corn- and soybean meal-based diet immediately after hatching. The specific activities of these two enzymes increase 2- to 3-fold between hatching and 35 days of age and decrease thereafter. In contrast, the specific activities of maltase-glucoamylase, lactase, and trehalase are greatest on Day 18 of embryonic development, and then gradually decrease. The specific activity of maltase-glucoamylase is high at hatching, declines until 18 days of age, and remains at the reduced level until 56 days of age. Lactase and trehalase are barely detectable in the proventriculus, the pancreas, and the mucosa (including enterocytes) of 1- to 7-day-old or older chickens. Thus, post-hatching chickens cannot digest lactose or trehalose and, therefore, cannot tolerate a large amount of these carbohydrates in their diets. However, an appropriate amount of dietary lactose (e.g., 0.5%–4% in a diet) has been used as an effective prebiotic for poultry (e.g., broilers and turkey) (Douglas et al. 2003; Simoyi et al. 2006). In the avian hindgut, the fermentation of ingested lactose by microbes produces lactic acid and SCFAs to lower the pH of the intestinal lumen, thereby inhibiting pathogenic bacteria, reducing infection, increasing the provision of energy substrates to the epithelial cells of the large intestine, and improving the growth performance of the birds.

## Absorption of Monosaccharides by the Small Intestine in Nonruminants

### Role of Glucose and Fructose Transporters in the Apical Membrane of Enterocytes

Monosaccharides are absorbed from the lumen of the small intestine into its enterocytes through specific carriers localized in the apical membrane of the cells (Table 5.2): (1) one or more of the 14 facilitative glucose transporters (GLUTs, the SLC2A family of proteins); and (2) sodium–glucose linked transporter-1 (SGLT1). They are all transmembrane proteins, with GLUTs 1-12 being $Na^+$-independent uniporters and SGLTs being $Na^+$-dependent symporters (Deng and Yan 2016). GLUT1 is ubiquitously expressed in animal cells, and GLUT3 is widely distributed in animal cells. These two transporters provide the cells with their basal glucose needs. In addition to its predominant localization in the basolateral membrane, GLUT2 is also present at a low level in the apical membranes of the enterocyte for glucose and fructose transport into or out of the cell. It is recruited into the apical membrane when intraluminal concentrations of glucose and $Ca^{2+}$ in the small intestine rise (e.g., after a meal). However, the role of GLUT2 in the transport of glucose from the intestinal lumen into enterocytes remains minor in comparison with SGLT1, which is responsible for the intestinal absorption of most diet-derived glucose (Ferraris et al. 1999). Except for GLUT5, all apical membrane GLUTs transport D-glucose, D-galactose, and D-xylose from the lumen of the small

**TABLE 5.2**
**Facilitative Glucose Transporters (GLUTs) in Animal Cells**

| GLUT[a] | Distribution in Animal Cells and Tissues |
|---|---|
| GLUT-1 | Ubiquitously expressed in cells; particularly abundant in blood–brain barrier, glial cells, red blood cells, placenta, and mammary tissue; provides cells with their basal glucose requirement |
| GLUT-2 | The major glucose transporter isoform expressed in hepatocytes, pancreatic ß-cells, and the basolateral membrane of enterocytes; also found to a lesser extent in kidney; also present in the apical membrane of enterocytes when intraluminal concentrations of glucose and $Ca^{2+}$ in the small intestine rise; responsible for the unidirectional transport of glucose, galactose, and fructose from enterocytes into the lamina propria and for the bidirectional transport of glucose, galactose, and fructose by the liver; absorbs dietary dehydroascorbic acid |
| GLUT-3 | Distributed in many tissues; particularly abundant in placenta, neurons of brain, kidneys, and fetal skeletal muscle; low levels in adult skeletal muscle |
| GLUT-4 | The major glucose transporter isoform in tissues that exhibit insulin-stimulated glucose uptake, such as skeletal muscle, heart, and adipose tissue; also present in brown adipose tissue; absent from avian skeletal muscle |
| GLUT-5 | A fructose transporter which is abundant in spermatozoa, testes, and small intestine; expressed to a lesser extent in adipose tissue, skeletal muscle, heart, brain, kidneys, mammary tissue, and placenta (unidirectional from maternal site to fetus); nearly absent from hepatocytes of nonruminant mammals; significant mRNA levels in avian and bovine livers |
| GLUT-6 | Present in spleen, leukocytes, and brain |
| GLUT-7 | Present in the endoplasmic reticulum membrane of hepatocytes, and in brain, small intestine, colon, and testis |
| GLUT-8 | Present in testes, blastocytes, brain, skeletal muscle, heart, adipocytes, and the apical membrane of enterocytes; transport trehalose in mammalian hepatocytes; absorbs dietary dehydroascorbic acid |
| GLUT-9 | Present in liver and kidneys |
| GLUT-10 | Present in liver and pancreas |
| GLUT-11 | Present in heart and skeletal muscle |
| GLUT-12 | Present in mammary tissue, skeletal muscle, heart, adipose tissue, and small intestine |
| GLUT13 | Present in animal cells for myoinositol transport |
| GLUT14 | Present in animal cells for glucose and fructose transport |

*Sources:* Aschenbach, J.R. et al. 2009. *J. Physiol. Biochem.* 65:251–266; Deng, D. and N. Yan. 2016. *Protein Sci.* 25:546–558; Gilbert, E.R. et al. 2007. *Poult. Sci.* 86:1739–1753; Zhao, F.Q. and A.F. Keating. 2007. *J. Dairy Sci.* 90(E. Suppl.):E76–E86.

[a] Glucose transporters belong to the SLC2A family of solute carriers. Their corresponding gene names are: SLC2A1 for GLUT-1 to SLC2A14 for GLUT-14.

intestine into the enterocytes. GLUT5 is a specific transporter of D-fructose in the apical membrane of the small intestine, as well as in the seminal vesicles, sperm, conceptus, and muscles.

As noted previously, the apical membrane SGLT1 is the major transporter of glucose and galactose on the luminal surface of the small intestine for their absorption into the enterocytes (Table 5.3). This transporter also transports $Na^+$ into the cells. $Na^+$ exits the enterocyte into the lamina propria through its basolateral $Na^+$-$K^+$ pump (an ATPase), which transports 3 $Na^+$ ions out of the cell in exchange for the entry of 2 $K^+$ ions into the cell (Chapter 1). One $Cl^-$ ion is pumped out of the enterocyte by the $Na^+$-$K^+$ ATPase into the lamina propria to maintain intracellular electroneutrality. The $Na^+$-dependent glucose transport system affects electric potential across the plasma membrane. Thus, when α-D-glucose is added to the mucosal side of the small intestine, the electric current of the plasma membrane is substantially increased as the sugar moves through the enterocyte. For comparison, sodium–glucose cotransporter-2 (SGLT2) is responsible for glucose reabsorption from the lumen of the proximal tubule of the nephron into the blood.

**TABLE 5.3**
**Sodium–Glucose Linked Transporters (SGLTs) in Animal Cells**

| SGLT | Distribution in Animal Cells and Tissues |
|---|---|
| SGLT1 | Apical membrane of the enterocyte in the small intestine (major glucose transporter for absorbing glucose from the intestinal lumen into the enterocyte) |
| SGLT2 | Luminal membrane of the proximal renal tubules (major glucose transporter for absorbing glucose from kidney tubules into the blood) |
| SGLT3 | Cholinergic neurons of the submucosal and myenteric plexi, and in skeletal muscle (possibly serving as a glucose sensor) |
| SGLT4 | Apical membrane of the enterocyte in the small intestine and luminal membrane of the proximal renal tubules (monosaccharide transporter for absorbing mannose and fructose from the intestinal lumen into the enterocyte, or from kidney tubules into the blood) |
| SGLT5 | Apical membrane of the enterocyte in the small intestine and luminal membrane of the proximal renal tubules (monosaccharide transporter for absorbing mannose, fructose, glucose, and galactose from the intestinal lumen into the enterocyte, or from kidney tubules into the blood) |
| SGLT6 | Apical membrane of the enterocyte in the small intestine and luminal membrane of the proximal renal tubules (monosaccharide transporter for absorbing myoinositol from the intestinal lumen into the enterocyte, or from kidney tubules into the blood) |

*Sources:* Gilbert, E.R. et al. 2007. *Poult. Sci.* 86:1739–1753; Deng, D. and N. Yan. 2016. *Protein Sci.* 25:546–558.

### Role of Basolateral Membrane GLUT2 in the Exit of Monosaccharides from Enterocytes into the Lamina Propria

GLUT2 is the major GLUT isoform in the tissues of the digestive system. In the small intestine, GLUT2 is constitutively localized mainly in the basolateral membrane of the enterocyte. After D-glucose, D-galactose, and D-fructose enter the enterocytes from the intestinal lumen, they are transported by the basolateral membrane GLUT2 from the cytoplasm of the cells into the extracellular space (interstitial fluid) of the lamina propria. Since GLUT2 is a high-capacity glucose transporter, it allows for a large flux of glucose out of the enterocytes into the lamina propria. The basolateral membrane GLUT2 also transports D-mannose and 2-deoxy-D-glucose from the enterocytes into the lamina propria (Gilbert et al. 2007; Deng and Yan 2016). Its various cell types use only a small amount of dietary glucose and other monosaccharides.

### Trafficking of Monosaccharides from the Lamina Propia into the Liver

Monosaccharides (e.g., D-Glucose, D-galactose, D-fructose, D-mannose, and 2-deoxy-D-glucose) present in the interstitial fluid of the lamina propria traffic from the lumen of the small intestine into the intestinal venule via a series of coordinated steps, as alluded to previously. Through the blood circulation, these simple sugars ultimately enter the portal vein for uptake by hepatocytes. In the liver, GLUT2 is primarily responsible for both taking up and releasing glucose. The net flux of glucose through this organ depends on the glucose concentration gradient across the plasma membrane. In the fed state, when the concentrations of glucose in the plasma are greater than the intracellular concentrations of glucose in the liver, glucose is taken up by hepatocytes. Under this condition, only a relatively small percentage of glucose in the blood is utilized by the liver (Kristensen and Wu 2012). Conversely, under fasting conditions, when the intracellular concentrations of glucose in the liver are greater than the concentrations of glucose in the plasma, glucose is released into the venous blood (Williamson and Brosnan 1974).

In nonruminants, approximately 5% of diet-derived glucose is catabolized in the small intestine and the remaining 95% enters the portal vein (Watford 1988). Glucose metabolism provides only 5%–10% of energy for this tissue in the fed state. As noted previously, approximately 10%–15% of glucose in the portal vein blood is extracted by the liver for glycogen synthesis and limited catabolism, and the remaining portion (85%–90%) enters the systematic circulation for metabolism in extrahepatic tissues (e.g., the heart, brain, skeletal muscle, and lymph nodes). Catabolism of glucose is necessary to provide NADPH that is required for syntheses of AAs and fatty acids in the small intestine.

## Developmental Changes of Intestinal Monosaccharide Transport in Nonruminants

### *Nonruminant Mammals*

Proteins for apical membrane GLUT1 and SGLT1, as well as basolateral GLUT2, are present in the fetal small intestine during the first trimester in mammals with a long gestation period (e.g., pigs, cattle, and sheep) or during the last trimester in mammals with a short gestation period (e.g., rats and mice) (Ferraris et al. 1999). These glucose transporters function to absorb D-glucose, D-galactose, and D-xylose before and immediately after birth. The specific activities (the amount of glucose transported per unit mucosal mass) of intestinal glucose transporters in nonruminant mammals are highest at birth and then progressively decline to lower levels at 21 days of age, that is, weaning (30% and 50% of values at birth for pigs and rats, respectively [Ferraris et al. 1999]). However, the total activities of the intestinal glucose transporters increase progressively during the suckling period, because of a marked increase in the intestinal mucosal mass (Drozdowski et al. 2010). Likewise, basolateral membrane GLUT2 is present in the mammalian small intestine at birth, and its protein abundance is enhanced by 2- to-3-fold in response to the onset of suckling. The total activity of the basolateral membrane GLUT2 increases between birth and weaning to transport D-glucose and D-galactose from the enterocytes to the interstitial space of the lamina propria.

Intestinal GLUT5 is virtually absent from the mammalian gut at birth and is expressed at a low level during the first week of postnatal life to absorb a small amount of D-fructose from the small-intestinal lumen. For example, in rats, apical membrane GLUT 5 is not detected in the small intestine until weaning. In piglets, apical membrane GLUT5 is barely detectable in the small intestine at 0–7 days of age and is expressed at a low level at 2-weeks of age. Thus, much of the orally administered fructose is not absorbed by the neonatal small intestine before weaning. Consequently, feeding a large amount of fructose to mammalian neonates (e.g., pigs) can result in intestinal dysfunction, malabsorption, and diarrhea. This is called the toxicity of fructose, like the toxicity of sucrose for mammalian neonates. After weaning, mammals have a high capacity to absorb dietary fructose due to the increased expression of the apical membrane GLUT5.

### *Avian Species*

In chickens, apical membrane GLUT5 and SGLT1 are expressed in the small intestine 5 days before hatching, and their mRNA levels increase by 2- to 3-fold between birth and 14 days (Ferraris et al. 1999; Gilbert et al. 2007). The expression of these two transporters allows for the absorption of luminal D-fructose, D-glucose, D-galactose, and D-xylose by the avian small intestine immediately after birth. In contrast, intestinal mRNA levels for apical membrane SGLT5, which is expressed on embryonic day 18 and then is increased by 2-fold at hatching, do not differ between birth and 14 days of age. Of note, basolateral membrane GLUT2 is expressed on embryonic day 18, increased by 10-fold at hatching, and further augmented 2-fold between birth and 14 days (Gilbert et al. 2007). The changes in mRNA levels do not always match the changes in monosaccharide transport. For example, in chickens, the specific activity of intestinal glucose transport (amount/g of intestinal mucosal mass) increases approximately 3-fold between birth and 1 day of age, then progressively declines to approximately 85% and 35% of the peak value (at 1 day of age) by 7 and 21 days of age, respectively, and remains at the reduced level throughout the adult life (Ferraris et al. 1999). This illustrates the physiological and nutritional importance of measuring the actual rate of substrate transport by the intestine rather than merely relying on data on the mRNA levels for transport proteins. Since the small-intestinal mucosal mass increases more than 10-fold between birth and

6 weeks of age, the total transport of glucose, galactose, and fructose by the gut increases during this period of growth. The ability of the avian small intestine to absorb D-fructose immediately after hatching helps to explain the interesting finding that dietary supplementation with D-fructose (as 15% high-fructose corn syrup) increases the growth performance of broilers without affecting their feed intake (Miles et al. 1987).

## DIGESTION AND ABSORPTION OF CARBOHYDRATES IN PRE-RUMINANTS

### Digestion of Carbohydrates in Pre-Ruminants

When pre-ruminants (e.g., preweaning calves and lambs) consume a liquid diet (e.g., milk), almost all of it bypasses the reticulo-rumen and instead passes through the omasum into the abomasum as a result of the reflex closure of the esophageal groove (Chapter 1). Like young monogastric mammals, pre-ruminants rapidly digest milk lactose in the small intestine, with the lactose digestibility being 99%. However, these animals have a limited or no ability to hydrolyze sucrose due to the underdevelopment of the small-intestinal sucrase, and cannot break down the cell walls of cereal grains due to the lack of enzymes to degrade cellulose and hemicellulose. In addition, owing to little or low secretion of salivary and pancreatic α-amylase, young pre-ruminants cannot use starch in either purified diets or unprocessed cereal grains (Porter 1969). Thus, oral administration of sucrose or starch to pre-ruminant calves does not increase the concentrations of glucose or fructose in the plasma. As the animals grow older (e.g., 80 kg calves), they can digest a small amount of dietary pregelatinized starch (e.g., $<5\%$ in the diet) with a high digestibility coefficient (e.g., 95%) (Gerrits et al. 1997).

### Absorption of Monosaccharides in Pre-Ruminants

D-glucose and D-galactose (products of lactose hydrolysis), as well as D-xylose, are absorbed rapidly into the enterocytes of the small intestine in all pre-ruminants, as in preweaning monogastric mammals. In sheep, the protein abundant of the apical membrane SLGT1 per unit of the small-intestinal mucosa is high at birth but is decreased by 50% at 3 weeks of age and to a minimal level at 11 weeks of age (Ferraris et al. 1999). This corresponds to a large flux of glucose and galactose from the lumen of the small intestine into the enterocytes during the suckling period in lambs. Generally, except for GLUT5, intestinal SGLT1, GLUT1, and GLUT2 transport D-glucose at higher rates than other simple sugars. In calves, GLUT5 is virtually absent from the small intestine at 0–10 days of age, but is expressed at a low level at 30–50 days of age (Porter 1969). Thus, pre-ruminant calves cannot tolerate a large amount of D-fructose in their diets. Consequently, much of orally administered D-fructose is unabsorbed and just passes through the small intestine. Consequently, like sucrose, feeding D-fructose to young calves can result in severe scouring.

## DIGESTION AND ABSORPTION OF CARBOHYDRATES IN RUMINANTS

### Fermentative Digestion of Carbohydrates in Ruminants

#### Major Dietary Complex Carbohydrates in the Rumen

In forages, plant cell walls are composed of β-1-4-linked polysaccharides which are complexed with lignin. Mature cereal grains consist of the outer surface pericarp (bran; 3%–8% of kernel weight; containing β-1-4-linked cellulose and pentosans), the starchy endosperm (60%–90% of kernel weight), and the germ (embryo; 2%–3% of kernel weight). In addition to the pericarp, barley and oats are surrounded by a fibrous hull (90% fiber and highly lignified; up to 25% of total kernel weight). The cell walls are composed of a cellulose skeleton filled with arabinoxylans, xylans, and β-glucans (e.g., mainly arabinoxylans in wheat and corn, but primarily β-glucans oats and barley).

Within the endosperm, starch granules are embedded in a protein matrix. Starch granules are associated with the protein tightly in corn, but only loosely in barley and wheat.

The pericarp of cereal grains is the foremost barrier to their digestion in the rumen. Thus, refining or destruction of the pericarp through physical processing (e.g., grinding and rolling) or mastication is essential for efficient starch utilization in ruminants. After the endosperm is exposed, endosperm cell walls can be readily digested in the rumen. Once the starch granules are dissociated from the protein matrix through proteolysis, there is little difference in the fermentative digestion of starch granules in the rumen among different grain types. The breakdown of the protein complex is a prerequisite for enzymic attack on the starch granules.

Plant-source carbohydrates can be broadly classified as structural and nonstructural. Structural carbohydrates (e.g., cellulose and hemicellulose) are less digestible in the ruminant digestive tract than nonstructural carbohydrates (NSCs) (sugars, starches, and other carbohydrates found inside the cells of plants). Carbohydrates usually comprise 60%–70% of the total diet for postweaning ruminants and are the major source of energy for these animals and their ruminal microbes. The compositions of carbohydrates (e.g., neutral detergent fiber [NDF] and acid detergent fiber [ADF]) differ among feedstuffs (Chapter 2). In general, roughages contain more NDF than non-fiber carbohydrates (e.g., starch), and vice versa for grains, barley, and soybean meal. Pectin is the most abundant soluble non-starch polysaccharides (NSPs) in roughages. Grains, corn silage, and barley contain much more starch than free sugars and pectin.

### Retention Times of Feed Particles and Carbohydrates in the Rumen

The rumen exhibits selective retention of ingested feed particles. The rate of passage of feed particles through the rumen is inversely related to their retention time in the rumen and, therefore, the rate of their digestion by ruminants. The greater the rumen retention time, the greater the rate of DM (including fiber) digestion. Rumen retention times of dietary carbohydrates are affected by many factors, including lag-rumination pool, feed intake, dietary nutrient content, the size of feed particles, the rate of escape of feed particles from the rumen, ruminal microbial ecosystems for nutrient fermentation, and animal species (Ellis et al. 1979). The mean retention time of fluid in the rumen of forage-fed cattle, sheep, and goats is approximately 10 h (Lechner-Doll et al. 1991). The mean retention times of feed particles in the rumen of the roughage-fed ruminants are: approximately 10 h for a large particle pool and approximately 25 h for a small particle pool (~28 h for cattle and 20 h for sheep and goats) (Lechner-Doll et al. 1991). For comparison, the transit times of digesta along the other parts of the gastrointestinal tract in ruminants are: omasum, 4 h (mixing flow); abomasum and small intestine, 4 h (tubular flow); cecum and proximal colon, 5 h (mixing flow); and distal colon, 4 h (tubular flow) (Huhtanen et al. 2008).

### Extracellular Hydrolysis of Complex Carbohydrates into Monosaccharides by Ruminal Microbes

Bacteria play the predominant role in the extracellular hydrolysis of dietary complex carbohydrates in the rumen, but fungi and protozoa also contribute to this process. Specifically, complex carbohydrates in the plant cell walls are hydrolyzed extracellularly by cellulases, hemicellulases, and xylanases to their monosaccharides. These enzymes are of primarily bacterial origin, and are also released at high levels by the anaerobic fungi (Akin and Borneman 1990). The main cellulolytic bacteria are *Fibrobacter succinogenes, Ruminococcus flavefacians*, and *Ruminococcus albus* (Chapter 1). Thus, the ruminal bacteria and fungi are essential to break down plant cell walls through the hydrolysis of β-1-4 glycosidic bonds in membrane polysaccharides. The lysis of the plant cell walls releases cellular soluble carbohydrates (e.g., monosaccharides) and also exposes the protein–starch granule matrix of grains. The rhizoids in ruminal fungi (e.g., *Orpinomyces joyonii, Neocallimastix patriciarum,* and *Piromyces communis*) are capable of penetrating directly through the protein matrix to allow for enhanced microbial colonization and enhanced proteolysis, so as to release the encased starch granules (McAllister et al. 1993). The starch granules and soluble forms of starch are hydrolyzed extracellularly to monosaccharides by microbial α-amylases and oligosaccharidases. These enzymes are of primarily bacterial origin, but are also produced by fungi (Mountfort and Asher 1988).

### Intracellular Hydrolysis of Complex Carbohydrates into Monosaccharides Ruminal Protozoa

Ruminal protozoa also produce cellulases, hemicellulases, xylanases, and α-amylase like bacteria and fungi. The protozoa engulf bacteria, as well as water-insoluble feed particles and starch granules through pinocytosis. The engulfment of bacteria is a way for the rumen to control the number of its bacteria. Within the protozoa, the above enzymes act in concert to hydrolyze the polysaccharides in the engulfed materials to the constituent monosaccharides. The number of protozoa in the rumen increases when the content of grains in the diet is increased from 0% to 40%. Owing to their ability to take up starch granules and predate on amylolytic bacteria, protozoa can substantially reduce the rate of starch digestion in the rumen (which may take up to 36 h) and, therefore, the risk for the development of clinical or subclinical acidosis in the host. Jouany and Ushida (1999) estimated that protozoa may be responsible for as much as 40% of the starch digestion in the rumen.

### Intracellular Degradation of Monosaccharides in Ruminal Microbes

Bacteria are the principal microbes to metabolize monosaccharides to SCFAs in the rumen, but fungi also possess the enzymes required for the intracellular biochemical processes. In addition, protozoa can modulate SCFA production in the rumen by engulfing and controlling the number of bacteria. Specifically, monosaccharides (e.g., glucose, fructose, and xylose) are taken up by bacteria and fungi for extensive fermentation by a series of enzymes to produce pyruvate (the precursor of SCFAs), as well as $CO_2$, methane, and $H_2$ in the rumen (Figure 5.2). Microbial fermentation is the only way to digest dietary fibers. In adult ruminants fed either only hay (Heald 1951) or a maintenance diet with a mixture of 50% hay and 50% grain (Bergman et al. 1974), little carbohydrates (including glucose), except for small amounts of cellulose, reach the duodenum (Heald 1951; Macrae and Armstrong 1969). However, in adult cattle and sheep fed all-concentrate diets, as much as 30% of starches may escape rumen fermentation and enter the small intestine (MacRae and Armstrong 1969; Symonds and Baird 1975). This may result from the reduced ability of rumen microbes to degrade dietary carbohydrates as a result of changes in rumen pH, as well as the numbers and species of rumen bacteria. Emerging evidence shows that ruminal AAs stimulate the growth of fibrolytic bacteria, particularly those involved in the degradation of hemicelluloses (Firkins et al. 2007). This indicates an important role for protein nutrition in ruminal utilization of dietary fiber and the efficiency of ruminant production.

### Generation and Utilization of NADH and NADPH in the Rumen

In ruminal microbes, starch- and fiber-derived glucose, fructose, and pentoses are metabolized to pyruvate through the enzymes of the glycolysis pathway, with the production of NADH and $H^+$ (Downs 2006). Through the pentose cycle, glucose is metabolized to produce NADPH and $H^+$. In addition, the NADP-linked malic enzyme converts malate into pyruvate and forms NADPH. The NADH is used by bacteria to generate methane and $H_2$ (see the following sections), reduce pyruvate into lactate, and convert acetate into butyrate, thereby regenerating $NAD^+$ to allow for glycolysis (Kandler 1983). The NADPH is required to reduce unsaturated fatty acids into saturated fatty acids, sulfate into sulfide, oxidized glutathione into reduced glutathione, nitrate into nitrite, and nitrite into ammonia; these reactions regenerate $NADP^+$, permitting the pentose cycle to proceed. Rates of NADH and NADPH production must be equal to rates of their utilization to maintain ruminal homeostasis. Owing to the extensive fermentation of carbohydrates in the rumen to SCFA, there is little glucose present in the lumen of the small intestine of ruminants (Table 5.1).

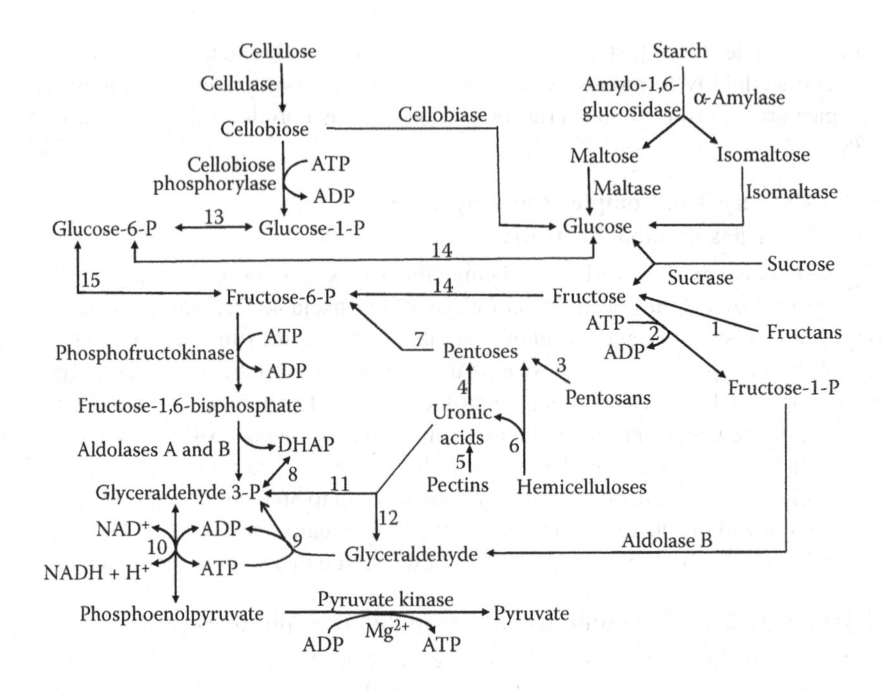


**FIGURE 5.2** Fermentation of carbohydrates to pyruvate in the rumen. The enzymes that catalyze the indicated reactions are: (1) β-fructan fructanohydrolases (e.g., exoinulinase and endoinulinase); (2) fructokinase (ketohexokinase); (3) enzymes that hydrolyze the polymers of pentoses (e.g., xylose and arabinose), including arabinosidase (hydrolyzing arabinoxylan to arabinose and xylan), endoxylanase (hydrolyzing xylan dextrins to xylose), exoxylanase, and β-xylopyranosidase (hydrolyzing xylobiose to xylose); (4) the enzymes that degrade galacturonic acid (the main constituent of pectin) to pentose (2-ketoglutarate) are: D-galacturonate dehydrogenase, galactarate dehydratase, 5-dehydro-4-deoxyglucarate dehydratase (decarboxylating), and 2,5-dioxovalerate dehydrogenase; (5) pectinases (e.g., pectin lyases) and polygalacturonase (pectin hydrolase), which hydrolyze the α-1,4 glycosidic bonds between galacturonic acid residues; (6) hemicellulases (e.g., endo-β-1,-4-xylanase [xylanase]), which hydrolyze interior β-1,-4 glycosidic linkages of the xylan backbone in hemicellulose to oligomers of different lengths; β-xylosidases, which hydrolyze the xylose oligomers to xylose; arabinase, which hydrolyzes the polymers of arabinose; glucanase, which hydrolyzes the polymers of glucose; glucuronidase, which releases glucuronic acid from glucuronoxylans; acetylxylan esterase, which hydrolyzes acetylester bonds in acetylxylans; and ferulic acid esterase, which hydrolyzes lignin–feruloylester bonds in xylans; (7) enzymes of the pentose cycle; (8) phosphotriose isomerase; (9) glyceraldehyde kinase; (10) enzymes of glycolysis, which include glyceraldehyde-3-phosphate dehydrogenase, phosphoglycerate kinase ($Mg^{2+}$), phosphoglycerate mutase, and enolase ($Mg^{2+}$); (11) the enzymes that degrade galacturonic acid to D-glyceraldehyde 3-phosphate are: uronate isomerase, D-tagaturonate reductase, D-altronate dehydratase, 2-keto-3-deoxy-D-gluconate kinase, and 2-keto-3-deoxy-6-phosphogluconate aldolase; (12) the enzymes that degrade galacturonic acid to 2-ketoglutarate are: D-galacturonate reductase, L-galactonate dehydratase, and 3-deoxy-L-*threo*hex-2-ulosonate aldolase; (13) phosphoglucomutase; (14) hexokinase and fructokinase; and (15) phosphohexose isomerase. *Notes*: DHAP, dihydroxyacetone phosphate. (Adapted from Downs, D.M. 2006. *Annu. Rev. Microbiol.* 60:533–559; Kandler, O. 1983. *Antonie Van Leeuwenhoek*. 49:209–224; McDonald, P. et al. 2011. *Animal Nutrition*, 7th ed. Prentice Hall, New York, NY.)

## Production of SCFAs in the Rumen

There are fundamental differences between ruminants and nonruminants in carbohydrate digestion (Weimer 1998). This is because the rumen provides a continuous culture system for large amounts of anaerobic bacteria, protozoa, and fungi. Fermentative properties of ruminal bacteria are summarized in Table 5.4. Most of the dietary carbohydrates are fermented in the rumen to form SCFAs, namely, acetic acid, propionic acid, and butyric acid due to the action of microbial enzymes. The breakdown of carbohydrates to SCFAs in the rumen can be divided into two stages: (I) the extracellular

**TABLE 5.4**
**Fermentative Properties of Ruminal Bacteria**

| Species | Function | Products |
|---|---|---|
| *Bacteroides succinogenes* | Cellulolytic, amylolytic | Formate, acetate, succinate |
| *Ruminococcus albus* | Cellulolytic, xylanolytic | Formate, acetate, ethanol, $H_2$, $CO_2$ |
| *Ruminococcus flavefaciens* | Cellulolytic, xylanolytic | Formate, acetate, succinate, $H_2$ |
| *Butyrivibrio fibrisolvens* | Cellulolytic, xylanolytic, PR | Formate, acetate, butyrate, lactate, ethanol, $H_2$, $CO_2$ |
| *Clostridium lochheadii* | Cellulolytic, PR | Formate, acetate, butyrate, ethanol, $H_2$, $CO_2$ |
| *S. bovis* | Amylolytic, PR, SS | Formate, acetate, lactate |
| *B. amylophilus* | Amylolytic, pectinolytic, PR | Formate, acetate, succinate |
| *B. ruminicola* | Amylolytic, pectinolytic, xylanolytic, PR | Formate, acetate, succinate, propionate |
| *Succinimonas amylolytica* | Amylolytic, dextrinolytic | Acetate, succinate |
| *Selenomonas ruminantium* | Amylolytic, PR, SS, GU, LU | Acetate, lactate, ropionate, $H_2$, $CO_2$ |
| *Lachnospira multiparus* | Amylolytic, pectinolytic, PR | Formate, acetate, lactate, ethanol, $H_2$, $CO_2$ |
| *Succinivibrio dextrinosolvens* | Pectinolytic, dextrinolytic | Formate, acetate, succinate, lactate |
| *Methanobrevibacter ruminantium* | Methanogenic, $H_2$-utilizer | Methane |
| *Methanosarcina barkeri* | Methanogenic, $H_2$-utilizer | Methane, $CO_2$ |
| *Spirochete species* | Pectinolytic, SS | Formate, acetate, lactate, succinate, ethanol |
| *M. elsdenii* | SS, LU | Acetate, propionate, butyrate, valerate, caproate, $H_2$, $CO_2$ |
| *Lactobacillus* sp. | SS | Lactate |
| *Anaerovibrio lipolytica* | Lipolytic, GU | Acetate, priopionate, succinate |
| *Eubacterium ruminantium* | SS | Formate, acetate, butyrate, $CO_2$ |

*Source:* Adapted from Stevens, C.E. and I.D. Hume. 1998. *Physiol. Rev.* 78:393–427.
*Note:* GU, glycerol-utilizing; LU, lactate-utilizing; PR, proteolytic; and SS, soluble sugar fermenter.

hydrolysis of carbohydrates (e.g., starch, cellulose, hemicellulose, and pectin) to monosaccharides, including pyruvate, as noted previously; and (II) the intracellular conversion of the monosaccharides into pyruvate (Figure 5.2) and its intracellular metabolism to form SCFAs (Figure 5.3). All of these reactions require specific enzymes, including those which hydrolyze β-1,4- and β-1,6-glycosidic linkages, as well as acetylester and lignin–feruloylester bonds (Richard and Hilditch 2009; Tanaka and Johnson 1971). In the rumen of cattle fed a roughage diet, rates of fermentation for starch, pectin, and cellulose (mmol/h) peak around 2.5, 5, and 10 h after the initiation of feeding, respectively (Baldwin et al. 1977). The ruminal fermentation of starch and pectin is completed by 5 and 15 h after the initiation of feeding. In contrast, rates of fermentation for cellulose (mmol/h) remain constant between 10 and 15 h after the initiation of feeding and decline slightly thereafter (Baldwin et al. 1977).

Acetate is the major SCFA in the rumen of ruminants fed on a variety of roughages and concentrates (Table 5.5). Concentrations of SCFAs in the rumen depend on the balance between their rates of production and absorption into the rumen epithelial cells. Total SCFAs in the rumen vary widely with the diets of animals and with the time that has elapsed since the previous meal, but are normally in the range of 75–150 mM (Balwin et al. 1977). The relative proportions of SCFAs are affected by the ratio of soluble carbohydrates to insoluble fibers in the diet. For example, mature fibrous forages give rise to a mixture of SCFAs containing a high proportion (~70%) of acetate, 20% propionate, and 10% butyrate, but less mature forages tend to yield a lower proportion of acetate and a higher proportion of propionate. The addition of concentrates to a forage diet also increases

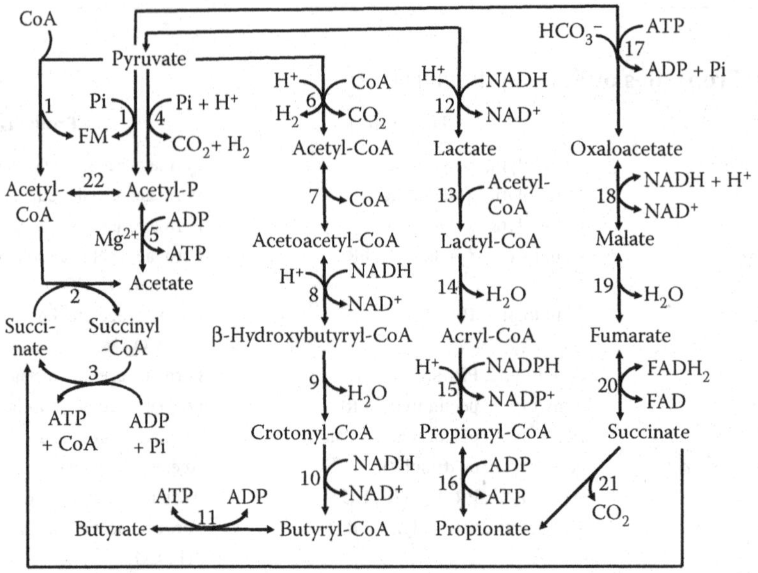

CoA
Pyruvate
1 Pi 1 4 Pi + $H^+$
FM $CO_2$ + $H_2$
$H^+$ 6 CoA
$H_2$ $CO_2$
Acetyl-CoA
$H^+$ 12 NADH
$NAD^+$
Lactate
$HCO_3^-$ 17 ATP
ADP + Pi
Oxaloacetate
Acetyl-CoA 22 Acetyl-P
$Mg^{2+}$ 5 ADP
ATP
Acetate
7 CoA
Acetoacetyl-CoA
$H^+$ 8 NADH
$NAD^+$
β-Hydroxybutyryl-CoA
9 $H_2O$
Crotonyl-CoA
10 NADH
$NAD^+$
13 Acetyl-CoA
Lactyl-CoA
14 $H_2O$
Acryl-CoA
$H^+$ 15 NADPH
$NADP^+$
Propionyl-CoA
16 ADP
ATP
Propionate
18 NADH + $H^+$
$NAD^+$
Malate
19 $H_2O$
Fumarate
20 $FADH_2$
FAD
Succinate
21 $CO_2$
2
Succi-nate Succinyl -CoA
3
ATP + CoA ADP + Pi
ATP ADP
Butyrate 11 Butyryl-CoA

**FIGURE 5.3** Formation of formate (FM) and SCFAs from pyruvate in ruminal bacteria. The enzymes that catalyze the indicated reactions are: (1) pyruvate formate-lyase (acetyl-CoA:formate C-acetyltransferase; ATP-dependent enzyme); (2) acetate:succinate CoA transferase; (3) succinate thiokinase; (4) pyruvate oxidase; (5) acetate kinase; (6) pyruvate:ferredoxin oxidoreductase; (7) thiolase; (8) β-hydroxybutyryl-CoA dehydrogenase; (9) β-hydroxybutyryl-CoA dehydratase; (10) crotonyl-CoA reducase; (11) butyrate kinase; (12) lactate dehydrogenase; (13) CoA transphorase; (14) lactyl-CoA dehydratase; (15) acrylyl-CoA reductas; (16) propionate kinase; (17) pyruvate carboxylase; (18) malate dehydrogenase; (19) fumarase; (20) succinate dehydrogenase; (21) succinate decarboxylase; and (22) phosphotransacetylase. CoA, coenzyme A; Pi, inorganic phosphate. (Adapted from Downs, D.M. 2006. *Annu. Rev. Microbiol.* 60:533–559; Kandler, O. 1983. *Antonie Van Leeuwenhoek.* 49:209–224; McDonald, P. et al. 2011. *Animal Nutrition*, 7th ed. Prentice Hall, New York, NY.)

the proportion of propionate at the expense of acetate. With all-concentrate diets, the proportion of propionate may exceed that of acetate in the rumen. The underlying biochemical mechanisms are complex, but involve changes in the ruminal bacteria and their metabolism. Specifically, rapid fermentation of starch and monosaccharides in concentrate diets results in a sudden drop in ruminal fluid pH due to lactic acid production via glycolysis, possibly causing metabolic acidosis (rumen pH $< 5.5$). A low ruminal pH inhibits the growth of ruminal cellulolytic bacteria and acetate-producing bacteria but promotes the growth of propionate-producing bacteria, thereby reducing the digestibility of roughages and acetate concentration but stimulating propionate production (Chesson and Forsberg 1997). The opposite is true when ruminants are fed a diet containing a high percentage of fiber and a low percentage of starch. Thus, the NRC (2001) recommends a maximum content of dietary non-fiber carbohydrate to be 44% for ruminants. Besides the ratio of forage to concentrate, the ruminal production of SCFAs is influenced by many other factors (e.g., the physical forms, water and fat content, and intake of the feed, as well as feeding methods) through their effects on physical fill and rumination (regurgitation, chewing, salivation, and swallowing) (Weimer 1998).

### Entry of SCFAs from the Rumen into Blood

The SCFAs produced in the rumen enter the blood primarily through three routes: approximately 75% are absorbed directly through the rumen wall, 20% from the omasum and abomasum, and 5% pass along with the digesta into the small intestine where they are absorbed into the portal vein. The absorption of SCFAs occurs through passive transport, and its rate depends on a concentration gradient. The uptake of SCFAs by the cell is accompanied by the efflux of intracellular bicarbonate via an antiporter (also called exchanger). The rate of absorption of SCFAs from the rumen into

**TABLE 5.5**
**Concentrations of SCFAs in the Rumen of Ruminants Fed Various Diets**

| Diet | Total (mM) | Molar Ratios (mol/mol) | | |
|---|---|---|---|---|
| | | Acetate | Propionate | Butyrate |
| **Cattle Fed Roughages or Concentrates** | | | | |
| Mature ryegrass herbage | 137 | 0.64 | 0.22 | 0.11 |
| Grass silage | 108 | 0.74 | 0.17 | 0.07 |
| Barley (no ciliate protozoa in rumen) | 146 | 0.48 | 0.28 | 0.14 |
| Barley (ciliates present in rumen) | 105 | 0.62 | 0.14 | 0.18 |
| Long hay/concentrates (0.4:0.6; g/g) | 96 | 0.61 | 0.18 | 0.13 |
| Pelleted hay/concentrates (0.4:0.6; g/g) | 140 | 0.50 | 0.30 | 0.11 |
| Hay/concentrates (g/g) | | | | |
| 1:0 | 97 | 0.66 | 0.22 | 0.09 |
| 0.8:0.2 | 80 | 0.61 | 0.25 | 0.11 |
| 0.6:0.4 | 87 | 0.61 | 0.23 | 0.13 |
| 0.4:0.6 | 76 | 0.52 | 0.34 | 0.12 |
| 0.2:0.8 | 70 | 0.40 | 0.40 | 0.15 |
| **Sheep Fed Roughages** | | | | |
| Young ryegrass herbage | 107 | 0.60 | 0.24 | 0.12 |
| Chopper lucerne hay | 113 | 0.63 | 0.23 | 0.10 |
| Ground lucerne hay | 105 | 0.65 | 0.19 | 0.11 |

*Source:* Adapted from McDonald, P. et al. 2011. *Animal Nutrition*, 7th ed. Prentice Hall, New York, NY.

the blood increases as the pH of the rumen fluid decreases. This has led to the concept that non-dissociated acids pass through the rumen wall more rapidly than their anions. During their passage from the rumen into the blood, some of the butyrate and propionate are metabolized to form β-hydroxybutyrate and lactate, respectively, in the rumen epithelium.

SCFAs play an important role in ruminant nutrition. First, acetate, propionate, and butyrate are the major sources of energy in ruminants. As noted previously, butyrate is the major substrate for ATP production in the epithelial cells of the large intestine and thus for maintaining the health of the hindgut in both ruminants and nonruminants. The rumen of the cow or sheep produces 3–4 kg or 0.3–0.4 kg SCFAs per day. Thus, SCFAs can effectively replace a bulk of glucose and long-chain fatty acids as metabolic fuels in the large intestine, liver, skeletal muscle, and kidneys. Similarly, SCFAs can substitute substantial amounts of glucose as oxidative substrates in the brains of ruminants. Second, propionate is used to synthesize glucose in the livers of ruminants. Third, acetate and butyrate are converted into acetoacetate and β-hydroxybutyrate in the rumen wall and colonocytes. These ketone bodies are utilized as metabolic fuels by extrahepatic tissues, including the brain, small intestine, heart, skeletal muscle, and kidneys. Third, SCFAs, along with $NH_3$, maintain ruminal fluid pH at 5.5–6.8. This is critical for bacterial growth and metabolism in the rumen.

## Production of Methane in the Rumen

Methane is produced by microbes known as methanogens, which belong to the domain *Archaea* and the phylum *Euryarchaeota*. The formation of methane does not require $O_2$, and is actually inhibited by $O_2$. Substrates for methane-producing enzymes are $CO_2$ (or $HCO_3^-$) + hydrogen gas ($H_2$), acetate, methanol, formate, and methylamines (e.g., mono-, di-, and trimethylamines) (Figure 5.4). $HCO_3^- + H^+$ are formed from $CO_2 + H_2O$ spontaneously, but this reaction is greatly facilitated by carbonic anhydrase. Carbohydrate fermentation is the major source of both $CO_2$ and $H_2$ in the

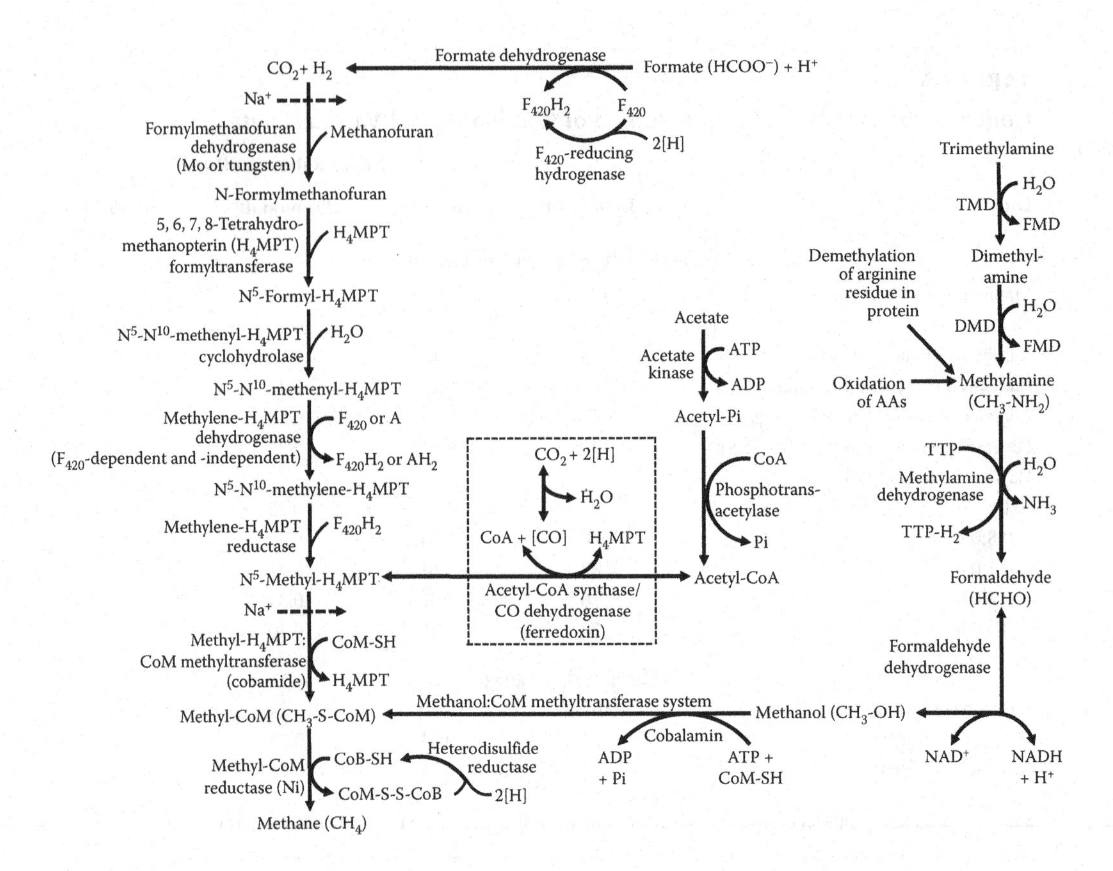


**FIGURE 5.4** Production of methane from carbon dioxide plus hydrogen gas, as well as from acetate, methanol, formate, and methylamines in ruminal bacteria. CoM (coenzyme M; 2-mercaptoethanesulfonate; $HS–CH_2–CH_2–SO_3^-$) is a coenzyme required for methyl-transfer reactions. CoB (coenzyme B; 7-mercapto-heptanoyl-threonine-phosphate) and $F_{420}$ (8-hydroxy-5-deazaflavin) are coenzymes required for redox reactions. A, receptor of electrons; AAs, amino acids; DMD, dimethylamine dehydrogenase (flavoprotein); FMD, formaldehyde; $F_{420}H_2$, reduced $F_{420}$; $H_4$MPT, 5,6,7,8-tetrahydro-methanopterin; TMD, trimethylamine dehydrogenase (flavoprotein); TTP, tryptophan tryptophylquinone. (Adapted from Hook, S.E. et al. 2010. *Archaea* Article ID 945785; Shima, S. et al. 2002. *J. Biosci. Bioeng.* 93:519–530.)

rumen. These two gases are also produced from the cleavage of formate by $F_{420}$-dependent formate dehydrogenase (FAD and molybdenum as cofactors) or NAD-dependent formate dehydrogenase. $F_{420}$, a coenzyme for hydride transfer, is a deazaflavin derivative exhibiting blue–green fluorescence when irradiated with UV light. Acetate is generated from the decarboxylation of pyruvate, which is derived primarily from carbohydrates and, to a lesser extent, AAs. In the rumen, methanol is produced mainly from the metabolism of the methyl esters of pectins and is exclusively converted to methane. Formate is formed from pyruvate by pyruvate-formate lyase (Figure 5.4). Methylamines are produced from AA degradation by bacteria and demethylation of arginine residues in protein.

In the rumen, the reduction of $CO_2$ by $H_2$ is the major pathway for methane production, where carbon is the terminal electron receptor. A smaller amount of methane is formed directly from acetate in the rumen. Some methanogens of the genus *Methanosarcina*, which grow slowly on $H_2$ and $CO_2$, utilize methanol and methylamines to produce methane.

The conversion of $CO_2 + H_2O$ to methane requires several unique cofactors (e.g., coenzymes M, G, and $F_{420}$, and tetrahydromethanopterin) and a series of complex reactions catalyzed by 10 enzymes (Figure 5.4). These coenzymes are either synthesized by the bacteria or supplied from an external source. As indicated in Figure 2.18, the formation of acetate and butyrate from pyruvate results in the production of $H_2$ and metabolic hydrogen in the form of reducing equivalents (e.g., NADH and NADPH), whereas propionate synthesis consumes the reducing equivalents and therefore is a competitive pathway for hydrogen utilization in the rumen. Thus, excessive $H_2$ is generated along with the production of acetate and butyrate, but not with that of propionate. Diets which have a lower proportion of fiber but a higher proportion of starch can increase the proportion of propionate among SCFAs in the rumen, resulting in reduced production of methane per mole of substrate fermented. The electrochemical gradient of sodium across the cell membrane provides energy to drive methane production from $CO_2$ and $H_2$.

Since methane cannot be utilized by animal tissues, and its synthesis is an energy-dependent process, methane production results in the irreversible loss of reducing equivalents and the reduced conversion of dietary energy into milk, skeletal muscle, or wool in ruminants. Thus, decreasing methane production is an important means to improving the efficiency of energy utilization in ruminant production. In addition, since methane is a contributor to the greenhouse effect, mitigation of methane emission is environmentally sustainable in animal agriculture. Methods for inhibiting methanogenesis include: (1) direct inhibition by halogenated methane analogs and related compounds (e.g., chloroform [not practical], chloral hydrate [not practical], amichloral [safe for *in vivo* feeding], trichloroacetamide, trichloroethyl adipate, bromochloromethane, 2-bromoethanesulfonic acid, and 9,10-anthraquinone); (2) use of ionophores (e.g., monensin and salinomycin) to alter bacterial population; (3) enhancers of propionate production (e.g., malate, fumarate); (4) rechanneling of substrates for methane production into the formation of alternative products by reducing the availability of cofactors, prosthetic groups, reducing equivalents (e.g., through biohydrogenation with polyunsaturated fatty acids as hydrogen acceptors), electron acceptors (carbon sources), and electron carriers (e.g., cytochromes); (5) the removal of protozoa from the rumen (defaunation) with use of phytochemicals (e.g., saponins); and (6) manipulation of microbial population and activity by nutrients (e.g., long-chain saturated fatty acids and lipids), plant extracts (e.g., condensed tannins and essential oils), probiotics (e.g., yeast and fungal probiotics), and other substances (e.g., formate). Significant challenges are that ruminal bacteria may adapt to these manipulation methods and render their effects only transient *in vivo*.

### Ruminal Metabolic Disorders

1. *Lactic acidosis.* When a large amount of highly fermentable carbohydrates is fed to ruminants, the rate of glycolysis to yield lactic acid in the rumen is much greater than the rate of lactic acid utilization, resulting in a rapid drop in ruminal fluid pH and the onset of lactic acidosis. In the rumen, major lactate-producing bacteria (e.g., *Streptococcus bovis*) are tolerant to low pH, whereas the growth and metabolic activity of major lactic acid utilizers (e.g., *Megasphaera elsdenii* and the *Selenomonads*) are inhibited by low pH (Fellner 2002). Thus, there is a lack of effective feedback inhibition of glycolysis in the rumen, such that ruminal lactic acidosis develops and becomes more severe, as the dietary intake of concentrate increases markedly beyond its maximum threshold (e.g., 50% concentrate in the diets of lactating cows; DM basis). A minimum of 50% roughage in the diet (DM basis) is recommended for feeding ruminants. Adapting the rumen to the increased concentrations of grains in diets over a period of weeks can reduce the incidence of acidosis in feeding ruminants (e.g., lactating dairy cows and feedlot beef). This is because the gradual adaptation to dietary concentrates can allow for the simultaneous growth of both lactic acid producing and utilizing microbes in the rumen. In addition, dietary supplementation with antimicrobial agents (e.g., ionophores) can be also effective in limiting the growth of lactic acid producing bacteria in the rumen and alleviating lactic acidosis in ruminants. Since ruminal acidosis reduces feed intake, growth performance, milk production, and profitability, while increasing culling rate and death loss, this metabolic disorder must be avoided in ruminant nutrition.
2. *Ruminal bloat in ruminants.* Under normal conditions, nearly all the methane and $H_2$, as well as most of the $CO_2$ produced in the rumen are removed by eructation. When the rate of gas production greatly exceeds the rate of eructation, the normal elimination of the

ruminal gases is impaired. This results in a disorder called bloat, which occurs in the form of a persistent foam mixed with either the ruminal contents (called primary bloat) or gases separated from the digesta (called secondary bloat). Bloat is characterized by the severe distention of the abdomen, the severe compression of the heart and lungs, and, therefore, impairment of blood circulation. With this metabolic disease, death rates can be up to 20% in cattle grazing bloat-prone pastures. The susceptibility of individual animals to bloat is affected by their genotypes and diets. For example, this disorder occurs primarily in cattle and, to a lesser extent, in sheep and goats. Pasture bloat is often observed in cattle grazing on legume pasture. This is possibly because products of rapid degradation of high amounts of soluble plant proteins (e.g., ammonia, $CO_2$, and $H_2S$), along with the high content of phospholipids in legumes, contribute to the formation and stabilization of the foam in the rumen. In contrast, feedlot bloat in cattle fed diets consisting of high percentages of grain concentrates and alfalfa or clovers results from the production of soft and adhesive slime by amylolytic bacteria, which leads to the formation of stable foam. Feedlot bloat in cattle fed high-concentrate or all-concentrate rations can be reduced through dietary management by the addition of coarsely chopped roughage.

#### Species Differences in Carbohydrate Digestion among Ruminants

There are species differences in digestion of carbohydrates among ruminants. For example, the digestibility of DM in a moderately high fiber diet is greater for cattle than deer, with the value for sheep and goats being intermediate (Huston et al. 1986). In addition, the rate of DM digestion is influenced more by diet than animal species, such that rumen residence time is shorter for concentrate particles than that for forages. In ruminants, the digestibility of total carbohydrates varies widely with the type of diet, ranging from 95% for molasses, to 75% for grass, 60% for hay, and 40% for straw. As in nonruminants, the digestibility of starch in the gastrointestinal tract is much higher than that of fibers. For example, the digestibility of alfalfa hay fiber is 44% in cattle, 45% in sheep, and 41% in goats (Huston et al. 1986). Thus, species differences in gastrointestinal dynamics of carbohydrate digestion are a major factor affecting the utilization of forages by ruminants.

### Absorption of Monosaccharides by the Small Intestine in Ruminants

The enterocytes of the ruminant small intestine express glucose and fructose transporters and therefore have the ability to absorb glucose, galactose, and fructose present in the lumen of the small intestine. The mechanisms of intestinal monosaccharide transport in ruminants are the same as those in nonruminants. However, in forage-fed ruminants, little glucose enters the lumen of the small intestine from the stomach due to the extensive ruminal fermentation. Thus, under normal feeding conditions, virtually no glucose is absorbed from the small intestine into the portal vein in cattle, sheep, goats, and other ruminant species.

In ruminants, the rate of glucose utilization by the small intestine is low. For example, in nonpregnant, non-lactating adult sheep fed lucerne hay at 0.5 h intervals, the arterial blood supplies 56.7 g glucose/h to the portal-drained viscera (primarily the small intestine) but only 0.6 g glucose/h is extracted, and the portal vein and the hepatic artery supply 56.1 and 9.5 g glucose/h to the liver, respectively, but only 0.8 g glucose/h is extracted (Bergman 1983). Thus, in contrast to nonruminants, only 1.4% of the glucose in portal vein blood is extracted by the liver in ruminants, and the remaining portion (98.6%) enters the systematic circulation for metabolism in extrahepatic tissues.

## FERMENTATION OF CARBOHYDRATES IN THE LARGE INTESTINE OF NONRUMINANTS AND RUMINANTS

The large intestine contains relatively large amounts of microorganisms (including bacteria and protozoa), compared with the small intestine (Chapter 1). If starch grains and dietary fibers escape the small intestine, they will be fermented in the large intestine. The processes for microbial fermentation and absorption of carbohydrates in the large intestine of nonruminants and ruminants are similar to those in the rumen of ruminants. However, hindgut fermentation in all animals is less effective than rumen fermentation. This is because the numbers of microorganisms are much lower and the transition time of chyme is much shorter in the large intestine than in the rumen. Nonetheless, concentrations of total SCFAs are found up to 150 mM in the lumen of the cecum and colon. Butyrate is the major source of energy for the epithelial cells of the large intestine and therefore is important for maintaining the health of the hindgut in ruminants and nonruminants.

In horses and rabbits, the enlarged colon and cecum contain microorganisms that ferment food constituents (including dietary fibers) via biochemical reactions similar to those in the rumen. In horses, 4%–30% of the ingested grain starch can escape the prececal digestion and enter the large intestine where its digestion is almost complete (Julliand et al. 2006). Regardless of methods for processing grains, the apparent digestibilities of their starch in the total gastrointestinal tract of horses are 98.8%, 96.8%, 97.9%, and 99.5%, respectively, for corn, oats, barley, and wheat (Julliand et al. 2006). The hindgut fermentation contributes to the utilization of 15%–30% of dietary soluble carbohydrates and 75%–85% of cell wall carbohydrates. However, high intakes of sugar and starch by horses (e.g., >12% and 20% NSCs for sensitive and less sensitive horses, respectively) may result in high rates of glycolysis in the hindgut to generate excess lactic acid, thereby adversely disturbing bacterial and protozoal activities (including the fermentation of dietary fiber) (Brøkner et al. 2012; Jensen et al. 2014). Thus, horses cannot tolerate large amounts of NSCs in one meal, and frequent feeding of small amounts of high sugar/starch diets (grains and concentrates) is recommended to prevent metabolic and intestinal disorders (e.g., colic or laminitis). With hay and concentrates, the entire digestive tract of horses can digest approximately 85% of the organic matter (including carbohydrates, protein, and fats) in their diets (Brøkner et al. 2016; Jensen et al. 2014). As a result, postweaning horses can grow by consuming forages, although their growth rate may be suboptimal. In contrast, the fermentability of dietary fiber in the large intestine of rabbits is not particularly high (e.g., only 14% for alfalfa hay fiber) (Yu and Chiou 1996), but their very high capacity to consume forages provides the physiological basis for them to survive and grow on grass.

In pigs, the hindgut is less enlarged in comparison with horses, and forages are poorly fermented (e.g., the digestibility of alfalfa hay fiber in diets with 5% alfalfa being ~20% only). However, postweaning pigs can ferment up to 50% of dietary cellulose and hemicellulose in young plants, cereal grains, and their byproducts when they are included as ingredients of conventional diets. Thus, green leafy vegetables can be used to feed pigs. In the large intestine of growing–finishing pigs, the fermentable fiber contributes 8 kJ/g (e.g., resistant starch [8.8 kJ/g], fructo-oligosaccharides [8.4 kJ/g], and inulin [8.8 kJ/g]) (Eswaran et al. 2013).

## DIGESTION AND ABSORPTION OF CARBOHYDRATES IN FISH

### DIETARY CARBOHYDRATES FOR FISH

The use of dietary carbohydrates by fish depends on species. Omnivorous fish (e.g., the common carp and channel catfish) can digest relatively large amounts of starch and glycogen, and herbivorous fish (e.g., the grass carp) can utilize a primarily vegetarian diet. In addition, hybrid striped bass can efficiently use 25% starch in the diet as a source of glucose and energy (Wu et al. 2015). In contrast, carnivorous fish (e.g., the Atlantic salmon and the Japanese yellowtail) consume little starch, but they do ingest a small amount of glycogen from their diets. The carnivorous fish digest carbohydrates less efficiently than omnivorous or herbivorous fish and cannot tolerate significant quantities of dietary complex carbohydrate. Besides nutritional and metabolic functions, carbohydrates are used to manufacture fish diets, because (1) starch enhances floatability and integrity of extruded pellets due to their expansion and gelatinization during extrusion; and (2) water-insoluble fiber (e.g., cellulose, hemicellulose, or their derivatives) is an effective binding agent to keep feed particles together and maintain pellet quality.

## Digestion of Carbohydrates in Fish

### Digestion of Starch and Glycogen

The fish do not have salivary glands or salivary α-amylase (Rønnestad et al. 2013). Thus, there is little digestion of starch or glycogen in their mouth. In all species of fish, the pancreas synthesizes and secretes α-amylase into the lumen of the intestine to digest starch and glycogen, as in terrestrial animals. However, its enzymatic activity differs greatly among fish species (Bakke et al. 2011). For example, the activity of α-amylase is generally greatest in herbivores, where it is widespread throughout the entire digestive tract. In carnivorous fish (e.g., the Atlantic salmon, rainbow trout, and sea perch), α-amylase activity is low possibly because of its gene mutation. Of note, Frøystad et al. (2006) reported that a peptide segment is deleted from the Atlantic salmon α-amylase and that its specific activity in the intestine is only 0.67% of that for the common carp. In omnivorous fish (e.g., most types of freshwater tilapia), α-amylase activity is generally intermediate between herbivores and carnivores, and its activity is much greater in the pancreas than in the upper part of the intestine. In addition to the pancreas, intestinal bacteria may be a source of α-amylase in the gut of aquatic animals. As for mammals, the products of carbohydrate digestion by α-amylase in fish are di- and oligosaccharides, which are further hydrolyzed by sucrase-isomaltase and maltase-glucoamylase to form monosaccharides (e.g., glucose, fructose, galactose, mannose, xylose, and arabinose).

Dietary intake of starch increases the secretion of pancreatic α-amylase in herbivorous and omnivorous fish, but has little effect in carnivorous fish (Bakke et al. 2011). The digestion of starch and dextrin by carnivorous fish decreases progressively if the content of dietary carbohydrates is >20%. However, the carnivores can utilize up to 60% glucose, sucrose, or lactose in the diet, indicating high disaccharidase activity in their intestine. Thus, like herbivorous and omnivorous fish, carnivorous fish can efficiently digest disaccharides. As reported for land animals, studies with channel catfish and rainbow trout have shown that fish have a higher ability to digest dietary carbohydrates after the ingredients (e.g., corn, wheat) are cooked to alter their structures and matrixes, resulting in complete hydration and swelling. Taken together, it is evident that pancreatic α-amylase activity is the major factor limiting the digestion of dietary starch and glycogen in fish.

### Digestion of β-(1-4)-Linked Carbohydrates

In some species of fish (e.g., carnivores), the gastric and intestinal mucosae synthesize and secrete chitinase (Bakke et al. 2011). This enzyme may also be produced by bacteria present in the gastrointestinal tract. Chitinase cleaves β-(1-4) linkages in chitin to release *N*-acetyl-D-glucosamine. The presence of endogenous chitinase provides an adaptation for certain fish to break down chitin-containing exoskeletons of their prey animals.

Cellulase and β-galactosidase of bacterial origin are present in the gut of most species of carps. However, fish are virtually incapable of hydrolyzing dietary fiber, because they lack cellulase and β-galactosidase in the intestine, just like the stomach and the small intestine of terrestrial animals. This explains the poor ability of fish to digest dietary soybean meal which contains significant levels of the galactosidic oligosaccharides raffinose and stachyose. The nutritive value of soybean meal and other legume seeds can be enhanced if they undergo enzymatic hydrolysis before meal production. It should also be pointed out that the nutritive value of pulses and other legume seeds can likewise be improved for fish since oligosaccharides constitute a large portion of the carbohydrates in legume seeds.

### Overall Digestibility of Starch

In fish, the digestibility of dietary starch is affected by many factors, including: (1) its molecular complexity, origin, degree of gelatinization, and content; (2) species, breeds, age, and health of fish;

and (3) environmental temperatures. For example, in 10 to 25 g rainbow trout raised in 15°C fresh water, the apparent digestibilities of 20% potato starch and 20% dextrin in diets are 69% and 77%, respectively; in 80 g Atlantic salmons raised in 10.2°C sea water, the apparent digestibilities of 10.5%, 14.5%, and 21.3% wheat starch are 88%, 82%, and 75%, respectively; and in 28 g European sea bass raised in 25°C sea water, the apparent digestibilities of 20% raw starch and 20% gelatinized starch in diets are 66% and 95%, respectively (NRC 2011).

### Absorption of Monosaccharides by the Intestine of Fish

Monosaccharides released from the hydrolysis of starch, glycogen, and other complex carbohydrates in the gut are absorbed through transmembrane glucose or fructose transporters into the intestinal epithelial cells in fish, as in mammals (Ferraris 2001). For example, as shown for carnivorous fish (Polakof and Soengas 2013), the gilthead sea bream (Sala-Rabanal et al. 2004), and zebrafish (Castillo et al. 2009), the apical membrane SGLT1 plays a major role in the intestinal absorption of glucose, galactose, xylose, and arabinose into the enterocytes. As in mammals, GLUT1 is also expressed in the apical membrane of fish intestinal enterocytes to absorb some of the luminal glucose (Teerijoki et al. 2000). GLUT5 has been reported to be expressed in the apical membrane of the intestinal enterocytes to absorb D-fructose from the intestinal lumen in fish (Sundell and Rønnestad 2011). The absorbed monosaccharide (e.g., glucose, fructose, galactose, mannose, xylose, or arabinose) exits the enterocytes through their basolateral membrane GLUT2 into the lamina propria where they are taken up into the intestinal venule. Through the blood circulation, the simple sugars move from the venule to the small vein and then to the portal vein. Depending on the species of fish as well as their developmental stage, living environment, and dietary composition, the efficiency of absorption of the monosaccharides from the intestinal lumen into the enterocytes is 95%–99%.

## GLUCOSE METABOLISM IN ANIMAL TISSUES

### Glucose Turnover in the Whole Body

Glucose is actively utilized by all animals. This sugar enters different tissues at different rates and through different major transporters (e.g., GLUT4 in skeletal muscle [except for birds], heart, and adipose tissue; GLU3 in the placenta; and GLUT2 in the liver and pancreas). At a physiologically steady state, the rate of whole-body glucose utilization is equal to the rate of whole-body glucose synthesis. The continuous utilization and synthesis of glucose in the body is known as glucose turnover. Expressed per metabolic body weight ($kg^{0.75}$), rates of whole-body glucose turnover are fairly constant among mammals but relatively high in avian species (Table 5.6). Rates of whole-body glucose turnover are reduced in response to food deprivation because of the lack of exogenous provision of substrates, but are increased under the conditions of pregnancy and lactation due to augmented demands for glucose. This is graphically illustrated from studies with sheep (Table 5.7).

Pathways for glucose metabolism in tissues are the same in animals (including ruminants, nonruminants, and fish), and thus these pathways are highlighted in this section. While catabolism refers to nutrient degradation, anabolism is characterized by nutrient biosynthesis. However, a degradation pathway for one substance can be viewed as a synthetic pathway for another substance. For example, glutamine catabolism in the liver or kidney results in glucose synthesis. While the pathways of glycolysis, glycogen synthesis, and the pentose cycle are present in all tissues, gluconeogenesis is restricted to the liver and kidneys in animals. At present, the quantitative aspects of glucose metabolism in fish are poorly understood, although glucose does not appear to be a major energy source for fish.

**TABLE 5.6**
**Rates of Whole-Body Glucose Turnover in Animals[a]**

| Species | Body Weight (kg) | Concentration of Glucose in Plasma (mM) | Whole-Body Glucose Turnover (g/h) | (g/h/kg BW) | (g/h/kg $BW^{0.75}$) |
|---|---|---|---|---|---|
| Rat | 0.2 | 5.5 | 0.9 | 4.5 | 5.36 |
| Laying hen | 2 | 12 | 1.6 | 0.80 | 0.85 |
| Dog | 15 | 5.0 | 2.5 | 0.17 | 0.26 |
| Sheep | 40 | 3.3 | 4.4 | 0.11 | 0.19 |
| Pig | 59 | 5.5 | 11.8 | 0.20 | 0.30 |
| Human | 71 | 5.0 | 9.1 | 0.13 | 0.22 |
| Horse | 186 | 5.0 | 15.3 | 0.082 | 0.15 |
| Cow | 500 | 3.3 | 30 | 0.060 | 0.12 |

*Source:* Adapted from Bergman, E.N. et al. 1974. *Proc. Fed. Am. Soc. Exp. Biol.* 33:1849–1854; Bergman, E.N. 1983. *World Animal Science*, Vol. 3. Elsevier, New York, NY, 173–196.

*Note:* BW, body weight; $BW^{0.75}$ = metabolic body weight.

[a] The values were obtained from nonruminant mammals and laying hens in the postabsorptive state or from sheep and cows in the fed state.

## Pathway of Glycolysis

### Definition of Glycolysis

Glycolysis is defined as the conversion of glucose into pyruvate. This pathway was discovered by Otto F. Meyerhof, who received the Nobel Prize in Physiology or Medicine in 1922. Glycolysis occurs in the cytosol of all animal cells. In the liver, glycolysis takes place primarily in perivenous

**TABLE 5.7**
**Effects of Fasting, Pregnancy, or Lactation on Whole-Body Glucose Turnover in Sheep[a]**

| Sheep | Body Weight (kg) | Concentrations of Glucose in Plasma (mM) | Glucose Turnover in the Whole Body (g/h) | (g/h/kg BW) | (g/h/kg $BW^{0.75}$) |
|---|---|---|---|---|---|
| | | **Nonpregnant** | | | |
| Fed | 53 | 3.3 | 4.6 | 0.087 | 0.16 |
| Fasted[b] | 53 | 3.0 | 3.0 | 0.057 | 0.12 |
| | | **Pregnant[c]** | | | |
| Fed | 68 | 2.6 | 7.5 | 0.110 | 0.19 |
| Fasted[b] | 71 | 1.6 | 4.6 | 0.064 | 0.13 |
| | | **Lactating (wk 2–4)** | | | |
| Fed | 61 | 3.2 | 13.3 | 0.218 | 0.32 |

*Source:* Adapted from Bergman, E.N. et al. 1974. *Proc. Fed. Am. Soc. Exp. Biol.* 33:1849–1854; Bergman, E.N. 1983. *World Animal Science*, Vol. 3. Elsevier, New York, NY, 173–196.

*Note:* BW, body weight; $BW^{0.75}$ = metabolic body weight.

[a] Nonpregnant or pregnant sheep were not in the lactating state.

[b] Fasted for 3–4 days.

[c] During the last month of twin pregnancy.

hepatocytes. In cells without mitochondria (e.g., mammalian red blood cells and bacteria), pyruvate is reduced by NADH + $H^+$ to lactate (Murray et al. 2001). Under conditions of limited $O_2$ provision, large amounts of lactate are produced in cells with mitochondria. This is also true for certain cells (e.g., lymphocytes, macrophages, and tumors) even though $O_2$ is not limiting. In animals, pyruvate is oxidized to $CO_2$ and water.

### Entry of Glucose into Cells via Different Transporters

Glucose transport is the first step in glucose utilization by the cell. Thus, it is important to understand the systems of glucose transport as described previously. Specifically, the entry of glucose into animal cells occurs via facilitated diffusion, which is an energy-independent process down a concentration gradient. Among 12 distinct facilitative glucose transporters (GLUT1 to GLUT12), GLUT2, GLUT3, and GLUT4 are known to be relatively tissue specific. In polarized epithelial cells such as the enterocyte of the small intestine and the proximal tubule of the kidney, glucose transport across the apical membrane (facing the lumen) into the cell is also carried out by SGLT1 and SGLT2, respectively. In the small intestine and kidneys, glucose is transported from the cytoplasm into the extracellular space mainly by GLUT2, which is located on the basolateral membrane. As a result, SGLT1 and GLUT2 work together to efficiently absorb luminal glucose into venous blood circulation in the small intestine, and SGLT2 and GLU2 to efficiently reabsorb the filtered luminal glucose back to the venous blood in the kidneys. In the livers of animals (including mammals, birds, and fish [Ferraris 2001; Krasnov et al. 2001]), GLUT2 is primarily responsible for both taking up and releasing glucose, depending on the glucose concentration gradient across the plasma membrane. GLUT3 is the major transporter of glucose in the placenta and the neurons of the brain, but is also distributed in some animal tissues (e.g., brain, liver, heart, skeletal muscle, and kidneys). GLUT4 is the major GLUT isoform in the skeletal muscle, heart, and white adipose tissue of mammals and fish (Hall et al. 2006). In these tissues, GLUT4 expression is regulated by insulin at the mRNA and protein levels, and the GLUT4 protein translocates to the plasma membrane in response to insulin. Interestingly, GLUT4 is absent from the skeletal muscle of birds, contributing to elevated concentrations of glucose in their plasma. GLUT-5 (the fructose transporter) is expressed primarily in the small intestine, testes, and placenta but is also present in skeletal muscle, kidneys, brain, and white adipose tissue.

It is difficult to determine the kinetics of glucose transport by individual transport isoforms because of the lack of mammalian cells expressing only a single isoform, with the exception of human erythrocytes. Human erythrocytes express only GLUT1. To overcome the problem of having multiple isoforms of GLUT present in most mammalian cells, *Xenopus laevis oocytes*, which have low levels of endogenous glucose transport and are amenable to the expression of specific transport proteins, have been widely used for measuring the kinetics of glucose transport catalyzed by a single GLUT isoform. Since glucose is readily metabolized by mammalian cells, various nonmetabolizable glucose analogs have been used to measure glucose transport kinetics. For example, 2-deoxyglucose, which can be phosphorylated by hexokinase but not further metabolized, is useful under conditions where phosphorylation is not rate limiting. 3-*O*-Methylglucose is neither phosphorylated nor metabolized by mammalian cells, and thus is the preferred substrate for kinetics analysis. The $K_M$ values (mM) of various glucose transporters for 3-*O*-methylglucose are as follows: GLUT1, 16.9–26.2; GLUT2, 40; GLUT3, 10.6; GLUT4, 1.8–4.8 (Olson and Pessin 1996). Although $K_M$ measurements in oocytes are quantitatively different from those determined for the endogenous glucose transporters, the above data suggest that GLUT3 and GLUT4 have a higher affinity for glucose than GLUT1 and GLUT2. Among the known GLUTs, GLUT2 has the highest $K_M$ for D-glucose, which allows for this transporter to function as a glucose sensor.

### Pathway of Glycolysis

The pathway of glycolysis (also known as the Embden–Meyerhof pathway) is outlined in Figure 5.5. The nonequilibrium reactions of glycolysis are catalyzed by the glucose transport system,

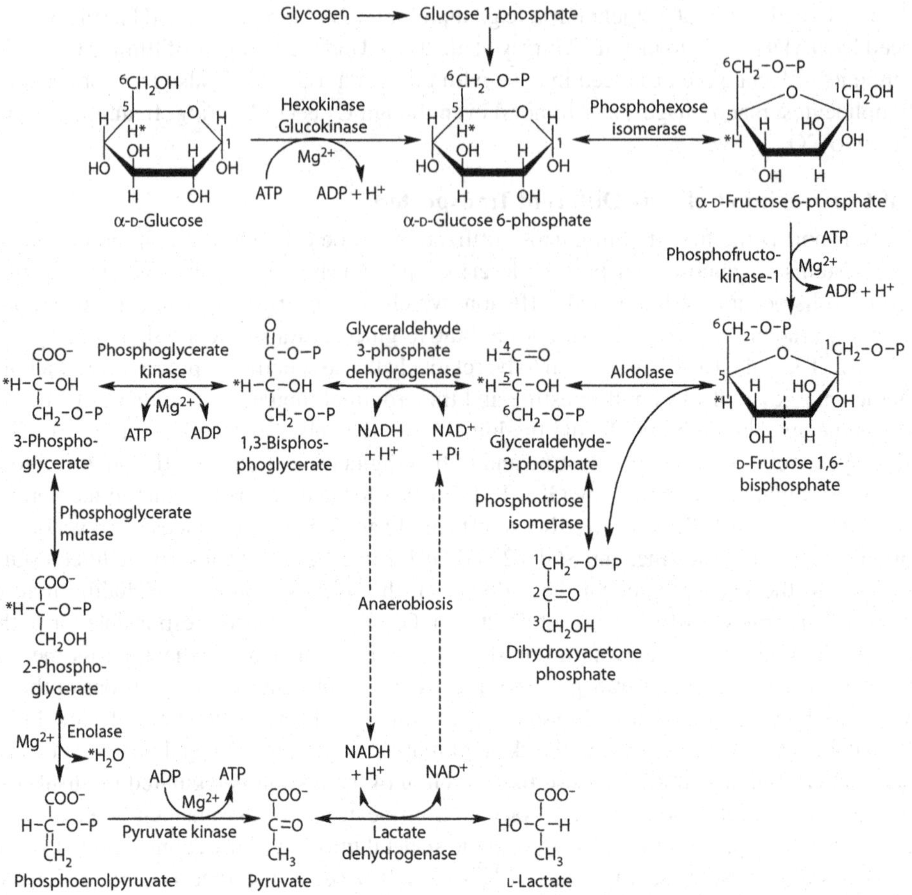

**FIGURE 5.5** Pathway of glycolysis in animal cells. Glycolysis occurs in the cytosol of all animal cells or microorganisms. The conversion of pyruvate to lactate in the cytosol or the oxidation of pyruvate to acetyl-CoA in mitochondria is required to regenerate $NAD^+$ so that glycolysis can proceed. Glycolysis is the sole source of ATP for mammalian red blood cells and a major source of ATP for some animal cells (e.g., cells of the immune system) under aerobic conditions, while providing significant amounts of energy for all animal cells under anaerobic conditions. This pathway is obligatory for complete oxidation of glucose to $CO_2$ and water. Note that glucokinase is also known as hexokinase IV, which is present in the livers of humans, pigs, rats, and many other single-stomached mammals, but is virtually absent from the livers of ruminants, many birds (including chickens), and certain fish species. The numbers 1–6 indicate the position of carbons in molecules. The sign "*" denotes a specific hydrogen atom. (Adapted from Devlin, T.M. 2011. *Textbook of Biochemistry with Clinical Correlations*. John Wiley & Sons, New York, NY.)

hexokinase, phosphofructokinase-1, and pyruvate kinase. The flux-generating step for glycolysis has been considered to be the absorption of glucose from the small intestine or, when glucose arises endogenously, the breakdown of glycogen in the liver. Key regulatory steps of the glycolysis are outlined as follows.

1. *Hexokinase*. In mammalian cells, the phosphorylation of glucose to glucose 6-phosphate is catalyzed by a family of closely related enzymes, called hexokinases. $Mg^{2+}$ is a cofactor for all hexokinase isozymes. Four mammalian hexokinases have been characterized. They are designated as hexokinase (HK) I, II, III, and IV, on the basis of their relative mobility following starch gel electrophoresis (Table 5.8). HK-I is ubiquitous in animal cells, whereas HK-II is primarily present in the skeletal muscle, heart, and adipose tissue. Expression of

**TABLE 5.8**
**Comparison of Enzymatic Kinetics among Hexokinases**

| | GK (HK-IV) | HK I, II, and III |
|---|---|---|
| $K_M$ for glucose | 5–12 mM | 0.02–0.13 mM |
| $K_M$ for ATP | ~ 0.5 mM | 0.2–0.5 mM |
| Ki for G-6-P | 60 mM | 0.2–0.9 mM |
| Molecular weight | 52 kDa | ~100 kDa |
| | **Substrate Preference** | |
| Glucose | 1 | 1 |
| Mannose | 0.8 | 1–1.2 |
| 2-Deoxyglucose | 0.4 | 1–1.4 |
| Fructose | 0.2 | 1.1–1.3 |

*Source:* Adapted from Olson, A.L. and J.E. Pessin. 1996. *Annu. Rev. Nutr.* 16:235–256.

HK-III is relatively low in most tissues, including the lungs, kidneys, and liver. HK I, II, and III can phosphorylate both glucose and fructose, but their enzymatic activity toward fructose is 88% of that toward glucose (Weinhouse 1976).

HK-IV (also known as glucokinase) is specifically expressed in the liver and pancreatic ß-cells, and converts glucose into glucose-6-P as HK I, II and III do, has very low activity toward fructose (Table 5.8), and is inactive toward galactose, allose, sorbitol, xylose, 3-methylglucose, and glucosamine (Weinhouse 1976). There are species differences in the hepatic expression of glucokinase: present at relatively high levels of activity in the livers of common frogs, dogs, guinea pigs, hamsters, humans, mice, monkeys, pigs, rabbits, rats, and turtles; very low or negligible in the livers of cats, goldfish, and finch; and absent from the livers of chickens, nine species of birds, rattlesnake, rainbow trout, and ruminants (e.g., cattle and sheep) (Weinhouse 1976). In those animals that have negligible or no glucokinase activity, their livers have a low ability to catabolize glucose under physiological conditions. For example, only 1.2% of the glucose supplied to the ruminant liver by the combined blood of the portal vein and the hepatic artery is extracted by this organ even under fed conditions (Bergman 1983). This is nutritionally significant for sparing glucose in ruminants which have no absorption of glucose by the small intestine when fed a roughage diet.

HK I, II, and III have relatively low $K_M$ values (<0.2 mM) for glucose and would be saturated by physiological concentrations of this sugar in most cell types, whereas HK-IV has a high $K_M$ value (5–12 mM) for glucose and would respond to elevated glucose concentrations in the plasma after feeding. The differences in tissue expression and kinetics of HK I–IV suggest that each isozyme has a distinct metabolic role. For example, in cattle and sheep, the lack of glucokinase in hepatocytes results in the negligible uptake of glucose by the liver. For nonruminants, since the $K_M$ value of HK-IV for glucose is much higher than that of HK I, II, and III, rates of glucose utilization by the liver are lower than those in skeletal muscle. Thus, when physiological plasma concentration rises in response to feeding, intracellular glucose in skeletal muscle, heart, and adipose tissue is readily phosphorylated by HK-II to form glucose-6-P. This reaction traps glucose inside the cell, because the plasma membrane is not permeable to glucose-6-P. Similarly, during and immediately after consumption of a carbohydrate meal, HK-IV converts glucose into glucose-6-P in the liver of nonruminants. In contrast, when the plasma glucose concentration is reduced during fasting, hepatic HK-IV activity is reduced and the liver is a net producer of glucose from glucogenic substrates. Therefore, HK-IV is a "glucose sensor" in liver, as GLUT2 is in liver and gastrointestinal tissues. This is also true in pancreatic ß-cells.

2. *Phosphofructokinase-1 (PFK-1).* This enzyme catalyzes the conversion of fructose 6-P to fructose 1,6-bisphosphate, and plays a major role in the regulation of the rate of glycolysis (Han et al. 2016). Phosphofructokinase-1 is an allosteric and inducible enzyme. As noted in Chapter 1, an allosteric enzyme is an enzyme whose activity at the catalytic site may be modulated by the presence of allosteric effectors at an allosteric site. "Allosteric" means "occupy another space."
3. *Pyruvate kinase.* Pyruvate kinase catalyzes the transfer of a phosphate group from phosphoenolpyruvate (PEP) to ADP, generating one molecule of pyruvate and one molecule of ATP. This enzyme requires $Mg^{2+}$ as a cofactor and has two isoforms: type M (muscle) and type L/R (liver and erythrocyte). The isozymes differ in their primary structures.

### Energetics and Significance of Glycolysis

The conversion of 1 mol of glucose to 2 mol of pyruvate is accompanied by the net production of 2 mol of ATP (see the calculations below), and by the reduction of 2 mol of $NAD^+$ to NADH + $H^+$. As noted previously, glycolysis is the only metabolic pathway for ATP production by all cells without mitochondria regardless of oxygen supply. In mitochondria-containing cells, glycolysis allows for the catabolism of glucose into pyruvate. The energetic efficiency of glycolysis is low.

Overall reaction of glycolysis:

$$\text{D-Glucose} + 2\,P_i + 2\,\text{ADP} + 2\,\text{NAD}^+ \rightarrow 2\,\text{Pyruvate} + 2\,\text{NADH} + 2\,H^+ + 2\,\text{ATP} + 2\,H_2O$$

1 mol of ATP is required for phosphorylation of D-glucose:

$$\text{Glucose} + \text{ATP} \rightarrow \text{Glucose 6-phosphate} + \text{ADP (Hexokinase)}$$

1 mol of ATP is required for phosphorylation of D-fructose 6-phosphate:

$$\text{Fructose 6-phosphate} + \text{ATP} \rightarrow \text{Fructose 1,6-bisphosphate} + \text{ADP (PFK-1)}$$

2 mol of ATP are produced from conversion of 2 mol of 1,3-bisphosphoglycerate to 3 phosphoglycerate (catalyzed by phosphoglycerate kinase):

$$2\,\text{(1,3-Bisphosphoglycerate)} + 2\,\text{ADP} \leftrightarrow 2\,\text{(3-Phosphoglycerate)} + 2\,\text{ATP}$$

2 mol of ATP are produced from conversion of 2 mol of PEP to pyruvate:

$$2\,\text{PEP} + 2\,\text{ADP} \rightarrow 2\,\text{Pyruvate} + 2\,\text{ATP}$$

Net production of ATP from the conversion of 1 mol of glucose to 2 mol of pyruvate:

$$2 + 2 - 1 - 1 = 2\text{ mol of ATP}$$

Glycolysis is of nutritional and physiological significance for animals. Specifically, this pathway provides ATP for: (1) all animal cells under hypoxic conditions; (2) microorganisms under anaerobic conditions; (3) some animal cells (e.g., cells of the immune system) under aerobic conditions; and (4) red blood cells of mammals as the sole source of energy. Glycolysis is also obligatory for complete oxidation of glucose to $CO_2$ and water and plays a role in regulating glucose homeostasis in mitochondria-containing cells. Furthermore, 2,3-bisphosphoglycerate, which is an intermediate in glycolysis, stabilizes the tetrameric structure of hemoglobin and modulates its binding affinity for $O_2$. Finally, glycolysis supplies intermediates for synthetic pathways: (1) glucose-6-P, which is a precursor of ribose-5-P required for synthesis of purine and pyrimidine nucleotides; (2) glycerol-3-P and dihydroxyacetone phosphate, which are precursors for the synthesis of triacylglycerols and phosphoglycerols; and (3) fructose-6-P, which is a precursor for the synthesis of glucosamine-6-P by glutamine:fructose-6-P amidotransferase (cytosolic). This enzyme is now referred to as glutamine:fructose-6-P transaminase. Glucosamine-6-P is the substrate for the synthesis of

UDP-*N*-acetylglucosamine, a precursor for the formation of all macromolecules containing amino sugars in cells. In postnatal animals, glucosamine-6-P may mediate tissue insensitivity to insulin in type II-diabetes mellitus and diabetes-associated cardiovascular abnormalities.

$$\text{Fructose 6-P} + \text{Glutamine} \rightarrow \text{Glucosamine 6-P} + \text{Glutamate}$$

### Conversion of Pyruvate into Lactate and the Cori Cycle

In cells without mitochondria, pyruvate is converted into lactate by lactate dehydrogenase, with the oxidation of NADH to $NAD^+$. This reaction also takes place in mitochondria-containing cells (e.g., immunocytes and tumors) under anaerobic conditions. The conversion of pyruvate to lactate allows for the regeneration of $NAD^+$ so that glycolysis proceeds in cells.

$$\text{D-Glucose} + 2\ \text{ADP} + 2\ P_i \rightarrow 2\ \text{L-Lactate} + 2\ \text{ATP} + 2\ H_2O$$

$$\text{Pyruvate} + \text{NADH} + H^+ \leftrightarrow \text{Lactate} + NAD^+$$

In 1929, G.F. Cori and G. Cori proposed that the lactate is released from the skeletal muscle and is taken up by the liver where it is converted to glucose. The lactate-derived glucose is taken up by the muscle. This pathway was named the Cori cycle and recognized with the Nobel Prize in Physiology or Medicine in 1947. It is now known that cells other than skeletal muscle, including lymphocytes and macrophages, also actively convert glucose into lactate and release lactate. There is no net production of glucose from lactate via the Cori cycle.

### Conversion of Pyruvate into Lactate or Ethanol

Under anaerobic conditions, pyruvate is converted to lactate by lactate dehydrogenase, and to ethanol by pyruvate decarboxylase (cytosolic and mitochondrial) and alcohol dehydrogenase in yeast, with the oxidation of NADH to $NAD^+$. The conversion of pyruvate to ethanol allows for the regeneration of $NAD^+$ so that glycolysis proceeds to increase ethanol production.

$$\text{Pyruvate} \rightarrow \text{Acetaldehyde} + CO_2 \quad \text{(Yeast)}$$

$$\text{Acetaldehyde} + \text{NADH} + H^+ \leftrightarrow \text{Ethanol} + NAD^+ \quad \text{(Yeast)}$$

### Cytosolic Redox State in Animal Cells

L-Lactate dehydrogenase (a cytosolic enzyme) catalyzes the interconversion of L-lactate and pyruvate. The equilibrium constant ($K_{eq}$) of this reaction is calculated as follows:

$$\text{Pyruvate} + \text{NADH} + H^+ \leftrightarrow \text{L-Lactate} + NAD^+$$

$$K_{eq} = ([\text{L-Lactate}] \times [NAD^+])/([\text{Pyruvate}] \times [\text{NADH}] \times [H^+])$$

Since $K_{eq}$ is a constant and intracellular pH is constant under normal physiological conditions, an increase in the ratio of [L-Lactate]/[Pyruvate] is equivalent to that of [NADH]/[$NAD^+$]. Since this reaction occurs in the cytosol, the [L-lactate]/[Pyruvate] ratio is a useful indicator of the cytosolic redox state (i.e., [NADH]/[$NAD^+$] ratio) in animal cells. When intracellular pH fluctuates considerably, [$H^+$] must be included in the calculation of $K_{eq}$.

### Glycolysis and Cell Proliferation

All cultured cells have a high rate of glycolysis even in the presence of adequate amounts of oxygen, which is referred to as aerobic glycolysis. Cell proliferation is associated with an enhanced rate of glycolysis and, therefore, $H^+$ production. Cells cannot divide or grow in the absence of glucose. In mitogen-stimulated lymphocytes (e.g., thymocytes) with a rapid rate of proliferation, increased cytosolic regeneration of $NAD^+$ by enhanced expression of lactate dehydrogenase effectively competes with the transport of NADH into the mitochondrion. Since glycolysis does not generate reactive oxygen species (ROS), highly proliferating cells can avoid oxidative stress.

### Pasteur Effect in Animal Cells

A Pasteur effect refers to the inhibition of glycolysis by aerobic oxidation in mitochondria-containing cells. This phenomenon, which was discovered in 1857 by Louis Pasteur, results from the inhibition of phosphofructokinase-1 by ATP and citrate that are produced by aerobic oxidation via the Krebs cycle. In other words, when oxygen concentration is low, glucose-derived pyruvate is converted into lactate (or ethanol plus carbon dioxide). When oxygen concentration is high, pyruvate is oxidized to acetyl-CoA that enters the Krebs cycle for oxidation to $CO_2$ and water, thereby inhibiting glycolysis.

### Warburg Effect

Some cells (e.g., tumors, activated macrophages, and proliferating lymphocytes) prefer to metabolize glucose through glycolysis even in the presence of ample oxygen. This phenomenon is known as the Warburg effect. In cancer cells, drivers for the metabolic derangements include: (1) adaptation to the extracellular microenvironment (low pH and low $pO_2$); and/or (2) aberrant signaling of oncogene activation (p53, Myc, Ras, Akt, and HIF). Metabolic advantages are to (1) increase rates of biosynthesis of nucleotides, lipids, and proteins; (2) avoid apoptosis by reducing the production of ROS through the mitochondrial electron transport system; and (3) participate in local metabolite-based paracrine and autocrine signaling. Adverse outcomes of the Warburg effect are the production of large amounts of metabolites (e.g., lactate from glucose) and the wasting of body energy reserves (e.g., formation of glucose from proteins and AAs, such as glutamine and alanine).

### Quantification of Glycolysis in Animal Cells

Under anaerobic conditions, the accumulation of lactate is a valid indicator of the rate of glycolysis. Under aerobic conditions, glycolysis is usually measured with use of [5-$^3$H]glucose (Wu and Thompson 1988). This is based on the principle that (1) 1 mole of $^3H_2O$ is produced from 1 mole of [5-$^3$H]glucose via glycolysis; and (2) the $^3H_2O$ produced is extensively diluted by intracellular and extracellular $H_2O$, so that reincorporation of $^3H_2O$ into metabolic pathways is negligible. Note that the use of [2-$^3$H]glucose to measure glycolysis is invalid, because [2-$^3$H]glucose-6-P loses its $^3$H in its conversion to Fructose-6-P catalyzed by phosphoglucoisomerase. Indeed, the rate of detritiation of [2-$^3$H]glucose is commonly used to estimate the rate of glucose phosphorylation in intact cells (Van Schaftingen 1995).

### Regulation of Glycolysis

Glycolysis can be regulated at the steps of glucose transport, hexokinase, PFK-1, and pyruvate kinase (Table 5.9). This is an excellent example for the concept of "distributive metabolic control." For example, fructose-1,6-bisphosphate is an allosteric activator of pyruvate kinase in tissues (e.g., liver and skeletal muscle), therefore serving as a positive feed-forward regulator. Since a persistent high concentration of glucose in the plasma of fasting subjects (hyperglycemia, >6.1 mM) is a diagnostic indicator of diabetes mellitus (a serious metabolic disease), extensive research has been conducted on glucose metabolism in mammalian cells. The near absence of glucose-stimulated insulin secretion is the common feature of insulin-dependent (Type 1) diabetes mellitus (IDDM), whereas patients with noninsulin-dependent (Type 2) diabetes mellitus (NIDDM) can still produce insulin or even more insulin early in the disease. The discovery of insulin and its role in stimulating glycolysis led to the award of the Nobel Prize in Physiology or Medicine to Frederick G. Banting in 1921.

### Transfer of NADH from the Cytosol into Mitochondria

Under aerobic conditions that favor the oxidation of pyruvate, the NADH generated from the pathway of glycolysis enters mitochondria for oxidation. Since NADH cannot penetrate the inner mitochondrial membrane, it is transported into the mitochondria via the glycerophosphate shuttle

**TABLE 5.9**
**Regulation of Glycolysis in Animal Cells**

| | Activation or Induction | Inhibition or Suppression |
|---|---|---|
| GLUT-1 | Phorbol esters, sulfonylureas, vanadate, butyrate, glucose, hypoxia, cAMP, serum, thyroid hormones, insulin, IGF-1, PDFG, FGF, growth hormone, TGF-ß, oncogenes | Rubusoside (a phytochemical), forskolin, cytochalasin B |
| GLUT-2 | Glucose, protein kinase C | Diabetes, forskolin, cytochalasin B |
| GLUT-4 | Insulin, muscle contraction, cAMP | Diabetes, food deprivation, forskolin, cytochalasin B |
| GLUT-5 | Fructose, glucocorticoids, thyroid hormones | Phytochemicals (rubusoside and astragalin-6-glucoside) |
| HK-1, 2, 3 | Hypoxia-inducible factors and Akt | Glucose-6-P and Pi |
| Glucokinase | Insulin, carbohydrate feeding | Glucagon, cAMP, diabetes, food deprivation, glucosamine |
| PFK-1 | Insulin, carbohydrate feeding, AMP, Pi, fructose-6-P, fructose-2,6-bisphosphate | Citrate, ATP, cAMP glucagon, diabetes, fast |
| Pyruvate kinase | Insulin, carbohydrate feeding, fructose, fructose-1-6-bisphosphate | ATP, alanine, glucagon, diabetes, food deprivation |

*Note:* Akt, protein kinase B; IGF-1: insulin-like growth factor-1; PDFG: platelet-derived growth factor; FGF: fibroblast growth factor; TGF-ß: transforming growth factor-ß.

(Figure 5.6) and the malate shuttle (Figure 5.7). In the glycerophosphate shuttle, mitochondrial glycerol 3-phosphate dehydrogenase is a flavoprotein with FAD rather than NAD as the cofactor, and the formation of $FADH_2$ from FAD is coupled with the conversion of glycerol-3-P to dihydroxyacetone-P. As a result, only 1.5 rather than 2.5 mol of ATP are produced for oxidation of 1 mol of cytosolic NADH. This shuttle is present at high activity in insect flight muscles. However, in mammals and birds, the expression of mitochondrial glycerol 3-phosphate dehydrogenase is highly variable in tissues, as the activity of this enzyme is present in the brain, brown adipose tissue, liver, and white skeletal muscle but is deficient in the heart and many other tissues (Mráček et al. 2013). The malate shuttle involves malate, glutamate, and aspartate, and the complexity of this system is

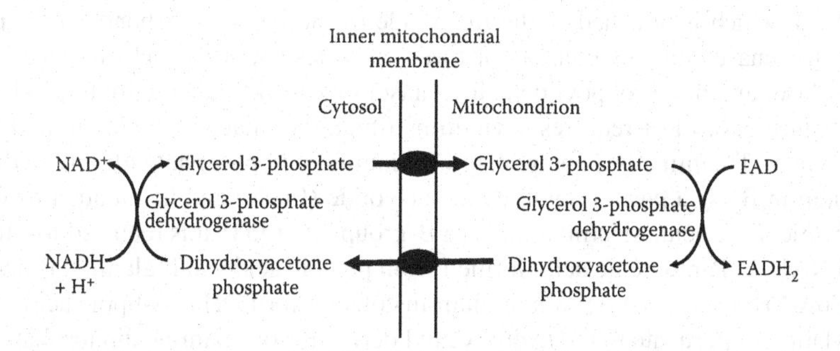


**FIGURE 5.6** The glycerophosphate shuttle for the transport of NADH from the cytosol into mitochondria in animal cells. This shuttle requires cytosolic and mitochondrial glycerol 3-phosphate dehydrogenases, which are different proteins and are encoded by different genes. The glycerophosphate shuttle is highly active in insect flight muscles, but occurs in mammals and birds in a tissue-specific manner. In these vertebrates, expression of mitochondrial glycerol 3-phosphate dehydrogenase is highly variable, with its enzyme activity being present in the liver, brain, brown adipose tissue, white adipose tissue, and white skeletal muscle, but being deficient in the heart and many other tissues.

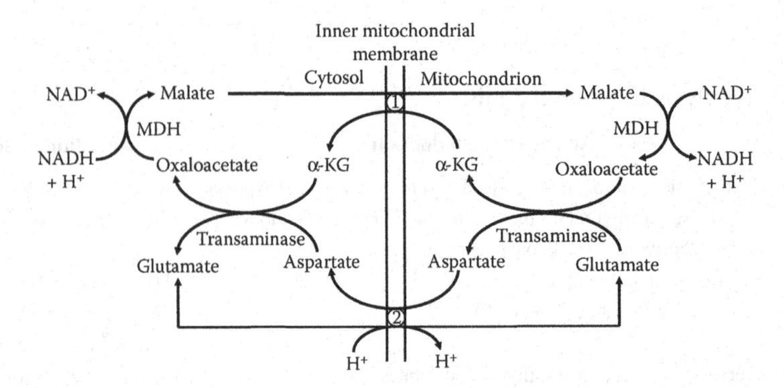


**FIGURE 5.7** The malate shuttle for the transport of NADH from the cytosol into mitochondria in animal cells. This shuttle requires glutamate and aspartate, as well as cytosolic and mitochondrial malate dehydrogenases (MDH), and is widely present at high activity in the cells and tissues of all animals. In vertebrates (e.g., mammals and birds), the malate shuttle is of more universal utility than the glycerophosphate shuttle for transporting NADH from the cytosol into mitochondria. α-KG, α-ketoglutarate.

due to the impermeability of the mitochondrial membrane to OAA. The malate shuttle is widely present in cells and tissues of all animals and is considered to be of more universal utility than the glycerophosphate shuttle in vertebrates (Ying 2008). In the heart, the malate shuttle is the dominant pathway for transporting NADH from the cytosol into mitochondria, with its activity being 10-fold or greater than that of the glycerophosphate shuttle. When NADH is transported into mitochondria via the malate shuttle, it is oxidized via the electron transport system to produce 2.5 mol of ATP per mol NADH. However, when NADH is transported into mitochondria via the glycerophosphate shuttle, it is oxidized via the electron transport system to produce 1.5 mol of ATP per mol NADH.

## Mitochondrial Oxidation of Pyruvate to Acetyl-CoA

Pyruvate can be produced from glucose, lactate, and most AAs (e.g., alanine, serine, cysteine, threonine, glycine, glutamine, glutamate, aspartate, and asparagine). If pyruvate is formed in the cytosol (e.g., in glycolysis), it must be transported into the mitochondria via a pyruvate or monocarboxylic acid transporter. Within the mitochondrion, pyruvate undergoes oxidative decarboxylation to acetyl-CoA by the pyruvate dehydrogenase complex (often simply referred to as pyruvate dehydrogenase, PDH), which is attached to the inner side of the inner mitochondrial membrane. The pyruvate dehydrogenase complex consists of three enzymes (pyruvate dehydrogenase, dihydrolipoyl transacetylase, and dihydrolipoyl dehydrogenase) that work sequentially to produce $CO_2$ and acetyl-CoA (Figure 5.8). PDH requires 4 vitamins (thiamine, niacin, riboflavin, and pantothenic acid) as coenzymes. Thiamine is a component of thiamine pyrophosphate (thiamine diphosphate). Riboflavin (vitamin $B_2$) is a part of flavin mononucleotide (FMN) and flavin adenine dinucleotide (FAD). Niacin (nicotinic acid, nicotinamide) is a B-group vitamin that is required for the formation of $NAD^+$ and $NADP^+$. Pantothenic acid (formed from pantoic acid and ß-alanine) is needed for the synthesis of CoA-SH (coenzyme A). A non-vitamin cofactor for PDH is α-lipoic acid.

Decarboxylation of pyruvate to the hydroxyethyl derivative of thiamine diphosphate (TPP):

$$\text{Pyruvate} + \text{TPP} \rightarrow CO_2 + \text{Hydroxyethyl-TPP (Pyruvate dehydrogenase)}$$

Transfer of acetyl group from hydroxyethyl-TDP to CoA-SH to from acetyl-CoA:

$$\text{Hydroxyethyl-TDP} + \text{Oxidized lipoamide} \rightarrow \text{Acetyl lipoamide}$$

$$\text{Acetyl lipoamide} + \text{CoA-SH} \rightarrow \text{Acetyl CoA} + \text{Dihydrolipoamide (reduced lipoamide)}$$

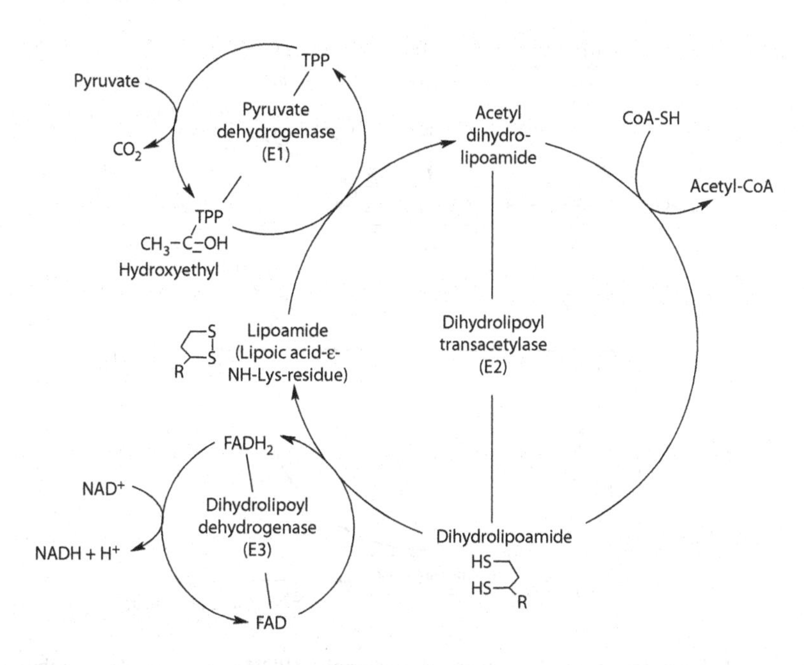


**FIGURE 5.8** The pyruvate dehydrogenase complex in animal cells. This enzyme complex consists of three different proteins that work together to decarboxylate pyruvate and generate acetyl-CoA in mitochondria. Thiamine, $NAD^+$, FAD, and CoA are required as cofactors for the indicated enzymes. TPP, thiamine pyrophosphate (thiamine diphosphate). E1–E3, enzymes 1–3. (Adapted from Murray, R.K. et al. 2001. *Harper's Review of Biochemistry*. Appleton & Lange, Norwalk, Connecticut.)

The above two steps are catalyzed by dihydrolipoyl transacetylase.

Dihydrolipoamide is converted to oxidized lipoamide by dihydrolipoyl dehydrogenase that requires FAD and $NAD^+$ as coenzymes:

$$\text{Dihydrolipoamide} + \text{FAD} \rightarrow \text{Oxidized lipoamide} + \text{FADH}_2$$

$$\text{FADH}_2 + \text{NAD}^+ \rightarrow \text{FAD} + \text{NADH} + \text{H}^+$$

$$\text{Net reaction: Pyruvate} + \text{NAD}^+ + \text{CoA} \rightarrow \text{CO}_2 + \text{Acetyl-CoA} + \text{NADH} + \text{H}^+$$

Pyruvate dehydrogenase in cells is regulated by end-product inhibition and covalent protein modification via cAMP-dependent phosphorylation and phosphatase-catalyzed dephosphorylation (Figure 5.9). The conversion of dephosphorylated PDH (active form) to phosphorylated PDH (inactive form) is catalyzed by PDH kinase. PDH phosphatase converts the inactive form to the active form of PDH. PDH is inactive in a phosphorylated form but is active in its dephosphorylated form. Thus, glucagon inhibits pyruvate oxidation by PDH, thereby promoting the conversion of pyruvate into glucose in hepatocytes.

## Oxidation of Acetyl-CoA via the Mitochondrial Krebs Cycle and ATP Synthesis

### Overall Reaction of the Krebs Cycle

As indicated in Chapter 1, a metabolic cycle is defined as the process in which an overall chemical change is brought about by a cyclic reaction sequence. A metabolic cycle has a high efficiency, because there is no production of "wasteful" byproducts. The Krebs cycle is a great example. This metabolic cycle was discovered by Dr. Hans Krebs in 1937, for which he was awarded the Nobel Prize in Physiology or Medicine in 1953.

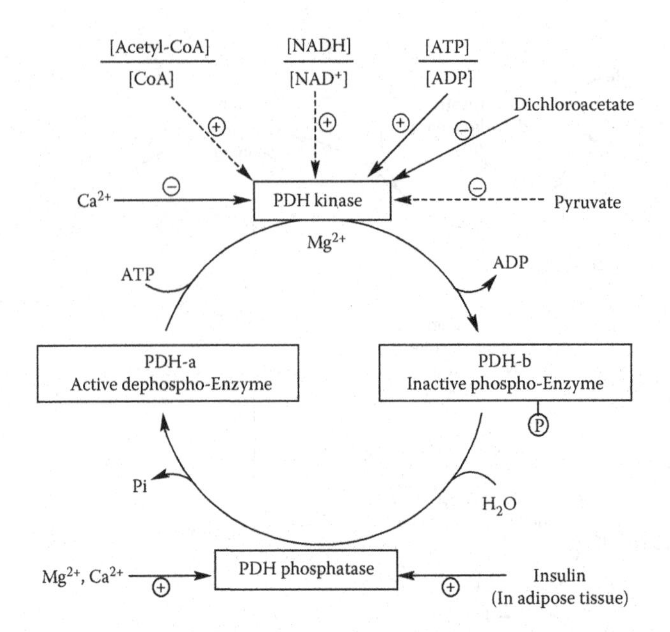


**FIGURE 5.9** Regulation of the pyruvate dehydrogenase complex (PDH) by end-product inhibition and covalent protein modification in animal cells. PDH activity is regulated by protein phosphorylation (inactive state, b form) by PDH kinase and dephosphorylation (active state, a form) by PDH phosphatase. Factors (e.g., insulin, $Mg^{2+}$, and $Ca^{2+}$) that activate PDH phosphatase, as well as factors (e.g., pyruvate, $Ca^{2+}$, and dichloroacetate) that inhibit PDH kinase and enhance pyruvate decarboxylation. In contrast, factors (e.g., high ratios of ATP/ADP, NADH/$NAD^+$, and acetyl-CoA/CoA, which are indicators of high-energy levels in cells) reduce pyruvate decarboxylation by stimulating PDH kinase. The signs (+) and (–) denote activation and inhibition, respectively. (Adapted from Devlin, T.M. 2011. *Textbook of Biochemistry with Clinical Correlations*. John Wiley & Sons, New York, NY.)

The Krebs cycle was worked out with the use of *in vitro* preparations of pigeon pectoral muscle. All the constituent enzymes of the Krebs cycle are located within the matrix of the mitochondria, with the exception of succinate dehydrogenase which is located on the inner surface of the inner mitochondrial membrane. Thus, all reactions of the Krebs cycle occur in the mitochondria, with oxaloacetate (OAA) combining acetyl-CoA to form citrate (Chapter 1). The overall reaction of the Krebs cycle is summarized as follows:

$$\text{Acetyl-CoA} + 3NAD^+ + FAD + GDP + Pi + 2H_2O \rightarrow 2CO_2 + 3NADH + FADH_2 + GTP + CoA + 3H^+$$

where $NAD^+$ is the oxidized form of nicotinamide adenine dinucleotide, FAD is flavin adenine dinucleotide, and CoA (or simply CoA) is coenzyme A. The intermediates of the Krebs cycle are neither formed nor destroyed in the net operation of the cycle. For the net oxidation of glucose, AAs and fatty acids, they have to be converted to acetyl-CoA. Note that some of the intermediates can exit the mitochondria into the cytosol for participation in other metabolic pathways, such as glucose and AA synthesis.

## Production of ATP and Water in Mitochondria

NADH and $FADH_2$ are produced from acetyl-CoA oxidation in the Krebs cycle. These reducing equivalents are oxidized via the mitochondrial respiratory chain to produce ATP and water, as described in Chapter 1. Briefly, oxidation and phosphorylation are tightly coupled in the respiratory chain, which contains three sites for the synthesis of ATP from ADP plus Pi by ATP synthase.

According to Mitchell's chemiosmotic theory on the mechanism of oxidative phosphorylation, oxidation of reducing equivalents in the respiratory chain generates protons ($H^+$) that are ejected from the mitochondrial matrix into the intermembrane space. The electrochemical potential difference resulting from the asymmetric distribution of $H^+$ across the mitochondrial membrane is used to drive the formation of ATP from ADP plus Pi. At the terminal step of the electron transport system, two $H^+$ ions accept ½ $O_2$ to generate $H_2O$.

Oxidation of 1 mol of NADH to $H_2O$ results in production of 2.5 mol of ATP:

$$\text{NADH} + \text{H}^+ + 1/2\ \text{O}_2 + 2.5\ \text{ADP} + 2.5\ \text{Pi} \rightarrow \text{NAD}^+ + \text{H}_2\text{O} + 2.5\ \text{ATP};$$

$$\text{P/O ratio} = 2.5$$

Oxidation of 1 mol of $FADH_2$ to $H_2O$ results in production of 1.5 mol of ATP:

$$\text{FADH}_2 + 1/2\ \text{O}_2 + 1.5\ \text{ADP} + 1.5\ \text{Pi} \rightarrow \text{FAD} + \text{H}_2\text{O} + 1.5\ \text{ATP};$$

$$\text{P/O ratio} = 1.5$$

## Energetics of Acetyl-CoA Oxidation

The reactions for the generation of NADH and $FADH_2$ via the Krebs cycle are as follows:

Isocitrate + $NAD^+$ ↔ α-KG + $CO_2$ + NADH + $H^+$ (2.5 ATP)
α-KG + $NAD^+$ + CoASH → Succinyl-CoA + $CO_2$ + NADH + $H^+$ (2.5 ATP)
Succinyl-CoA + GDP + Pi ↔ Succinate + CoASH + GTP
GTP + ADP ↔ ATP + GDP (1 ATP)
Succinate + FAD ↔ Fumarate + $FADH_2$ (1.5 ATP)
Malate + $NAD^+$ ↔ OAA + NADH + $H^+$ (2.5 ATP)

Thus, net 10 mol ATP are produced from the oxidation of 1 mol acetyl-CoA in cells.

## Energetics of Glucose Oxidation in Aerobic Respiration

In aerobic respiration, the complete oxidation of 1 mol of glucose to 6 mol of $CO_2$ and 6 mol of $H_2O$ produces 30 mol of ATP when the cytosolic NADH is transported into mitochondria via the glycerophosphate shuttle. The amount of ATP produced is 32 mol per 1 mol of glucose when the cytosolic NADH is transported into the mitochondria via the malate shuttle. To be more conservative, nutritionists usually use the value of 30 mol ATP/mol glucose to calculate the energetic efficiency of glucose oxidation in animals (McDonald et al. 2011).

1 mol of Glucose → 2 mol of Pyruvate via glycolysis (2 ATP, net)
Oxidation of 2 mol of NADH produced from glucose via glycolysis (3 or 5 ATP)
2 mol Pyruvate → 2 mol Acetyl-CoA (5 ATP)
Oxidation of 2 mol of acetyl-CoA in the Krebs cycle (20 ATP)

## Nutritional and Physiological Significance of the Krebs Cycle in Animals

1. *Oxidation of glucose, fatty acids, and AAs to $CO_2$.* When amounts of dietary carbohydrates, fats, and proteins plus AAs exceed the needs for synthetic pathways in animals, these nutrients are oxidized to $CO_2$ by conversion to acetyl-CoA and its subsequent oxidation via the Krebs cycle. $CO_2$ is then expelled from the body through respiration. This is the major mechanism for the irreversible loss of energy substrates from organisms. Thus, the major function of the Krebs cycle is to oxidize acetyl-CoA.

2. *ATP production.* ATP is the major form of chemical energy in cells. Oxidation of acetyl-CoA via the Krebs cycle produces not only $CO_2$ but also NADH, $FADH_2$, and GTP. GTP and ATP are interconverted by nucleoside diphosphate kinase (GTP + ADP ↔ GDP + ATP). The oxidation of NADH and $FADH_2$ via the mitochondrial respiratory chain results in the generation of ATP, with $O_2$ serving as the final oxidant of reducing equivalents to produce $H_2O$. This reaction eliminates the hydrogen atoms in dietary carbohydrates, fats, and proteins plus AAs. The mitochondrial oxidation of acetyl-CoA is the major source of energy in all animal cells with aerobic respiration. Thus, in aerobic respiration, the Krebs cycle plays an essential role in converting food energy into biological energy (ATP) for animals. Of note, glucose is the exclusive metabolic fuel for the brain in both fed and postabsorptive states. Interestingly, concentrations of glucose in plasma are positively correlated with the size of the brain (Table 5.10). The absence (anoxia) or partial deficiency (hypoxia) of $O_2$ causes total or partial inhibition of the Krebs cycle.

   AMP is a good indicator of cellular energy deficiency, as increased hydrolysis of ATP results in the rapid accumulation of ADP and then AMP in cells (ATP → ADP + Pi → AMP + 2Pi). The energy charge of the adenylate pool is a better measure of energy status in cells than the concentration of a single nucleotide. ADP can be converted by adenylate kinase (also called myokinase) into ATP (2ADP ↔ ATP + AMP). Thus, based on the metabolism of these nucleotides, adenylate energy charge in cells can be calculated as (ATP + 0.5 ADP)/(ATP + ADP + AMP).
3. *Central role in cell metabolism.* Acetyl-CoA is a common metabolite of glucose, AAs, and fatty acids in intracellular compartmentalized reactions. Thus, the Krebs cycle is at the center of metabolism in animals. Some metabolic pathways end with the formation of constituents of the Krebs cycle, while other pathways originate from the cycle. Examples include gluconeogenesis, fatty acid synthesis, as well as the transamination, deamination, and synthesis of AAs. Therefore, the Krebs cycle plays an important role in both oxidative and synthetic processes; specifically, it is an amphibolic pathway that involves both catabolism and anabolism in the same cell.

### Metabolic Control of the Krebs Cycle

Oxidation of acetyl-CoA via the Krebs cycle is regulated by the availability of OAA and at several other stages, which include citrate synthase, isocitrate dehydrogenase, and α-KG dehydrogenase (Chapter 1).

**TABLE 5.10**
**The Size of the Brain Is Inversely Correlated with Glucose Concentration in the Plasma of Healthy, Postabsorptive Animals**

| Species | Size of Brain (% of Body Weight) | Concentrations of Glucose in Plasma (mM) |
|---|---|---|
| Chicken | 6 | 12–15 |
| Pig | 2 | 5.0–5.5 |
| Human | 2 | 5.0–5.5 |
| Cattle | 0.2 | 2.5–3.4 |
| Sheep | 0.2 | 2.5–3.4 |

*Source:* Adapted from Bell, D.J. and B.M. Freeman. 1971. *Physiology and Biochemistry of the Domestic Fowl*, Vol. 2. Academic Press, New York, NY; Bergman, E.N. 1983. *World Animal Science*, Vol. 3. Elsevier, New York, NY, 173–196; Swenson, M.J. and W.O. Reece. 1984. *Duke's Physiology of Domestic Animals*. Cornell University Press, Ithaca, New York

Like PDH, the activity of α-KG dehydrogenase is also regulated by protein phosphorylation (inactive state) and dephosphorylation (active state). The factors that regulate the activity of these enzymes include citrate, $Ca^{2+}$, ADP, $NAD^+$/NADH, ATP, and CoA. When the production of acetyl-CoA from glucose exceeds its oxidation, the acetyl-CoA is diverted to the synthesis of fatty acids in the liver and adipose tissue. If the production of acetyl-CoA from fatty acids exceeds its oxidation, the acetyl-CoA is used for the synthesis of ketone bodies in the liver. When the liver produces excessive amounts of ketone bodies, severe ketoacidosis occurs, as in cows during the first month of lactation and in sheep during late (e.g., the last four weeks) gestation. In both cases, reduced voluntary feed intake by the mothers, despite an increased demand for energy to support milk production or fetal growth, results in the increased mobilization of maternal fats to generate ketone bodies. The ketoacidosis in ruminants can be treated with the intravenous administration of propionate, OAA, or glucose.

### Isotopic Tracing of the Krebs Cycle

Labeled tracers are essential to study energy-substrate oxidation via the Krebs cycle. Therefore, it is imperative to understand the patterns of labeling in intermediates and products. When [1-$^{14}$C] acetyl-CoA (meaning that the C-1 of acetyl-CoA is labeled with $^{14}$C) is introduced into the Krebs cycle only once, it is condensed with OAA to form [5-$^{14}$C]citrate, [5-$^{14}$C]cis-aconitate, [5-$^{14}$C]isocitrate, [5-$^{14}$C]α-ketoglutarate (α-KG), [4-$^{14}$C]succinyl-CoA, [4-$^{14}$C]succinate, and [1,4-$^{14}$C]succinate. [1,4-$^{14}$C]Succinate is formed due to the "isotope randomization" of this molecule, because it is a symmetric compound and succinate dehydrogenase does not differentiate between its two carboxyl groups. [1,4-$^{14}$C]Succinate leads to [1,4-$^{14}$C]fumarate, [1,4-$^{14}$C]malate, and [1,4-$^{14}$C]OAA formation. Thus, during the first turn of the cycle, there is no $^{14}CO_2$ produced. Note that two carbon atoms are lost as $CO_2$ in one revolution of the Krebs cycle. However, they are not derived from the acetyl-CoA that has immediately entered the cycle, but from the portion of the citrate molecule that is derived from OAA. After the first turn of the cycle, the OAA that is regenerated is now labeled as [1,4-$^{14}$C] OAA. [1,4-$^{14}$C]OAA is condensed with unlabeled acetyl-CoA to form [1,6-$^{14}$C]citrate, [1,6-$^{14}$C]oxalosuccinate, and [1-$^{14}$C]α-KG, with 50% of $^{14}CO_2$ being lost as $^{14}$CO. [1-$^{14}$C]α-KG is decarboxylated to succinyl-CoA with another 50% of $^{14}$C being lost as $^{14}CO_2$. Thus, 100% of $^{14}$C is lost as $^{14}CO_2$ during the second turn of the Krebs cycle.

When [2-$^{14}$C]acetyl-CoA (labeled in the methyl group) is introduced into the Krebs cycle only once, it is condensed with OAA to form [4-$^{14}$C]citrate, [4-$^{14}$C]cis-aconitate, [4-$^{14}$C]isocitrate, [4-$^{14}$C] oxalosuccinate, [4-$^{14}$C]α-KG, [3-$^{14}$C]succinyl-CoA, [2,3-$^{14}$C]succinate, [2,3-$^{14}$C]fumarate, [2,3-$^{14}$C] malate, and [2,3-$^{14}$C]OAA. Thus, there is no loss of $^{14}$C as $^{14}CO_2$ during the first turn of the cycle. During the second turn of the cycle, [2,3-$^{14}$C]OAA is condensed with unlabeled acetyl-CoA to yield [2,3-$^{14}$C]citrate, [2,3-$^{14}$C]oxalosuccinate, [2,3-$^{14}$C]α-KG, [1,2-$^{14}$C]succinyl-CoA, [1,2-$^{14}$C]succinate, and [1,2,3,4-$^{14}$C]succinate (due to isotope randomization). [1,2,3,4-$^{14}$C]Succinate leads to [1,2,3,4-$^{14}$C]fumarate, [1,2,3,4-$^{14}$C]malate, and [1,2,3,4-$^{14}$C]OAA. Thus, during the second turn of the Krebs cycle, there is still no loss of $^{14}$C as $^{14}CO_2$. During the third turn of the cycle, [1,2,3,4-$^{14}$C]OAA is condensed with unlabeled acetyl-CoA to form [1,2,3,6-$^{14}$C]citrate, [1,2,3,6-$^{14}$C]isocitrate, [1,2,3,6-$^{14}$C]oxalosuccinate, and [1,2,3-$^{14}$C]α-KG, with 25% of $^{14}$C being lost as $^{14}CO_2$. The decarboxylation of [1,2,3-$^{14}$C]α-KG to [1,2-$^{14}$C]succinyl-CoA results in the loss of another 25% of $^{14}$C as $^{14}CO_2$. This leads to [1,2-$^{14}$C]succinate, [1,2,3,4-$^{14}$C]succinate (due to isotope randomization), and [1,2,3,4-$^{14}$C] OAA. Thus, during the third turn of the cycle, 50% of $^{14}$C is lost as $^{14}CO_2$. By the end of the 15th cycle, all $^{14}$C in [2-$^{14}$C]acetate is lost as $^{14}CO_2$ (Table 5.11).

The labeling pattern of intermediates of the Krebs cycle depends on the labeled compounds introduced into the cycle. This complexity has caused problems in the interpretation of data obtained from isotope tracing studies. For example, in dairy cows, the appearance of $^{14}$C from [$^{14}$C]acetate in glucose due to the isotope randomization should not be taken as evidence for net synthesis of glucose from acetate. In contrast, net synthesis of glucose from acetate is possible in plants and many microorganisms due to the presence of the glyoxylate cycle. This metabolic cycle, however, is absent in animals.

**TABLE 5.11**
**The Loss of $^{14}C$ in [2-$^{14}C$]Acetyl-CoA as $^{14}CO_2$ in the Krebs Cycle**

| Turn of the Krebs Cycle | Loss of $^{14}C$ as $^{14}CO_2$ | Accumulated Loss of $^{14}C$ as $^{14}CO_2$ |
|---|---|---|
| 1st | 0% | 0% |
| 2nd | 0% | 0% |
| 3rd | 50% | 50% |
| 4th | 25% | 75% (50% + 25%) |
| 5th | 12.5% | 87.5% (75% + 12.5%) |
| 6th | 6.25% | 93.75% (87.5% + 6.25%) |
| 7th | 3.125% | 96.88% (93.75% + 3.125%) |
| 8th | 1.56% | 98.44% (96.88% + 1.56%) |
| 9th | 0.78% | 99.22% (98.44% + 0.78%) |
| 10th | 0.39% | 99.61% (99.22% + 0.39%) |
| 11th | 0.195% | 99.81% (99.61% + 0.195%) |
| 12th | 0.10% | 99.91% (99.81% + 0.10%) |
| 13th | 0.05% | 99.96% (99.91% + 0.05%) |
| 14th | 0.025% | 99.99% (99.96% + 0.025%) |
| 15th | 0.0125% | 100% (99.99% + 0.0125%) |

*Source:* Weinman, E.O. et al. 1957. *Physiol. Rev.* 37:252–272.

*Note:* When [2-$^{14}C$]acetyl-CoA (labeled in the methyl group) is introduced into the Krebs cycle only once, it is condensed with OAA to form [4-$^{14}C$]citrate. There is no loss of $^{14}C$ as $^{14}CO_2$ during the first and second turns of the cycle. Starting at the third turn of the cycle, 50% of the labeled carbon at the end of the previous cycle is lost. By the end of the 15th cycle, all $^{14}C$ in [2–$^{14}C$] acetate has been lost as $^{14}CO_2$.

## Mitochondrial Redox State

ß-Hydroxybutyrate dehydrogenase (a mitochondrial enzyme) catalyzes the interconversion of ß-hydroxybutyrate and acetoacetate. Thus, the ratio of [ß-hydroxybutyrate]/[acetoacetate] can be used as an indicator of the mitochondrial redox state. This enzyme is present in nearly all extrahepatic tissues with mitochondria, including the skeletal muscle, heart, liver, intestine, kidneys, and brain. Since $K_{eq}$ is a constant and intracellular pH is constant under normal physiological conditions, an increase in the ratio of [ß-Hydroxybutyrate]/[Acetoacetate] is equivalent to that of [NADH]/[NAD$^+$]. When intracellular pH fluctuates considerably, [H$^+$] must be included in the calculation of $K_{eq}$.

$$\text{Acetoacetate} + \text{NADH} + \text{H}^+ \leftrightarrow \text{ß-Hydroxybutyrate} + \text{NAD}^+$$

$$K_{eq} = ([\text{ß-Hydroxybutyrate}] \times [\text{NAD}^+])/([\text{Acetoacetate}] \times [\text{NADH}] \times [\text{H}^+])$$

## Crabtree Effect in Animal Cells

The Crabtree effect refers to the inhibition of oxygen consumption by the addition of glucose in animal cells. This results from decreased oxidation of acetyl-CoA via the Krebs cycle by increasing aerobic glycolysis (the production of lactate despite the presence of mitochondria and oxygen). The Crabtree effect was first described in tumor cells by Crabtree in 1929. It has also been demonstrated in noncancer tissues or cells such as pig platelets, coronary epithelium, thymocytes, and guinea pig sperm. A major role of the Crabtree effect has been suggested to spare endogenous fuels and minimize oxidative metabolism and, therefore, ROS production.

## Cytosolic Pentose Cycle

### Reactions of the Pentose Cycle

The pentose cycle (also known as the pentose phosphate pathway or hexose monophosphate shunt) is an alternative route for the oxidation of glucose in animal cells (Figure 5.10). It is quantitatively the second most important pathway for glucose oxidation to form $CO_2$ in the body. Unlike the oxidation of glucose via glycolysis and the Krebs cycle, there is no production of ATP from glucose metabolism via the pentose cycle. Like the pathway of glycolysis, the pentose cycle occurs in the cytosol (Wamelink et al. 2008). However, in contrast to glycolysis, $NADP^+$, but not $NAD^+$, is used as a hydrogen acceptor in the pentose cycle.

The sequence of reactions of the pentose cycle can be viewed as consisting of two phases: (1) an oxidative nonreversible phase and (2) a non-oxidative reversible phase. In the oxidative nonreversible phase, glucose-6-P undergoes dehydrogenation and decarboxylation to generate pentose, ribulose-5-P, $CO_2$, and NADPH. Of note, decarboxylation of 6-phosphogluconate to ribulose-5-P is the only reaction for the production of $CO_2$ in the pentose cycle. The carbon of the $CO_2$ molecule originates from the carbon-1 of glucose-6-P. As indicated previously, the carbon-1 of glucose-6-P can also be oxidized to $CO_2$ via glycolysis and the Krebs cycle. In contrast, the carbon-6 of glucose-6-P is oxidized to $CO_2$ only via the Krebs cycle.

In the non-oxidative reversible phase, ribulose-5-P is converted back to fructose-6-P through a series of reactions involving the four main types of enzymes: epimerase, ketoisomerase, transketolase, and transaldolase. Although the individual reactions involved in the conversion of ribulose-5-P to hexose phosphate are straightforward, it is impossible to depict them in a simple linear sequence. When the pentose cycle starts with three molecules of glucose-6-P, two molecules of fructose-6-P and one molecule of glyceraldehyde are generated as end products. Thus, if the cycle starts with six molecules of glucose-6-P, four molecules of fructose-6-P and two molecules of glyceraldehyde are generated. Fructose-6-P can be converted to glucose-6-P by phosphohexose isomerase, whereas two molecules of glyceraldehyde can form one molecule of glucose-6-P via the reversed reactions of the glycolysis, which are present in all animal cells. The overall reaction of the pentose cycle can be written as follows:

$$6\ \text{G-6-P} + 12\ \text{NADP}^+ + 6\ \text{H}_2\text{O} \rightarrow 6\ \text{CO}_2 + 5\ \text{F-6-P} + 12\ \text{NADPH} + 12\ \text{H}^+ \quad (5.1)$$

$$(\text{G-6-P} = \text{glucose-6-P};\ \text{F-6-P} = \text{fructose-6-P})$$

Since F-6-G can be converted to G-6-P, reaction (5.1) can be rearranged as follows:

$$6\ \text{G-6-P} + 12\ \text{NADP}^+ + 6\ \text{H}_2\text{O} \rightarrow 6\ \text{CO}_2 + 5\ \text{G-6-P} + 12\ \text{NADPH} + 12\ \text{H}^+ \quad (5.2)$$

Thus, the net reaction of the pentose phosphate pathway is as follows:

$$\text{G-6-P} + 12\ \text{NADP}^+ + 6\ \text{H}_2\text{O} \rightarrow 6\ \text{CO}_2 + 12\ \text{NADPH} + 12\ \text{H}^+ \quad (5.3)$$

As written, reaction (5.3) erroneously suggests that a single glucose molecule is completely oxidized to six molecules of $CO_2$ via the pentose cycle. However, this is not the case. Reaction (5.3) only simply indicates the efficiency of NADPH production from glucose via the pentose cycle.

### Activity of the Pentose Cycle in Animal Tissues and Cells

The pentose cycle is active in the liver, adipose tissue, adrenal cortex, thyroid, erythrocytes, testis, lactating mammary gland, activated phagocytes (macrophages and monocytes), activated neutrophils, and enterocytes. For example, in neonatal-pig enterocytes and activated rat-macrophages, approximately 15% and 25%–30% of glucose are utilized via the pentose cycle, respectively (Wu 1996; Wu and Marliss 1993). In contrast, the pentose cycle has a low activity in the non-lactating mammary gland, resting macrophages, other resting mononuclear cells (e.g., lymphocytes),

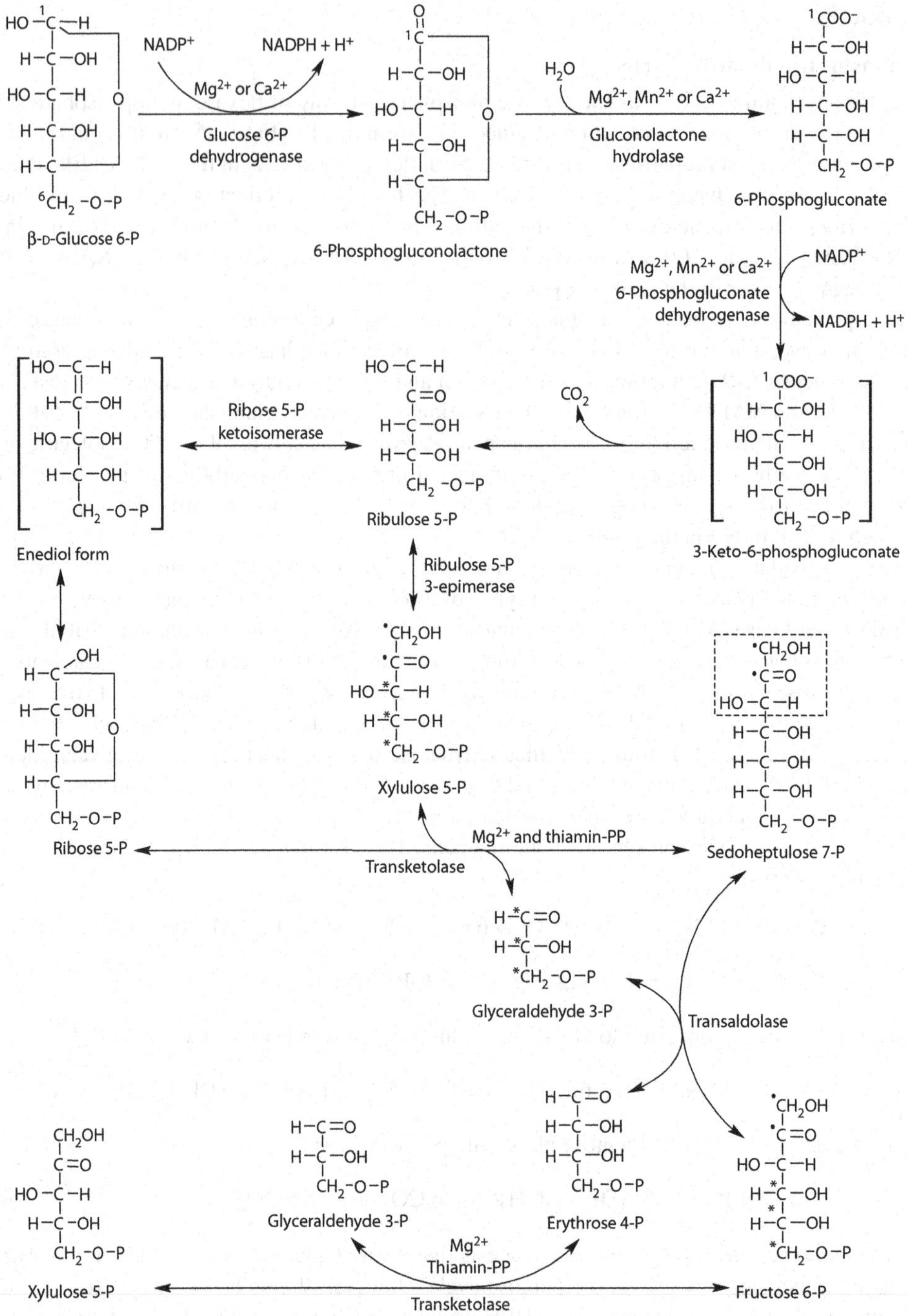

**FIGURE 5.10** The pentose cycle in animal cells. The pentose cycle, which is also known as the pentose phosphate pathway or hexose monophosphate shunt, is present in the cytosol of all animal cells. This pathway consists of an oxidative nonreversible phase and a non-oxidative reversible phase. In the oxidative nonreversible phase, glucose-6-P undergoes dehydrogenation and decarboxylation to generate pentose, ribulose-5-P, $CO_2$, and NADPH. In the non-oxidative reversible phase, ribulose-5-P is converted back to glucose-6-P. When NADPH is not oxidized via the mitochondrial electron system, no ATP is produced from glucose catabolism through the pentose cycle. The numbers 1 and 6 indicate the position of carbons in molecules. The signs "." and "*" denote specific carbon atoms.

endothelial cells, and skeletal muscle. Thus, in resting rat-macrophages and endothelial cells, only approximately 5% and 2%–3% of glucose taken up by the cells are metabolized via the pentose cycle, respectively (Wu and Marliss 1993; Wu et al. 1994). A relatively low activity of the pentose cycle in cells such as endothelial cells does not necessarily indicate a minor role of this pathway in cell function. For example, NADPH is essential for NO synthesis in endothelial cells.

The tissues or cells which possess a relatively high level of pentose cycle activity have one or more of the following characteristics: (1) active synthesis of fatty acids (e.g., liver, adipose tissue, and lactating mammary gland) and steroids (e.g., liver, placenta, and adrenal cortex); (2) active synthesis of superoxide anion ($O_2^-$) from $O_2$ via the non-mitochondrial respiratory chain (e.g., phagocytes); (3) active synthesis of NO from arginine (e.g., activated macrophages [probably with the exception of guinea-pig macrophages] and activated hepatocytes). All of these synthetic processes require NADPH and play important roles in either storing energy (adipose tissue) or host defense (macrophages).

### Physiological Significance of the Pentose Cycle

Glucose metabolism via the pentose cycle produces Ribose-5-P, which is converted into PRPP (5-phosphoribosyl-1-pyrophosphate). The latter is required for the synthesis of purine and pyrimidine nucleotides (RNA and DNA) (Chapter 4). In addition, the pentose cycle is the major metabolic pathway for the generation of NADPH from $NADP^+$ (Wu et al. 2001). Many biochemical reactions are dependent on NADPH, and some of them are outlined as follows:

1. Fatty acid synthesis (e.g., liver, adipose tissue, and mammary tissue) in the cytosol (Chapter 6).
2. Synthesis of cholesterol and steroid hormones from acetyl-CoA in specific tissues (e.g., the liver, adrenal cortex, testis, and ovary) (Chapter 6).
3. Synthesis of dopamine, epinephrine (adrenaline), and norepinephrine (noradrenaline) in the cytosol of adrenal medulla and nervous tissue (Chapter 7).
4. Reduction of GSSG (oxidized glutathione) to 2 GSH (reduced glutathione) in the cytosol, which helps to convert $H_2O_2$ to $H_2O$ in some tissues (e.g., red blood cells, red muscle, lens, and cornea) (Chapter 7).
5. Participation in the cytosolic sorbitol (polyol) pathway for the synthesis of D-fructose (see below).
6. Synthesis of proline from pyrroline-5-carboxylate (P5C) in the cytosol. The proline-P5C cycle has been proposed as a mechanism for transferring NADPH from the cytosol to mitochondria (Chapter 7).

$$\text{P5C} + \text{NADPH} + H^+ \rightarrow \text{Proline} + \text{NADP}^+$$

7. Synthesis of superoxide anion ($O_2^-$) by NADPH oxidase in phagocytes. This enzyme is located in both the cytosol and the plasma membrane. Consumption of $O_2$ and production of both $O_2^-$ and $H_2O_2$ by macrophages and neutrophils are increased in response to immunological stimulation, which is referred to as respiratory burst. Increased respiratory burst has been found to be associated with enhanced killing of microorganisms by phagocytes.

$$2O_2 + \text{NADPH} + H^+ \rightarrow 2O_2^- + \text{NADP}^+ + 2\,H^+ \quad \text{(NADPH oxidase)}$$

$$2O_2^- + 2\,H^+ \rightarrow H_2O_2 + O_2 \quad \text{(Superoxide dismutase)}$$

$$O_2^- + H_2O_2 \rightarrow O_2 + HO^- + HO \quad \text{(Haber–Weiss reaction)}$$

8. Synthesis of NO from L-arginine by NO synthase in the cytosol, plasma membrane, and mitochondria. NO synthase requires tetrahydro-L-biopterin, $FAD^+$, FMN, $Ca^{2+}$, and calmodulin.

$$\text{L-Arginine} + O_2 + 1.5\ \text{NADPH} + 1.5\ H^+ \rightarrow \text{L-Citrulline} + \text{NO} + 1.5\ \text{NADP}^+$$

9. Synthesis of P5C from glutamate in the mitochondria of enterocytes of most mammals (including pigs, rats, sheep, cattle, and humans). P5C synthase is almost exclusively located in the mitochondria of the mammalian small intestine. This indicates the importance of the small intestine in citrulline and arginine metabolism in mammals. P5C synthase is absent in the small intestine of chicks.

$$\text{Glutamate} + \text{NADPH} + \text{H}^+ + \text{ATP} \rightarrow \text{P5C} + \text{NADP}^+ + \text{ADP} + \text{Pi} \quad \text{(P5C synthase)}$$

10. Synthesis of glucuronic acid, ascorbic acid (vitamin C), and pentoses via the uronic acid pathway, another cytosolic pathway for the metabolism of glucose-6-phosphate (see below).
11. Conversion into NADH in mitochondria. NADPH can be converted into NADH by mitochondrial nicotinamide nucleotide transhydrogenase (Hoek and Rydstrom 1988):

$$\text{NADP}^+ + \text{NADH} + \text{H}^+_{\text{out}} \leftrightarrow \text{NADPH} + \text{NAD}^+ + \text{H}^+_{\text{in}}$$

In mammalian cells, nicotinamide nucleotide transhydrogenase is an integral protein of the mitochondrial inner membrane. The forward reaction above (transfer of electrons from NADH to $NADP^+$) is coupled to the translocation of protons from the cytosolic side to the matrix side of the mitochondrial inner membrane to generate NADPH in mitochondria. Wu (1996) reported that this reaction is not sufficient for the intramitochondrial provision of NADPH from NADH for citrulline synthesis from glutamine in pig enterocytes. In the reverse reaction of the nicotinamide nucleotide transhydrogenase, the transfer of electrons from NADPH to $NAD^+$ is coupled to the translocation of protons from the matrix side to the cytosolic side of the mitochondrial inner membrane to produce NADH. This allows for the oxidation of the cytosolic NADPH to produce ATP after the nucleotide enters the mitochondria from the cytosol through the malate shuttle or the glycerophosphate shuttle.

## Quantification of the Pentose Cycle

The yields of $^{14}CO_2$ from [1-$^{14}$C]glucose and [6-$^{14}$C]glucose have been used to estimate the activity of the pentose cycle in animal cells (e.g., hepatocytes and adipocytes). This is based on the assumptions that $^{14}CO_2$ is produced from [1-$^{14}$C]glucose via both the pentose cycle and the Krebs cycle and that $^{14}CO_2$ is produced from [6-$^{14}$C]glucose only via the Krebs cycle. Note that glucose has to be converted to pyruvate before its carbons are oxidized via the Krebs cycle.

1. *Katz and Wood's equation.* In 1963, Katz and Wood (1963) developed the following classic equation for estimating the flux of glucose through the pentose cycle:

$$\frac{\text{G1}_{\text{CO}_2} - \text{G6}_{\text{CO}_2}}{1 - \text{G6}_{\text{CO}_2}} = \frac{3\,\text{PC}}{1 + 2\,\text{PC}}$$

$G1_{CO_2}$: $^{14}CO_2$ produced from [1-$^{14}$C]glucose at steady state
$G6_{CO_2}$: $^{14}CO_2$ produced from [6-$^{14}$C]glucose at steady state
PC: Fraction of glucose that is metabolized to $CO_2$ and glyceraldehyde 3-P via the pentose cycle

In deriving the above equation, Katz and Wood made the following important assumptions: (1) isotopic steady states for the production of $^{14}CO_2$ from both [1-$^{14}$C]glucose and [6-$^{14}$C]glucose; (2) cell homogeneity in a tissue; specifically, the tissue can be treated mathematically as if it were a single cell, or all cells are metabolically identical; (3) gluconeogenesis is absent in the tissue or cells; and (4) complete mixing of fructose-6-P produced by the pentose cycle with a pool of hexose-P formed from the entering glucose.
2. *Larrabee's approach.* The assumptions used to derive Katz and Wood's equation may make it not applicable to many tissues or cells, including macrophages, endothelial

cells, enterocytes, and chicken embryos. Also, considerable amounts of time are often required for the production of $^{14}CO_2$ from [6-$^{14}$C]glucose to reach an isotopic steady state. Unfortunately, many investigators have used Katz and Wood's equation to estimate the pentose cycle activity with no statement of the assumptions implicit in its use or even though the implicit assumptions cannot be validated. Owing to these concerns about Katz and Wood's equation, Larrabee (1989, 1990) proposed that the difference in $^{14}CO_2$ production from [1-$^{14}$C]glucose and [6-$^{14}$C]glucose can be used to estimate the activity of the pentose cycle in metabolically homogenous or nonhomogenous cells (tissues), under isotopic steady or non-steady state, and in the presence or absence of gluconeogenesis in tissues or cells. The lower and upper values for the flux of glucose through the PC can be optimized by following the time-course of the difference in $^{14}CO_2$ from [1-$^{14}$C]glucose and [6-$^{14}$C]glucose, but useful values can be obtained when the time-course data are not available.

During any time period, the flux of glucose to the pentose cycle is as follows:

Glucose to PC flux $\geq$*C1–*C6
*C1: $^{14}CO_2$ produced from [1−$^{14}$C]glucose
*C6: $^{14}CO_2$ produced from [6−$^{14}$C]glucose
Lower limit of glucose to PC flux $\geq$*C1–*C6
Upper limit of glucose to PC flux $\leq$*C1 at steady state

Thus, a lack of difference in $^{14}CO_2$ production from [1-$^{14}$C]glucose and [6-$^{14}$C]glucose is not necessarily evidence of the absence of the pentose phosphate pathway in animal cells. Also, when *C1 is much greater than *C6, the true value of glucose to PC flux approaches *C1. Larrabee (1989) has reported that, in the peripheral ganglia of chicken embryos, the lower limit of glucose to PC flux is 34 μmol/g/h and the upper limit is 46 μmol/g/h. Thus, the flux of glucose to PC lies between 34 and 46 μmol/g/h. Based on the rate of glucose uptake (125 μmol/g/h), 27%–37% of the glucose utilized by these cells is metabolized via the pentose cycle.

### Regulation of the Pentose Cycle

Activity of the pentose cycle in animal cells is regulated by the availability of $NADP^+$, which is a cofactor for glucose-6-P dehydrogenase and 6-phosphogluconate dehydrogenase. Thus, oxidation of NADPH to $NADP^+$ through NADPH-dependent reactions plays an important role in controlling the oxidative phase and, therefore, the entire phase of the pentose cycle. On the other hand, glucose-6-P dehydrogenase is subject to feedback inhibition by NADPH, allosteric inhibition by long-chain fatty acyl-CoA (e.g., palmitoyl-CoA) and dehydroepiandrosterone, competitive inhibitors (e.g., glucosamine-6-P for glucose-6-P and gallated catechins for $NADP^+$), and uncompetitive inhibitors (thienopyrimidine and quinazolinone derivatives) (Figure 5.11). Therefore, the pentose cycle can be stimulated when utilization of NADPH is augmented in cells. In addition, expression of glucose-6-P dehydrogenase is enhanced by insulin, glucocorticoids, thyroid hormones, high carbohydrate diet, hypoxia, and $H_2O_2$ at transcriptional and/or translational levels (Kletzien et al. 1994). Since both the pentose cycle and glycolysis involve glucose-6-P as a common substrate, these two pathways may compete in the cytosol, depending on metabolic needs for NADPH or NADH. Insulin enhances glucose metabolism through the pentose cycle in cells (e.g., endothelial cells; Wu et al. 1994) likely via mechanisms involving increases in glucose uptake, hexokinase activity, $Ca^{2+}$ influx into cells, and NADPH oxidation.

## Metabolism of Glucose via the Uronic Acid Pathway

Besides the pentose cycle and glycolysis, glucose-6-P is utilized through the uronic acid pathway in animal cells, which involves the conversion of glucose-6-P to glucuronic acid, ascorbic acid

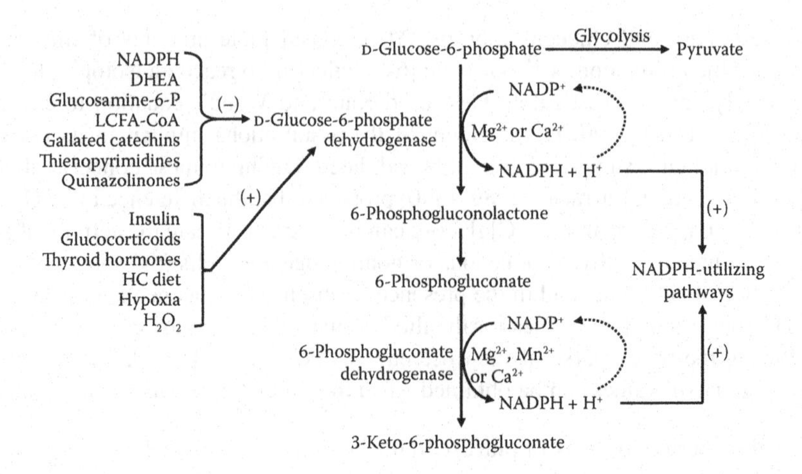


**FIGURE 5.11** Regulation of the pentose cycle in animal cells. Glucose-6-P dehydrogenase is a key rate-controlling enzyme in glucose metabolism via the pentose cycle. In short-term regulation, this enzyme is inhibited by NADPH, DHEA, glucosamine-6-P, LCFA-CoA, gallated catechins, as well as synthetic thienopyrimidine and quinazolinone derivatives. In long-term regulation, expression of this enzyme is activated by insulin, glucocorticoids, thyroid hormones, a high carbohydrate diet, hypoxia, and $H_2O_2$ at transcriptional and/or translational levels. Oxidation of NADPH via NADPH-dependent reactions regenerates NADP+, so that the dehydrogenation of D-glucose-6-P and 6-phosphogluconate can proceed. DHEA, dehydroepiandrosterone; LCFA-CoA, long-chain fatty acyl-CoA. The signs (+) and (–) denote activation and inhibition, respectively.

(vitamin C), and pentoses (Figure 5.12). Although the uronic acid pathway is quantitatively a minor pathway for glucose metabolism in animal cells, glucuronic acid is involved in the excretion of toxic metabolites and foreign chemicals (xenobiotics) as glucuronides. UDP-glucuronate is the active form of glucuronate for reactions involving the incorporation of glucuronic acid into proteoglycans and heteropolysaccharides (e.g., hyaluronic acid) or for reactions in which glucuronate is conjugated to such substrates as steroid hormones, certain drugs, and bilirubin (the metabolite of heme). In humans and other primates, as well as guinea pigs, ascorbic acid cannot be synthesized from glucose because of the absence of L-gulonolactone oxidase. Like the pentose cycle, the uronic acid pathway does not produce ATP.

## Gluconeogenesis

### Definition of Gluconeogenesis

Gluconeogenesis is defined as the metabolic process by which glucose is formed from non-carbohydrate, including lactate, pyruvate, glycerol, propionate, AAs, and odd-numbered long-chain fatty acids. Propionate (a $C_3$ SCFA) is the major substrate for gluconeogenesis in ruminants. In mammals and birds, gluconeogenesis occurs only in the liver and kidneys, because they possess glucose-6-phosphatase. The newly synthesized glucose is released and transported via the blood circulation to other tissues. Thus, gluconeogenesis is a biosynthetic process, because a 3-carbon substance is converted into the 6-carbon glucose.

Plasma glucose concentrations are determined by the balance between the rates of glucose production and utilization in the body. Partly due to impaired glucose synthesis, hypoglycemia can occur in neonates (e.g., piglets and preterm infants), late pregnancy in ruminants, small-for-gestational-age infants, and patients with sepsis or tumors. In contrast, intensive exercise enhances hepatic gluconeogenesis and, therefore, the plasma concentration of glucose in healthy animals. Similarly, hyperglycemia occurs

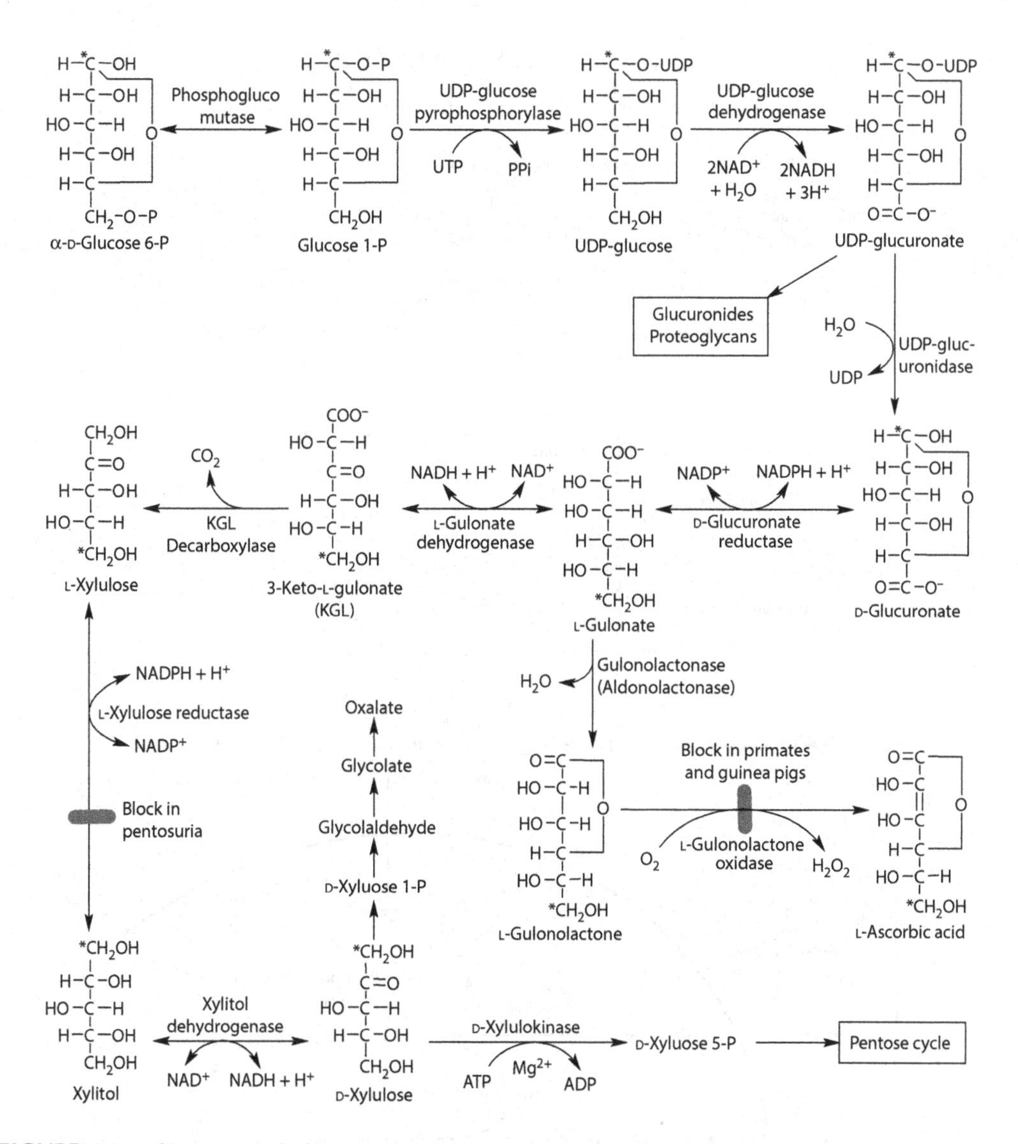


**FIGURE 5.12** Glucose metabolism via the uronic acid pathway in the cytosol of animal cells. The initial molecule of this pathway is D-glucose-6-P, which is produced from D-glucose by hexokinases I, II, and III, or glucokinase. The hydroxyl group of the terminal carbon in glucose-6-P is oxidized to a carboxyl group. The uronic acid pathway generates glucuronic acid, pentose, and ascorbic acid (vitamin C). Glucuronic acid plays an important role in: (1) the excretion of toxic metabolites and foreign chemicals (xenobiotics) as glucuronides, and (2) the synthesis of proteoglycans and heteropolysaccharides (e.g., hyaluronic acid). In primates (e.g., humans and monkeys) and guinea pigs, as well as some species of insects, birds, fish, and invertebrates, vitamin C cannot be synthesized from glucose due to the lack of L-gulonolactone oxidase.

in diabetic patients not treated with insulin because of both increased gluconeogenesis and reduced glucose catabolism in the whole body.

## Pathway of Gluconeogenesis

Gluconeogenesis is considered as a partial reversal of the glycolytic pathway because many of the reactions of glycolysis participate in gluconeogenesis (Figure 5.13). The reactions common to both glycolysis and gluconeogenesis are near-equilibrium ones in which a small increase in product

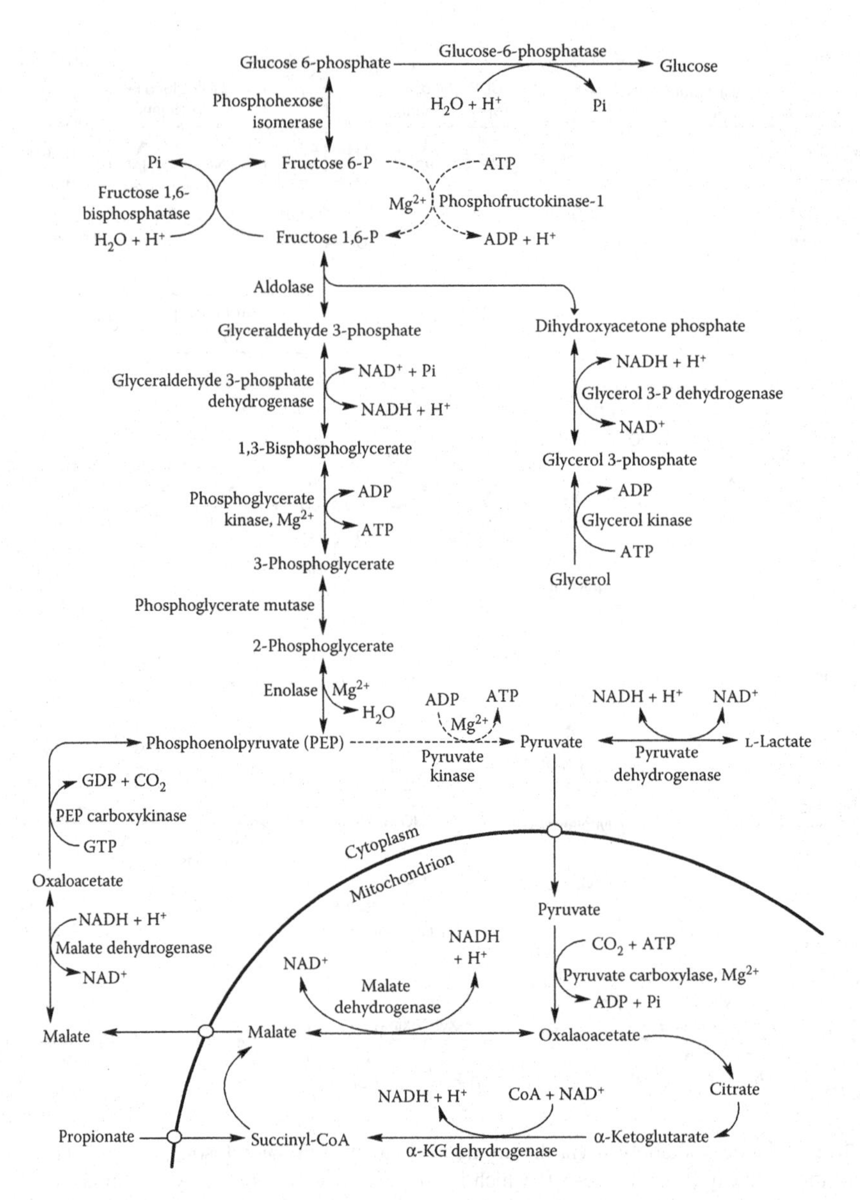


**FIGURE 5.13** Gluconeogenesis from pyruvate, lactate, glycerol, and glucogenic AAs in the liver and kidneys of animals. Synthesis of glucose from pyruvate, lactate, glycerol, and glucogenic AAs involves reversal reactions of glycolysis. The irreversible reactions of glycolysis between phosphoenolpyruvate (PEP) and pyruvate, between fructose-6-P and fructose-1,6-bisphosphate, and between glucose and glucose-6-P are circumvented by different reactions catalyzed by pyruvate carboxylase, PEP carboxykinase, fructose-1,6-bisphosphatase, and glucose-6-phosphatase. The latter enzyme is expressed almost exclusively in the liver and kidneys. The intracellular location of PEP carboxykinase affects the formation of glucose from AAs and glycerol, but not from lactate or pyruvate.

concentrations or a decrease in substrate concentrations can reverse the direction of the metabolic flux. However, there are three nonequilibrium reactions in glycolysis:

1. Between phosphoenolpyruvate and pyruvate ($\Delta G = -26.4$ kJ·mol$^{-1}$) (pyruvate kinase)
2. Between fructose-6-P and fructose-1,6-bisphosphate ($\Delta G = -24.5$ kJ·mol$^{-1}$) (PFK-1)
3. Between glucose and glucose-6-P ($\Delta G = -32.9$ kJ·mol$^{-1}$) (hexokinase)

Reversal of the direction of flux through the nonequilibrium reactions would require very large changes in the concentrations of substrates and products, and such large changes in intracellular metabolites would not be physiologically feasible. Thus, these reactions are described as the "energy barriers" to gluconeogenesis (Krebs 1964), and are circumvented by different reactions catalyzed by the following four enzymes: pyruvate carboxylase, phosphoenolpyruvate carboxykinase (PEPCK), fructose-1,6-bisphosphatase, and glucose-6-phosphatase (Van de Werve et al. 2000). The latter enzyme is expressed almost exclusively in the liver and kidneys.

1. Conversion of pyruvate to phosphoenolpyruvate (PEP)

   $$\text{Pyruvate} + CO_2 + \text{ATP} \rightarrow \text{Oxaloacetate} + \text{ADP} + \text{Pi} \quad \text{(Pyruvate carboxylase)}$$

   Pyruvate carboxylase requires vitamin B, biotin, and $Mg^{2+}$. In the liver and kidneys, this enzyme is located exclusively in the mitochondrion.

   $$\text{OAA} + \text{GTP} \rightarrow \text{PEP} + CO_2 + \text{GDP} \quad \text{(PEPCK)}$$

   In rats, mice, and golden hamsters, PEPCK is located exclusively in the cytosol. However, PEPCK is almost entirely a mitochondrial enzyme in the liver of pigeons, chickens, and rabbits, and in these species PEP is transported from the mitochondria to the cytosol for conversion into fructose-1,6-bisphosphate (Table 5.12). The intracellular distribution of PEPCK in the mitochondria and cytosol of chicken kidneys varies with nutritional and physiological status: mitochondria ≫ cytosol (fed), mitochondria > cytosol (48 h starved), mitochondria = cytosol (96 h starved and acidotic). In humans, cattle, sheep, pigs, guinea pigs, and frogs, PEPCK is equally distributed in the cytosol and mitochondria. The location of PEPCK in the mitochondria of the chicken liver explains why chicken hepatocytes have a limited ability to synthesize glucose from AAs (Watford et al. 1981).
2. Conversion of fructose-1,6-bisphosphate into fructose-6-P

$$\text{Fructose-1,6-bisphosphate} + H_2O + H^+ \rightarrow \text{Fructose-6-P} + \text{Pi} \quad \text{(Fructose-1,6-bisphosphatase)}$$

**TABLE 5.12**
**Species Differences in Intracellular Distribution of Phosphoenolpyruvate Carboxykinase (PEPCK) in the Liver and Kidney of Animals**

| Species | Tissue | Intracellular Distribution |
|---|---|---|
| Rat, mouse, hamster | Liver | Primarily cytosolic |
| | Kidney | PEPCK-M = PEPCK-C |
| Chicken, pigeon, rabbit | Liver | Exclusively mitochondrial |
| | Kidney | Both mitochondrial and cytosolic |
| | | PEPCK-M >> PEPCK-C (Fed) |
| | | PEPCK-M > PEPCK-C (48 h fasted) |
| | | PEPCK-M = PEPCK-C (96 h fasted or acidotic) |
| Human, pig, cattle, | Liver | PEPCK-M = PEPCK-C |
| sheep, frog | Kidney | PEPCK-M = PEPCK-C |
| Guinea pig | Liver | PEPCK-M > PEPCK-C |
| | Kidney | PEPCK-M > PEPCK-C |

*Source:* Adapted from Watford, M. 1985. *Fed. Proc.* 44:2469–2074; Yang, J.Q. et al. 2009. *J. Biol. Chem.* 284:27025–27029.
*Note:* PEPCK-M, mitochondrial isoform of PEPCK; PEPCK-C, cytosolic isoform of PEPCK.

This enzyme is present in the cytosol of the liver and kidney, and has been demonstrated in skeletal muscle. Fructose-1,6-bisphosphatase is inhibited by fructose-2,6-bisphosphate, a molecule discovered in 1980 (Van Schaftingen et al. 1980). Fructose-2,6-bisphosphate plays an important role in the regulation of glycolysis and gluconeogenesis.

3. Conversion of glucose-6-P into glucose

$$\text{Glucose-6-P} + H_2O + H^+ \rightarrow \text{Glucose} + \text{Pi} \quad \text{(Glucose-6-phosphatase)}$$

This enzyme is present in the cytosol of the liver and kidney, but is absent from skeletal muscle, heart, and adipose tissue.

4. Net reaction of gluconeogenesis from pyruvate

$$\text{2Pyruvate} + \text{4ATP} + \text{2GTP} + \text{2NADH} + 2H^+ + 2H_2O \rightarrow \text{Glucose} + \text{4ADP} + \text{2GDP} + \text{6Pi} + 2NAD^+$$

Thus, six molecules of ATP are required to synthesize one molecule of glucose from two molecules of pyruvate. Gluconeogenesis requires large amounts of ATP, which is supplied by fatty acid oxidation.

## Physiological Substrates for Gluconeogenesis

1. *Lactate.* Large amounts of lactate are produced primarily from glucose animals. It has been estimated that about 120 g of lactate is produced each day by a normally active man. Of this, about 40 g is produced by tissues which are virtually anaerobic in their metabolism (e.g., red blood cells, kidney medulla, and retina). The contribution of other tissues and cells (e.g., skeletal muscle, small intestine, brain, skin, cells of the immune system) will vary depending on physiological and pathological conditions. Normally, plasma concentration of lactate is about 1 mM, which represents a steady-state concentration that reflects the balance between rates of lactate production and utilization.

   The principal tissue for lactate utilization is the liver, where lactate is converted mainly to glucose and glycogen and, to a lesser extent, to triacylglycerol. However, other tissues, such as skeletal muscle and the heart, can both oxidize lactate and convert it to glycogen. The conversion of lactate into glucose or glycogen removes the proton ($H^+$) produced via glycolysis and therefore plays a role in maintaining acid–base balance in the body. In fed and 3-day fasted adult sheep, lactate contributes to approximately 15% and 10% of glucose synthesis in the whole body, respectively (Bergman 1983).

$$\text{2 Lactate} + 2\ NAD^+ \leftrightarrow \text{2 Pyruvate} + \text{2 NADH} + 2\ H^+ \rightarrow \text{Glucose}$$

2. *Glycerol.* In mammals and birds, glycerol is formed primarily from the hydrolysis of triglyceride by lipoprotein lipase, adipose triglyceride lipase, and hormone-sensitive lipase in white adipose tissue and skeletal muscle that do not express glycerol kinase. The mammary gland of mammals is also a source of glycerol as this organ does not contain glycerol kinase. Thus, the concentration of glycerol in plasma is often used as an indicator of lipolysis. During fasting and intensive exercise when lipolysis is enhanced, glycerol is an important substrate for gluconeogenesis during prolonged starvation. For example, a fasting, resting man generates 19 g of glycerol each day and almost all of the glycerol is converted to glucose. In fed and 3-day fasted adult sheep, glycerol contributes to approximately 5% and 25% of glucose synthesis in the whole body, respectively (Bergman 1983). Interestingly, while concentrations of glycerol in the plasma of mammals and birds do not normally exceed 0.25 mM, those in the rainbow smelt, which lives in the waters of the North Atlantic, can reach 0.4 M in the winter when the ambient sea temperatures approach 0°C (Driedzic et al. 2006). In these aquatic animals, glycerol serves as an "antifreeze" and it is produced almost exclusively from glycerol-3-phosphate (an intermediate of glucose and serine metabolism) by glycerol-3-phosphatase in the liver. This process is known as

glyceroneogenesis, which refers to the formation of glycerol via non-lipolysis pathways. There is evidence that glyceroneogenesis also occurs in mammals and birds.

Glycerol + ATP → Glycerol-3-P + ADP (Glycerol kinase; liver and kidney)

Glycerol-3-P + $NAD^+$ → Dihydroxyacetone-P + NADH + $H^+$ (Glycerol-3-P dehydrogenase)

Dihydroxyacetone-P ↔ Glyceraldehyde-3-P (Phosphotriose isomerase)

Dihydroxyacetone-P + Glyceraldehyde-3-P ↔ Fructose-1,6-P (Aldolase)

3. *AAs.* Experiments in the 1930s demonstrated that, based on their capacity for gluconeogenesis or ketogenesis, AAs could be divided into three classes: glucogenic, ketogenic, and glucogenic-plus-ketogenic (Table 5.13). Glucogenic AAs (Ala, Arg, Asp, Cys, Gln, Glu, Gly, His, Met, Pro, Ser, and Val) are those AAs whose metabolites can be converted to glucose through the production of pyruvate or one of the intermediates in the Krebs cycle. Ketogenic AAs (Leu and Lys) are those AAs whose metabolism gives rise solely to acetyl-CoA (the precursor of ketone bodies) which cannot be converted to glucose in animals. Glucogenic-plus-ketogenics AAs (Ile, Phe, Thr, Trp, and Tyr) are those AAs whose metabolism generates intermediates that can be converted to both glucose and acetyl-CoA. Alanine and glutamine are major glucogenic AAs in the mammalian liver. In addition, serine plays an important role in hepatic glucose production by ruminants, particularly during sepsis and pregnancy. Renal gluconeogenesis is low in fed animals (e.g., sheep and pigs) but is increased in food-deprived animals, with glutamine being the most important substrate. In fed and 3-day fasted adult sheep, AAs contribute to approximately 30% and 45% of glucose synthesis in the whole body, respectively (Bergman 1983).
4. *Propionate.* Propionate is the major source of glucose in ruminants (e.g., cattle, sheep, and goats), and enters the main gluconeogenic pathway via the Krebs cycle after conversion to succinyl-CoA (Figure 5.14). In this pathway, propionyl-CoA carboxylase requires vitamin biotin and methylmalonyl-CoA isomerase requires vitamin $B_{12}$ (cobalamin). Wilson et al. (1983) reported that, in fed ewes, the contribution of propionate to glucose synthesis increased from 37% in the nonpregnant state and in mid-pregnancy to 55% in late pregnancy and to 60% during lactation. In 3-day fasted sheep with no detectable uptake of propionate by the liver and kidneys, there is little synthesis of glucose from the SCFA (Bergman 1983).

**TABLE 5.13**
**Glucogenic and Ketogenic AAs in Animals**

| Glucogenic AA | Ketogenic Amino Acids | Glucogenic-Plus-Ketogenic |
|---|---|---|
| Ala→Pyruvate | Lys→Acetyl-CoA | Ile→Propionyl-CoA, Acetyl-CoA |
| Arg→α-Ketoglutarate | Leu→Acetyl-CoA | Phe→Fumarate, Acetoacetate |
| Asp→OAA | | Thr→Propionyl-CoA, Acetyl-CoA |
| Cys→Pyruvate | | Trp→Pyruvate, Acetyl-CoA |
| Gln→α-Ketoglutarate | | Tyr→Fumarate, Acetoacetate |
| Glu→α-Ketoglutarate | | |
| Gly→Pyruvate | | |
| His→α-Ketoglutarate | | |
| Met→Succinyl-CoA | | |
| Pro→α-Ketoglutarate | | |
| Ser→Pyruvate | | |
| Val→Succinyl-CoA | | |

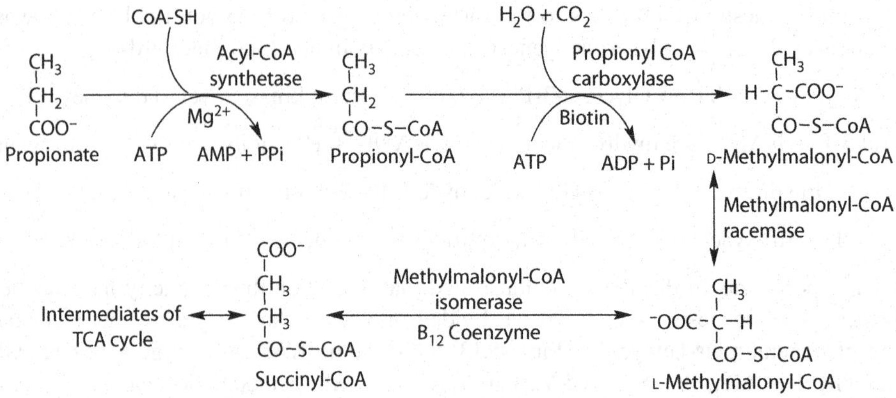

CoA-SH
Acyl-CoA synthetase
$Mg^{2+}$
ATP AMP + PPi
Propionate ($CH_3$–$CH_2$–$COO^-$) → Propionyl-CoA ($CH_3$–$CH_2$–CO–S–CoA)
$H_2O + CO_2$
Propionyl CoA carboxylase
Biotin
ATP ADP + Pi
→ D-Methylmalonyl-CoA ($CH_3$–H–C–$COO^-$, CO–S–CoA)
Methylmalonyl-CoA racemase
L-Methylmalonyl-CoA ($^-OOC$–C–H, $CH_3$, CO–S–CoA)
Methylmalonyl-CoA isomerase
$B_{12}$ Coenzyme
Succinyl-CoA ($COO^-$–$CH_2$–$CH_2$–CO–S–CoA)
Intermediates of TCA cycle

**FIGURE 5.14** Conversion of propionate into succinyl-CoA that enters the main pathway of gluconeogenesis in the liver of ruminants. Propionate, which is produced from the fermentation of carbohydrates in the rumen, is quantitatively the single most important substrate for hepatic synthesis in fed ruminants. This pathway requires vitamin biotin and $B_{12}$ as cofactors. Gluconeogenesis plays an important role in maintaining glucose homeostasis in ruminants.

5. *Acetate* in organisms other than animals. Conversion of acetate to glucose occurs via the glyoxylate cycle, which is widely found in microorganisms (including bacteria in the rumen), yeasts, fern spores, and plant seeds (Figure 5.15). In addition to the typical Krebs cycle enzymes (citrate synthase, aconitase, and malate dehydrogenase), the glyoxylate cycle includes two unique enzymes, isocitrate lyase, and malate synthase. This pathway circumvents the decarboxylation steps of the Krebs cycle, and produces one molecule of succinate from two molecules of acetyl-CoA, thereby allowing for the conversion of fatty acids to glucose in organisms other than animals. All attempts to demonstrate the glyoxylate cycle in insects have so far failed. Much evidence shows that this metabolic pathway is absent from animal cells (Ward 2000).

## Regulation of Gluconeogenesis

Glucogenogenesis is limited in animals fed a high-starch and adequate protein diet (Kristensen and Wu 2012). During fasting, the concentrations of glucagon in the blood increase, whereas those of insulin and glucogenic AAs decrease despite the increased release of AAs from skeletal muscle. In addition, the release of glycerol from white adipose tissue is enhanced in food-deprived animals. During exercise, both the release of lactate and AAs from skeletal muscle and the release of glycerol from white adipose tissue are elevated, as are the concentrations of glucagon and epinephrine in the blood. All of these metabolic changes during fasting and exercise favor gluconeogenesis.

1. *Intracellular compartmentation.* In the liver, gluconeogenesis occurs in periportal hepatocytes, as does fatty acid oxidation. The presence of both pathways in the same cell confers the following metabolic advantages to: (1) efficiently couple ATP produced from fatty acid oxidation with glucose synthesis; and (2) facilitate metabolic control of gluconeogenesis by products of fatty acid oxidation: acetyl-CoA, citrate, and ATP. In the kidneys with cytosolic PEPCK, catabolism of Gln or Asp provides OAA and malate in mitochondria, and the malate enters the cytosol for efficient conversion into glucose (Watford 1985).
2. *Provision of glucogenic precursors, ATP and NADH.* Since the flux-generating steps for gluconeogenesis are the concentrations of its substrates, AAs, glycerol, lactate, and propionate, rates of production of these precursors in animals are one important factor for determining hepatic and renal gluconeogenesis (Neese et al. 1995). Likewise, the availability of ATP (particularly from oxidation of long-chain fatty acids and AAs) and NADH in the

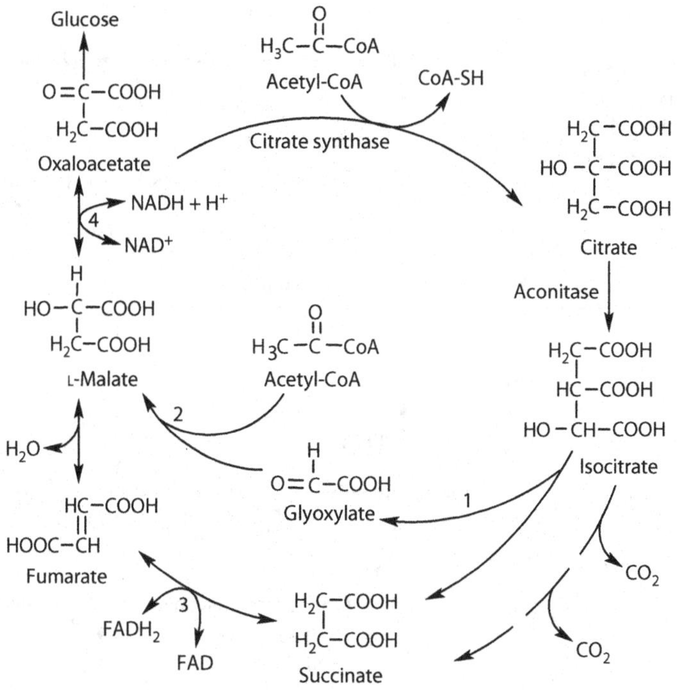

**FIGURE 5.15** The glyoxylate cycle in organisms other than animals. In microorganisms (including bacteria in the rumen), yeasts, fern spores, and plant seeds, acetate is converted into glucose via the glyoxylate cycle. In this pathway, isocitrate is cleaved into glyoxylate and succinate. Glyoxylate combines with acetyl-CoA to form L-malate, whereas succinate undergoes dehydrogenation to yield fumarate. The enzymes that catalyze the indicated reactions are: (1) isocitrate lyase; (2) malate synthase; and (3) succinate dehydrogenase. The glyoxylate cycle is absent from animals, which do not contain isocitrate lyase or malate synthase.

liver and kidneys can limit glucose synthesis from potential substrates. Let us use birds to exemplify a key role of NADH in gluconeogenesis (Figure 5.16). In chicken hepatocytes where PEPCK is localized exclusively in the mitochondria, the metabolism of glucogenic AAs does not generate NADH in the cytosol and, therefore, no glucose even under conditions of 48-h fasting (Watford et al. 1981). In contrast, in chicken kidney tubules where PEPCK is localized in the cytosol, metabolism of glucogenic AAs generates NADH in this compartment and, therefore, glucose under both fed and fasting conditions (Watford et al. 1981).

3. *Intracellular concentrations of acetyl-CoA, citrate, and adenine nucleotides.* Gluconeogenesis is also regulated by concentrations of acetyl-CoA, citrate, and adenine nucleotides in hepatocytes and renal tubules (Figure 5.17). Specifically, acetyl-CoA activates pyruvate carboxylase and therefore increases the conversion of pyruvate to OAA. In addition, acetyl-CoA inhibits pyruvate dehydrogenase, thereby enhancing the availability of pyruvate for glucose production. Citrate (derived from acetyl-CoA) and ATP also inhibit PFK-1. These changes explain why the oxidation of fatty acids, which produces acetyl-CoA, inhibits glycolysis and stimulates gluconeogenesis. Furthermore, the oxidation of fatty acids provides ATP that is required for gluconeogenesis, as noted previously. Both gluconeogenesis and fatty acid oxidation occur in periportal hepatocytes. Thus, impairment of fatty acid oxidation causes hypoglycemia in mammals. Likewise, under conditions where mitochondrial ATP production is reduced and cytosolic ADP or AMP concentration is elevated, gluconeogenesis in hepatocytes and the kidneys is decreased. This is because ADP and AMP inhibit pyruvate carboxylase and fructose-1,6-bisphosphatase, respectively.

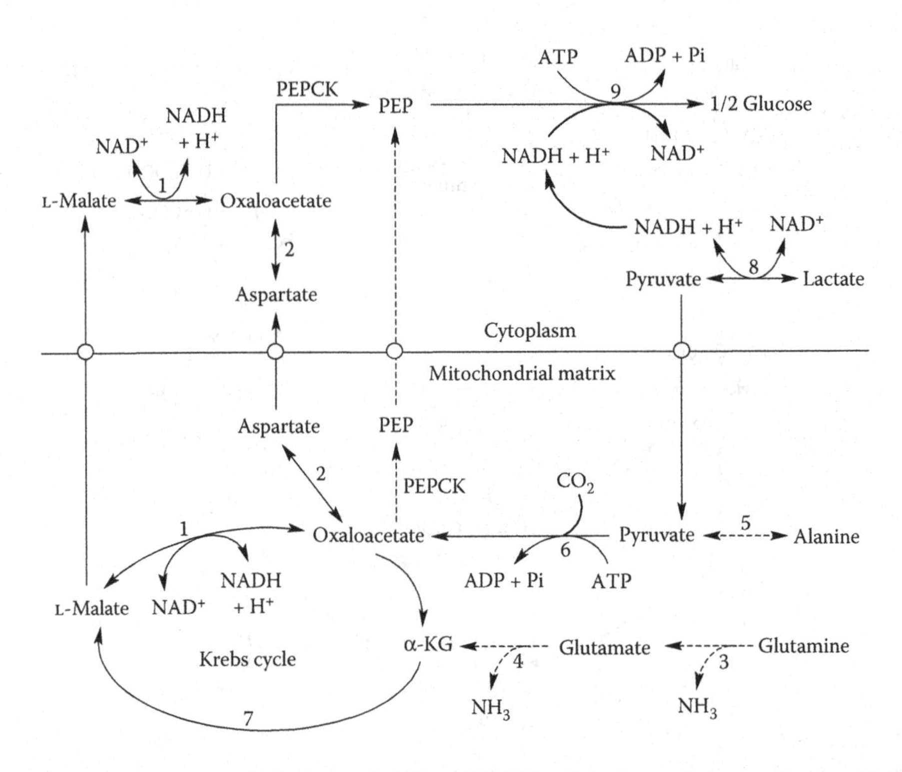


**FIGURE 5.16** An important role for the availability of NADH and the intracellular localization of phosphoenolpyruvate carboxykinase (PEPCK) in gluconeogenesis. For cells where PEPCK is localized exclusively in mitochondria, the metabolism of glucogenic AAs does not generate NADH in the cytosol and therefore produces no glucose. In contrast, in cells where PEPCK is localized in the cytosol, the metabolism of glucogenic AAs (e.g., alanine, glutamine, and glutamate) produces NADH in the cytosol and, therefore, glucose. Stoichiometrically, 0.5 mol of glucose is synthesized from 1 mol of alanine. α-KG, α-ketoglutarate; PEP, phosphoenolpyruvate. (Adapted from Watford, M. 1985. *Fed. Proc.* 44:2469–2074.)

4. *Glucagon and fructose-2,6-bisphosphate (F-2,6-P).* Glucagon inhibits glycolysis and stimulates gluconeogenesis, whereas the opposite is true for F-2,6-P, which is the most potent activator of PFK-1 and inhibitor of F-1-6-Pase (Hers and Van Schaftingen 1982). By increasing the intracellular concentration of cAMP, glucagon promotes the phosphorylation of pyruvate kinase, thereby reducing its enzymatic activity and favoring the conversion of pyruvate into glucose. In addition, cAMP-dependent kinase phosphorylates phosphofructokinase-2/fructose-2,6-bisphosphatase (a bifunctional enzyme; i.e., one protein having two different enzymatic activities), resulting in an increase of fructose-2,6-bisphosphatase activity but a decrease in phosphofructokinase-2 (Figure 5.18). This leads to a reduction in the intracellular concentration of F-2,6-P, which favors gluconeogenesis. Such a mechanism also explains why an excess or deficiency of glucose in blood inhibits or promotes gluconeogenesis, respectively (Figure 5.19). Specifically, the concentration of F-2,6-P in hepatocytes and renal tubules is elevated in response to an abundant supply of glucose, thereby enhancing glycolysis to form pyruvate. Conversely, the concentration of F-2,6-P in hepatocytes and kidneys is lowered in response to an inadequate provision of glucose, thereby stimulating the conversion of OAA and pyruvate into glucose.
5. *Insulin and gluconeogenesis.* In healthy animals, high concentrations of blood glucose after consumption of a carbohydrate or protein meal stimulate the release of insulin from pancreatic ß-cells, whereas the blood concentration of insulin is decreased during fasting. High circulating levels of insulin antagonize the action of glucagon and inhibit hepatic

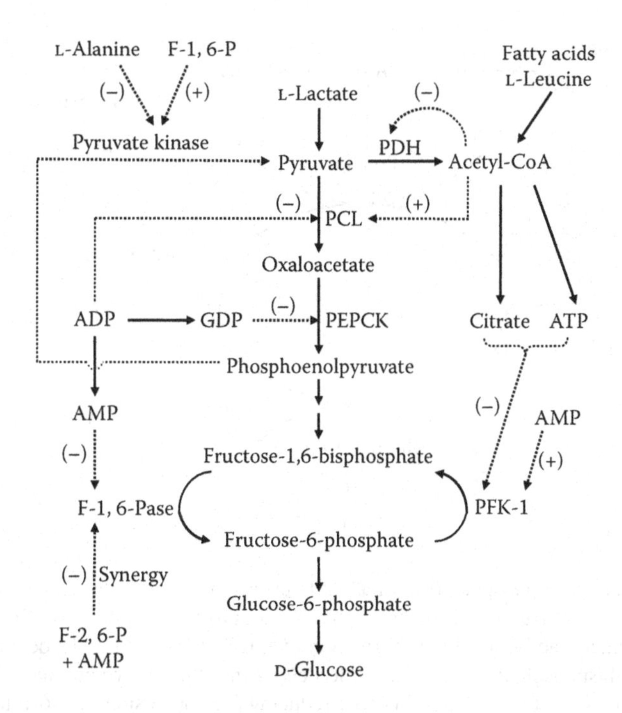


**FIGURE 5.17** Regulation of hepatic and renal gluconeogenesis by intracellular concentrations of acetyl-CoA, citrate, alanine, and adenine nucleotides. Factors (e.g., enhanced activity of F-1,6-Pase, PCL, and PEPCK, as well as reduced activity of PFK-1, pyruvate kinase, and PDH) that increase intracellular F-6-P concentration favor gluconeogenesis. Conversion of F-1,6-P to fructose-6-P not only provides the substrate for glucose synthesis but also relieves an allosteric effect of F-1,6-P on activating pyruvate kinase. Citrate, ATP, acetyl-CoA, and alanine promote glucose synthesis, whereas F-2,6-P, and AMP suppress this pathway through synergic inhibition of F-1,6-Pase. F-1,6-P, fructose-1,6-bisphosphate; F-2,6-P, fructose-2,6-bisphosphate; F-1,6-Pase, fructose-1,6-bisphosphatase; PCL, pyruvate carboxylase; PDH, pyruvate dehydrogenase; PEPCK, phosphoenolpyruvate carboxykinase; PFK-1, phosphofructokinase 1. The signs (+) and (−) denote activation and inhibition, respectively.

gluconeogenesis by decreasing (1) intracellular concentration of cAMP due to the activation of 3′-5′-cyclic nucleotide phosphodiesterase in hepatocytes; (2) uptake of lactate by the liver; (3) the concentrations of glucogenic AAs in the blood; and (4) expression of glucogenic enzymes in the liver and kidneys. Thus, glucose synthesis from AAs and other substrates is limited in the liver of growing pigs fed a high-starch and 16%-CP diet (Figure 5.20). Partly through its effect on inhibiting hepatic gluconeogenesis, insulin plays a role in stimulating food intake by animals (Nizielski et al. 1986).

$$\text{ATP} \rightarrow \text{cAMP} + \text{PPi} \quad \text{(Adenylate cyclase)}$$

$$\text{cAMP} + \text{H}_2\text{O} \rightarrow \text{AMP} \quad \text{(3}'\text{-5}'\text{-cyclic nucleotide phosphodiesterase)}$$

6. *Glucocorticoids and gluconeogenesis.* Glucocorticoids are steroid hormones that promote gluconeogenesis in the liver via increasing protein degradation in skeletal muscle to provide glucogenic AAs, intracellular cAMP concentration, and expression of glucogenic genes (Devlin 2011). Notably, through activating CCAAT/enhancer-binding protein-β and cAMP regulatory element-binding protein, glucocorticoids enhance the transcription of the PEPCK gene for promoting hepatic gluconeogenesis. In a concerted response, glucocorticoids reduce glucose uptake and utilization by skeletal muscle and white adipose tissue through antagonizing insulin's action, thereby providing glucose for hepatic glucose

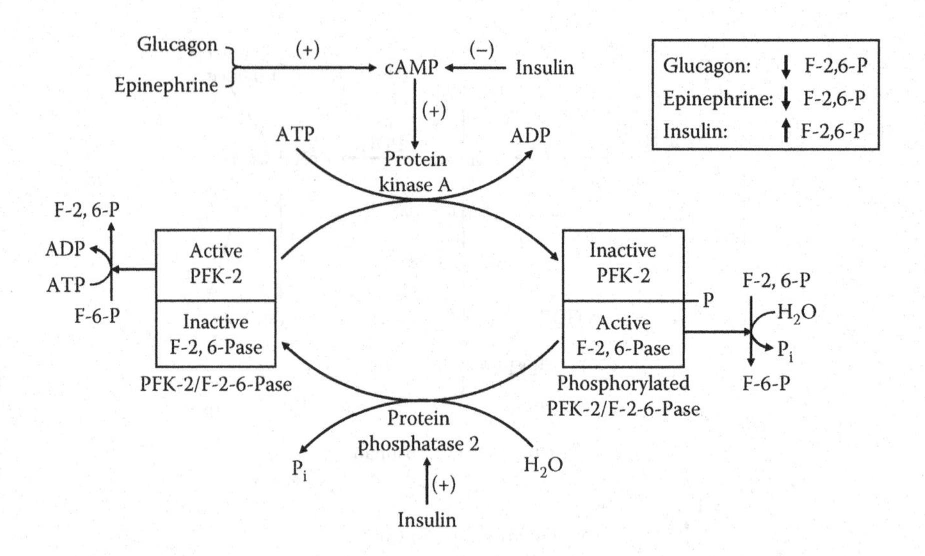


**FIGURE 5.18** Regulation of phosphofructokinase 2/fructose-2,6-bisphosphatase by fructose-2,6-bisphosphate. Phosphofructokinase 2/fructose-2,6-bisphosphatase is a bifunctional enzyme, that is, one protein having two different enzymatic activities. Phosphorylation of this enzyme by cAMP-dependent protein kinase increases fructose-2,6-bisphosphatase activity, while decreasing phosphofructokinase-2 activity. Glucagon and epinephrine increase cAMP production, thereby reducing the conversion of F-6-P to F-2,6-P (an inhibitor of F-1,6-Pase) and stimulating glucose synthesis. In contrast, insulin has an opposite effect and plays an important role in suppressing hepatic gluconeogensis. F-6-P, fructose-6-phosphate; F-2,6-P, fructose-2,6-bisphosphate; F-2,6-Pase, fructose-2,6-bisphosphatase; PFK-2, phosphofructokinase 2. The signs (+) and (–) denote activation and inhibition, respectively.

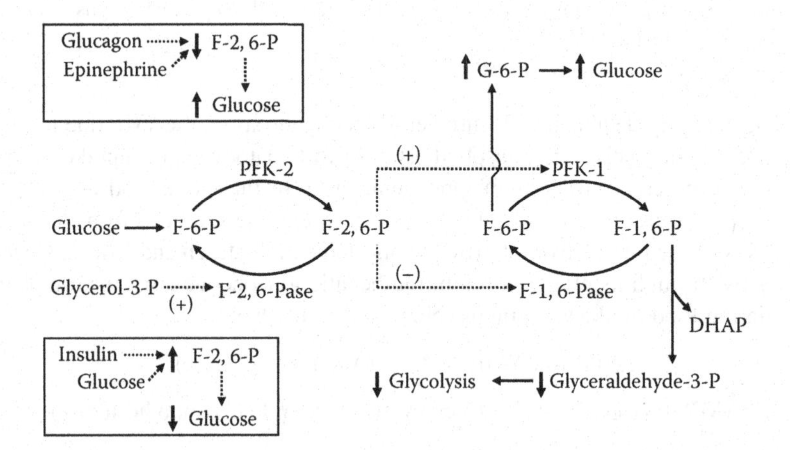


**FIGURE 5.19** Regulation of hepatic and renal gluconeogenesis by glucose availability and hormones through a change in the intracellular concentration of fructose-2,6-bisphosphate. When the circulating levels of glucose and insulin are high, concentrations of F-2,6-P (an inhibitor of F-1,6-Pase) in the liver and kidneys are increased, thereby inhibiting glucose synthesis. In contrast, when the circulating levels of glucagon and epinephrine are elevated, concentrations of F-2,6-P (an inhibitor of F-1,6-Pase) in the liver and kidneys are decreased, thereby promoting glucose synthesis. DHAP, dihydroxyacetone phosphate; F-6-P, fructose-6-phosphate; F-2,6-P, fructose-2,6-bisphosphate; F-2,6-Pase, fructose-2,6-bisphosphatase; G-6-P, glucose-6-P; PFK-2, phosphofructokinase 2. The signs (+) and (–) denote activation and inhibition, respectively.

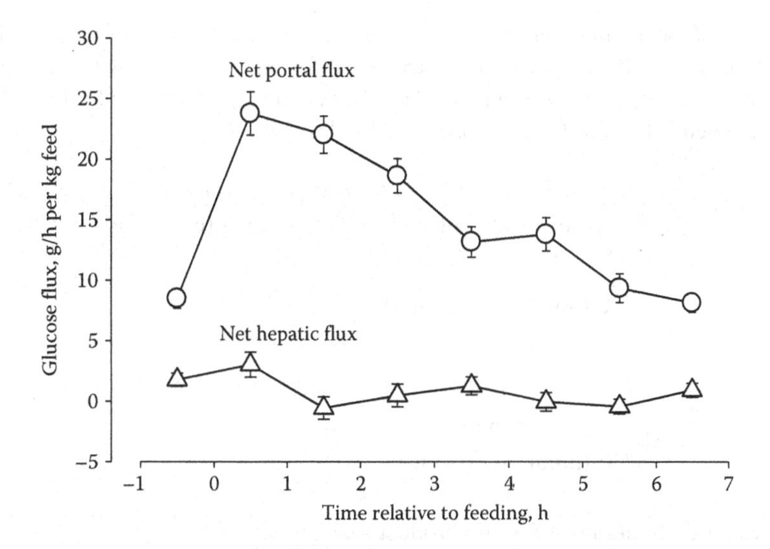


**FIGURE 5.20** Net portal flux (open bar) and net hepatic flux (filled bar) of glucose in 60 kg growing pigs fed a high-starch and 16%-CP diet at the rate of 3.6% of body weight per day. Feed was divided into three equally sized meals per day at 8 h intervals. A positive flux denotes net release, and a negative flux denotes net uptake across the tissues. Each data point represents mean ± SEM, $n = 16$. (From Kristensen, N.B. and G. Wu. 2012. In: *Nutritional Physiology of Pigs*, Chapter 13. Edited by K.E. Bach, N.J. Knudsen, H.D. Kjeldsen, and B.B. Jensen. Danish Pig Research Center, Copenhagen, Denmark, pp. 1–17. With permission.)

synthesis. Therefore, excess glucocorticoids result in hyperglycemia and insulin resistance in animals.

7. *Ethanol and gluconeogenesis.* High concentrations of ethanol (e.g., 10 mM) inhibit hepatic gluconeogenesis from lactate, glycerol, dihydroxyacetone, proline, serine, alanine, fructose, and galactose (Krebs et al. 1969). In contrast, ethanol does not affect glucose synthesis from pyruvate in the liver. When ethanol is oxidized by alcohol dehydrogenase to form acetaldehyde, $NAD^+$ is reduced to NADH + $H^+$, thereby lowering the ratio of [free $NAD^+$]/[free NADH] in hepatocytes. The disturbance of the intracellular [free $NAD^+$]/[free NADH] ratio is exacerbated when acetaldehyde is oxidized by $NAD^+$-dependent acetaldehyde dehydrogenase to acetic acid. This leads to decreases in the formation of pyruvate and, therefore, glucose from lactate. Since conversion of pyruvate into glucose does not require $NAD^+$, this pathway is not suppressed by alcohol. Ethanol inhibits gluconeogenesis from glycerol, dihydroxyacetone, glucogenic AAs, fructose, and galactose, likely through reducing their uptake by the liver.

$NAD^+$ → NADH + $H^+$; $NAD^+$ → NADH + $H^+$
$CH_3CH_2OH$ (ethanol) → [Ethanol dehydrogenase] → $CH_3CHO$ (acetaldehyde) → [Acetaldehyde dehydrogenase] → Acetyl-CoA

## Quantification of Gluconeogenesis

1. *In vitro incubation of cells.* Hepatocytes are incubated with physiological concentrations of glucogenic substrates (labeled or unlabeled) to determine the production of glucose (labeled or unlabeled). Specifically, an appropriately labeled substrate is used to measure the formation of glucose from the particular substrate. For example, if hepatocytes are incubated in 1 mL of buffer containing 1 mM L-lactate plus L-[U-$^{14}$C]lactate ($3 \times 10^6$ dpm), and [$^{14}$C]glucose (6000 dpm) is formed, the amount of glucose synthesized by the cells can be calculated

on the basis of the assumption that intracellular specific radioactivity of L-[U-$^{14}$C]lactate is similar to its extracellular specific radioactivity. First, we need to know the concept of the specific radioactivity (SA) of a radiolabeled compound (e.g., $^{14}$C-labeled L-lactate), or isotope enrichment (IE) of a stable isotope (e.g., $^{13}$C-labeled L-lactate).

$$SA = \frac{\text{Amount of radioactive isotope (dpm)}}{\text{Mass of labeled plus unlabeled isotopes (e.g., nmol)}} = \frac{^{14}C\text{ (dpm)}}{^{14}C\text{ (nmol)} + {}^{12}C\text{(nmol)}}$$

$$IE = \frac{\text{Mass of stabel isotope (e.g., }\mu\text{mol)}}{\text{Mass of labeled plus unlabeled isotopes (e.g., }\mu\text{mol)}} = \frac{^{13}C\ (\mu\text{mol})}{^{13}C\ (\mu\text{mol}) + {}^{12}C(\mu\text{mol})}$$

Examples for calculations of SA and product production:

$$\text{Specific activity (SA) of lactate} = 3\times10^6\ \text{dpm/1000 nmol} = 3000\ \text{dpm/nmol lactate} = 3000/3 = 1000\ \text{dpm/nmol C}$$

$$\text{Glucose synthesis from lactate} = \frac{\text{Labeled glucose produced (dpm)}}{\text{SA of [U-}^{14}\text{C]lactate (dpm/nmol C)}} \times \frac{1}{6} = \frac{6000\ \text{dpm}}{1000\ \text{dpm/nmol C}} \times \frac{1}{6} = 1\ \text{nmol glucose}$$

2. *Perfused organs.* An isolated, perfused liver is often used to study gluconeogenesis (Ekberg et al. 1995). The liver is perfused with physiological concentrations of glucogenic substrates (labeled or unlabeled), and effluent perfusate is collected for the determination of the production of glucose (labeled or unlabeled). The calculation of glucose synthesis is the same as that for *in vitro* cell incubation.
3. *In vivo study.* Labeled isotopes must be used to study gluconeogenesis *in vivo* to distinguish the sources of potential substrates (Chung et al. 2015). Animals or humans are often intravenously infused with a suitable radioactive or stable isotope, and labeled glucose is measured by a liquid scintillation counter (for radioactive isotopes) or mass spectroscopy (for stable isotopes). Of course, *in vivo* experiments are much more complex than *in vitro* incubation and organ perfusion studies, in terms of calculation and data interpretation.

## Nutritional and Physiological Significance of Gluconeogenesis

1. *Maintenance of glucose homeostasis in animals.* It must be recognized that a constant supply of glucose is necessary as the dominant source of energy for the nervous system when the circulating levels of ketone bodies are low (e.g., <0.15 mM) and as the sole source of energy for red blood cells under all conditions. This is particularly important for strict carnivores (e.g., cats, tigers, carnivorous fish, and certain marine mammals [sea lion, seal, and white whale]) who ingest a limited amount of carbohydrate from diets. Gluconeogenesis is also essential for ruminants who absorb little or no glucose in the small intestine under normal feeding conditions. In adult sheep fed Lucerne hay at 0.5 h intervals, the rates of glucose production by the liver and kidney are 4.5 and 0.7 g/h, respectively.

The rate of gluconeogenesis matches the rate of glucose utilization in the sheep, which is 1.4 and 3.8 g/h in the splanchnic bed (the portal-drained viscera + liver) and other tissues (including skeletal muscle, brain, heart, blood, kidneys, and adipose tissue), respectively (Bergman 1983). Thus, a failure of gluconeogenesis is usually fatal for animals (Yang et al. 2009).

Normal concentrations of glucose in plasma are approximately 5.0–5.5 mM in postabsorptive dogs, cats, humans, pigs, and rats, approximately 2.5–3.4 mM in ruminants, and approximately 12–15 mM in chickens. Below a critical glucose concentration in plasma (e.g., 3.5 mM in pigs and 1 mM in sheep), animals exhibit brain dysfunction, which can lead to coma and death. Since nonruminants are capable of gluconeogenesis, they do not have specific dietary requirements for carbohydrates. This is consistent with experimental results from studies involving pigs, rats, poultry, fish, and marine mammals. However, it should be noted that (1) dietary fiber is beneficial for maintaining the intestinal health of nonruminants (particularly gestating and lactating sows); and (2) total dependence of glucose provision on endogenous synthesis from AAs will not only increase the cost of animal production, but also will have negative impacts on the function of the liver, kidneys, and possibly other organs.

2. *Low-carbohydrate diets or high demands for glucose.* In nonruminants, whenever the carbohydrate content of diets is low or demands for carbohydrate by those tissues that depend exclusively on glucose for energy are high, gluconeogenesis becomes particularly important. If gluconeogenesis is insufficient, hypoglycemia occurs in animals. Although most diets are rich in carbohydrates, some (e.g., the traditional diet of the Eskimos and carnivores) are low in carbohydrates. Under these feeding conditions, animals require a high level of gluconeogenesis to maintain normal glucose concentrations in plasma.
3. *Fasting.* During fasting, carbohydrate intake is absent and after endogenous glycogen reserves have been utilized within 12 h, gluconeogenesis plays an important role in maintaining glucose homeostasis in animals (Brosnan 1999). Before plasma concentrations of ketone bodies are sufficiently increased, the neurons in the brain depend on glucose for energy provision. This necessitates gluconeogenesis in response to fasting. Of note, rates of whole-body glucose production in fasted animals depend on the availability of glucogenic substrates and, therefore, the stage of food deprivation.
4. *Neonates.* Hypoglycemia usually occurs in neonates (e.g., piglets with limited white adipose tissue), and particularly in the newborn infants of diabetic mothers. High levels of glucose in maternal blood lead to hyperglycemia in the fetus, which activates the release of insulin by fetal pancreatic β-cells. At birth, the newborn continues to increase insulin production but no longer receives an increased transfer of glucose from the maternal blood. Thus, within the first days after birth, hypoglycemia usually develops in neonates with prenatal exposure to hyperglycemia.
5. *Lactation.* During lactation, large amounts of glucose are used for the synthesis of both lactose and triacylglycerol by mammary glands. Thus, gluconeogenesis is markedly enhanced in a mother nursing her offspring. This is particularly important for lactating ruminants which face an additional nutritional problem, namely, the extensive fermentation of carbohydrates by ruminal microorganisms and little absorption of glucose by the small intestine. Propionate is the principal glucogenic substrate for ruminants, as noted previously.
6. *Acid–base balance.* Conversion of some substrates (e.g., lactate) to glucose consume $H^+$, thus playing a role in regulating the acid–base balance. This is of particular importance during intensive exercise when the high rates of glycolysis in skeletal muscle produce large amounts of lactate. Synthesis of glucose from lactate can conserve the glucose carbons (particularly in ruminants), in contrast to the irreversible oxidation of lactate to $CO_2$ and water. Since lactate is derived from glucose, gluconeogenesis from lactate does not result in a net production of glucose in animals. Similarly, conversion of glutamate and aspartate

into glucose in the liver and kidneys is also associated with the removal of $H^+$. Likewise, the use of glutamine as a glucogenic precursor in the kidneys during starvation generates ammonia to aid in buffering the $H^+$ which is produced through hepatic ketogenesis.

$$\text{Lactate oxidation to } CO_2\text{:} \quad C_3H_5O_3^- + H^+ + 3O_2 \rightarrow 3CO_2 + 3H_2O$$

$$\text{Lactate} \rightarrow \text{Glucose:} \quad 2C_3H_5O_3^- + 2H^+ \rightarrow C_6H_{12}O_6$$

## Glycogen Metabolism

### Glycogen as a Hydrophilic Macromolecule

Excess glucose is stored as glycogen in animals and as starch in plants. Glycogen is a highly branched polysaccharide molecule, with α-glucose residues linked by α-1,4 glycosidic bonds (main chain) and by α-1,6 glycosidic bonds. Glycogen can have a molecular weight of $10^8$, a mass equivalent to $6 \times 10^5$ glucose residues. Although almost all animal cells contain glycogen, the liver, skeletal muscle, and heart are the major sites of glycogen synthesis and deposition in animals (Chapter 2). Glycogen is a hydrophilic macromolecule associated with water in a ratio of 1:2. Thus, deposition of 1 g glycogen in skeletal muscle retains 2 g water. Muscle (skeletal muscle plus heart) and liver are the major sites of glycogen storage in animals.

### Pathway of Glycogen Synthesis

The liver, skeletal muscle, and heart are all major sites for glycogen synthesis (glycogenesis) in animals. There are both direct and indirect pathways for this metabolic pathway. The direct pathway utilizes glucose as a substrate, whereas the indirect pathway depends on C-3 units, such as alanine and lactate. Glycogenesis occurs in the cytosol and its pathway is outlined in Figure 5.21. Glucose is first phosphorylated to glucose-6-P, catalyzed by hexokinase in muscles and glucokinase in the liver. (Note that glucose-6-P is also the initial substrate of the pentose cycle.) Glucose-6-P is converted to glucose-1-P by phosphoglucomutase. In this reaction, phosphoglucomutase itself is phosphorylated, and the phospho-group participates in a reversible reaction in which glucose-1,6-bisphosphate is an intermediate.

$$\text{Enz-P} + \text{G-6-P} \leftrightarrow \text{Enz} + \text{G-1,6-P} \leftrightarrow \text{Enz-P} + \text{G-1-P}$$

Subsequently, glucose-1-P reacts with uridine triphosphate (UTP) to form uridine diphosphate glucose (UDPGlc), which is catalyzed by UDPGlc pyrophosphorylase. The subsequent hydrolysis of inorganic pyrophosphate (PPi) by inorganic pyrophosphatase pulls the reaction to the right side of the equation.

$$\text{UTP} + \text{G-1-P} \leftrightarrow \text{UDPGlc} + \text{PPi}$$

Glycogenin (a protein with a molecular weight of 37,000–38,000 Daltons) serves as the physiological primer for glycogen synthesis (Figure 2.34). About eight glucose residues (in the form of UDPGlc) are added to tyrosine-194 of glycogenin to form fully glucosylated glycogenin (protein primer for synthesis of proglycogen). The fully glucosylated glycogenin serves as the protein primer for the synthesis of proglycogen (M.W. 400,000 Daltons) in the presence of proglycogen synthase, branching enzyme, and UDPGlc. Glucose residues (in the form of UDPGlc) are further added to proglycogen to form macroglycogen (M.W. $10^7$ Daltons) in the presence of macroglycogen synthase and branching enzyme.

As noted previously, glycogen is a highly branched molecule with α-(1,4) and α-(1,6) linkages. The branching results from the action of the branching enzyme [amylo α-(1,4) → (1,6)-transglucosidase. This enzyme transfers a part of the α-1,4-chain (minimum length of six glucose residues)

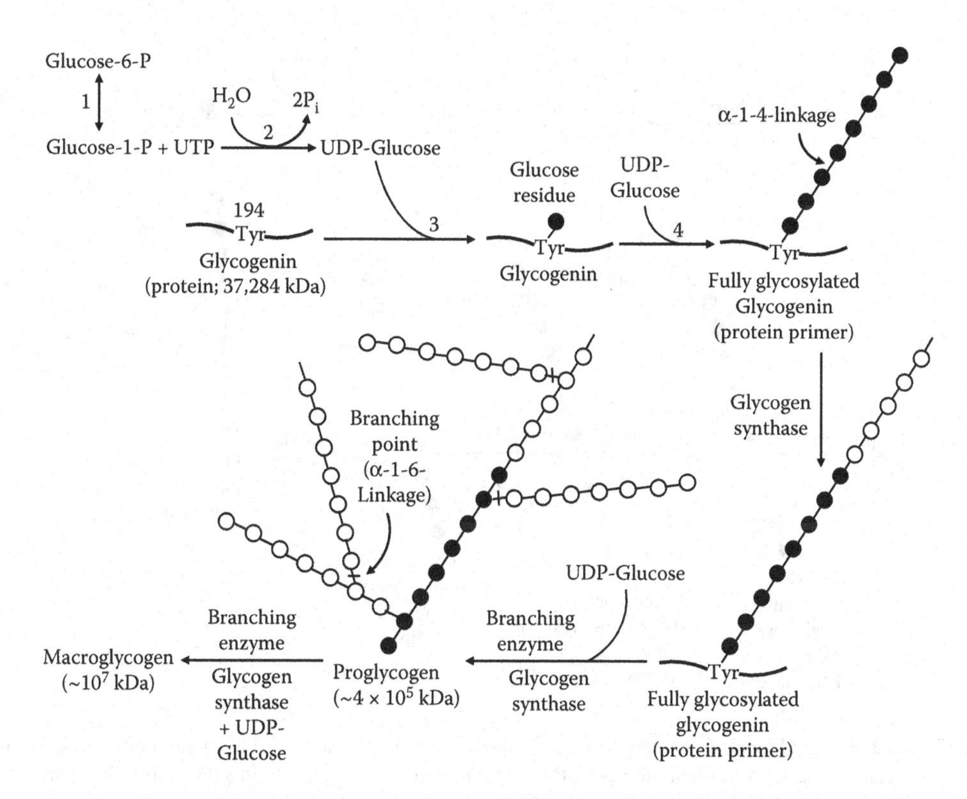


**FIGURE 5.21** Synthesis of glycogen (glycogenesis) in animals. Glycogenin is the primer for glycogen synthesis in animal cells. The glucose moiety from UDP-glucose is attached to the tyrosine-194 of glycogen, followed by the formation of glucose polymers in the α-1,4 linkage (main chain). The branching enzyme forms α-1,6 linkages of glucose molecules at the branch. The enzymes that catalyze the indicated reactions are: (1) phosphoglucomutase; (2) UDP-glucose pyrophosphorylase; (3) glycogenin's tyrosine glucosyltransferase; and (4) spontaneous autocatalysis, adding seven glucose residues to the existing glucose residue linked to Tyr-194 of glycogenin.

to a neighboring chain to form an α-1,6-linkage, thus establishing a branch point in the molecule. The branches in glycogen grow by further additions of α-1,4-glucosyl units and further branching.

The discovery of glycogenin in 1985 as a self-glucosylating protein that primes glycogen synthesis has significantly increased our understanding of the mechanism of glycogen synthesis. This discovery was based on the original finding that a liver pellet could synthesize from UDPGlc a glycogen-like product that can be precipitated by trichloroacetic acid and their postulated hypothesis (Krisman and Barengo 1975). This finding changed the traditional view that preexisting glycogen was required as the primer for glycogen synthesis in animals (Alonso et al. 1995).

## Pathway of Glycogen Degradation (Glycogenolysis)

Glycogen degradation is also known as glycogenolysis, which occurs in the cytosol. This metabolic pathway is not the reverse of glycogenesis, but involves separate enzymes and a debranching mechanism (Figure 5.22). The first and rate-controlling step of glycogenolysis is catalyzed by glycogen phosphorylase.

$$\text{Glycogen } (C_6)_n + \text{Pi} \rightarrow \text{Glycogen } (C_6)_{n-1} + \text{Glucose-1-P} \quad \text{(Glycogen phosphorylase)}$$

Glycogen phosphorylase is specific for breaking the 1 → 4-linkages of glycogen to form glucose-1-P. The terminal glucosyl residues from the outermost chains of the glycogen molecule are removed

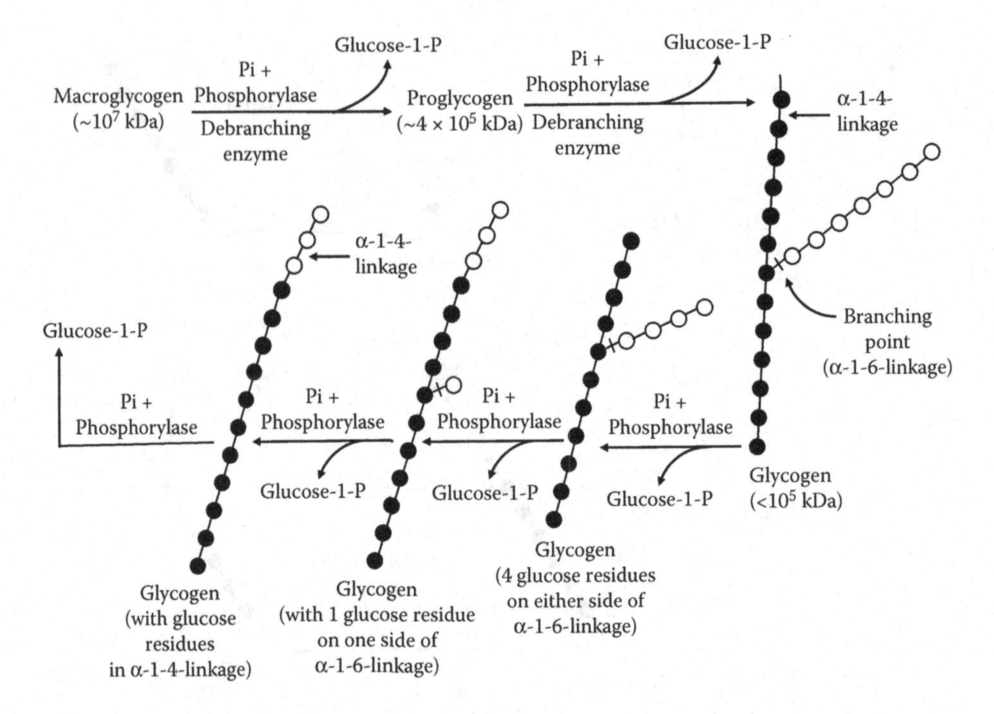


**FIGURE 5.22** Degradation of glycogen (glycogenolysis) in animals. Activated glycogen phosphorylase initiates glycogen degradation to form glucose-1-P. The branching α-1,6 linkages in side chains are hydrolyzed by the debranching enzyme to produce chains of glucose residues in α-1,4 linkages, followed by their cleavage through the action of glycogen phosphorylase. Note that Pi is required for glycogen phosphorylase activity.

sequentially until approximately four glucose residues remain on either side of the α-1,6 branches. Glucan transferase transfers a trisaccharide unit (three glucose residues) from one branch of a glycogen molecule to the other branch, thus exposing the α-1,6 branch point. The hydrolytic splitting of the α-1,6 linkages requires a specific debranching enzyme [amylo(1,6)-glucosidase]. Note that the eukaryotic glycogen debranching enzyme, a bifunctional protein, possesses two different catalytic activities (oligo-1,4 → 1,4-glucantransferase/amylo-1,6-glucosidase) on a single polypeptide chain (Nakayama et al. 2001). With the removal of the branch, further action by glycogen phosphorylase can proceed to release glucose-1-P. Thus, the combined actions of glycogen phosphorylase and the glycogen debranching enzyme lead to the complete breakdown of glycogen. As noted previously, glucose-1-P can be converted to glucose-6-P. The presence of glucose-6-phosphatase in the liver and kidneys (but not in skeletal muscle or heart) enables the formation of glucose from glucose-6-P and glycogen.

## Regulation of Glycogenesis

The principal enzyme regulating glycogen synthesis is glycogen synthase. This enzyme exists in either a dephosphorylated state (a form, active form) or a phosphorylated state (b form, inactive form). Glycogen synthase is phosphorylated by a protein kinase (mainly protein kinase A), whereas glycogen synthase phosphatase (also known as protein phosphatase-1) catalyzes its dephosphorylation (Figure 5.23). Several protein kinases can phosphorylate glycogen synthase, thereby inhibiting its activity. These kinases are known as cAMP-dependent protein kinase, $Ca^{2+}$/calmodulin-dependent protein kinase, and glycogen synthase kinases-3, -4, and -5. Glycogen synthase phosphatase is inhibited by inhibitor-1-phosphate upon its activation by cAMP-dependent protein kinase. Some hormones and metabolites also affect glycogenesis. For example, insulin increases glycogenesis by promoting dephosphorylation of glycogen synthase b (inactive) to form glycogen synthase a

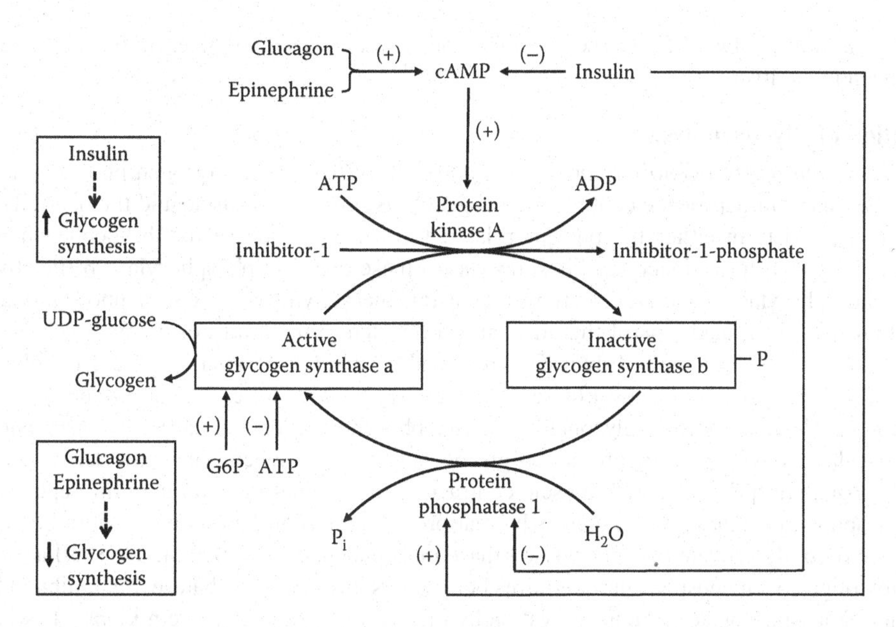


**FIGURE 5.23** Regulation of glycogen synthase through protein phosphorylation and dephosphorylation, as well as allosteric control, in animals. Glycogen synthase exists in a dephosphorylated state (active form) or phosphorylated state (inactive form). This enzyme is phosphorylated by protein kinase A, whereas protein phosphatase-1 catalyzes its dephosphorylation. Protein kinase A also phosphorylates inhibitor-1, which is an inhibitor of protein phosphatase 1. Protein kinase A itself is activated by cAMP. By increasing cAMP concentration in cells, glucagon and epinephrine suppress glycogenesis. The opposite effect is true for insulin. Glycogen synthase is allosterically activated by glucose-6-P (G6P) and inhibited by ATP. The signs (+) and (–) denote activation and inhibition, respectively.

(active), whereas fasting, epinephrine, norepinephrine, and glucagon decrease glycogenesis by promoting phosphorylation of glycogen synthase a (active) to glycogen synthase b (inactive) by stimulating cAMP production. Note that concentrations of these three hormones in plasma are elevated during intensive exercise, contributing to elevated concentrations of glucose in plasma.

Glucocorticoids modulate glucose homeostasis in animals partly through control of glycogenesis in a tissue-specific manner. Specifically, glucocorticoids increase glycogen synthesis and storage in the liver by enhancing the availability of glucose as well as expression of glucogenic enzymes and glycogen synthase (Devlin 2011). In contrast, glucocorticoids inhibit insulin-stimulated glycogen synthesis in skeletal muscle by antagonizing insulin signaling. Moreover, glucocorticoids inhibit the secretion of insulin from pancreatic β cells and also antagonize the action of insulin in the liver, skeletal muscle, heart, and white adipose tissue.

Glucose-6-P (an allosteric activator of glycogen synthase) and glucose (a precursor of glucose-6-P) promote, but ATP (an allosteric inhibitor of glycogen synthase) reduces, glycogenesis in eukaryotic cells (e.g., myocytes and hepatocytes) (Palm et al. 2013). There is evidence that arginine stimulates glycogen formation in white adipocytes (Egan et al. 1995). In contrast, a high concentration of glycogen reduces glycogenesis through a feedback inhibition mechanism, particularly in hepatocytes. Glycogen synthase is also allosterically inhibited by ATP. The discovery of cAMP as a second messenger in the cell led to the award of the Nobel Prize in Physiology or Medicine to Earl W. Sutherland in 1971.

Intracellular compartmentalization of glycogenesis is another factor regulating this pathway in the liver. Specifically, glycogen synthesis from lactate and AAs, as well as luconeogenesis, occurs mainly in periportal hepatocytes, whereas glycogen is synthesized from glucose predominantly in perivenous hepatocytes just like the degradation of glycogen into pyruvate. The separation of these opposing pathways in two different hepatocyte populations makes it possible for the net production of glycogen in the liver.

## Regulation of Glycogenolysis

1. *Regulation of glycogenolysis in skeletal muscle and the heart.* Glycogen phosphorylase is the major target for the control of glycogenolysis in skeletal muscle and the heart. This enzyme exists in either the phosphorylated form (a form, active) or the dephosphorylated form (b form, inactive). Phosphorylase kinase converts phosphorylase b (inactive) to phosphorylase a (active), thereby increasing the activity of glycogen phosphorylase (Figure 5.24). Elucidation of this mechanism resulted in the award of the Nobel Prize in Physiology or Medicine to Edwin G. Krebs and Edmond H. Fischer in 1992. Like glycogen synthase, phosphorylase kinase is also phosphorylated by cAMP-dependent protein kinase. However, unlike glycogen synthase, phosphorylation increases glycogen phosphorylase activity, thereby promoting glycogenolysis. $Ca^{2+}$ synchronizes the activation of glycogen phosphorylase with muscle contraction by stimulating a calmodulin-dependent phosphorylase kinase. It is noteworthy that protein phosphorylation and calcium binding each partially activate phosphorylase kinase independent of the other, and the full activation of glycogen phosphorylase requires both events. Protein phosphatase-1 is inhibited by inhibitor-1-phosphate upon its activation by the cAMP-dependent protein kinase. Fasting, epinephrine, and norepinephrine enhance glycogenolysis in skeletal and cardiac muscles by elevating intracellular cAMP concentrations. Of note, glucocorticoids play a permissive role for catecholamine-induced glycogenolysis in skeletal muscle (Devlin 2011). In contrast, insulin suppresses intramuscular glycogenolysis by inhibiting glycogen phosphorylase activity. In skeletal muscle, this enzyme is allosterically stimulated by AMP

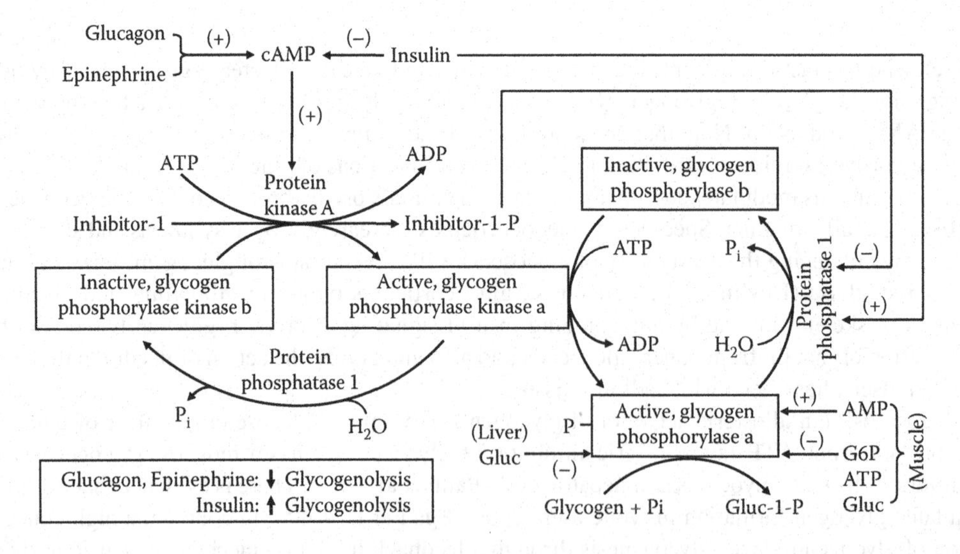


**FIGURE 5.24** Regulation of glycogen phosphorylase by protein phosphorylation and dephosphorylation in animals. Glycogen phosphorylase exists in a dephosphorylated state (inactive form) or phosphorylated state (active form). This enzyme is phosphorylated by protein kinase A, whereas protein phosphatase-1 catalyzes its dephosphorylation. Protein kinase A also phosphorylates inhibitor-1, which is an inhibitor of protein phosphatase 1. Protein kinase A itself is activated by cAMP. By increasing cAMP concentration in cells, glucagon and epinephrine stimulate glycogenolysis. The opposite effect is true for insulin. Note that allosteric regulation by metabolites (e.g., glucose [Gluc]) differs between skeletal muscle and liver. The signs (+) and (−) denote activation and inhibition, respectively.

(the intramuscular concentration of which increases during strenuous exercise), but inhibited by glucose-6-P and ATP (the intramuscular concentration of which increases after feeding).

2. *Regulation of glycogenolysis in the liver.* Hepatic glycogen phosphorylase also exists in either the phosphorylated form (a form, active) or the dephosphorylated form (b form, inactive), like its isozyme in muscles (Figure 5.24). However, liver glycogen phosphorylase is immunologically and genetically distinct from muscle phosphorylase. Insulin inhibits glycogenolysis by decreasing intracellular cAMP concentration, whereas fasting, glucagon, epinephrine, and norepinephrine promote glycogenolysis by increasing intracellular cAMP concentration (Devlin 2011). Epinephrine and norepinephrine can also increase hepatic glycogenolysis by mobilizing $Ca^{2+}$ from mitochondria to the cytosol, followed by the stimulation of a $Ca^{2+}$/calmodulin-sensitive phosphorylase kinase. Thus, cAMP integrates the regulation of glycogenesis and glycogenolysis in the liver through cAMP-dependent protein kinase. Hepatic glycogen phosphorylase activity is allosterically inhibited by glucose, but is not sensitive to allosteric control by glucose-6-P, AMP, or ATP. The difference in the allosteric regulation of glycogen phosphorylase between liver and skeletal muscle reflects their different roles as a producer and a utilizer of glucose, respectively, under various physiological conditions.

### Determination of Glycogenesis and Glycogenolysis

Glycogenesis and glycogenolysis can be measured in incubated cells and perfused organs (Ekberg et al. 1995). For example, glycogenesis can be measured in the presence of D-[U-$^{14}$C]glucose. On the other hand, glycogenolysis can be measured from the production of $^{14}CO_2$ plus [$^{14}$C]lactate from prelabeled [$^{14}$C]glycogen. *In vivo* measurements of glycogenesis and glycogenolysis are technically difficult due to the multiple pathways for the metabolism of their intermediates in animals (Chung et al. 2015).

### Nutritional and Physiological Significance of Glycogen Metabolism

The major function of glycogenesis is to store glucose as glycogen immediately after the consumption of a starch-containing meal or when the dietary supply of glucose is in excess. This helps prevent a marked increase in extracellular and intracellular osmolarity that would result from a high concentration of free glucose. In producing ducks, forced-feeding with excess starch for a couple of weeks before marketing helps produce the liver with a large amount of glycogen. However, too much glycogen can impair the function of both the liver and muscles. Hepatic glycogenolysis can immediately provide glucose to maintain the blood glucose concentration during fasting, short-periods of starvation (e.g., the diurnal fast), exercise, as well as in other conditions that might result in hypoglycemia (e.g., transient overproduction of insulin or injury). Likewise, muscle glycogenolysis supplies energy during exercise and fasting. Assuming that energy expenditure for a physically active 70 kg man is 3000 kcal/day, the complete oxidation of all the glycogen and glucose in the body can provide at most 1341 kcal or less than half of the energy needed for a day. However, at times when blood glucose is reduced (e.g., starvation) or energy needs are increased (e.g., exercise), muscle and/or liver glycogen can be mobilized to provide glucose or glucose-6-P for metabolic utilization.

## FRUCTOSE METABOLISM IN ANIMAL TISSUES

### Synthesis of Fructose from Glucose in a Cell-Specific Manner

In animals, D-fructose is synthesized from D-glucose via aldose reductase and sorbitol dehydrogenase (SD) in a tissue-dependent manner (Figure 5.25). These enzymes are located in the cytosol. The liver, ovaries, placenta (trophoblast cells), seminal vesicles, kidney, red blood cells, and eyes (lens, retina, and Schwann cells) all express aldose reductase. This enzyme requires NADPH as the

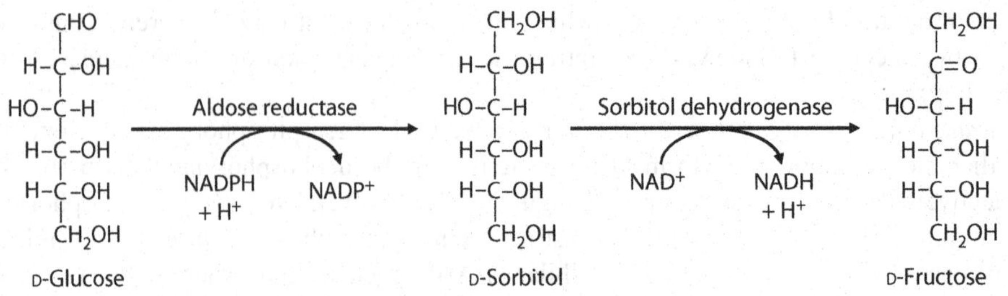

D-Glucose —(Aldose reductase; NADPH + $H^+$ → $NADP^+$)→ D-Sorbitol —(Sorbitol dehydrogenase; $NAD^+$ → NADH + $H^+$)→ D-Fructose

**FIGURE 5.25** Synthesis of D-sorbitol and D-fructose from D-glucose in certain animal tissues. The liver, ovaries, placenta, and male seminal vesicles can convert D-glucose into D-fructose in the cytosol via aldose reductase and SD. This sorbitol (polyol) pathway requires NADPH and $NAD^+$ as cofactors. SD is also known as iditol dehydrogenase.

essential cofactor. Thus, the pentose cycle plays an important role in the conversion of D-glucose to D-sorbitol and, therefore, into D-fructose. Among these tissues and cells, only the liver, ovaries, placenta, and seminal vesicles also have SD activity, and therefore they are capable of synthesizing D-fructose from D-glucose. On the basis of the high abundance of fructose in the semen of nearly all mammals studied and in fetal fluids (including fetal blood, allantoic fluid, and amniotic fluid), the net rates of fructose synthesis are likely high in the seminal vesicles and placentae.

Synthesis of fructose from glucose is upregulated by reproductive hormones. There is evidence that 17 beta-estradiol and progesterone enhance the expression of aldose reductase in animal tissues. This is consistent with the increased abundance of fructose in fetal fluids during pregnancy (Chapter 2). The concentrations of fructose in fetal blood, allantoic fluid, and amniotic fluid are high, partly due to the lack of transport of fructose from the fetus to the mother. In males, several lines of evidence show that testosterone plays a key role in inducing fructose production (Gonzales 2001; Schirren 1963). First, no fructose is detected in the seminal glands of various male domestic animals while they are infantile. Second, fructose is present in pubescent animals with the significant production of testosterone. Third, the castration of pubescent animals results in reduced concentrations of fructose in the seminal vesicles and semen, while the administration of testosterone to these males restores fructose concentrations in both seminal vesicles and semen.

### Pathways for Fructose Catabolism

The overall pathways for fructose catabolism to produce glycerol, 3-phophoglycerate, and glucose in the cytosol of animal cells are shown in Figure 5.26. It should be borne in mind that the metabolic fate of fructose is highly cell specific. For example, much of the fructose metabolized in the liver of mammals is recovered as glucose, whereas glucosamine-6-P, but not glucose, is formed from fructose in trophectoderm cells (Kim et al. 2012). In tissues (e.g., pig endometrium and placenta) that lack gluconeogenesis, there is no detectable production of pyruvate, lactate, or $CO_2$ from 1 or 5 mM D-fructose. It remains to be determined whether fructose catabolism occurs in various compartments of the cell.

Entry of fructose into cells, which is mediated primarily by GLUT2 in hepatocytes and by GLUT5 in extrahepatic cells, is the first step for fructose utilization. Of note, the GLUT5 protein is barely detectable in hepatocytes of nonruminant mammals (e.g., humans, rats, and pigs; Aschenbach et al. 2009), but significant GLUT5 mRNA levels are present in avian and bovine hepatocytes (Gilbert et al. 2007). Insulin stimulates fructose uptake by skeletal muscle, but has no effect in the liver. Thus, whole-body clearance of this sugar is impaired in diabetic patients or subjects with insulin resistance. Upon entering into the cell, the catabolism of fructose can be initiated by three enzymes: fructokinase, hexokinase, and SD (Figure 5.25). Of note, the expression of these enzymes is also cell specific, and the direction of the net reaction is dependent on the intracellular

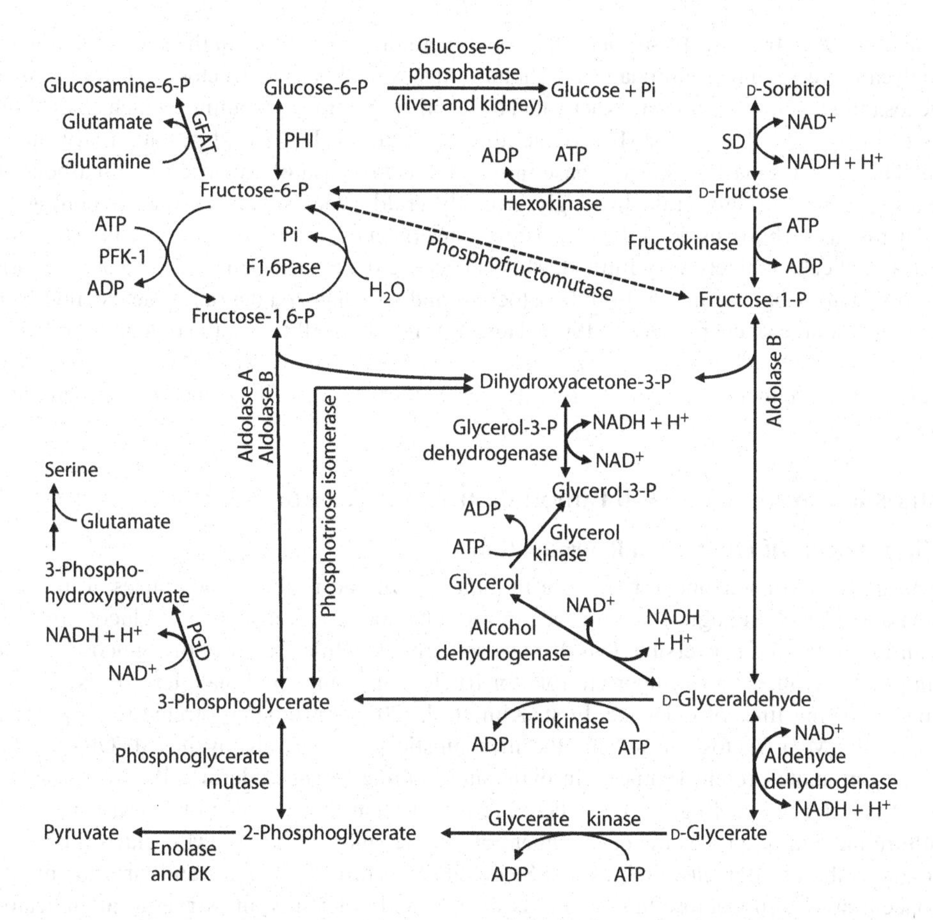


**FIGURE 5.26** Catabolism of D-fructose in animals. Catabolism of fructose is initiated by fructokinase, hexokinase, and SD in a cell-specific manner. The liver is the principal organ for degrading fructose in all animals, whereas glucosamine-6-P is formed from fructose in placentae. These three enzymes convert fructose into fructose-1-P, fructose-6-P, and sorbitol, respectively. Fructose-1-P and fructose-6-P may be interconverted by phosphofructomutase. Fructose-1-P is cleaved by aldolase B into dihydroxyacetone-3-P and D-glyceraldehyde, whereas fructose-6-P is degraded by aldolases A and B to dihydroxyacetone-3-P and 3-phosphoglycerate. Fructose-6-P can also be converted into glucose-6-P or fructose-1-6-bisphosphate and therefore participate in the synthesis of glycosaminoglycans (including hyaluronan and chondroitins) via glutamine:fructose-6-P transaminase (GFAT). In the liver and kidneys, the 3-carbon intermediates of fructose (e.g., glyceraldehyde, glycerol, glyceraldehyde-3-P, and serine) can be converted into glucose. Both hepatocytes and spermatozoa degrade fructose into lactate and $CO_2$ as a source of energy (Jones 1998). However, in other cell types, the oxidation of fructose into lactate and $CO_2$ is limited. F1,6Pase, fructose-1,6-bisphosphatase; PGD, 3-phosphoglycerate dehydrogenase; PFK1, phosphofructokinase 1; PHI, phosphohexose isomerase; PK, pyruvate kinase.

concentrations of glucose and related metabolites. The liver is the principal organ to degrade fructose in mammals, birds, and fish.

Fructose-1-P is generated by fructokinase, whereas fructose-6-P is produced by hexokinases. Fructose-1-P and fructose-6-P may be interconverted in animal tissues by phosphofructomutase. This would be analogous to the interconversion between glucose-6-P and glucose-1-P by phosphoglucomutase, which is widely expressed in animal tissues. Although phosphofructomutase is not known to be present in animals, this enzyme has been reported for bacteria and its expression is induced by elevated levels of D-fructose or D-mannose (Binet et al. 1998). Fructose-1-P is cleaved by aldolase B into dihydroxyacetone-3-P and D-glyceraldehyde, whereas fructose-6-P is degraded by aldolases A and B to dihydroxyacetone-3-P and 3-phosphoglycerate. Fructose-6-P is also converted into glucose-6-P or fructose-1-6-bisphosphate, and therefore participates in the synthesis of glycosaminoglycans (including hyaluronan and chondroitins) via glutamine:fructose-6-P transaminase. The hexosamine-synthetic pathway is activated by its other substrate, glutamine, which is also highly abundant in the fetus [e.g., 25 mM in ovine allantoic fluid on Day 60 of gestation (Kwon et al. 2003)]. Thus, fructokinase and hexokinase initiate the catabolism of fructose into 3-carbon intermediates (e.g., possibly glyceraldehyde, glycerol, glyceraldehyde-3-P, and serine). In contrast, SD traps fructose as sorbitol inside of the cell, as the conversion of sorbitol into glucose in extrahepatic and extrarenal cells is likely very limited. This is because the equilibrium of SD favors the formation of D-sorbitol from D-glucose. Both hepatocytes and spermatozoa degrade fructose into lactate and $CO_2$ as a source of energy (Jones 1998). However, in other cell types, the oxidation of fructose into lactate and $CO_2$ is limited, thereby conserving fructose carbons. Much research is warranted to quantify fructose metabolism in animal cells, particularly those in male and female reproductive systems.

### Nutritional, Physiological, and Pathological Significance of Fructose

#### Beneficial Effects of Fructose in Reproduction

The unusually high abundance of fructose in male semen and in fetal fluids raises an intriguing question about its physiological significance in reproduction. The conversion of glucose into fructose can minimize the irreversible loss of glucose carbons, while fructose, like glucose, can help sustain protein synthesis. An important role for fructose in female and male fertility is consistent with the following lines of evidence. First, Kim et al. (2012) have demonstrated that, like 4 mM D-glucose, 4 mM D-fructose stimulates the mechanistic target of rapamycin (MTOR) signaling pathway to promote protein synthesis in ovine and porcine trophectoderm cells, as well as their proliferation, and remodeling. Second, there are reports that the presence of 2 mM D-fructose in the culture medium improves the development of bovine embryos but 2 mM D-glucose is toxic to the bovine embryos (Barceló-Fimbres and Seidel 2008). Third, in humans and farm mammals, a low concentration of D-fructose in semen is associated with infertility and serves as an indicator of poor-quality spermatozoa (Schirren 1963). Fourth, adding 10 mM D-fructose to semen enhances the fertility of artificially inseminated buffalo from 25% to 40% (Akhter et al. 2014). Collectively, these results indicate that D-fructose is essential for mammalian fertility.

#### Pathological Effects of Excess Fructose

High intake of fructose or sucrose may result in the development of insulin resistance and obesity in postnatal animals (Gaby 2005). The underlying mechanisms are multifactorial and include the impaired utilization of glucose by the skeletal muscle, heart, and white adipose tissue due to defects in cell signaling. In diabetic subjects, sorbitol accumulation increases intracellular osmolality, and therefore this sugar is a significant factor that contributes to retinal damage and renal abnormalities. It is possible that fructose itself is not toxic to animal cells. However, by inducing insulin resistance and interfering with glucose oxidation, excess fructose has adverse effects on the health of postnatal mammals. Interestingly, this problem does not occur in the fetus likely because: (1) fetal glucose, but not fructose, returns to the mother for disposal; (2) the production of ROS in the fetus is minimized because glucose and AAs, rather than fatty acids, are the main metabolic fuels; and (3) high concentrations of glutathione and glycine in the conceptus protect the fetus from oxidative injury.

## GALACTOSE METABOLISM IN ANIMAL TISSUES

### Pathway of UDP-Galactose Synthesis from D-Glucose in Animal Tissues

D-Galactose is a C-4 epimer of D-glucose. Although the spontaneous epimerization of D-glucose yields D-galactose, this reaction occurs at a very slow rate. In animal tissues, including the

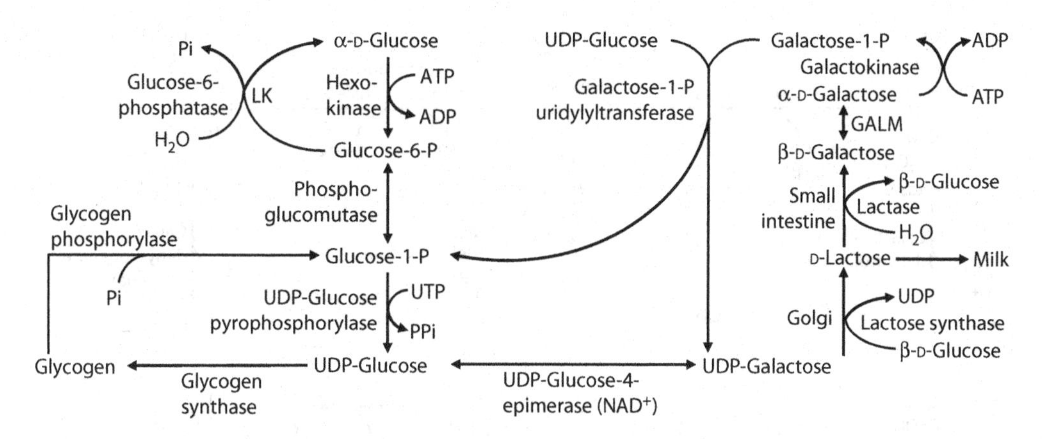


**FIGURE 5.27** Conversion of D-glucose into D-lactose and D-galactose in lactating mammals. This series of cytosolic reactions is called the Leloir pathway. The epithelial cells of lactating mammary glands contain lactose synthase in the Golgi lumen to synthesize D-lactose from UDP-galactose and β-D-glucose. However, this enzyme is absent from other tissues. UDP-glucose-4-epimerase is also called UDP-galactose-4-epimerase, and requires $NAD^+$ as the cofactor. GALM, galactose mutarotase; LK, liver and kidneys.

lactating mammary gland, UDP-galactose is formed from D-glucose by several cytosolic enzymes. Specifically, D-glucose is phosphorylated by hexokinase into glucose-6-P, which is converted into glucose-1-P by phosphoglucomutase. In addition, UDP-pyrophosphorylase catalyzes the formation of UDP-glucose from glucose-1-P and UTP. UDP-glucose-4-epimerase (also known as UDP-galactose 4-epimerase) converts UDP-glucose into UDP-galactose (Figure 5.27). UDP-galactose in the cytosol is transported into the Golgi lumen by an active transporter for the synthesis of glycolipids, phospholipids, proteoglycans, and glycoproteins in all cells.

The epithelial cells of lactating mammary glands contain lactose synthase in the Golgi lumen to synthesize D-lactose from UDP-galactose and β-D-glucose, but this enzyme is absent from other tissues (Rezaei et al. 2016). Thus, there is no biosynthesis of D-lactose or D-galactose from D-glucose in cells other than mammary epithelial cells. Lactose synthase is a complex of galactosyltransferase and α-lactalbumin (the regulatory subunit of the enzyme complex). α-Lactalbumin is only synthesized by epithelial cells of the lactating mammary gland, indicating an important role for AAs (as the precursors of proteins) in lactose production by lactating mammals. In non-mammary epithelial cells, the lack of α-lactalbumin does not allow for the formation of a functional lactose synthase complex from galactosyltransferase, and therefore no lactose is produced (Permyakov et al. 2016). Lactose synthesis is triggered by prolactin, and is enhanced by growth hormone and insulin-like growth factor-I (Rezaei et al. 2016).

## Pathway of Galactose Catabolism

Galactose exists in both α- and β-configurations in nature. This sugar is present in milk and other dairy products, as well as plant-source materials (e.g., sugar beets and mucilages). In the small intestine, lactase (bound to the surface of enterocytes) hydrolyzes D-lactose into β-D-galactose and β-D-glucose. The initial step for galactose catabolism is the conversion of β-D-galactose to α-D-galactose by galactose mutarotase. The metabolism of α-D-galactose to UDP-glucose is catalyzed sequentially by galactokinase, galactose-1-phosphate uridyltransferase, and UDP-galactose-4-epimerase (Figure 5.27). This series of reactions, which take place in the cytosol, is called the Leloir pathway. Specifically, galactokinase phosphorylates α-D-galactose into galactose-1-P. Galactose-1-phosphate uridyltransferase transfers a UMP group from UDP-glucose to galactose-1-P to form UDP-galactose (Yager et al. 2004). Finally, UDP galactose-4-epimerase interconverts

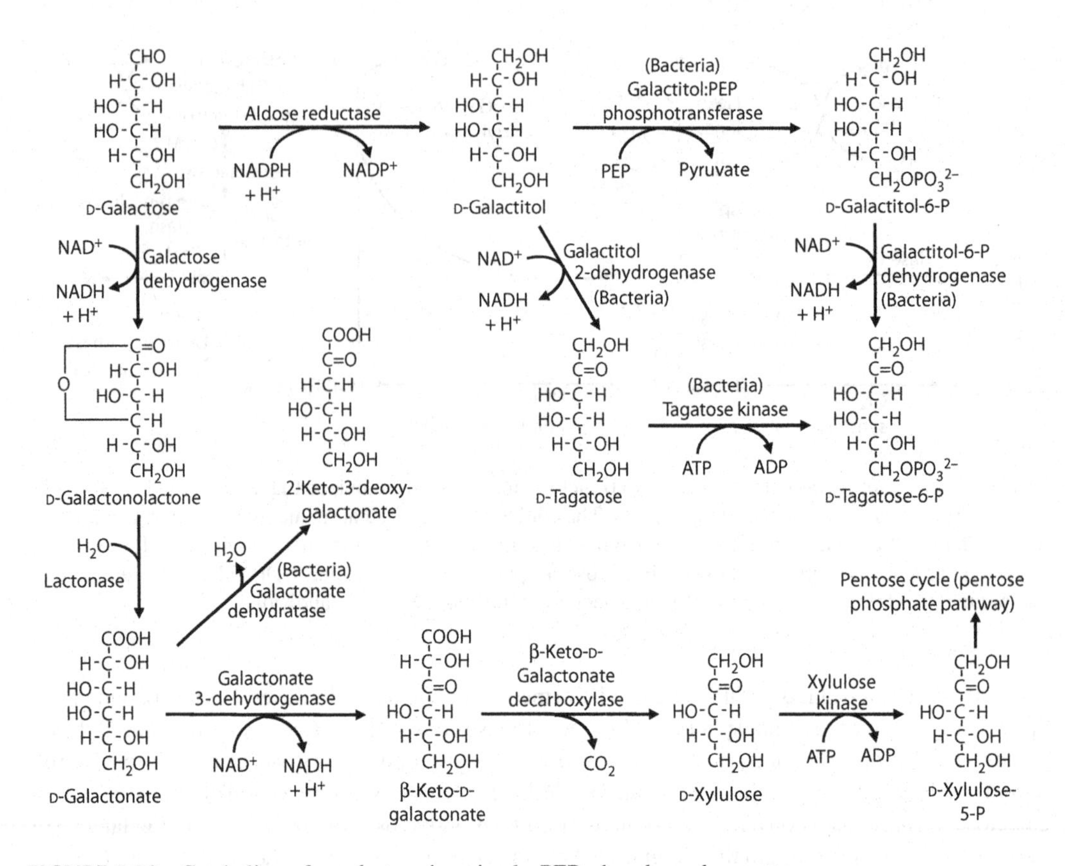


**FIGURE 5.28** Catabolism of D-galactose in animals. PEP, phosphoenolpyruvate.

UDP-galactose and UDP-glucose. UDP-Glucose is the substrate for glycogen synthesis in all cell types. The degradation of glycogen by glycogen phosphorylase generates glucose-1-P, which is converted into glucose-6-P by phosphoglucomutase. In the liver and kidneys, glucose-6-phosphatase catalyzes the formation of D-glucose from glucose-6-P. In all cells, glucose-6-P is metabolized into pyruvate and lactate. In mitochondria, pyruvate can be further oxidized through the Krebs cycle and the respiratory chain to $CO_2$ and $H_2O$.

Besides the reactions described above, D-galactose can be degraded by additional pathways. For example, D-galactose is reduced by aldose reductase into D-galactitol in the cytosol of most animal cells (Figure 5.28). D-Galacitol can be accumulated in tissues when the extracellular concentration of D-galactose is high, because animals lack enzymes to degrade D-galacitol. In addition, the livers of animals express enzymes to sequentially convert D-galactose into D-galactonolactone, D-galactonate, β-keto-D-galactonate, and D-xylulose (Cuatrecasas and Segal. 1966). D-Xylulose is then phosphorylated by xylulose kinase into D-xylulose-6-P, which enters the pentose cycle for metabolism into ribose-5-P and NADPH (Figure 5.27). These reactions also take place in bacteria and fungi for galactose utilization. These microbes also contain aldose reductase to convert D-galactose into D-tagatose-6-P.

## Physiological and Pathological Significance of Galactose

Galactose is required for lactose synthesis and milk production by the lactating mammary glands of nearly all terrestrial mammals (Rezaei et al. 2016). Thus, this monosaccharide plays an important role in the nutrition and growth of suckling neonates. Such a notion is true for some, but not all, sea mammals, depending on lactose concentrations in their milk. Besides lactose synthesis, galactose participates in the galactosylation of proteins and lipids in the Golgi (Coelho et al. 2015). For example, galactosyl transferase catalyzes the conversion of UDP-galactose and *N*-acetyl-D-glucosamine into galactosyl-*N*-acetyl-D-glucosamine, which is used for glycoprotein production. In addition, within the endoplasmic reticulum, ceramides are galactosylated by UDP-galactose:ceramide galactosyltransferase into galactosylated ceramides. These compounds play important roles in glycosphingolipid synthesis, the regulation of axon conductance in the nervous system, and cell signaling. In animals with an inherited deficiency of a key enzyme (e.g., galactokinase or galactose-1-P uridylyltransferase) in the pathway of D-galactose degradation, a metabolic disorder known as galactosemia occurs. This disease is characterized by such syndromes as an enlarged liver, cirrhosis, renal failure, cataracts, vomiting, seizure, and brain damage (McAuley et al. 2016). Evidence shows that excessive galactitol induces cataract formation in the lens and contributes to cell damage in the central nervous system, whereas excessive galactose-1-P impairs hepatic metabolism and causes liver dysfunction. Interestingly, chickens, which have a low activity of hepatic galactokinase (Gordon et al. 1971), are very susceptible to the galactose toxicity syndrome. Thus, 10 or 15% of galactose in a diet causes high mortality in broiler chicks (Douglas et al. 2003). This illustrates another difference in carbohydrate metabolism between mammals and birds.

## NUTRITIONAL AND PHYSIOLOGICAL EFFECTS OF DIETARY NSPS IN ANIMALS

### Nonruminants

#### Effects of NSPs on Feed Intake by Animals

High dietary water-soluble or insoluble NSPs reduce feed intake by nonruminants (e.g., pigs and poultry) via different mechanisms (Bedford and Morgan 1996; Lindberg 2014). Soluble NSPs (e.g., pectin, guar gum, arabinoxylans, β-glucans, and sodium alginate) readily dissolve in water to become gelatinous and viscous substances, which increase viscosity (fluid resistance to flow) in the lumen of the stomach and small intestine. This leads to decreases in gastric emptying, small-intestinal contractions, and digesta transit through the small intestine. Note that some readily fermentable fibers are not gel formers and some viscous fibers are not all readily fermented. There is evidence that via sensory mechanisms in the mucosae of the gastrointestinal smooth muscle and the gut–brain signaling pathway, dietary soluble NSPs stimulate the release of peptide YY and glucagon-like peptide-1 (GLP-1), but inhibit the release of ghrelin by the gastrointestinal tract (Greenway et al. 2007; Zijlstra et al. 2007). Since peptide YY and GLP-1 suppress, but ghrelin promotes, food consumption, the effects of soluble NSPs on their release help explain how these NSPs reduce appetite and feed intake by animals.

In contrast to soluble NSPs, insoluble NSPs (e.g., cellulose and hemicellulose) are nonviscous, have negligible effects on gastric emptying, and increase the rate of small intestine transit. There is evidence that insoluble NSPs reduce appetite and feed intake at the initial level of the small intestine. Specifically, insoluble NSPs reduce the absorption of glucose by the small intestine, leading to an increase in its concentration at the terminal ileum and, therefore, the secretion of GLP-1. In addition, insoluble NSPs stimulate the secretion of CCK (Holt et al. 1992). Both GLP-1 and CCK are known to contribute to satiety and food intake suppression (Flint et al. 1998).

#### Effects of NSPs on Nutrient Digestibility, Growth, and Feed Efficiency

High intake of either water-soluble or insoluble NSPs reduces nutrient digestibility, growth rate, and feed efficiency in nonruminants (e.g., pigs and poultry) through common and also different mechanisms (Bedford and Morgan 1996; Lindberg 2014). Both soluble and insoluble NSPs bind to and entrap lipids, protein, starch, vitamins, and minerals to form fibrous complexes. These effects of the NSPs result in: (1) dilution of digestive enzymes and their substrates, (2) interference of enzyme–substrate interaction, (3) reduced digestion of nutrients, and (4) reduced and delayed absorption of nutrients (including glucose, lipids, and AAs) in the small intestine. In addition, the soluble

NSPs-induced increase in viscosity within the lumen of the small intestine, as noted previously, further impairs nutrient digestion and absorption through (1) decreasing small-intestinal contractions and (2) increasing the thickness of the unstirred water layer. Furthermore, through mechanical stimulation, insoluble NSPs shorten the time of the transit of digesta through the small intestine, thereby reducing nutrient digestion and absorption. For example, feed intake, DM digestibility, and daily weight gain were 4.8%, 3.2%, and 16% lower in postweaning young pigs fed a 15.2% NDF diet (containing 5% bamboo meal) than those fed a 11.9% NDF diet (Yu et al. 2016). Similarly, high inclusion levels of soluble or insoluble NSPs suppress feed intake, nutrient digestibility, and weight gains in growing pigs (Longland et al. 1994), as well as rainbow trout, tilapia, and Atlantic salmon (Refstie et al. 1999; Shiau et al. 1988). Of note, in obese animals, dietary supplementation with soluble or insoluble NSPs increases the fecal excretion of nitrogen, ash, and fat, while reducing postprandial glycemic response, blood lipid concentrations, and risk for cardiovascular disease (Blaak et al. 2012).

### Effects of NSPs on Intestinal and Overall Health

Although a high percentage of NSPs in the diet is an anti-nutritional factor, their adequate intake is very important for the intestinal health of animals. While all NSPs undergo little degradation in the small intestine, they are either fully or partially fermented in the large intestine to generate SCFAs. Thus, the effects of dietary NSPs on intestinal health are affected by their physical and chemical properties, including the degree of their solubility in water (Bach Knudsen et al. 2017). Soluble NSPs are also highly fermentable in the large bowel to produce SCFAs, which are major metabolic fuels for colonocytes and regulators of their gene expression. The hydrolysis of soluble NSPs and proteins in plant ingredients provides both carbon and nitrogen sources for bacteria to grow. Therefore, bacteria, lipids, fermentation products (including SCFAs, $NH_4^+$, and gases), and other biomass (e.g., endogenous secretions and undigested material) are the major contributors to the increase in stool bulk with the intake of rapidly fermented soluble NSPs (e.g., those in oat bran), while decreasing the risk for colon cancer in animals (Turner and Lupton 2011).

Insoluble NSPs (e.g., wheat bran) have no appreciable water holding capacity. They are only partially digestible in the colon and cecum, and thus have a lesser effect on SCFA production than soluble NSPs. However, insoluble NSPs provide a bulking effect, increase fecal mass, shorten the time of the transit of luminal contents through the large intestine, and alleviate constipation (Bach Knudsen et al. 2017). Insoluble NSPs act as effective laxatives by binding to luminal undigested material and stimulating the gut mucosa through mechanoreceptors, thereby inducing secretion and peristalsis. Large, coarse particles provide a greater laxative efficacy than fine, smooth particles (no or little effect) (Blaak et al. 2012). Stool weight is generally increased by adding insoluble NSPs to the diet.

The proportions of water-soluble NSPs in sugar beet pulp, oat bran, barley, rye, and beans are higher than those in alfalfa hay, wheat straw, wheat bran, palm kernel expeller, bamboo meal, as well as the hulls of wheat, oats, corn, and rice. In all these products, insoluble NSPs are more abundant than soluble NSPs. Of interest, comparable amounts of NSPs from wheat and oat brans have the same effect on daily fecal output, even though >90% and only 50%–60% of their NSPs are water insoluble, respectively. However, wheat bran is more effective than oat bran in the prevention and treatment of constipation, whereas oat bran can lower blood concentrations of glucose, TAGs, and cholesterol in animals to a greater extent than wheat bran. A low level of either soluble or insoluble NSPs in the diet can cause constipation, colonic inflammation, and the occurrence of hemorrhoids in nonruminants (Bach Knudsen et al. 2017).

As herbivores, horses have evolved to consume diets that are low in starch but rich in NSPs. These diets usually consist of forages (e.g., hay, haylage, and grass) which are vital to the health of the digestive system. There are reports that inclusion of soluble fiber in diets increased the concentrations of total cecal SCFA and propionic acid, which resulted in stable and constant plasma glycemic and insulinemic responses in horses (Brøkner et al. 2016).

## RUMINANTS

### Effects of NDF on Rumen pH and Environment

A term commonly used in ruminant nutrition is NDF, which primarily refers to the amount of cellulose, hemicellulose, and lignin in the feedstuff. Thus, the NDF is equivalent to water-insoluble NSPs in nonruminant nutrition, but is an essential nutrient to postweaning ruminants. In both grazing and feedlot ruminants (e.g., cattle), the NDF plays a vital role in maintaining their ruminal health by preventing the occurrence of ruminal acidosis through the following mechanisms: (1) promoting rumination to allow for a greater amount buffer to reach the rumen environment via saliva and digestion; (2) slowing down the fermentation of starches and NSPs to form SCFAs to maintain ruminal pH; (3) decreasing the concentration of acetic acid in the rumen; and (4) facilitating the fermentation of dietary protein and nonprotein nitrogenous substances to yield $NH_3$, which takes up $H^+$ as $NH_4^+$. Individual roughage sources can influence the frequency of rumination, but ruminal NDF content rarely negatively affects beef cattle consuming an appropriate amount of high-concentrate diet (Galyean and Defoor 2003).

### Effects of NDF on Intestinal Health

SCFAs have the same physiological functions in the hindgut of ruminants as in nonruminants, as noted previously. Since not all dietary fibers are fermented in the rumen, those that escape the rumen enter the large intestine, where they are extensively fermented by bacteria to affect the metabolism and health of colonocytes, as well as fecal formation, bulking, and excretion. These effects of NDF vary with its types, the ratio of cellulose to hemicellulose, and lignification of the plant cell wall. Although the fiber carbohydrate portion is positively correlated with rumen fill or physical fill, it rarely has a negative effect on intestinal health in grazing beef cattle supplemented with a high-concentrate feed (Galyean and Defoor 2003). Rather, in ruminants, inadequate intake of NSPs adversely affects gastrointestinal function.

### Effects of NDF on Lactation and Growth Performance

NDF must be fermented in the rumen to exert its major nutritional effect on the lactation and growth performance of ruminants. Thus, digestibility of NDF is an important indicator of forage quality, particularly because the content and rumen degradability of NDF in forages vary widely with their species, maturity, growing environment, and lignification. A greater amount of rumen-fermentable NDF results in a greater amount of metabolizable energy available to ruminants, ultimately enhancing feed efficiency and performance in both dairy and beef cattle production systems. For example, owing to reduced acetate synthesis by ruminal bacteria, a diet containing $<25\%$ NDF or $<16\%$ NDF from forage, despite an adequate amount of total carbohydrate, reduces milk fat content in lactating cows (Clark and Armentano 1993). A one-unit increase in *in vitro* or *in situ* NDF digestibility (within the range of 54.5%–62.9%) was found to be associated with a 0.17 kg increase in DMI and a 0.25-kg increase in 4% fat-corrected milk (Oba and Allen 1999). Rations for dairy cows must generally contain at least 25% dietary NDF and a large proportion (at least 76%) of dietary NDF should come from forages (i.e., minimum forage NDF being 19%). As noted previously, the concentration of NDF from forage in the diet, which is closely related to chewing activity, is a determinant of rumen pH of ruminants (including dairy cows). Thus, these animals require sufficient NDF in diets to maximize growth rate and milk yield (NRC 2001).

### Effects of NDF on Feed Intake

Feed intake positively influences the production performance of ruminants. Adequate dietary NDF is necessary for maintaining proper rumen function. However, excess dietary NDF can limit voluntary feed intake because of physical fill in the rumen. Much evidence shows that the relationship between dietary NDF content and feed intake is complex and nonlinear (Arelovich et al. 2008). Depending on the amount and quality of dietary NDF, it can either enhance or reduce feed intake by ruminants. For example, DM intake by beef cattle can increase with increasing dietary NDF content from 7.5% to 22%, but can decrease sharply when dietary NDF content increases from 22% to 46%. Digestibility of dietary NDF also affects DM intake. In dairy cows fed silages with similar NDF and CP contents but a higher NDF digestibility, DM intake and milk yield are increased in comparison with the control group of cows fed a diet with a lower NDF digestibility (Oba and Allen 1999). The underlying mechanisms likely involve a series of cell signaling cascade in the gastrointestinal tract-brain axis.

## SUMMARY

The gastrointestinal tract is the first site for initiating the utilization of dietary carbohydrates by animals in a species- and age-dependent manner. At birth and during the suckling period, neonatal mammals (both pre-ruminants and nonruminants) have a high activity of intestinal lactase to convert milk lactose into β-D-galactose and β-D-glucose, but have a very low or no activity of intestinal α-amylase, sucrase-isomaltase, and maltase-glucoamylase for utilizing starch, glycogen, sucrose, and maltose. In contrast, birds cannot tolerate a large amount of lactose in a diet but can consume and utilize cereal grains immediately after hatching. In postweaning mammals, the intestinal activity of lactase is sharply reduced, but the amounts of salivary and pancreatic α-amylases as well as intestinal α-amylase, sucrase-isomaltase, and maltase-glucoamylase are progressively increased until the small intestine becomes fully mature. Thus, after weaning, mammals can effectively utilize diets containing: (1) starch and glycogen, which are hydrolyzed into α-D-glucose in the small intestine under the combined actions of α-amylase, sucrase-isomaltase, and maltase-glucoamylase; and (2) disaccharides (e.g., sucrose which is hydrolyzed into α-D-glucose and β-D-fructose; and maltose which is hydrolyzed into two units of α-D-glucose). In non-carnivorous fish whose pancreas produces and secretes a significant quantity of pancreatic α-amylase, dietary starch or glycogen can serve as a low-cost energy source. In all animals, monosaccharides are absorbed into enterocytes of the small intestine by SGLT1 (glucose and galactose) and GLUT5 (fructose), and the simple sugars enter the portal circulation. While the enterocytes of all postnatal animals can effectively absorb D-glucose and D-galactose and the enterocytes of post-hatching birds can also absorb D-fructose well, the enterocytes of mammals can significantly take up D-fructose only after weaning. Thus, sucrose and fructose in diets are toxic to neonatal mammals, and a large amount of lactose in diets causes morbidity in poultry.

In nonruminants (e.g., pigs, poultry, fish, and humans), nearly all indigestible dietary fibers enter the large intestine for fermentation into SCFAs. In contrast, both water-soluble and insoluble complex carbohydrates (e.g., starch, cellulose, and hemicellulose) are extensively fermented into SCFAs, and, to a lesser extent, $CO_2$ and methane, in the rumen of ruminants, such that little glucose is absorbed into enterocytes in cattle, sheep, goats, and deer. Since butyrate is the major metabolic fuel for colonocytes, dietary fiber is crucial for intestinal health in both ruminants and nonruminants. Dietary fiber (NDF) has an additional role in maintaining proper rumen pH and functions and is considered to be a nutritionally essential carbohydrate for ruminants.

After D-glucose is absorbed by enterocytes, it is metabolized via multiple pathways. In the cytosol of all animal cells, D-glucose is utilized through glycolysis to yield pyruvate and NADH. Pyruvate is converted into L-lactate in cells without mitochondria or in cells with mitochondria when glycolysis produces NADH faster than the electron transport chain can oxidize it, such as under hypoxic conditions or during intense exercise. When oxygen supply is adequate, pyruvate and NADH are transported, via specific transporter systems, from the cytosol into mitochondria, where pyruvate is oxidized by PDH into acetyl-CoA and then, through the Krebs cycle, into $CO_2$, $FADH_2$, and NADH. The reducing equivalents ($FADH_2$ and NADH) are oxidized, through the mitochondrial respiratory chain, into $H_2O$, with the production of 1.5 and 2.5 molecules of ATP per 1 molecule of $FADH_2$ and NADH, respectively. Of note, D-glucose is converted into

D-fructose in the liver, ovaries, placenta, and male seminal vesicles. In the reproductive tract, D-fructose activates mTOR cell signaling, promotes conceptus development, and maintains sperm vitality. In all animals, excess D-Glucose is stored as glycogen primarily in the liver and skeletal muscle through glycogenesis, and glycogen is mobilized rapidly to eventually generate glucose, when glycogen phosphorylase is activated by cAMP-dependent protein kinase (e.g., fasting and intensive exercise). D-Glucose is also metabolized through the pentose cycle to produce NADPH and ribose-5-P, and through the uronic acid pathway to generate glucuronic acid, ascorbic acid (vitamin C in some species), and pentoses.

Besides its catabolism, D-glucose is synthesized from glucogenic substrates (e.g., alanine, glutamine, serine, glycerol, lactate, pyruvate, and propionate) by the liver and kidneys of animals in a species- and nutritional status-dependent manner. When dietary intake of glucose or glucose-containing carbohydrates is limited or there is no feed intake, glucose synthesis from glucogenic AAs and glycerol is highly active to provide glucose for tissues of both ruminants and nonruminants, particularly the brain and red blood cells. In addition, dietary carbohydrates (e.g., starch, glycogen, and oligosaccharides) are extensively fermented to form SCFAs in the rumen, and gluconeogenesis from propionate is particularly important in fed ruminants. Thus, these animals must synthesize glucose to survive and grow. In the epithelial cells of lactating mammary glands, glucose is used for the synthesis of galactose and lactose. Dietary galactose is utilized through its initial conversion into glucose. The pathways of glucose metabolism are regulated by hormones (e.g., insulin, glucagon, catecholamines, and prolactin), cellular energy status, and cellular concentrations of metabolites to maintain glucose homeostasis in the blood. Of particular note, glycolysis and gluconeogenesis are reciprocally controlled by fructose-2,6-bisphosphate in the liver. Such well-coordinated metabolic control is essential for the efficient utilization of dietary carbohydrates and glucose homeostasis, as well as growth, development, and health for all animals. Otherwise, hypoglycemia results in nervous dysfunction and eventually coma and death in all animals. Likewise, impaired utilization of glucose by skeletal muscle results in diabetes, and reduced catabolism of galactose causes mortality, with chickens being highly susceptible to galactosemia. Thus, exquisite regulation of carbohydrate metabolism is vital to the growth, development and survival of animals.

## REFERENCES


Akhter, S., M.S. Ansari, B.A. Rakha, S.M.H. Andrabi, M. Qayyum, and N. Ullah. 2014. Effect of fructose in extender on fertility of buffalo semen. *Pakistan J. Zool.* 46:279–281.

Akin, D.E. and W.S. Borneman. 1990. Role of rumen fungi in fiber degradation. *J. Dairy Sci.* 73:3023–3032.

Alonso, M.D., J. Lomako, W.M. Lomako, and W.J. Whelan. 1995. A new look at the biogenesis of glycogen. *FASEB J.* 9:1126–1137.

Arelovich, H.M., C.S. Abney, J.A. Vizcarra, and M.L. Galyean. 2008. Effects of dietary neutral detergent fiber on intakes of dry matter and net energy by dairy and beef cattle: Analysis of published data. *Prof. Anim. Sci.* 24:375–383.

Aschenbach, J.R., K. Steglich, G. Gäbel, and K.U. Honscha. 2009. Expression of mRNA for glucose transport proteins in jejunum, liver, kidney and skeletal muscle of pigs. *J. Physiol. Biochem.* 65:251–266.

Bach Knudsen, K.E. 2001. The nutritional significance of "dietary fiber" analysis. *Anim. Feed Sci. Technol.* 90:3–20.

Bach Knudsen, K.E., N.P. Nørskov, A.K. Bolvig, M.S. Hedemann, and H.N. Laerke. 2017. Dietary fibers and associated phytochemicals in cereals. *Mol. Nutr. Food Res.* 61(7):1–15.

Bakke, A.M., C. Glover, and A. Krogdahl. 2011. Feeding, digestion and absorption of nutrients. *Fish Physiol.* 30:57–110.

Baldwin, R.L., L.J. Koong, and M.J. Ulyatt. 1977. Model of ruminant digestion. *Agr-Bio. Syst.* 2:282.

Barceló-Fimbres, M. and G.E. Seidel. 2008. Effects of embryo sex and glucose or fructose in culture media on bovine embryo development. *Reprod. Fertil. Dev.* 20:141–142.

Bedford, M.R. and A.J. Morgan. 1996. The use of enzymes in poultry diets. *World's Poult. Sci. J.* 52:61–68.

Bergman, E.N. 1983. The pool of cellular nutrients: Glucose. In: *World Animal Science*, Vol. 3. Edited by P.M. Riis, Elsevier, New York, pp. 173–196.

Bergman, E.N., R.P. Brockman, and C.F. Kaufman. 1974. Glucose metabolism in ruminants: Comparison of whole-body turnover with production by gut, liver, and kidneys. *Proc. Fed. Am. Soc. Exp. Biol.* 33:1849–1854.

Binet, M.R., M.N. Rager, and O.M. Bouvet. 1998. Fructose and mannose metabolism in *Aeromonas hydrophila*: Identification of transport systems and catabolic pathways. *Microbiology.* 144:1113–1121.

Blaak, E.E., J.-M. Antoine, D. Benton, I. Björck, L. Bozzetto, F. Brouns, M. Diamant et al. 2012. Impact of postprandial glycaemia on health and prevention of disease. *Obesity Rev.* 13:923–984.

Bondi, A.A. 1987. *Animal Nutrition.* John Wiley & Sons, New York, NY.

Brøkner, C., D. Austbø, J.A. Næsset, D. Blache, K.E. Bach Knudsen, and A.H. Tauson. 2016. Metabolic response to dietary fibre composition in horses. *Animal.* 10:1155–1163.

Brøkner, C., D. Austbø, J.A. Næsset, K.E. Knudsen, and A.H. Tauson. 2012. Equine pre-caecal and total tract digestibility of individual carbohydrate fractions and their effect on caecal pH response. *Arch. Anim. Nutr.* 66:490–506.

Brosnan, J.T. 1999. Comments on metabolic needs for glucose and the role of gluconeogenesis. *Eur. J. Clin. Nutr.* 53(Suppl. 1):S107–S111.

Castillo, J., D. Crespo, E. Capilla, M. Díaz, F. Chauvigné, J. Cerdà, and J.V. Planas. 2009. Evolutionary structural and functional conservation of an ortholog of the GLUT2 glucose transporter gene (SLC2A2) in zebrafish. *Am. J. Physiol. Regul. Integr. Comp. Physiol.* 297:R1570–R1581.

Chesson, A. and C.W. Fossberg. 1997. Polysaccharides degradation by rumen microorganisms. In: *The Rumen Microbial Ecosystem*, 2nd ed. Edited by P.N. Hobson and C.S. Stewart. Blackie, London, UK, pp. 329–381.

Chotinsky, D., E. Toncheva, and Y. Profirov. 2001. Development of disaccharidase activity in the small intestine of broiler chickens. *Br. Poult. Sci.* 42:389–393.

Chung, S.T., S.K. Chacko, A.L. Sunehag, and M.W. Haymond. 2015. Measurements of gluconeogenesis and glycogenolysis: A methodological review. *Diabetes.* 64:3996–4010.

Clark, P.W. and L.E. Armentano. 1993. Effectiveness of neutral detergent fiber in whole cottonseed and dried distillers grains compared with alfalfa haylage. *J. Dairy Sci.* 76:2644–2650.

Coelho, A.I., G.T. Berry, and M.E. Rubio-Gozalbo. 2015. Galactose metabolism and health. *Curr. Opin. Clin. Nutr. Metab. Care.* 18:422–427.

Cuatrecasas, P. and S. Segal. 1966. Galactose conversion to D-xylulose: An alternate route of galactose metabolism. *Science.* 153:549–551.

Deng, D. and N. Yan. 2016. GLUT, SGLT, and SWEET: Structural and mechanistic investigations of the glucose transporters. *Protein Sci.* 25:546–558.

Devlin, T.M. 2011. *Textbook of Biochemistry with Clinical Correlations.* John Wiley & Sons, New York, NY.

Douglas, M.W., M. Persia, and C.M. Parsons. 2003. Impact of galactose, lactose, and Grobiotic-B70 on growth performance and energy utilization when fed to broiler chicks. *Poult. Sci.* 82:1596–1601.

Downs, D.M. 2006. Understanding microbial metabolism. *Annu. Rev. Microbiol.* 60:533–559.

Drozdowski, L.A. and A.B.R. Thomson. 2006. Intestinal sugar transport. *World J. Gastroenterol.* 12:1657–1670.

Driedzic, W.R., K.A. Clow, C.E. Short, and K.V. Ewart. 2006. Glycerol production in rainbow smelt (*Osmerus mordax*) may be triggered by low temperature alone and is associated with the activation of glycerol-3-phosphate dehydrogenase and glycerol-3-phosphatase. *J. Exp. Biol.* 209:1016–1023.

Drozdowski, L.A., T. Clandinin, and A.B.R. Thomson. 2010. Ontogeny, growth and development of the small intestine: Understanding pediatric gastroenterology. *World J. Gastroenterol.* 16:787–799.

Egan, J.M., T.E. Henderson, and M. Bernier. 1995. Arginine enhances glycogen synthesis in response to insulin in 3T3-L1 aipocytes. *Am. J. Physiol.* 269:E61–E66.

Ekberg, K., V. Chandramouli, K. Kumaran, W.C. Schumann, J. Wahren, and B.R. Landau. 1995. Gluconeogenesis and glucuronidation in liver *in vivo* and the heterogeneity of hepatocyte function. *J. Biol. Chem.* 270:21715–21717.

Ellis, W.C., J.H. Matis, and C. Lascano. 1979. Quantitating ruminal turnover. *Fed. Proc.* 38:2702–2706.

Eswaran, S., J. Muir, and W.D. Chey. 2013. Fiber and functional gastrointestinal disorders. *Am. J. Gastroenterol.* 108:718–727.

Fang, Y.Z., S. Yang, and G. Wu. 2002. Free radicals, antioxidants, and nutrition. *Nutrition* 18:872–879.

Fellner, V. 2002. Rumen microbes and nutrient management. *Proceedings of American Registry of Professional Animal Scientists—California Chapter Conference*, October 2002, Coalinga, California.

Ferraris, R.P. 2001. Dietary and developmental regulation of intestinal sugar transport. *Biochem. J.* 360:265–276.

Ferraris, R.P., R.K. Buddington, and E.S. David. 1999. Ontogeny of nutrient transporters. In: *Development of the Gastrointestinal Tract.* Edited by I.R. Sanderson and W.A. Walker. B.C. Decker Inc., Hamilton, Canada, pp. 123–146.

Firkins, J.L., Z. Yu, and M. Morrison. 2007. Ruminal nitrogen metabolism: Perspectives for integration of microbiology and nutrition for dairy. *J. Dairy Sci.* 90(E. Suppl.):E1–E16.

Flint, A., A. Raben, A. Astrup, and J.J. Holst. 1998. Glucagon-like peptide 1 promotes satiety and suppresses energy intake in humans. *J. Clin. Invest.* 101:515–520.

Frøystad, M.K., E. Lilleeng, A. Sundby, and A. Krogdahl. 2006. Cloning and characterization of alpha-amylase from Atlantic salmon (*Salmo salar* L.). *Comp. Biochem. Physiol. A* 145:479–492.

Gaby, A.R. 2005. Adverse effects of dietary fructose. *Altern. Med. Rev.* 10:294–306.

Galyean, M.L. and P.J. Defoor. 2003. Effects of roughage source and level on intake by feedlot cattle. *J. Anim. Sci.* 81(E. Suppl. 2):E8–E16.

Gerrits, W.J.J., J. Dijkstra, and J. France. 1997. Description of a model integrating protein and energy metabolism in preruminant calves. *J. Nutr.* 127:1229–1242.

Gilbert, E.R., H. Li, D.A. Emmerson, K.E. Webb Jr., and E.A. Wong. 2007. Developmental regulation of nutrient transporter and enzyme mRNA abundance in the small intestine of broilers. *Poult. Sci.* 86:1739–1753.

Gonzales, G.F. 2001. Function of seminal vesicles and their role on male fertility. *Asian J. Androl.* 3:251–258.

Gordon, M., H. Wells, and S. Segal. 1971. Enzymes of the sugar nucleotide pathway of galactose metabolism in chick liver. *Enzyme* 12:513–522.

Greenway, F., C.E. O'Neil, L. Stewart, J. Rood, M. Keenan, and R. Martin. 2007. Fourteen weeks of treatment with Viscofiber (R) increased fasting levels of glucagon-like peptide-1 and peptide-YY. *J. Med. Food.* 10:720–724.

Hall, J.R., C.E. Short, and W.R. Driedzic. 2006. Sequence of Atlantic cod (*Gadus morhua*) GLUT4, GLUT2 and GPDH: Developmental stage expression, tissue expression and relationship to starvation-induced changes in blood glucose. *J. Exp. Biol.* 209:4490–4502.

Han, H.S., G. Kang, J.S. Kim, B.H. Choi, and S.H. Koo. 2016. Regulation of glucose metabolism from a liver-centric perspective. *Exp. Mol. Med.* 48:e218.

Heald, P.J. 1951. The assessment of glucose-containing substances in rumen microorganisms during a digestion cycle in sheep. *Br. J. Nutr.* 5:84–93.

Hers, H.G. and M. Van Schaftingen. 1982. Fructose 2,6-bisphosphate 2 years after its discovery. *Biochem. J.* 206:1–12.

Hoek, J.B. and J. Rydstrom. 1988. Physiological roles of nicotinamide nucleotide transhydrogenase. *Biochem. J.* 254:1–10.

Holt, S., J. Brand, C. Soveny, and J. Hansky. 1992. Relationship of satiety to postprandial glycaemic, insulin and cholecystokinin responses. *Appetite* 18:129–141.

Hook, S.E., A.G. Wright, and B.W. McBride. 2010. Methanogens: Methane producers of the rumen and mitigation strategies. *Archaea* 2010: Article ID 945785.

Huhtanen, P., S. Ahvenjärvi, M.R. Weisbjerg, and P. NØrgaard. 2008. Digestion and passage of fibre in ruminants. In: *Ruminant Physiology.* Edited by K. Sejrsen, T. Hvelplund, and M.O. Nielsen. Wageninger Academic, Wageningen, The Netherlands, pp. 87–135.

Huston, J.E., B.S. Rector, W.C. Ellis, and M.L. Allen. 1986. Dynamics of digestion in cattle, sheep, goats and deer. *J. Anim. Sci.* 62:208–215.

Jensen, R.B., D. Austbø, K.E. Bach Knudsen, and A.H. Tauson. 2014. The effect of dietary carbohydrate composition on apparent total tract digestibility, feed mean retention time, nitrogen and water balance in horses. *Animal.* 8:1788–1796.

Jones, A.R. 1998. Chemical interference with sperm metabolic pathways. *J. Reprod. Fertil. Suppl.* 53:227–234.

Jouany, J.P. and K. Ushida. 1999. The role of protozoa in feed digestion—Review. *Asian Australas. J. Anim. Sci.* 12:113–128.

Julliand, V., A. De Fombelle, and M. Varloud. 2006. Starch digestion in horses: The impact of feed processing. *Livest. Sci.* 100:44–52.

Kandler, O. 1983. Carbohydrate metabolism in lactic acid bacteria. *Antonie Van Leeuwenhoek* 49:209–224.

Katz, J. and H.G. Wood. 1963. The use of $C^{14}O_2$ yields from glucose-1- and -6-$C^{14}$ for the evaluation of the pathways of glucose metabolism. *J. Biol. Chem.* 238:517–523.

Kim, J.Y., G.W. Song, G. Wu, and F.W. Bazer. 2012. Functional roles of fructose. *Proc. Natl. Acad. Sci. USA.* 109:E1619–E1628.

Kletzien, R.F., P.K. Harris, and L.A. Foellmi. 1994. Glucose-6-phosphate dehydrogenase: A "housekeeping" enzyme subject to tissue-specific regulation by hormones, nutrients, and oxidant stress. *FASEB J.* 8:174–181.

Krasnov, A., H. Teerijoki, and H. Mölsä. 2001. Rainbow trout (*Onchorhynchus mykiss*) hepatic glucose transporter. *Biochim. Biophys. Acta.* 1520:174–178.

Krebs, H.A. 1964. Gluconeogenesis. *Proc. R. Soc. (Biol).* 159:545.

Krebs, H.A., R.A. Freedland, R. Hems, and M. Stubbs. 1969. Inhibition of hepatic gluconeogenesis by ethanol. *Biochem. J.* 112:117–124.

Krisman, C.R. and R. Barengo. 1975. A precursor of glycogen biosynthesis: Alpha-1,4-glucan-protein. *Eur. J. Biochem.* 52:117–123.

Kristensen, N.B. and G. Wu. 2012. Metabolic functions of the porcine liver. In: *Nutritional Physiology of Pigs*, Chapter 13. Edited by K.E. Bach, N.J. Knudsen, H.D. Kjeldsen, and B.B. Jensen. Danish Pig Research Center, Copenhagen, Denmark, pp. 1–17.

Kwon, H., T.E. Spencer, F.W. Bazer, and G. Wu. 2003. Developmental changes of amino acids in ovine fetal fluids. *Biol. Reprod.* 68:1813–1820.

Larrabee, M.G. 1989. The pentose cycle (hexose monophosphate shunt). *J. Biol. Chem.* 264:15875–15879.

Larrabee, M.G. 1990. Evaluation of the pentose phosphate pathway from $^{14}CO_2$ data. *Biochem. J.* 272:127–132.

Lechner-Doll, M., M. Kaske, and W. van Engelhardt. 1991. Factors affecting the mean retention time of particles in the forestomach of ruminants and camelids. In: *Physiological Aspects of Digestion and Metabolism in Ruminants.* Edited by T. Tsuda, Y. Sasaki, and R. Kawashima. Academic Press, Inc., New York, NY, pp. 455–482.

Lindberg, J.E. 2014. Fiber effects in nutrition and gut health in pigs. *J. Anim. Sci. Biotechnol.* 5:15.

Longland, A.C., J. Carruthers, and A.G. Low. 1994. The ability of piglets 4 to 8 weeks old to digest & perform on diets containing two contrasting sources of non-starch polysaccharide. *Anim. Prod.* 58:405–410.

Macrae, J.C. and D.G. Armstrong. 1969. Studies on intestinal digestion in sheep. II. Digestion of carbohydrate constituents in hay, cereal, and hay-cereal rations. *Br. J. Nutr.* 23:377–387.

Manners, M.J. 1976. The development of digestive function in the pig. *Proc. Nutr. Soc.* 35:49–55.

McAllister, T.A., Y. Dong, L.J. Yanke, H.D. Bae, and K.-J. Cheng. 1993. Cereal grain digestion by selected strains of ruminal fungi. *Can. J. Microbiol.* 39:113–118.

McAuley, M., H. Kristiansson, M. Huang, A.L. Pey, and D.J. Timson 2016. Galactokinase promiscuity: A question of flexibility? *Biochem. Soc. Trans.* 44:116–122.

McDonald, P., R.A. Edwards, J.F.D. Greenhalgh, C.A. Morgan, and L.A. Sinclair. 2011. *Animal Nutrition*, 7th ed. Prentice Hall, New York, NY.

Miles, R.D., D.R. Campbell, J.A. Yates, and C.E. White. 1987. Effect of dietary fructose on broiler chick performance. *Poult. Sci.* 66:1197–1201.

Mountfort, D.O. and R.A. Asher. 1988. Production of α-amylase by the ruminal anaerobic fungus *Neocallimastix frontalis. Appl. Environ. Microbiol.* 54:2293–2299.

Mráček, T., Z. Drahota, and J. Houštěk. 2013. The function and the role of the mitochondrial glycerol-3-phosphate dehydrogenase in mammalian tissues. *Biochim. Biophys. Acta.* 1827:401–410.

Murray, R.K., D.K. Granner, P.A. Mayes, and V.W. Rodwell. 2001. *Harper's Review of Biochemistry.* Appleton & Lange, Norwalk, Connecticut.

Nakayama, A., K. Yamamoto, and S. Tabata. 2001. Identification of the catalytic residues of bifunctional glycogen debranching enzyme. *J. Biol. Chem.* 276:28824–28828.

National Research Council (NRC). 2001. *Nutrient Requirements of Dairy Cattle.* National Academy Press, Washington, DC.

National Research Council (NRC). 2011. *Nutrient Requirements of Fish and Shrimp.* National Academy Press, Washington, DC.

Neese, R.A., J.M. Schwarz, D. Faix, S. Turner, A. Letscher, D. Vu, and P. Hellerstein. 1995. Gluconeogenesis and intrahepatic triose phosphate flux in response to fasting or substrate loads. *J. Biol. Chem.* 270:14452–14463.

Nizielski, S.E., J.E. Morley, T.J. Bartness, U.S. Seal, and A.S. Levine. 1986. Effects of manipulations of glucoregulation on feeding in the ground squirrel. *Physiol. Behav.* 36:53–58.

Noy, Y. and D. Sklan. 1995. Digestion and absorption in the young chick. *Poult. Sci.* 74:366–373.
Oba. M. and M.S. Allen. 1999. Evaluation of the importance of the digestibility of neutral detergent fiber from forage: Effects on dry matter intake and milk yield of dairy cows. *J. Dairy Sci.* 82:589–596.
Olson, A.L. and J.E. Pessin. 1996. Structure, function, and regulation of the mammalian facilitative glucose transporter gene family. *Annu. Rev. Nutr.* 16:235–256.
Palm, D.C., J.M. Rohwer, and J.S. Hofmeyr. 2013. Regulation of glycogen synthase from mammalian skeletal muscle—A unifying view of allosteric and covalent regulation. *FEBS J.* 280:2–27.
Permyakov, E.A., S.E. Permyakov, L. Breydo, E.M. Redwan, H.A. Almehdar, and V.N. Uversky. 2016. Disorder in milk Proteins: α-lactalbumin. *Curr. Protein Pept. Sci.* 17:352–367.
Polakof, S. and J.L. Soengas. 2013. Evidence of sugar sensitive genes in the gut of a carnivorous fish species. *Comp. Biochem. Physiol. B* 166:58–64.
Pond, W.G., D.C. Church, and K.R. Pond. 1995. *Basic Animal Nutrition and Feeding*, 4th ed. John Wiley & Sons, New York, NY.
Porter, J.W.G. 1969. Digestion in the pre-ruminant animal. *Proc. Nutr. Soc.* 28:115–121.
Refstie, S., B. Svihus, K.D. Shearer, and T. Storebakken. 1999. Nutrient digestibility in Atlantic salmon and broiler chickens related to viscosity and non-starch polysaccharide content in different soybean products. *Aquaculture.* 79:331–345.
Rezaei, R., Z.L. Wu, Y.Q. Hou, F.W. Bazer and G. Wu. 2016. Amino acids and mammary gland development: nutritional implications for neonatal growth. *J. Anim. Sci. Biotechnol.* 7:20.
Richard, P. and S. Hilditch. 2009. D-Galacturonic acid catabolism in microorganisms and its biotechnological relevance. *Appl. Microbiol. Biotechnol.* 82:597–604.
Rønnestad, I., M. Yúfera, B. Ueberschär, L. Ribeiro, Ø. Sæle, and C. Boglione. 2013. Feeding behaviour and digestive physiology in larval fish: Current knowledge, and gaps and bottlenecks in research. *Rev. Aquaculture.* 5(Suppl. 1):S59–S98.
Sala-Rabanal, M., M.A. Gallardo, J. Sánchez, and J.M. Planas. 2004. Na-dependent D-glucose transport by intestinal brush border membrane vesicles from gilthead sea bream (*Sparus aurata*). *J. Membr. Biol.* 201:85–96.
Schirren, C. 1963. Relation between fructose content of semen and fertility in man. *J. Reprod. Fertil.* 5:347–358.
Shiau, S.Y., H.L. Yu, S. Hwa, S.Y. Chen, and S.I. Hsu. 1988. The influence of carboxymethylcellulose on growth, digestion, gastric emptying time and body composition of tilapia. *Aquaculture.* 70:345–354.
Shima, S., E. Warkentin, R.K. Thauer, and U. Ermler. 2002. Structure and function of enzymes involved in the methanogenic pathway utilizing carbon dioxide and molecular hydrogen. *J. Biosci. Bioeng.* 93:519–530.
Simoyi, M. F., M. Milimu, R. W. Russell, R. A. Peterson, and P. B. Kenney. 2006. Effect of dietary lactose on the productive performance of young turkeys. *J. Appl. Poult Res.* 15:20–27.
Stevens, C.E. and I.D. Hume. 1998. Contributions of microbes in vertebrate gastrointestinal tract to production and conservation of nutrients. *Physiol. Rev.* 78:393–427.
Sundell, K.S. and I. Rønnestad. 2011. Intestinal absorption. In: *Encyclopedia of Fish Physiology.* Edited by A.P. Farrell, Elsevier, New York, NY, pp. 1311–1321.
Svihus, B. 2014. Starch digestion capacity of poultry. *Poult. Sci.* 93:2394–2399.
Swenson, M.J. and W.O. Reece. 1984. *Duke's Physiology of Domestic Animals.* Cornell University Press, Ithaca, New York.
Symonds, H.W. and G.D. Baird. 1975. Evidence for the absorption of reducing sugar from the small intestine of the dairy cow. *Br. Vet. J.* 131:17–22.
Tanaka, N. and M.J. Johnson. 1971. Equilibrium constant for conversion of pyruvate to acetyl phosphate and formate. *J. Bacteriol.* 108:1107–1111.
Teerijoki, H., A. Krasnov, T. Pitkänen, and H. Mölsä. 2000. Cloning and characterization of glucose transporter in teleost fish rainbow trout (*Oncorhynchus mykiss*). *Biochim. Biophys. Acta.* 1494:290–294.
Thompson, J.R., G. Weiser, K. Seto, and A.L. Black. 1975. Effect of glucose load on synthesis of plasma glucose in lactating cows. *J. Dairy Sci.* 58:362–370.
Turner, N.D. and J.R. Lupton. 2011. Dietary fiber. *Adv. Nutr.* 2:151–152.
Van de Werve, G., A. Lang, C. Newgard, M.C. Mechin, Y. Li, and A. Berteloot. 2000. New lessons in the regulation of glucose metabolism taught by the glucose 6-phosphatase system. *Eur. J. Biochem.* 267:1533–1549.

Van Schaftingen, E. 1995. Glucosamine-sensitive and -insensitive detritiation of [2-$^3$H]glucose in isolated rat hepatocytes: A study of the contributions of glucokinase and glucose-6-phosphatase. *Biochem. J.* 308:23–29.

Van Schaftingen, E., Hue, L. and Hers, H.G. 1980. Fructose 2,6-bisphosphate, the probably structure of the glucose- and glucagon-sensitive stimulator of phosphofructokinase. *Biochem. J.* 192:897–901.

Wamelink, M.M., E.A. Struys, and C. Jakobs. 2008. The biochemistry, metabolism and inherited defects of the pentose phosphate pathway: A review. *J. Inherit. Metab. Dis.* 31:703–717.

Ward, K.A. 2000. Transgene-mediated modifications to animal biochemistry. *Trends Biotechnol.* 18:99–102.

Watford, M. 1985. Gluconeogenesis in the chicken: Regulation of phosphoenolpyruvate carboxykinase gene expression. *Fed. Proc.* 44:2469–2074.

Watford, M. 1988. What is the metabolic fate of dietary glucose? *Trends Biochem. Sci.* 13:329–330.

Watford, M., Y. Hod, Y.B. Chiao, M.F. Utter, and R.W. Hanson. 1981. The unique role of the kidney in gluconeogenesis in the chicken. The significance of a cytosolic form of phosphoenolpyruvate carboxykinase. *J. Biol. Chem.* 256:10023–10027.

Weimer, P.J. 1998. Manipulating ruminal fermentation: A microbial perspective. *J. Anim. Sci.* 76:3114–3122.

Weinhouse, S. 1976. Regulation of glucokinase in liver. *Curr. Top Cell. Regul.* 11:1–50.

Weinman, E.O., E.H. Strisower, and I.L. Chaikoff. 1957. Conversion of fatty acids to carbohydrate: Application of isotopes to this problem and role of the Krebs cycle as a synthetic pathway. *Physiol. Rev.* 37:252–272.

Williamson, D.H. and J.T. Brosnan. 1974. Concentrations of metabolites in animal tissues. In: *Methods of Enzymatic Analysis*. Edited by H.U. Bergmeyer, Academic Press, New York, pp. 2266–2292.

Wilson, S., J.C. MacRae, and P.J. Buttery. 1983. Glucose production and utilization in non-pregnant, pregnant and lactating ewes. *Br. J. Nutr.* 50:303–316.

Wu, G. 1996. An important role for pentose cycle in the synthesis of citrulline and proline in porcine enterocytes. *Arch. Biochem. Biophys.* 336:224–230.

Wu, G., C.J. Field and E.B. Marliss. 1991. Glutamine and glucose metabolism in thymocytes from normal and spontaneously diabetic BB rats. *Biochem. Cell Biol.* 69:801–808.

Wu, G., T.E. Haynes, H. Li, W. Yan, and C.J. Meininger. 2001. Glutamine metabolism to glucosamine is necessary for glutamine inhibition of endothelial nitric oxide synthesis. *Biochem. J.* 353:245–252.

Wu, G., S. Majumdar, J. Zhang, H. Lee, and C.J. Meininger. 1994. Insulin stimulates glycolysis and pentose cycle activity in bovine microvascular endothelial cells. *Comp. Biochem. Physiol.* 108C:179–185.

Wu, G. and E.B. Marliss. 1993. Enhanced glucose metabolism and respiratory burst in peritoneal macrophages from spontaneously diabetic BB rats. *Diabetes*. 42:520–529.

Wu, G. and J.R. Thompson. 1988. The effect of ketone bodies on alanine and glutamine metabolism in isolated skeletal muscle from the fasted chick. *Biochem. J.* 255:139–144.

Wu, X., S. Castillo, M. Rosales, A. Burns, M. Mendoza, and D.M. Gatlin III. 2015. Relative use of dietary carbohydrate, non-essential amino acids, and lipids for energy by hybrid striped bass, Morone chrysops ♀? × M. saxatilis ♂. *Aquaculture* 435:116–119.

Yager, C., C. Ning, R. Reynolds, N. Leslie, and S. Segal. 2004. Galactitol and galactonate accumulation in heart and skeletal muscle of mice with deficiency of galactose-1-phosphate uridyltransferase. *Mol. Genet. Metab.* 81:105–111.

Yang, J.Q., S.C. Kalhan, and R.W. Hanson. 2009. What is the metabolic role of phosphoenolpyruvate carboxykinase? *J. Biol. Chem.* 284:27025–27029.

Yen, J.T. 2001. Digestive system. In: *Biology of the Domestic Pig*. Edited by W.G. Pond and H.J. Mersmann. Cornell University Press, Ithaca, New York, pp. 390–453.

Yin, F., Z. Zhang, J. Huang, and Y.L. Yin. 2010. Digestion rate of dietary starch affects systemic circulation of amino acids in weaned pigs. *Br. J. Nutr.* 103:1404–1412.

Ying, W. 2008. $NAD^+$/NADH and $NADP^+$/NADPH in cellular functions and cell death: Regulation and biological consequences. *Antioxid. Redox Signal.* 10:179–206.

Yu, B. and P.W.S. Chiou. 1996. Effects of crude fibre level in the diet on the intestinal morphology of growing rabbits. *Lab. Anim.* 30:143–148.

Yu, C., S. Zhang, Q. Yang, Q. Peng, J. Zhu, X. Zeng, and S. Qiao. 2016. Effect of high fibre diets formulated with different fibrous ingredients on performance, nutrient digestibility and faecal microbiota of weaned piglets. *Arch. Anim. Nutr.* 70:263–277.

Zhang, W., D. Li, L. Liu, J. Zang, Q. Duan, W. Yang, and L. Zhang. 2013. The effects of dietary fiber level on nutrient digestibility in growing pigs. *J. Anim. Sci. Biotechnol.* 4(1):17.
Zhao, F.Q. and A.F. Keating. 2007. Expression and regulation of glucose transporters in the bovine mammary gland. *J. Dairy Sci.* 90(E. Suppl.):E76–E86.
Zijlstra, N., M. Mars, D.E. Wijk, R.M. Westerterp-Plantenga, and C. de Graaf. 2007. The effect of viscosity on ad libitum food intake. *Int. J. Obesity.* 32:676–683.

# 6 Nutrition and Metabolism of Lipids

Lipids are highly reduced molecules, including fats (triacylglycerols [TAGs]; also called triglycerides), fatty acids, phospholipids, cholesterol, and related metabolites (Chapter 3). The lipids are soluble in organic solvents (e.g., benzene, ether, or chloroform). Except for short- and medium-chain fatty acids, lipids are only sparingly soluble in water. Thus, fats and free lonvag-chain fatty acids (LCFAs, also known as nonesterified fatty acids) circulate in the blood as an albumin complex (Goldberg et al. 2009). Within cells, these nutrients and their hydrophobic derivatives are attached to specific TAGs or fatty acid-binding proteins (FABPs) (Pepino et al. 2014). Thus, "free" fatty acids in an animal are actually not free so as to prevent their toxic effects. In proximate feed analysis, all kinds of lipids are determined together as the ether extract (Li et al. 1990). Because of their major role as energy substrates, fats and fatty acids are the focus of this chapter regarding the lipid nutrition and metabolism.

Lipids are main dietary macronutrients and comprise important signaling molecules in nutrient metabolism (Field et al. 1989; Hou et al. 2016). In the small intestine, lipids are emulsified by bile salts, undergo enzymatic hydrolysis to free fatty acids and monoacylglycerols (MAGs), and are then assembled into mixed micelles. Lipid digestion products are transported from the mixed micelles into the enterocyte where they are reassembled with apolipoproteins (Apo) into chylomicrons and other lipoproteins for export into lymphatic vessels and return into the blood circulation (Besnard et al. 1996). During their transport in the blood, the lipoproteins are hydrolyzed extracellularly by lipoprotein lipases (LPLs) localized on the endothelial surface of the vasculature within extrahepatic tissues (e.g., skeletal muscle and white adipose tissue [WAT]) (Kersten 2014; Thomson and Dietschy 1981). When the dietary intake of fats is greater than the amount of fats broken down between meals, *de novo* synthesis of fatty acids will be attenuated, but the excess amount of dietary energy is stored as TAGs in the body (Jobgen et al. 2006). In contrast, when an animal consumes a low-fat but high-starch diet, excess carbohydrates are used for the synthesis of fatty acids and TAGs in a tissue-specific manner. When deficiencies of nutritionally essential ω3 and ω6 unsaturated fatty acids occur, animals exhibit numerous syndromes, such as skin lesions, growth restriction, and reproductive failure (Spector and Kim 2015). Under the conditions of no or inadequate energy intake (e.g., fasting and early lactation), TAGs are mobilized from tissues (especially WAT but also including the liver) through the action of hormone-sensitive lipases (HSLs) to generate metabolic fuels (e.g., LCFAs, ketone bodies, and glycerol) (Yeaman 1990). Ketone bodies are crucial for the function of the brain when the concentration of glucose in the plasma is reduced, as the brain does not take up saturated or monounsaturated LCFAs from the blood due to the blood–brain barrier.

Quantitatively, LCFAs are the major energy substrates for the liver, skeletal muscle, heart, and kidneys in both fed and fasting states and therefore play an important role in the function of these tissues (Jobgen et al. 2006). Fatty acids are oxidized to $CO_2$ and $H_2O$ primarily in the mitochondria of cells via the pathway of β-oxidation. Chain shortening of very-long-chain fatty acids can also occur in peroxisomes, and the resulting acyl-CoAs subsequently enter the mitochondria for β-oxidation (Reddy and Hashimoto 2001). Like fatty acid synthesis, fatty acid oxidation is regulated by hormones (e.g., insulin, glucocorticoids), metabolites (e.g., acetyl-CoA and malonyl-CoA), and peroxisome proliferator-activated receptors (PPARs; members of the nuclear hormone receptor superfamily). While fats fulfill essential physiological function, their excessive intake contributes to a variety of metabolic disorders and chronic diseases, including obesity, diabetes, and cardiovascular disease in animals (Beitz 1993). However, in beef cattle, a certain level of intramuscular fats (especially monounsaturated fatty acids [MUFAs]) is necessary to improve meat quality (Smith 2013). Thus, studies of lipid nutrition and metabolism are of great importance for both animal agriculture and medicine.

## DIGESTION AND ABSORPTION OF LIPIDS IN NONRUMINANTS

### Overall View

Swine diets usually contain 5% lipids, but pigs can digest at least 20% lipids (including TAGs) in diets (on an as-fed basis). Lipid content (on an as-fed basis) in chicken diets is usually 5%, 6%, and 8%, respectively, for starters (1–21 days of age), growers (22–35 days of age), and finishers (36–49 days of age). Equine diets usually contain 4%–5% lipids, but horses can digest up to 20% lipids (including TAGs) in diets (on a dry matter [DM] basis) without the risk of developing diarrhea. Fish diets usually contain 5%–15% lipids, but some fish (e.g., salmon) can digest 30% lipids (including TAGs) in diets (on an as-fed basis). In nonruminant animals, some digestion of lipids begins in the mouth (lingual lipase) and stomach (gastric lipase), but most digestion occurs in the small intestine. The products of lipid digestion are absorbed into the enterocytes of the small intestine (Phan and Tso 2001). Events of lipid digestion and absorption in all nonruminant mammals include: (1) hydrolysis of lipids by lipases (from the pancreas and enterocytes); (2) the micellar solubilization of lipid digestion products in the small intestine; (3) the uptake of the solubilized products by enterocytes through the apical membrane; (4) the resynthesis of TAGs, as well as the assembling of chylomicrons, nascent very-low-density lipoproteins (VLDLs), and premature high-density lipoproteins (HDLs) in enterocytes; and (5) the secretion of the lipoproteins into the lymphatic circulation (most of nonruminants) or the portal vein (poultry). An overview of lipid digestion and absorption is outlined in Figure 6.1.

#### Digestion of Lipids in the Mouth and Stomach

A total of 98%–99% of lipids in the diets of most nonruminant animals (e.g., pigs, dogs, rodents, birds, and fish) are TAGs. However, herbivorous animals (e.g., horses and rabbits) consume large amounts of galactolipids from vegetative material (Drackley 2000). In nonruminants, the digestion of lipids starts in the oral cavity through the action of lingual lipases, which are secreted by glands in the tongue to hydrolyze TAGs (Doreau and Chilliard 1997). Lipid digestion continues in the stomach through (1) proteases in the stomach that release lipids from feed matrices; (2) the formation of a coarse lipid emulsion due to gastric acidic medium and motility (i.e., peristalsis or churning action); and (3) the actions of lingual and gastric lipases (Thomson and Dietschy 1981). The latter are secreted by the fundic region of the stomach. Both lingual and gastric lipases attack primarily short- and medium-chain fatty acid linkages on the *sn*-3 position of TAGs (Velazquez et al. 1996). Gastric lipase activity is higher in suckling neonates than in adults and is higher toward milk TAGs than pancreatic lipase (Drackley 2000). In both the young and adults, the crude emulsions of lipids formed in the stomach enter the duodenum as fine lipid droplets. Overall, the hydrolysis of TAGs into fatty acids, MAGs, and glycerol is quantitatively limited in the mouth and stomach of nonruminants.

#### Digestion of Lipids in the Small Intestine

##### General Process

The digestion of lipids in nonruminants occurs predominantly in the small intestine. This process requires secretions from the liver (bile via the gallbladder) and the pancreas, the formation of lipid micelles, as well as the enzymatic hydrolysis of TAGs to fatty acids, MAGs, phospholipids, and cholesteryl esters. The primary components of the bile are bile salts and phospholipids, whereas TAG lipases, pro-colipase, phospholipases (including pro-phospholipase $A_2$), and $NaHCO_3$ (for pH

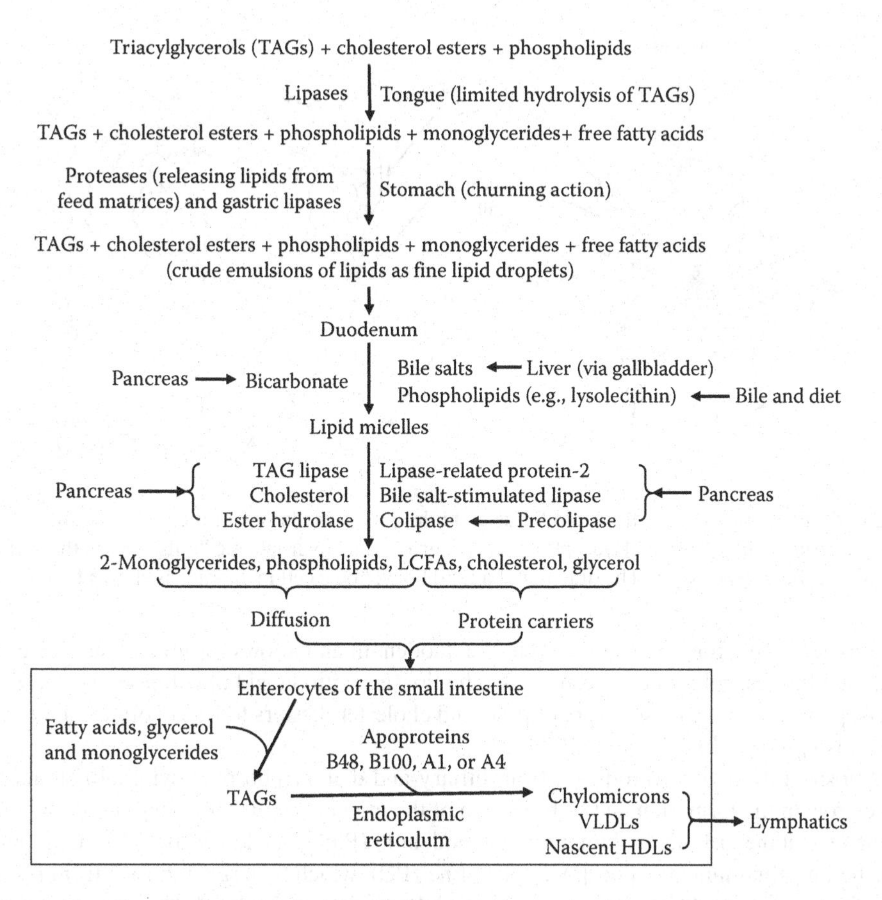


**FIGURE 6.1** An overview of lipid digestion and absorption in the gastrointestinal tract of nonruminant animals. The digestion of lipids begins within the mouth and then the stomach and is completed primarily in the small intestine. The products of lipid digestion are absorbed into the enterocytes. The jejunum is the major site for the digestion and absorption of lipids. HDLs, high-density lipoproteins; LCFAs, long-chain fatty acids; VLDLs, very-low-density lipoproteins.

adjustment in the small intestine) are constituents of pancreatic juice necessary for lipid digestion (Drackley 2000). Pro-colipase and pro-phospholipase $A_2$ are activated in the lumen of the duodenum by trypsin through limited proteolysis to form the active colipase and pro-phospholipase $A_2$. Pro-colipase may also be activated by a pancreatic pro-colipase activation peptide, which is a pentapeptide. Thus, interorgan cooperation is required for complete lipid digestion. Impaired digestion and absorption of fats can result from (1) deficiencies of taurine, glycine, protein, and phospholipids, leading to the impaired formation of micelles; (2) diseases that impair the secretion of bile acids, such as biliary obstruction or liver diseases; and (3) diseases that influence the secretion of TAG lipase, colipase, and bicarbonate from the pancreas, such as pancreatic cancer and cystic fibrosis (Goldstein and Brown 2015). In these cases, medium-chain TAGs can be better tolerated as a source of dietary energy. For both mammals and birds, lipid digestion takes place mainly in the jejunum, and to a lesser extent, in the duodenum and the ileum (Iqbal and Hussain 2009).

## Formation of Lipid Micelles

Gastric lipid emulsions that enter the duodenum mix well with bile salts and pancreatic juice (including lipase) to undergo marked changes in chemical and physical forms. Specifically, TAGs, MAGs, fatty acids, cholesterol, and phospholipids aggregate with bile salts to form small emulsion particles (Figure 6.2). The emulsion particles are coated with bile salts. Emulsion increases the surface area

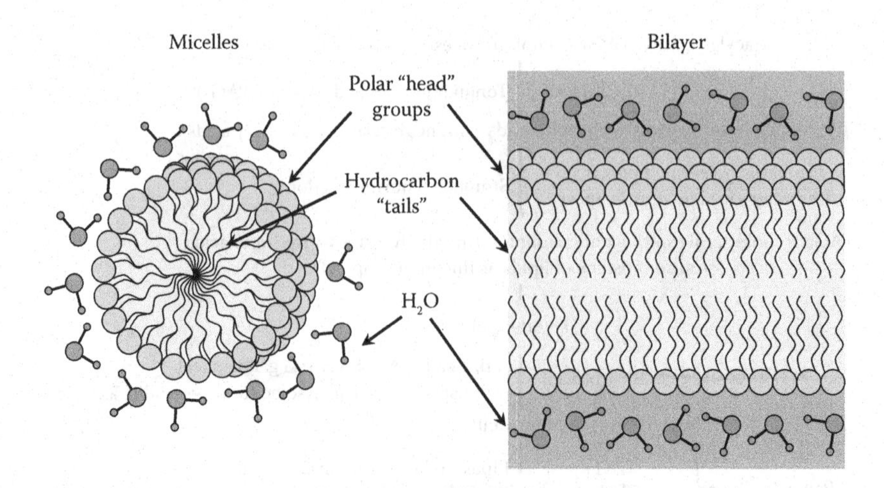


**FIGURE 6.2** Formation of micelles from lipids and bile salts in the lumen of the small intestine. The lipid micelles are coated with bile salts. Hydrophilic "head" groups and hydrophobic "tails" are on the surface and the core of micelles, respectively. The drawing of a lipid bilayer on a cell membrane is shown for comparison.

of the fat that arrives from the stomach into the duodenum and allows for greater surface exposure to pancreatic lipases, colipase, and esterases. The lipases, with the aid of colipase, hydrolyze TAGs to MAGs, phospholipids to lysophospholipids, and cholesterol esters to free cholesterol; all of these reactions also produce LCFAs.

Lysophosphatidylcholine (produced from biliary and dietary phosphatidyl choline) and MAGs play a key role in the formation and stabilization of the micelles, which are very small globules that are formed spontaneously in the lumen of the duodenum (Phan and Tso 2001). The major phospholipid in the intestinal lumen is phosphatidylcholine (PC), which is derived mostly from bile (80%) but also from the diet (10%). The micelles are globules with polar heads (groups) at the globule surface to interact with water and nonpolar tails (hydrocarbon chains) being sequestered inside the globule to exclude water. Bile salts and MAGs contain portions of molecules that can interact with water and other portions that can interact with lipids. The formation of micelles increases the solubility of the lipid complex in an aqueous solution and reduces the cytotoxicity of free fatty acids and bile salts. Micelles serve to transport their lipid components to the endothelial cells of blood vessels. As noted in Chapter 3, bile salts, which are the conjugates of bile acids with taurine and/or glycine, are synthesized from cholesterol in the liver and secreted into the duodenum. There are both taurine and glycine bile salts (chenodeoxycholic acid) in pigs, but only the bile acid (cholic acid)–taurine conjugate in poultry. The bile salts (primarily cholic acid) of ruminants (e.g., cattle and sheep) contain glycine as the predominant amino acid (AA) but also a large amount of taurine.

## Digestion of TAGs, Phospholipids, and Cholesterol Esters

The pancreatic enzymes primarily responsible for lipid digestion are TAG lipase, lipase-related protein-2, bile salt-stimulated lipase (also known as carboxyl ester lipase), precolipase, and cholesteryl esterase (Lowe 2002). Pancreatic TAG lipase hydrolyzes (a) the *sn*-1 and *sn*-3 linkages of long-chain TAGs to produce 2-MAGs and two molecules of LCFAs; and (b) the *sn*-1, *sn*-2, and *sn*-3 linkages of medium-chain TAGs to produce three molecules of LCFAs plus one molecule of glycerol (Figure 6.3). This enzyme does not hydrolyze the *sn*-2 linkage of long-chain TAGs and, thus, lipolysis stops at the 2-MAG stage. There is only a small amount of diacylglycerols (DGAs) produced from the degradation of TAGs in the nonruminant small intestine. The action of pancreatic lipases generates a liquid–crystalline interface at the surface of the emulsion particles.

Pancreatic lipase-related protein-2 has broad substrate specificity and acts preferentially on MAGs, phospholipids, and galactolipids. Similarly, bile salt-stimulated lipase has broad substrate

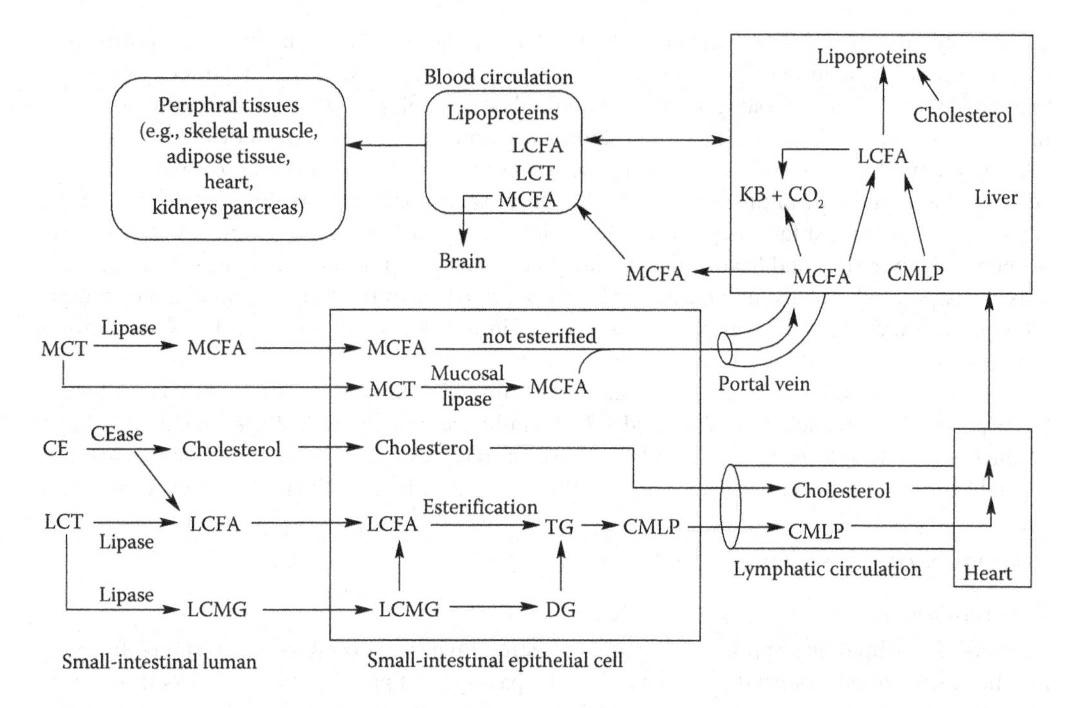


**FIGURE 6.3** Digestion and absorption of lipids in the small intestine of nonruminants. Hydrolysis of medium-chain triacylglycerol (MCT) and long-chain triacylglycerol (LCT) by pancreatic lipases and of cholesterol esters (CE) by cholesterol esterase (Cease) occurs in the lumen of the nonruminant small intestine. Enterocytes take up medium-chain fatty acids (MCFAs), long-chain fatty acids (LCFAs), cholesterol, long-chain monoacylglycerol (LCMG), and cholesterol. MCFAs are not actively esterified into TAGs in the cells and are absorbed directly into the portal vein. In the endoplasmic reticulum of enterocytes, LCFAs and LCMG are re-esterified to triacylglycerol (TG) through the formation of diacylglycerols (DG). TG is incorporated into chylomicrons plus other lipoproteins (CMLP) for export into lacteals. CMLP and MCFA are catabolized by the liver and peripheral tissues.

specificity and is capable of hydrolyzing TAGs, phospholipids, and cholesteryl esters, as well as the esters of ω3 and ω6 PUFAs (Thomson and Dietschy 1981). In addition, phospholipids are hydrolyzed by phospholipase $A_2$ to produce mainly lysophospholipids and free fatty acids. For example, PC is hydrolyzed in the lumen to form lysophosphatidylcholine. Cholesteryl esters are also hydrolyzed by pancreatic cholesteryl esterase to yield cholesterol and LCFAs (Lowe 2002). Colipase is a small protein required for the optimal enzyme activity of pancreatic lipase. By binding to the C-terminal, noncatalytic domain of pancreatic lipase, colipase prevents the inhibitory effect of bile salts on the lipase-catalyzed intraduodenal hydrolysis of dietary long-chain TAGs.

Emulsification of the hydrophobic products of lipids continues actively in the small intestine in preparation for their efficient absorption across the enterocyte via micelles. The micelles are needed to move the water-insoluble lipids (e.g., fatty acids, MAGs, and cholesterol) across the unstirred water layer outside the brush-border membrane of enterocytes to the surface of these cells for absorption.

### Digestibility of Dietary Lipids

Neonatal mammals efficiently digest milk fats. For example, the digestibility of sow's milk fat by 2-day-old pigs is 95% and is even higher in older pigs (Manners 1976). The digestibility of TAGs in grain cereals or added lipids is high in postweaning nonruminant mammals (e.g., often 90%–95% in pigs) and in posthatching poultry (e.g., 82% at Day 2, 89% at Day 21, and 90%–95% after 3 weeks of age) (Doreau and Chilliard 1997; Li et al. 1990). The digestibility of dietary TAGs is 90%–95% in horses and 85%–95% in fish. Efficient absorption of lipids by enterocytes ensures that dietary fat is maximally available to be used as a major source of energy for supporting cellular functions. In addition, TAGs serve as reservoirs for energy storage, lipoprotein trafficking, bile acid synthesis, and steroidogenesis in animals. The rates of digestion and absorption of dietary lipids are enhanced by the presence of unsaturated fatty acids in diets. Much evidence shows that intestinal TAG digestibility increases with increasing unsaturation and decreases with increasing chain length in saturated or unsaturated LCFAs. Three reasons can explain this nutritional phenomenon. First, unsaturated fatty acids (e.g., oleic, linoleic, and α-linolenic acids) readily form mixed micelles with bile salts and have a higher solubility in bile acid micelles than long-chain saturated fatty acids. Second, MAGs and unsaturated fatty acids act synergistically to promote the incorporation of saturated fatty acids in diets into micelles in the small intestine. Third, the solubility of saturated or unsaturated LCFAs in micelles decreases as the hydrocarbon chain length increases. These principles can guide the practice of animal feeding. For example, the digestibility of saturated fats is poor in young chicks (e.g., 40% and 79% for tallow at Days 1 and 7 of age), due to the limited production of bile salts (Carew et al. 1972). However, the presence of unsaturated fatty acids (e.g., vegetable oil) in the diet enhances the digestibility of saturated fats in the birds (Carew et al. 1972).

## Absorption of Lipids by the Small Intestine

### General Process

The process of lipid absorption in the small intestine involves several steps: (a) the diffusion of micelles through the unstirred water layer; (b) the passage of lipid digestion products through the plasma membrane of enterocytes via simple diffusion (protein carrier–independent), passive transport (protein carrier–independent; e.g., several fatty acid transporters), or active transport (protein carrier–dependent); (c) cytosolic activation and esterification of fatty acids; (d) the formation of chylomicrons and lipoproteins, and (e) the exocytosis of chylomicrons, VLDLs, and HDLs from enterocytes into the lamina propria. For nonruminant mammals and birds, the absorption of lipids occurs primarily in the jejunum, and to a lesser extent, in the duodenum and ileum (Iqbal and Hussain 2009). Absorption of lipids from the small intestine can be reduced by a high intake of dietary fibers. Any damage to the pancreas or small intestine can result in lipid malabsorption.

### Absorption of Lipids into Enterocytes

MAGs (e.g., primarily 2-MAGs), phospholipids, and a small amount of TAGs enter enterocytes primarily by simple diffusion through the lipid membrane (Figure 6.3). The absorption of LCFAs from the small-intestinal lumen occurs via both simple diffusion and protein carriers (e.g., CD36) in an energy-independent manner (Chen et al. 2001; Pepino et al. 2014). Genetic deletion of CD36 (a multiligand receptor) reduces the uptake of LCFAs by enterocytes (Goldberg et al. 2009). Expression of fatty acid transporters is upregulated by the presence of dietary fat or some forms of genetic obesity. In contrast, the absorption of cholesterol requires a transporter possibly in an energy-dependent process. A protein carrier, named Niemann–Pick C1-like 1 (NPC1L1) protein, has been identified at the apical membrane of enterocytes as a cholesterol uptake transporter, which plays a crucial role in the ezetimibe-sensitive cholesterol absorption pathway (Kawase et al. 2015). Expression of *Npc1l1* is enhanced in the cholesterol-depleted porcine intestine and suppressed in mice fed a cholesterol-rich diet. Of note, ATP-binding cassette (ABC) transporters, ABCG5 and ABCG8, which are also localized at the apical membrane of enterocytes as cholesterol efflux transporters, promote the active efflux of cholesterol and plant sterols from enterocytes back into the intestinal lumen for excretion (Kawase et al. 2015). Thus, the net absorption of cholesterol is determined by the balance between the influx and efflux of intraluminal cholesterol molecules crossing the brush-border membrane of the enterocyte. In animals, there is net absorption of dietary cholesterol (~50%; with the remainder being excreted in feces), but virtually no absorption of plant sterols under physiological conditions. Fatty acids of <14 carbons are not actively esterified into TAGs in enterocytes and are absorbed directly into the portal vein (Figure 6.4).

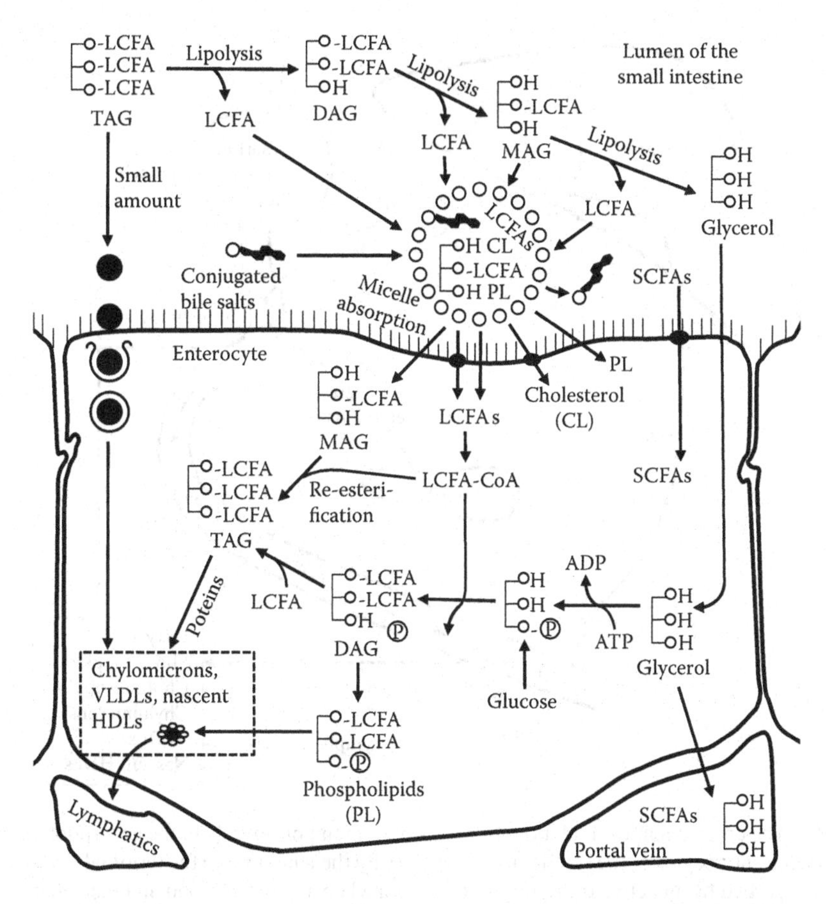


**FIGURE 6.4** Uptake of lipids in micelles by enterocytes of nonruminants. These cells take up (1) monoacylglycerol (MAG; primarily 2-monoacylglycerol) and phospholipids (PL) through simple diffusion; (2) cholesterol (CL) and short-chain fatty acids (SCFAs) through specific transmembrane protein carriers; and (3) long-chain fatty acids (LCFAs) through both simple diffusion and transmembrane protein carriers. Chylomicrons, very-low-density lipoproteins (VLDLs), and nascent high-density lipoproteins (HDLs) are assembled from triacylglycerol (TAG), proteins, phospholipids, and cholesterol. Through the lamina propria of the small-intestinal mucosa, SCFAs and glycerol enter the portal vein, whereas lipoproteins move into the lymphatics.

Bile salts are released from the disruption of the micelles at the duodenum, jejunum, and ileum after the products of lipid digestion are absorbed by the enterocytes. In the terminal ileum, most (95%) bile salts are absorbed by an active transport system into the hepatic portal blood and enter the liver for re-secretion into the lumen of the duodenum. This is called "enterohepatic circulation" (Figure 6.5), which is active in animals (including pigs, fowls, and humans). The small amount (5%) of bile salts in the ileum that is not absorbed from the terminal ileum flows to the large intestine where they are converted into products called "secondary bile salts" by microbes and are excreted in the feces. The enterohepatic circulation helps to conserve bile salts in the body.

## Resynthesis of TAGs in Enterocytes

In the endoplasmic reticulum of enterocytes, lysophosphatidyl choline is reacylated to form PC, whereas LCFAs are reversibly and noncovalently bound to cytosolic FABPs and activated by long-chain acyl-CoA synthetase (ACS) to yield acyl-CoA (Phan and Tso 2001). The acyl-CoA is either metabolized in the endoplasmic reticulum, mitochondria, and peroxisomes, or bound to acyl-CoA-binding proteins to constitute an intracellular acyl-CoA pool (Figure 6.3). Most acyl-CoA esters

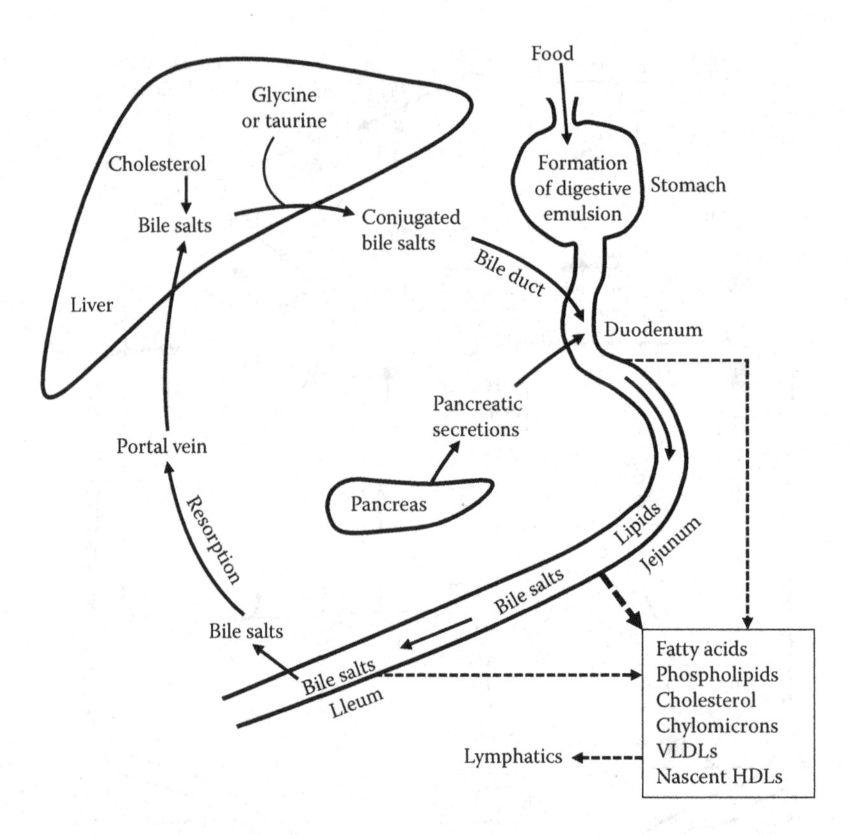


**FIGURE 6.5** The enterohepatic circulation. Bile salts play an important role in the absorption of lipid digestion products into enterocytes of the small intestine (primarily the jejunum). In the terminal ileum, most (95%) bile salts are absorbed by an active transport system into the hepatic portal blood and then enter the liver for re-secretion into the lumen of the duodenum.

are used for esterification with MAGs for the resynthesis of TAGs. The MAG pathway is primarily responsible for the resynthesis of TAGs from fatty acids, but the glycerol 3-phosphate pathway also plays a role, especially in ruminants (see a section on TAG synthesis in this chapter). Oxidation of fatty acids to $CO_2$ and water is limited in the small intestine (Jobgen et al. 2006).

### Assimilation of Wax Esters

Wax esters (long-chain fatty alcohols esterified to LCFAs) are significant dietary neutral lipids for birds, including seabirds and some passerines (Chapter 3). These animals can assimilate the wax esters in enterocytes with higher efficiencies (greater than 90%) than those attainable by mammals (<50%). This feature of lipid digestion can be explained by the following reasons, as proposed by Place (1992). First, the concentrations of bile salts in the small-intestinal lumen (~50 mM) and gallbladder (>600 mM) in birds are much greater than those in mammals. Second, birds possess the ability of regular retrograde movement of duodenal contents to the gizzard, which aids in further digestion of wax esters. Third, birds have a high capacity to hydrolyze wax esters as effectively as TAGs. Therefore, despite the similar processes of lipid digestion between birds and mammals, birds can utilize dietary wax esters more efficiently than mammals.

### Assembly of Chylomicrons, VLDLs, and HDLs in Enterocytes

Apoproteins B (predominantly ApoB48 and a trace amount of ApoB100) and microsomal triglyceride transfer protein (MTP) participate in the efficient assembly and secretion of lipoproteins in enterocytes (Iqbal and Hussain 2009). ApoB48, which is a truncated form of Apo100, is produced by the posttranscriptional editing of the mRNA for ApoB100 (Davidson and Shelness 2000). In the endoplasmic reticulum of these cells, TAGs, cholesterol, and phospholipids are assembled, along with apoproteins, primarily into chylomicrons (containing ApoB48 and ApoA4), and, to a much lesser extent, VLDLs (also containing ApoB48), and nascent HDLs (containing ApoA1). Esterification of cholesterol as cholesteryl esters is crucial for the assembly of these lipoproteins. About 70% of the cholesterol in lipoproteins exists in the form of cholesterol esters, and 30% in the free form. In enterocytes, the formation of cholesteryl esters in lipoproteins is catalyzed by (1) lecithin:cholesterol acyltransferase (LCAT, also known as phosphatidylcholine acyltransferase [PCAT]; Figure 6.6) and (2) acyl-CoA:cholesterol acyltransferase (ACAT; Figure 6.7). LCAT and ACAT convert free cholesterol into cholesteryl ester (a more hydrophobic form of cholesterol), which is then sequestered into the core of a lipoprotein particle (Figure 6.3). The transfer of cholesterol esters generated by LCAT and ACAT to the core of the lipoprotein particles and the subsequent maturation of the lipoproteins requires the action of a phospholipid transfer protein, which provides phospholipids to allow for surface expansion of the particles. LCAT is present in multiple tissues (including the small intestine and liver) and is released from the liver into the blood circulation. On the other hand, ACAT (a membrane-bound protein) utilizes long-chain fatty acyl-CoA and cholesterol as substrates to form a cholesteryl ester in the cytosol. In mammals, two isoenzymes, ACAT1 and ACAT2, which are encoded by two different genes, regulate cholesterol homeostasis in tissues. Defects in LCAT and ACAT result in abnormal packaging of lipoproteins.

Chylomicrons are very heterogeneously sized particles that consist of a core of TAGs and cholesteryl esters, as well as a monolayer of phospholipids, cholesterol, and apolipoproteins (Wang et al. 2015). In animals, the chylomicrons are formed exclusively in the small intestine. These intestinal lipoproteins are processed in the Golgi apparatus before being released by the enterocytes through exocytosis. In nonruminant mammals, chylomicrons, VLDLs, and HDLs are too large to pass directly into the venous blood stream draining the small intestine, but instead are secreted into the intestinal lymphatics, which drain into the venous system (Chapter 1). In poultry with a poorly developed lymphatic system, the very large lipoprotein particles (called portomicrons), which are assembled inside enterocytes and have a much lower proportion of TAGs than mammalian chylomicrons, are absorbed across the basolateral membrane into the portal vein (Fraser et al. 1986). The avian small intestine does not appear to release VLDLs or HDLs. In reptiles, chylomicrons and

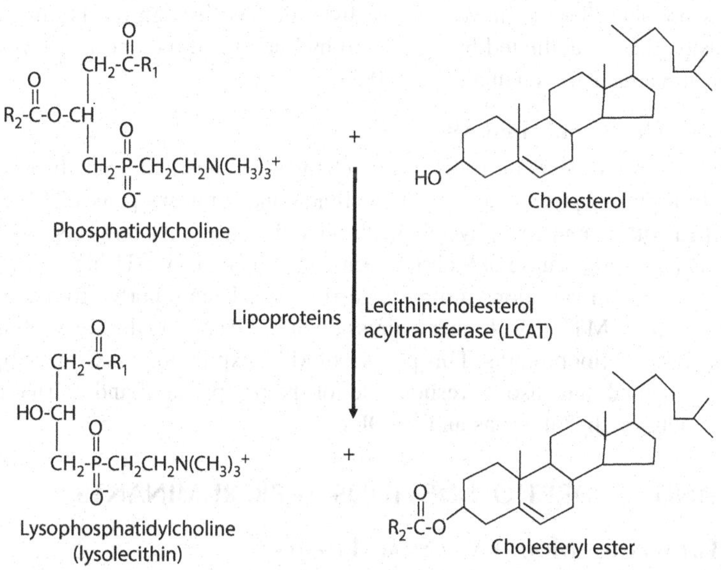

Phosphatidylcholine + Cholesterol → (Lipoproteins; Lecithin:cholesterol acyltransferase (LCAT)) → Lysophosphatidylcholine (lysolecithin) + Cholesteryl ester

**FIGURE 6.6** Formation of cholesteryl esters from cholesterol and phosphatidylcholine in lipoproteins by lecithin:cholesterol acyltransferase (LCAT). This enzyme is expressed in enterocytes and other cell types to catalyze the esterification of cholesterol.

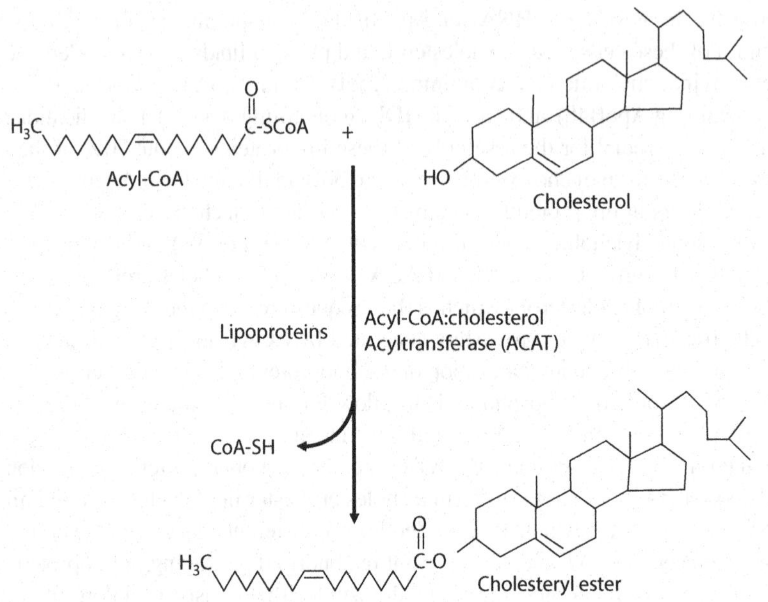

**FIGURE 6.7** Formation of cholesteryl esters from cholesterol and acetyl-CoA in lipoproteins by acyl-CoA:cholesterol acyltransferase (ACAT). This enzyme is expressed in enterocytes and other cell types to catalyze the esterification of cholesterol.

VLDLs enter the lymphatics and then the bloodstream (Price 2017). Short- and medium-chain fatty acids in the lumen of the small intestine enter the portal circulation. Thus, the intestine-derived lipoproteins transport dietary TAGs, cholesterol, and phospholipids to extraintestinal tissues.

Although the output of lipoproteins from the enterocytes is known to be required for the complete absorption of dietary lipids, the movement of these lipid–protein complexes from the intercellular space through the basement membrane to the lamina propria is not fully understood (Kohan et al. 2010). It is possible that the movement of chylomicrons through the lamina propria occurs via simple diffusion that is facilitated by interstitial hydration and the one-way directional flow of lymph in the intestinal lacteals (Phan and Tso 2001).

### Diurnal Changes in Intestinal Lipid Absorption

Results from studies with rodents indicate diurnal changes in intestinal lipid absorption (Iqbal and Hussain 2009). In postabsorptive rodents, plasma lipid concentrations peak at 1–2 h after feeding and are maintained within a narrow physiological range thereafter. Also in rats, lipid absorption is higher at 2400 than at 1200 because of their nocturnal feeding behavior. Using *in situ* loops and isolated enterocytes, circadian variations in lipid digestion have been reported to result from changes in intestinal expression of MTP (e.g., higher expression of MTP at 2400 than at 1200) and, therefore, the intestinal assembly of lipoproteins. This pattern of MTP expression maximizes lipid absorption at the time of feeding and may also be responsible for the postprandial and diurnal changes in the plasma concentrations of chylomicrons and VLDLs.

## DIGESTION AND ABSORPTION OF LIPIDS IN PRERUMINANTS

### Digestion of Lipids in the Mouth and Small Intestine

#### Limited Digestion by Salivary Lipase in Mouth, Forestomaches, and Abomasum

The content of lipids in milk varies greatly among species, such as 16% for horses, 37% for ruminants (cattle and sheep), 40% for pigs, 47% for rats, and 49% for rabbits. The saliva of preruminants contains lipase (known as pregastric esterase) to allow for limited hydrolysis of dietary TAGs. This enzyme also acts in their abomasum in a manner similar to that of pancreatic lipase in the small intestine to cleave butyrate and other fatty acids from milk TAGs. The activity of pregastric esterase decreases with age and normally disappears by three months of age in calves fed a whole milk (Drackley 2000). The decrease in the secretion of the pregastric esterase is more rapid in calves consuming liquid skim milk or high roughage diets than in cow-nursed neonates. Because the rumen of preruminants is underdeveloped in its function and microbiota, unsaturated fatty acids in the diet can escape hydrogenation during their passage from the mouth to the small intestine. Thus, the tissues of preruminants contain more unsaturated fatty acids than adult ruminants. Overall, the rate of lipid digestion is low in the mouth, forestomaches, and abomasum of preruminants, and the immature reticulorumen can absorb a small amount of SCFAs from the milk and its limited microbial fermentation.

#### Extensive Digestion of Lipids in the Small Intestine

The small intestine is the primary site for lipid digestion in preruminants. The processes of intestinal lipid digestion in these animals (e.g., suckling calves and lambs) with a nonfunctional rumen are the same as those in preweaning monogastric mammals. Specifically, the pancreas of preruminants secretes pancreatic lipase and colipase into the lumen of the duodenum. The activity of these enzymes is high at birth and may double during the first weeks of postnatal life (Porter 1969). Thus, young ruminants digest milk TAGs well, with a true digestibility of 95%–99% (Gerrits et al. 1997), as well as other animal and vegetable fats which are emulsified to particle sizes of <4 μm in diameter. The digestibility of TAGs in well-used nonmilk foods is generally also high in preruminants (e.g., 90%–95%) (Bauchart 1993). However, these young animals have a lower ability to hydrolyze fats predominantly as tristearin than the natural milk fats.

### Absorption of Lipids by the Small Intestine

Dietary lipids and their digestion products are absorbed by the small intestine in preruminants, as in preweaning nonruminant mammals. As noted previously, there is little esterification of MCFAs within enterocytes. Thus, when preruminants are either nursed by their mothers or fed replacer liquid milk, MCFAs (water-soluble) present in the lumen of the small intestine are absorbed through the apical and basolateral membrane MCFA transporters of enterocytes into the interstitial space of the lamina propria. MCFAs then enter the intestinal venule and, through the small vein, the portal vein. LCFAs (lipid-soluble) and MAGs are absorbed through the apical and basolateral membrane of specific transporters of enterocytes, or simple diffusion, into the cells. Preruminants secrete relatively large amounts of bile salts and lysophospholipids into the lumen of the duodenum for solubilizing dietary lipids and, therefore, exhibit high rates of absorption of saturated fatty acids in milk (95%–99%). Inside the enterocytes, the absorbed lipids are assembled into chylomicrons (predominantly ApoB48), VLDLs, and nascent HDLs, which are exported into the lamina propria and then enter either the intestinal lymphatic vessel or the portal vein in preruminants (Bauchart et al. 1989). In preruminants, 80% of lipids in the intestinal lymph are present in the form of TAGs (Laplaud et al. 1990).

## DIGESTION AND ABSORPTION OF LIPIDS IN RUMINANTS

There are marked differences in lipid digestion and absorption between ruminant and nonruminant animals (Nafikov and Beitz 2007). Specifically, ruminants exhibit (1) a negligible activity of salivary lipase activity; (2) significant hydrolysis of TAGs in the rumen; (3) a relatively low ability of ruminal microbes to degrade dietary lipids in comparison with carbohydrates; (4) a high capacity for the ruminal biohydrogenation of unsaturated fatty acids; and (5) a relatively low pancreatic lipase activity in the small intestine (Palmquist 1988). This limits the inclusion of fats in ruminant diets (a maximum of 7% on a DM basis). In ruminants, there is virtually no absorption of long- and

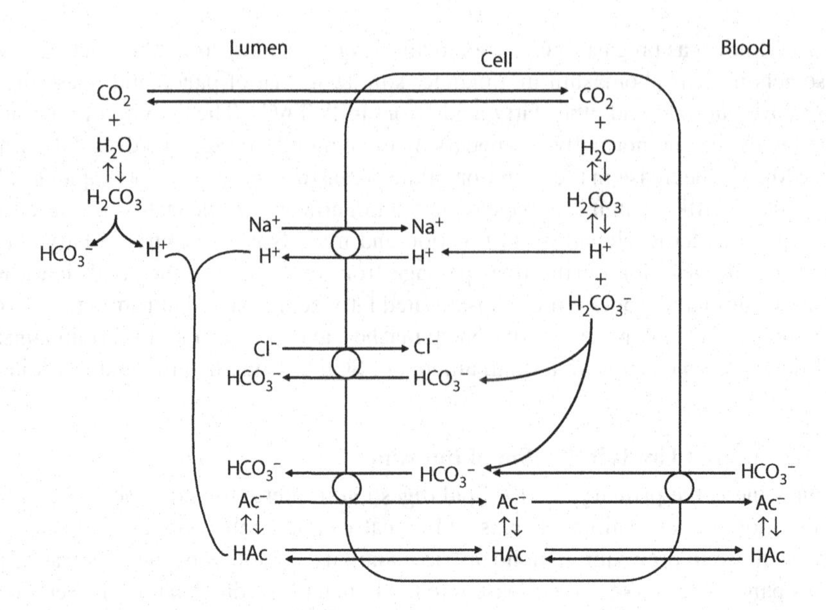


**FIGURE 6.8** Absorption of SCFAs from the lumen of the rumen into the blood circulation. The epithelial cells of the rumen express protein transporters to take up SCFAs from the ruminal lumen. This process is associated with the secretion of $H^+$ from the cells, as well as of $HCO_3^-$ from both the cells and the blood. $AC^-$, acetic acetate; HAc, acetic acid.

medium-chain fatty acids in the rumen, omasum, or abomasum, and no modification of long- and medium-chain fatty acids in the omasum or abomasum (Bauchart 1993). In contrast, large amounts of SCFAs are absorbed from the rumen through its epithelium into the blood circulation (Figure 6.8). Thus, the absorbed fatty acids in the small intestine are more saturated than dietary fatty acids. This explains why although the diets of ruminants naturally contain high proportions of unsaturated fatty acids (particularly linoleic and α-linolenic acids), their fat deposits are very rich in stearic acid. Dietary lipids that escape the rumen and microbial lipids are further hydrolyzed in the small intestine. Overall, the true digestibility of dietary esterified lipids (including TAGs) in the entire digestive tract of ruminants is 70%–75%.

## Digestion of Lipids in the Rumen

### Roles of Microorganisms

Bacteria are primarily responsible for lipid digestion in the rumen. There is little evidence for a nutritionally significant role of rumen protozoa and fungi, or salivary and plant lipases in this process (Palmquist 1988). However, protozoa play a role in the hydrolysis and isomerization of dietary phospholipids. Of note, the hydrolysis and isomerization of lipids are extracellular processes. Rumen microorganisms synthesize fatty acids from SCFAs that are derived from their metabolism of dietary TAGs or carbohydrates and produce branched-chain fatty acids from branched-chain AAs. These newly formed fatty acids are incorporated primarily into microbial cell membrane phospholipids and TAGs for digestion in the abomasum and small intestine. Note that the anaerobic conditions in the rumen are not favorable for the oxidation of fatty acids to $CO_2$ and water. Therefore, in the rumen, unesterified fatty acids are either incorporated into microbial lipids or hydrogenated by the microbes.

### Products of Lipid Hydrolysis

The lipids in the diets of ruminants exist mainly in the esterified forms of mono- and di-galactoglycerides in forages, and as TAGs in concentrates and, to a lesser extent, phospholipids in all plant-based feedstuffs (Drackley 2000). The hydrolysis of the ester linkages in TAGs, phospholipids, and glycolipids is the initial step of lipid digestion by bacterial enzymes in the rumen. Specifically, digalacto-diglycerides are hydrolyzed by bacterial α-galactosidase to yield galactose and monogalacto-diglycerides, which are then hydrolyzed by bacterial β-galactosidase to generate galactose and diglycerides. Extensive hydrolysis of esterified dietary lipids is carried out by bacterial lipases (Bauman and Griinari 2003). For example, *Anaerovibrio lipolytica* is responsible for the hydrolysis of TAGs, as *Butyrivibrio fibrisolvens* is for the hydrolysis of phospholipids and glycolipids. Bacterial lipases attack *sn*-1, *sn*-2, and *sn*-3 linkages of TAGs, and thus there is little production of MAGs in the rumen, in contrast to lipid digestion in nonruminants. Glycerol and galactose, which are released from lipid hydrolysis, are fermented to primarily yield SCFAs. Approximately 85%–95% of esterified lipids are hydrolyzed to their constituent components (e.g., LCFAs, glycerol, and galactose) in the rumen of ruminants.

### Biohydrogenation of Unsaturated Fatty Acids

Because the rumen lacks molecular oxygen, the oxidation of fatty acids to $CO_2$ and water by ruminal microbes is absent, as noted previously. Thus, the disposal of hydrogen atoms occurs through the reduction of double bonds in unsaturated fatty acids to yield saturated fatty acids, which serves as a defense mechanism for the survival and activity of the microbes (Jenkins 1993). These unsaturated fatty acids, which are released from TAG hydrolysis, are first isomerized and then hydrogenated extensively by bacteria and protozoa to yield saturated fatty acids. The forages of grazing ruminants typically contain 2%–3% fatty acids, with a higher ratio of unsaturated fatty acids to saturated fatty acids than the diets for nonruminants. For example, α-linolenic acid ($C_{18:3}$; *cis*-9, *cis*-12, *cis*-15) accounts for 61% of total fatty acids in pasture grass (Palmquist 1988). In contrast, linoleic acid ($C_{18:2}$; *cis*-9, *cis*-12) is the predominant fatty acid in cereal grains and seeds (e.g., 47% in corn grain). Indeed, the major substrates for biohydrogenation are linoleic and linolenic acids. The rate of rumen biohydrogenation of fatty acids is typically faster with increased unsaturation. For most diets, linoleic acid and linolenic acid are hydrogenated to the extent of 70%–95% and 85%–100%, respectively, with stearic acid ($C_{18:0}$) as a major product (Beam et al. 2000).

The process of biohydrogenation also involves isomerization as the initial reaction, resulting in the formation of many intermediate compounds with *trans* double bonds or conjugated fatty acids (e.g., production of conjugated linoleic acid and vaccenic acid from linoleic acid) and saturated fatty acids (Figure 6.9). For example, an isomerization of the *cis*-12 double bond to a *trans*-11 configuration generates a conjugated di- or trienoic fatty acid. Then, a reduction of the *cis*-9 double bond yields a *trans*-11 fatty acid. Finally, the hydrogenation of the *trans*-11 double bond produces stearic acid (linoleic and linolenic acid pathways) or *trans*-15 18:1 (linolenic acid pathway). Of note, two key biohydrogenation intermediates are (1) *trans*-11 18:1 (vaccenic acid), which is formed from linoleic and linolenic acids; and (2) *cis*-9, *trans*-11 conjugated linoleic acid, which is formed from linoleic acid. Eight positional isomers of CLA are possible, but the predominant product in the rumen is the *cis*-9, *trans*-11 isomer. In the rumen, >90% of polyunsaturated fatty acids are hydrogenated, and <10% of them escape the rumen (Drackley 2000). Because unsaturated LCFAs are toxic to many species of bacteria, particularly those involved in fiber digestion, and because there is excess hydrogen in the rumen, biohydrogenation is favorable for the formation of methane from $CO_2$ and [$2H^+$], as well as the production of propionate. However, large amounts of unsaturated LCFAs can exceed the capacity of biohydrogenation to bring about undesirable effects on the rumen microbial population and dietary fiber digestion. Thus, because lipolysis is a prerequisite for biohydrogenation to proceed in the rumen and because the isomerases for converting a *cis* to a *trans* double bond act only on unesterified fatty acids with a free carboxyl group, the feeding of rumen-protected lipids helps to minimize lipolysis in the rumen and maximize their passage to the small intestine.

## Digestion of Lipids in the Abomasum

As noted previously, the long-chain fatty acids in the rumen are not absorbed into its epithelial cells, but rather will enter the abomasum. The lipids that leave the rumen (pH 5.5–6) consist

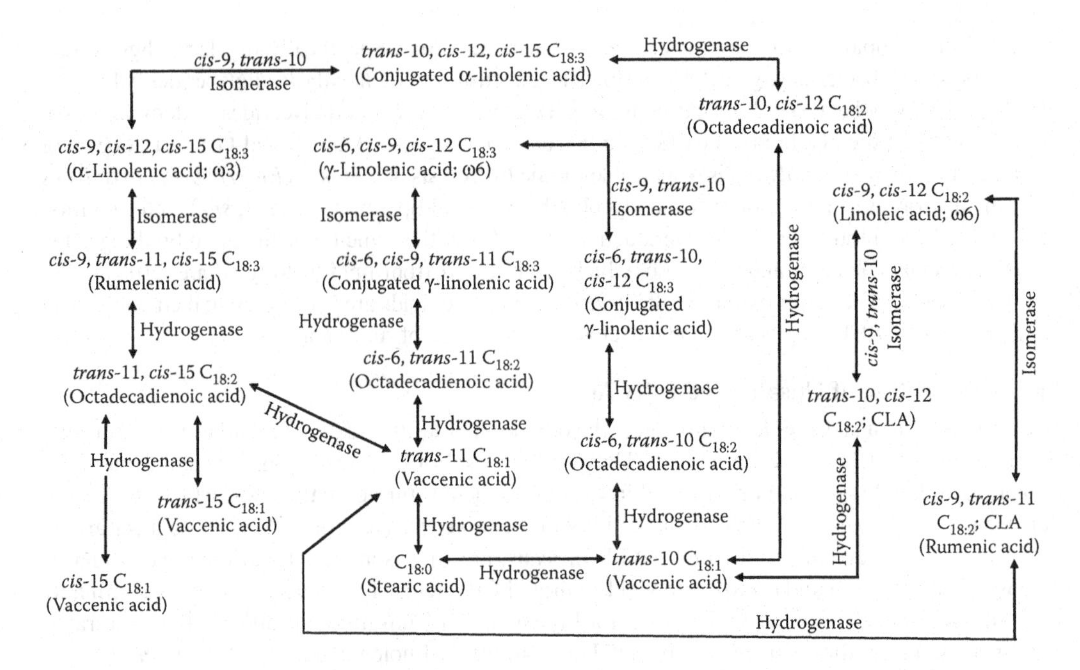


**FIGURE 6.9** Formation of conjugated fatty acids by ruminal bacteria. Through the isomerization and hydrogenation of *cis* and *trans* PUFAs, a variety of conjugated fatty acids are produced in ruminal bacteria. Examples include the formation of conjugated linoleic acid (CLA) from linoleic acid and of conjugated α-linolenic acid from α-linolenic acid.

predominantly of (1) free fatty acids (85%–90%) as their potassium, sodium, or calcium salts; and (2) phospholipids (10%–15%) as part of microbial cell membranes. In the abomasum (~pH 2), the fatty acid salts are dissociated to release free fatty acids, which then flow into the small intestine, the primary site for their absorption. The profile of fatty acids that reach the small intestine is very different from that in the diet consumed by the animals (Drackley 2000).

## Digestion of Lipids in the Small Intestine

Approximately 85% (80%–90%) of the lipids (excluding SCFAs) that enter the small intestine are free LCFAs attached to dietary feed particles, with the remaining lipids being microbial phospholipids, as well as a small amount of TAGs and glycolipids from residual feed material (Palmquist 1988). These esterified fatty acids are hydrolyzed by pancreatic lipases in the ruminant small intestine, as described for the nonruminant small intestine. Compared with nonruminants, lipid digestion in the small intestine of ruminants is only moderate due primarily to the limited amounts of bile salts and pancreatic lipases released to the small intestine of ruminants (Bergen and Mersmann 2005).

### Digestibility of Dietary Lipids in the Small Intestine

The ruminal microbial lipases that enter the small intestine and the pancreatic lipases that are secreted into the small intestine have relatively low activities to hydrolyze highly saturated (or hydrogenated) TAGs in ruminants. Thus, the digestibility of fats (6%–8% of dry digesta) entering the small intestine of these animals is ~80%, which is usually lower than that in nonruminants (Doreau and Chilliard 1997). Intestinal digestibility of fats is similar between 16- and 18-carbon fatty acids (~75%–80%), and is slightly greater for fats with unsaturated fatty acids than for those with saturated fatty acids (Avila et al. 2000). The extent of intestinal TAG hydrolysis is reduced as the dietary level of fat is increased or when factors such as low rumen pH and ionophores inhibit the activity and growth of bacteria. For example, in dairy cows, true fat digestibility in the small intestine decreases progressively from 95% to 78% when dietary fat intake increases from 200 g/day (1% fat on the DM basis) to 1,400 g/day (8% fat on the DM basis) (Bauchart 1993; Drackley 2000). This is due to a relatively low activity of ruminal lipase. There is evidence that when dietary fat content in the diet exceeds 7% (DM basis), the number and activity of ruminal bacteria are reduced substantially to impair the hydrolysis of dietary fats, protein, and fibers, as well as AA and SCFA synthesis, in the rumen (Nafikov and Beitz 2007). Thus, although fat supplementation has become a common practice to increase the energy density of diets for high producing dairy cows, a total fat content of >7% in diets (DM basis) is not recommended for ruminants, such as cattle, goats, and sheep (Drackley 2000).

### Absorption of Lipids by the Small Intestine

#### Absorption of Lipids into Enterocytes

The absorption of fatty acids, phospholipids, and cholesterol by the small intestine (primarily the jejunum) of ruminants is the same as that in nonruminants, except that lysophosphatidylcholine replaces MAG (which is not an end product of lipid hydrolysis in the rumen) as an emulsifying agent (Doreau and Chilliard 1997). In the upper small intestine of ruminants, lysophosphatidylcholine is produced from lecithin (the main phospholipid in rumen microbial cells, pancreatic juice, and bile) by phospholipase secreted from the pancreas. Pancreatic juice and bile salts, which enter the duodenum through the common bile duct, are essential for lipid absorption. Bile salts are also essential for dissociating fatty acids from feed particles. In ruminants, there is more taurine- than glycine-conjugated bile salts, because the taurine conjugates are more soluble at the low pH found in their small intestine. In ruminants fed conventional diets, 15%–25% of total fatty acids in the digesta are absorbed in the upper jejunum and 55%–65% are absorbed in the middle and the lower jejunum (Bauchart 1993).

The fatty acids absorbed by the small intestine are transported to various tissues, including mammary glands, skeletal muscle, heart, and adipose tissue (Bergen and Mersmann 2005). Of note, some fatty acids with a *trans* double bond between the 10th and 11th carbons, which are produced in relatively large amounts by the rumen of lactating cows that are fed an excessive amount of grains or a low-fiber diet, may inhibit milk fat synthesis and, therefore, may result in milk fat depression (Bauman and Griinari 2003).

#### Resynthesis of TAGs in Enterocytes

The synthesis of TAGs from free fatty acids and glycerol in the endoplasmic reticulum of ruminant enterocytes occurs via the glycerol 3-phosphate pathway (see the section on TAG synthesis in this chapter). The 2-MAG pathway for TAG synthesis is absent because little 2-MAG enters the small intestine from the abomasum. Oxidation of fatty acids to $CO_2$ and water is limited in the small intestine, as compared to that of glutamate, glutamine and aspartate (Wu 2013).

#### Assembly of Chylomicrons and VLDL in Enterocytes

ApoB and MTP are essential for the assembly and secretion of chylomicrons and VLDLs in the endoplasmic reticulum of ruminant enterocytes, as described previously for nonruminants. The chylomicrons in ruminants are analogous to those in nonruminants, but have a lower proportion of TAGs and, therefore, are better classified as VLDLs (Drackley 2000). This reflects a regularly lower content of TAGs in ruminant feedstuffs than in most nonruminant diets.

## DIGESTION AND ABSORPTION OF LIPIDS IN FISH

### Digestion of Lipids in the Intestine

The diets of fish may contain 6%–40% lipids as TAGs, phospholipids, waxes, and free fatty acids, all of which generally have a high content of unsaturated fatty acids. As in nonruminant mammals, the digestion of lipids in fish requires emulsifiers (proteins, phospholipids, and bile salts) and pancreatic juices (including sodium bicarbonate, as well as pancreatic lipase, colipase, and cholesteryl ester hydrolase) in the proximal part of the intestine digestive tract. Lipase is present in fish, but its activity varies markedly among different species (e.g., Atlantic salmon, rainbow trout, hybrid bass, and zebrafish) (Bakke et al. 2011; Tocher and Sargent 1984). For example, colipase-dependent pancreatic lipase (which has a high specificity and digestive efficiency for TAGs) and bile salt-dependent carboxyl ester lipase (which has a broad specificity for lipids including wax esters) are the main lipases in freshwater fishes and marine fishes, respectively. Fish synthesize phospholipases to efficiently hydrolyze phospholipids. In these aquatic animals, dietary content and types of lipids can affect the secretion of pancreatic lipase, colipase, and cholesteryl ester hydrolase from the pancreas to adapt to the different sources of foods. The digestibility of lipids in fish is 85%–99%, depending on various factors (Bakke et al. 2011). These factors include species, breeds, developmental stage, feeding rate, water temperature, lipid source and type, and dietary composition of all other nutrients (particularly protein and PC). For example, lipid digestibility is decreased as the chain length of fatty acids in TAGs increases, but is enhanced as the degree of desaturation of fatty acids in TAGs increases. Also, given the important roles of many different proteins in the hydrolysis of TAGs and phospholipids, protein malnutrition impairs dietary lipid digestibility in fish, as in mammals.

#### Absorption of Lipids in the Intestine

In fish with pyloric ceca (the blind appendages attached to the proximal intestine), the primary site of lipid absorption is the ceca, rather than the proximal intestine (Sire et al. 1981). Specifically, the products of lipid digestion (including MAGs, free fatty acids, and glycerol) are mixed as micelles with bile salt, lysophosphatidylcholine, cholesterols, and fat-soluble vitamins. As the intestine contracts, the mixed micelles move through the luminal unstirred water layer into the surface of the intestinal enterocytes for absorption through specific transporters and diffusion. For example, intestinal-membrane SCFA exchangers have been recognized for herbivorous teleosts (Titus and Ahearn 1991), whereas intestinal FABP has been identified in both zebrafish (*Danio rerio*) and common carp (Bakke et al. 2011). Water-soluble short- and medium-chain fatty acids exit the basolateral membrane of the enterocyte into the lamina propria, and then enter the intestinal venule and the portal vein. Within the enterocytes, the absorbed LCFAs are esterified with MAGs or glycerol to form TAGs, which are packaged primarily as chylomicrons and VLDLs (Sire et al. 1981; Tocher and Glencross 2015).

Although dietary lipids (including LCFAs) are efficiently absorbed ultimately into the blood of fish (Tocher and Glencross 2015), the processes of the trafficking of dietary fats and LCFAs from the enterocytes into the systemic circulation are poorly understood. The lymphatic system in fish is not as well developed as in mammals (Steffensen and Lomholt 1992). Thus, there have been suggestions that the intestine-derived chylomicrons and VLDLs enter both the lymphatics and portal circulation (Rust 2002). In their studies with rainbow trout, Sire et al. (1981) found only a trace amount of gastrically administered $^{14}$C-labeled linoleic and palmitic acids in the liver and blood within 6 h after administration despite the appearance of a large amount of the tracers at the intestine (44% and 56% of the administered dose, respectively, in the caeca). These authors concluded that postprandially, lipids are absorbed slowly into the lymph rather than the portal vein. In agreement with these results, Eliason et al. (2010) reported that the concentrations of total lipids and TAGs in the portal vein of rainbow trout fed a lipid-containing meal (1% of body weight) did not differ at 0, 3, 6, and 12 h after feeding. Collectively, available evidence shows that the intestine-derived chylomicrons and VLDLs exit the basolateral membrane of the enterocytes into the intestinal lymphatics.

The factors which affect lipid digestion also influence lipid absorption in fish. For example, in these animals, SCFAs and MCFAs, which are soluble in water, are absorbed faster in the intestine than saturated LCFAs, which have a high degree of hydrophobicity and a low micellar solubility and which must pass through the luminal unstirred water layer to reach the enterocytes (Bakke et al.

2011). In addition, free (nonesterified) fatty acids and PC are absorbed at higher rates than TAGs, because the former have a smaller size and a lower hydrophobicity than the latter. Furthermore, as in mammals, high levels of dietary neutral TAGs lead to their accumulation in the enterocytes of fish, therefore reducing their export across the basolateral membrane of the enterocytes and, consequently, the absorption of lipids into the cells across their apical membrane. This may explain why the bioavailability of dietary lipids to the extraintestinal tissues of fish decreases as dietary TAG content increases.

## LIPOPROTEIN TRANSPORT AND METABOLISM IN ANIMALS

The chemical composition and secretion of intestinal lipoproteins affect dietary lipid utilization by animals and, therefore, their growth and production performance, as well as the quality of their meats, eggs, and milk. Efficient use of dietary lipids for lean tissue gains and the formation of high-quality products depend on the knowledge of lipoprotein transport and metabolism among key organs, such as the small intestine, liver, skeletal muscle, and WAT. These processes are qualitatively similar among various animal species, although quantitative differences are noted.

### Release of Lipoproteins from the Small Intestine and Liver

#### Overall View

TAGs are the predominant lipids in chylomicrons and VLDLs, but cholesterol and phospholipids are the main lipids in LDLs and HDLs, respectively (Puri 2011). LDLs contain about 10%–15% TAGs. These lipoproteins are so large in size that they cannot pass through the endothelial cells of the capillaries without prior hydrolysis. There is tremendous interest in lipoprotein metabolism in animals, because its abnormality causes fatty livers and chronic diseases (e.g., diabetes, hypercholesterolemia, hypertriacylglycerolemia, and atherosclerosis) and contributes to obesity in animals. The pathways of lipid transport and the metabolism of lipoproteins are similar between ruminants and nonruminant mammals; the small intestine releases chylomicrons into the portal vein rather than the lymphatic system. In the lymphatics of fed nonruminant mammals (e.g., pigs and humans) and ruminants, chylomicrons and VLDLs are the major lipid fractions, respectively. This is consistent with the finding that the small intestine (diet)-derived lipids are mainly chylomicrons in nonruminants and VLDLs in ruminants. The release of chylomicrons and nascent VLDLs from the mammalian small intestine (or portomicrons from avian small intestine) and the release of nascent VLDLs and mature HDLs from the liver of animals (including birds) all increase with the intestinal load of TAGs absorbed. In mammals, through the lymphatic circulation, chylomicrons and VLDLs enter the systemic blood circulation and their remnants are taken up primarily by the liver through the ApoE receptor and the LDL receptor, respectively (Figure 6.10). The liver synthesizes and releases nascent VLDLs and mature HDLs. Of note, LPL is absent from the liver of adult animals (including humans) but is expressed in this organ only during the perinatal period (Table 6.1). In healthy animals, fatty acids and glycerol, which are produced from the hydrolysis of lipoprotein TAGs by LPL, are efficiently oxidized to $CO_2$ and water, providing energy for tissue metabolism, and glycerol can also be utilized for glucose synthesis. The liver is the final organ for the catabolism of lipoprotein cholesterol to form bile acids, whereas the kidneys play a major role in the degradation of the protein components of the lipoproteins by peripheral tissues.

#### Metabolism of Chylomicrons, VLDLs, and LDLs

1. *Synthesis and release of chylomicrons and VLDLs from the small intestine and of VLDLs from the liver.* After a meal containing lipids, chylomicrons (containing ApoB48) and nascent VLDLs (containing ApoB100 and ApoA4) are synthesized from fatty acids, glycerol, 2-monoglycerides, cholesteryl esters, free cholesterol, phospholipids, and many different proteins (including apoproteins) in the endoplasmic reticulum of enterocytes (Tso et al. 2001). Thereafter, the chylomicrons and VLDLs are transported to the Golgi apparatus

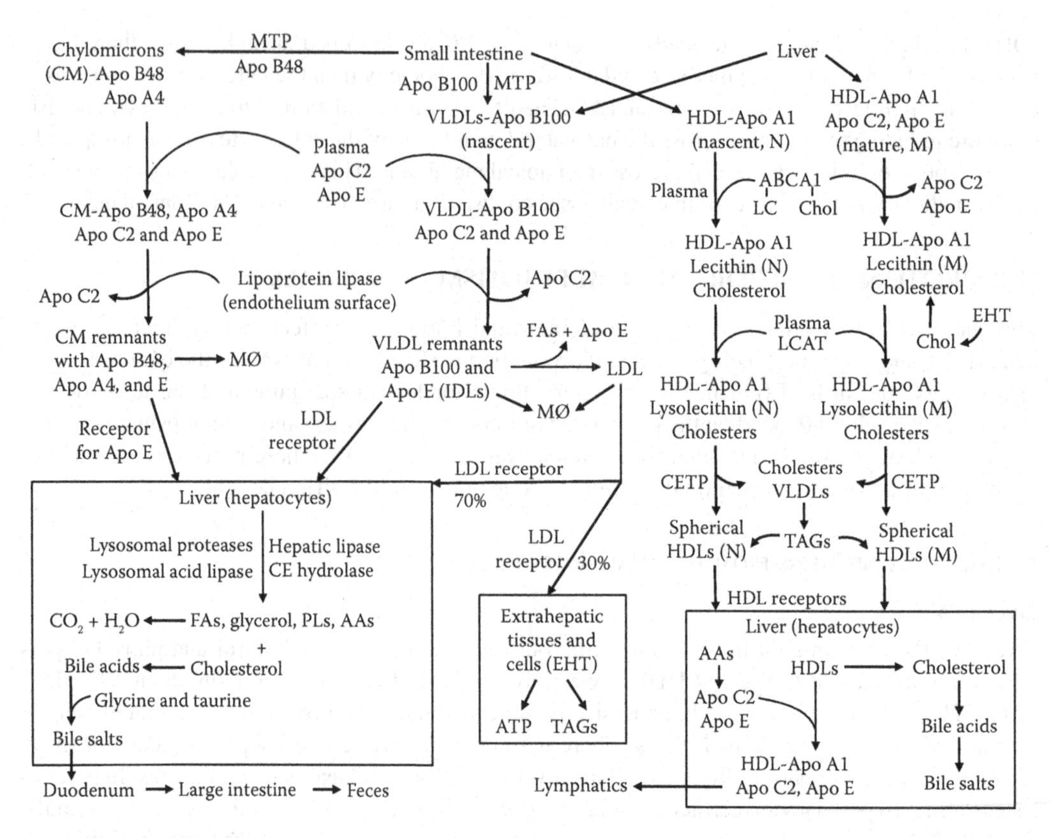


**FIGURE 6.10** Interorgan metabolism of lipoproteins in animals. The small intestine releases chylomicrons, very-low-density lipoproteins (VLDLs), and nascent high-density lipoproteins (HDLs), whereas the liver releases VLDLs and mature HDLs. During their transport through the blood circulation, chylomicrons and VLDLs acquire apolipoprotein (Apo) C2 and E from HDLs and lose TAGs to become chylomicron remnants and VLDL remnants (intermediate-density lipoproteins [IDLs] and low-density lipoproteins [LDLs]). Chylomicron remnants are taken up mainly by the liver through the ApoE receptor, whereas the VLDL remnants are taken up primarily by the liver and, to a less extent, peripheral tissues, through the LDL receptor. During their transport in the blood circulation, nascent HDLs from the small intestine (N) and mature HDLs from the liver (M) receive lecithin (LC) and free cholesterol (Chol) from a plasma lipid transporter (known as ATP-binding cassette transporter A1 [ABCA1]; released from the liver and intestine). Thereafter, the plasma lecithin:cholesterol acyltransferase (LCAT), which is activated by ApoA1, converts lecithin and free cholesterol on the HDLs into lysolecithin and cholesteryl esters, respectively, yielding spherical HDLs. Through the action of the plasma cholesteryl ester transfer protein (CETP), one-third of the LCAT-derived cholesteryl esters are transferred from the spherical HDLs to VLDLs to promote VLDL catabolism. The spherical HDLs are taken up by the liver. Free fatty acids (FAs) from lipoproteins are oxidized to $CO_2$ and water by the liver and peripheral tissues, whereas cholesterol is converted into bile acid in hepatocytes for ultimate excretion into the feces. MØ, macrophage.

for final processing and assembly, such as the addition and glycosylation of many proteins (including apoproteins). The Golgi vesicles containing chylomicrons and VLDLs migrate toward the basolateral membrane of enterocytes, and these two lipoproteins are discharged into the intercellular space of the lamina propria through exocytosis (reverse pinocytosis) (Besnard et al. 1996). The composition of fatty acids in the TAGs of chylomicrons closely resembles that of the dietary lipids consumed by animals. Chylomicrons are the major lipoproteins secreted by the small intestine in the fed state, whereas VLDLs are the only lipoproteins released by the gut during fasting (Yen et al. 2015). The release of chylomicrons and VLDLs from the small intestine is enhanced by high-fat feeding, and their ratios in the intestinal lymph are increased by the amount of PUFAs (e.g., linoleic acid)

**TABLE 6.1**
**Tissue- and Cell-Specific Distribution of Enzymes That Degrade Lipoproteins**

| Enzyme | Hepatocytes | Adipose Tissue | Skeletal Muscle | Heart | Kidneys | Smooth Muscle | Macrophages |
|---|---|---|---|---|---|---|---|
| HSL | Negligible | High | High | High | Medium | Low | Low |
| LPL | Absent | High | High | High | Medium | Low | Low |
| LAL | High | Low | Low | Low | High | Low | Medium |
| HL | High | Absent | Absent | Absent | Absent | Absent | Low |
| Proteases | High | Low | Medium | Medium | High | Low | Medium |
| LCEH | High | Low | Low | Low | Medium | Low | Medium |

*Source:* Fried, S.K. et al. 1993. *J. Clin. Invest.* 92:2191–2198; Jobgen, W.S. et al. 2006. *J. Nutr. Biochem.* 17:571–588; Yeaman, S.J. 1990. *Biochim. Biophys. Acta* 1052:128–132.

*Note:* High, high activity; low, low activity; medium, medium activity; HL, hepatic lipase (extracellular); HSL, hormone-sensitive lipase (intracellular); LAL, lysosomal acid lipase; LCEH, lysosomal cholesteryl ester hydrolase (cholesteryl esterase); LPL, lipoprotein lipase (extracellularlly localized on the endothelium surface of the microvasculature within extrahepatic tissues to hydrolyze both lipoproteins and cholesteryl esters to produce fatty acids and glycerol).

entering the duodenum. ApoA4 in chylomicrons may mediate lipid-induced satiety in animals through cell signaling in the hypothalamus of the brain (Tso and Liu 2004).

In fowl, the small intestine releases portomicrons (equivalent to mammalian chylomicrons) into the portal vein. These particles are likely too large to pass through the endothelium of the hepatic capillary bed of birds or to be ultimately taken up by their hepatocytes (Hermier 1997). Therefore, the intestine-derived lipoproteins are not catabolized by the avian liver (Hermier 1997). The portomicrons are absent from the plasma of fasted birds and are present only at a very low concentration in the plasma of fed neonatal birds due to the relatively low amounts of fats in most poultry diets and the rapid catabolism of portomicrons in extrahepatic tissues.

In preruminants, most of the intestine-derived VLDLs are exported into the intestinal lymphatics but some are taken into the portal vein, and the livers release an appreciable amount of HDLs and a small amount of VLDLs (Laplaud et al. 1990). In lymph samples obtained 10 h after a meal (i.e., at peak lipid absorption), the molar ratio of chylomicrons to VLDL is ~4:1. Of note, VLDLs represent only 5% of the total lipoproteins in the plasma of young calves and are absent from fetal calves (Bauchart 1993). In preruminants with limited ruminal fermentation and biohydrogenation, the compositions of fatty acids in chylomicrons and VLDLs are greatly influenced by dietary lipid intake.

In all animals, the liver does not produce or release chylomicrons. However, hepatocytes of the liver synthesize VLDLs from TAGs, cholesterol, phospholipids, ApoB100, and other proteins and then release the VLDLs. The VLDLs released from the liver travel through the lymphatics to the blood circulation (Goldstein and Brown 2015). In the fed state, the liver is the major source of VLDLs in the plasma. Under physiological conditions, hepatic assembly and secretion of VLDLs, as well as hepatic release of free fatty acids, are suppressed by insulin. The underlying mechanisms are that (1) insulin reduces the availability of free fatty acids in the plasma for hepatic uptake due to an increase in their use by the WAT for TAG synthesis and a decrease in whole-body lipolysis; and (2) insulin activates the PI3-kinase signaling, which inhibits the addition of TAGs to the precursor apoproteins by the ADP-ribosylation factor. This is consistent with the role of insulin acting as an anabolic hormone to enhance energy storage as TAGs in both the liver and WAT. In contrast, in obesity and Type-II diabetes mellitus with insulin resistance, a major feature of metabolic syndrome is hepatic hypersecretion of VLDLs, leading to hypertriglyceridemia.

2. *Metabolism of chylomicrons and VLDLs during their transport in the blood.* After the intestine-derived chylomicrons, as well as the intestine- and liver-derived VLDLs, exit the lymphatics, they sequentially enter the microvasculature, venous blood circulation, right heart, lungs, left heart, aorta, and arterial blood vessels (Chapter 1). During their transport in the blood, chylomicrons and VLDLs acquire ApoC2 and ApoE from the mature HDLs in the plasma that are released by the liver (Figure 6.10). Thereafter, most of the TAGs on the chylomicrons and VLDLs are hydrolyzed extracellularly by the LPLs localized on the luminal surface of the endothelium within extrahepatic tissues (particularly skeletal muscle and WAT) (Fried et al. 1993). The LPL reaction removes ~80% of TAGs from chylomicrons to form their remnants; subsequently, ApoC2 (the activator of the LPL) is released from chylomicrons to terminate the hydrolysis of their TAGs by the endothelium surface-bound LPL. The LPL reaction also removes ~60% of TAGs from VLDLs, and this hydrolysis, along with the terminal release of ApoC2 from the VLDLs, yields IDLs. The removal of ~60% TAGs from IDLs by the endothelium surface-bound LPL, along with the release of ApoE from the IDLs, generates LDLs (Goldstein and Brown 2015). Thus, the VLDL remnants are IDLs and LDLs. Of note, the hydrolysis of chylomicrons and VLDLs by the LPL also produces fatty acids, glycerol, phospholipids, and free cholesterol. Approximately 7.5%, 2.5%, and 90% of ApoB100 in the plasma are found in VLDLs, IDLs, and LDLs, respectively. LDLs are the major carrier of cholesterol in humans, pigs, rabbits, sheep, and guinea pigs. The chylomicron and VLDL remnants are ~50% smaller in diameter than their parent lipoproteins and can pass, along with fatty acids, phospholipids, cholesterol, and glycerol, through the endothelial cells of the capillaries into interstitial space for uptake by the liver and/or peripheral (nonhepatic) tissues.
3. *Uptake and metabolism of chylomicron and VLDL remnants by the liver and peripheral (nonhepatic) tissues.* Through the blood circulation, the liver and, to a much less extent, macrophages take up the chylomicron remnants (containing both ApoB48 and ApoE) through a receptor specific to ApoE (Figure 6.10). This organ and, to a lesser extent, certain extrahepatic tissues and cells (e.g., skeletal muscle, heart, adipose tissue, kidneys and macrophages) also take up LDLs (containing ApoB100) through the LDL receptor for catabolism (Goldstein and Brown 2015). Furthermore, the liver takes up a small amount of IDLs (containing ApoB100) through the LDL receptor. The rate of internalization of chylomicron remnants, IDLs, and LDLs through receptor-mediated endocytosis is determined by the amount and activity of their respective receptors, rather than by the concentrations of the lipoproteins (Goldstein and Brown 2015). Hepatic lipase, which is synthesized and released by hepatocytes, is crucial for extracellular lipoprotein metabolism in the liver. This is because hepatic lipase is strategically localized at the surface of liver sinusoid capillaries and the surface of hepatocytes to hydrolyze extracellular TAGs, cholesteryl esters, and phospholipids in the chylomicron remnants, IDLs, and LDLs entering the liver.

   In both the liver and extrahepatic tissues, lysosomal acid lipase (LAL) can hydrolyze intracellular TAGs and cholesteryl esters in the endocytosed lipoproteins, and lysosomal cholesteryl ester hydrolase (cholesteryl esterase) can degrade intracellular cholesteryl esters (Table 6.1). HSL hydrolyzes intracellular TAGs in extrahepatic tissues (particularly skeletal muscle and adipose tissue) (Yeaman 1990). The products of the catabolism of chylomicron remnants, IDLs, and LDLs are fatty acids, glycerol, phospholipids, free cholesterol, and AAs. These metabolites have different metabolic fates depending on the type of tissue. For example, fatty acids are oxidized to $CO_2$ and $H_2O$ in hepatocytes and skeletal muscle. In contrast, free cholesterol is converted into bile acids in hepatocytes but is transferred to HDL particles in extrahepatic tissues.The physiological significance of the LDL receptor for LDL metabolism is epitomized by the finding that a defect in familial hypercholesterolemia greatly contributes to dyslipidemia in affected subjects (Goldstein and Brown 2015). The liver and kidneys are the major extrahepatic sites to degrade lipoproteins in chylomicron remnants and LDLs, respectively. Approximately 70% and 30% of LDLs are degraded in the liver and extrahepatic tissues, respectively (Puri 2011). Thus, the liver plays a central role in the catabolism of chylomicrons, VLDLs, and LDLs.

4. *Uptake and metabolism of LCFAs by the liver and peripheral (nonhepatic) tissues.* The LCFAs released from the partial degradation of chylomicrons and VLDLs in the plasma by the endothelium surface-bound LPL are taken up into the liver, as well as peripheral (nonhepatic) tissues and cells, such as skeletal muscle, heart, WAT, kidneys, and macrophages through simple diffusion and membrane-bound transporters (Figure 6.3). Deletion of a major LCFA transporter, CD36, greatly impairs the transport of LCFAs by these tissues and cells, as well as the clearance of lipoproteins from the blood (Goldberg et al. 2009). In skeletal muscle, the abundance of the CD36 protein is chronically upregulated by insulin, muscle contraction, and PPAR-δ to increase the uptake of LCFAs (Nahle et al. 2008). Fatty acids are the major metabolic fuels in the liver, skeletal muscle, and heart and contribute substantially to ATP production in the kidneys. PUFAs are also signaling molecules in cells. All fatty acids can be used for the synthesis of TAGs in tissues, particularly the liver and WAT in a species-dependent manner (Jobgen et al. 2006), and participate in cell metabolism including the assembly of membrane lipid bilayers.
5. *Turnover and functions of chylomicrons and VLDLs.* Chylomicrons released from the small intestine, as well as nascent VLDLs released from the small intestine and liver, are rapidly metabolized in animals. For example, the labeled TAG fatty acids in chylomicrons administered intravenously have a half-life of 8–9 min in small animals (e.g., rats) and <60 min in large animals (e.g., 14 min in healthy humans and 51 min in hypertriglyceridemic subjects) (Cortner et al. 1987). About 80% of the fatty acid label is found in the adipose tissue, heart, and skeletal muscle, whereas 20% of the label is in the liver. In contrast, the half-life of ApoB100 in IDLs or LDLs (~2 days) is much longer than that of chylomicrons or VLDLs. Chylomicrons and VLDLs mainly transport TAGs to the liver and peripheral (nonhepatic) tissues to either be used for energy or stored. In contrast, LDLs primarily deliver cholesterol to various tissues (e.g., liver and adrenal cortex) for the synthesis of bile acids and steroid hormones in a cell-specific manner.
6. *Regulation of LPL activity.* Different isoforms of LPL are synthesized and secreted into the endothelial surface of the capillaries by the parenchymal (the main part) cells of different tissues (e.g., adipocytes in the WAT, myofibers in skeletal muscle, and myocytes in heart) (Lee et al. 2014; Macfarlane et al. 2008). LPL is activated by ApoC2 (a component of HDLs) but inhibited by ApoC3 (a component of VLDLs) and Angptl4 (protein angiopoietin-like 4) (Goldberg et al. 2009). Regulation of LPL expression and activity by hormones, nutritional status, and other factors (e.g., cytokines and exercise) is tissue specific (Table 6.2), depending on the nutritional state and physiological needs of animals. For example, in response to physiological levels of insulin, LPL activity is enhanced in the WAT but reduced in skeletal muscle. In contrast, the opposite is true during fasting. This reflects the different functions of these two tissues in TAG metabolism. Specifically, LPL in the WAT facilitates the extracellular hydrolysis of blood TAGs to LCFAs and glycerol for uptake by adipocytes, where LCFAs and glycerol are re-esterified into TAGs for storage (Kersten 2014). On the other hand, LPL in skeletal muscle promotes the intravascular conversion of extracellular (blood) TAGs into LCFAs as major metabolic fuels. Overall, insulin stimulates TAG deposition in the WAT in the fed state, whereas TAGs in the blood are utilized by skeletal muscle for ATP production to spare glucose during fasting. Thus, LPL controls the partitioning of dietary and endogenous TAGs into storage or oxidation in animals, thereby playing an important role in whole-body fat homeostasis.

In the mammary gland, LPL expression is enhanced during late pregnancy and lactation through the effects of prolactin to provide fatty acids for milk TAG synthesis (Rezaei et al. 2016). This enzyme converts blood-borne TAGs into LCFAs and glycerol for uptake by

**TABLE 6.2**
**Effects of Hormones, Nutritional Status, and Other Factors on Expression and Activities of Lipoprotein Lipase and Hormone-Sensitive Lipase (HSL) in White Adipose Tissue (WAT) and Skeletal Muscle (SKM)**

| | Lipoprotein Lipase | | HSL | |
|---|---|---|---|---|
| | WAT | SKM | WAT | SKM |
| Hormones | | | | |
| Catecholamines | ↓ | ↑ | ↑ | ↑ |
| Glucagon | ↓ | ↑ | ↑ | ↑ |
| Glucocorticoids | | | | |
| Short term | ↑ | ↑ | ↑ | ↑ |
| Long term | ↑ | ↑ | ↓ | ↓ |
| Growth hormone | ↓ | ↑ | ↑ | ↑ |
| Insulin | ↑ | ↓ | ↓ | ↓ |
| Parathyroid hormones | ↓ | ↑ | ↑ | ↑ |
| Thyroid hormones | ↓ | ↑ | ↑ | ↑ |
| Nutritional status | | | | |
| Fasting (vs. fed state) | ↓ | ↑ | ↑ | ↑ |
| Feeding (vs. fasting) | ↑ | ↓ | ↓ | ↓ |
| High-fat diet (vs. low-fat diet) | ↑ | ↑ | ↓ | ↓ |
| High-starch diet (vs. low-starch diet) | ↑ | ↓ | ↓ | ↓ |
| High-protein diet (vs. normal-protein diet) | NC | ↑ | ↑ | ↑ |
| ω3-Polyunsaturated fatty acids | ↓ | ↑ | ↑ | ↑ |
| Other factors | | | | |
| AMP-activated protein kinase | ↓ | ↑ | ↑ | ↑ |
| Exercise | ↓ | ↑ | ↑ | ↑ |
| Interferon-α | ↓ | ↓ | ↑ | ↑ |
| Interferon-γ | ↓ | ↓ | ↑ | ↑ |
| Interleukin-1 | ↓ | ↓ | ↑ | ↑ |
| Lipopolysaccharide | ↓ | ↓ | ↑ | ↑ |
| Peroxisome proliferator-activated receptor-α | – | ↑ | – | ↑ |
| Peroxisome proliferator-activated receptor-γ | ↑ | NC | ↓ | NC |
| Peroxisome proliferator-activated receptor-δ/β | ↓ | ↑ | ↑ | ↑ |
| Tumor necrosis factor-α | ↓ | ↓ | NC | ↑ |

*Source:* Bijland, S. et al. 2013. *Clin. Sci.* 124:491–507; Donsmark, M. et al. 2004. *Proc. Nutr. Soc.* 63:309–314; Goldberg, I.J. et al. 2009. *J. Lipid Res.* 50:S86–S90; Huang, C.W. et al. 2016. *Int. J. Mol. Sci.* 17:1689; Lee, M.J. et al. 2014. *Biochim. Biophys. Acta* 1842:473-481; Macfarlane, D.P. et al. 2008. *J. Endocrinol.* 197:189–204; Picard, F. et al. 2002. *Clin. Vaccine Immunol.* 9:4771–4776.

*Note:* ↓, decrease; ↑, increase; NC, no change.

mammary epithelial cells. Although LPL is not directly activated by a cAMP-dependent kinase, the expression and abundance of this enzyme are increased in brown adipose tissue, WAT, heart, skeletal muscle, and the adrenal glands during cold exposure (Goldberg et al. 2009). Likely mediators for the enzyme induction are elevated levels of thyroid hormones and catecholamines in the plasma to promote the transcription of target genes. This is physiologically important to provide fatty acids for nonshivering heat production by the various tissues.

In the liver, LPL is expressed during fetal and early postnatal life, but thereafter is suppressed by a novel transcription factor, termed RF-1-LPL that binds to an NF-1-like site in the region of the glucocorticoid response element (Semenkovich et al. 1989). The hepatic expression of LPL during the perinatal period is also induced by thyroid hormones and glucocorticoids. The loss of LPL in the liver of adult animals maximizes the delivery of both dietary and endogenous lipids (e.g., TAGs and cholesterol) to extrahepatic tissues. The replacement of LPL in the liver is hepatic lipase, as noted previously.

7. *Regulation of hepatic lipase activity.* Hepatic lipase is expressed almost exclusively in hepatocytes, and its mRNA is not detected in other tissues, including the pancreas, WAT, lung, heart, skeletal muscle, mammary gland, adrenal gland, and ovary (Semenkovich et al. 1989). The expression of lipase is enhanced by growth hormone, androgens, and glucocorticoids, but inhibited by estrogens, ω3 PUFAs, and cholesterol to control TAG uptake by hepatocytes and the concentrations of free fatty acids in the plasma (Perret et al. 2002). Results of recent studies indicate that sphingomyelin is also an inhibitor of hepatic lipase activity, such that this enzyme is most active when sphingomyelin is depleted from lipoprotein substrates (Yang and Subbaiah 2015). This stimulation of hepatic lipase is greater with LDL and VLDL than with HDL.

## Metabolism of HDLs

1. *Release of nascent HDLs from the small intestine and of mature HDLs from the liver.* HDL metabolism begins in both the small intestine and the liver (Figure 6.10). HDLs, which have different proportions of apolipoproteins, cholesterol, and phospholipids than chylomicrons and VLDLs, take part in the metabolism of lipoprotein TAGs and cholesterol. Enterocytes of the small intestine synthesize and release, into the lymphatic circulation, a small amount of newly formed HDLs (called nascent HDLs), which contain ApoA1, but not ApoC2 or ApoE (Goldstein and Brown 2015). In contrast, hepatocytes of the liver synthesize and release a large amount of mature HDLs with ApoA1, ApoC2, and ApoE. The HDLs released from the liver travel through the lymphatics to the blood circulation. In mammals, birds, and fish, the liver is the predominant source of HDLs in the plasma.
2. *Metabolism of intestine-derived HDLs during transport in the blood.* After entering the blood, ApoA1 in the intestine-derived HDLs interacts extracellularly (the plasma) with a lipid transporter (known as ATP-binding cassette transporter A1 [ABCA1]), which is released primarily from the liver (70%) and, to a lesser extent, from the small intestine (30%) (Lee et al. 2012). This interaction promotes the transfer of phospholipids and free cholesterol from ABCA1 to ApoA1, generating discoidal nascent HDLs. Thus, ABCA1 mediates the assembly of free cholesterol and phospholipids with ApoA1. Thereafter, the plasma LCAT, which is activated by ApoA1, converts PC and free cholesterol on the HDLs into lysophosphatidylcholine and cholesteryl esters, respectively, yielding spherical HDLs (Puri 2011). Through the action of the plasma cholesteryl ester transfer protein (CETP), one-third of the LCAT-derived cholesteryl esters are transferred from the spherical HDLs to VLDLs to promote VLDL catabolism. This reaction also results in the exchange of TAGs to the HDL particles. The spherical HDLs have a surface layer of polar lipids and apolipoproteins and are recognized by the liver.
3. *Metabolism of liver-derived HDLs during transport in the blood.* As noted previously, the liver releases mature HDLs containing ApoA1, ApoC2, and ApoE into the blood. These mature HDLs transfer ApoC2 and ApoE to chylomicrons and VLDLs, yielding smaller HDL particles (Semenkovich et al. 1989). The metabolism of the liver-derived HDLs during transport in the blood resembles that of the intestine-derived nascent HDLs, except that the liver-derived HDLs collect more free cholesterol from peripheral (nonhepatic) tissues and cells than the intestine-derived nascent HDLs. Ultimately, the liver-derived spherical HDLs containing high proportions of lysophosphatidylcholine and cholesteryl esters are

generated and return to the liver. In the plasma, these HDLs make up the majority (90%) of all the HDLs, which are heterogeneous in size, shape, and protein/lipid content. The process of cholesterol transport from peripheral tissues and cells to the liver is known as "reverse cholesterol transport" (Krieger 1998).

Through its release of ApoC2 and ApoE, the liver-derived mature HDLs are required for the metabolism of chylomicrons and VLDLs. This is because ApoC2 is an activator of LPL in tissues and the ApoE-containing chylomicron remnants are recognized by their ApoE-specific receptors in hepatocytes. Thus, the mature HDLs released by the liver act as a repository for ApoC2 and ApoE. The liver is also the ultimate organ for the degradation of HDL cholesteryl esters via the synthesis of bile acids, which is then excreted in the feces.

4. *Uptake and metabolism of plasma spherical HDLs by the liver.* The plasma spherical HDLs, which are generated from the intestine- and liver-derived HDLs, are taken up by the liver through HDL receptors (e.g., scavenger receptor class B type I). Once inside the hepatocytes, the spherical HDLs have two metabolic fates: (1) binding to ApoC2 and ApoE to form mature, fully active HDLs for release from the liver; or (2) being hydrolyzed by hepatic lipase, LAL, lysosomal cholesteryl ester hydrolases, and lysosomal proteases to produce fatty acids, glycerol, cholesterol, lysophosphatidylcholine, and AAs.
5. *Turnover and functions of HDLs.* Proteomic studies have identified the presence of more than 50 different proteins that are associated with the mature HDLs, some of which are proteins that are implicated in the anti-inflammatory functions of HDLs (Iqbal and Hussain 2009). The average half-life of the HDLs is 5 days (Puri 2011). HDL lipids are also heterogeneous and include a wide variety of bioactive lipids, including phosphosphingolipids (e.g., sphingosine 1 phosphate), oxysterols, and lysolipids. HDLs serve as (1) a reservoir of apoproteins that can be transferred to other lipoproteins; (2) an acceptor of unesterified cholesterol (because the high content of phospholipids in HDLs can solubilize cholesterol); (3) the site for esterification of cholesterol (through the action of LCAT); and (4) a reverse transport of cholesterol from peripheral tissues and cells to the liver for the final disposal of cholesterol as bile acid. Thus, because of their antioxidative and cholesterol efflux roles, HDLs inhibit the development of atherosclerosis, which is the primary underlying cause of cardiovascular disease (Goldstein and Brown 2015).

## Important Role for HDLs in Cholesterol Metabolism

Cholesterol metabolism requires esterification reactions, which occur in both cells and the plasma (Puri 2011). In nearly all animal cells, ACAT promotes the formation of cholesteryl esters (e.g., cholesteryl oleate) from cholesterol and fatty acids in the endoplasmic reticulum. This enzyme is activated by free cholesterol and plays a key role in hepatic bile acid biosynthesis. Thus, ACAT regulates the intracellular homeostasis of free cholesterol and its release from cells. In the blood, cholesterol is esterified by LCAT, which is released from the liver. The cholesteryl esters are substrates for CETP, which is attached to HDLs in the plasma. CETP accepts TAGs from VLDLs or LDLs and exchanges TAGs for cholesteryl esters from HDLs, and vice versa. In other words, CETP facilitates the transport of cholesteryl esters and TAGs between lipoproteins in the blood. Therefore, HDLs play an important role in the reverse transport of cholesterol from peripheral tissues to the liver.

## Species Differences in Lipoprotein Metabolism

There are species differences in plasma concentrations of lipoproteins. For example, pigs and humans have high levels of LDLs in plasma, and LDLs are the major lipoproteins in plasma (Puri 2011). In horses and ruminants, HDLs are the major lipoproteins and there is considerable overlap in the density range of LDLs and HDLs (Drackley 2000). Thus, it is more difficult to separate LDLs and HDLs using the conventional ultracentrifugal methods. In animals with familial hypercholesterolemia, IDL cannot be taken up into the liver and is converted into LDL. Therefore, plasma levels of LDL are high in these patients. A defect in LPL may account for high plasma levels of TAGs in some patients.

# FATTY ACID SYNTHESIS IN TISSUES

## Synthesis of Saturated Fatty Acids from Acetyl-CoA

Acetyl-CoA is the principal building block of fatty acids in the cytosol of nearly all animal cells. In the liver, this metabolic pathway occurs primarily in perivenous hepatocytes (Jobgen et al. 2006). If acetyl-CoA is formed from the oxidation of pyruvate, AAs, or fatty acids in the mitochondria, acetyl-CoA is transported into the cytosol via the formation of citrate from oxaloacetate (OAA). The use of mitochondria-generated acetyl-CoA for fatty acid synthesis is a complex biochemical process. First, acetyl-CoA is converted into citrate in the mitochondria, which enters the cytosol through the citrate transporter (Figure 6.11). In the cytosol, citrate is cleaved to form OAA and acetyl-CoA by ATP-citrate lyase in the presence of ATP and CoA. If short-chain fatty acyl-CoAs are formed from SCFAs in the cytosol, the acyl-CoAs are directly used for local fatty acid synthesis. Of note, it was previously thought that the low activity of ATP-citrate lyase limited the use of glucose for fatty acid biosynthesis in ruminant adipose tissue. However, it has been established that, like many other tissues, the uptake and utilization of glucose for fatty acid synthesis is limited by the activity of 6-phosphofructokinase (Smith and Prior 1981).

### Formation of Malonyl-CoA from Acetyl-CoA by Acetyl-CoA Carboxylase

The conversion of acetyl-CoA into malonyl-CoA by acetyl-CoA carboxylase (ACC) is the initial and rate-controlling step in fatty acid synthesis from acetyl-CoA (Figure 6.12). This multisubunit enzyme is localized in the endoplasmic reticulum and requires NADPH, ATP, $Mn^{2+}$, biotin, and $HCO_3^-$ as cofactors. The ACC-catalyzed reaction involves two steps: the carboxylation of biotin and the transfer of the carboxyl biotin to acetyl-CoA to form malonyl-CoA.

Animals have two isoforms of ACC (ACC1 and ACC2), which differ in tissue distribution and function. ACC1 is expressed primarily in lipogenic tissues (e.g., adipose tissue and lactating

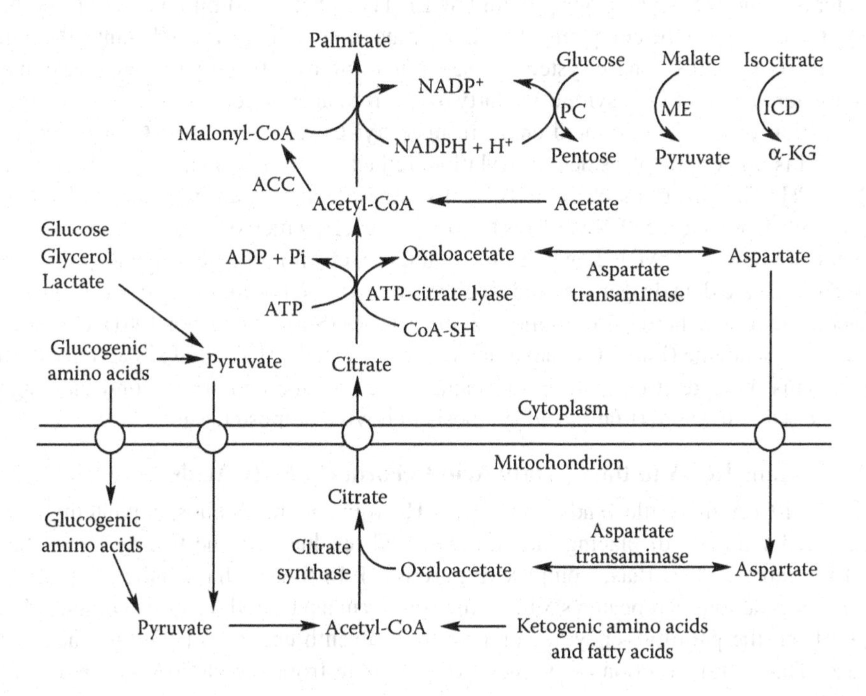


**FIGURE 6.11** Translocation of acetyl-CoA from mitochondria into the cytosol. Acetyl-CoA and OAA are converted into citrate by citrate synthase in mitochondria. The citrate leaves the mitochondria through the citrate transporter into the cytosol, where citrate is cleaved by ATP-citrate lyase into acetyl-CoA and OAA. ACC, acetyl-CoA carboxylase; ICD, isocitrate dehydrogenase; ME, malic enzyme; PC, pentose cycle.

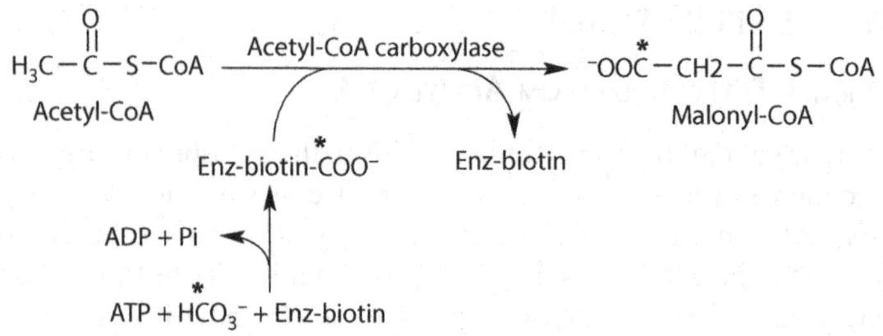

$H_3C-C(=O)-S-CoA$ (Acetyl-CoA) —Acetyl-CoA carboxylase→ $^{-}OOC^{*}-CH_2-C(=O)-S-CoA$ (Malonyl-CoA)

Enz-biotin-$COO^{-}$* → Enz-biotin

ATP + $HCO_3^-$* + Enz-biotin → Enz-biotin-$COO^{-}$* + ADP + Pi

**FIGURE 6.12** The conversion of acetyl-CoA into malonyl-CoA by acetyl-CoA carboxylase in the cytosol. This is the initial and rate-controlling step in fatty acid synthesis from acetyl-CoA.

mammary glands), where the *de novo* synthesis of fatty acids is nutritionally and physiologically important. In contrast, ACC2 is present mainly in oxidative tissues (e.g., skeletal muscle and heart), where the β-oxidation of fatty acids provides the bulk of ATP for metabolic utilization. Of note, both ACC1 and ACC2 are highly expressed in the liver, where both the synthesis and oxidation of fatty acids are important, depending on nutritional status and physiological needs. Thus, ACC1 is mainly involved in fatty acid synthesis.

### Formation of $C_4$ Fatty Acid Chain from Acetyl-CoA and Malonyl-CoA by Fatty Acid Synthase

In mammals, birds, fish, and yeast, fatty acid synthase is a multienzyme complex (Figure 6.13). The fatty acid synthase complex is a dimer, consisting of two identical monomers in a "head–tail" arrangement. Each monomer (polypeptide) contains seven different enzyme activities (ketoacyl synthase, acetyl transacylase, malonyl transacylase, hydratase, enoyl reductase, ketoacyl reductase, and thioesterase) and the acyl carrier protein (ACP). The functional unit consists of one-half of a monomer interacting with the complementary half of the other. In bacteria and plants, the individual enzymes of the fatty acid synthase system are separate proteins. The fatty acid synthase in eukaryotes is an efficient metabolon to synthesize fatty acids from acetyl-CoA.

The formation of the $C_4$ fatty acid chain from acetyl-CoA and malonyl-CoA is illustrated in Figure 6.14. This process involves decarboxylation, reduction by NADPH, dehydration, and reduction by NADPH. The two units of the fatty acid synthase complex are represented by 1 and 2 in Figure 6.14. The major source of NADPH is the pentose cycle, which occurs in the cytosol (Bauman 1976). Other sources of NADPH, which are quantitatively minor ones, include malic enzyme (NADP-linked malate dehydrogenase) and isocitrate dehydrogenase in the cytosol (Figure 6.11). In ruminant adipose tissue, there is low malic enzyme activity (Smith and Prior 1981). However, malic enzyme activity in bovine (but not ovine) adipose tissue exceeds ACC and FAS activity (Smith and Prior 1981). This indicates that there is sufficient malic enzyme activity to contribute significant amounts of NADPH to support fatty acid synthesis in bovine adipose tissue.

### Addition of Malonyl-CoA to the $C_4$ Fatty Acid to Form $C_{16}$ Fatty Acids

A new malonyl-CoA molecule binds with the –SH group of the 4′-phosphopantetheine (unit 2) of the fatty acid synthase, displacing the saturated acyl residue onto the free cysteine –SH group (unit 1) of the fatty acid synthase complex (Figure 6.14). In tissues that synthesize palmitate, the sequence of the reactions is repeated six more times to form a palmityl–enzyme complex. Palmitate is liberated from the palmityl–enzyme complex by a seventh enzyme of the fatty acid synthase, thioesterase. The overall reaction of synthesis of palmitate from acetyl-CoA and malonyl-CoA is shown as follows:

$$\text{Acetyl-CoA} + 7\ \text{Malonyl-CoA} + 14\ \text{NADPH} + 14\ H^+ \rightarrow \text{Palmitate} + 7\ CO_2 + 6\ H_2O + 8\ \text{CoA} + 14\ \text{NADP}^+$$

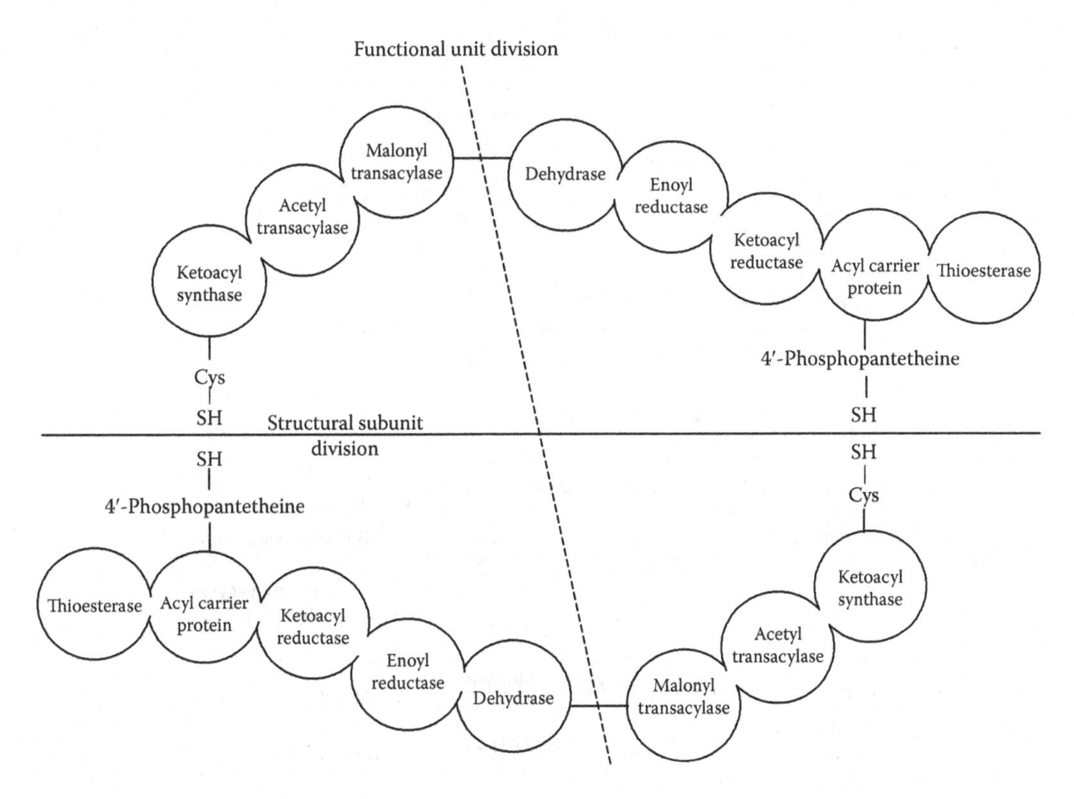


**FIGURE 6.13** The fatty acid synthase in mammals, birds, fish, and yeast. This enzyme is a dimer, consisting of two identical monomers in a "head–tail" arrangement. Each monomer (polypeptide) contains seven different enzymatic activities (ketoacyl synthase, acetyl transacylase, malonyl transacylase, hydratase, enoyl reductase, ketoacyl reductase, and thioesterase) and the acyl carrier protein. The functional unit consists of one-half of a monomer interacting with the complementary half of the other. (Adapted from Mayes, P.A. 1996a. *Harper's Biochemistry*. Edited by R.K. Murray, D.K. Granner, and V.W. Rodwell. Appleton & Lange, Stamford, CT, pp. 216–223.)

## Metabolic Fate of Palmitate

Under physiological and nutritional conditions that favor lipogenesis, free palmitate is activated to palmitoyl-CoA by palmitoyl-CoA synthetase in the cytosol. The resulting palmitoyl-CoA is esterified to TAGs and cholesteryl esters and undergoes chain elongation and desaturation in the smooth endoplasmic reticulum. Palmitoyl-CoA may also participate in the palmitoylation of cysteine residues of proteins by protein palmitoyltransferases (transmembrane proteins) to regulate their biological activities. Elongation of the fatty acid chain beyond C16 occurs in the endoplasmic reticulum, and this metabolic pathway requires the addition of acetyl-CoA as malonyl-CoA to the hydrocarbon chain, as well as NADPH (Figure 6.15).

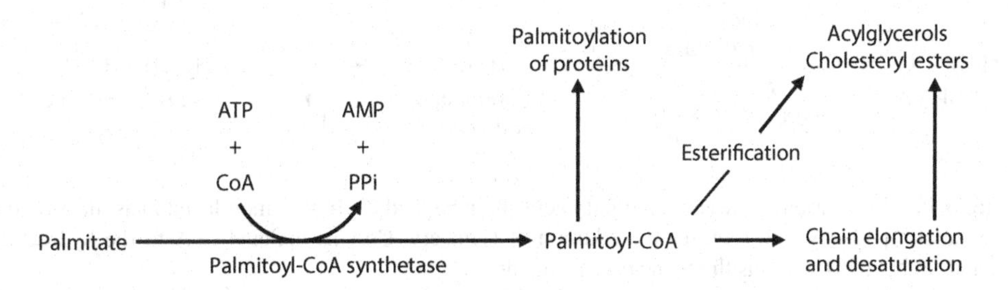

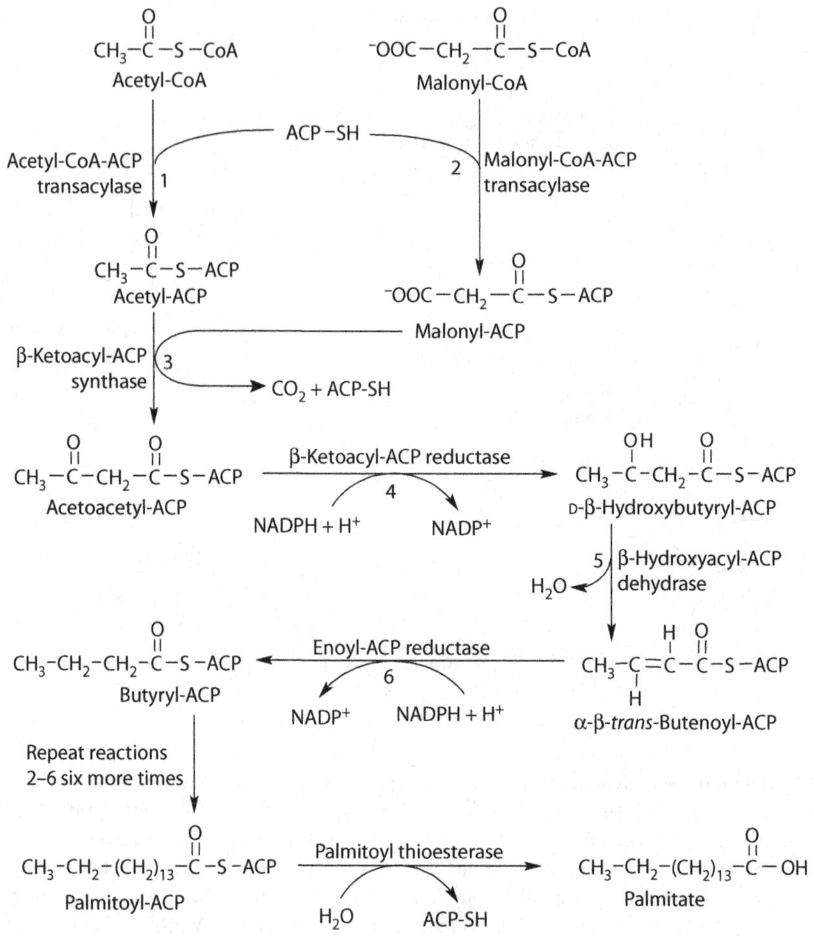

$CH_3-C(=O)-S-CoA$
Acetyl-CoA

$^-OOC-CH_2-C(=O)-S-CoA$
Malonyl-CoA

ACP−SH

Acetyl-CoA-ACP transacylase 1

2 Malonyl-CoA-ACP transacylase

$CH_3-C(=O)-S-ACP$
Acetyl-ACP

$^-OOC-CH_2-C(=O)-S-ACP$
Malonyl-ACP

β-Ketoacyl-ACP synthase 3

$CO_2$ + ACP-SH

$CH_3-C(=O)-CH_2-C(=O)-S-ACP$
Acetoacetyl-ACP

β-Ketoacyl-ACP reductase
4
NADPH + $H^+$
$NADP^+$

$CH_3-C(OH)-CH_2-C(=O)-S-ACP$
D-β-Hydroxybutyryl-ACP

5 β-Hydroxyacyl-ACP dehydrase
$H_2O$

$CH_3-C(H)=C(H)-C(=O)-S-ACP$
α-β-*trans*-Butenoyl-ACP

Enoyl-ACP reductase
6
$NADP^+$
NADPH + $H^+$

$CH_3-CH_2-CH_2-C(=O)-S-ACP$
Butyryl-ACP

Repeat reactions 2–6 six more times

$CH_3-CH_2-(CH_2)_{13}-C(=O)-S-ACP$
Palmitoyl-ACP

Palmitoyl thioesterase
$H_2O$
ACP-SH

$CH_3-CH_2-(CH_2)_{13}-C(=O)-OH$
Palmitate

**FIGURE 6.14** The synthesis pathway of long-chain fatty acid (e.g., palmitate) from acetyl-CoA in animal cells. These reactions take place in the smooth endoplasmic reticulum. ACP, acyl carrier protein.

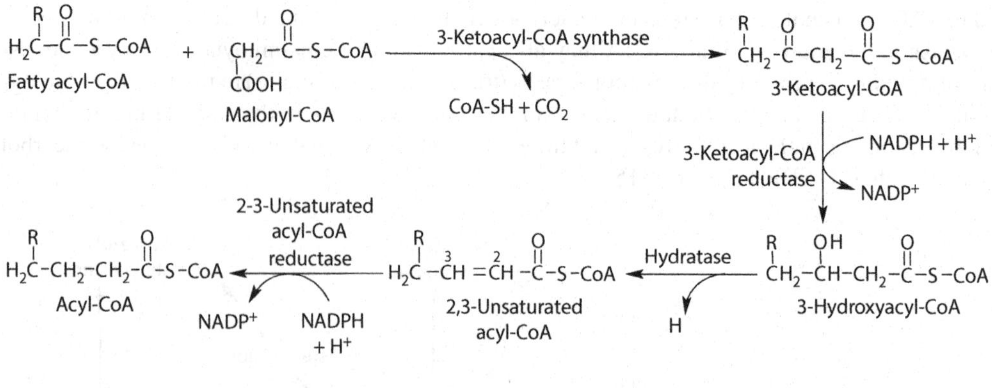

$H_2C(R)-C(=O)-S-CoA$
Fatty acyl-CoA

+

$CH_2(COOH)-C(=O)-S-CoA$
Malonyl-CoA

3-Ketoacyl-CoA synthase
CoA-SH + $CO_2$

$CH_2(R)-C(=O)-CH_2-C(=O)-S-CoA$
3-Ketoacyl-CoA

3-Ketoacyl-CoA reductase
NADPH + $H^+$
$NADP^+$

$CH_2(R)-CH(OH)-CH_2-C(=O)-S-CoA$
3-Hydroxyacyl-CoA

Hydratase
H

$H_2C(R)-{}^3CH={}^2CH-C(=O)-S-CoA$
2,3-Unsaturated acyl-CoA

2-3-Unsaturated acyl-CoA reductase
$NADP^+$
NADPH + $H^+$

$H_2C(R)-CH_2-CH_2-C(=O)-S-CoA$
Acyl-CoA

**FIGURE 6.15** Elongation of the saturated fatty acid chain beyond $C_{16}$ in the smooth endoplasmic reticulum. This metabolic pathway also requires the addition of (1) acetyl-CoA as malonyl-CoA to the hydrocarbon chain; and (2) NADPH + $H^+$ as the reducing equivalent.

## Synthesis of Saturated Fatty Acids from Propionyl-CoA or Butyryl-CoA plus Acetyl-CoA

In addition to acetyl-CoA, the primer for fatty acid synthesis can also be propionyl-CoA or butyryl-CoA. The addition of all the subsequent $C_2$ units is also via malonyl-CoA incorporation, and this malonyl-CoA is synthesized from acetyl-CoA. The pathway for the synthesis of saturated fatty acids from propionyl-CoA or butyryl-CoA plus acetyl-CoA is the same as described previously for the synthesis of fatty acids from acetyl-CoA. In ruminants, large amounts of propionate are formed in the rumen, which contributes to the formation of fatty acids with an odd carbon number.

## Synthesis of Short-Chain Fatty Acids

Short-chain fatty acids are the $C_{2-5}$ organic fatty acids, which are produced primarily in the rumen of ruminants and in the intestine (mainly the large intestine) of nonruminants as a result of anaerobic bacterial fermentation of dietary fats, protein, and carbohydrates (including nonstarch fibers) (Chapter 5). In the hindgut of animals, acetate, propionate, and butyrate account for 83% of short-chain fatty acids and can amount to 100–150 mM. Acetate is an important energy substrate, and propionate is a major substrate for gluconeogenesis in ruminants. Butyrate is the preferred energy substrate for colonocytes and modulates their growth and differentiation. A slowly fermentable fiber, such as wheat bran, is more effective than a completely fermentable fiber, such as oat bran, in producing high levels of butyrate throughout the proximal and distal colon (Turner and Lupton 2011). The fact that different dietary substrates are preferentially fermented to different short-chain fatty acids may be important in the relationship between diet and intestinal health. Thus, through increased production of butyrate, enhanced gut motility, and dilution of fecal toxic substances, high intake of dietary fibers may protect against colon cancer in animals. Conversely, inadequate intake of dietary fibers may contribute to intestinal dysfunction and colon cancer.

## Synthesis of MUFAs in Animals

### Synthesis of $\Delta^9$ MUFAs

All animals have acyl-CoA $\Delta^9$ desaturase in the endoplasmic reticulum to convert a saturated acyl-CoA to a monosaturated acyl-CoA. Subsequently, an acyl-CoA thioesterase hydrolyzes the acyl-CoA ester to the corresponding free acid and CoA. Acyl-CoA $\Delta^9$ desaturase requires cytochrome $b_5$, NADH (P)-cytochrome $b_5$ reductase, and molecular oxygen and introduces a double bond at the $\Delta^9$ position into a saturated LCFA (Ntambi 1999). Therefore, mammals, birds, and fish can synthesize the ω9 (oleic acid; $C_{18:1}$ ω9) and ω7 (palmitoleic acid; $C_{16:1}$ ω7) families of unsaturated fatty acids from saturated LCFAs (e.g., palmitate; $C_{16:0}$) by a combination of chain elongation and desaturation. Thus, oleic acid and palmitoleic acid are not classified as nutritionally essential for animals, meaning that these fatty acids are not needed in diets.

$$\text{Saturated fatty acyl-CoA} + 2\ \text{Ferrocytochrome}\ b_5 + O_2 + 2\ H^+ \rightarrow \text{Unsaturated fatty acyl-CoA} + 2\ \text{Ferricytochrome}\ b_5 + 2\ H_2O\ (\text{Acyl-CoA}\ \Delta^9\ \text{desaturase})$$

$$\text{Stearoyl-CoA} + 2\ \text{Ferrocytochrome}\ b_5 + O_2 + 2\ H^+ \rightarrow \text{Oleoyl-CoA} + 2\ \text{Ferricytochrome}\ b_5 + 2\ H_2O\ (\text{Stearoyl-CoA desaturase})$$

$$\text{Acyl-CoA} + H_2O \rightarrow \text{Free fatty acid} + \text{CoA}\ (\text{Acyl-CoA thioesterase})$$

A nutritionally important acyl-CoA $\Delta^9$ desaturase is stearoyl-CoA desaturase (SCD), which was named for its ability to convert stearic acid into oleic acid (Koeberle et al. 2016). SCD also converts other saturated fatty acids into their MUFA counterparts. This enzyme is expressed in many tissues, but its expression varies greatly among animal species. For example, the SCD activity of the rodent liver is two orders of magnitude greater than that of the WAT. In cattle, sheep, and pigs, SCD activity is highest in the WAT, followed by skeletal muscle, intestinal mucosa, and liver in descending order (Kouba et al. 1997; Smith 2013). Indeed, SCD is nearly absent from the bovine liver (Smith 2013). In chickens, SCD activity is much higher in the liver than in the WAT. The tissue distribution of SCD provides a biochemical basis to explain differences in tissue oleic acid concentrations among different species. For example, stearic acid accounts for 12% and 25% of hepatic lipids, respectively, in mice and livestock species (cattle, sheep, and pigs). There is evidence that SCD is the only desaturase whose expression and activity in animal tissues can be substantially modified by diet (Smith 2013).

### Introduction of Double Bonds between $\Delta^9$ Carbon and $\Delta^1$ Carbon

In most animals (e.g., cattle, goats, sheep, pigs, rats, dogs, chickens, and many fish species), additional double bonds in unsaturated LCFAs can be introduced between the $\Delta^9$ carbon and the $\Delta^1$ carbon (the carboxyl group), such that the unsaturated LCFAs have double bonds at the $\Delta^4$, $\Delta^5$, and $\Delta^6$ carbon positions in addition to the double bond at the $\Delta^9$ carbon position. The double bonds at the $\Delta^4$, $\Delta^5$, and $\Delta^6$ carbon positions are formed by $\Delta^4$, $\Delta^5$, and $\Delta^6$ desaturases, respectively. Mammals, birds, Atlantic salmon, and many of other fish species (including freshwater and marine fish) possess separate genes for $\Delta^5$ (*FADS1*) and $\Delta^6$ (*FADS2*) desaturases (Nakamura and Nara 2004). In zebrafish, a bifunctional protein contains both $\Delta^5$ and $\Delta^6$ desaturase activities (Hastings et al. 2001). $\Delta^6$ desaturase catalyzes the first and rate-limiting step for the desaturation and elongation of linoleic acid ($C_{18:2}$; ω6) and α-linolenic acid ($C_{18:3}$; ω3). Thus, ω3, ω6, and ω9 PUFAs are synthesized from their respective precursors by introducing one or more double bonds between the $\Delta^9$ carbon and the $\Delta^1$ carbon, as well as chain elongation, in animal cells (Figure 6.16). There is evidence that the synthesis of PUFAs from linoleic acid and arachidonic acid in the liver and brain of young pigs is inhibited by dietary CLA in pigs, and this effect is more pronounced in the neonates fed a low-fat (3% fat) diet than those fed a high-fat (25% fat) diet (Lin et al. 2011).

In contrast to other mammals, the cat family of animals has $\Delta^5$ desaturase activity but little or no $\Delta^6$ desaturase activity in tissues (e.g., the liver), and, therefore, cannot convert (1) linoleic acid into

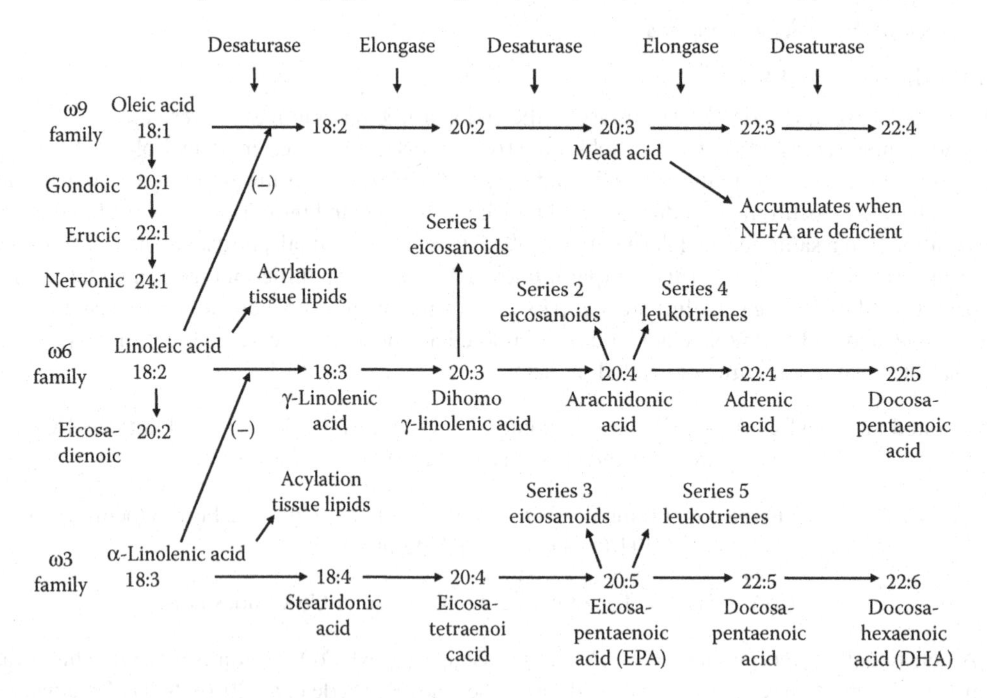


**FIGURE 6.16** Formation of eicosanoids of series 1, 2, 3, and 4, as well as leukotrienes of series 4 and 5, from polyunsaturated fatty acids (PUFAs) in animal cells.

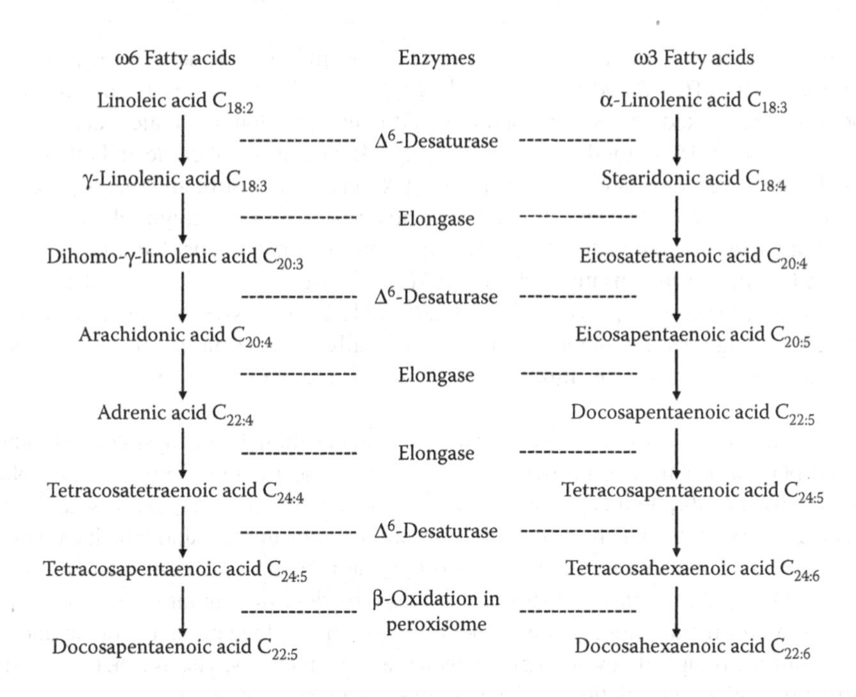


**FIGURE 6.17** Elongation of the unsaturated fatty acid chain beyond $C_{18}$ in the smooth endoplasmic reticulum. This metabolic pathway also requires the addition of acetyl-CoA as malonyl-CoA to the hydrocarbon chain, as well as NADPH. The shortening of a polyunsaturated fatty acid chain from C24 to C22 through β-oxidation in the peroxisome is also shown.

arachidonic acid and ω6 docosapentaenoic acid or (2) α-linolenic acid into EPA and DHA (Sinclair et al. 1979). Because carnivores have very limited ability to synthesize long-chain PUFAs, these animals need a supply of preformed LCFAs (e.g., $C_{20}$ and $C_{22}$ PUFAs) in diets (Rivers et al. 1975, 1976).

A separate gene for $\Delta^4$ desaturase has not been found for mammals or birds. However, in mammalian cells, $\Delta^6$ desaturase has $\Delta^4$ desaturase activity, which allows for a limited conversion of EPA into DHA (Park et al. 2015). Of interest, there is a gene for $\Delta^4$ desaturase in a lower eukaryote, *Thraustochytrium* sp. (Qiu et al. 2001) and in the herbivorous, primitive marine teleost fish (*Siganus canaliculatus*) (Li et al. 2010). Thus, most animals are capable of synthesizing (1) arachidonic acid ($C_{20:4}$ ω6) and n-6 docosapentaenoic acid ($C_{22:5}$ ω6) from linoleic acid ($C_{18:2}$ ω6); and (2) eicosapentaenoic acid (EPA, $C_{20:5}$ ω3), n-3 docosapentaenoic acid ($C_{22:5}$ ω3), and docosahexaenoic acid (DHA, $C_{22:6}$ ω3) from α-linolenic acid ($C_{18:3}$ ω3) (Figure 6.17).

### Failure of Animals to Introduce Double Bonds beyond $\Delta^9$ Carbon

All animals (including mammals, birds, and fish) lack enzymes to introduce a double bond in a saturated or unsaturated LCFA beyond the $\Delta^9$ carbon position and, therefore, cannot synthesize linoleic acid or α-linolenic acid from acetyl-CoA or palmitate. These two fatty acids are classified as nutritionally essential for animals. Polyunsaturated LCFAs, EPA, and DHA are abundant in the liver and adipose tissue of deep-sea fish, because the marine animals consume algae that contain these fatty acids. In contrast, plants and bacteria can introduce bonds at the $\Delta^6$, $\Delta^9$, $\Delta^{12}$, and $\Delta^{15}$ carbon positions and, therefore, can synthesize the nutritionally essential fatty acids.

## Differences between *Trans* Unsaturated Fatty Acids and PUFAs in Animal Nutrition

*Trans* unsaturated fatty acids are uncommon in nature but are generated mainly as a side product when vegetable oils are hydrogenated in food processing for their conversion from liquids to solids through chemical reactions. Elaidic acid ($C_{18:1}$ ω9, a *trans* isomer of oleic acid) is the principal *trans* unsaturated fatty acid often found in partially hydrogenated vegetable oils for use in margarine, snack food, packaged baked goods, and fried food. Of note, the amount of elaidic acid is negligible (accounting for only ~0.1% of total fatty acids) in the milk and meats of cattle and other ruminants (Alonso et al. 1999). Vaccenic acid is the major MUFA in ruminant milk and meats. *Trans* unsaturated fatty acids (chemically still unsaturated fatty acids) have a similar straight-chain conformation to saturated fatty acids and are metabolized more like saturated fatty acids than like the *cis* unsaturated fatty acids. Thus, *trans* unsaturated fatty acids can raise LDLs and lower HDLs in humans (Abbey and Nestel 1994). *Trans* polyunsaturated fatty acids do not possess essential fatty acid activity and can even antagonize the metabolism of nutritionally essential fatty acids and worsen their deficiencies in animals. Thus, *trans* unsaturated fatty acids are of concern in both animal nutrition and food safety.

The composition of dietary unsaturated fatty acids is of nutritional and physiological importance because (1) it plays a role in determining the fatty acid composition of membrane phospholipids, membrane fluidity, membrane receptors and enzymes, and membrane transporters; and (2) it provides ω6 and ω3 fatty acids, which are essential for normal cell function and which cannot be synthesized by the body. For example, SCD activity is present in virtually all cell types and is essential for membrane fluidity. Also, arachidonic acid and DHA are deposited in large amounts in the non-myelin membranes of the developing central nervous system. Inadequate intake of ω6 and ω3 fatty acids may impair neurological development, learning ability, memory, visual function, cardiac and skeletal structures, blood circulation, cell membrane integrity, nutrient absorption and transport, skin integrity, and immune response (Field et al. 2008; Gimenez et al. 2011). In addition, ω3 PUFAs enhance the oxidation of saturated and monounsaturated LCFAs to $CO_2$ and $H_2O$, thereby reducing the concentrations of fatty acids and TAGs in the plasma. Animal diets must contain ω3 PUFAs for optimal growth and health. A desirable ratio of ω3 to ω6 fatty acids in diets may be 2:1.

### Measurements of Fatty Acid Synthesis

The *de novo* synthesis of fatty acids in cells and tissues can be measured with the use of (1) [$^{14}$C]-labeled acetate, glucose, and AAs, which can be converted into $^{14}$C-labeled LCFAs (e.g., palmitate); or (2) $^3H_2O$, which can be incorporated into $^3$H-labeled LCFAs (Smith and Prior 1986). The labeled fatty acid product is then separated from its labeled precursor through extraction by organic solvents. The rate of fatty acid production is calculated as the amount of radioactivity in the labeled fatty acid product divided by the specific radioactivity of the labeled precursor.

### Species Differences in the Use of Substrates for *De Novo* Fatty Acid Synthesis

Substrates (e.g., glucose, lactate, pyruvate, glycerol, and AAs) that are metabolized to form acetyl-CoA can serve as precursors for fatty acid synthesis (Prior et al. 1981). However, there are species differences in this synthetic pathway (Table 6.3). For example, glucose is the major substrate for fatty acid synthesis in nonruminants. For example, 40% of absorbed glucose is used for fatty acid synthesis in 80-kg pigs. In contrast, glucose is poorly utilized for fatty acid synthesis in ruminants (Smith and Prior 1981) because of the following reasons. First, ATP-citrate lyase activity is very low in ruminant adipose tissue, as compared with nonruminant adipose tissue. Second, there is a low rate of production of pyruvate from glucose due to a low activity of hexokinase in ruminant tissues (Table 6.4). In ruminants, short-chain fatty acids are the major substrates for fatty acid synthesis. In such cases, acetate, propionate, and butyrate are first activated to form acetyl-CoA, propionyl-CoA, and butyryl-CoA in the cytosol, respectively, thus bypassing the mitochondria and the ATP-citrate lyase step. Because large amounts of propionate are produced in the rumen, there are relatively high amounts of fatty acids with an odd carbon number in ruminant plasma, tissues, and milk (Bergen and Mersmann 2005). In addition, because branched-chain fatty acids are produced from BCAAs in

**TABLE 6.3**
**Species Differences in *De Novo* Fatty Acid Synthesis in the Liver and White Adipose Tissue**

| | *De Novo* Fatty Acid Synthesis | |
|---|---|---|
| **Species** | **Liver** | **White Adipose Tissue** |
| Cat | Yes | Yes |
| Chicken | Yes | No |
| Dog | Yes | Yes |
| Human | Yes | No |
| Mouse | Yes | Yes |
| Pig | No | Yes |
| Rabbits | Yes | Yes |
| Rat (adult) | Yes | No |
| Rat (young) | Yes | Yes |
| Ruminants[a] | No | Yes |

*Source:* Jobgen, W.S. et al. 2006. *J. Nutr. Biochem.* 17:571–588.
[a] Ruminants: cattle, goats, and sheep.

**TABLE 6.4**
**Activities of Some Enzymes Involved in Lipogenesis in Bovine Subcutaneous Adipose Tissue[a]**

| **Enzyme** | **Maximal Activity (nmol/min per g Wet Weight)** |
|---|---|
| Hexokinase | 18 |
| Phosphofructosekinase-1 | 84 |
| Pyruvate kinase | 44 |
| ATP-citrate lyase | 79 |
| NADP-malate dehydrogenase | 207 |
| Pyruvate carboxylase | 42 |
| Aconitase hydratase | 49 |
| NADP-isocitrate dehydrogenase | 1976 |
| Acetyl-CoA carboxylase | 54 |

*Source:* Smith, S.B. and R.L. Prior. 1981. *Arch. Biochem. Biophys.* 211:192–201.
[a] The rate of incorporation of L-lactate at the extracellular concentration of 10 mM into fatty acids was 48 nmol/min per g wet weight.

the rumen, there are relatively large amounts of medium-chain and long-chain, branched fatty acids in ruminant plasma, tissues, and milk.

## Tissue Differences within the Same Animal in the Use of Substrates for *De Novo* Fatty Acid Synthesis

Although all tissues can synthesize fatty acids from acetyl-CoA, the major site of this metabolic pathway within the same animal is highly dependent on the tissues (Table 6.3). For example, WAT is the major site for lipid synthesis in nonlactating cattle, sheep, goats, pigs, dogs, and cats (Jobgen et al. 2006). In poultry, humans, and adult rats, the liver is the major site of *de novo* fatty acid synthesis and lipogenesis (Bergen and Mersmann 2005). In mice, rabbits, and young rats, both the liver and WAT are the major lipogenic sites. The absence of fatty acid synthesis in the WAT of adult rats is due to its lack of ACC activity. In lactating mammals, mammary glands actively synthesize fatty acids and other lipids for milk production. In response to immune activation, macrophages synthesize and release large amounts of fatty acids and their metabolites.

## Nutritional and Hormonal Regulation of Fatty Acid Synthesis

Regulation of fatty acid synthesis by nutrients and hormones (Table 6.5) involves both short-term and long-term mechanisms. The energy status of the cells, the intracellular concentration of acetyl-CoA, malonyl-CoA, and NADPH, and the activities of ACC, fatty acid synthase, and the enzymes of the pentose cycle are the important factors affecting the synthesis of saturated straight-chain fatty acid synthesis (Bauman 1976). The activity of ACC is regulated by protein phosphorylation and dephosphorylation, allosteric factors, and the abundance of the enzyme protein. $\Delta^9$ desaturase is the rate-controlling enzyme in the synthesis of MUFAs from saturated fatty acids.

### Short-Term Mechanisms

The short-term mechanisms for the regulation of fatty acid synthesis are mainly through the allosteric and covalent modification of ACC and CPT-I. Activated ACC converts acetyl-CoA into malonyl-CoA (an inhibitor of CPT-I), thereby promoting fatty acid synthesis and inhibiting fatty acid oxidation. ACC activity is inhibited by the phosphorylation of the ACC protein (catalyzed by cAMP-dependent PKA) and is stimulated by the dephosphorylation of ACC protein. Eventually, cAMP activates PKA, which phosphorylates HSL and perilipin to elicit the intracellular hydrolysis of TAGs. Therefore, factors that enhance or reduce intracellular cAMP concentration promote or suppress lipogenesis, respectively (Table 6.5).

1. *ACC.* This enzyme is inactivated by acyl-CoA (the product of fatty acid synthesis) through feedback inhibition, suggesting that an abundant provision of fatty acids reduces the conversion of acetyl-CoA into fatty acids, thereby favoring the oxidation of acetyl-CoA and, thus, fatty acids to $CO_2$ and water.
2. *Hormones.* Insulin is a major hormone regulating fatty acid synthesis in the WAT and liver through (a) the activation of ACC via protein dephosphorylation; (b) the enhanced uptake of LCFAs by hepatocytes and adipocytes through increases in the expression of fatty acid transport protein 1 (FATP1; a member of the FATP/Slc27 protein family) and blood flow. In contrast to insulin, ACC is inhibited by glucagon, epinephrine, and norepinephrine (as occurring during fasting and exercise) via cAMP-dependent phosphorylation.

   Anabolic and catabolic hormones alter intracellular cAMP concentrations through different mechanisms. For example, catecholamines bind to G-coupled β-adrenergic receptors on the plasma membrane to activate adenylate cyclase, such that cAMP is formed from ATP. Thyroid hormones bind to the nuclear thyroid hormone receptors, resulting in enhanced expression of target genes, including adenylate cyclase. Glucagon binds to receptors on the plasma membrane that are coupled to the G protein located on the cytoplasmic side of the plasma membrane. With conformational changes of the G protein, GDP in its α-subunit is replaced with GTP, causing the release of the α-subunit from the β- and γ-subunits of the G protein. This α-subunit then interacts with adenylate cyclase, resulting in the activation of the enzyme. Growth hormone binds to its plasma membrane receptor, leading to the dimerization of the receptor. Conformational changes in the growth hormone receptor cause the phosphorylation and activation of intracellular Janus kinase (a tyrosine kinase; JAK) and the latent cytoplasmic transcription factors, called signal transducer and activator of transcription (STAT) proteins, STAT1, STAT3, and STAT5. Such a series of signal transduction promotes the expression of target genes, including adenylate cyclase. Glucocorticoids

**TABLE 6.5**
**Effects of Hormones, Nutritional Status, and Other Factors on Fatty Acid Synthesis and Oxidation in Adipose Tissue (WAT), Skeletal Muscle (SKM), and Liver**

| | Fatty Acid (FA) Synthesis | | | FA Oxidation | | Net Effect in the Body | |
|---|---|---|---|---|---|---|---|
| | WAT | SKM | Liver | SKM | Liver | TAG Synthesis | TAG Deposition |
| Hormones | | | | | | | |
| Catecholamines | ↓ | ↓ | ↓ | ↑ | ↑ | ↓ | ↓ |
| Glucagon | ↓ | ↓ | ↓ | ↑ | ↑ | ↓ | ↓ |
| Glucocorticoids | | | | | | | |
| Short-term | ↑ | ↑ | ↑ | ↑ | ↑ | ↓ | ↓ |
| Long-term | ↑ | ↑ | ↑ | ↓ | ↓ | ↑ | ↑ |
| Growth hormone | ↓ | ↓ | ↓ | ↑ | ↑ | ↓ | ↓ |
| Insulin | ↑ | ↑ | ↑ | ↓ | ↓ | ↑ | ↑ |
| Parathyroid hormones | ↓ | ↓ | ↓ | ↑ | ↑ | ↓ | ↓ |
| Thyroid hormones | ↓ | ↓ | ↓ | ↑ | ↑ | ↓ | ↓ |
| Nutritional status | | | | | | | |
| Fasting (vs. feeding) | ↓ | ↓ | ↓ | ↑ | ↑ | ↓ | ↓ |
| Feeding (vs. fasting) | ↑ | ↑ | ↑ | ↑ | ↑ | ↑ | ↑ |
| High-fat diet (vs. low-fat diet) | ↓ | ↓ | ↓ | ↑ | ↑ | ↓ | ↑ |
| High-starch diet[a] | ↑ | ↑ | ↑ | ↓ | ↓ | ↑ | ↑ |
| High-protein diet[b] | ↓ | ↓ | ↓ | ↑ | ↑ | ↓ | ↓ |
| ω3-Polyunsaturated fatty acids | ↓ | ↓ | ↓ | ↑ | ↑ | ↓ | ↓ |
| Other factors | | | | | | | |
| AMP-activated protein kinase | ↓ | ↓ | ↓ | ↑ | ↑ | ↓ | ↓ |
| Exercise | ↓ | ↓ | ↓ | ↑ | ↑ | ↓ | ↓ |
| Interferon-α | ↓ | ↓ | ↓ | ↑ | ↑ | ↓ | ↓ |
| Interferon-γ | ↓ | ↓ | ↓ | ↑ | ↑ | ↓ | ↓ |
| Interferon-tau | ↓ | ↓ | ↓ | ↑ | ↑ | ↓ | ↓ |
| Interleukin-1 | ↓ | ↓ | ↓ | ↑ | ↑ | ↓ | ↓ |
| Lipopolysaccharide | ↓ | ↓ | ↓ | ↓ | ↓ | ↓ | ↓ |
| PPAR-α | – | ↓ | ↓ | ↑ | ↑ | ↓ | ↓ |
| PPAR-γ | ↑ | NC | NC | NC | NC | ↑ | ↑ |
| PPAR-δ/β | ↓ | ↓ | ↓ | ↑ | ↑ | ↓ | ↓ |
| Tumor necrosis factor-α | ↓ | ↓ | ↓ | ↑ | ↑ | ↓ | ↓ |

*Source:* Bijland, S. et al. 2013. *Clin. Sci.* 124:491–507; Donsmark, M. et al. 2004. *Proc. Nutr. Soc.* 63:309–314; Goldberg, I.J. et al. 2009. *J. Lipid Res.* 50:S86–S90; Huang, C.W. et al. 2016. *Int. J. Mol. Sci.* 17:1689; Lee, M.J. et al. 2014. *Biochim. Biophys. Acta* 1842:473–481; Macfarlane, D.P. et al. 2008. *J. Endocrinol.* 197:189–204; Minnich, A. et al. 2001. *Am. J. Physiol. Endocrinol. Metab.* 280:E270–E279; Picard, F. et al. 2002. *Clin. Vaccine Immunol.* 9:4771–4776; Tekwe, C.D. et al. 2013. *BioFactors* 39:552–563.

*Note:* ↓, decrease; ↑, increase; AMPK, AMP-activated protein kinase; NC, no change; PPAR, peroxisome proliferator-activated receptor.

[a] Compared with low-starch diet.

[b] Compared with normal-protein diet.

downregulate the expression of cyclic-nucleotide phosphodiesterase 3B (PDE3B; an enzyme that hydrolyzes cAMP to AMP), thereby elevating cellular cAMP concentration (Xu et al. 2009). In contrast, insulin brings about an opposite effect by promoting protein kinase B (PKB)-mediated phosphorylation after the binding of the hormone to its plasma membrane receptor, leading to the activation of PDE3B to break down cAMP.

The concentrations of glucagon and epinephrine in the plasma are increased during exercise and in response to "fight/flight" stress, cold stress, and high protein intake. The ratio of glucagon to insulin is higher in Type-I diabetic patients and during fasting. Growth hormone decreases fatty acid synthesis and lipogenesis in tissues by inhibiting expression of the fatty acid synthase complex and increasing the production of cAMP. Along with its effect on promoting lipolysis, growth hormone decreases fat deposition in animals. Growth hormone is among the most potent hormones for causing an increase in plasma fatty acid concentrations *in vivo* and is the only pituitary hormone to produce such an effect within 3.5 h after administration (Goodman 1968).

3. *Citrate*. This metabolite activates ACC. Cytosolic citrate concentrations are increased in the well-fed state. Thus, citrate is an indicator of a plentiful supply of acetyl-CoA from dietary glucose and AAs as energy substrates in animals. Under these nutritional conditions, enhanced fatty acid synthesis helps to store dietary energy in TAGs.
4. *Long-chain acyl-CoAs*. These derivatives of LCFAs inhibit ACC. This is a good example of metabolic feedback inhibition by a product of a reaction sequence. Long-chain acyl-CoAs also inhibit pyruvate dehydrogenase (PDH) by inhibiting the ATP–ADP exchange transporter of the inner mitochondrial membrane. Subsequently, an increase in the mitochondrial [ATP]/[ADP] ratio activates PDH kinase, converting PDH from an active form (dephosphorylated) to an inactive form (phosphorylated). This reduces the formation of acetyl-CoA from pyruvate for fatty acid synthesis.
5. $HCO_3^-$. Bicarbonate is required for ACC activity. Carbonic anhydrase converts $CO_2 + H_2O$ into $HCO_3^- + H^+$. When the availability of $HCO_3^-$ is reduced during metabolic acidosis (e.g., ketosis during lactation and pregnancy), fatty acid synthesis in animals is reduced.

### Long-Term Mechanisms

Long-term mechanisms for the regulation of fatty acid synthesis mainly involve changes in rates of synthesis and degradation of the related enzymes, as well as insulin sensitivity (Jump et al. 2013). This accompanies the normal daily cycle of feeding–fasting and, therefore, involves complex biochemical processes. Insulin is an important hormone for causing the induction of enzyme biosynthesis, but glucagon and glucocorticoids have the opposite effect. At the gene level, the expression of ACC is upregulated by sterol regulatory element-binding protein-1c (SREBP-1c). SREBP-1c is a transcription factor that upregulates the transcription of key genes in the pathways for the biosynthesis of fatty acids and cholesterol. Notably, feeding a high-starch diet stimulates SREBP-1c expression in the liver and WAT. In contrast, PUFAs inhibit SREBP-1c expression in the lipogenic tissues to reduce fatty acid synthesis by antagonizing ligand-dependent activation of the LXR: $C_{20:5}\ \omega 3 = C_{20:4}\ \omega 6 > C_{18:2}\ \omega 6 > C_{18:1}\ \omega 9$ (Jump et al. 2013).

The tissue-specific expression of ACC1 primarily in the WAT and lactating mammary gland and of ACC2 mainly in skeletal and cardiac muscles suggests that ACC1 and ACC2 play an important role in regulating the synthesis and oxidation of fatty acids in response to chronic nutritional and hormonal alterations. Finally, the expression of SCD is inhibited by fasting, diabetes, or high dietary intake of PUFAs (e.g., linoleic acid), but enhanced by insulin administration, high dietary intake of starch, saturated fatty acids, or high cholesterol (Ntambi 1999). These long-term mechanisms take several days to become fully manifested. Partly because of increased expression of the genes for fatty acid synthesis in the liver and WAT, the activity of this metabolic pathway is generally increased with age.

## Cholesterol Synthesis and Cellular Sources

### Cholesterol Synthesis from Acetyl-CoA in Liver

Ever since cholesterol was first isolated from gallstones in 1784, it has received much attention from scientists in the chemical and biomedical fields. In the livers (hepatocytes) of all mammals, birds, and fish, cholesterol is synthesized from acetyl-CoA through three phases: (1) the synthesis of isopentenyl pyrophosphate, an activated isoprene unit from acetyl-CoA; (2) the condensation of six molecules of isopentenyl pyrophosphate to form squalene; and (3) the cyclizing of squalene to form a tetracyclic product, which is subsequently converted into cholesterol (Figure 6.18). In trout and goldfish, both the liver (the major site) and the intestine are capable of *de novo* synthesis of cholesterol. However, insects and some marine invertebrates (e.g., whiteleg shrimp [also called Pacific white shrimp, *Litopenaeus vannamei*], lobsters, crabs, oysters, and crayfish) cannot synthesize

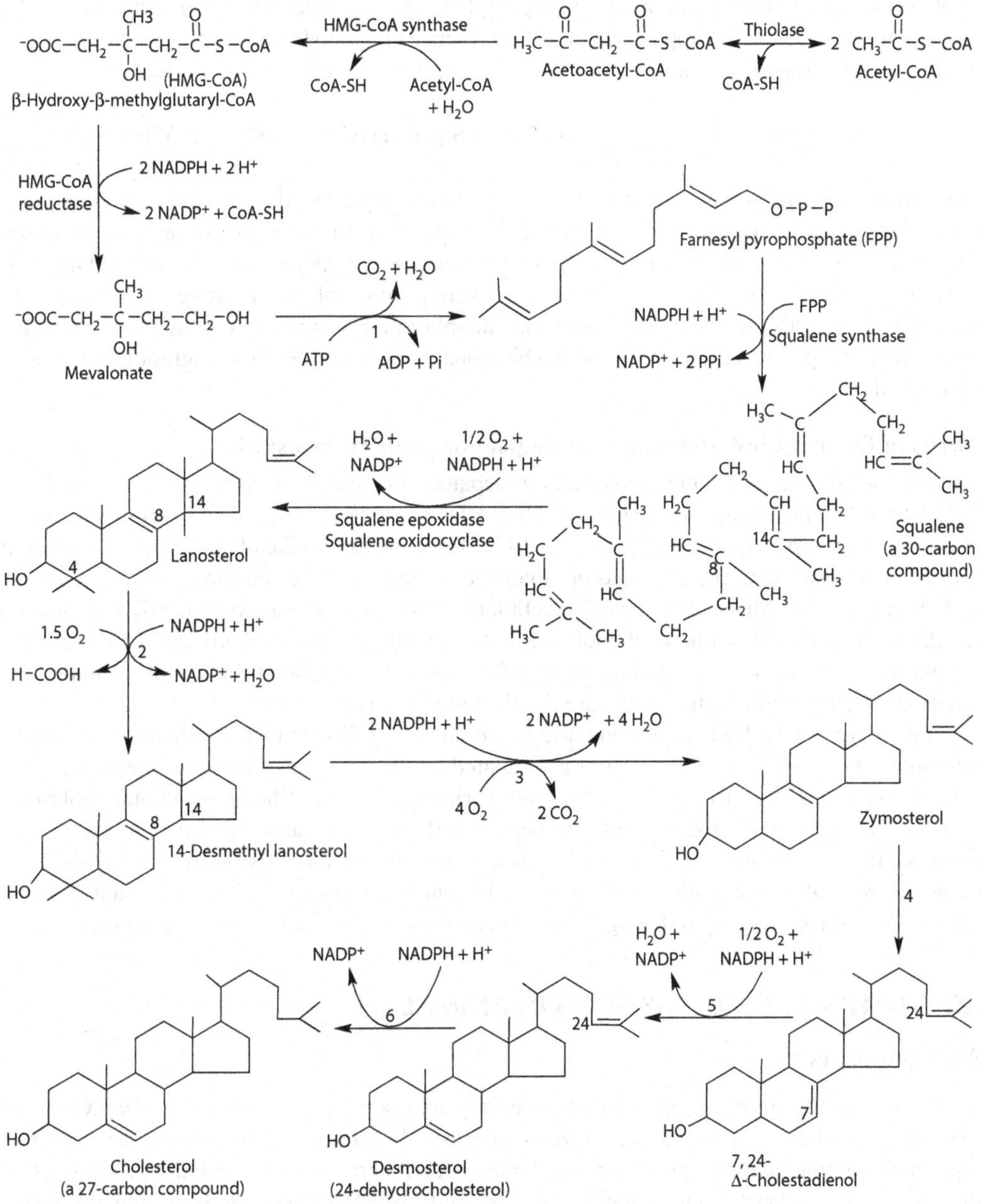

**FIGURE 6.18** Synthesis of cholesterol from acetyl-CoA in the liver of animals. This metabolic pathway occurs via three phases: (1) the synthesis of isopentenyl pyrophosphate, an activated isoprene unit from acetyl-CoA; (2) the condensation of six molecules of isopentenyl pyrophosphate to form squalene; and (3) the cyclizing of squalene to form a tetracyclic product, which is subsequently converted into cholesterol.

cholesterol or other sterols from acetate (Teshima and Kanazawa 1971); therefore, these animals must consume cholesterol from their diets for survival, growth, and development.

The first-phase reactions take place in the cytosol, where HMG-CoA synthase catalyzes the formation of HMG-CoA from acetyl-CoA and acetoacetyl-CoA, followed by the reduction of this intermediate to mevalonate by HMG-CoA reductase and the conversion of mevalonate into 3-isopentenyl pyrophosphate by three consecutive ATP-dependent reactions. The HMG-CoA reductase, which is an integral protein of the endoplasmic reticulum membrane, is a rate-controlling enzyme in cholesterol synthesis. The second-phase reactions begin in the endoplasmic reticulum, where isopentenyl pyrophosphate is isomerized to dimethylallyl pyrophosphate ($C_5$ unit). The latter condenses with a $C_{10}$ compound (isopentenyl pyrophosphate) in the presence of geranyl transferase to yield a $C_{15}$ compound (farnesyl pyrophosphate), which is reduced by squalene synthase to form squalene.

$$2 \text{ Farnesyl pyrophosphate } (C_{15}) + \text{NADPH} \rightarrow \text{Squalene } (C_{30}) + 2 \text{ PPi} + \text{NADP}^+ + \text{H}^+$$

The third-phase reactions start with the cyclization of squalene through the formation of an intermediate squalene epoxide by $O_2^-$ and NADPH-dependent squalene epoxidase, which is bound to the membrane of the endoplasmic reticulum. The squalene epoxide is then cyclized to lanosterol by oxidosqualene cyclase. Finally, lanosterol is converted into cholesterol through a series of reactions catalyzed by enzymes associated with the endoplasmic reticulum membrane: the removal of three methyl groups, the reduction of one double bond by NADPH, and the migration of the other double bond.

#### Sources of Cellular Cholesterol and the Regulation of Its Homeostasis

There are four sources of cellular cholesterol in hepatocytes: chylomicrons from the diet, extracellular LDLs from small intestine-derived VLDLs, HDLs from the intestine and peripheral tissues, and *de novo* synthesis (Goldstein and Brown 2015). Thus, dietary intake of cholesterol can directly affect its concentration in the liver and plasma. The sources of cholesterol in extrahepatic tissues are chylomicrons from diets, as well as extracellular LDLs from intestine- and liver-derived VLDLs and HDLs. Through the synthesis of cholesterol, dietary intakes of fatty acids, carbohydrates, and AAs indirectly influence the circulating levels of cholesterol in the blood. In healthy animals, concentrations of cholesterol in the plasma are tightly controlled (Puri 2011).

As noted previously, HMG-CoA synthase is the rate-controlling enzyme in hepatic cholesterol synthesis from acetyl-CoA. This pathway is regulated by the amounts of cholesterol which is present in chylomicrons and carried to the liver from peripheral tissues. When intracellular cholesterol levels are increased in hepatocytes and extrahepatic cells, the abundance of their LDL receptors is decreased, thereby reducing the uptake of extracellular LDLs by these tissues (primarily the liver) and increasing LDL concentrations in the plasma. In contrast, lovastatin and statins inhibit cytosolic HMG-CoA synthase, thereby reducing the plasma cholesterol and LDL levels in animals.

## TAG SYNTHESIS AND CATABOLISM IN ANIMALS

### TAG Synthesis in Animals

As lipid-soluble oils, high concentrations of free fatty acids are toxic to animals. While LCFAs are transported by albumin in the plasma, there is a limit to the capacity of the protein for carrying a large amount of lipid-soluble material in the bloodstream. Esterification of medium- and long-chain fatty acids derived from diets or synthesized *de novo* to form TAGs (highly reduced and anhydrous) in WAT is the main means for the transport and storage of fatty acids in the body. TAGs are a component of animal growth and are used to sustain animals during fasting (Etherton and Walton 1986). While all cell types are capable of synthesizing TAGs, the small intestine, liver, and WAT are the major sites for the occurrence of TAG synthesis in nonlactating animals. In lactating mammals, mammary glands also actively synthesize and release milk TAGs. In animals, two major pathways for TAG synthesis in the endoplasmic reticulum involve either MAG or glycerol-3-phosphate (G3P) as the initial acyl acceptor (Coleman and Mashek 2011). Both pathways use fatty acyl-CoA thioesters as donors of acyl groups, and they converge on the final acylation step (Figure 6.19). The quantitative importance of each pathway depends on specific tissues.

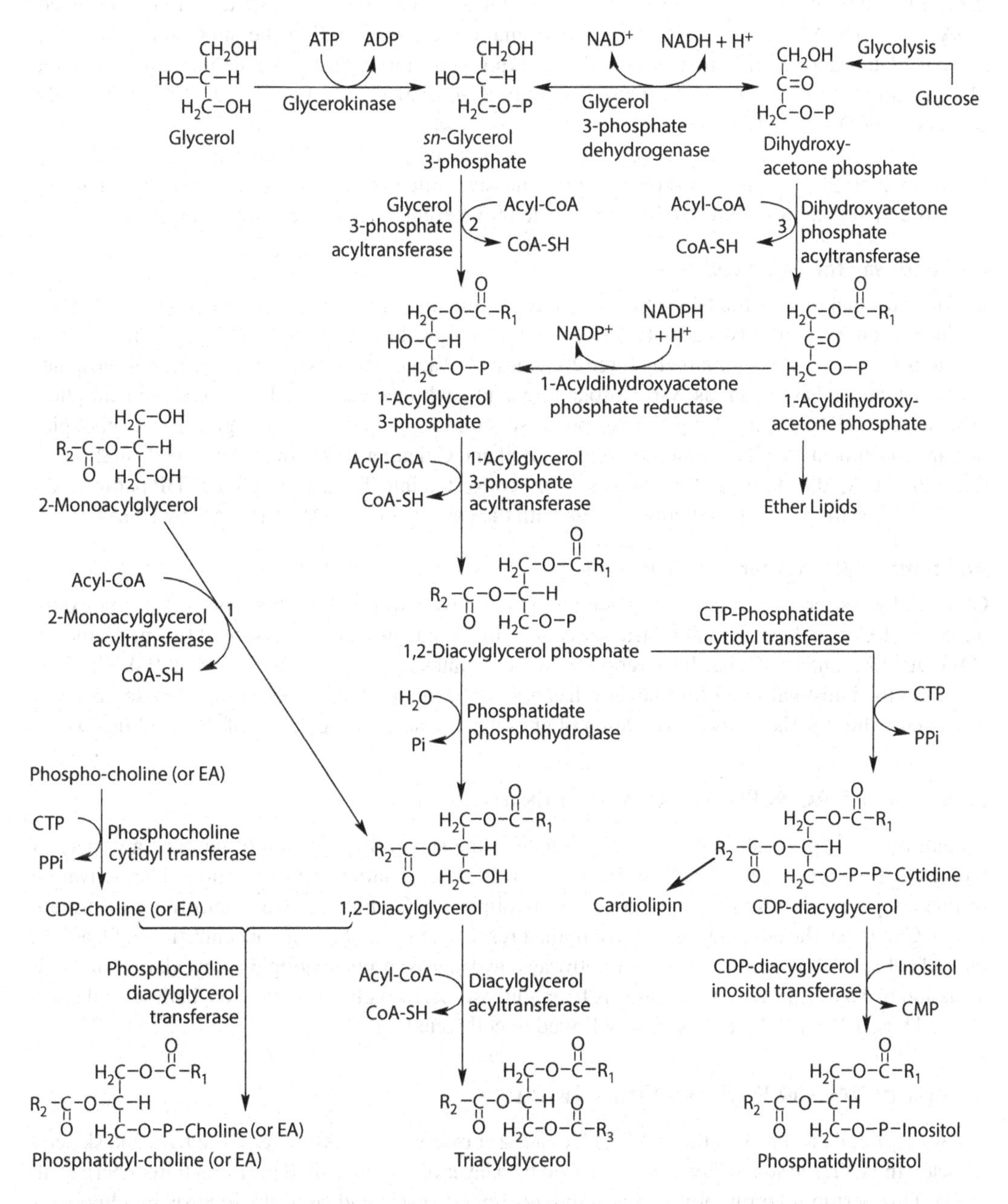


**FIGURE 6.19** Synthesis of TAGs in the endoplasmic reticulum of animal cells. TAGs are synthesized from LCFAs and glycerol via two major pathways involving either MAG or glycerol-3-phosphate (G3P) as the initial acyl acceptor. Both pathways use fatty acyl-CoA thioesters as donors of acyl groups, and they converge on the final acylation step. CDP, cytidine diphosphate; CMP, cytidine monophosphate; CTP, cytidine triphosphate; EA, ethanolamine.

### MAG Pathway for TAG Synthesis

The MAG pathway is primarily responsible for the synthesis of TAGs in enterocytes of the nonruminant small intestine, but is also present in extraintestinal tissues (Bell and Coleman 1980). Inside the cells, LCFAs are bound to FABPs at each stage of TAG synthesis (Storch and Corsico 2008). In the MAG pathway, 2-MAG and fatty acyl-CoA are covalently joined to form DAGs in a reaction catalyzed by MAG acyltransferases (MGATs). Further acylation of DAGs by DAG acyltransferase (DGAT) results in the synthesis of TAGs. Two DGATs have been identified and characterized: DGAT1 and DGAT2. DGAT1 is expressed in many tissues (including the small intestine, liver, adrenal gland, and skin), whereas DGAT2 is expressed mainly in the small intestine and liver. MGAT2 and MGAT3 also exhibit DGAT activity (Cao et al. 2007). Finally, DGAT catalyzes the conversion of DAGs to TAGs. In the postprandial state when fatty acids and MAGs are taken up by the enterocytes, the MAG pathway accounts for more than 75% of TAG synthesis in the small intestine (Yen et al. 2015). Through processing the massive influx of substrates after a lipid-containing meal, the MAG pathway plays an important role in the efficient absorption of dietary fats.

### G3P Pathway for TAG Synthesis

In extraintestinal tissues, the biosynthesis of TAG occurs through the G3P pathway, in which DAG is produced from G3P after two acylation steps and the removal of the phosphate group. This series of reactions is catalyzed sequentially by three enzymes: G3P acyltransferase, 1-acylglycerol-3-phosphate acyltransferase (also known as lysophosphatidic acid acyltransferase), and phosphatidic acid phosphatase. The G3P pathway also generates precursors for the synthesis of major glycerophospholipids that are constituents of all cellular membranes (Bell and Coleman 1980). In the ruminant small intestine with few MAGs, fatty acids and glycerol are converted into TAGs through the G3P pathway. As in the MAG pathway, the G3P pathway ends with the conversion of DAG into TAG by DGAT.

### Additional Pathways for TAG Synthesis

Other pathways for TAG synthesis, which are quantitatively minor, have been proposed. For example, an acyl-CoA-independent DAG transacylase, which catalyzes the conversion of two molecules of DAG into TAG and MAG, has been reported in the rat intestine (Lehner and Kuksis 1993). The gene encoding the intestinal DAG transacylase has not yet been identified. The synthesis of some TAGs also occurs through the dephosphorylation of phosphatidic acid and acylation of the resulting DAGs.

## Function of DAG in Protein Kinase C Signaling

Protein kinase C plays an important role in membrane signal transduction to mediate a variety of biological functions, such as cell proliferation, cell differentiation, and secretion. The activation of this enzyme requires $Ca^{2+}$ and acidic phospholipid. DAG enhances $Ca^{2+}$-sensitivity of protein kinase C to make the enzyme fully active in the presence of physiological concentrations of $Ca^{2+}$. In animal cells, DAG is produced by four pathways: hydrolysis of phospholipids, deacylation of TAG, acylation of MAG, and *de novo* synthesis from glucose-derived glycerol via phosphatidic acid (Puri 2011). Thus, TAG metabolism is closely linked to cell signaling.

## Storage of TAGs in WAT and Other Tissues

TAGs are stored primarily in the WAT and, to a lesser extent, other tissues (e.g., the liver and skeletal muscle). In WAT, the stored TAGs are enclosed by a layer of protein called perilipin (Greenberg et al. 1991). This perilipin family of proteins stabilizes lipid droplets and controls lipolysis in adipocytes (Brasaemle 2007). Phosphorylation of perilipin by cAMP-dependent protein kinase is essential for the mobilization of fats from the WAT. In the fatty liver, excess TAGs result in its multiple metabolic dysfunctions. Although an appropriate amount of TAGs between muscle fibers (called intramuscular fats) can enhance meat taste, excess amounts of intermuscular fats reduce meat quality and value.

## MOBILIZATION OF TAGS FROM TISSUES TO RELEASE GLYCEROL AND FATTY ACIDS

### INTRACELLULAR LIPOLYSIS BY HSL IN ANIMAL TISSUES

#### Tissue Distribution and Function of HSL

When animals have a need for energy beyond that provided from the diet, intracellular TAGs (particularly in skeletal muscle) are hydrolyzed by lipases to yield fatty acids and glycerol (Figure 6.20). This process is called intracellular lipolysis. HSL is the major enzyme to hydrolyze the first fatty acid from TAG, yielding a fatty acid and DAG. The name HSL was coined to indicate the potent effect of certain hormones (e.g., catecholamines, glucagon, growth hormone, and testosterone) on stimulating HSL activity. As an intracellular neutral lipase, HSL is capable of hydrolyzing not only TAGs, but also DAGs and MAGs, as well as cholesteryl and retinyl esters (Kraemer and Shen 2002). Thus, HSL has broad substrate specificity. Of note, the hydrolytic activity of HSL against DAGs and MAGs is not affected by protein phosphorylation (Yeaman 1990). This feature of HSL differentiates it from other lipases (e.g., LPL and hepatic lipase). The hydrolysis of TAGs in white adipocytes is shown as follows:

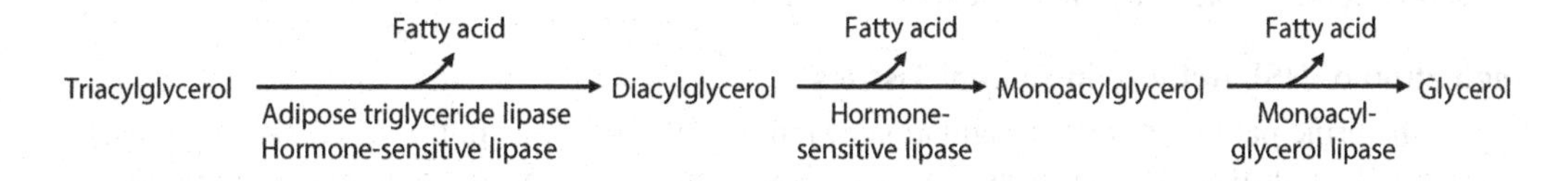


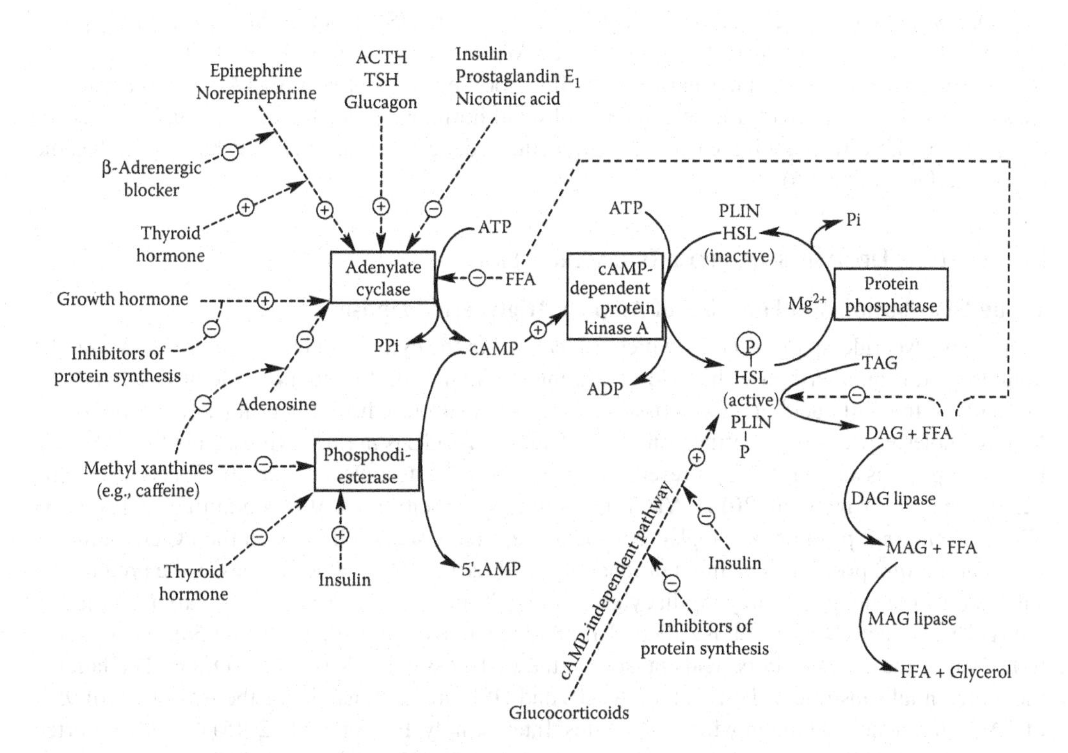


**FIGURE 6.20** Mobilization of TAGs from tissues through cAMP-dependent phosphorylation of hormone-sensitive lipase (HSL) and perilipin (PLIN) to release glycerol and fatty acids. In tissues (e.g., skeletal muscle and WAT) that do not have glycerol kinase activity, glycerol is not re-used locally for TAG synthesis. ACTH, adrenocorticotropic hormone; DAG, diacylglycerol; FFA, free fatty acids; MAG, monoacylglycerol; TAG, triacylglycerol; TSH, thyroid-stimulating hormone.

Glycerol from TAG hydrolysis is utilized to generate either TAGs through the action of glycerol kinase in tissues other than WAT and muscle, or glucose in the liver and kidneys (Doreau and Chilliard 1997). Depending on nutritional and physiological conditions, the metabolic fate of fatty acids is either mitochondrial oxidation to produce $CO_2$, water, and ATP production or hepatic ketogenesis to generate acetoacetate and β-hydroxybutyrate.

$$\text{Glycerol} \xrightarrow[\text{Glycerol kinase}]{\text{ATP} \rightarrow \text{ADP}} \text{Glycerol-3-phosphate} \xrightarrow[\text{Glycerol-3-P dehydrogenase}]{\text{NAD}^+ \rightarrow \text{NADH} + \text{H}^+} \text{Dihydroxyacetone 3-phosphate}$$

HSL is highly expressed in the WAT and steroidogenic tissues and, to a lesser extent, is found in a variety of other tissues and cell types, including the heart, skeletal muscle, kidneys, pancreatic islets, testes, ovaries, and macrophages. In contrast, HSL is normally expressed at a very low level in hepatocytes, but its hepatic expression is upregulated by the activation of PPARγ (Reid et al. 2008). Under physiological conditions, HSL plays a key role in regulating lipolysis primarily in adipocytes and also contributes to steroidogenesis and spermatogenesis, as well as possibly insulin secretion and action in the whole body (Kraemer and Shen 2002).

### Regulation of HSL Activity in Animal Tissues

HSL is the principal target for the regulation of intracellular lipolysis in the WAT, skeletal muscle, and heart (Lee et al. 2014). This enzyme is regulated by both short-term (minutes to hours) and long-term (days to weeks) mechanisms. The short-term regulation involves the phosphorylation of proteins, particularly the cAMP-dependent PKA to convert HSL from an inactive form (dephosphorylated) into an active form (phosphorylated). Without activation by PKA, HSL is inactive in tissues. PKA also phosphorylates perilipin to allow for the access of HSL to TAGs for their hydrolysis. Catecholamines, thyroid hormones, parathyroid hormone, growth hormone, and glucocorticoids activate HSL through increasing the intracellular concentration of cAMP, but insulin has the opposite effect (Table 6.5).

## Intracellular Lipolysis by Adipose Triglyceride Lipase

### Tissue Distribution and Function of Adipose Triglyceride Lipase

Adipose triglyceride lipase (ATGL), which is localized in the cytosol and tightly associated with the lipid droplet, is another lipase that hydrolyzes intracellular TAG to one molecule of DAG and one molecule of free fatty acid in animal tissues. This TAG hydrolase has little or no activity for DAGs, MAGs, cholesteryl esters, or retinyl esters as substrates. ATGL is mainly expressed in the WAT and brown adipose tissue, but is also present at low levels in the testicles, pancreatic islets, heart, and skeletal muscle (Nagy et al. 2014). ATGL has strong specificity for TAGs containing LCFA esters ($C_{16-20}$) in the *sn*-2 position of the glycerol backbone. Likewise, ATGL acts on the PC containing a PUFA at the *sn*-2 position. The main product of ATGL is 1,3-DAG, which serves as the preferential substrate of the lipogenic enzyme diacylglycerol acyltransferase 2. Interestingly, after binding to the ATGL's co-activator, which is called CGI-58 (comparative gene identification 58), ATGL starts to hydrolyze the esters of fatty acids present in the *sn*-1 position, releasing 2,3-DAGs. The latter is the preferential substrate of HSL. Thus, ATGL and HSL are responsible for the hydrolysis of 95% of TAGs in rodent and human white adipocytes. Interestingly, Fowler et al. (2015) recently reported that ATGL, not HSL, is the primary lipolytic enzyme in the WAT of fasting elephant seals.

### Regulation of ATGL Activity

ATGL is activated by CGI-58, as noted previously. The role of CGI-58 is epitomized by the findings that its genetic deficiency causes Chanarin–Dorfman syndrome, a rare neutral lipid-storage disease which is characterized by an abnormal accumulation of TAG in nonlipid-storing cell types (e.g., skeletal muscle, heart, and skin), as well as skeletal myopathy and exercise intolerance. The enzymatic activity of ATGL is inhibited by insulin and long-chain fatty acyl-CoA but enhanced by glucocorticoids (Nagy et al. 2014; Perret et al. 2002). ATGL gene expression and protein abundance in the WAT are enhanced by fasting and downregulated by refeeding. Furthermore, ATGL expression is reduced in animal models (mice and rats) of obesity and Type-II diabetes mellitus.

## Intracellular Lipolysis by Diacylglyceol Lipase and Monoacylglycerol Lipase in Animal Tissues

### Functions of Diacylglyceol Lipase and Monoacylglycerol Lipase

While HSL can hydrolyze DAGs and MAGs, these esters of fatty acids are degraded by diacylglyceol lipase (DGL) and monoacylglycerol lipase (MGL), respectively, in a tissue-dependent manner. In adipocytes which express little DGL, HSL is the only enzyme catalyzing DAG hydrolysis to form MAG and fatty acid, and the rate of this reaction is 10- to 30-fold greater than that of TAG hydrolysis. In other cell types, DAG is degraded by both HSL and DGL to release one molecule of MAG plus one molecule of free fatty acid. For example, in the brain, DGL degrades the DAG containing arachidonic acid at the *sn*-2 position to generate one molecule of fatty acid and one molecule of 2-arachidonoylglycerol. The latter is the most abundant ligand for the cannabinoid receptors in the brain to regulate axonal growth and development, as well as the generation and migration of new neurons. 2-Arachidonoylglycerol is also a precursor of arachidonic acid in tissues.

MGL was first isolated from rat adipose tissue and is now known to be present in all other tissues, including the liver, skeletal muscle, heart, brain, lung, stomach, kidney, spleen, adrenal gland, and testes. This enzyme specifically hydrolyzes the *sn*-1 and *sn*-2 ester bonds of MAGs at equal rates but has no catalytic activity against DAGs, TAGs, or cholesteryl esters. In tissues (e.g., the brain), MGL is responsible for the hydrolysis of 85% of endocannabinoid 2-arachidonoylglycerol. Such a biochemical reaction regulates the concentration of endogenous cannabinoids (endocannabinoids), which are lipid molecules for mediating retrograde signaling at central synapses and other forms of short-range neuronal communication. The activities of DGL and MGL for hydrolyzing their respective substrates (DAGs and MAGs) are 10–30 times greater than the activities of HSL for TAGs, DAGs, and MAGs in the WAT and other tissues (Yang and Subbaiah 2015).

### Regulation of DGL and MGL Activities

DGL is constitutively active, and its enzymatic activity has been reported to be increased by cAMP-dependent protein phosphorylation and palmitoylation in animal tissues (Reisenberg et al. 2012). Palmitoylation, which involves the covalent linkage of a LCFA to a cysteine residue in a protein, can enhance the hydrophobicity of the enzyme, association with the membrane, protein–protein interaction, sub-cellular trafficking, and substrate access. Available evidence shows that MGL activity is not regulated by protein phosphorylation, but the expression of the MGL gene in the WAT and other tissues is enhanced by glucocorticoids and PPAR-$\alpha$.

## Intracellular Lipolysis by Lysosomal Acid Lipase (LAL)

LAL is present in the lysosomes of hepatocytes and nonhepatic tissues. This enzyme can hydrolyze intracellular TAGs and cholesteryl esters at an acidic pH and, therefore, is an acidic lipase. LAL is the only lipase that catalyzes intracellular degradation of TAGs in the liver and is the primary enzyme that hydrolyzes cholesteryl esters derived from LDLs (Dubland and Francis 2015). The resulting cholesterol leaves the lysosome to enter the endoplasmic reticulum for re-esterification and formation of cytosolic lipid droplets. A deficiency of LAL results in the accumulation of fats in various tissues, such as the liver, small intestine, spleen, adrenal glands, lymph nodes, and the walls of blood vessels. Affected individuals, particularly neonates, exhibit digestive disorders and malabsorption, liver dysfunction or failure, and coronary artery disease.

## OXIDATION OF FATTY ACIDS IN ANIMALS

### Metabolic Fate of Fatty Acids: $CO_2$ Production and Ketogenesis

All animals can readily oxidize fatty acids to $CO_2$ and water in fed and fasting states. However, not all animals have a high rate of oxidizing fatty acids to ketone bodies (acetoacetate, β-hydroxybutyrate, and acetone), even during a prolonged period of food deprivation. Acetoacetate and β-hydroxybutyrate fulfill physiological functions as metabolic fuels and signals, but acetone is a metabolic waste with an unpleasant odor (Robinson and Williamson 1980). The formation of ketone bodies from acetyl-CoA is known as ketogenesis. In the mitochondria of the liver, whether acetyl-CoA produced from the β-oxidation of LCFAs is oxidized to $CO_2$ or ketone bodies depends on intracellular concentrations of OAA and malonyl-CoA, CPT-I activity, and HMG-CoA synthase activity. An increase in the hepatic oxidation of fatty acids does not necessarily enhance the production of both $CO_2$ and ketone bodies from the substrates in the liver. For example, in the liver of rats fed a fat-containing diet, the oxidation of fatty acids to $CO_2$ and water is augmented but ketogenesis is suppressed, such that the concentrations of acetoacetate and β-hydroxybutyrate are relatively low (<0.2 mM). In contrast, food deprivation results in increased oxidation of fatty acids to $CO_2$ and the formation of ketone bodies in the liver of most animals (including rats and ruminants). Furthermore, consumption of a balanced diet containing adequate digestible carbohydrates suppresses ketogenesis, while promoting the oxidation of fatty acids to $CO_2$ and water. These lines of evidence show the complex mechanisms responsible for the regulation of fatty acid oxidation to form $CO_2$ or ketone bodies.

### Mitochondrial β-Oxidation of Fatty Acids to $CO_2$ and Water

Under normal feeding and fasting conditions, fatty acids are a major source of energy for many tissues, including the liver, heart, and skeletal muscle. An increase in fatty acid oxidation to generate $CO_2$ and water occurs when dietary fat intake is increased. Thus, dietary supplementation with fats can improve lactation performance in sows under the conditions of high ambient temperatures (Rosero et al. 2012). During fasting, increased β-oxidation of fatty acids provides acetyl-CoA for the synthesis of large amounts of ketone bodies in most animal species. The ketone bodies serve as important metabolic fuels for the brain, heart, skeletal muscle, intestine, and kidneys when food intake is absent or severely inadequate. Thus, fatty acid β-oxidation occurs under conditions of both food deprivation and regular feeding.

Fatty acids with $<C_{20}$ (e.g., short-, medium-, and long-chain fatty acids) are β-oxidized to $CO_2$ and water in the mitochondria. This pathway occurs in animal cells with mitochondria. Long-chain and very-long-chain fatty acids ($\geq C_{20}$) are β-oxidized in peroxisomes and the smooth endoplasmic reticulum to generate shorter-chain fatty acids (e.g., $C_{16}$ or $C_{18}$), which are then β-oxidized in the mitochondria. On the basis of tissue mass and the rate of fatty acid β-oxidation, the liver, heart, skeletal muscle, and kidneys are the major tissues of fatty acid oxidation in animals. In the liver, this metabolic pathway occurs primarily in periportal hepatocytes, as does ketogenesis.

#### Pathway of Mitochondrial β-Oxidation of Fatty Acids

Early in the twentieth century, Knoop (1904) fed rats with fatty acid (even carbon number) derivatives with a phenyl group attached to the ω carbon and found that phenylacetic acid was a final product of the oxidation process. However, when fatty acid (odd carbon number) derivatives with a phenyl group attached to the ω carbon were fed to rats, benzoic acid was a final product of the oxidation process. Fifty years later, Lynen and Reichert (1951) discovered that the two-carbon fragment from β-oxidation was acetyl-CoA, but not acetate.

$$C_6H_5\text{-}CH_2(CH_2)_{16}COOH \xrightarrow[\text{Rat}]{O_2} C_6H_5\text{-}CH_2\text{-}COOH + 8\,CH_3\text{-}COOH$$

Fatty acid with even carbon number — Phenylaceticacid — Acetic acid

$$C_6H_5\text{-}CH_2(CH_2)_{15}COOH \xrightarrow[\text{Rat}]{O_2} C_6H_5\text{-}COOH + 8\,CH_3\text{-}COOH$$

Fatty acid with odd carbon number — Benzoic acid — Acetic acid

It is now known that fatty acids are oxidized in the mitochondria, which facilitates the oxidation of its product, acetyl-CoA, via the Krebs cycle and the electron transport system. The major pathway of fatty acid oxidation is β-oxidation, in which two carbons are cleaved at a time from acyl-CoA. This cleavage of $C_2$ units starts at the carboxyl end, with the chain being broken down between the α ($C_2$) and β ($C_3$) carbon atoms, hence the name of β-oxidation. The pathway of mitochondrial fatty acid β-oxidation includes the activation of a fatty acid to acyl-CoA, the transfer of acyl-CoA from the cytosol into the mitochondrial matrix, and the β-oxidation of acyl-CoA to form acetyl-CoA (Bartlett and Eaton 2004).

### *Activation of a Fatty Acid to Acyl-CoA*

The first step in fatty acid oxidation is the conversion of a fatty acid into acyl-CoA by acyl-CoA synthase (ACS, also called thiokinase). Activation of LCFAs to acyl-CoA by ACS for LCFAs ($ACS_L$) occurs on either the outer mitochondrial membrane or the surface of the endoplasmic reticulum. This is an ATP-dependent reaction, with two high-energy bonds in one ATP molecule being hydrolyzed to provide energy. The amount of energy needed by ACS is equivalent to the conversion of 2 ATP into 2 ADP + 2 Pi. The long-chain acyl-CoA formed in the cytosol will enter the mitochondrial matrix for β-oxidation to yield acetyl-CoA.

$$\text{Long-chain fatty acid} + \text{ATP} + \text{CoA} \rightarrow \text{Long-chain acyl-CoA} + \text{AMP} + \text{PPi}$$
$$(\text{ACS}_\text{L} \text{ in the cytosol})$$

Short- and medium-chain fatty acids are transported from the cytosol into the mitochondria, where these fatty acids are activated to form thiol ester bonds with CoA by mitochondrial ACSs for short- and medium-chain fatty acids, respectively (i.e., $ACS_S$ and $ACS_M$). For example, acetate and butyrate are converted by ACS to form acetyl-CoA and butyryl-CoA, respectively. Through the mitochondrial β-oxidation, 1 mol butyryl-CoA is cleaved into 2 mol acetyl-CoA, with the generation of 1 mol $FADH_2$ and 1 mol NADH.

$$\text{Short-chain fatty acid} + \text{ATP} + \text{CoA} \rightarrow \text{Short-chain acyl-CoA} + \text{AMP} + \text{PPi}$$
$$(\text{ACS}_\text{S} \text{ in mitochondria})$$

$$\text{Medium-chain fatty acid} + \text{ATP} + \text{CoA} \rightarrow \text{Medium-chain acyl-CoA} + \text{AMP} + \text{PPi}$$
$$(\text{ACS}_\text{M} \text{ in mitochondria})$$

### *Transfer of Long-Chain Acyl-CoA from the Cytosol into the Mitochondrial Matrix*

The second step in LCFA oxidation is the transfer of long-chain acyl-CoA as acylcarnitine from the outer mitochondrial membrane into the mitochondrial matrix. This process involves carnitine palmitoyltransferase I (CPT-I, in the outer membrane of mitochondria), carnitine palmitoyltransferase II (CPT-II, on the inside of the inner membrane of mitochondria), and carnitine-acylcarnitine translocase (Figure 6.21). Carnitine is synthesized from lysine and methionine in the liver and kidneys. Without carnitine, LCFAs and long-chain acyl-CoA cannot enter the mitochondria. However, short- and medium-chain fatty acids can penetrate mitochondria without the need for carnitine. CPT-I represents the main site of control for the entry of LCFAs into the mitochondria. CPT-I is the rate-controlling step of the CPT system and of liver fatty acid oxidation. In rats and pigs, the

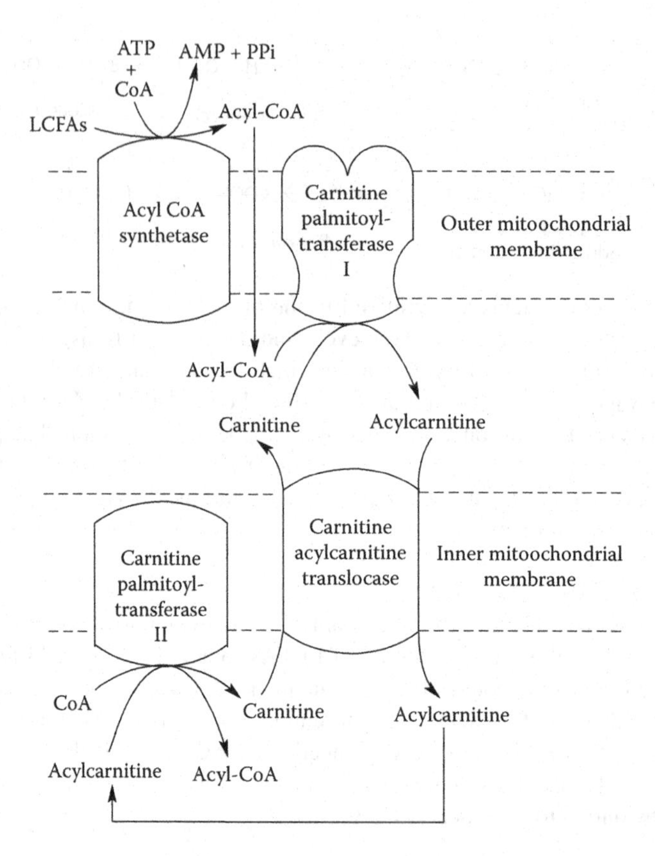


**FIGURE 6.21** Transport of long-chain acyl-CoA from the cytosol into the mitochondrial matrix. This process requires carnitine palmitoyltransferase I (CPT-I, in the outer membrane of mitochondria), carnitine palmitoyltransferase II (CPT-II, on the inside of the inner membrane of mitochondria), and carnitine-acylcarnitine translocase. LCFAs, long-chain fatty acids. (Adapted from Mayes, P.A. 1996b. *Harper's Biochemistry*. Edited by R.K. Murray, D.K. Granner, and V.W. Rodwell. Appleton & Lange, Stamford, CT, pp. 224–235.)

expression of CPT-I in the liver and extrahepatic tissues (e.g., skeletal muscle) is low at birth but is increased rapidly after birth. In contrast, the expression of CPT-II in the tissues is high during the fetal stage and does not seem to undergo a postnatal change.

The mammalian CPT-1 subfamily of proteins consists of three members: CPT-1A, 1B, and 1C (Price et al. 2003). CPT-1C is restricted to the central neural tissues and its function is unknown. CPT-1A (also known as the liver isoform) is expressed in the liver, kidney, pancreatic islets, and intestine, whereas CPT-1B (also known as the muscle isoform) is present at high activity in the heart, skeletal muscle, testes, and brown adipocytes (Brown et al. 1997). Compared with the muscle type of CPT-I, the liver isoform of CPT-I has a lower $K_m$ for carnitine and is less sensitive, but still highly sensitive, to inhibition by malonyl-CoA.

### *β-Oxidation of Acyl-CoA to Form Acetyl-CoA*

The third step in fatty acid oxidation is the β-oxidation of acyl-CoA ($C_{4-19}$) to form acetyl-CoA (Figure 6.22). This involves four reactions catalyzed by acyl-CoA dehydrogenase (FAD-linked), enoyl-CoA hydratase, 3-hydroxyacyl-CoA dehydrogenase ($NAD^+$-linked), and 3-ketoacyl-CoA thiolase. In animals, the activities of enoyl-CoA hydratase, 3-hydroxyacyl-CoA dehydrogenase, and 3-ketoacyl-CoA thiolase are contained in the same protein, which is called the mitochondrial trifunctional protein. For the cleavage of 1 $C_2$ unit to form 1 mol of acetyl-CoA, 1 mol of NADH and 1 mol of $FADH_2$ are produced. The overall reaction of β-oxidation of palmitate is as follows:

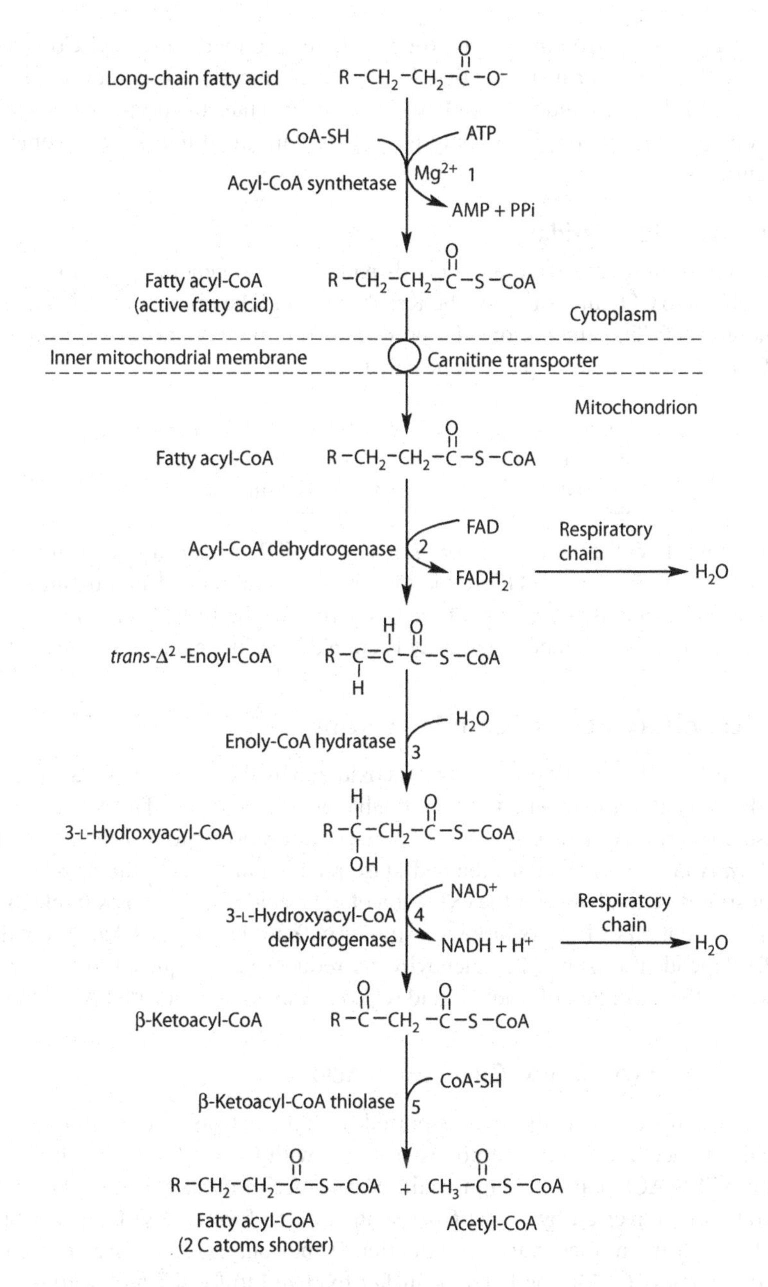


**FIGURE 6.22** The β-oxidation of long-chain acyl-CoA to form acetyl-CoA in the mitochondria of animal cells. In the cytosol, acyl-CoA synthetase converts a long-chain fatty acid into acyl-CoA, which is transported into the mitochondrial matrix through a carnitine-dependent transport system. During each cycle of the acyl-CoA oxidation, a 2-carbon unit (acetyl-CoA), 1 $FADH_2$, and 1 NADH + $H^+$ are generated. This biochemical process is called β-oxidation.

$$\text{Palmitate} + 8\ \text{CoA} + \text{ATP} + 7\ \text{FAD} + 7\ \text{NAD}^+ \rightarrow 8\ \text{Acetyl-CoA} + \text{AMP} + \text{PPi} + 7\ \text{FADH}_2 + 7\ \text{NADH} + 7\text{H}^+$$

Fatty acids with an odd carbon number are oxidized in a manner similar to that of those with an even carbon number, until the three-carbon molecule, propionyl-CoA, is generated. This product is further degraded via a series of three enzymes, the ATP-dependent propionyl-CoA carboxylase (using biotin as a cofactor), methylmalonyl-CoA racemase, and methylmalonyl-CoA mutase (using vitamin $B_{12}$ as a cofactor) to form succinyl-CoA. The latter enters the Krebs cycle for oxidation in various tissues or is utilized for glucose synthesis in the liver. Thus, the propionyl residue from fatty acids with an odd carbon number is the only part of the fatty acid that is glucogenic in animals, particularly ruminants.

### Energetics of Fatty Acid β-Oxidation

The major function of mitochondrial fatty acid β-oxidation is to generate acetyl-CoA. The acetyl-CoA is then oxidized to $CO_2$ and water via the Krebs cycle and the mitochondrial electron transport system, producing ATP. The amount of ATP produced from the complete oxidation of fatty acids (e.g., 1 mol of palmitate as an example) can be calculated as follows:

| | | |
|---|---|---|
| 7 $FADH_2$ | → | 10.5 ATP ($7 \times 1.5 = 10.5$) |
| 7 NADH + $H^+$ | → | 17.5 ATP ($7 \times 2.5 = 17.5$) |
| 8 Acetyl-CoA | → | 80 ATP ($8 \times 10 = 80$) |

The total amount of ATP produced is 108. Because 2 ATP are consumed during the activation of palmitate to palmityl-CoA, net ATP production for the oxidation of 1 mol palmitate is 106 mol. The oxidation of fatty acids is the major source of energy for the liver, heart, skeletal muscle, and kidneys. In hepatocytes, this metabolic pathway is coupled to gluconeogenesis during fasting.

## Oxidation of Long-Chain Unsaturated Fatty Acids

A MUFA (i.e., a fatty acid with one double bond) is oxidized by the same set of reactions as saturated fatty acids with even carbon numbers, until the double bond is reached. The enzyme *cis*-$\Delta^3$-enoyl-CoA isomerase converts the double bond in the *cis* configuration into a *trans* configuration. The newly formed *trans* fatty acid bypasses the hydratase reaction and enters the β-oxidation pathway. Figure 6.23 illustrates the pathway for the oxidation of oleic acid ($C_{18:1}$) as an example for MUFAs to acetyl-CoA. The oxidation of PUFAs follows a similar path to that of MUFAs, except that an additional NADPH-dependent enzyme, 2,4-dienoyl-CoA reductase, is required to reduce one double bond, as shown for the oxidation of linoleic acid ($C_{18:2}$) as an example for PUFAs in Figure 6.24.

## Oxidation of Short- and Medium-Chain Fatty Acids

Short- and medium-chain fatty acids are transported from the cytosol into the mitochondria, where these fatty acids are activated to form thiol ester bonds with CoA by mitochondrial ACSs. There are short-chain ACSs ($ACS_S$) and medium-chain ACSs ($ACS_M$) in animal cells. For example, acetate and butyrate are converted by acetyl-CoA synthetase to form acetyl-CoA and butyryl-CoA, respectively. Through the mitochondrial β-oxidation, 1 mol butyryl-CoA is converted into acetoacetyl-CoA (a β-ketoacyl-CoA). The latter is further oxidized to form 2 mol acetyl-CoA, with the generation of 1 mol $FADH_2$ and 1 mol NADH. Alternatively, butyrate can be metabolized to D-β-hydroxybutyrate via the formation of acetoacetyl-CoA and then of HMG-CoA (by HMG-CoA synthase), as described in the following section on ketogenesis.

Short-chain fatty acid + ATP + CoA → Short-chain acyl-CoA + AMP + PPi
($ASC_S$ in mitochondria)

Medium-chain fatty acid + ATP + CoA → Medium-chain acyl-CoA + AMP + PPi
($ASC_M$ in mitochondria)

Propionate is converted into succinyl-CoA via a series of enzymes, as described in Chapter 5. Succinyl-CoA is metabolized to pyruvate through the following reactions. Depending on physiological

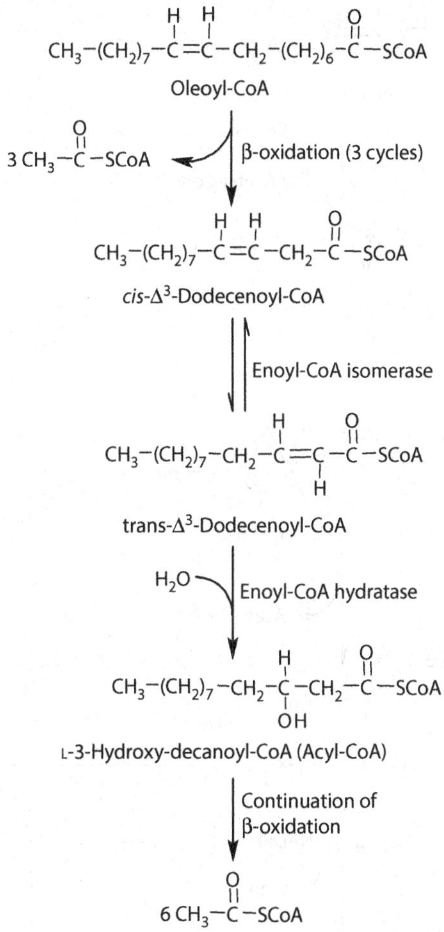

$CH_3-(CH_2)_7-CH=CH-CH_2-(CH_2)_6-C(=O)-SCoA$

Oleoyl-CoA

↓ β-oxidation (3 cycles) → $3\ CH_3-C(=O)-SCoA$

$CH_3-(CH_2)_7-CH=CH-CH_2-C(=O)-SCoA$

*cis*-$\Delta^3$-Dodecenoyl-CoA

⇅ Enoyl-CoA isomerase

$CH_3-(CH_2)_7-CH_2-CH=CH-C(=O)-SCoA$

trans-$\Delta^3$-Dodecenoyl-CoA

↓ $H_2O$, Enoyl-CoA hydratase

$CH_3-(CH_2)_7-CH_2-CH(OH)-CH_2-C(=O)-SCoA$

L-3-Hydroxy-decanoyl-CoA (Acyl-CoA)

↓ Continuation of β-oxidation

$6\ CH_3-C(=O)-SCoA$

**FIGURE 6.23** Oxidation of oleic acid ($C_{18:1}$) as an example for monounsaturated fatty acids to generate acetyl-CoA in the mitochondria of animal cells. Enoyl-CoA isomerase (a mitochondrial enzyme) catalyzes the conversion of a *cis* or *trans* double bond of a fatty acid at the γ-carbon (position 3) to a *trans* double bond at the β-carbon (position 2).

conditions, pyruvate is either oxidized to $CO_2$ plus $H_2O$ or is used for hepatic glucose production (Chapter 5). Under physiological conditions, propionate is the major substrate for gluconeogenesis in ruminants.

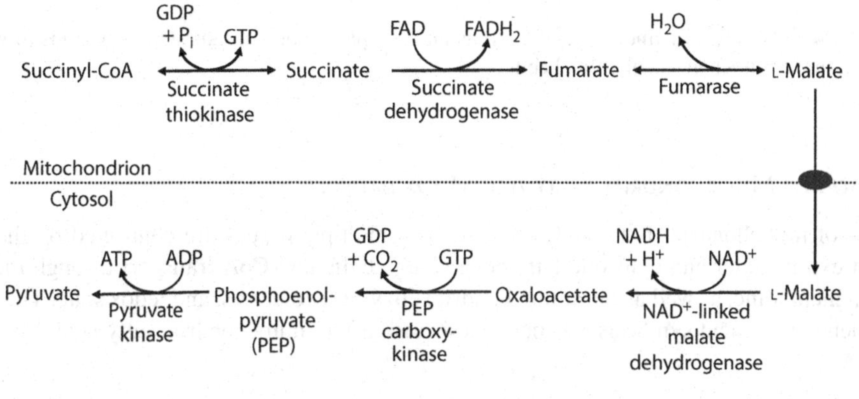

Succinyl-CoA ⇄ Succinate (Succinate thiokinase; GDP + $P_i$ → GTP) → Fumarate (Succinate dehydrogenase; FAD → $FADH_2$) ⇄ L-Malate (Fumarase; $H_2O$)

Mitochondrion

Cytosol

L-Malate → Oxaloacetate (NAD⁺-linked malate dehydrogenase; $NAD^+$ → NADH + $H^+$) → Phosphoenol-pyruvate (PEP) (PEP carboxy-kinase; GTP → GDP + $CO_2$) → Pyruvate (Pyruvate kinase; ADP → ATP)

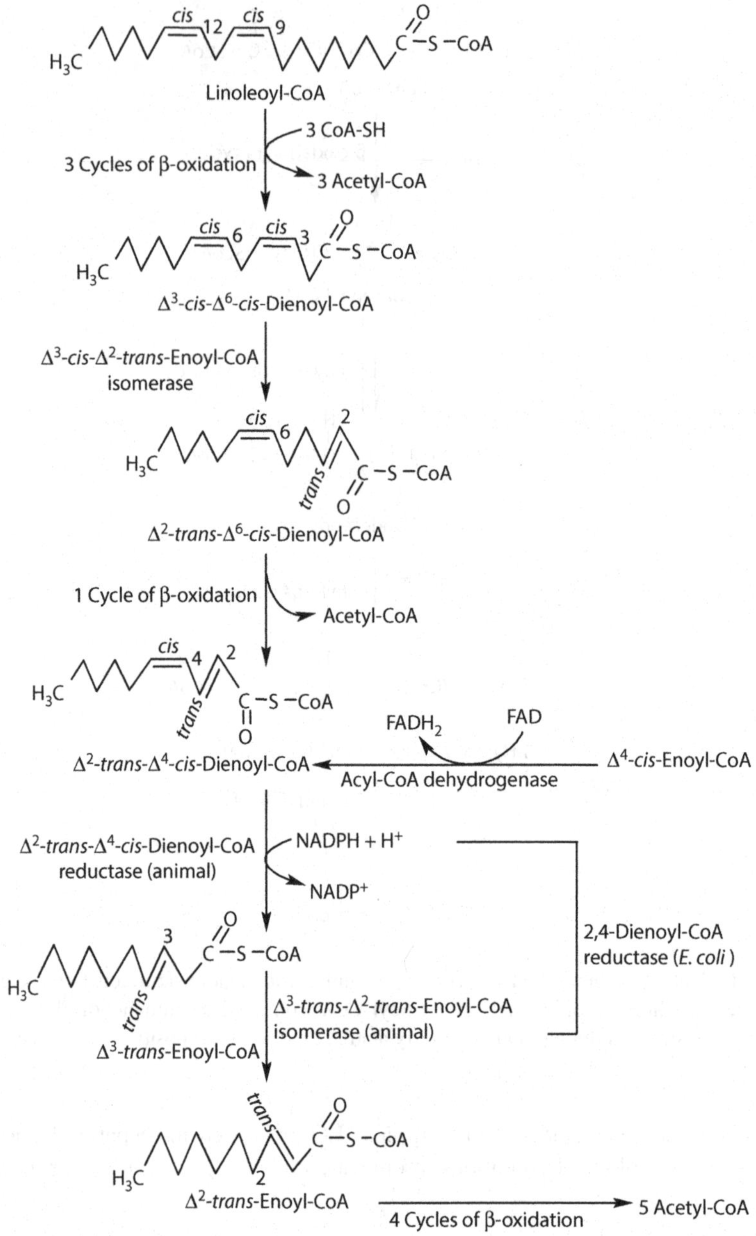

cis 12 cis 9
$H_3C$ C−S−CoA
Linoleoyl-CoA
3 Cycles of β-oxidation
3 CoA-SH
3 Acetyl-CoA
cis 6 cis 3
$H_3C$ C−S−CoA
$\Delta^3$-*cis*-$\Delta^6$-*cis*-Dienoyl-CoA
$\Delta^3$-*cis*-$\Delta^2$-*trans*-Enoyl-CoA isomerase
cis 6 2
$H_3C$ trans C−S−CoA
$\Delta^2$-*trans*-$\Delta^6$-*cis*-Dienoyl-CoA
1 Cycle of β-oxidation
Acetyl-CoA
cis 4 2
$H_3C$ trans C−S−CoA
$FADH_2$ FAD
$\Delta^2$-*trans*-$\Delta^4$-*cis*-Dienoyl-CoA ← Acyl-CoA dehydrogenase — $\Delta^4$-*cis*-Enoyl-CoA
$\Delta^2$-*trans*-$\Delta^4$-*cis*-Dienoyl-CoA reductase (animal)
NADPH + $H^+$
$NADP^+$
2,4-Dienoyl-CoA reductase (*E. coli*)
3
$H_3C$ trans C−S−CoA
$\Delta^3$-*trans*-Enoyl-CoA
$\Delta^3$-*trans*-$\Delta^2$-*trans*-Enoyl-CoA isomerase (animal)
trans
$H_3C$ 2 C−S−CoA
$\Delta^2$-*trans*-Enoyl-CoA → 4 Cycles of β-oxidation → 5 Acetyl-CoA

**FIGURE 6.24** Oxidation of linoleic acid ($C_{18:2}$) as an example for polyunsaturated fatty acids to generate acetyl-CoA in the mitochondria of animal cells.

## Regulation of Mitochondrial Fatty Acid β-Oxidation

The rates of mitochondrial fatty acid β-oxidation in multiple tissues are controlled by the availability of extracellular and cytosolic fatty acids, long-chain acyl-CoA transport through the mitochondrial membrane, as well as intramitochondrial enzymes, cofactors, and redox state. The factors that influence fatty acid synthesis and lipogenesis also affect mitochondrial fatty acid β-oxidation (Table 6.5).

1. *ACC, CPT-I, hormones, and AMPK.* CPT-I is required for the entry of long-chain acyl-CoA from the cytosol into the mitochondrial matrix. Thus, the activity of CPT-I is a rate-controlling factor for mitochondrial β-oxidation (McGarry 1995). In the liver and possibly other insulin-sensitive tissues (e.g., heart and skeletal muscle), CPT-I exerts ~80% of control over the β-oxidation of LCFAs under normal conditions (Bartlett and Eaton 2004). As discussed previously, glucagon, epinephrine, norepinephrine, growth hormone, thyroid hormones, and glucocorticoids inhibit ACC, thereby decreasing the availability of malonyl-CoA (an allosteric inhibitor of CPT-I) and promoting LCFA oxidation in animal tissues. Similarly, AMPK inhibits ACC by phosphorylating this protein, leading to reduced malonyl-CoA availability and enhanced oxidation of LCFAs. In contrast, insulin activates ACC to inhibit fatty acid oxidation. Furthermore, cGMP-dependent protein kinase G activates AMPK and inhibits ACC through protein phosphorylation, thereby promoting the oxidation of fatty acids (Jobgen et al. 2006).

   Under the conditions of fasting, the concentration of malonyl-CoA in the liver, skeletal muscle, and heart is reduced to promote fatty acid oxidation (Saha et al. 1995). Similar metabolic changes are observed in Type-I diabetic patients with severe insulin deficiency. In contrast, the concentration of malonyl-CoA in skeletal muscle is elevated in obese and Type-II diabetic subjects due to increased ACC activity, contributing to impaired oxidation of LCFAs, their intramuscular accumulation, and insulin resistance. Likewise, elevated levels of glucose induce a rise in hepatic and muscular malonyl-CoA, thereby attenuating the fatty acid oxidation.
2. *The availability of metabolites.* Cofactors and substrates (e.g., OAA, CoA, NADH, $NAD^+$, FAD, and acyl-CoA) which can affect the activities of dehydrogenases, reductases, citrate synthase, and oxidases can influence the rate of mitochondrial β-fatty acid oxidation. For example, if mitochondrial $NAD^+$ and FAD are limited, and if the reoxidation of NADH and $FADH_2$ via the mitochondrial electron transport system (e.g., due to reduced coenzyme Q pool, enzyme deficiency, enzyme inhibition, a high ratio of ATP/ADP, or hypoxia) is reduced, β-oxidation itself will be inhibited. Any accumulation of 3-hydroxyacyl-CoA esters following the inhibition of the 3-hydroxyacyl-CoA dehydrogenases will cause feedback inhibition of the 2-enoyl-CoA hydratases and then the acyl-CoA dehydrogenases, leading to impaired production of acetyl-CoA. Furthermore, because mitochondrial CoA concentration is low, intramitochondrial accumulation of acyl-CoA can reduce the availability of free CoA for 3-ketoacyl-CoA thiolase, leading to the accumulation of 3-ketoacyl-CoA, which inhibits 3-hydroxyacyl-CoA dehydrogenase, 2-enoyl-CoA hydratase, and acyl-CoA dehydrogenase. Finally, because acetyl-CoA is also an inhibitor of 3-ketoacyl-CoA thiolase, an increase in the ratio of acetyl-CoA/CoA will result in the inhibition of 3-ketoacyl-CoA thiolase, the accumulation of 3-ketoacyl-CoA, and then the inhibition of β-oxidation.

## Peroxisomal β-Oxidation Systems I and II

In animals, very long straight-chain fatty acids ($\geq C_{20}$), very long branched-chain fatty acids ($\geq C_{20}$), dicarboxylic acids, and bile acid derivatives are β-oxidized through peroxisomal pathways I and II (Van Veldhoven 2010). Peroxisomal fatty acid β-oxidation was discovered initially in germinating castor bean seedlings in 1969 and was subsequently found in the rat liver in 1976. It is now known that peroxisomal β-oxidation of very-long-chain fatty acids takes place in the kidneys and other tissues. The products of this metabolic pathway are medium-chain and long-chain acyl-CoA, as well as $H_2O_2$ and acetyl-CoA.

### Activation of Very-Long-Chain Fatty Acids into Very-Long-Chain Acyl-CoA

In this metabolic pathway, very-long-chain fatty acids are first activated by very-long-chain ACS to form very-long-chain acyl-CoA in the cytosol. Peroxisomal system I (also known as the classical peroxisomal β-oxidation system) is responsible for the β-oxidation of straight, very-long-chain fatty acids, whereas peroxisomal system II is responsible for the oxidation of branched, very-long-chain fatty acids (Reddy and Hashimoto 2001). Peroxisomal fatty acid β-oxidation is of minor importance for ATP production, but its related disorders can result in diseases, such as neurological abnormalities.

### Transport of Very-Long-Chain Acyl-CoA from the Cytosol into the Peroxisome

Very long fatty acyl-CoA enters the peroxisome from the cytosol via an ABC transporter protein. This transport system does not require carnitine but is facilitated by ATP which changes the conformation of the protein transporter. In mammalian peroxisomes, the ABC transport protein is called ALD (adrenoleukodystrophy) protein. The significance of the ALD protein is epitomized by the finding that its inborn deficiency causes damage to the myelin sheath (an insulating membrane that surrounds nerve cells in the brain) and death.

### Shortening of Very-Long-Chain Fatty Acyl-CoA

The subsequent peroxisomal reactions for the peroxisomal β-oxidation of very-long-chain fatty acyl-CoA include dehydrogenation, hydration, a second dehydrogenation, and the thiolytic cleavage (Figure 6.25), which are equivalent to mitochondrial fatty acid β-oxidation. However, the first step of the peroxisomal pathway is catalyzed by acyl-CoA oxidase (not by acyl-CoA dehydrogenase like the mitochondrial β-oxidation pathway). In addition, L-bifunctional protein (enoyl-CoA hydratase and L-3-hydroxyacyl-CoA dehydrogenase) catalyzes the conversion of enoyl-CoA into L-3-ketoacyl-CoA in system I, whereas D-bifunctional protein (enoyl-CoA hydratase and D-3-hydroxyacyl-CoA dehydrogenase) catalyzes the conversion of enoyl-CoA into D-3-ketoacyl-CoA in system II. In both systems I and II, the peroxisomal β-oxidation of very-long-chain fatty acids generates acetyl-CoA, as well as medium- and long-chain fatty acyl-CoA, which are subsequently transported into the mitochondria for further β-oxidation.

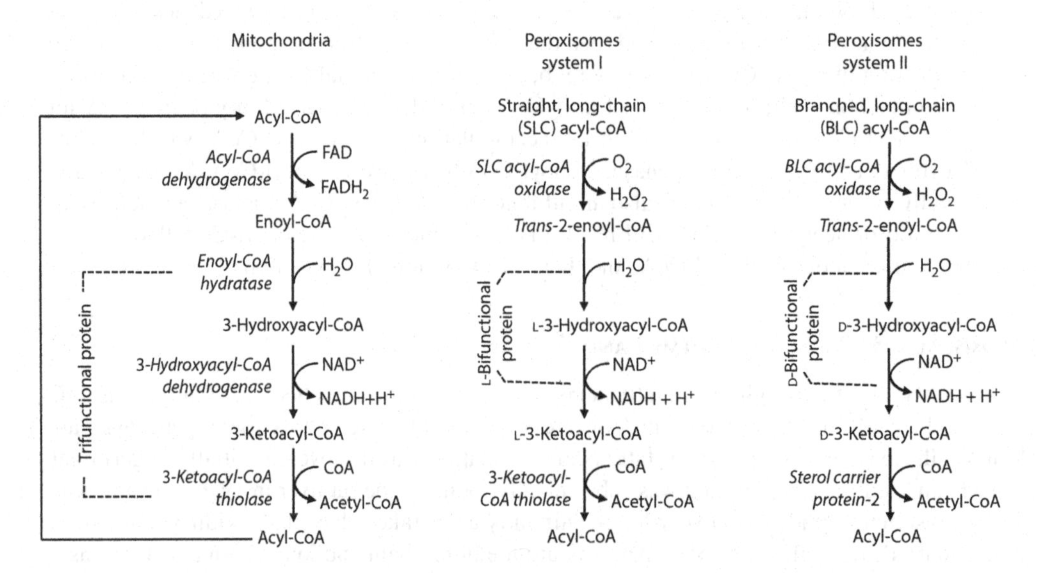


**FIGURE 6.25** Peroxisomal β-oxidation of long and very-long-chain fatty acids in comparison with mitochondrial β-oxidation. In animals, long- and very-long-chain fatty acids ($\geq C_{20}$), as well as dicarboxylic acids, branched long-chain and very-long-chain fatty acids, and bile acid derivatives, are β-oxidized by two peroxisomal pathways. The resulting shorter-chain fatty acyl-CoA products enter the mitochondria for final oxidation to $CO_2$ and water.

### Regulation of Peroxisomal β-Oxidation

Peroxisomal β-oxidation is regulated by a variety of PPAR ligands through their binding to various PPARs, such as PPAR-α, PPAR-β (also called PPAR-δ), and PPAR-γ (1, 2, and 3) (Table 6.6). PPAR-α, which promotes fatty acid oxidation, is expressed mainly in the liver and skeletal muscle. PPAR-γ1 is present in all tissues, PPAR-γ2 (upregulating fat storage) is predominant in the WAT, and PPAR-γ3 (anti-inflammatory) is highly expressed in M2-macrophages and the WAT. Among animal tissues, PPAR-δ/β (mimicking the effect of exercise) is most abundant in skeletal muscle. PPAR ligands, which are designated as peroxisome proliferators, include a broad spectrum of synthetic and naturally occurring compounds, as well as biochemical metabolites of eicosanoids. They enter the nucleus of the cell to exert their physiological or pharmacological effects.

Peroxisomal system I is transcriptionally induced by PPAR-α ligands. As a member of the nuclear hormone receptor superfamily, PPAR-α is highly expressed in hepatocytes, brown adipose tissue, enterocytes, proximal tubular epithelium of the kidneys, adrenal gland, and heart muscle, and, to a lesser extent, in skeletal muscle. Synthetic PPAR-α ligands include hypolipidemic drugs (e.g., fenofibrate or Tricor, and gemfibrozil), certain food flavors, and leukotriene $D_4$ receptor antagonists. Natural/biological PPAR-α ligands include long-chain and very-long-chain fatty acids (particularly ω3-PUFAs), a high-fat diet, the adrenal steroid dehydroepiandrosterone, and eicosanoids derived from arachidonic acid via the lipoxygenase and cyclooxygenase pathways (Puri 2011). In general, PPAR-α ligands exhibit little obvious structural similarity, and the only shared chemical feature is that they have the potential to be transformed into a carboxylic acid derivative. Activated PPAR-α interacts with 9-*cis*-retinoic acid receptor (RXR) to form PPAR-α/RXR heterodimers, which then bind with the peroxisome proliferator response elements localized in numerous gene promoters to increase the expression of all enzymes of peroxisomal system I. PPAR-α is activated under conditions of energy deprivation to β-oxidize fatty acids and produce ketone bodies by promoting the uptake, utilization, and catabolism of fatty acids. As a result, synthetic PPAR-α ligands, such as fenofibrate and gemfibrozil, can reduce plasma concentrations of triglycerides and total cholesterol.

**TABLE 6.6**
**Expression and Ligands of Peroxisome Proliferator-Activated Receptors in Animal Tissues**

| PPAR | Expression in Tissues | Ligands |
|---|---|---|
| PPAR-α | Mainly in hepatocytes and skeletal muscle; also in the heart, proximal tubular epithelium of kidney, brown adipose tissue, adrenal gland, and small intestine<br>Upregulation of fatty acid oxidation and ketogenesis during fasting, and of fatty acid oxidation in the fed state | Fenofibrate (Tricor), glitazones, and gemfibrozil (synthetic); ω3-PUFAs, other long-chain fatty acids, high-fat diet; adrenal steroid dehydroepiandrosterone; and eicosanoids derived from arachidonic acid (natural) |
| PPAR-β (PPAR-δ) | Most abundant in skeletal muscle; widely expressed in animal tissues, such as heart, liver, kidneys, and adipose tissue<br>Increasing cell differentiation; decreasing cell proliferation; promoting glucose and fatty acid oxidation | GW1516 (synthetic) (now abandoned due to its carcinogenic effect); ω3-PUFAs and their metabolites (natural) |
| PPAR-γ1 | Virtually all tissues<br>Increasing epithelial cell differentiation | Thiazolidinediones (TZDs) (glitazones; synthetic), ω3-PUFAs |
| PPAR-γ2 | Mainly in white adipose tissue<br>Increasing adipogenesis; improving insulin sensitivity | Thiazolidinediones (TZDs) (glitazones, synthetic), ω3-PUFAs |
| PPAR-γ3 | Mainly in M2-macrophages and white adipose tissue (anti-inflammatory) | Thiazolidinediones (TZDs) (glitazones, synthetic), ω3-PUFAs |

*Source:* Puri, D. 2011. *Textbook of Medical Biochemistry*. Elsevier, New York, NY, pp. 235–266; Reddy, J.K. and T. Hashimoto. 2001. *Annu. Rev. Nutr.* 21:193–230; Van Veldhoven, P.P. 2010. *J. Lipid Res.* 51:2863–2895.

In addition to PPAR-α, PPAR-γ and PPAR-δ (all are nuclear receptors) have been identified in animals. There are three PPARγ proteins (PPAR-γ1, PPAR-γ2, and PPAR-γ3) which differ at their 5-prime ends, with each under the control of its own promoter. PPAR-γ is expressed predominantly in the WAT, liver, mammary glands, urinary bladder, colonic mucosa, and M2-macrophages and may play an important role in adipogenesis, epithelial differentiation, and anti-inflammatory response. Thus, PPAR-γ can improve insulin sensitivity in obese subjects. PPAR-δ is widely expressed in most tissues, and its function may be to promote epithelial cell development and cell proliferation, as well as glucose and fatty acid oxidation.

#### Role of Peroxisomal β-Oxidation in Ameliorating Metabolic Syndrome

The primary function of the peroxisomal β-oxidation is to shorten very-long-chain fatty acids so that they can be further degraded to $CO_2$ and water in mitochondria. Physiologically or pharmacologically active PPAR ligands promote the deposition of plasma fatty acids as TAGs in the WAT, the oxidation of fatty acids in the liver and skeletal muscle, and anti-inflammatory reactions in macrophages and the circulatory system. For example, some antidiabetic drugs (e.g., glitazones) bind PPAR-α and PPAR-γ, causing a marked increase in peroxisomes and a decrease in the circulating levels of TAGs, VLDLs, and LDLs (Puri 2011). These drugs can also attenuate the long-chain fatty acyl-CoA-induced activation of NFκB in skeletal muscle, thereby improving the insulin signaling pathway (DeFronzo 2010). Thus, like metformin and sulfonylureas, PPAR ligands or agonists aid in reducing the circulating levels of glucose and ameliorating dyslipidemia in obese and diabetic animals, reducing the risk for the development of cardiovascular disease.

### Production and Utilization of Ketone Bodies in Animals

#### Production of Ketone Bodies Primarily by Liver

Under certain metabolic conditions (e.g., fasting, a low ratio of insulin/glucagon, underfeeding, or energy deficits as occurring during lactation, pregnancy, and exercise), most animal species (e.g., cattle, sheep, goats, rats, dogs, and chicks) are capable of producing large amounts of ketone bodies from fatty acid-derived acetyl-CoA (Beitz 1993). This mitochondrial process is illustrated in Figure 6.26, with HMG-CoA synthase being a rate-controlling enzyme (Hegardt 1999). The conversion of acetyl-COA to acetoacetate involves the formation of acetoacetyl-CoA and HMG-CoA by thiolase, HMG-CoA synthase, and HMG-CoA lyase. Finally, acetoacetate is reduced by D-β-hydroxybutyrate dehydrogenase to form β-hydroxybutyrate, and this reversible reaction is present in all cells with mitochondria. Note that β-hydroxybutyrate is technically not a ketone according to the International Union of Pure and Applied Chemistry (IUPAC) nomenclature, although this metabolite has been so called for historical reasons.

$$\text{Acetoacetate} + \text{NADH} + \text{H}^+ \leftrightarrow \beta\text{-Hydroxybutyrate} + \text{NAD}^+$$

Ketogenesis occurs primarily in the same periportal hepatocytes of the liver as fatty acid β-oxidation and, to a much lesser extent, in colonocytes. Ruminal epithelial cells are also capable of producing both acetoacetate and β-hydroxybutyrate. The synthesis of ketone bodies is associated with the production of $H^+$. Thus, a high rate of ketogenesis in uncontrolled diabetes, during early lactation in cows and during late pregnancy, results in severe ketosis (Beitz 1993). If the $H^+$ is not buffered or removed, a low pH in the blood is life-threatening as in patients with Type-I diabetes. In animal production, ketosis causes a decreased milk yield in cattle, as well as pregnancy toxemia in sheep and goats (particularly multifetal pregnancies).

Interestingly, ketogenesis in young or adult pigs is very limited due to a low or negligible activity of HMG-CoA synthase (Duée et al. 1994). The mitochondrial HMG-CoA synthase protein in the liver of 48 h-old unsuckled pigs is barely detectable. Thus, the concentrations of ketone bodies

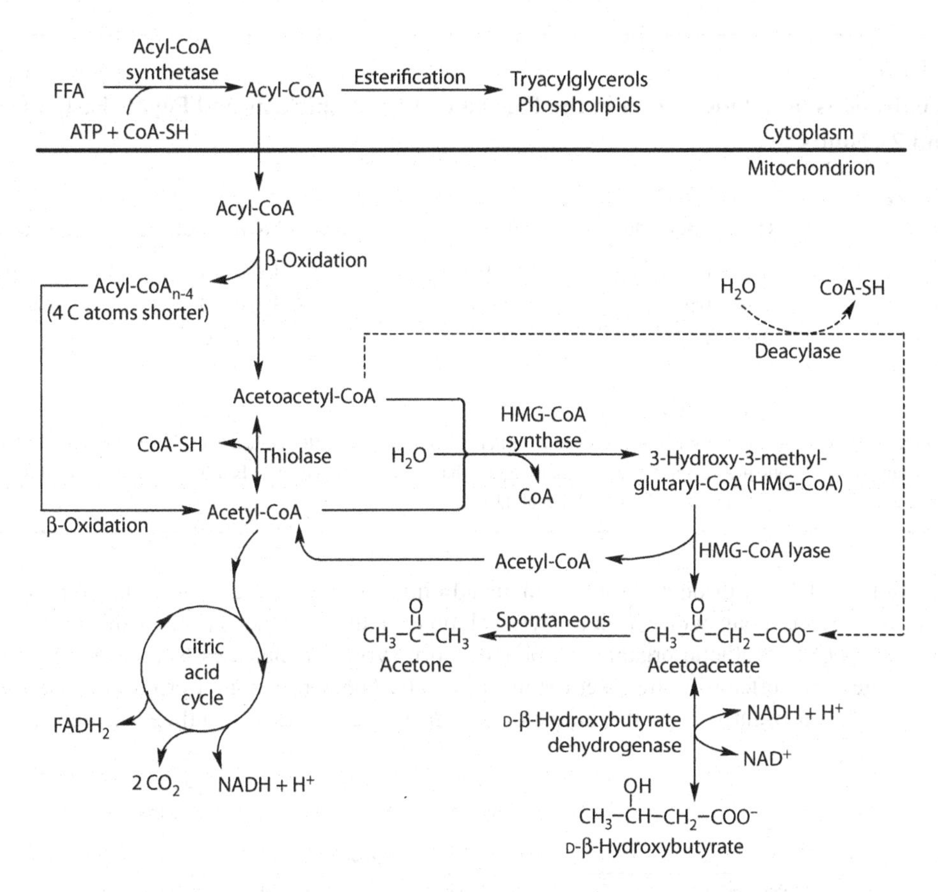


**FIGURE 6.26** Mitochondrial production of ketone bodies (acetoacetate, D-β-hydroxybutyrate, and acetone) from acetyl-CoA in animals. All these reactions occur in the mitochondria of mammals, birds, and fish. In pigs, ketogenesis is limited due to a very low activity of HMG-CoA synthase.

are very low in the plasma of pigs (<0.2 mM) even during a 2-day or longer period of food deprivation (Gentz et al. 1970), although these metabolites are also produced from the catabolism of ketogenic AAs. Fasting for 12 or 24 h did not affect the circulating levels of acetoacetate or D-β-hydroxybutyrate in young pigs (Table 6.7). This metabolic feature in pigs, coupled with their lack of brown adipose tissue, increases the risks for hypoglycemia as well as high rates of morbidity and mortality during the neonatal period.

## Regulation of Hepatic Ketogenesis

Regulation of hepatic ketogenesis involves multiple tissues: (1) the WAT, which supplies free fatty acids to the liver; (2) the liver, which either oxidizes fatty acids or synthesizes TAGs; and (3) the skeletal muscle and other tissues (e.g., heart, kidneys, brain, and small intestine) that oxidize ketone bodies. At the cellular level, ketogenesis is affected by (1) the intracellular concentrations of fatty acids, acetyl-CoA, OAA, and malonyl-CoA; and (2) activities of CPT-I and HMG-CoA synthase. All of these factors are subject to metabolic control by insulin, glucagon, and the ratio of insulin to glucagon (Figure 6.27).

A substantial increase in the production of ketone bodies does not occur *in vivo* unless blood levels of free fatty acids produced from the lipolysis of TAGs in the WAT are markedly elevated, as occurs during food deprivation (Prior and Smith 1982). As shown in Table 6.7, 12- and 24-h fasting in 10-day-old chickens increases the plasma concentration of acetoacetate by 6.1- and 7.1-fold, respectively, and of D-β-hydroxybutyrate by 7.9- and 16.5-fold, respectively. Increasing intracellular

**TABLE 6.7**

**Concentrations of Ketone Bodies in the Plasma of Young Chickens and Piglets Fasted for 12 and 24 Hours**

| Nutritional Status | Chickens[a] | | Piglets[b] | |
|---|---|---|---|---|
| | D-β-Hydroxybutyrate | Acetoacetate | D-β-Hydroxybutyrate | Acetoacetate |
| Fed | 0.15 ± 0.002 | 0.11 ± 0.01 | 0.071 ± 0.004 | 0.054 ± 0.003 |
| 12-h fast | 1.34 ± 0.01 | 0.78 ± 0.04 | 0.073 ± 0.005 | 0.056 ± 0.004 |
| 24-h fast | 2.63 ± 0.02 | 0.89 ± 0.05 | 0.076 ± 0.005 | 0.058 ± 0.004 |

*Source:* Wu, G. and J.R. Thompson. 1987. *Int. J. Biochem.* 19:937–943.

*Note:* Values (mM) are means ± SEM, $n = 10$.

[a] Blood samples were obtained from 10-day-old male broiler chickens that were fed or had been fasted for 12 h or 24 h.

[b] Blood samples were obtained from 7-day-old male piglets that were fed by sows or had been fasted for 12 h or 24 h. Ketone bodies were analyzed as described by Wu et al. (1991).

concentrations of OAA through the intravenous administration of sodium pyruvate, sodium propionate, or glucose along with an electrolyte solution, or through dietary supplementation with propylene glycol (a synthetic organic compound), corn syrup, or molasses (sources of digestible carbohydrates), can effectively treat ketosis in ruminants. The conversion of propylene glycol into L-lactate and then D-glucose for the inhibition of hepatic ketogenesis is outlined in Figure 6.28.

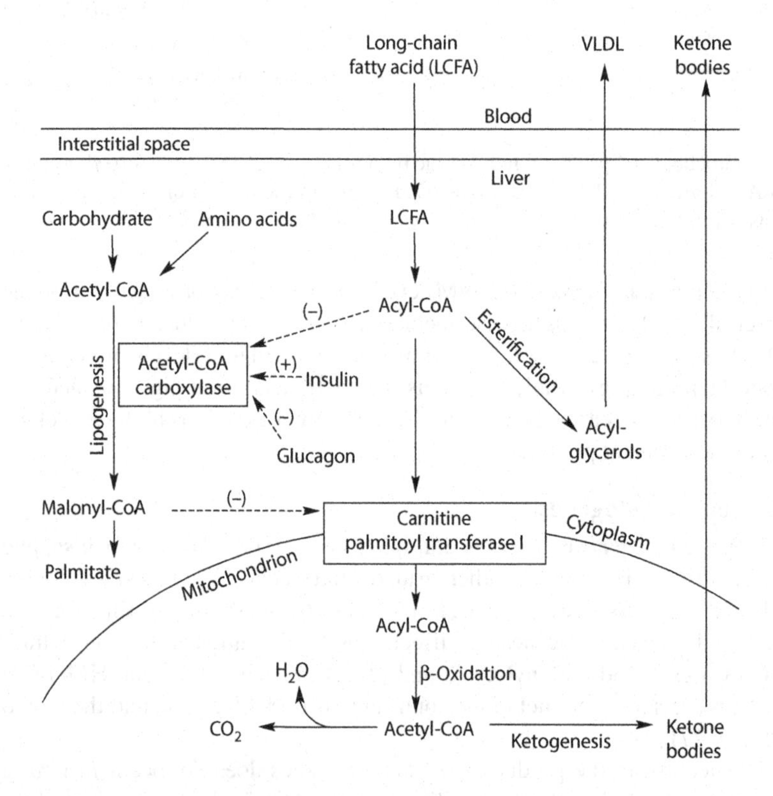


**FIGURE 6.27** Regulation of mitochondrial ketogenesis in animals. The rates of hepatic ketogenesis are affected by the concentrations of free fatty acids in the plasma; hepatic oxidation of fatty acids to form acetyl-CoA; and expression of the required proteins. All of these factors are influenced by insulin, glucagon, and the ratio of insulin to glucagon. LCFA, long-chain fatty acids; VLDL, very-low-density lipoproteins.

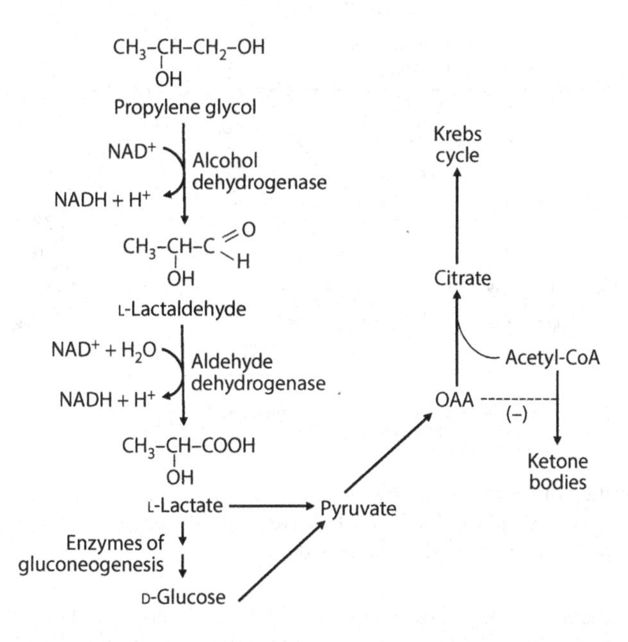


**FIGURE 6.28** Metabolism of propylene glycol to pyruvate and glucose for inhibiting hepatic ketogenesis in ruminants.

A reduction in the availability of malonyl-CoA due to the inhibition of acetyl-CoA carboxylase promotes the oxidation of LCFAs and the production of ketone bodies. Finally, intravenous or intramuscular administration of insulin reduces hepatic ketogenesis and the circulating levels of ketone bodies in patients with Type-I diabetes. The relationship between metabolic states and hepatic ketogenesis is summarized in Table 6.8.

## Utilization of Ketone Bodies by Extrahepatic Tissues

The liver of animals cannot oxidize ketone bodies to acetyl-CoA, because of the lack of enzymes (3-ketoacid-CoA transferase [also known as succinyl-CoA:3-ketoacid-CoA transferase] and acetoacetyl-CoA synthetase) for the conversion of acetoacetate to acetoacetyl-CoA (Robinson and Williamson 1980). In contrast, many extrahepatic tissues, which include the brain, skeletal muscle, heart, kidney, WAT, and small intestine, possess one or both of these two enzymes for the activation of acetoacetate to form acetoacetyl-CoA (Figure 6.29). The 3-ketoacid-CoA transferase and

**TABLE 6.8**
**Nutritional and Hormonal Regulation of Hepatic Ketogenesis**

| Feeding | Hormone | Malonyl-CoA Level | Fatty Acid Synthesis | Fatty Acid Oxidation | Ketogenesis |
|---|---|---|---|---|---|
| Carbohydrate | ↑ Insulin<br>↓ Glucagon | ↑ | ↑ | ↓ | ↓ |
| Starvation | ↓ Insulin<br>↑ Glucagon | ↓ | ↓ | ↑ | ↑ |
| Uncontrolled diabetes | ↓ Insulin<br>↑ Glucagon | ↓ | ↓ | ↑ | ↑ |

*Note:* ↓, decrease; ↑, increase.

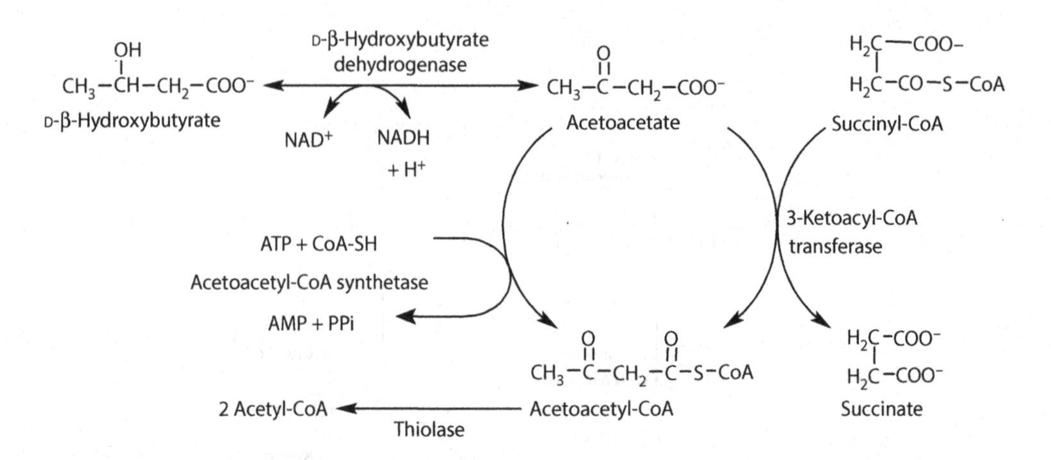


**FIGURE 6.29** Utilization of ketone bodies by extrahepatic tissues. All these reactions occur in the tissues of mammals, birds, and fish, except for the livers. The liver lacks the enzyme for converting acetoacetate to acetyl-CoA and, therefore, cannot utilize the ketone bodies.

acetoacetyl-CoA synthetase are localized in the mitochondrial matrix and the cytosol of all extrahepatic tissues, respectively. Thus, in the presence of CoA-SH, acetoacetate and D-β-hydroxybutyrate are extensively oxidized in the extrahepatic tissues.

Ketone bodies are not metabolic wastes. They are the major energy source for the brain during prolonged fasting when blood glucose concentrations are low. Ketone bodies inhibit the catabolism of protein, AAs, and glucose in extrahepatic tissues to spare these nitrogen reserves and nutrients in the case of starvation (Thompson and Wu 1991). Ketone bodies can be regarded as important metabolic fuels and signals. For example, β-hydroxybutyrate can protect neurons against the toxicity induced by the administration of 1-methyl-4-phenylpyridinium (heroin analog) or a fragment of amyloid protein (Kashiwaya et al. 2000). Also, high circulating levels of acetoacetate and β-hydroxybutyrate, which are achieved through the consumption of ketogenic diets, can protect individuals with epilepsy from seizures (Clanton et al. 2017).

## α-Oxidation of Fatty Acids

Although the mitochondrial β-oxidation is the major pathway for the oxidation of short-, medium-, and long-chain fatty acids in animals, α-oxidation of fatty acids can occur in the brain, liver, kidneys, and skin as a quantitatively minor pathway (Van Veldhoven 2010). In α-oxidation, one carbon is removed at a time from the carboxyl end of the molecule. The α-oxidation of fatty acids occurs primarily in the peroxisome and, to a lesser extent, the smooth endoplasmic reticulum, and does not require CoA intermediates or generate high-energy phosphate compounds (Jansen and Wanders 2006). The discovery of high amounts of phytanic acid in the kidney, liver, and brain of patients suffering from *Refsum's syndrome* prompted extensive research on its catabolism via the α-oxidation pathway.

Phytanic acid (3,7,11,15-tetramethylhexadecanoic acid; a multibranched $C_{20}$ fatty acid containing four methyl residues on a $C_{16}$ backbone) was known to be a component of cow's milk in the 1950s (Hansen and Shorland 1951). Phytanic acid is formed from phytol (3,7,11,15-tetramethyl-hexadec-*trans*-2-ene-1-ol) by bacteria. The steps of α-oxidation of phytanic acid include: (1) the activation of the fatty acid to phytanoyl-CoA by long-chain ACS and the transport of the acyl-CoA into peroxisomes; (2) 2-hydroxylation of phytanoyl-CoA by phytanoyl-CoA hydroxylase ($Fe^{2+}$) to 2-hydroxyphytanoyl-CoA; (3) the conversion of 2-hydroxyphytanoyl-CoA into pristanal and formyl-CoA by 2-hydroxyphytanoyl-CoA lyase (thiamine pyrophosphate, $Mg^{2+}$); and (4) the dehydrogenation of pristanal by an $NAD^+$-linked aldehyde dehydrogenase (Jansen and Wanders 2006).

Formyl-CoA is hydrolyzed to formic acid and CoA-SH. It is now known that *Refsum's syndrome* results from impaired catabolism of phytanic acid via the α-oxidation in affected patients.

### ω-Oxidation of Fatty Acids

Another minor pathway for fatty acid oxidation is known as ω-oxidation, which is brought about by hydroxylase enzymes involving cytochrome P-450 in the endoplasmic reticulum and production of $H_2O_2$ (Van Veldhoven 2010). In ω-oxidation, the $-CH_3$ group of fatty acids is converted to a $-CH_2OH$ group that is subsequently oxidized to $-COOH$, thus producing a dicarboxylic acid. The enzymes for ω-oxidation are localized in the smooth endoplasmic reticulum of the liver and kidneys, instead of the mitochondria for the β-oxidation (Kroetz and Xu 2005). The three steps of ω-oxidation are (1) hydroxylation by mixed function oxidase; (2) oxidation by $NAD^+$-linked alcohol dehydrogenase; and (3) oxidation by $NAD^+$-linked aldehyde dehydrogenase. The long-chain dicarboxylic acid is usually β-oxidized (primarily in peroxisomes) to form adipic ($C_6$) and suberic ($C_8$) acids, which are excreted in the urine. ω-Oxidation is normally a minor catabolic pathway for fatty acids, but becomes more important when β-oxidation is defective.

### Measurements of Fatty Acid Oxidation and Lipolysis

The oxidation of fatty acids in cells and tissues can be measured with the use of [$^{14}C$] or [$^3H$]-labeled fatty acid as a substrate, followed by the collection of $^{14}CO_2$ or $^3H_2O$. The carbon-1 and other carbons of fatty acids can be labeled with $^{14}C$, but a labeled $^3H$ should not be in the carboxyl group as it can be exchanged with $H^+$ in water. The radioactivity of $^{14}C$ or $^3H$ is measured by a liquid scintillation counter. The rate of fatty acid oxidation is calculated as the amount of radioactivity in the labeled product of fatty acid oxidation ($^{14}CO_2$ or $^3H_2O$) divided by the specific radioactivity of the labeled precursor. When mass spectrometry is available as an analytical tool, $^{14}C$ and $^3H$ can be replaced by $^{13}C$ and $^2H$ in labeled substrates, respectively.

In adipocytes and muscle cells that lack glycerol kinase, the release of glycerol by the cells is a useful indicator of lipolysis. However, this approach is not valid for measuring lipolysis in the liver which contains a high level of glycerol kinase activity. Whole-body lipolysis can be quantified with the use of a glycerol tracer. Regional lipolysis in the WAT and skeletal muscle of live animals can be determined by arteriovenous sampling or microdialysis techniques for glycerol measurement.

## METABOLISM AND FUNCTIONS OF EICOSANOIDS

### Synthesis of Bioactive Eicosanoids from PUFAs

Bioactive eicosanoids are mainly synthesized from arachidonic acid ($C_{20:4}$ ω6), but minor eicosanoids are formed from α-linolenic acid or EPA ($C_{20:5}$ ω3), or dihomo-γ-linolenic acid ($C_{20:3}$ ω6, a metabolite of linoleic acid), in the endoplasmic reticulum. These precursor fatty acids are normally bound to the cell membrane and nuclear membrane and must be released from their membrane sites by phospholipase (e.g., phospholipase $A_2$) to be metabolized through various pathways for the synthesis of bioactive eicosanoids (Field et al. 1989; Hou et al. 2016).

While animal cells constitutively generate many kinds of eicosanoids, their biosynthesis is enhanced when the cells are exposed to pathogens, trauma, ischemia, chemotactic factors, cytokines, or growth factors (Christmas 2015). Four families of enzymes initiate the metabolism of arachidonic acid to eicosanoids: (1) cyclooxygenases (COX): COX-1 (constitutive) or COX-2 (inducible), which convert arachidonic acid into prostanoids (Figure 6.30); (2) lipoxygenases, which convert arachidonic acid into 5-HETE, 5-oxo-ETE, leukotrienes, and lipoxins; (3) cytochrome P450 monooxygenases, which convert arachidonic acid into 20-HETE and 19-HETE; and (4) epoxygenases, which convert arachidonic acid into nonclassic eicosanoid epoxides (e.g., 5,6-EET and 14,15-EET). COX, the lipoxygenases, and the phospholipases are tightly regulated, as oxidation by COX or lipoxygenase

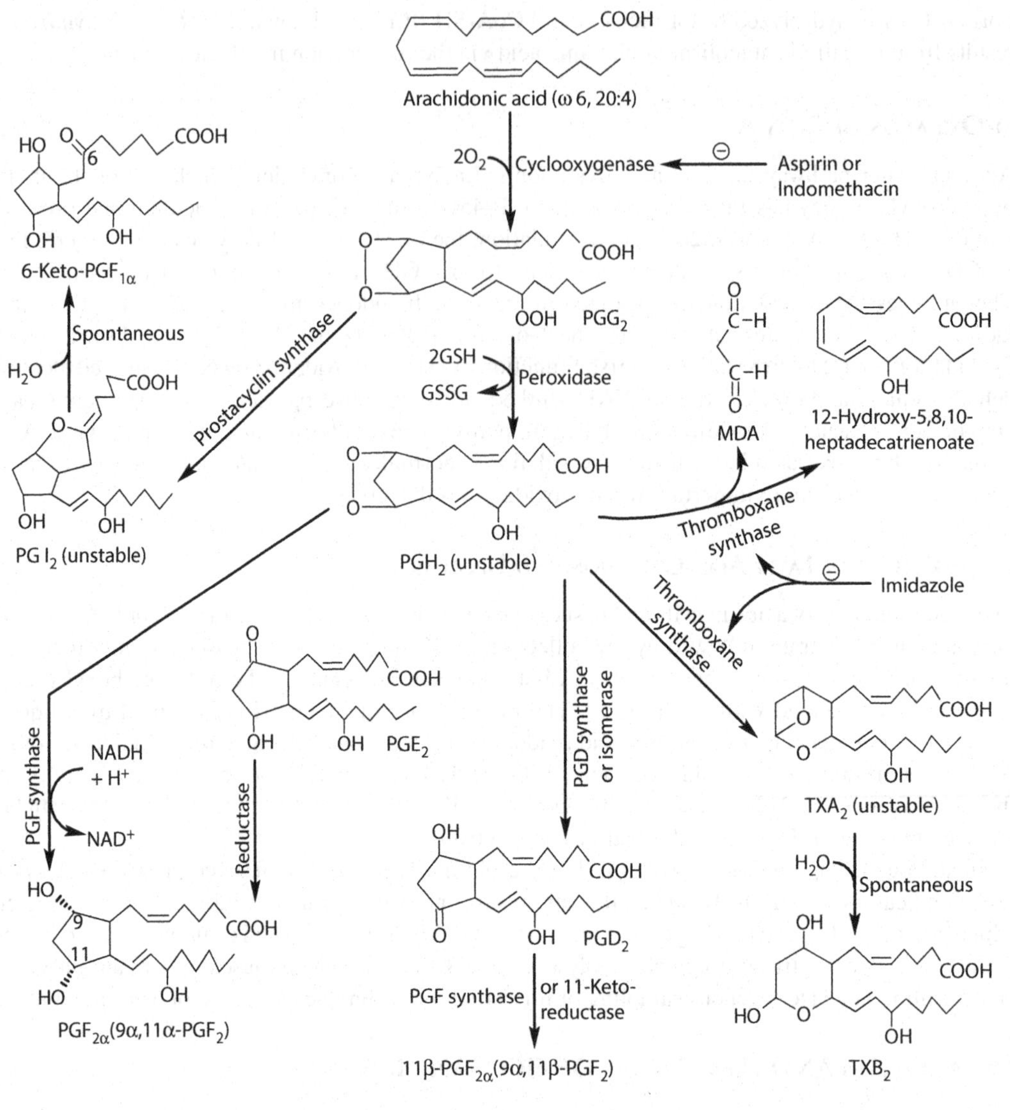

**FIGURE 6.30** Metabolism of eicosanoids to arachidonic acid in animals through cyclooxygenases.

generates highly reactive oxygen species and peroxides. Aspirin and indomethacin are potent inhibitors of COXs (Powell and Rokach 2015). The metabolites of arachidonic acid have two double bonds (2-series eicosanoids). EPA and dihomo-γ-linolenic acid are metabolized by pathways similar to those for arachidonic acid to produce eicosanoid metabolites with three double bonds (3-series eicosanoids; e.g., $PGE_3$, $PGF_{3\alpha}$, and $TXA_3$) and one double bond (1-series eicosanoids; e.g., $PGE_1$, $PGF_{1\alpha}$, and $TXA_1$), respectively. In addition, the metabolism of EPA and DHA generates, respectively, E and D series resolvins with three hydroxyl groups, whereas the metabolism of DHA also produces protectins and maresins with two hydroxyl groups (Serhan 2014). Lipoxins, resolvins, protectins, and maresins are collectively coined as specialized pro-resolving mediators (Serhan 2014).

## Degradation of Bioactive Eicosanoids

Bioactive eicosanoids are rapidly degraded by animal cells via modification (e.g., hydroxylation of the hydrocarbon chain) through the cytochrome P450 detoxification system, conjugation with glutathione (GSH) or glucuronides for excretion, and oxidation via the peroxisomal β-oxidation pathway (Turgeon et al. 2003). Among all tissues, the lungs have the highest rates of degradation of the eicosanoids. In animals, the plasma half-lives of most eicosanoids range from a few seconds to a few minutes. This is important to minimize the circulating levels of inflammatory eicosanoids and prevent any pathological effects of other eicosanoids.

Cytochrome P450 enzymes are crucial for converting PUFAs into some biologically active eicosanoids as noted previously and can also metabolize the eicosanoids into inactive compounds for excretion (Christmas 2015; Xu et al. 2016). Cytochromes P450 are hemoproteins containing heme as a cofactor. The term P450 is derived from the spectrophotometric peak of the cytochrome protein at the wavelength of its absorption maximum (450 nm) in the reduced state and bound with carbon monoxide. The cytochrome P450 system refers to a series of enzymes (e.g., cytochrome P450 ω-hydroxylase [a subset of monooxygenases], cytochrome P450 monooxygenase, and epoxygenase) in an NADPH-dependent electron transfer chain. The most common reaction in the cytochrome P450 system is catalyzed by monooxygenase (either cytochrome P450 ω-hydroxylase or cytochrome P450 monooxygenase), which inserts one oxygen atom from $O_2$ into the aliphatic position of an organic substance and the other oxygen atom into water (Powell and Rokach 2015). After eicosanoids are deactivated by the cytochrome P450 enzymes, the metabolites are excreted primarily in urine and, to a lesser extent, in feces.

$$\text{Organic substance} + O_2 + \text{NADPH} + H^+ \rightarrow \text{Organic substance-OH} + H_2O + \text{NADP}^+$$

Conjugation of eicosanoids with GSH and glucuronic acid occurs primarily in the liver and results in the formation of mercapturates (Figure 6.31) and glucuronides, respectively. The GSH conjugates are formed through the actions of GSH *S*-transferase, γ-glutamyl transpeptidase, cysteinyl glycine dipeptidase, and *N*-acetyl transferase. The glucuronide-conjugation (glucuronidation) reaction is catalyzed by UDP-glucuronosyltransferase, which transfers the glycosyl group from a nucleotide sugar (UDP-glucuronic acid) to a wide variety of compounds (including eicosanoids) to form water-soluble derivatives (e.g., glucuronides). The end products of GSH conjugation and glucuronidation are excreted mainly in urine and, to a lesser extent, in feces.

Gly–Cys–Glu
Glutathione
Glutathione S-transferase
R
Gly–Cys–Glu
R
Glutathione conjugate
γ-Glutamyl transpeptidase
Glutamate
Gly–Cys
R
Glycyl-cysteine conjugate
Cysteinyl glycine dipeptidase
Glycine
R—S—CH₂—CH(COOH)—NH₂
Cysteine conjugate
N-Acetyl transferase
Acetyl-CoA
R—S—CH₂—CH(COOH)—NH—C(=O)—CH₃
Mercapturate
Deacetylase

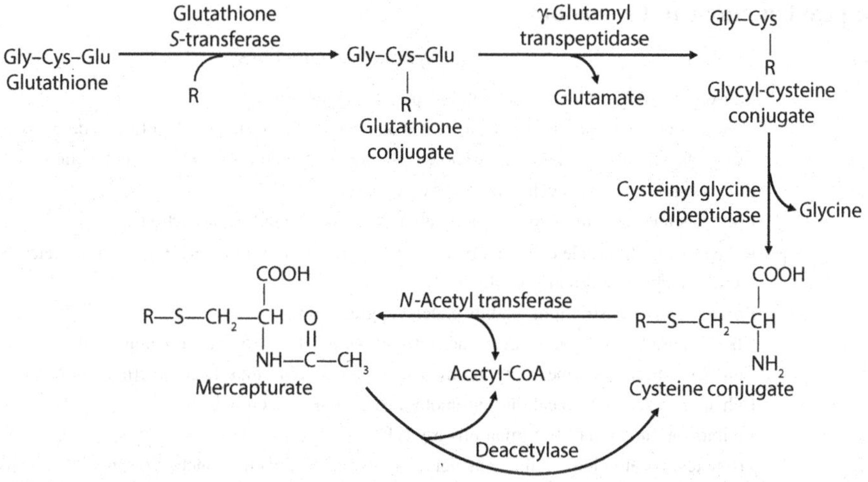

**FIGURE 6.31** Conjugation of eicosanoids with glutathione (GSH) to form mercapturate in the liver. R = substances (e.g., various electrophiles, physiological compounds and metabolites [estrogen, prostaglandins, leukotrienes, and melanins], and xenobiotics [e.g., bromobenzene and acetaminophen] that can conjugate with glutathione in hepatocytes for excretion in urine and feces).

As very-long-chain fatty acids, eicosanoids and their metabolites (including prostaglandins, epoxy fatty acids, thromboxanes, and leukotrienes) can be degraded via the peroxisomal β-oxidation pathway to generate shorter-chain CoA and acetyl-CoA (Van Veldhoven 2010). These products then enter the mitochondria for β-oxidation to $CO_2$ and water. Thus, through the cooperation of both peroxisomes and mitochondria, eicosanoids can be completely oxidized in animals. This assumes physiological importance when the activities of cytochrome P450, GSH conjugates, and glucuronidation pathways are reduced.

## Physiological Functions of Eicosanoids

The eicosanoids have specific effects on target cells close to the site of their production (Hou et al. 2016). These compounds are considered "local hormones," which participate in intercellular and intracellular signal cascades to exert effects on inflammation, fever, hemodynamics, blood clotting, immune system modulation, reproduction, cell growth, and biological clock (Table 6.9). Prostaglandins bind to (1) plasma membrane G protein-coupled receptors, stimulating the formation of cAMP (e.g., $PGE_1$, $PGI_2$, and $PGD_2$), the phosphatidylinositol-4,5-bisphosphate signal pathway ($TXA_2$, $PGE_2$, and $PGF_{2\alpha}$), and intracellular $Ca^{2+}$ release; or (2) PPAR-γ, influencing gene transcription, depending on cell type and eicosanoid. Some leukotrienes also act via specific G protein-coupled receptors on the plasma membrane. Besides the receptor-mediated actions of eicosanoids, ω3 and ω6 PUFAs affect their respective metabolism, thereby eliciting diverse biological responses. For example, ω3 PUFAs can inhibit the synthesis of pro-inflammatory eicosanoids from arachidonic acid, and vice versa (Clandinin et al. 1993). Thus, excess ω6 PUFAs promote inflammation, but ω3 PUFAs suppress inflammation in animals. The interlinking mechanisms responsible for the anti-inflammatory actions of ω3 PUFAs include: (1) altered cell membrane composition of phospholipid fatty acids, (2) disruption of lipid rafts, (3) inactivation of the pro-inflammatory transcription factor NFκB to reduce the expression of inflammatory genes, (4) activation of the anti-inflammatory transcription factor PPARγ, and (5) binding to the G protein-coupled receptor GPR120 to decrease the production of PGE2 and other pro-inflammatory cytokines (Calder 2015).

**TABLE 6.9**
**Physiological Functions of Eicosanoids**

| Eicosanoid | Physiological Functions |
|---|---|
| PG-$I_2$ | Relaxes arterial smooth muscle; inhibits platelet aggregation |
| TX-$A_2$ | Contracts arterial smooth muscle; activates platelet aggregation; blood clotting; allergic reactions |
| PG-$E_2$ | Contracts smooth muscle cells; promotes inflammation; induces fever; pain perception |
| PG-$E_1$ | Relaxes smooth muscle cells; improves erectile function |
| PG-$F_{2\alpha}$ | Promotes uterine contraction; induces labor; enhances bronchoconstriction |
| PG-$D_2$ | Relaxes smooth muscle cells; inhibits platelet aggregation; inhibits neurotransmitter release; allergic reactions; promotes hair growth |
| 20-HETE | Promotes vasoconstriction; inhibits platelet aggregation |
| LT-B4 | Chemotactic factor for leukocytes; activator of leukocytes; promotes inflammation |
| LT-C4, D4 | Enhances vascular permeability; promotes vascular smooth muscle contraction; allergic reactions |
| LT-E4 | Enhances vascular permeability; promotes airway mucin secretion |
| Lx-A4, B4 | Inhibits the function of pro-inflammatory cells |
| 14,15-EET | Promotes vasodilation; inhibits platelet aggregation; inhibits the function of pro-inflammatory cells |
| SPMs | Evokes anti-inflammatory responses and contributes to inflammation resolution |

*Note:* EET, epoxyeicosatrienoic acids; HEPE, hydroxy-eicsapentaenoic acid; HETE, hydroxyeicosatetraenoic acid; LT, leukotriene; Lx, lipoxin; PG, prostaglandin; SPM, lipoxins, resolvins, protectins, and maresins; TX, thromboxane.

# PHOSPHOLIPID AND SPHINGOLIPID METABOLISM

## Phospholipid Metabolism

As noted in Chapter 1, phospholipids consist of a glycerol molecule, two fatty acids, and a phosphate group. They are amphipathic molecules in the lipid bilayer of the plasma membrane and contribute to the physicochemical properties of the membrane (e.g., the membrane fluidity). Therefore, phospholipids influence the conformation and function of membrane-bound proteins (e.g., hormone receptors, ion channels, and nutrient transporters). In addition, as precursors for the synthesis of signaling molecules, phospholipids regulate gene expression and nutrient metabolism. Dietary intakes of nutrients, such as protein, fatty acids (both saturated and polyunsaturated), vitamins (e.g., A, E, and folate), and microminerals (e.g., zinc and magnesium), affect the composition and metabolism of phospholipids in animals (Gimenez et al. 2011).

### Synthesis of Phospholipids

In bacteria (as those in the digestive tract of animals) and yeast, the *de novo* synthesis of phospholipids involves the formation of phosphatidate (DAG-3-phosphate) from dihydroxyacetone phosphate (an intermediate of glycolysis) and fatty acyl-CoA, leading to the generation of cytidine diphosphate (CDP)-DAG (Figure 6.32). Because bacteria and yeast contain the $Mn^{2+}$- and CDP-DAG-dependent phosphatidylserine (PS) synthase, they are capable of synthesizing PS from CDP-DAG and serine. This enzyme, however, is absent from mammals, birds, and fish. Thus, despite the presence of enzymes for converting glucose, fatty acyl-CoA, and serine into CDP-DAG in their endoplasmic reticulum, animal cells do not synthesize PS, phosphatidylethanolamine (PE), or PC from CDP-DAG. However, in animals, CDP-DAG is the precursor for the synthesis of cardiolipin (an abundant phospholipid in mitochondrial membranes) in the mitochondrial inner membrane and of phosphatidylinositol (PI) in the endoplasmic reticulum (Figure 6.33).

In animals, there are two pathways for PE production: (1) *de novo* synthesis from ethanolamine and DAG in the endoplasmic reticulum; and (2) the decarboxylation of PS to form PE in the inner membrane of mitochondria (Tatsuta et al. 2014). PE serves as the common precursor for the synthesis of PS, PC, and sphingomyelin (Figure 6.32). Specifically, PE is converted into PC by PE *N*-methyltransferase, which requires *S*-adenosylmethionine (a metabolite of methionine) as the cofactor. For PS synthesis, PS synthase 1 exchanges serine in PC for choline, whereas PS synthase 2 exchanges serine in PE for ethanolamine. These two distinct enzymes are not related to the $Mn^{2+}$- and CDP-DAG-dependent PS synthase in bacteria and yeast (Vance and Tasseva 2013). PC is hydrolyzed by various phospholipases and lysophospholipases to form choline and phosphatidate. The latter is recycled to CDP-DAG in the endoplasmic reticulum, as noted previously. This, along with the conversion of PC-derived sphingomyelin into phosphocholine, helps to conserve phospholipids in the body.

The majority of lipids (including phospholipids) are synthesized in the endoplasmic reticulum and transported to the mitochondria. However, cardiolipin is formed from CDP-DAG, and PS is converted into PE, in the inner membrane of mitochondria. Thus, the intracellular transport of phospholipids from the sites of their synthesis to their destinations is essential for the formation and function of all cell membranes. It appears that, under physiological conditions, *de novo* synthesis of phospholipids cannot meet the needs of animals, including calves, cats, dogs, fish, fur animals, horses, mice, pigs, poultry, and rats (Gimenez et al. 2011). Therefore, diets must supply these nutrients to the animals to ensure their optimal growth, development, and health.

### Sources of Ethanolamine and Choline in Animals

Plants and algae can produce ethanolamine from serine via a soluble serine decarboxylase. In contrast, animal cells and bacteria lack serine decarboxylase and, therefore, cannot directly decarboxylate serine to form ethanolamine. However, in both animals and bacteria, serine and palmitoyl-CoA

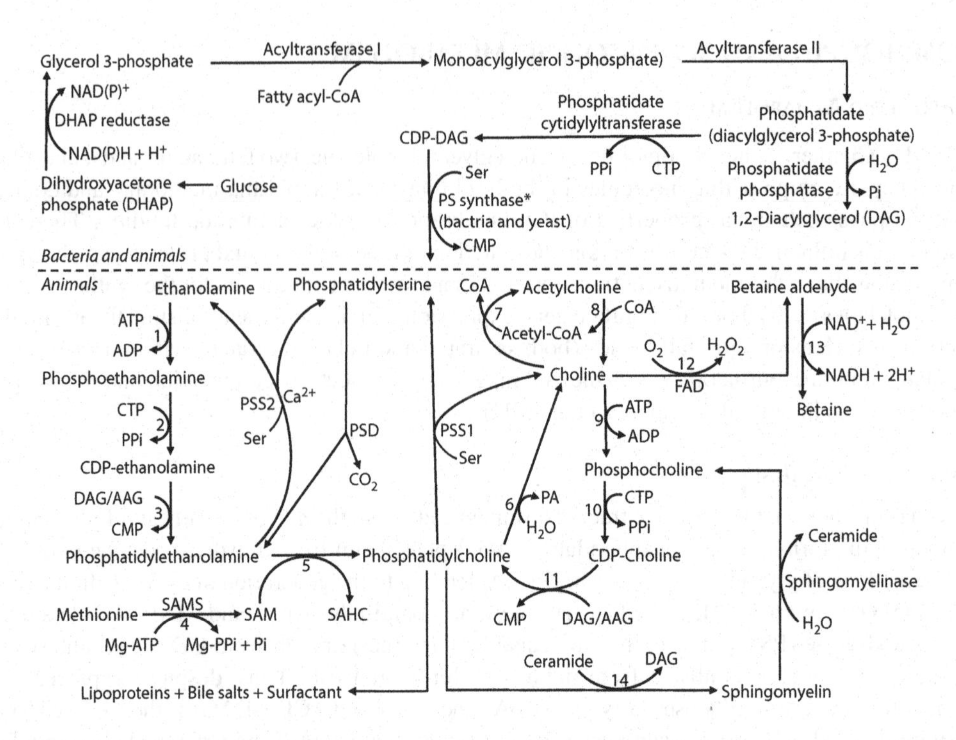


**FIGURE 6.32** Phospholipid metabolism in animals and yeast. The reactions below the broken line occur in animal cells, whereas those above the broken line take place in bacteria and animal cells except for the $Mn^{2+}$- and CDP-DAG-dependent PS synthase. This enzyme is absent from animal cells, as indicated by the sign "*." The enzymes catalyzing the indicated reactions are as follows: 1, ethanolamine kinase; 2, CTP:phosphoethanolamine cytidylyltransferase; 3, CDP-ethanolamine:1,2-diacylglycerol ethanolamine-phosphotransferase; 4, *S*-adenosylmethionine synthase; 5, phosphatidylethanolamine *N*-methyltransferase; 6, various phospholipases and lysophospholipases; 7, choline acetyltransferase; 8, choline acetyltransferase; 9, choline kinase; 10, CTP:phosphocholine cytidylyltransferase; 11, CDP-choline:1,2-diacylglycerol cholinephosphotransferase; 12, choline oxidase; 13, betaine aldehyde dehydrogenase; and 14, phosphatidylcholine:ceramide cholinephosphotransferase. With the exception of PSD (which is located in the inner mitochondrial membrane), the enzymes for phospholipid synthesis are present in the endoplasmic reticulum. AAG, 1-*O*-alkyl-2-acetyl-*sn*-glycerol; CTP, cytidine triphosphate; CDP, cytidine diphosphate; CMP, cytidine monophosphate; DAG, diacylglycerol; PA, phosphatidate; PSD, phosphatidylserine decarboxylase; PSS1, phosphatidylserine synthase 1; PSS2, phosphatidylserine synthase 1; SAHC, *S*-adenosylhomocysteine; SAM, *S*-adenosylmethionine; SAMS, *S*-adenosylmethionine synthase.

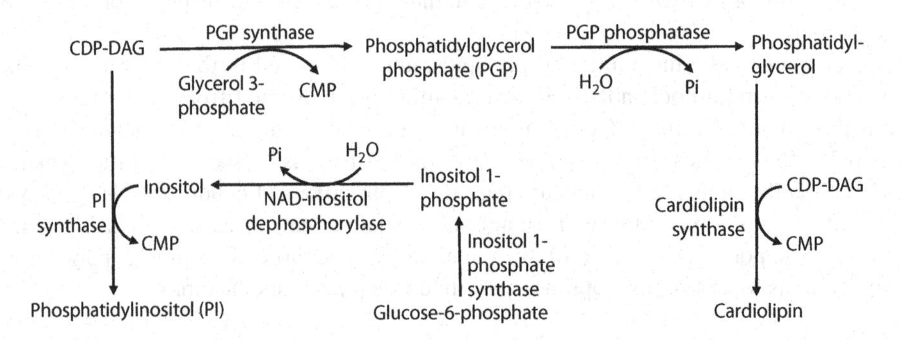


**FIGURE 6.33** Synthesis of cardiolipin and phosphatidylinositol from CDP-DAG in animal cells. The reactions for the conversion of CDP-DAG into cardiolipin occur in the inner membrane of mitochondria, whereas phosphatidylinositol is generated from glucose-6-phosphate in the endoplasmic reticulum. CDP, cytidine diphosphate; CMP, cytidine monophosphate; DAG, diacylglycerol.

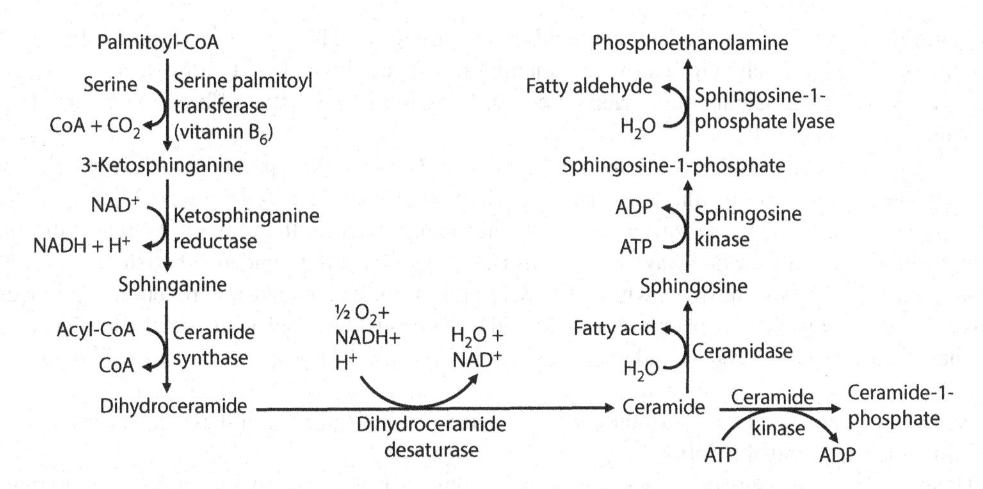


**FIGURE 6.34** *De novo* synthesis of ceramide from palmitoyl-CoA and L-serine, as well as ceramide degradation in animal cells. These reactions occur in the endoplasmic reticulum.

are converted into ceramide through a series of enzyme-catalyzed reactions in the endoplasmic reticulum, where ceramide is metabolized to form fatty aldehyde and phosphoethanolamine (Figure 6.34). PS synthase 2 converts PE and serine into PS and ethanolamine. Bacteria can also synthesize PS from glucose, serine, and acyl-CoA, and the PS is metabolized to PE and then ethanolamine (Figure 6.32). Note that although a small amount of ethanolamine can be generated via the breakdown of sphingolipids by sphingosine-1-phosphate lyase, this reaction does not result in a net *de novo* synthesis of ethanolamine from endogenous sphingolipids. Furthermore, dietary phospholipids and ethanolamine can be additional sources of ethanolamine in animals. The concentration of ethanolamine in the plasma of nonruminants is usually low (2–10 μM; Wu 2013). In ruminants, because ruminal bacteria can *de novo* synthesize ethanolamine from glucose, fatty acids, and serine, the concentrations of ethanolamine in the plasma range from 30 to 100 μM, depending on diets, age, and physiological status (Kwon et al. 2003).

PC, which is formed from PE and PS, is the endogenous source of choline (Figure 6.32). Ultimately, serine and methionine are required for the synthesis of choline in animals. This pathway is most active in the liver among animal tissues. Under physiological conditions, the *de novo* synthesis of choline cannot meet the needs of animals and, therefore, their diets must provide choline (Zeisel 1981). This is particularly important for fetuses and neonates (including preruminants), because their small-intestinal microbial activity is either absent or too low to synthesize a significant amount of choline. Because choline is a substrate for the syntheses of PC and acetylcholine, a deficiency of choline impairs neurological development, cognitive function, and nerve impulse transmission, as well as muscle damage and the abnormal deposition of TAGs in the liver (called nonalcoholic fatty liver disease). Good dietary sources of choline are eggs, meat, poultry, fish, cruciferous vegetables, peanuts, and dairy products.

## Sphingolipid Metabolism

Sphingolipids have an important role in nutrition and physiology, because their metabolism produces diverse molecules that serve as structural components (sphingomyelin and glycosphingolipids in cell membranes) and in signal transduction (e.g., sphingosine, ceramide, and sphingosine-1-phosphate) in cells. In animals, the brain is particularly enriched in sphingolipids (Denisova and Booth 2005). These lipids are formed from phospholipids and such raw materials as serine and fatty acids. Specifically, PC:ceramide cholinephosphotransferase converts PC and ceramide into sphingomyelin. Additionally, animal cells can *de novo* synthesize sphingolipids (e.g., ceramide) from serine and palmitoyl-CoA in the endoplasmic reticulum (Figure 6.34). The synthesized sphingolipids are then imported into mitochondrial and other membranes. These lipids help to provide a water-proof skin layer and also participate in a variety of cellular signaling to regulate differentiation, proliferation, and apoptosis of cells.

Hydrolysis of sphingolipids is initiated in lysosomes. For example, sphingomyelin is hydrolyzed by the lysosomal sphingomyelinase to form phosphocholine and ceramide (Figure 6.32). A complex sphingolipid is ultimately broken down into sphingosine, which is then reused by reacylation to form ceramide (the salvage pathway). Of note, a critical step in sphingolipid metabolism is catalyzed by sphingosine-1-phosphate lyase, which is widely present in the endoplasmic reticulum of tissues. This enzyme cleaves the phosphorylated sphingoid bases to yield PE and a fatty aldehyde. The latter is either hexadecenal or hexadecanal in the case of sphingosine-1-phosphate or dihydrosphingosine-1-phosphate as the substrate, respectively. The intracellular concentrations of sphingolipids depend on the balance between the rates of their synthesis and catabolism, as well their dietary intake and intestinal digestion and absorption.

There is no known nutritional requirement for sphingolipids by animals. The ingested sphingolipids are hydrolyzed in the intestine to ceramides and sphingoid bases for absorption into the enterocytes (Vesper et al. 1999). Results of animal studies indicate that dietary supplementation with sphingolipids can suppress colon carcinogenesis, reduce serum LDL, and elevate serum HDL. Thus, sphingolipids may be a "functional" constituent of food for improvement of animal health. In the absence of sphingolipid intake from diets, animals cannot maintain the homeostasis of these lipids.

## METABOLISM OF STEROID HORMONES

### SYNTHESIS OF PROGESTERONE AND GLUCOCORTICOIDS

The cytochrome P450 (CYP) enzymes, as well as hydroxysteroid dehydrogenases (HSDs) and steroid reductases, are responsible for the synthesis of steroid hormones from cholesterol in a cell-specific manner (e.g., adrenal gland, testes, and ovaries) (Figure 6.35). These enzymes are highly substrate-selective and include NADPH-dependent steroid dehydrogenases and reductases. The initial step of the synthetic pathways, that is, the conversion of cholesterol into pregnenolone, is catalyzed by CYP11A1 (cholesterol monooxygenase; cholesterol side-chain cleavage). This enzyme is bound to the mitochondrial inner membrane of all steroidogenic tissues. Pregnenolone is converted to (1) progesterone by 3β-hydroxysteroid dehydrogenase (3β-HSD), a non-CYP450 enzyme present in both mitochondria and the endoplasmic reticulum of the placenta and steroidogenic tissues; and (2) 17α-hydroxy-pregnenolone by CYP17, which is a single protein with both 17α-hydroxylase and 17,20-lyase activities, and is expressed in the ovaries, testes, and adrenal cortex (Sanderson 2006). In the adrenal cortex, progesterone is metabolized to corticosterone, aldosterone, and cortisol, while 17α-hydroxy-pregnenolone is converted into cortisol. The circulating levels of the adrenal hormones vary with species. For example, cortisol and corticosterone are the predominant glucocorticoids in the plasma of pigs and chickens, respectively. The production of glucocorticoids in the context of the adrenal gland is stimulated by adrenocorticotropic hormone (ACTH) or under stress conditions (e.g., heat stress). High levels of glucocorticoids induce a catabolic response in animals, which can be ameliorated by dietary supplementation with the structural analogs of the hormones, such as the the extracts of *Yucca schidigera*.

### SYNTHESIS OF TESTOSTERONE AND ESTROGEN

Cholesterol-derived 17α-hydroxy-pregnenolone is the common intermediate for the synthesis of testosterone by Leydig cells in the testes and of estrogen by granulosa cells in the ovaries. These are anabolic hormones that promote protein synthesis and cell growth. Luteinizing hormone (LH)

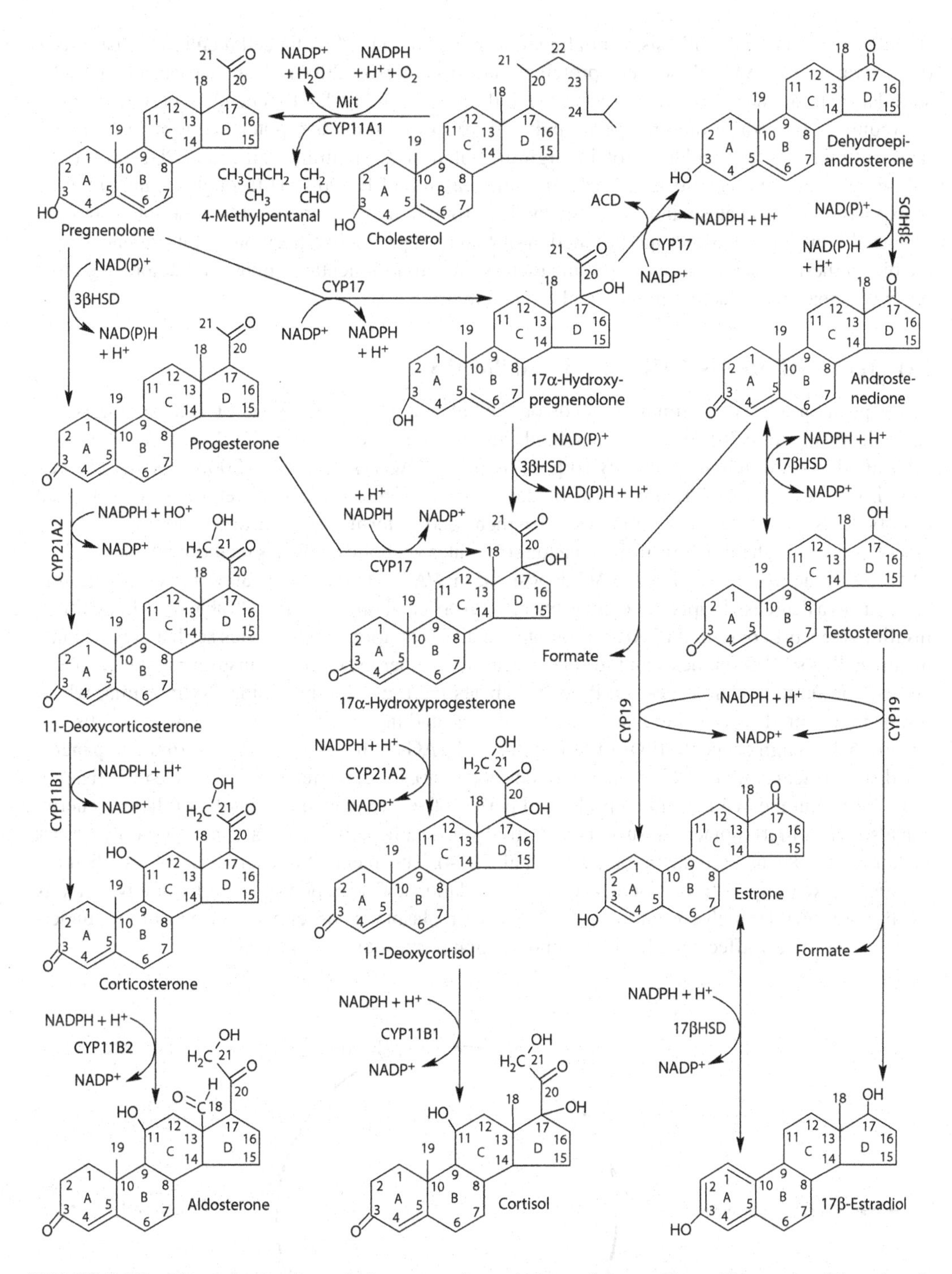


**FIGURE 6.35** Biosynthesis of steroid hormones from cholesterol in a cell-specific manner. The adrenal cortex produces glucocorticoids (corticosterone, aldosterone, and cortisol) and progesterone. The production of the adrenal hormones in the context of the adrenal gland is stimulated by adrenocorticotropic hormone (ACTH) or under stress conditions (e.g., heat stress). High levels of glucocorticoids induce a catabolic response in the animal, which can be ameliorated by dietary supplementation with their structural analogs, such as *Yucca* extracts.

stimulates testosterone synthesis by binding to its receptor on the Leydig cell membrane that causes the activation of cAMP-dependent protein kinase (Sanderson 2006). Testosterone and follicle-stimulating hormone (FSH), which act through the activation of cAMP-dependent protein kinases, are required to produce mature sperm and achieve full reproductive potential in males. Dietary intake of nutrients (particularly protein, arginine, vitamin A, vitamin E, zinc, and PUFAs) is critical for spermatogenesis. Estrogen synthesis is increased by LH and FSH through the upregulation of expression of aromatase and 17β-HSD, which promote the conversion of estrone into estradiol. Maternal nutrition can affect the production of female reproductive hormones. Interferences with the biosynthesis of sex hormones by some dietary and environmental nonnutrient factors (e.g., toxins) will impair reproduction in both males and females.

## FAT DEPOSITION AND HEALTH IN ANIMALS

The deposition of fats in animals depends on the balance between the rates of TAG synthesis and catabolism (Figure 6.36). When dietary lipids are not completely oxidized to $CO_2$ and water, fatty acids are deposited in tissues (mainly adipose tissue) as TAGs (Jobgen et al. 2006). Likewise, when there is excess acetyl-CoA relative to its oxidation via the Krebs cycle, the acetyl-CoA is converted to fatty acids and cholesterol. Fatty acids are then used to form TAGs for deposition in WAT and other tissues. A high ratio of insulin/glucagon stimulates anabolic pathways including those for TAG synthesis in the liver or WAT and TAG deposition in WAT, while a lower ratio of insulin/glucagon (e.g., due to a decreased supply of dietary energy) favors catabolic responses (Table 6.5). In addition, insulin, glucocorticoids, and PPAR-γ promote the differentiation of adipocytes so that they become mature cells for TAG synthesis and storage. Because of hyperglycemia and insulin resistance, obese animals or animals with Type-I or Type-II diabetes mellitus usually exhibit dyslipidemia, which results in impaired LDL metabolism, oxidative stress, and increased risk for cardiovascular disease (Figure 6.37). High concentrations of fatty acids and TAGs in the plasma can contribute to pancreatic disorders (e.g., inflammation and tumor development). Like overfeeding, excessive mobilization of LCFAs from the WAT during a prolonged period of severe inadequate intake of dietary energy can also result in dyslipidemia, such as the fatty liver (i.e., hepatic lipidosis) that commonly occurs in dairy cows during early lactation (Bode et al. 2004). This metabolic disorder develops when the hepatic uptake of lipids from blood exceeds the oxidation and secretion of lipids by the liver, and is usually preceded by high concentrations of LCFAs in plasma. Thus, either over-nutrition or under-nutrition negatively affects the health and production performance of animals.

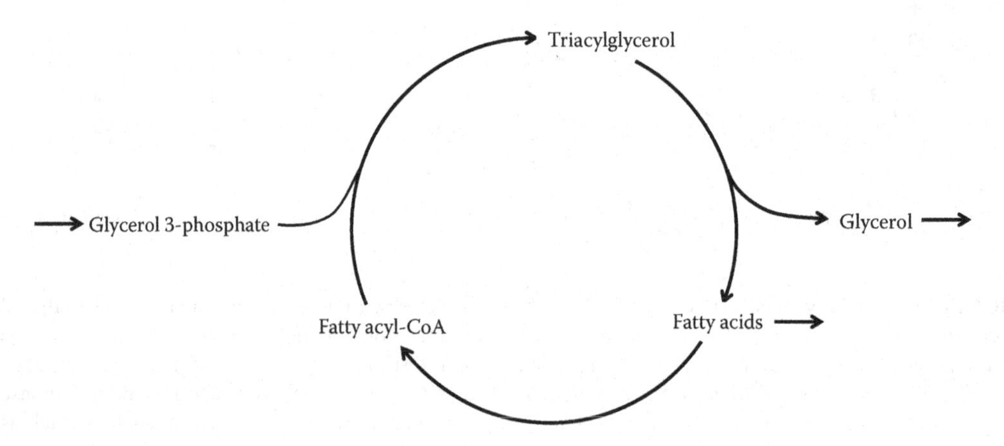


**FIGURE 6.36** Intracellular turnover of TAGs in animals. The balance between the rates of fat synthesis and catabolism determines the deposition of TAGs in cells and the whole body.

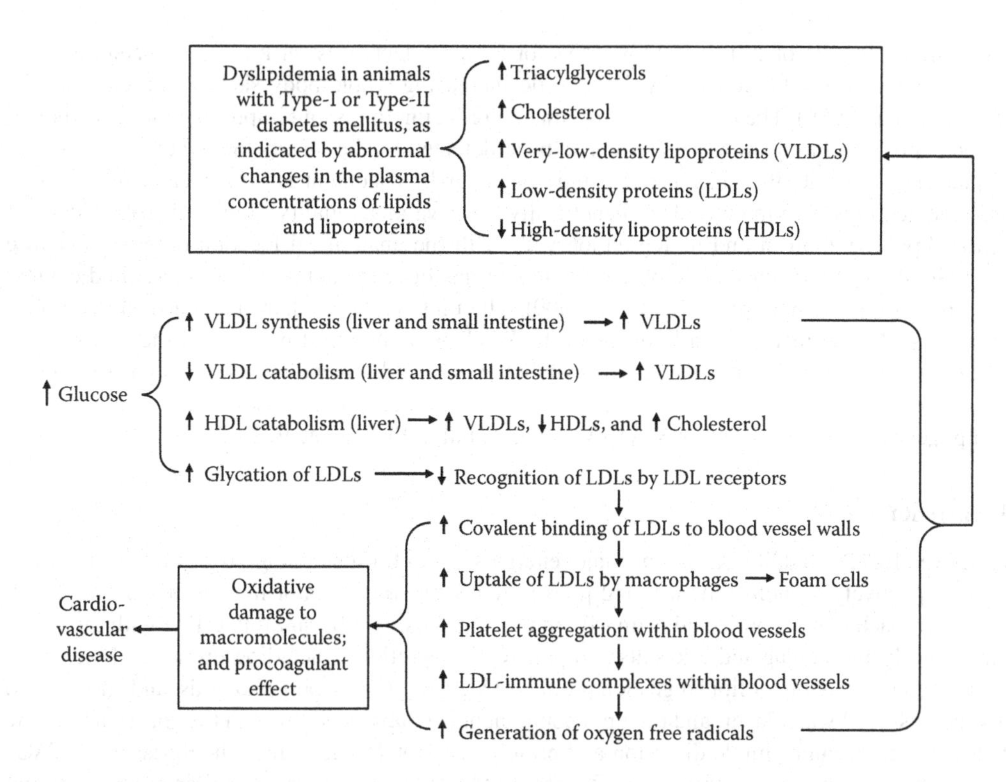


**FIGURE 6.37** Dyslipidemia in animals with Type-I or Type-II diabetes mellitus. Glycosylated LDL proteins are not recognized by their receptors, resulting in high levels of LDLs in the blood, as well as oxidative stress and increased risk for cardiovascular disease.

A major issue in the production of livestock and poultry is that excessive amounts of subcutaneous WAT (e.g., backfat and abdominal fat) are deposited in their market-weight bodies (Etherton and Walton 1986). Let us use the pig as an example. Pigs start to accumulate large amounts of body fat beginning at 45 kg body weight and that fat content increases disproportionately 10-fold between 45 and 115 kg (market weight) body weights. Strikingly, in market-weight pigs, the subcutaneous adipose tissue represents 70% of the carcass lipid. Because consumers are demanding low fat meats, excessive subcutaneous adipose tissue is trimmed at slaughter to meet government and/or consumers' requirements. The more backfat a market-weight pig has, the lower the price or grade. Deposition of subcutaneous adipose tissue not only decreases the proportion of lean tissue in the carcass and economic returns but also potentially reduces the use of dietary energy for muscle protein accretion. Therefore, minimizing excess subcutaneous and abdominal WAT is of enormous importance for improving the quality and economic returns of the swine industry worldwide. This also applies, in many countries, to the production of ruminants, poultry, and fish.

Hormonal and nutritional means have been explored to regulate fat content in farm animals. Specifically, increasing the circulating level of growth hormone or dietary intake of protein and AAs can potentially reduce fat deposition in animals (Bergen and Mersmann 2005; McKnight et al. 2010; Wray-Cahen et al. 2012). For example, intramuscular administration of recombinant porcine somatotropin to 74 kg barrows (50 μg/kg body weight per day) for 24 days increases the percentage of protein and water in the body and skeletal muscle, while reducing the percentage of fats in the whole body and WAT (Kramer et al. 1993). Compared with pigs fed a 14%-CP diet, feeding a high-protein diet (20% CP) enhances protein gain and reduces TAG accretion in growing pigs. Furthermore, diets containing unsaturated fatty acids can enhance the beta-oxidation of LCFAs, while reducing abdominal fat deposition and fatty acid synthesis in animals (e.g., pigs and chickens), as compared to diets containing saturated fats (Sanz et al. 2000). Finally, supplementing 1%

L-arginine to the diet of 110-day-old barrows for 60 days decreases serum TAG concentration by 20% and whole-body fat content by 11%, while increasing whole-body skeletal muscle mass by 5.5% (Tan et al. 2009). The effects of L-arginine on reducing lipids and improving the efficiency of protein deposition in finishing pigs have also been detected by the metabolomic analysis of serum samples (He et al. 2009). Unexpectedly, intramuscular lipid content is 70% greater in arginine-supplemented pigs than in controls to beneficially improve meat quality (Tan et al. 2009), indicating that lipid metabolism and its regulation vary with the anatomical location of WAT. Because muscle lipid represents only ~3% of carcass fats, it has little impact on whole-body lipid content in arginine-supplemented pigs (Tan et al. 2009). The underlying mechanisms are likely complex, but may involve (1) increases in lipolysis in the WAT, mitochondrial biogenesis, the oxidation of fatty acids to $CO_2$ and water in tissues (primarily the liver and skeletal muscle), and partitioning of dietary energy toward protein synthesis in skeletal muscle; and (2) decreases in fatty acid synthesis and lipogenesis in the liver and/or WAT (McKnight et al. 2010; Tan et al. 2012).

## SUMMARY

Fat-derived LCFAs and SCFAs are the major energy sources for the monogastric animals and ruminants, respectively. In nonruminants and preruminants, the digestion of lipids starts in the mouth and the stomach and is completed primarily in the upper part of the small intestine with the aid of taurine or glycine-conjugated bile salts and pancreatic secretions (including lipases and bicarbonate). Micelles consisting of lipid digestion products (MAGs, LCFAs, phospholipids, and cholesterol) pass the unstirred water layer, and the lipid components are absorbed through the apical membrane of enterocytes through simple diffusion and protein carriers. In ruminants, the digestion of TAGs in the rumen is limited (a maximum of 7% fats in the diet) but generates similar products but no MAG, and the resulting LCFAs (containing many biohydrogenated and conjugated LCFAs) are absorbed in the small intestine as in nonruminants. In all animals, the absorption of glycerol as well as SCFAs and medium-chain fatty acids into enterocytes is mediated by protein carriers.

Once inside enterocytes, TAGs are resynthesized for the assembling of chylomicrons, nascent VLDLs, and premature HDLs. These lipoproteins are secreted into the lacteals (most nonruminants and all ruminants) or the portal vein (poultry), and then enter the blood circulation at the junction of the jugular and subclavian veins. During their transport in the blood, mature HDLs released from the liver transfer ApoC-II and ApoE to chylomicrons and VLDLs, and these fat-rich lipoproteins are then hydrolyzed extracellularly by LPLs localized on the luminal surface of the microvascular endothelium within extrahepatic tissues, such as skeletal muscle, heart, WAT, kidneys, and macrophages. The resulting chylomicron remnants are taken up mainly by the liver and, to a lesser extent, by macrophages, whereas the resulting VLDL remnants (LDLs primarily plus IDLs) are mainly taken up by the liver and, to a lesser extent, by peripheral tissues (e.g., skeletal muscle, heart, WAT, and kidneys) for catabolism in a tissue-dependent manner. Because the liver lacks LPL, hepatic lipase plays an important role in the clearance of TAGs from the blood. HDLs, released from the small intestine and liver, collect cholesterol from the peripheral tissues into the liver. In the liver, cholesterol is synthesized from acetyl-CoA and converted into bile acids or bile alcohols for excretion in the feces. Cholesterol is also used for the synthesis of all steroid hormones. Phospholipids, particularly PC, play an important role in TAG digestion, as well as interorgan cholesterol and lipoprotein metabolism. In all animal cells, PUFAs can be metabolized to produce eicosanoids with diverse physiological functions, such as vasodilation, smooth muscle contraction, and mediation of pro- or anti-inflammatory responses.

In the fed and fasting states of animals, fatty acids are oxidized to $CO_2$ and water primarily via the mitochondrial β-oxidation pathway. Minor pathways for the catabolism of LCFAs and very-long-chain fatty acids are the β-oxidation and ω-oxidation pathways in the peroxisome and the endoplasmic reticulum, respectively. In most animals, except for pigs, under the conditions of fasting, energy deficits (e.g., lactation, late pregnancy, and intensive exercise), and Type-I diabetes mellitus, fatty acids are oxidized to acetoacetate and D-β-hydroxybutyrate, which serve as major

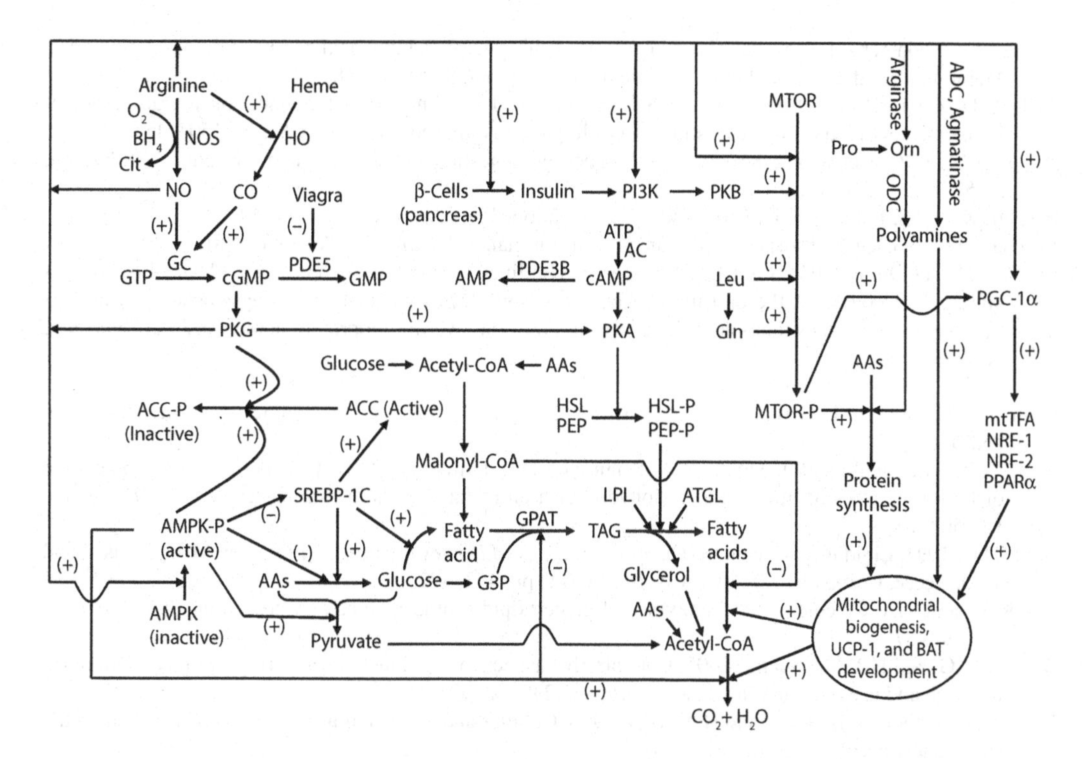


**FIGURE 6.38** Regulation of fat deposition in animals through cell signaling involving cAMP- and cGMP-dependent protein kinases. AC, adenylyl cyclase; ACC, acetyl-CoA carboxylase; ADC, arginine decarboxylase; AMPK, AMP-activated protein kinase; ATGL, adipose triglyceride lipase; BAT, brown adipose tissue; BH4, tetrahydrobiopterin; Cit, citrulline; GC, guanylyl cyclase; G3P, glycerol-3-phosphate; GPAT, glycerol-3-phosphate acyltransferase; HO, heme oxygenase; HSL, hormone-sensitive lipase; LPL, lipoprotein lipase; MTOR, mechanistic target of rapamycin; mtTFA, mitochondrial transcription factor A; NO, nitric oxide; NOS, nitric oxide synthase; NRF, nuclear respiration factor; ODC, ornithine (Orn) decarboxylase; PDE5, phosphodiesterase 5; PDE3B, phosphodiesterase 3B; PEP, perilipins; PGC-1a, peroxisome proliferator-activated receptor-γ (PPAR-γ) coactivator 1α; PKA, cAMP-dependent protein kinase A; PKG, cGMP-dependent protein kinase G; PPAR-α, peroxisome proliferator-activated receptor-α; Pro, proline; SREBP-1C, sterol regulatory element-binding protein-1c; TAG, triacylglycerols; UCP-1, uncoupling protein-1. (Adapted from Wu, G. 2013. *Amino Acids: Biochemistry and Nutrition*. CRC Press, Boca Raton, FL.)

energy substrates for the brain and extrahepatic tissues, as well as cell signaling molecules. In the fed state, saturated and monounsaturated LCFAs are synthesized primarily from glucose and AAs in nonruminants, but from SCFAs and lactate in ruminants, in a tissue-dependent manner. When dietary intake of energy exceeds energy expenditure, TAGs are accumulated in the WAT and liver. The deposition of TAGs in the body depends on the balance between their synthesis and catabolism, which are under regulation by hormones (insulin, growth hormone, and glucocorticoids), AAs (e.g., arginine), and metabolites (e.g., NO and CO) via cell signaling involving protein kinases A and G (Figure 6.38). Excess deposition of TAGs in tissues results in obesity and can lead to insulin resistance and dyslipidemia, as well as increased risk for cardiovascular disease, fatty liver, and pancreatic disorders. Interorgan metabolism of lipids plays an important role in the maintenance of their whole-body homeostasis in the health of mammals, birds, and fish.

## REFERENCES


Abbey, M. and P.J. Nestel. 1994. Plasma cholesteryl ester transfer protein activity is increased when trans-elaidic acid is substituted for cis-oleic acid in the diet. *Atherosclerosis* 106:99–107.

Alonso, L., J. Fontecha, L. Lozada, M.J. Fraga, and M. Juárez. 1999. Fatty acid composition of caprine milk: Major, branched-chain, and trans fatty acids. *J. Dairy Sci.* 82(5):878–884.

Avila, C.D., E.J. DePeters, H. Perez-Monti, S.J. Taylora, and R.A. Zinn. 2000. Influences of saturation ratio of supplemental dietary fat on digestion and milk yield in dairy cows. *J. Dairy Sci.* 83:1505–1519.

Bakke, A.M., C. Glover, and A. Krogdahl. 2011. Feeding, digestion and absorption of nutrients. *Fish Physiol.* 30:57–110.

Bartlett, K. and S. Eaton. 2004. Mitochondrial β-oxidation. *Eur. J. Biochem.* 271:46–49.

Bauchart, D. 1993. Lipid absorption and transport in ruminants. *J. Dairy Sci.* 76:3864–3881.

Bauchart, D., D. Durand, P.M. Laplaud, P. Forgez, S. Goulinet, and M.J. Chapman. 1989. Plasma lipoproteins and apolipoproteins in the preruminant calf, *Bos* spp.: Density distribution, physicochemical properties, and the *in vivo* evaluation of the contribution of the liver to lipoprotein homeostasis. *J. Lipid Res.* 30:1499–1514.

Bauman, D.E. 1976. Intermediary metabolism of adipose tissue. *Fed. Proc.* 35:2308–2313.

Bauman, D.E. and J.M. Griinari. 2003. Nutritional regulation of milk fat synthesis. *Annu. Rev. Nutr.* 23:203–227.

Beam, T.M., T.C. Jenkins, P.J. Moate, R.A. Kohn, and D.L. Palmquist. 2000. Effects of amount and source of fat on the rates of lipolysis and biohydrogenation of fatty acids in ruminal contents. *J. Dairy Sci.* 83:2564–2573.

Beitz, D.C. 1993. Lipid metabolism. In: *Dukes' Physiology of Domestic Animals*. Edited by M.J. Swenson and W.O. Reece. Cornell University Press, Ithaca, NY, pp. 453–472.

Bell R.M. and R.A. Coleman. 1980. Enzymes of glycerolipid synthesis in eukaryotes. *Annu. Rev. Biochem.* 49:459–487.

Bergen, W.G. and H.J. Mersmann. 2005. Comparative aspects of lipid metabolism: Impact on contemporary research and use of animal models. *J. Nutr.* 135:2499–2502.

Besnard, P., I. Niot, A. Bernard, and H. Carlier. 1996. Cellular and molecular aspects of fat metabolism in the small intestine. *Proc. Nutr. Soc.* 55:19–37.

Bijland, S., S.J. Mancini, and I.P. Salt. 2013. Role of AMP-activated protein kinase in adipose tissue metabolism and inflammation. *Clin. Sci.* 124:491–507.

Bobe, G., J.W. Young, and D.C. Beitz. 2004. Invited review: Pathology, etiology, prevention, and treatment of fatty liver in dairy cows. *J. Dairy Sci.* 87:3105–3124.

Brasaemle, D.L. 2007. The perilipin family of structural lipid droplet proteins: Stabilization of lipid droplets and control of lipolysis. *J. Lipid Res.* 48:2547–2559.

Brown, M.S., J. Herz, and J.L. Goldstein. 1997. LDL-receptor structure. Calcium cages, acid baths and recycling receptors. *Nature* 388:629–630.

Calder, P.C. 2015. Marine omega-3 fatty acids and inflammatory processes: Effects, mechanisms and clinical relevance. *Biochim. Biophys. Acta* 1851:4694–4684.

Cao J., L. Cheng, and Y. Shi. 2007. Catalytic properties of MGAT3, a putative triacylglycerol synthase. *J. Lipid Res.* 48:583–591.

Carew, L.B., Jr., R.H. Machemer, Jr., R.W. Sharp, and D.C. Foss. 1972. Fat absorption by the very young chick. *Poult. Sci.* 51:738–742.

Chen, M., Y. Yang, E. Braunstein, K.E. Georgeson, and C.M. Harmon. 2001. Gut expression and regulation of FAT/CD36: Possible role in fatty acid transport in rat enterocytes. *Am. J. Physiol. Endocrinol. Metab.* 281:E916–E923.

Christmas, P. 2015. Role of cytochrome P450s in inflammation. *Adv. Pharmacol.* 74:163–192.

Clandinin, M.T., S. Cheema, C.J. Field, and V.E. Baracos. 1993. Dietary lipids influence insulin action. *Ann. N.Y. Acad. Sci.* 683:151–163.

Clanton, R.G., G. Wu, G. Akabani, and R. Aramayo. 2017. Control of seizures by ketogenic diet-induced modulation of metabolic pathways. *Amino Acids* 49:1–20.

Coleman, R.A. and D.G. Mashek. 2011. Mammalian triacylglycerol metabolism: Synthesis, lipolysis, and signaling. *Chem. Rev.* 111:6359–6386.

Cortner, J.A., P.M. Coates, N.A. Le, D.R. Cryer, M.C. Ragni, A. Faulkner, and T. Langer. 1987. Kinetics of chylomicron remnant clearance in normal and in hyperlipoproteinemic subjects. *J. Lipid Res.* 28:195–206.

Davidson, N.O. and G.S. Shelness. 2000. Apolipoprotein B: mRNA editing, lipoprotein assembly, and presecretory degradation. *Annu. Rev. Nutr.* 20:169–193.

DeFronzo, R.A. 2010. Insulin resistance, lipotoxicity, type 2 diabetes and atherosclerosis: The missing links. *Diabetologia* 53:1270–1128.

Denisova, N.A. and S.L. Booth. 2005. Vitamin K and sphingolipid metabolism: Evidence to date. *Nutr. Rev.* 63:111–121.

Donsmark, M., J. Langfort, C. Holm, T. Ploug, and H. Galbo. 2004. Regulation and role of hormone-sensitive lipase in rat skeletal muscle. *Proc. Nutr. Soc.* 63:309–314.

Doreau, M. and Y. Chilliard. 1997. Digestion and metabolism of dietary fat in farm animals. *Br. J. Nutr.* 78:S15–S35.

Drackley, J.K. 2000. Lipid metabolism. In: *Farm Animal Metabolism and Nutrition*. Edited by J.P.F. D'Mello. CAPI Publishing, Wallingford, UK, pp. 97–119.

Dubland, J.A. and G.A. Francis. 2015. Lysosomal acid lipase: At the crossroads of normal and atherogenic cholesterol metabolism. *Front. Cell Dev. Biol.* 3:1–11 (Article 3).

Duée, P.H., J.P. Pégorier, P.A. Quant, C. Herbin, C. Kohl, and J. Girard. 1994. Hepatic ketogenesis in newborn pigs is limited by low mitochondrial 3-hydroxy-3-methylglutaryl-CoA synthase activity. *Biochem. J.* 298:207–212.

Eliason, E.J., B. Djordjevic, S. Trattner, J. Pickova, A. Karlsson, A.P. Farrell, and A.K. Kiessling. 2010. The effect of hepatic passage on postprandial plasma lipid profile of rainbow trout (*Oncorhynchus mykiss*) after a single meal. *Aquacult. Nutr.* 16:536–543.

Etherton, T.D. and P.E. Walton. 1986. Hormonal and metabolic regulation of lipid metabolism in domestic livestock. *J. Anim. Sci.* 63:76–88.

Field, C.J., M. Toyomizu, and M.T. Clandinin. 1989. Relationship between dietary fat, adipocyte membrane composition and insulin binding in the rat. *J. Nutr.* 119:1483–1489.

Field, C.J., J.E. Van Aerde, L.E. Robinson, and M.T. Clandinin. 2008. Effect of providing a formula supplemented with long-chain polyunsaturated fatty acids on immunity in full-term neonates. *Br. J. Nutr.* 99:91–99.

Fowler, M.A., D.P. Costa, D.E. Crocker, W.J. Shen, and F.B. Kraemer. 2015. Adipose triglyceride lipase, not hormone-sensitive lipase, is the primary lipolytic enzyme in fasting elephant seals (*Mirounga angustirostris*). *Physiol. Biochem. Zool.* 88:284–294.

Fraser, R., V.R. Heslop, F.E. Murray, and W.A. Day. 1986. Ultrastructural studies of the portal transport of fat in chickens. *Br. J. Exp. Pathol.* 67:783–791.

Fried, S.K., C.D. Russell, N.L. Grauso, and R.E. Brolin. 1993. Lipoprotein lipase regulation by insulin and glucocorticoids in subcutaneous and omental adipose tissues of obese women and men. *J. Clin. Invest.* 92:2191–2198.

Gentz, J., G. Bengtsson, J. Hakkarainen, R. Hellström, and B. Persson. 1970. Metabolic effects of starvation during neonatal period in the piglet. *Am. J. Physiol.* 218:662–668.

Gerrits, W.J., J. France, J. Dijkstra, M.W. Bosch, G.H. Tolman, and S. Tamminga. 1997. Evaluation of a model integrating protein and energy metabolism in preruminant calves. *J. Nutr.* 127:1243–1252.

Gimenez, M.S., L.B. Oliveros, and N.N. Gomez. 2011. Nutritional deficiencies and phospholipid metabolism. *Int. J. Mol. Sci.* 12:2408–2433.

Goldberg, I.J., R.H. Eckel, and N.A. Abumrad. 2009. Regulation of fatty acid uptake into tissues: Lipoprotein lipase- and CD36-mediated pathways. *J. Lipid Res.* 50:S86–S90.

Goldstein, J.L. and M.S. Brown. 2015. A century of cholesterol and coronaries: From plaques to genes to statins. *Cell* 161:161–172.

Goodman, H.M. 1968. Growth hormone and the metabolism of carbohydrate and lipid in adipose tissue. *Ann. N.Y. Acad. Sci.* 148:419–440.

Greenberg, A.S., J.J. Egan, S.A. Wek, N.B. Garty, E.J. Blanchette-Mackie, and C. Londos. 1991. Perilipin, a major hormonally regulated adipocyte-specific phosphoprotein associated with the periphery of lipid storage droplets. *J. Biol. Chem.* 266:11341–11346.

Hansen, R.P. and F.B. Shorland. 1951. The branched chain fatty acids of butterfat II. Isolation of a multi-branched C20 saturated fatty acid fraction. *Biochem. J.* 50:358–360.

Hastings, N., M. Agaba, D.R. Tocher, M.J. Leaver, J.R. Dick, J.R. Sargent, and A.J. Teale. 2001. A vertebrate fatty acid desaturase with Δ5 and Δ6 activities. *Proc. Natl. Acad. Sci. USA* 98:14304–14309.

He, Q.H., X.F. Kong, G. Wu, P.P. Ren, H.R. Tang, F.H. Hao, R.L. Huang et al. 2009. Metabolomic analysis of the response of growing pigs to dietary L-arginine supplementation. *Amino Acids* 37:199–208.

Hegardt, F.G. 1999. Mitochondrial 3-hydroxy-3-methylglutaryl-CoA synthase: A control enzyme in ketogenesis. *Biochem. J.* 338:569–582.

Hermier, D. 1997. Lipoprotein metabolism and fattening in poultry. *J. Nutr.* 127:805S–808S.

Hou, T.Y., D.N. McMurray, and R.S. Chapkin. 2016. Omega-3 fatty acids, lipid rafts, and T cell signaling. *Eur. J. Pharmacol.* 785:2–9.

Huang, C.W., Y.S. Chien, Y.J. Chen, K.M. Ajuwon, H.M. Mersmann, and S.T. Ding. 2016. Role of n-3 polyunsaturated fatty acids in ameliorating the obesity-induced metabolic syndrome in animal models and humans. *Int. J. Mol. Sci.* 17:1689.

Iqbal, J. and M.M. Hussain. 2009. Intestinal lipid absorption. *Am. J. Physiol. Endocrinol. Metab.* 296:E1183–E1194.
Jansen, G.A. and R.J. Wanders. 2006. Alpha-oxidation. *Biochim. Biophys. Acta* 1763:1403–1412.
Jenkins, T.C. 1993. Lipid metabolism in the rumen. *J. Dairy Sci.* 76:3851–3863.
Jobgen, W.S., S.K. Fried, W.J. Fu, C.J. Meininger, and G. Wu. 2006. Regulatory role for the arginine-nitric oxide pathway in metabolism of energy substrates. *J. Nutr. Biochem.* 17:571–588.
Jump, D.B., S. Tripathy, and C.M. Depner. 2013. Fatty acid-regulated transcription factors in the liver. *Annu. Rev. Nutr.* 33:249–269.
Kashiwaya, Y., T. Takeshima, N. Mori, K. Nakashima, K. Clarke, and R.L. Veech. 2000. D-ß-hydroxybutyrate protects neurons in models of Alzheimer's and Parkinson's disease. *Proc. Natl. Acad. Sci. USA* 97:5440–5444.
Kawase, A., S. Hata, M. Takagi, and M. Iwaki. 2015. Pravastatin modulate Niemann-Pick C1-like 1 and ATP-binding cassette G5 and G8 to influence intestinal cholesterol absorption. *J. Pharm. Pharm. Sci.* 18:765–772.
Kersten, S. 2014. Physiological regulation of lipoprotein lipase. *Biochim. Biophys. Acta.* 1841:919–933.
Knoop, F. 1904. Der Abbau aromatischer Fettsäuren im Tierkörper. *Beitr. Chem. Physiol. Pathol.* 6:150–162.
Koeberle, A., K. Löser, and M. Thürmer. 2016. Stearoyl-CoA desaturase-1 and adaptive stress signaling. *Biochim. Biophys. Acta* 1861:1719–1726.
Kohan, A., S. Yoder, and P. Tso. 2010. Lymphatics in intestinal transport of nutrients and gastrointestinal hormones. *Ann. N.Y. Acad. Sci.* 1207 (Suppl. 1):E44–E51.
Kouba, M., J. Mourot, and P. Peiniau. 1997. Stearoyl-CoA desaturase activity in adipose tissues and liver of growing large white and Meishan pigs. *Comp. Biochem. Physiol. B* 118:509–514.
Kraemer, F.B. and W.J. Shen. 2002. Hormone-sensitive lipase: Control of intracellular tri-(di-) acylglycerol and cholesteryl ester hydrolysis. *J. Lipid Res.* 43:1585–1594.
Kramer, S.A., W.G. Bergen, A.L. Grant, and R.A. Merkel. 1993. Fatty acid profiles, lipogenesis, and lipolysis in lipid depots in finishing pigs treated with recombinant porcine somatotropin. *J. Anim. Sci.* 71:2066–2072.
Krieger, M. 1998. The "best" of cholesterols, the "worst" of cholesterols: A tale of two receptors. *Proc. Natl. Acad. Sci. USA* 95:4077–4080.
Kroetz, D.L. and F. Xu. 2005. Regulation and inhibition of arachidonic acid omega-hydroxylases and 20-HETE formation. *Annu. Rev. Pharmacol. Toxicol.* 45:413–438.
Kwon, H., T.E. Spencer, F.W. Bazer, and G. Wu. 2003. Developmental changes of amino acids in ovine fetal fluids. *Biol. Reprod.* 68:1813–1820.
Laplaud, P.M., D. Bauchart, D. Durand, and M.J. Chapman. 1990. Lipoproteins and apolipoproteins in intestinal lymph of the preruminant calf, 60s spp., at peak lipid absorption. *J. Lipid Res.* 31:1781–1792.
Lee, J., Y. Park, and S.I. Koo. 2012. ATP-binding cassette transporter A1 and HDL metabolism: Effects of fatty acids. *J. Nutr. Biochem.* 23:1–7.
Lee, M.J., P. Pramyothin, K. Karastergiou, and S.K. Fried. 2014. Deconstructing the roles of glucocorticoids in adipose tissue biology and the development of central obesity. *Biochim. Biophys. Acta* 1842:473–481.
Lehner, R. and Kuksis, A. 1993. Triacylglycerol synthesis by an sn-1,2(2,3)-diacylglycerol transacylase from rat intestinal microsomes. *J. Biol. Chem.* 268:8781–8786.
Li, D.F., R.C. Thaler, J.L. Nelssen, D.L. Harmon, G.L. Allee, and T.L. Weeden. 1990. Effect of fat sources and combinations on starter pig performance, nutrient digestibility and intestinal morphology. *J. Anim. Sci.* 68:3694–3704.
Li, Y., O. Monroig, L. Zhang, S. Wang, X. Zheng, J.R. Dick, C. You, and D.R. Tocher. 2010. Vertebrate fatty acyl desaturase with Δ4 activity. *Proc. Natl. Acad. Sci. USA* 107:16840–16845.
Lin, X., J. Bo, S.A. Oliver, B.A. Corl, S.K. Jacobi, W.T. Oliver, R.J. Harrell, and J. Odle. 2011. Dietary conjugated linoleic acid alters long chain polyunsaturated fatty acid metabolism in brain and liver of neonatal pigs. *J. Nutr. Biochem.* 22:1047–1054.
Lowe, M.E. 2002. The triglyceride lipases of the pancreas. *J. Lipid Res.* 43:2007–2016.
Lynen, F. and E. Reichert. 1951. Zur chemischen Struktur der, aktivierten Essigsäure. *Angew. Chem.* 63:47–48.
Macfarlane, D.P., S. Forbes, and B.R. Walker. 2008. Glucocorticoids and fatty acid metabolism in humans: Fuelling fat redistribution in the metabolic syndrome. *J. Endocrinol.* 197:189–204.
Manners, M.J. 1976. The development of digestive function in the pig. *Proc. Nutr. Soc.* 35:49–55.
Mayes, P.A. 1996a. Biosynthesis of fatty acids. In: *Harper's Biochemistry.* Edited by R.K. Murray, D.K. Granner, and V.W. Rodwell. Appleton & Lange, Stamford, CT, pp. 216–223.
Mayes, P.A. 1996b. Oxidation of fatty acids: Ketogenesis. In: *Harper's Biochemistry.* Edited by R.K. Murray, D.K. Granner, and V.W. Rodwell. Appleton & Lange, Stamford, CT, pp. 224–235.

McGarry, J.D. 1995. Malonyl-CoA and carnitine palmitoyltransferase I: An expanding partnership. *Biochem. Soc. Trans.* 23:481–485.

McKnight, J.R., M.C. Satterfield, W.S. Jobgen, S.B. Smith, T.E. Spencer, C.J. Meininger, C.J. McNeal, and G. Wu. 2010. Beneficial effects of L-arginine on reducing obesity: Potential mechanisms and important implications for human health. *Amino Acids* 39:349–357.

Minnich, A., N. Tian, L. Byan, and G. Bilder. 2001. A potent PPARalpha agonist stimulates mitochondrial fatty acid beta-oxidation in liver and skeletal muscle. *Am. J. Physiol. Endocrinol. Metab.* 280:E270–E279.

Nafikov, R.A. and D.C. Beitz. 2007. Carbohydrate and lipid metabolism in farm animals. *J. Nutr.* 137:702–705.

Nagy, H.M., M. Paar, C. Heier, T. Moustafa, P. Hofer, G. Haemmerle, A. Lass, R. Zechner, M. Oberer, and R. Zimmermann. 2014. Adipose triglyceride lipase activity is inhibited by long-chain acyl-coenzyme A. *Biochim. Biophys. Acta* 1841:588–594.

Nahle, Z., M. Hsieh, T. Pietka, C.T. Coburn, P.A. Grimaldi, M.Q. Zhang, D. Das, and N.A. Abumrad. 2008. CD36-dependent regulation of muscle FoxO1 and PDK4 in the PPAR delta/beta-mediated adaptation to metabolic stress. *J. Biol. Chem.* 283:14317–14326.

Nakamura, M.T. and T.Y. Nara. 2004. Structure, function, and dietary regulation of $\Delta^6$, $\Delta^5$, and $\Delta^9$ desaturases. *Annu. Rev. Nutr.* 24:345–376.

Ntambi, J.M. 1999. Regulation of stearoyl-CoA desaturase by polyunsaturated fatty acids and cholesterol. *J. Lipid Res.* 40:1549–1558.

Palmquist, D.L. 1988. The feeding value of fats. In: *Feed Science.* Edited by E.R. Ørskov. Elsevier Science Publishers B. V., New York, NY, pp. 293–311.

Park, H.G., W.J. Park, K.S. Kothapalli, and J.T. Brenna. 2015. The fatty acid desaturase 2 (*FADS2*) gene product catalyzes $\Delta^4$ desaturation to yield *n*-3 docosahexaenoic acid and *n*-6 docosapentaenoic acid in human cells. *FASEB J.* 29:3911–3919.

Pepino, M.Y., O. Kuda, D. Samovski, and N.A. Abumrad. 2014. Structure-function of CD36 and importance of fatty acid signal transduction in fat metabolism. *Annu. Rev. Nutr.* 34:281–303.

Perret, B., L. Mabile, L. Martinez, F. Tercé, R. Barbaras, and X. Collet. 2002. Hepatic lipase: Structure/function relationship, synthesis, and regulation. *J. Lipid Res.* 43:1163–1169.

Phan, C.T. and P. Tso. 2001. Intestinal lipid absorption and transport. *Front. Biosci.* 6:D299–D319.

Picard, F., D. Arsenijevic, D. Richard, and Y. Deshaies. 2002. Responses of adipose and muscle lipoprotein lipase to chronic infection and subsequent acute lipopolysaccharide challenge. *Clin. Vaccine Immunol.* 9:4771–4776.

Place, A.R. 1992. Comparative aspects of lipid digestion and absorption: Physiological correlates of wax ester digestion. *Am. J. Physiol.* 263:R464–R471.

Porter, J.W.G. 1969. Digestion in the pre-ruminant animal. *Proc. Nutr. Soc.* 28:115–121.

Powell, W.S. and J. Rokach. 2015. Biosynthesis, biological effects, and receptors of hydroxyeicosatetraenoic acids (HETEs) and oxoeicosatetraenoic acids (oxo-ETEs) derived from arachidonic acid. *Biochim. Biophys. Acta* 1851:340–355.

Price, E.R. 2017. The physiology of lipid storage and use in reptiles. *Biol. Rev. Camb. Philos. Soc.* 92:1406–1426. doi: 10.1111/brv.12288.

Price, N.T., V.N. Jackson, F.R. van der Leij, J.M. Cameron, M.T. Travers, B. Bartelds, N.C. Huijkman, and V.A. Zammit. 2003. Cloning and expression of the liver and muscle isoforms of ovine carnitine palmitoyltransferase 1: Residues within the N-terminus of the muscle isoform influence the kinetic properties of the enzyme. *Biochem. J.* 372:871–879.

Prior, R.L. and S.B. Smith. 1982. Hormonal effects on partitioning of nutrients for tissue growth: Role of insulin. *Fed. Proc.* 41:2545–2549.

Prior, R.L., S.B. Smith, and J.J. Jacobson. 1981. Metabolic pathways involved in lipogenesis from lactate and acetate in bovine adipose tissue: Effects of metabolic inhibitors. *Arch. Biochem. Biophys.* 211:202–210.

Puri, D., Ed. 2011. Lipid metabolism II: Lipoproteins, cholesterol and prostaglandins. In: *Textbook of Medical Biochemistry.* Elsevier, New York, NY, pp. 235–266.

Qiu, X., H. Hong, and S.L. MacKenzie. 2001. Identification of a $\Delta 4$ fatty acid desaturase from *Thraustochytrium* sp. involved in the biosynthesis of docosahexanoic acid by heterologous expression in *Saccharomyces cerevisiae* and *Brassica juncea. J. Biol. Chem.* 276:31561–31566.

Reddy, J.K. and T. Hashimoto. 2001. Peroxisomal ß-oxidation and peroxisome proliferator-activated receptor α: An adaptive metabolic system. *Annu. Rev. Nutr.* 21:193–230.

Reid, B.N., G.P. Ables, O.A. Otlivanchik, G. Schoiswohl, R. Zechner, W.S. Blaner, I.J. Goldberg, R.F. Schwabe, S.C. Chua, Jr., and L.S. Huang. 2008. Hepatic overexpression of hormone-sensitive lipase and adipose triglyceride lipase promotes fatty acid oxidation, stimulates direct release of free fatty acids, and ameliorates steatosis. *J. Biol. Chem.* 283:13087–13099.

Reisenberg, M., P.K. Singh, G. Williams, and P. Doherty. 2012. The diacylglycerol lipases: Structure, regulation and roles in and beyond endocannabinoid signaling. *Philos. Trans. R. Soc. Lond. B Biol. Sci.* 367:3264–3275.

Rezaei, R., Z.L. Wu, Y.Q. Hou, F.W. Bazer, and G. Wu. 2016. Amino acids and mammary gland development: Nutritional implications for neonatal growth. *J. Anim. Sci. Biotechnol.* 7:20.

Rivers, J.P.W., A.G. Hassam, M.A. Crawford, and M.R. Brambell. 1976. The inability of the lion (*Panthero leo*, L.) to desaturate linoleic acid. *FEBS Lett.* 67:269–270.

Rivers, J.P.W., A.J. Sinclair, and M.A. Crawford. 1975. Inability of the cat to desaturate essential fatty acids. *Nature* 258:171–173.

Robinson, A.M. and D.H. Williamson. 1980. Physiological roles of ketone bodies as substrates and signals in mammalian tissues. *Physiol. Rev.* 60:143–187.

Rosero, D.S., E. van Heugten, J. Odle, R. Cabrera, C. Arellano, and R.D. Boyd. 2012. Sow and litter response to supplemental dietary fat in lactation diets during high ambient temperatures. *J. Anim. Sci.* 90:550–559.

Rust, M.B. 2002. Nutritional physiology. *Fish Nutr.* 3:367–452.

Saha, A.K., T.G. Kurowski, and N.B. Ruderman. 1995. A malonyl-CoA fuel-sensing mechanism in muscle: Effects of insulin, glucose, and denervation. *Am. J. Physiol.* 269:E283–E289.

Sanderson, J.T. 2006. The steroid hormone biosynthesis pathway as a target for endocrine-disrupting chemicals. *Toxicol. Sci.* 94:3–21.

Sanz, M., C.J. Lopez-Bote, D. Menoyo, and J.M. Bautista. 2000. Abdominal fat deposition and fatty acid synthesis are lower and beta-oxidation is higher in broiler chickens fed diets containing unsaturated rather than saturated fat. *J. Nutr.* 130:3034–3037.

Semenkovich, C.F., S.H. Chen, M. Wims, C.C. Luo, W.H. Li, and L. Chan. 1989. Lipoprotein lipase and hepatic lipase mRNA tissue specific expression, developmental regulation, and evolution. *J. Lipid Res.* 30:423–431.

Serhan, C.N. 2014. Pro-resolving lipid mediators are leads for resolution physiology. *Nature* 510:92–101.

Sinclair, A.J., J.G. McLean, and E.A. Monger. 1979. Metabolism of linoleic acid in the cat. *Lipids* 14:932–936.

Sire, M.F., C. Lutton, and J.M. Vernier. 1981. New views on intestinal absorption of lipids in teleostan fishes: An ultrastructural and biochemical study in the rainbow trout. *J. Lipid Res.* 22:81–94.

Smith, S.B. 2013. Functional development of stearoyl-CoA desaturase gene expression in livestock species. In: *Stearoyl-CoA Desaturase in Lipid Metabolism.* Edited by J.M. Ntambi. Springer, New York, NY, pp. 141–160.

Smith, S.B. and R.L. Prior. 1981. Evidence for a functional ATP-citrate lyase:NADP-malate dehydrogenase pathway in bovine adipose tissue: Enzyme and metabolite levels. *Arch. Biochem. Biophys.* 211:192–201.

Smith, S.B. and R.L. Prior. 1986. Comparisons of lipogenesis and glucose metabolism between ovine and bovine adipose tissues. *J. Nutr.* 116:1279–1286.

Spector, A.A. and H.Y. Kim. 2015. Discovery of essential fatty acids. *J. Lipid Res.* 56:11–21.

Steffensen, J.F. and J.P. Lomholt. 1992. The secondary vascular system. *Fish Physiol.* 12A:185–217.

Storch, J. and B. Corsico. 2008. The emerging functions and mechanisms of mammalian fatty acid-binding proteins. *Annu. Rev. Nutr.* 28:73–95.

Tan, B.E., X.G. Li, Y.L. Yin, Z.L. Wu, C. Liu, C.D. Tekwe, and G. Wu. 2012. Regulatory roles for L-arginine in reducing white adipose tissue. *Front. Biosci.* 17:2237–2246.

Tan, B.E., Y.L. Yin, Z.Q. Liu, X.G. Li, H.J. Xu, X.F. Kong, R.L. Huang et al. 2009. Dietary L-arginine supplementation increases muscle gain and reduces body fat mass in growing-finishing pigs. *Amino Acids* 37:169–175.

Tatsuta, T., M. Scharwey, and T. Langer. 2014. Mitochondrial lipid trafficking. *Trends Cell Biol.* 24:44–52.

Tekwe, C.D., J. Lei, K. Yao, R. Rezaei, X.L. Li, S. Dahanayaka, R.J. Carroll, C.J. Meininger, F.W. Bazer, and G. Wu. 2013. Oral administration of interferon tau enhances oxidation of energy substrates and reduces adiposity in Zucker diabetic fatty rats. *BioFactors* 39:552–563.

Teshima, S. and A. Kanazawa. 1971. Biosynthesis of sterols in the lobster, *Panirlirus japonica*, the prawn, *Penaeus japonicus*, and the crab, *Porturius trituberculatus*. *Comp. Biochem. Physiol.* 38B:597–602.

Thompson, J.R. and G. Wu. 1991. The effect of ketone bodies on nitrogen metabolism in skeletal muscle. *Comp. Biochem. Physiol. B* 100:209–216.

Thomson, A.B.R. and J.M. Dietschy. 1981. Intestinal lipid absorption: Major extracellular and intracellular events. In: *Physiology of the Gastrointestinal Tract.* Edited by L.R. Johnson. Raven Press, New York, NY, pp. 1147–1220.

Titus, E. and G.A. Ahearn. 1991. Transepithelial acetate transport in a herbivorous teleost: Anion exchange at the basolateral membrane. *J. Exp. Biol.* 156:41–61.

Tocher, D.R. and B.D. Glencross. 2015. Lipids and fatty acids. In: *Dietary Nutrients, Additives, and Fish Health*. Edited by C.S. Lee, C. Lim, D.M. Gatlin, and C.D. Webster. John Wiley & Sons, Hoboken, NJ, pp. 47–94.

Tocher, D.R. and J.R. Sargent. 1984. Studies on triacylglycerol wax ester and sterol ester hydrolases in intestinal caeca of rainbow trout (*Salmo gairdneri*) fed diets rich in triacylglyceols and wax esters. *Comp. Biochem. Physiol.* 77B:561–571.

Tso, P., M. Liu, T.J. Kalogeris, and A.B. Thomson. 2001. The role of apolipoprotein A-IV in the regulation of food intake. *Annu. Rev. Nutr.* 21:231–254.

Tso, P. and M. Liu. 2004. Ingested fat and satiety. *Physiol. Behav.* 8:275–287.

Turgeon, D., S. Chouinard, P. Bélanger, S. Picard, J.F. Labbé, P. Borgeat, and A. Bélanger. 2003. Glucuronidation of arachidonic and linoleic acid metabolites by human UDP-glucuronosyltransferases. *J. Lipid Res.* 44:1182–1191.

Turner, N.D. and J.R. Lupton. 2011. Dietary fiber. *Adv. Nutr.* 2:151–152.

Van Veldhoven, P.P. 2010. Biochemistry and genetics of inherited disorders of peroxisomal fatty acid metabolism. *J. Lipid Res.* 51:2863–2895.

Vance, J.E. and G. Tasseva. 2013. Formation and function of phosphatidylserine and phosphatidylethanolamine in mammalian cells. *Biochim. Biophys. Acta* 1831:543–554.

Velazquez, O.C., R.W. Seto, and J.L. Rombeau. 1996. The scientific rationale and clinical application of short-chain fatty acids and medium-chain triacylglycerols. *Proc. Nutr. Soc.* 55:49–78.

Vesper, H., E.M. Schmelz, M.N. Nikolova-Karakashian, D.L. Dillehay, D.V. Lynch, and A.H. Merrill, Jr. 1999. Sphingolipids in food and the emerging importance of sphingolipids to nutrition. *J. Nutr.* 129:1239–1250.

Wang, F., A.B. Kohan, C.M. Lo, M. Liu, P. Howles, and P. Tso. 2015. Apolipoprotein A-IV: A protein intimately involved in metabolism. *J. Lipid Res.* 56:1403–1418.

Wray-Cahen, D., F.R. Dunshea, R.D. Boyd, A.W. Bell, and D.E. Bauman. 2012. Porcine somatotropin alters insulin response in growing pigs by reducing insulin sensitivity rather than changing responsiveness. *Domest. Anim. Endocrinol.* 43:37–46.

Wu, G. 2013. *Amino Acids: Biochemistry and Nutrition*. CRC Press, Boca Raton, FL.

Wu, G., A. Gunasekara, H. Brunengraber, and E.B. Marliss. 1991. Effects of extracellular pH, $CO_2$, and $HCO_3^-$ on ketogenesis in perfused rat liver. *Am. J. Physiol.* 261:E221–E226.

Wu, G. and J.R. Thompson. 1987. Ketone bodies inhibit leucine degradation in chick skeletal muscle. *Int. J. Biochem.* 19:937–943.

Xu, C., J. He, H. Jiang, L. Zu, W. Zhai, S. Pu, and G. Xu. 2009. Direct effect of glucocorticoids on lipolysis in adipocytes. *Mol. Endocrinol.* 23:1161–1170.

Xu, X., R. Li, G. Chen, S.L. Hoopes, D.C. Zeldin, and D.W. Wang. 2016. The role of cytochrome P450 epoxygenases, soluble epoxide hydrolase, and epoxyeicosatrienoic acids in metabolic diseases. *Adv. Nutr.* 7:1122–1128.

Yang, P. and P.V. Subbaiah. 2015. Regulation of hepatic lipase activity by sphingomyelin in plasma lipoproteins. *Biochim. Biophys. Acta* 1851:1327–1336.

Yeaman, S.J. 1990. Hormone-sensitive lipase—A multipurpose enzyme in lipid metabolism. *Biochim. Biophys. Acta* 1052:128–132.

Yen, C.E., D.W. Nelson, and M.I. Yen. 2015. Intestinal triacylglycerol synthesis in fat absorption and systemic energy metabolism. *J. Lipid Res.* 56:489–501.

Zeisel, S.H. 1981. Dietary choline: Biochemistry, physiology, and pharmacology. *Annu. Rev. Nutr.* 1:95–121.

# 7 Nutrition and Metabolism of Protein and Amino Acids

Protein, which consists of amino acids (AAs) linked by peptide bonds, is a major component of animals. The growth of organisms depends on the deposition of protein in their tissues, such as the placenta, skeletal muscle, and small intestine (Bergen 2008; Buttery 1983; Reeds et al. 1993). Dietary protein is hydrolyzed by proteases and peptidases (oligo-, tri-, and di-peptidases) to generate tripeptides, dipeptides, and free AAs in the lumen of the gastrointestinal tract. These digestion products are either utilized by bacteria in the small intestine or absorbed into enterocytes (Dai et al. 2011). The absorbed AAs that are not degraded by the small intestine enter the portal vein for utilization (including protein synthesis) by extraintestinal tissues. Except for the absorption of intact immunoglobulins by the small intestine of mammalian neonates, dietary protein has no nutritive value to animals unless it is digested. Thus, animals have dietary requirements for AAs but not protein (Chiba et al. 1991; Wu et al. 2014a). The content, digestibility, and proportions of AAs in dietary protein are the determinants of its nutritive quality.

AAs contain nitrogen and sulfur, as well as hydrocarbon skeletons, and cannot be replaced by any other nutrients (e.g., carbohydrates and lipids). Whether or not the hydrocarbon skeletons are synthesized *de novo* by animal cells depends on the AA and animal species (Baker 2009; Reeds et al. 2000). Adequate intake of dietary AAs is essential for the optimal growth, development, and health of all animals. Thus, protein undernutrition causes stunting, anemia, physical weakness, edema, vascular dysfunction, and impaired immunity (Waterlow 1995). However, excess protein intake results in wasting and environmental nitrogen pollution, as well as digestive, hepatic, renal, and vascular abnormalities. Therefore, optimizing the recommendations of dietary AA requirements for animals is important for maximizing their growth, production performance, and feed efficiency, while improving their health and resistance to infectious disease.

AAs were traditionally classified as nutritionally essential or nonessential for animals solely based on nitrogen balance or growth. The so-called "nutritionally nonessential AAs" (NEAAs) have not been considered by the U.S. National Research Council (NRC) for any species because they were tactically assumed to be sufficiently synthesized *de novo*. However, a growing body of the literature shows that this assumption is invalid, because the supply of the synthesizable AAs in diets cannot maximally support the survival, growth, reproduction, or lactation performance of animals (Hou et al. 2015; McKnight et al. 2010). The different functions of individual AAs beyond serving as the building blocks for proteins must be considered when formulating diets for livestock, avian, and aquatic species, as well as companion animals, to improve the efficiency of nutrient utilization and well being (Wang et al. 2017; Wu 2013). It is now recognized that animals do have dietary requirements of all proteinogenic AAs and that the long-standing term "NEAAs" is a misnomer in nutritional sciences (Hou and Wu 2017). These key aspects of AA nutrition and metabolism in animals are highlighted in this chapter. The standard abbreviations of all AAs (Chapter 4) are used throughout the text to facilitate its reading.

## DIGESTION AND ABSORPTION OF PROTEIN IN NONRUMINANTS

On an as-fed basis, swine diets usually contain 12%–20% crude protein (CP): for example, 20% at weaning (21 days of age); 14% during the finishing period; 12% during gestation; and 18% during lactation. CP content (on an as-fed basis) in chicken diets is usually 22%, 20%, and 18%, respectively, for starters (1–21 days of age), growers (22–35 days of age), and finishers (36–49 days of age).

Equine diets usually contain 12%–14% CP, but horses can digest 20% protein in diets (on a dry matter [DM] basis). Fish diets usually contain 30%–50% CP, depending on species. In nonruminants, some digestion of dietary protein starts in the stomach and most digestion occurs in the small intestine. Events of this process include: (1) denaturing of dietary protein and activation of zymogens by gastric acid in the stomach, followed by local digestion with active gastric proteases to form large peptides; and (2) hydrolysis of the large peptides and the undigested proteins in the small intestine by the pancreas- and enterocyte-derived proteases. Proteases are enzymes that degrade proteins by hydrolysis of peptide bonds, whereas oligo-, tri-, and di-peptidases hydrolyze oligo-, tri- and di-peptides, respectively. The protein digestion products are absorbed into the enterocytes via AA and peptide transporters (Matthews 2000). An overview of protein digestion and absorption is outlined in Figure 7.1. Among the different segments of the small intestine, the jejunum is the major site for terminal protein digestion and the absorption of the digestion products, but these processes also take place in the duodenum and ileum. The digestibility of dietary protein is affected by biological (e.g., species and strains of animals, physiological status, and individual variations), environmental (e.g., ambient temperatures, pollution, and noise), and dietary factors (e.g., the form, odor, texture, and particle size of feed) (Sauer et al. 2000).

## Digestion of Protein in the Stomach of Nonruminants

### Secretion of Gastric Hydrochloric Acid

In nonruminants, the digestion of dietary protein in the stomach requires not only active gastric proteases (pepsins and rennin) but also hydrochloric acid (HCl). This acid is produced from NaCl and

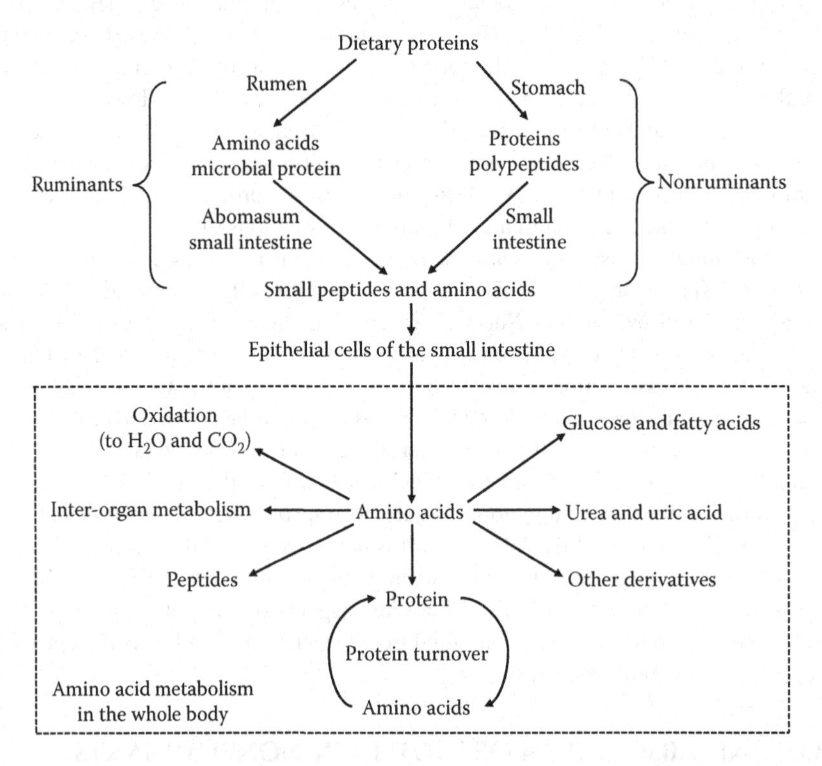


**FIGURE 7.1** Overall view of protein metabolism in animals. Ruminants digest dietary protein in the rumen, as well as rumen-escaped and microbial proteins in the abomasum and the small intestine. In nonruminants, the digestion of dietary protein is initiated in the stomach and completed in the small intestine. In all animals, the products of protein digestion (small peptides and free AAs) are absorbed into the epithelial cells (enterocytes) of the small intestine, and utilized by the whole body.

carbonic acid ($H_2CO_3$) by parietal cells in the gastric glands of the stomach to create an acidic environment (e.g., pH = 2–2.5 in adults; equivalent to $10^{-2}$–$10^{-2.5}$ M HCl). The stimulatory or inhibitory factors for the control of gastric acid secretion act primarily through affecting the production of gastrin (stimulatory) or somatostatin (inhibitory) in the mucosa of the stomach and duodenum (Figure 7.2).

1. *Stimuli of gastric acid secretion.* Neural, hormonal, and nutritional stimuli of gastric secretion enhance the generation of one or more of the following molecules: (1) gastrin (endocrine; secreted by gastrin G-cells; primary stimulus); (2) acetylcholine (neurocrine; released by the vagus nerve and enteric system); and (3) histamine (nutritional and paracrine; released from gastric enterochromaffin-like cells) (Cranwell 1995; Yen 2001). These signaling molecules bind to their respective receptors on the plasma membrane of the parietal cell to increase histamine release and cAMP production (Figure 7.2).
2. *Inhibitors of gastric acid secretion.* The factors inhibiting gastric HCl secretion include: (1) slow gastric emptying; (2) high $H^+$ concentrations in gastric and duodenal contents (stimulating secretin release); (3) some nutritional factors (e.g., dietary protein and fat intakes, and feed particle size); and (4) many gastrointestinal peptides of different sources

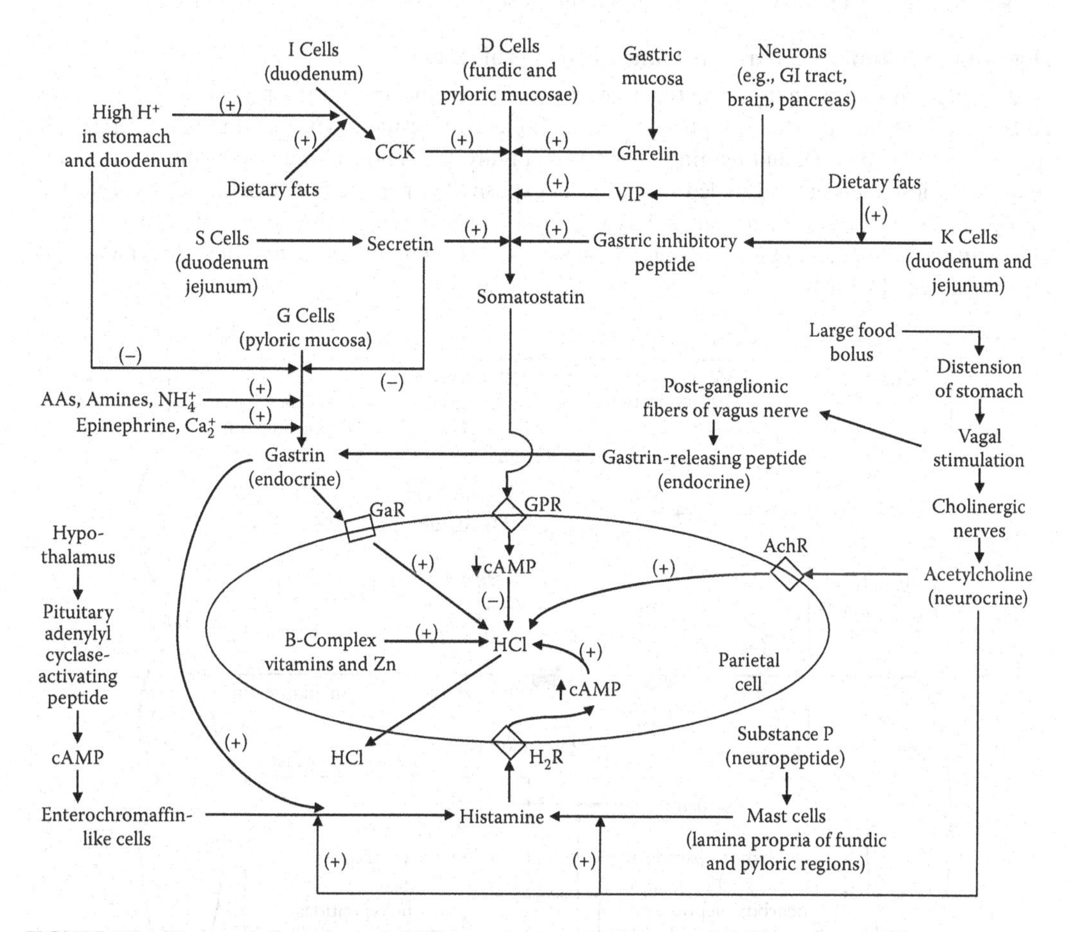


**FIGURE 7.2** The regulation of gastric HCl secretion by stimulatory or inhibitory factors. These factors act primarily through affecting the production of gastrin (stimulatory) or somatostatin (inhibitory) by the mucosae of the stomach and the duodenum. AAs, amino acids; AchR, acetylcholine receptor; CCK, cholecystokinin; GI, gastrointestinal; GaP, gastrin receptor; GPR, G protein-coupled receptor; VIP, vasoactive intestinal peptide. (+), stimulatory; (−), inhibitory.

(Figure 7.2). Examples of these peptides are secretin (released by D-cells in the duodenum and jejunum), gastric inhibitory peptide (GIP, also known as glucose-dependent insulinotropic peptide; released by K-cells in the duodenum and jejunum), vasoactive intestinal peptide (released by the gastrointestinal tract, brain, pancreas, heart, and many other tissues), peptide YY (released by L-cells of the ileal mucosa), and somatostatin (secreted by endocrine cells of the gastric epithelium; a primary inhibitor). Secretin, GIP, and vasoactive intestinal peptide all stimulate the release of somatostatin, which binds to the G protein-coupled receptor on the plasma membrane of parietal cells on the stomach mucosa and inhibits adenylyl cyclase activity (i.e., cAMP production).

Different dietary factors inhibit gastric HCl secretion through different mechanisms. Examples include: (1) food-induced distension through mechanoreceptors to stimulate secretin release; (2) high concentrations of fat digestion products through the activation of cholecystokinin (CCK) release from intestinal enteroendocrine I cells in the duodenum; (3) dietary deficiencies of protein, zinc, and B-complex vitamins by impairing various metabolic pathways; (4) a large size of feed particles due to their rapid passage out of the stomach and possible damage to its epithelium; and (5) a small size of feed particles because of their prolonged retention in the stomach (particularly the esophageal region) and damage to its epithelium (gastric ulceration) (Rojas and Stein 2017).

## Digestive Function of Gastric HCl and Gastric Proteases

Gastric HCl has two main digestive functions: (a) to convert inactive gastric proteases (pepsinogens A, B, C, and D, and pro-rennin [pro-chymosin]; collectively called zymogens) to active proteases (pepsins A, B, C, and D, and rennin [chymosin]) (Figure 7.3); and (b) to denature dietary proteins so that they lose their natural folded structures to expose their peptide bonds to the active proteases for hydrolysis. All these zymogens are synthesized and released by the chief cells of the gastric glands in the fundic and pyloric regions (Cranwell 1995). Rennin is a mammalian enzyme and is not synthesized by birds.

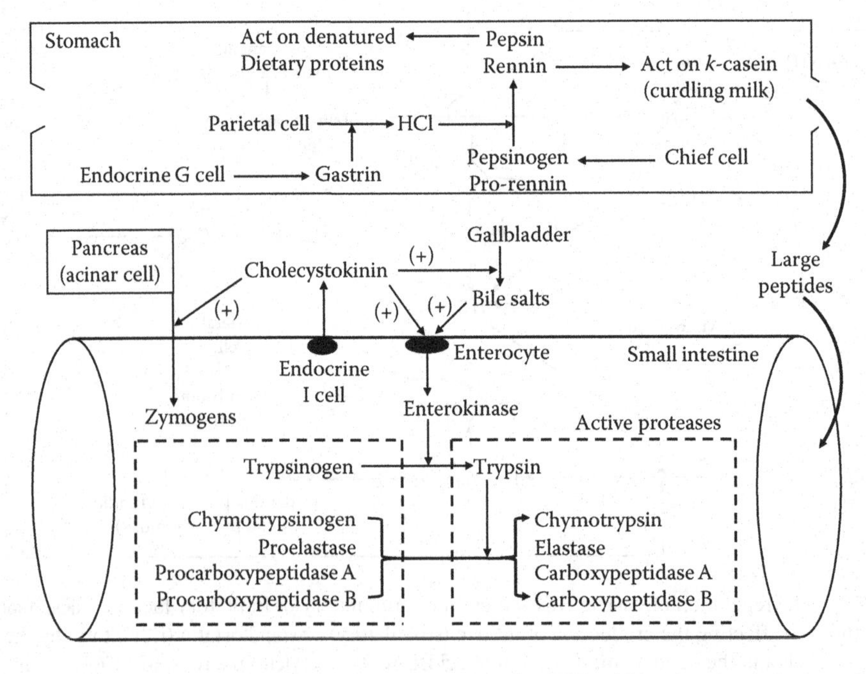


**FIGURE 7.3** Conversion of zymogens to active proteases by HCl within the stomach through limited auto-catalysis.

The pancreatic protease precursors are activated by gastric HCl through limited autocatalysis. Pepsin A (optimum pH = 2) is the major type of pepsin. As endopeptidases, pepsins break down peptide bonds between a hydrophobic AA and a preferably aromatic AA (e.g., Phe, Trp, or Tyr) from the inside of protein to generate large peptides (Figure 7.4). Pepsins are inhibited by high pH and by pepstatin. The latter is a hexapeptide that contains an unusual AA, statine [(3S,4S)-4-amino-3-hydroxy-6-methylheptanoic acid)], and was originally isolated from the cultures of *Actinomyces*.

## Developmental Changes of Gastric Proteases in Nonruminant Mammals

Not all aspects of developmental changes in gastric proteases are known for each species. Available data from most species studied to date indicate that the abundances of pepsinogens A, B, and C in the stomach are very low at birth but increase markedly after birth. For example, in pigs, pepsinogens A and C in the stomach are barely detectable at birth, but their concentrations (mg/g tissue) increase progressively in the entire mucosa of the gastric fundic region between birth and day 160 of age (Cranwell 1995). Likewise, in pigs, pepsinogen B in the entire mucosa of the fundic region of the stomach is negligible at birth and increases markedly between birth and day 30 of age. Of note, the concentration of the mucosal pepsinogen B (mg/g tissue) peaks at day 30 of age, then declines progressively to a medium level at day 60 of age, and thereafter remains at the medium level until day 160 of age. Starting from day 30 of age, pepsinogen A is the most abundant gastric protease in the gastric mucosa of pigs among all the zymogens.

Enteral feeding and glucocorticoids play an important role in the induction of gastric pepsinogens A, B, and C in postnatal animals. In contrast, the expression of gastric pro-rennin increases progressively in fetal pigs during the last trimester of gestation and peaks at birth (Yen 2001). As a result, in pigs, the concentration of pro-rennin (mg/g tissue) in the entire wall of the fundic region of the stomach is greatest at birth but declines progressively to a very low level at day 60 of age, and then remains at the minimal level until day 160 of age. These patterns in the development of gastric

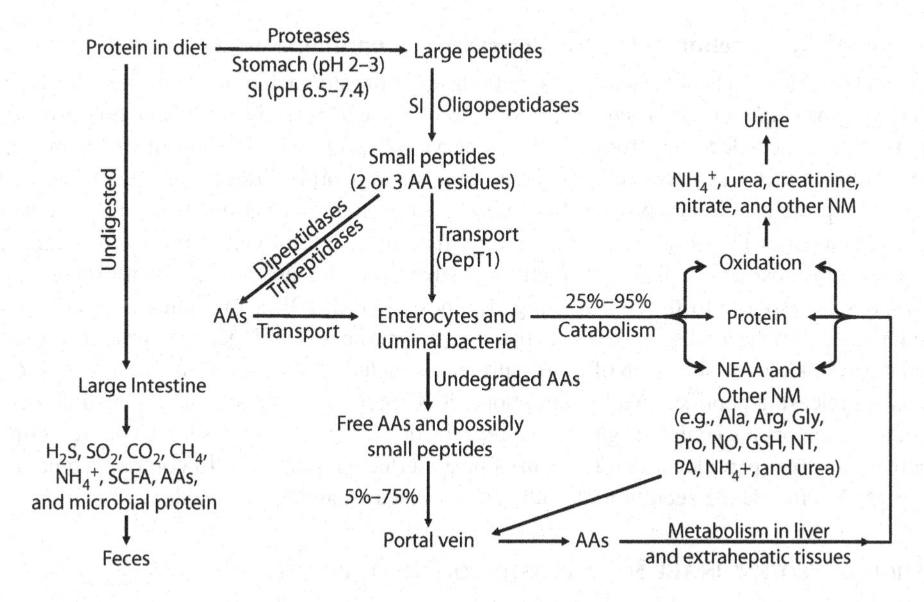


**FIGURE 7.4** Digestion of dietary protein in the gastrointestinal tract of the small intestine in monogastric animals, including humans. All diet-derived AAs undergo various degrees of catabolism by luminal bacteria and some of them are oxidized by enterocytes. For example, 95% of dietary glutamate is utilized by the small intestine, and only 5% of dietary glutamate enters the portal circulation. AA metabolites are excreted in feces and urine. AAs, amino acids; GSH, glutathione; NEAA, nutritionally nonessential AAs; NM, nitrogenous metabolites; NT, nucleotides; PepT1, $H^+$ gradient-driven peptide transporter 1; SCFA, short-chain fatty acids; SI, small intestine.

zymogens play an important role in the adaptation of mammals to the shift of dietary protein source from milk to primarily ingredients of plant origin.

As noted previously, the amount of rennin within the stomach of adult mammals is low or negligible. However, rennin (optimum pH = 3–4) plays a crucial role in curdling or coagulating milk proteins in the stomach of mammalian neonates. Rennin has a weak proteolytic activity. There are three isoforms for rennin, that is, rennins A, B, and C (Rampilli et al. 2004). The majority of milk protein is casein, which exists in four major types: α-s1, α-s2, β, and κ. In milk, κ casein interacts with α and β caseins to form water-soluble micelles. As an endopeptidase, rennin partially degrades the κ casein, converting it into para-κ casein and a smaller protein (Brinkhuis and Payens 1985). Consequently, para-κ casein cannot stabilize the micellar structure of caseins, resulting in the precipitation of the hydrophobic α and β caseins by $Ca^{2+}$ to form a curd. The casein curd is then degraded by pepsins to yield large peptides. If milk proteins are not coagulated in the stomach, they will rapidly flow out of the stomach and will not be subject to initial digestion by pepsins, and may also pass through the small intestine quickly. In animals that lack rennin, milk is partially coagulated by the action of pepsins.

### Developmental Changes of Gastric Proteases in Avian Species

Avian species exhibit a different pattern of changes in the development of gastric proteases than mammals. Studies with chickens and quails indicate that the specific activities of pepsinogens A, B, and C in the proventriculus (glandular stomach) increase progressively during embryonic development (Yasugi and Mizuno 1981) and reach a temporary peak several days before hatching. Interestingly, in both chickens and quails, the specific activities of the gastric acid proteases increase 30-fold within 24 h after hatching, in comparison with the values at birth, regardless of enteral feeding. The rapid shift in the expression of these gastric enzymes is likely mediated by hormones, such as glucocorticoids. This, along with the grinding function of the gizzard, prepares the birds for post-hatching consumption and utilization of solid foods.

### Regulation of the Secretion of Gastric Proteases in Nonruminants

The amounts and activities of proteases and peptidases in the stomach of nonruminants are affected by: (1) dietary protein intake, (2) gene expression in response to enteral feeding and glucocorticoids, (3) the release of acetylcholine from the vagus nerve, (4) acid concentration in the stomach, and (5) the secretion of CCK, gastrin, and other gastrointestinal peptides (Raufman 1992). Since gastric proteases are proteins, dietary provision of AAs has a profound effect on stimulating the synthesis of these enzymes by the chief cells of the gastric mucosa (San Gabriel and Uneyama 2013). For example, in most teleost fish, pancreatic digestive proteases are produced and secreted from the pancreas in response to the first feeding (Rønnestad et al. 2013). In addition, dietary protein intake increases gastric acid secretion to activate gastric proteases and facilitate protein hydrolysis. Factors that stimulate the secretion of gastric proteases include AAs, histamine, acetylcholine, gastrin, gastrin-releasing peptide, vagal stimulation, CCK, secretin, and vasoactive intestinal peptide. Most of these factors also enhance gastric acid production; some exceptions are CCK, secretin, and vasoactive intestinal peptide, which have an opposite effect (Figure 7.2). In contrast, somatostatin and peptide YY inhibit the secretion of both gastric proteases and gastric acid.

## Digestion of Proteins in the Small Intestine of Nonruminants

### Flow of Digesta from the Stomach into the Small Intestine for Proteolysis

Dietary proteins that are resistant to pepsins in the stomach, together with the large polypeptides resulting from the enzymatic hydrolysis by pepsins in the stomach, enter the duodenum. In the lumen of the duodenum, the proteins and the large polypeptides are further broken down by pancreas- and intestine mucosa-derived proteolytic enzymes in the alkaline medium (owing to bile salts, pancreatic juice, and duodenal secretions) (see the sections below). The extracellular proteolysis occurring in the duodenum is limited due to the short length of this intestinal segment in animals (Barrett 2014). The chyme moves into the jejunum, where most proteolysis takes place due to its long length and high protease activities. Continuous digestion of protein and polypeptides can occur in the ileum if their degradation is not completed in the jejunum.

### Release of Pancreactic Pro-Proteases into the Lumen of the Duodenum

The acinar cells of the pancreas secrete inactive proteases (pro-proteases) into the lumen of the duodenum. They are the zymogens of endopeptidases (trypsin, chymotrypsins A, B, and C, and elastase) and exopeptidases (carboxypeptidases A and B) (Table 7.1). These inactive enzymes become active in the duodenal lumen by a cascade of limited proteolysis (the removal of an N-terminal oligopeptide [2–6 AA residues] from each zymogen). First, enterokinase, which is synthesized and

**TABLE 7.1**
**Digestive Proteases and Peptidases in the Stomach and the Small Intestine**

| Enzyme | Site of Production | Recognized Amino Acid Residues in Peptide Bonds | pH of Optimal Activity |
|---|---|---|---|
| | **(1) Proteases in the Lumen of the Stomach** | | |
| Pepsins A, B, C, and D[a] | Mucosa of stomach | Aromatic and hydrophobic AAs (most efficient) | 1.8–2 |
| Renins A, B, and C[a] | Mucosa of stomach | Weak proteolytic activity; clot milk protein | 1.8–2 |
| | **(2) Proteases in the Lumen of the Small Intestine** | | |
| Trypsin[a] | Pancreas | Arginine and lysine | 8–9 |
| Chymotrypsins A, B, and C[a] | Pancreas | Aromatic AAs and methionine | 8–9 |
| Elastase[a] | Pancreas | Aliphatic AAs | 8–9 |
| Carboxypeptidase A[b] | Pancreas | Aromatic AAs | 7.2 |
| Carboxypeptidase B[b] | Pancreas | Arginine and lysine | 8.0 |
| Aminopeptidases[b] | Enterocytes (small intestine) | AAs with free $NH_2$ groups | 7.0–7.4 |
| | **(3) Oligopeptidases, Tripeptidases, and Dipeptidases in the Lumen of the Small Intestine** | | |
| Oligopeptidase A | Enterocytes | A broad spectrum of oligopeptides | 6.5–7.0 |
| Oligopeptidase B | Enterocytes | Basic AAs in oligopeptides | 6.5–7.0 |
| Oligopeptidase P | Enterocytes | Pro or OH-Pro In oligopeptides | 6.5–7.0 |
| Dipeptidases | Enterocytes | Dipeptides (not containing imino acids) | 6.5–7.5 |
| Tripeptidases | Enterocytes | Dipeptides (not containing imino acids) | 6.5–7.5 |
| Prolidase I (dipeptidase)[c] | Enterocytes | Proline or hydroxyproline | 7.2 |
| Prolidase II (dipeptidase)[d] | Enterocytes | X-Hydroxyproline | 8.0 |

[a] Endopeptidase (also called proteinase in the literature).

[b] Exopeptidase (a metalloprotease). Examples are aminopeptidases A, B, N, L, and P, which cleave an acidic AA (e.g., Asp or Glu), basic AA (e.g., Arg or Lys), neutral AA (e.g., Ala or Met), Leu, and Pro, respectively, from the N-terminus of a polypeptide. Aminopeptidase M removes any unsubstituted AA (including Ala and Pro) from the N-terminal position of a polypeptide; it is both an amino- and an imino-peptidase.

[c] Reacts with all imino dipeptides at high activity.

[d] Exhibits very low activity toward Gly-Pro, and reacts with X (a non-glycine AA; e.g., methionine or phenylalanine)-Hydroxyproline at high activity.

released by enterocytes of the duodenum, converts trypsinogen into trypsin (the active enzyme) through the removal of an N-terminal hexapeptide. Trypsin then converts other pancreatic zymogens into active forms, such as chymotrypsins A, B, and C, elastase, and carboxypeptidases A and B. This series of protease activations is controlled by bile acids and CCK, which stimulate the production of enterokinase by the duodenal enterocytes and of proteases by the pancreas (Figure 7.1). The active pancreatic proteases are present in the small-intestinal lumen, and some of them may be associated with the brush-border surface of the enterocyte.

### Release of Proteases and Oligopeptidases from the Small-Intestinal Mucosa into the Intestinal Lumen

The mucosae of the duodenum, jejunum, and ileum release the active forms of proteases and oligopeptidases into the brush-border surface, some of which are present in the intestinal lumen. Therefore, no activation of these enzymes is required for their proteolytic actions. Aminopeptidases are exopeptidases that hydrolyze a protein or large peptide from the N-terminus. While some of the intestinal aminopeptidases (e.g., aminopeptidases A, B, N, and P) have a broad substrate specificity, others (e.g., Ala aminopeptidase, Leu aminopeptidase, Met aminopeptidase, and *N*-formylmethionine aminopeptidase) are highly specific toward the N-terminus containing a specific AA (e.g., Ala, Leu, Met, or formylmethionine) (Giuffrida et al. 2014; Sherriff et al. 1992). Of note, *N*-formylmethionyl oligopeptides arise from N-terminal peptide sequences of bacterial precursor proteins. As their names imply, aminopeptidases A, B, and N cleave peptide bonds at the N-terminus adjacent to an anionic (A), basic (B), or neutral (N) AA, respectively. Aminopeptidase P cleaves a peptide bond at the N-terminus adjacent to proline or hydroxyproline. Many, but not all, of the aminopeptidases are zinc metalloenzymes.

Oligopeptidases hydrolyze peptide bonds in oligopeptides consisting of 2–20 AA residues (Giuffrida et al. 2014). Oligopeptidase A acts on a broad spectrum of oligopeptide substrates. However, Oligopeptidase B hydrolyzes a peptide bond containing a basic AA in an oligopeptide, and prolyl oligopeptidase (prolyl endopeptidase) cleaves Pro or OH-Pro from the inside of an oligopeptide. As alluded to previously, oligopeptidases are bound to the brush-border surface of enterocytes.

### Extracellular Hydrolysis of Proteins and Polypeptides in the Small Intestine

All the proteases and peptidases present in the small intestine have an optimum pH ranging from 6.5 to 9.0, which is similar to the luminal fluid pH of the duodenum (pH 6.5), jejunum (pH 7.0), and the terminal ileum (pH 7.4) in nonruminants, mammals, and birds, and of the intestine of many fish species (pH 6.5–7.4). Trypsin, chymotrypsins, and elastase (all endopeptidases) specifically cleave AA residues in peptide bonds residing inside a protein or polypeptide; namely, basic AAs, aromatic AAs plus Met, and aliphatic AAs, respectively (Figure 7.5). Carboxypeptidases A and B (exopeptidases) catalyze, respectively, the hydrolysis of an aromatic (or aliphatic) AA (e.g., Phe or Ala) and a basic AA (Lys, Arg, or His) from the C-terminal position of a protein or polypeptide (Figure 7.5). Aminopeptidases (exopeptidases) cleave an AA from the N-terminal position of a polypeptide. For example, aminopeptidases A, B, N, L, and P remove an acidic AA (e.g., Asp or Glu), basic AA (e.g., Arg or Lys), neutral AA (e.g., Ala or Met), Leu, or Pro, respectively, from the N-terminus of a polypeptide. Interestingly, aminopeptidase M (originally found in the so-called microsomes) cleaves any unsubstituted AA (including Ala and Pro) from the N-terminal position of a polypeptide and therefore acts as both an amino- and an imino-peptidase.

Through their collective actions, the proteases present in the small intestine ultimately generate oligopeptides. The latter are hydrolyzed by oligopeptidases into small peptides (consisting of 2–6 AA residues) and free AAs in the lumen of the small intestine. The small peptides containing 4–6 AA residues are further hydrolyzed by peptidases (primarily bound to the brush-border of enterocytes and, to a lesser extent, in the intestinal lumen) to form free AAs, dipeptides, and tripeptides (Giuffrida et al. 2014). Dipeptides (not containing imino acids, i.e., proline or hydroxyproline) and tripeptides are hydrolyzed by mucosa-derived dipeptidases and tripeptidases, respectively.

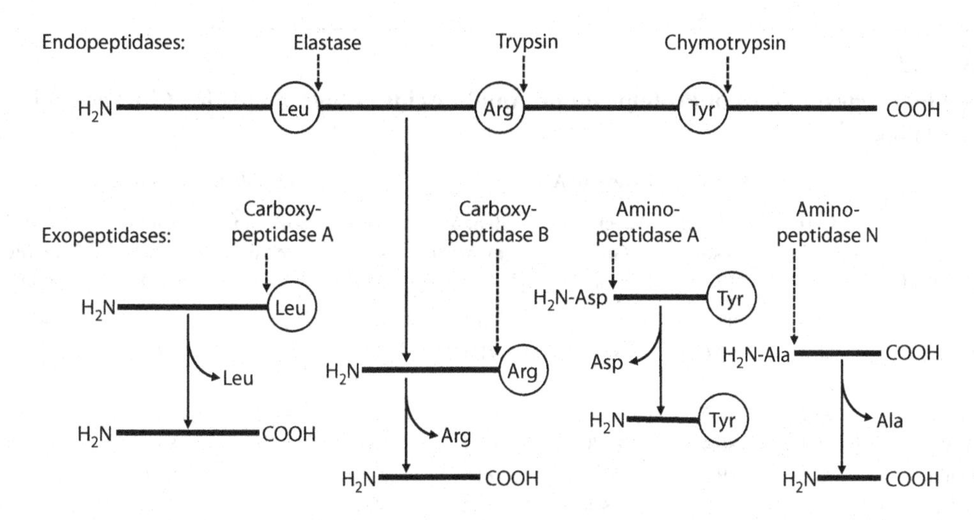


**FIGURE 7.5** Specific cleavage of peptide bonds by trypsin, chymotrypsins, and elastase (all endopeptidases), as well as carboxypeptidases (Carboxy) A and B (all exopeptidases).

Dipeptides containing an imino acid are cleaved by mucosa-derived prolidases. Prolidase I acts on all dipeptides containing an imino acid, whereas prolidase II has a stricter substrate requirement (i.e., acting on only dipeptides containing a non-glycine AA [e.g., Met or Phe] and an imino acid). All peptidases are highly active on the apical membrane of the enterocyte at birth and remain so throughout life (Austic 1985). The products of protein digestion in the lumen of the small intestine consist of approximately 20% free AAs and 80% di- plus tri-peptides.

## Developmental Changes in Extracellular Proteases in the Small Intestine of Nonruminant Mammals

Mammals (e.g., pigs) are born with relatively low activities of chymotrypsins A, B, and C, elastase, and carboxypeptidases A and B in the small intestine, but a well-developed intestinal peptidase capacity (Austic 1985; Cranwell 1995). After birth, the total activities of all pancreatic proteases measured in the whole small-intestinal contents increase with age before weaning, decrease markedly during the first 3–7 days postweaning, and rise again thereafter during the growing period, as shown for pigs, guinea pigs, and rabbits (Debray et al. 2003; Owsley et al. 1986; Tarvid 1992; Yen 2001). The intestine-derived proteases exhibit a pattern of changes similar to the pancreas-derived proteases (Austic 1985). The development of intestinal proteases has important implications for protein digestion. For example, young mammals effectively digest non-immunoglobulin proteins in colostrum (100%; Lin et al. 2009) and milk (92%; Mavromichalis et al. 2001). However, these animals have a lower ability to hydrolyze plant-source proteins than adults (Wilson and Leibholz 1981). This is because the young animals have underdevelopments in gastrointestinal mucosal and microbial proteases before weaning, and they do not possess strong teeth to grind solid materials (e.g., cereal grains). Young mammals cannot use any proteins that are entrapped inside cereal grains due to the lack of exposure of the proteins to digestive proteases. This is because the plant cell walls are barely broken down and the dietary non-starch polysaccharides (NSPs) that are bound to plant proteins are barely degraded (Yen 2001). However, as alluded to previously, young mammals can utilize processed plant-source proteins in the matrix of the ingredients containing little or none of the following hyper-allergic or anti-nutritional factors: trypsin inhibitors, glycinin, β-conglycinin, phytate, oligosaccharides (raffinose and stachyose), and saponins (Sauer and Ozimek 1986). After weaning, pigs adapt to solid diets and develop a relatively high ability to digest proteins in corn grains, soybean meal (SBM), sorghum grains, and meat & bone meal (MBM), with their true ileal digestibilities ranging from 85% to 90% (Table 7.2).

**TABLE 7.2**
**True Ideal Digestibilities of Protein-Bound Amino Acids in Ingredients for Chicken and Swine Diets[a]**

| | Broilers (21 Days of Age) | | | | Pigs (50–65 Days of Age) | | | |
|---|---|---|---|---|---|---|---|---|
| Amino Acid | Corn Grain (%) | Soybean Meal (%) | Sorghum Grain (%) | Meat & Bone Meal (%) | Corn Grain (%) | Soybean Meal (%) | Sorghum Grain (%) | Meat & Bone Meal (%) |
| Alanine | 87.6 | 88.9 | 85.4 | 90.2 | 88.5 | 89.0 | 87.2 | 90.5 |
| Arginine | 88.4 | 90.6 | 87.2 | 91.4 | 89.3 | 90.2 | 88.4 | 91.3 |
| Asparagine | 86.5 | 88.3 | 85.9 | 90.6 | 86.8 | 88.5 | 86.0 | 90.2 |
| Aspartate | 87.2 | 89.5 | 86.1 | 90.2 | 86.3 | 88.2 | 85.8 | 89.7 |
| Cysteine | 85.1 | 86.4 | 84.8 | 89.4 | 86.0 | 87.1 | 85.1 | 89.0 |
| Glutamine | 88.6 | 89.5 | 87.6 | 90.8 | 87.7 | 89.2 | 86.8 | 90.8 |
| Glutamate | 89.2 | 90.2 | 88.4 | 91.2 | 88.1 | 89.6 | 87.4 | 91.0 |
| Glycine | 86.4 | 88.3 | 85.7 | 90.5 | 86.6 | 88.0 | 85.7 | 89.5 |
| Histidine | 85.5 | 87.4 | 84.9 | 89.6 | 87.0 | 88.5 | 86.2 | 90.2 |
| Isoleucine | 88.7 | 89.3 | 88.0 | 90.8 | 88.2 | 88.9 | 87.6 | 90.5 |
| Leucine | 88.2 | 89.0 | 87.6 | 90.3 | 87.8 | 89.6 | 86.4 | 90.6 |
| Lysine | 85.0 | 88.4 | 84.3 | 90.0 | 84.5 | 89.8 | 83.7 | 90.4 |
| Methionine | 87.5 | 90.1 | 86.8 | 90.6 | 88.6 | 89.1 | 87.4 | 90.5 |
| Phenylalanine | 89.1 | 90.3 | 88.5 | 90.9 | 89.5 | 90.0 | 88.9 | 91.0 |
| Proline | 86.8 | 88.0 | 85.9 | 89.4 | 86.4 | 87.2 | 86.0 | 89.2 |
| Hydroxyproline | – | – | – | 88.7 | – | – | – | 88.4 |
| Serine | 88.4 | 90.2 | 87.5 | 91.1 | 88.6 | 89.0 | 87.9 | 90.6 |
| Threonine | 85.2 | 86.5 | 84.8 | 89.3 | 84.9 | 86.8 | 84.3 | 88.5 |
| Tryptophan | 86.0 | 87.2 | 85.3 | 89.0 | 85.2 | 88.1 | 84.6 | 89.7 |
| Tyrosine | 88.5 | 89.6 | 88.0 | 91.4 | 89.0 | 90.2 | 88.2 | 91.0 |
| Valine | 88.2 | 89.8 | 87.6 | 90.7 | 87.1 | 88.7 | 86.1 | 90.3 |

*Source:* Wu, G. 2014. *J. Anim. Sci. Biotechnol.* 5:34.
[a] Except for glycine, all AAs are L-isomers.

After weaning, horses gradually develop a high capacity for digesting dietary protein in the large intestine and are able to digest plant-source feed (e.g., forages, grasses, corn, soybean meal, wheat, and barley). In horses, total tract protein digestibility is 85%–90% for soybean meal and cereal grains (e.g., corn, oats, and sorghum), with prececal digestibility (occurring in the small intestine) being greater than 50%; 78% for alfalfa, with prececal digestibility being 28%; and 60% for coastal bermudagrass, with prececal digestibility being 17% (Spooner 2012). Thus, in these animals, dietary protein is hydrolyzed mainly in the small intestine when they consume cereal grains but in the large intestine when they consume forages. The process of protein digestion in the large intestine of horses is similar to that in the rumen.

#### Developmental Changes in Extracellular Proteases in the Small Intestine of Avian Species

Total protease activities in the avian small intestine increase markedly between birth and 21 days of age (Noy and Sklan 1995). For example, total trypsin activity is 5- to 6-fold greater at day 10 than at day 1 post hatching, and total chymotrypsin activity rises gradually from shortly after hatching to day 14 post-hatching and then remains constant until day 23 post-hatching (Nir et al. 1993; Nitzan et al. 1991). In chickens, total carboxypeptidase A activity peaks on the first day after hatching, declines during the first week post-hatching, and then remains at a constant level until 56 days post-hatching (Tarvid 1991). As in mammals, intestinal peptidase activity is high in poultry at birth (Tarvid 1992). This developmental pattern of intestinal proteases, coupled with a functional gizzard to grind the ingested cereal grains, allows newly hatched birds to utilize a solid corn- and soybean meal-based diet, albeit at a lower rate (e.g., compared with older animals). Accordingly, the true digestibility of plant-source CP in chickens is increased from 78% at 4 days of age to 92% at 21 days of age (Noy and Sklan 1995). Similarly, 3-week-old broiler chickens can effectively utilize plant-source proteins, as indicated by a digestibility coefficient of 85%–90% for individual AAs (Table 7.2). In birds, as reported for mammals, luminal bacteria in the small intestine can be a significant source of proteases and peptidases for the hydrolysis of dietary protein and peptides (Dai et al. 2015), and the feedstuff matrix can also greatly affect the digestibility of dietary protein (Moughan et al. 2014; Sauer et al. 2000).

### Regulation of the Activities of Small-Intestinal Proteases in Nonruminants

The amounts and activities of proteases and peptidases in the small-intestinal tract are affected by dietary factors through: (1) direct inhibition of proteases, (2) regulation of gene expression, and (3) regulation of CCK secretion. For example, increasing dietary protein levels stimulates the synthesis and secretion of proteolytic enzymes by the pancreas and small-intestinal mucosa (Yen 2001). In contrast, raw soybeans and other leguminous seeds contain inhibitors of proteases (e.g., trypsin and chymotrypsin), leading to the depression of protein digestion and animal growth. Since protease inhibitors are heat-sensitive, soybeans must be heated at an appropriate temperature before they are used to feed animals. Fatty acids with $\geq C_{12}$ (including oleic acid and linoleic acid) stimulate CCK production by intestinal enteroendocrine I cells (McLaughlin et al. 1998) and the small intestine in animals (Chelikani et al. 2004). An underlying mechanism responsible for the effect of fatty acids (e.g., linoleic acid) is the activation of the transient receptor potential channel type M5 (TRPM5) (Shah et al. 2012). Through the CCK-induced production of pancreatic proteases, dietary fatty acids, particularly ω6 and ω9 unsaturated fatty acids, can enhance the digestibility of dietary protein in animals.

### Protein Digestibility versus Dietary AA Bioavailability in Nonruminants

The small intestine is the terminal site for the digestion of dietary protein in nonruminants. As noted in Chapter 1, digestion is defined as chemical disintegrations of foodstuffs in the digestive tract into smaller molecules that are suitable for assimilation by the animal. In the small intestine, the digestion of dietary protein is a chemical process for the hydrolysis of di-, tri-, and poly-peptides. It should be pointed out that the term "AA digestibility," which has long been used in describing the hydrolysis of dietary protein, is a misnomer in animal nutrition. This is because "AA digestibility" actually does not refer to the process of AA breakdown into smaller molecules in the gastrointestinal tract. The term "AA digestibility" should be replaced by "protein digestibility" or "coefficient of AA release from protein." The concept of protein digestibility differs from that of dietary AA bioavailability. The latter represents the combined results of digestion, absorption, and metabolism of dietary protein and AAs in the gastrointestinal tract.

### Catabolism of Free AAs and Small Peptides by the Luminal Bacteria of the Small Intestine in Nonruminants

The lumen of the small intestine harbors many species of bacteria (Chapter 1), which can degrade free AAs and small peptides. Dai et al. (2011) reported high rates of the utilization of Gln, Lys, Arg, Thr, Leu, Ile, Val, and His by luminal bacteria from the pig small intestine. Except for the formation of Glu and its metabolites (Ala and Asp) from Gln, and of Orn from Arg, there was no net production of any AAs from Gln, Lys, Arg, Thr, Leu, Ile, Val, and His by pig intestinal microbes. These authors also found that small-intestinal bacteria, particularly *Streptococcus* sp., *Megasphaera elsdenii*, *Escherichia coli*, and *Klebsiella* sp., degraded AAs at different rates in a species-dependent manner and that protein synthesis was a major pathway for AA metabolism in all the bacteria studied. Of note, Yang et al. (2014) demonstrated that bacteria from the small-intestinal lumen of pigs degraded AAs, but bacteria that tightly adhered to the small-intestinal epithelial wall of pigs might be able to synthesize AAs, suggesting variations in AA metabolism by bacteria from different niches. Some *in vivo* studies indicate that 10%–30% of dietary AAs (in the form of free AAs and small peptides), particularly those that are not synthesized by eukaryotes, are degraded by the small-intestinal microbes in postweaning pigs (Stoll and Burrin 2006). This may also be true for other species, but experimental data remain to be obtained. Those free AAs and small peptides that are derived from protein digestion are utilized by the small-intestinal bacteria mainly for protein synthesis (Dai et al. 2010). The microbial protein enters the large intestine primarily for excretion in the feces.

## Absorption of Small Peptides and AAs by the Small Intestine of Nonruminants

Absorption refers to the movement of the products of digestion across the intestinal mucosa into the vascular system for utilization by an animal. The cells responsible for nutrient absorption are enterocytes, which contain the apical membrane and the basolateral membrane. There is a lateral space between two enterocytes. The apical membranes of the enterocytes form microvilli, which increase the area of absorption. Absorption of AAs can occur through two routes. (1) Nutrients may pass completely through the enterocytes, entering at the apical membrane and leaving through the basolateral membrane into the lateral space (transcellular absorption). (2) Alternatively, nutrients may move through the tight junctions directly into the lateral space (paracellular absorption). The latter is represented by the receptor-mediated absorption of intact proteins (e.g., immunoglobulins) by enterocytes in mammalian neonates before "*gut closure*" (Chapter 1). AAs and possibly a small amount of small peptides absorbed into the lamina propria enter the venule and then the portal vein (Figure 7.6).

### Transport of Di- and Tri-Peptides by Enterocytes

Absorption of tripeptides and dipeptides occurs through the apical-membrane $Na^+$-independent, $H^+$-driven peptide transporter 1 (PepT1), which is expressed primarily in the small intestine. However,

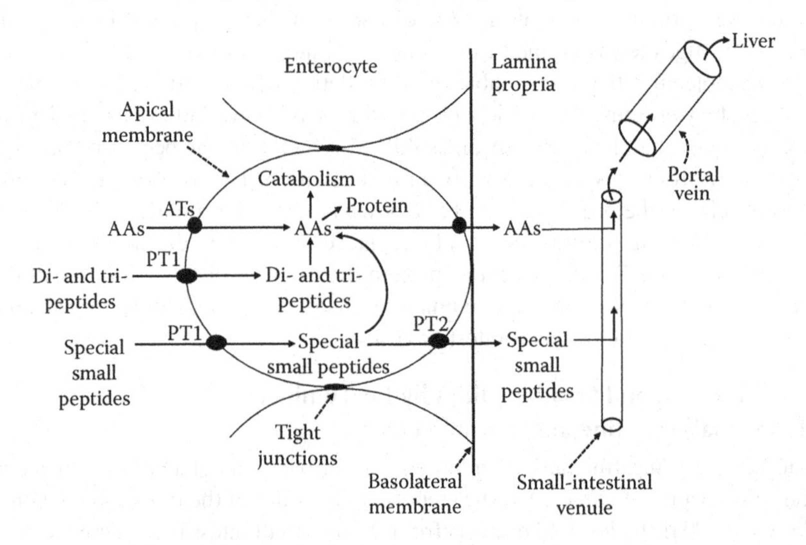


**FIGURE 7.6** Absorption of small peptides and free AAs by enterocytes of the small intestine. After entering enterocytes, free AAs are either used for protein synthesis or degraded, and the remaining AAs exit into the lamina propria of the intestinal mucosa. Enterocytes rapidly hydrolyze the absorbed di- and tri-peptides into free AAs. A significant amount of some special small peptides may escape catabolism inside the enterocytes and exit into the lamina propria. ATs, AA transporters; PT1, peptide transporter 1; PT2, peptide transporter 2.

peptide absorption is indirectly coupled to $Na^+$ transport into enterocytes, because the needed protons are provided by $Na^+/H^+$ exchange. Importantly, tripeptides and dipeptides are absorbed intact from the lumen of the small intestine into its enterocytes, where they are hydrolyzed by cytosolic peptidases to form free AAs (Zhanghi and Matthews 2010). PepT1 does not transport a peptide consisting of four or more AAs (Gilbert et al. 2008). The formation of small peptides in the small intestine can reduce its luminal osmolality and maintain the homeostasis of its enterocytes. Owing to the high activity of intracellular peptidases in the small intestine, it is unlikely that a nutritionally significant quantity of peptides in the lumen of the healthy gut can transcellularly enter the portal vein or the intestinal lymphatics. This is consistent with the absence of PepT1 from the basolateral membrane of the enterocytes (Matthews 2000). However, it is possible that a limited, but physiologically significant, amount of special small peptides may be absorbed intact from the luminal content to the bloodstream through M cells, exosomes, and enterocytes via transepithelial cell transport. Examples of these unique small peptides may include those containing an imino acid (e.g., Gly–Pro–OH–Pro, a degradation product of collagen) or a formyl AA (e.g., *N*-formyl–Met–Leu–Phe, a bacterial peptide serving as a chemotactic for leukocytes) (Dorward et al. 2015). Diet-derived peptides can exert their bioactive (e.g., physiological and regulatory) actions at the level of the small intestine, and the intestinally generated signals can be transmitted to the brain, the endocrine system, and the immune system to beneficially impact the whole body.

Di- and tri-peptides are absorbed into the enterocytes of the small intestine faster than their constituent free AAs (Matthews 2000). The high rate of transport of small peptides minimizes the time for their exposure to luminal bacteria for catabolism and improves the balance of free AAs in the portal vein. This indicates the importance of small peptides in animal nutrition. The concept of peptide transport was generally accepted by the scientific community only in the late 1970s after many years' considerable debate since the first observation of possible intestinal peptide absorption in the late 1950s. Animals will gain more protein and grow faster if they are fed a diet consisting of intact proteins or peptides, in comparison with animals fed the same diet, except that the AAs are provided in the free form. For example, the weight gain was 62% higher and urinary N excretion was 25% lower in young rats fed a 15% casein diet, in comparison with an isonitrogenous diet containing similar amounts of free AAs (Daenzer et al. 2001). Also, 5 to 20 kg pigs fed a diet containing 11.9% casein, 9.1% AAs, and 1% $NaHCO_3$ exhibited an 18% increase in daily weight gain and a 20% increase in gain:feed ratio, compared with pigs fed a 20% AA diet (Officer et al. 1997).

### Transport of Free AAs by Enterocytes

The absorption of AAs is rapid in the duodenum and jejunum but slower in the ileum. Different AAs are absorbed by enterocytes at different rates (Bröer and Palacín 2011). There are four mechanisms for the transport of AAs into the enterocytes through their apical membrane: (a) $Na^+$-independent system (facilitated system), (b) $Na^+$-dependent system (active transport), (c) simple diffusion (a passive, non-saturable transport system without a need for carrier proteins), and (d) the $\gamma$-glutamyl cycle. Simple diffusion and the $\gamma$-glutamyl cycle are insignificant for AA transport by enterocytes and other cell types under physiological conditions. In contrast, apical-membrane $Na^+$-dependent and $Na^+$-independent AA transporters (Table 7.3) are responsible for the uptake of ~60% and 40% of free AAs from the lumen of the small intestine into enterocytes, respectively. Examples of these apical-membrane AA transporters (transmembrane proteins) are given in Figure 7.7. The conventional names of AA transporters are based on their major substrates, whereas the Gene Nomenclature Committee groups AA transporters into solute carrier (SLC) families according to their gene sequence similarity. For example, SLC7A1, SLC7A2, and SLC7A3 encode the CAT (cationic AA transporter)-1, CAT-2, and CAT-3 proteins, respectively, in the conventional system $y^+$ for the transport of basic AAs by cells.

Several characteristics of the apical-membrane AA transport are noteworthy. First, one AA can be transported by multiple systems. For example, Gln is taken up by the apical and basolateral membranes of the enterocyte through $Na^+$-dependent systems N (SN1 and SN2), $B^0$, $B^{0,+}$, and A, as well

**TABLE 7.3**
**AA Transporters in the Apical Membrane of Enterocytes and in Other Cell Types of Animals**

| Transport System | Gene Name | Major Amino Acids | Note |
|---|---|---|---|
| | | **$Na^+$-Independent System** | |
| asc | SLC7A10 | Small AAs (Ala, Ser, Cys, Gly, and Thr) | Transports small neutral AAs and D-Ser |
| $b^{0,+}$ | SLC7A9 | Neutral (0) and basic (+) AAs | Also transports cystine |
| L | SLC7A5 | Large neutral AAs (e.g., Leu, Phe, and Met) | Also transports ABHDC and His |
| L | SLC7A8 | All neutral AAs except for Pro | Has a greater affinity for large neutral AAs |
| L | SLC43A1 | Large neutral AAs | Has a greater affinity for BCAAs |
| $X_c^-$ | SLC7A11 | Acidic AAs (Glu and Asp) | Also transports cystine |
| $y^+$ (CAT-1) | SLC7A1 | Cationic AAs (e.g., Arg, His, Lys, and Orn) | Also transports neutral AAs |
| $y^+$ (CAT-2) | SLC7A2 | Cationic AAs (e.g., Arg, His, Lys, and Orn) | Also transports neutral AAs |
| $y^+$ (CAT-3) | SLC7A3 | Cationic AAs (e.g., Arg, His, Lys, and Orn) | Also transports neutral AAs |
| $y^+L$ | SLC7A6 | Cationic AAs and large neutral AAs | Also transports Gln |
| $y^+L$ | SLC7A7 | Cationic AAs and large neutral AAs | Also transports Ala, Gln, and Cys |
| | | **$Na^+$-Dependent System** | |
| A | SLC38A1 | Small and neutral AAs (e.g., Ala and Met) | Also transports His, Asn, and Cys |
| A | SLC38A2 | Small and neutral AAs (e.g., Ala and Met) | Also transports His, Asn, Cys, and Pro |
| ASC | SLC1A4 | Small AAs (Ala, Ser, and Cys) | Also transports Thr |
| ASC | SLC1A5 | Small AAs (Ala, Ser, and Cys) | Also transports Cys, Gln, and Thr |
| BETA | SLC6A1 | γ-Aminobutyrate (GABA) | $Na^+$- and $Cl^-$-dependent transporter |
| BETA | SLC6A6 | Taurine transporter; also β-Ala and GABA | $Na^+$- and $Cl^-$-dependent transporter |
| BETA | SLC6A11 | GABA, betaine, and taurine | $Na^+$- and $Cl^-$-dependent transporter |
| $B^0$ | SLC6A15 | Neutral AAs (e.g., BCAAs, Met, and Pro) | $Na^+$- and $Cl^-$-dependent transporter |
| $B^{0,+}$ | SLC6A14 | All neutral and basic AAs and β-Ala | $Na^+$- and $Cl^-$-dependent transporter |
| Gly | SLC6A9 | Gly and sarcosine | Inhibited by lithium |
| IMINO | SLC6A20 | Pro and OH-Pro | Also transports neutral AAs (e.g., Gly) |
| N (SN1) | SLC38A3 | Gln, Asn, Cit, and His | Also transports Ala |
| N (SN2) | SLC38A5 | Gln, Asn, Cit, and His | Also transports Ala, Ser, and Gly |
| NBB | SLC6A19 | All neutral AAs (brush-border transporter) | Bound to apical membrane of enterocytes |
| Phe | Unknown | Phe and Met (brush-border transporter) | Bound to apical membrane of enterocytes |
| $X_{AG}^-$ | SLC1A1 | Asp and Glu | Also transports Cys, cysteine, and D-Asp |
| $X_{AG}^-$ | SLC1A2 | Asp and Glu | Also transports Cys, cysteine, and D-Asp |
| $X_{AG}^-$ | SLC1A3 | Asp and Glu | Also transports D-Asp |

ABHDC, 2-aminobicyclo[2,2,1]heptane-dicarboxylic acid; BCAAs, branched-chain AAs; SLC, solute carrier.

as $Na^+$-independent systems $b^{0,+}$, L, and $y^+L$ (Wu 2013). In addition, BCAAs are transported by systems L, $y^+L$, $B^0$, and $B^{0,+}$. The redundancy of transporters for any AA reduces risk for the absence of its uptake by cells which would occur if there were only one transporter for an AA. Second, AA transporters exhibit cell- and tissue-specific differences in their expression, which play an important role in the interorgan metabolism of AAs. The nutritional and physiological significance of this phenomenon can be illustrated by the findings that mammalian hepatocytes have a low abundance of cationic AA transporters (CAT-1, 2, and 3 proteins) and therefore a low ability to take up extracellular basic AAs. Since the mammalian hepatocytes have a very high ability to degrade the basic AAs, their limited uptake by these cells minimizes their irreversible loss in the liver, thereby maximizing their availability from the diet, the small intestine, and the blood to extrahepatic cells and

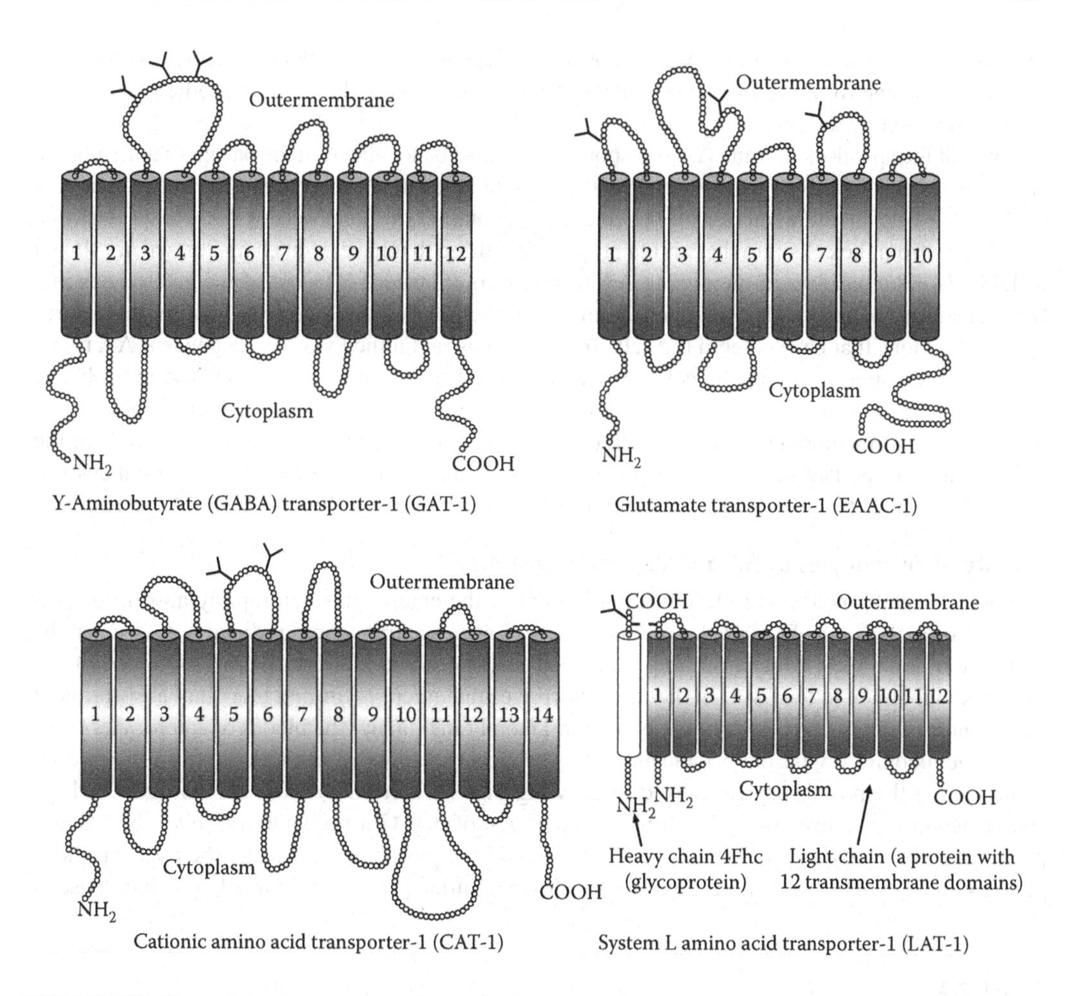


**FIGURE 7.7** Examples of transporters (transmembrane proteins) of acidic, basic, and neutral AAs in animal cells. (Adapted from Bröer, S. and M. Palacín, 2011. *Biochem. J.* 436:193–211; and Hyde, R. et al. 2003. *Biochem. J.* 373:1–18.)

tissues. Third, a physiological AA may not be transported by all cells in an animal. For instance, macrophages and endothelial cells readily take up extracellular L-citrulline (Cit), but there is little uptake of this AA by the mammalian liver. This ensures that the small intestine-derived Cit is fully available for Arg synthesis in extrahepatic tissues and cells. Fourth, the $Na^+$-dependent AA transport systems transport both AAs and $Na^+$ (all soluble in water) into the cell in an ATP-dependent manner, which affects electric potential across the plasma membrane and the influx of water (Hyde et al. 2003). The $Na^+$ which has entered the cell will exit the cell through the basolateral membrane $Na^+/K^+$-ATP pump (also called $Na^+/K^+$-ATPase), which transports 3 $Na^+$ ions out of the enterocyte in exchange for the influx of 2 $K^+$ ions. The energy that powers this transport process is provided by the hydrolysis of ATP into ADP plus Pi. The $Na^+$-dependent uptake of 1 mol AA from the intestinal lumen into the enterocytes requires 1 mol ATP. Thus, when Gln or Glu is added to the mucosal side of the small intestine, the electric current of the plasma membrane and water absorption are increased as the AA enters the cell.

An AA transporter binds $Na^+$ first and then an AA. The binding of the transporter to $Na^+$ increases its affinity for the AA substrate. The binding of the AA transporter to both the $Na^+$ and the AA results in a further conformational change of the transporter protein, leading to the entry of both substrates from the intestinal lumen into the cytoplasm of the enterocytes. Thus, the rapid and complete absorption of most AAs is absolutely dependent on the electrochemical gradient of $Na^+$ across the enterocytes and also contributes to the generation of the osmotic gradient that drives water absorption by the cells.

Some of the apical-membrane AA transporters may also be localized in the basolateral membrane of the enterocytes for the efflux of AAs from the cells into the interstitial space of the mucosal lamina propria. The basolateral membrane of the enterocyte contains additional sets of AA transporters that export AAs from the cells into the lamina propria, and those that have been characterized are shown in Table 7.4. The basolateral-membrane AA transporters transport AAs out of the enterocytes in a $Na^+$-dependent or independent manner. To maintain the balance of electrolytes within the enterocytes, 3 $Na^+$ ions that have entered the cells from the intestinal lumen via $Na^+$-dependent AA transporters are transported out of the cells by the basolateral membrane $Na^+/K^+$-ATPase in exchange for the influx of 2 $K^+$ ions. The basolateral membrane of the enterocytes is more permeable to AAs than their apical membrane or non-epithelial membranes. Thus, simple diffusion of AAs from the enterocytes into the lamina propria can occur, but is quantitatively minor for the intestinal absorption of AAs across the enterocytes, compared to that by the basolateral-membrane AA transporters.

### Polarity of Enterocytes in AA and Peptide Transport

The apical membrane (facing the intestinal lumen) of the enterocytes can rapidly absorb luminal AAs (Yen et al. 2004). During the digestion period after enteral feeding, dietary AAs enter the portal vein down their concentration gradients. Therefore, there is a positive influx of AAs from the intestinal lumen to the liver. In the postabsorptive state, there is limited intestinal absorption of AAs in nonruminants. In contrast, the basolateral membrane (facing the blood) of enterocytes takes up a large amount of Gln, but no nutritionally significant quantity of other AAs, from the arterial blood during the postabsorptive period in growing pigs (Wu et al. 1994b). This is due to a high abundance of Gln transporters, but limited expression of non-Gln transporters, in the basolateral membrane of the enterocyte. It is also possible that, in the postabsorptive state, the concentrations of non-Gln AAs in the interstitial fluid of the mucosal lamina propria are much lower than those in

**TABLE 7.4**
**AA Transporters in the Basolateral Membrane of Enterocytes**

| Transport System | Isoform | Major AAs | $Na^+$ Dependence | Notes |
|---|---|---|---|---|
| A | – | Neutral AAs (including Gln) | Yes | Efflux from enterocytes |
| ASC | – | Ala, Ser, and Cys | Yes | Efflux from enterocytes |
| asc-Like | – | Ala, Ser, and Cys | No | Efflux from enterocytes |
| Gly | GLY1 | Glycine | $Na^+$, $Cl^-$ | Efflux from enterocytes |
| L | LAT2-4F2hc | Large neutral AAs | No | Efflux from enterocytes |
| N | – | Gln, Asn, Cit, and His | Yes | Efflux from enterocytes |
| TAT1[a] | – | Aromatic AAs (Trp, Tyr, and Phe) | No | Efflux from enterocytes |
| SNAT2[b] | – | Neutral AAs | Yes | Efflux from enterocytes |
| $y^+L$ | $Y^+LAT1$ | Cationic AAs | No | Efflux from enterocytes |
| | | Large neutral AAs | Yes | Influx from blood to enterocytes |
| | $Y^+LAT2$[c] | Cationic AAs | No | Efflux from enterocytes |
| | | Large neutral AAs | Yes | Influx from blood to enterocytes |
| $y^+$ | CAT-1 | Cationic AAs | No | Efflux from enterocytes |

[a] *T*-type AA transporter-1.
[b] SNAT, sodium-coupled neutral AA transporter. SNAT1 and 4 are expressed in extraintestinal tissues.
[c] Expressed in both epithelial and non-epithelial tissues.

the cytosol of the enterocytes. This would hinder the transport of AAs via $Na^+$-dependent or independent transporters against the concentration gradients of the AAs. Thus, an enteral diet must be provided to postnatal animals, so that they will obtain adequate AAs to support the maintenance, growth, function, and health of the small-intestinal mucosa. Like adult rats, the small intestine of young pigs takes up 30% of Gln from the arterial blood in the postabsorptive state (Wu et al. 1994b), indicating an important role of the gut in whole-body Gln utilization.

The small-intestinal mucosa does not take up small peptides from the arterial blood. This is because the basolateral membrane of the enterocytes lacks PepT1. As noted previously, the basolateral membrane of the enterocytes may express other peptide transporters. For example, Shepherd et al. (2002) reported the presence of a peptide transporter in the basolateral membrane of the enterocytes in the rat small intestine. These authors observed the transepithelial transport of a non-hydrolyzable dipeptide, D-Phe–L-Gln (1 mM), from the lumen of the small intestine into the vascular perfusate. There is also evidence that the basolateral membrane of the colonocyte (the human intestinal cell line Caco-2) may contain an $Na^+$-independent peptide transporter to transport small peptides out of the cells into the lamina propria of the large intestine (Irie et al. 2004). A dipeptide [Gly-Sarcosine (*N*-methylglycine)] enters the Caco-2 cells through their apical membrane and exits the cells through their basolateral membrane in a pH-dependent manner. Interestingly, the $K_M$ for the efflux of the dipeptide is lower than that of its influx. The molecular characteristics of the peptide transporter in the rat small intestine or the Caco-2 cells have not been identified.

### Metabolism of AAs in Enterocytes

The available evidence shows: (a) no degradation of Asn, Cys, His, Phe, Lys, Thr, Trp, and Tyr; (b) a very low rate of degradation of Ala, Gly, Met, and Ser; (c) high rates of degradation of Arg (after weaning only), Pro, and three BCAAs; and (d) very high rates of degradation of Asp, Glu, and Gln as the major metabolic fuels in enterocytes from pigs, rats, sheep, and calves (Chen et al. 2007, 2009; Wu et al. 2005). In the intestinal mucosa, Met is metabolized to provide *S*-adenosylmethionine (SAM), which is decarboxylated in the cytosol to yield $CO_2$ and the decarboxylated SAM. The latter is used for polyamine synthesis, as well as DNA and protein methylation. In enterocytes, the rate of SAM (and thus Met) decarboxylation is quantitatively very low, and there is no oxidation of other Met carbons (Chen et al. 2009). In the intestinal mucosa, Pro is extensively oxidized by mitochondrial Pro oxidase to form pyrroline-5-carboxylate (P5C), which is the precursor of L-ornithine (Orn) and Cit. However, the oxidation of Pro to $CO_2$ in enterocytes is limited due to a very low activity of P5C dehydrogenase (Wu 1997). In porcine, rat, ovine, and bovine enterocytes, Cit is synthesized from Gln, Glu, and Pro via the formation of Orn, whereas Ala is generated from Gln and Glu (Wu 1997). Although mitochondria-generated Orn is effectively channeled for Cit production in these cells, extracellular Orn is not utilized by them for Cit synthesis and instead is metabolized to form Pro because of the complex compartmentalization of Orn degradation (Wu et al. 1994a). In contrast, chicken enterocytes do not synthesize Orn, Cit, or Arg from Gln, Glu, and Pro, and have a very low rate of Gln degradation (Wu et al. 1995). Thus, there are marked differences in intestinal mucosal AA metabolism between mammals and birds.

The studies with pigs graphically illustrate developmental changes in AA metabolism in the small-intestinal mucosa. For example, in porcine enterocytes, the rates of Cit and Arg synthesis from Gln are greatest at birth, decline progressively thereafter, reach the lowest level at 14–21 days of age, and are induced after weaning (Wu and Morris 1998). Between 0 and 21 days of age, Pro is a major substrate for Cit and Arg syntheses in these cells (Wu 1997). In neonatal pigs, their enterocytes convert almost all Cit into Arg due to high activities of argininosuccinate synthase (ASS) and argininosuccinate lyase (ASL), and release almost all the synthesized Arg due to the near absence of arginase activity. This helps to maximize the availability of the diet- and small intestine-derived Arg to extraintestinal tissues. In postweaning pigs, their enterocytes convert only a small percentage of the synthesized Cit (10%) into Arg because of the reduced activities of ASS and ASL, and instead release 90% of the synthesized Cit from the cells. After weaning, the kidneys express high activities of ASS and ASL to readily convert Cit into Arg in their proximal tubules with limited arginase activity, and release nearly all the synthesized Arg into the blood circulation. Such metabolic adaptation to weaning is of nutritional significance to spare the intestine-synthesized Cit, because arginase is induced in the enterocytes of postweaning mammals, including pigs (Wu 1995). Arginase hydrolyzes Arg into Orn and urea, which would contribute to a loss of the Cit synthesized from Glu, Gln, and Pro in the enterocytes of postweaning pigs. Although Pro and Arg are actively degraded by enterocytes of postweaning mammals, these two AAs support the growth and remodeling of the small intestine partly through polyamine synthesis. In the postweaning pigs, <20% of the extracted AAs are utilized for intestinal mucosal protein synthesis. Thus, not all AAs that enter enterocytes from the small-intestinal lumen exit into the portal circulation.

## DIGESTION AND ABSORPTION OF PROTEIN IN PRERUMINANTS

### Digestion of Proteins in the Abomasum and the Small Intestine in Preruminants

In preruminants, milk or a liquid diet largely bypasses the reticulorumen and flows from the mouth directly into the abomasum (Chapter 1). The processes for the digestion of dietary protein by proteases in the abomasum and the small intestine in preruminants are the same as those in preweaning nonruminant mammals. The concentrations of proteolytic enzymes in the gastric and small-intestinal contents of preruminants are similar between birth and weaning (Porter 1969). Young calves and lambs have sufficient activities of the digestive proteases to hydrolyze the ingested milk protein, and an addition of exogenous proteases to diets does not enhance its digestibility.

The pH of the gastrointestinal tract plays an important role in protein digestion in preruminants as in preweaning monogastric mammals. In preruminants, the abomasal contents have a pH ~2.0 before feeding (which aids in the activation of gastric proteases) and a pH ~6.0 immediately after milk consumption due to dilution by a large volume of the neutral milk. The gastric solution has a gradual reduction in pH to the pre-feeding value 5 h after milk consumption, because of gastric emptying and HCl secretion (Porter 1969). Since saliva and gastric mucosal secretions are continuously added to the abomasal fluid, the total volume of the chyme leaving the abomasum is about twice the volume of the consumed milk. In young calves, the rate of the flow of abomasal contents into the duodenum peaks in the first hour after feeding, and the flow of the chyme into the jejunum is greatest during the first 4–5 h after feeding. Since there is continuous secretion of the pancreatic juice and bile into the lumen of the duodenum, feeding has little effect on pH values (7.0–7.4) in the distal small intestine.

Like young nonruminant mammals, preruminants are well adapted to the digestion of milk protein. The true digestibility of natural milk protein in young calves is 100% (Gerrits et al. 1997). However, the proteins of overheated milk are less well digested than those of natural milk. Pasteurization of milk does not affect its protein digestibility in preruminants. In contrast to milk, preruminants cannot break down the cell walls of cereal grains and therefore cannot use the proteins in unprocessed cereal grains or in raw soybeans. These animals also have a limited ability to use even soy flour (finely ground, defatted soybean meal) if it contains trypsin inhibitor and other factors that cause depression in food intake and poor growth. Liquid soy flour is an ineffective source of protein for preruminants because such a diet is unpalatable to the animals and often causes severe diarrhea. Of interest, Colvin and Ramsey (1968) reported that the nutritive value of trypsin inhibitor-free soya flour could be improved by treatment with acid at pH 4 for 5 h at 37°C. This is likely due to the denaturation of plant-source proteins and the partial inhibition of non-trypsin anti-nutritional factors.

### Absorption of Protein Digestion Products by the Small Intestine in Preruminants

Healthy young preruminants have a high capacity for absorbing the products of protein digestion in the small intestine, particularly the jejunum (Porter 1969). As in preweaning monogastric mammals, di- and tri-peptides as well as free AAs are produced from the terminal digestion of dietary protein in the small intestine. These digestion products are absorbed into the enterocytes through the $H^+$-driven PepT1 for the small peptides and various AA transporters for free AAs (Table 7.3). There is evidence that large amounts of di- and tri-peptides in the lumen of the small intestine are absorbed rapidly into its enterocytes in young calves (Koeln et al. 1993). In these animals, as reported for non-ruminants, the apical membrane of the enterocytes has at least four classes of $Na^+$-dependent AA transporters, one each for acidic, basic, neutral, and β-AAs (Matthews 2000). Dietary sodium intake is necessary for the rapid and complete absorption of dietary AAs from the lumen of the small intestine into the lamina propria. Thus, since AA transport by the enterocytes drives the absorption of water across the cells into the blood, some AAs (e.g., Gly and Gln) are added, along with D-glucose and NaCl, to rehydration solutions to treat diarrhea in young calves (Naylor et al. 1997).

## DIGESTION AND ABSORPTION OF PROTEIN IN RUMINANTS

CP is an important concept in ruminant nutrition (Chapter 4). Utilization of dietary protein and non-protein nitrogen (NPN) in ruminants involves the rumen, abomasum, and the small intestine (Figure 7.8). Adequate intake of rumen-degraded CP (RDP) is critical for maximizing ruminal microbial growth, feed intake, and the digestibility of nutrients (particularly protein and fibers) (Firkins and Yu 2015). Depending on its type, protein may undergo extensive extracellular degradation by proteases and peptidases of bacterial origin (Wu 2013). The resultant products serve as precursors for intracellular AA and protein synthesis primarily in bacteria. Bacteria are either engulfed by protozoa or flow into the stomach along with the protozoa to provide the ruminant with bacterial and protozoal

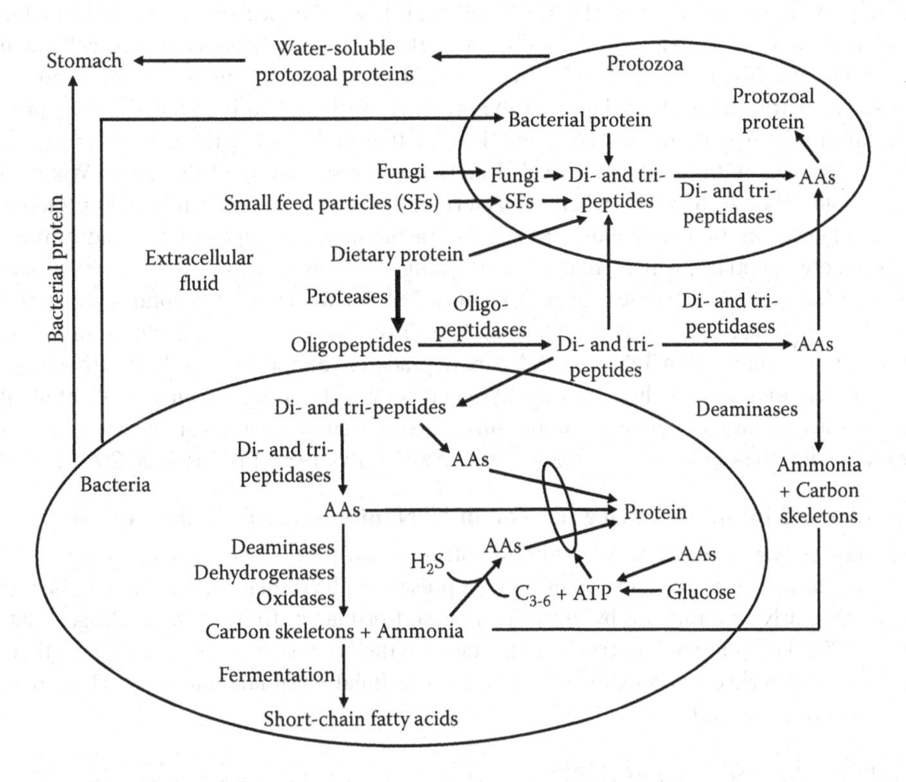


**FIGURE 7.8** Fermentative digestion of protein in the rumen. Dietary proteins are hydrolyzed by extracellular proteases and oligopeptidases of primarily bacterial origin to form di- and tri-peptides and some AAs. Some AAs can be degraded to form ammonia and the corresponding α-ketoacids. Bacteria use small peptides, AAs, and ammonia to synthesize new proteins. Protozoa engulf bacteria, fungi, small feed particles, and insoluble proteins, and use these substrates for synthesizing protozoal proteins.

proteins. The latter are hydrolyzed by proteases and peptidases in the stomach and the small intestine. In ruminants, the true digestibility of plant-source protein and rumen-protected high-quality protein in diets at the end of the ileum (after passing through the forestomachs, abosamum, duodenum, and jejunum) is 62%–66% and 85%–90%, respectively (Chalupa and Sniffen 1994). Much evidence shows that cost-effective ruminant production with high economic returns should be based on: (1) meeting the N needs of ruminal fermentation from low-CP diets; and (2) providing adequate and balanced amounts of AAs (the AA profile of microbes being complemented with rumen-undegraded protein) for absorption from the small intestine into the blood circulation (NRC 2001).

## Degradation of Dietary Protein in the Rumen

### Extracellular Proteolysis by Bacterial Proteases and Oligopeptidases

The rumen harbors various species and strains of anaerobic bacteria (including methanogenic archaea), protozoa, and fungi (Firkins and Yu 2015). Approximately 40% or more of the bacteria isolated from ruminal fluid have proteolytic activity toward extracellular protein, because they release high-activity proteases and peptidases. The major proteolytic bacteria are *Ruminobacter amylophilus*, *Butyrivibrio fibrisolvens*, and *Prevotella ruminicola*, with *P. ruminicola* being the most numerous proteolytic bacteria (Nagaraja 2016). In contrast, *R. amylophilus* is the most active proteolytic bacteria in cultures, but its number in the rumen is low. Note that feed proteins, large peptides, or oligopeptides (consisting of 5 or more AA residues) do not enter bacteria, because both gram-negative and positive bacteria have a size exclusion of ~ five AAs (Higgins and Gibson 1986).

Bacteria play a major role in the ruminal degradation of dietary protein, as well as other potential sources of proteins (Broderick et al. 1991; Russell et al. 1992; Wallace 1994). The latter include the endogenous proteins of saliva (e.g., 5.4 g/day in cattle fed forage diets), epithelial cells sloughed from the ruminal epithelium (e.g., 5 g/day in a cow and steer), and the remains of the lysed ruminal microbes. The extracellular degradation of the proteins in the rumen is initiated by the proteases of bacterial origin. Approximately 90% and 10% of the total proteolytic activity are associated with the cell surface of bacteria and the cell-free fraction, respectively (NRC 2001). Water-soluble proteins are adsorbed to bacteria, whereas bacteria are adsorbed to water-insoluble proteins. The hydrolysis of proteins by extracellular proteases (including carboxypeptidases and aminopeptidases) yields oligopeptides, which are degraded by oligopeptidases to form small peptides (consisting of 2–3 AA residues) and some free AAs (Figure 7.8). Some di- and tri-peptides are hydrolyzed by di- and tri-peptidases, respectively, into free AAs. The major sources of bacterial proteases and peptidases are summarized in Table 7.5. AAs are degraded to ammonia plus their carbon skeletons through AA deaminases, dehydrogenases, and oxidases (Wu 2013). Monensin and essential oils are known to reduce bacterial population in the rumen and inhibit AA deamination independent of, or concomitant with, their effects on protozoa (Bergen and Bates 1984; Firkins et al. 2007).

### Extracellular and Intracellular Degradation of NPN into Ammonia in the Rumen

NPN substances (e.g., ammonia, AAs, nitrate, nitrite, small peptides, nucleic acids [up to 20% of NPN], glucosamines, uric acid, and allantoin) are present in the rumen, where they can be metabolized extracellularly to ammonia by enzymes released primarily from bacteria (Vogels and Van der Driet 1976). The ruminal bacteria can also take up the NPN substances and convert them into ammonia. The bacteria convert extracellular and intracellular ammonia into AAs. These reactions are illustrated in Figure 7.9.

#### *Utilization of Urea, Nitrate, and Nitrite*

Urea is hydrolyzed into ammonia and $CO_2$ by urease. This enzyme is absent from animal cells (Wu 2013). Nitrate is reduced to nitrite by nitrate reductase, and nitrite is then converted into ammonia by nitrite reductase. These reactions consume $2H^+$ and, therefore, $H_2$, because $2H^+$ and $H_2$ are interconverted by bacterial hydrogenase and ferredoxin hydrogenase (Averill 1996).

**TABLE 7.5**
**The Major Sources of Bacterial Proteases and Peptidases in The Rumen**

1. Proteases: Protein → oligopeptides
*D. ruminantium, B. fibrisolvens*[a], and *E. caudatum*
*Clostridium* spp, *E. simplex,* and *E. budayi*
*E. caudatum ecaudatum, E. ruminantium,* and *E. maggii*
*Fusobacterium* spp., *E. medium*
*L. multipara, O. caudatus,* and *P. ruminicola*
*P. multivesiculatum, R. amylophilus*[b], and *S. ruminantium*
*O. joyonii, N. frontalis, S. bovis,* and *P. communis*

2. Oligopeptidases: Oligopeptides to Di- and tri-peptides → AAs
*S. bovis, R. amylophilus,* and *P. ruminicola*

3. Di- and tri-peptidases: Di- and tri-peptides → AAs
*D. ruminantium* and *E. caudatum*
*F. succinogenes, M. elsdenii,* and *P. ruminicola*[a]
*Isotricha* spp., *L. multipara,* and *S. ruminantium*

4. Deaminases: AAs → $NH_3$
*C. aminophilum*[b] and *C. sticklandii*
*P. anerobius, B. fibrisolvens,* and *P. ruminicola*
*M. elsdenii, S. ruminantium,* and *E. caudatum*

*Sources:* Broderick, G.A. et al. 1991. In: *Physiological Aspects of Digestion and Metabolism in Ruminants*. Edited by T. Tsuda and Y. Sasaki. Academic Press, Orlando, Florida, pp. 541–592; Russell, J.B. et al. 1992. *J. Anim. Sci.* 70:3551–3561; Wallace, R.J. 1994. In: *Principles of Protein Metabolism in Ruminants*. Edited by J.M. Asplund. CRC Press, Boca Raton, Florida, pp. 71–111.

[a] High numbers but low activity: *Butyrivibrio fibrisolvens, Megasphaera elsdenii, Prevotella ruminicola* (>60% of ruminal bacteria), *Selenomonas ruminantium,* and *Streptococcus bovis* ($>10^9$ cells/mL ruminal fluid; 10–20 nmol $NH_3$/min per mg protein). Quantitatively, they are the major fermenters of AAs in the rumen.

[b] Low numbers but high activity: *Clostridium aminophilum, Clostridium sticklandii,* and *Peptostreptococcus anaerobius* ($10^7$ cells/mL ruminal fluid; 300 nmol $NH_3$/min per mg protein).

In the rumen, nitrate-utilizing bacteria include *Wolinella succinogenes, Veillonella parvula,* and *Selenomonas ruminantium* (Yang et al. 2001). Thus, although $H_2$ is a major product of fermentation by isolated protozoa, fungi, and some bacteria, it does not accumulate in the rumen because of its immediate use by the mixed populations of microbes (Moss et al. 2000). Likewise, in the rumen, some nitrate and nitrite are reduced to nitric oxide (NO), $NH_3$, and $N_2O$ (Yang et al. 2016), and there is little production or fixation of $N_2$ (Nagaraja 2016; Pun and Satter 1975).

$$\begin{array}{ccccc} & & \text{NO (nitric oxide)} & \longrightarrow & N_2O \text{ (nitrous oxide)} \\ & & \uparrow & \nearrow & \\ NO_3^- \text{(nitrate)} & \longrightarrow & NO_2^- \text{(nitrite)} & \longrightarrow & NH_3 \text{ (ammonia)} \end{array}$$

$$NO_{3^-} + 2e^- + 2H^+ (\text{from NADPH} + H^+) \leftrightarrow NO_{2^-} + H_2O + NADP^+ \text{ (bacteria, nitrate reductase[Mo])}$$

$$NO_{2^-} + 2e^- + 2H^+ \leftrightarrow NO + H_2O \quad \text{(bacteria, nitrate reductase [heme])}$$

$$NO_{2^-} + 2e^- + 2H^+ \leftrightarrow NO + H_2O \text{ (bacteria, nitrate reductase [copper])}$$

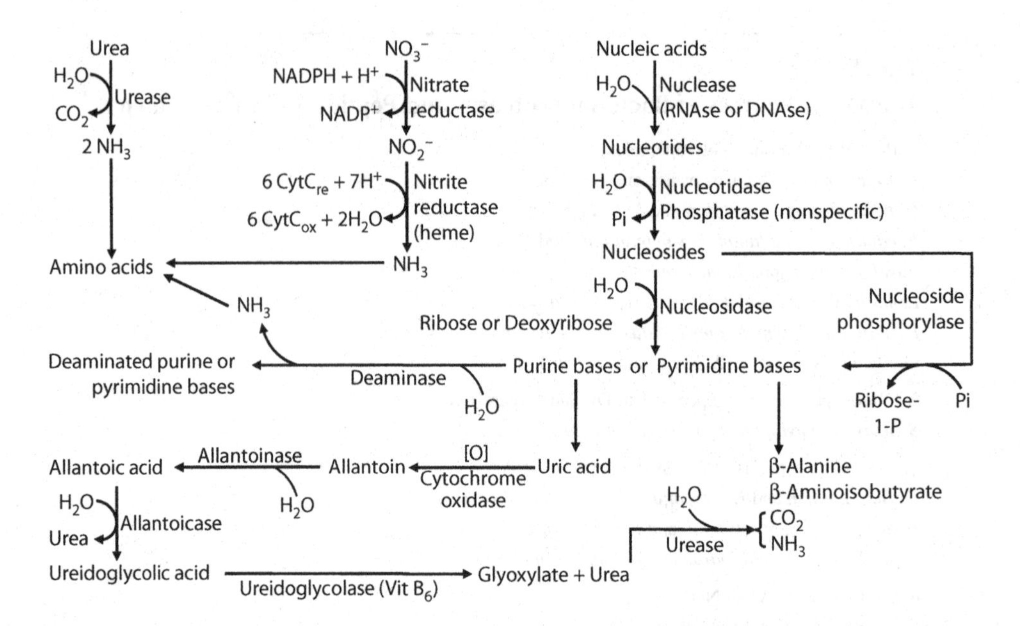


**FIGURE 7.9** Extracellular degradation of NPN substances into ammonia in the rumen. These reactions are catalyzed extracellularly by enzymes of primarily bacterial origin. $CytC_{ox}$, oxidized cytochdrome c; $CytC_{re}$, reduced cytochdrome c.

$$2NO_{2^-} + 4e^- + 3H_2O \leftrightarrow N_2O + 6OH^- \quad \text{(bacteria, nitrate reductase [copper])}$$

$$NO_{2^-} + 6e^- + 7H^+ \rightarrow NH_3 + 2H_2O \quad \text{(bacteria, nitrate reductase [cytochrome C])}$$

$$2NO + 2e^- + 2H^+ \leftrightarrow N_2O + H_2O \text{ (bacteria, nitric oxide reductase)}$$

$$2NO + 2e^- + 2H^+ \quad \text{(from NADPH+ H}^+\text{)} \leftrightarrow N_2O + H_2O\text{+NADP}^+ \quad \text{(fungi, nitric oxide reductase)}$$

$$H_2 + \text{Oxidized ferredoxin} \leftrightarrow 2H^+ + \text{Reduced ferredoxin}$$
$$\text{(bacteria, ferredoxin hydrogenase [Fe-S center])}$$

$$2H_2 + \text{NAD} + 2 \text{ Oxidizied ferredoxin} \leftrightarrow 2H^+ + \text{NADH} + H^+$$
$$+2 \text{ Reduced ferredoxin (bacteria, hydrogenase [Fe-S center])}$$

$$H_2 \leftrightarrow 2H^+ \text{ (bacteria,[Fe}-\text{Fe] hydrogenase [Fe}-\text{S center] or [Ni}-\text{Fe] hydrogenase [Fe}-\text{S center])}$$

$$H_2 \leftrightarrow 2H^+ \quad \text{(bacteria,[Fe] hydrogenase [containing no Fe}-\text{S center])}$$

The reduction potentials (E°) for the microbial production of $CH_4$, $HS^-$, nitrate, and ammonia at pH 7.0 (Lam and Kuypers 2011) are shown as follows. The greater the value of the reduction potential, the easier the reductive reaction.

$$CO_2 + 4H_2 \rightarrow CH_4 + 2H_2O \text{ (E}^\circ = -0.30 \text{ V)}$$

$$SO_4^{2-} \rightarrow HS^-(E^\circ = -0.23\,V)$$

$$NO_2^- \rightarrow NH_4^+(E^\circ = -0.34\,V)$$

$$NO_3^- \rightarrow NH_4^+(E^\circ = -0.36\,V)$$

$$NO_3^- \rightarrow NO_2^-(E^\circ = -0.42\,V)$$

Thus, the reduction of nitrate or nitrite to $NH_3$ is energetically more favorable than the reduction of $CO_2$ plus $H_2$ to $CH_4$. As a result, $CH_4$ production is substantially reduced when nitrate is added to the rumen (Moss et al. 2000). Since nitrate can act as an alternative $H_2$ sink in the rumen, dietary supplementation with appropriate doses of nitrate (<1.5% of DM) to ruminants can reduce $CH_4$ emissions and improve production performance (Lee and Beauchemin 2014). A disadvantage of this method is nitrate or nitrite poisoning because of a slow reduction process for nitrate or nitrite by ruminal bacteria (Nagaraja 2016). Specifically, when the rate of nitrate reduction to nitrite in the rumen is greater than the rate of nitrite reduction to $NH_3$, nitrite is accumulated and then absorbed across the rumen wall into the blood (Yang et al. 2016). In the blood, nitrite binds to red blood cells and converts the ferrous ($Fe^{2+}$) form of hemoglobin to its ferric ($Fe^{3+}$) form (methemoglobin), while nitrite itself is oxidized to nitrate. Since methemoglobin cannot carry oxygen, high levels of methemoglobin will result in toxicity syndromes, including reduced food intake, breathing difficulties, brain damage, or even death. To reduce nitrate or nitrite toxicity in ruminants, a strategy of acclimation over 2 weeks or longer has been implemented in some studies (Lee and Beauchemin 2014). Note that methylene blue (1 mg/kg BW, intravenous administration) can be used to treat nitrate or nitrite poinsoning by rapidly converting methemoglobin into hemoglobin (Van Dijk et al. 1983).

#### *Utilization of Nucleic Acids*

In the rumen, nucleic acids (5%–10% of dietary N) are degraded by nucleases (e.g., ribonucleases and deoxyribonucleases) into nucleotides, which are further hydrolyzed by nucleotidases and non-specific phosphatases into nucleosides and Pi (Nagaraja 2016). The nucleosides are degraded into: (1) purine or pyrimidine bases plus ribose or deoxyribose by nucleosidases; or (2) purine or pyrimidine bases plus ribose-1-P by nucleoside phosphorylase. Purines are converted sequentially into uric acid, allantoin, allantoic acid, ureidoglycolic acid, and urea plus glycoxylate. Pyrimidine bases are metabolized to β-alanine, β-aminoisobutyrate, ammonia, and $CO_2$. All these products have been found in the rumen of ruminants (Vogels and Van der Driet 1976). Indeed, 42% of the rumen coliform isolates are capable of growing on a medium that contains uric acid as the primary source of carbon and nitrogen. The predominant uricolytic organism is *Paracolobactrum aerogenoides*, but *S. ruminantium* can also use adenine and uric acid, but not allantoin, xanthine, or uracil, as nitrogen sources. The collective actions of ruminal bacteria benefit their ruminant hosts through the conversion of NPN into ammonia, AAs, and protein.

### **Intracellular Protein Synthesis from Small Peptides, AAs, and Ammonia in Microbes**

Extracellular di- and tri-peptides, free AAs, and ammonia in the rumen are taken up by the bacteria, which are quantitatively the major microbes for synthesizing protein (McDonal et al. 2011). Ruminal protozoa take up a small amount of extracellular di- and tri-peptides and free AAs but no extracellular ammonia, whereas ruminal fungi take up a small amount of extracellular di- and tri-peptides, free AAs, and ammonia. Before their use for protein synthesis in all the microbes, the small peptides must be hydrolyzed into free AAs, and ammonia converted into free AAs. Within the ruminal microorganisms, free AAs are used via multiple metabolic pathways for the production of: (1) proteins and peptides; (2) new AAs (including all L-AAs and, to a much lesser extent, some D-AAs); (3) ammonia, NO, and $H_2S$; (4) nucleic acids; (5) amines; (6) α-ketoacids (e.g., pyruvate, oxaloacetate [OAA], α-ketoglutarate [α-KG], and branched-chain α-ketoacids [BCKAs]); and (7) short-chain fatty acids (SCFAs). The energy required for AA and protein syntheses, as well as AA transport into the cells, is provided primarily from the fermentation of dietary carbohydrates and, to a lesser extent, AA catabolism. In addition, many minerals (e.g., magnesium, manganese, zinc, sulfur, and cobalt) participate in these synthetic processes. Thus, adequate intake of digestible carbohydrates and minerals is essential for maximum microbial protein synthesis in the rumen. In all microbes, protein synthesis is maximized when the release of AAs from dietary protein matches ATP production from the degradation of carbohydrates.

About 90% of the total N in the rumen content exists in an insoluble form (e.g., microbial proteins, smaller particles of undigested dietary protein, and sloughed rumen epithelial cells). N in the soluble pool (about 10% of the total rumen N) consists of ammonia N (~70%) and a mixture of free AAs and peptides. Ammonia N is present in the rumen in concentrations varying between 20 and 500 mg/L, depending on diet and time after feeding. A minimum concentration of ruminal ammonia (50 mg/L fluid) is necessary for bacteria to grow well in the rumen. Maximum concentrations of ammonia are usually reached about 2 h after ingestion of a protein-containing diet. AA- and peptide-N are present at much lower concentrations (usually <20 mg/L) than those of ammonia in the rumen (McDonal et al. 2011). The proportion of microbial protein from ammonia in the rumen depends on N sources: e.g., ranging from 26% when high concentrations of peptides and free AAs are present (as in steers fed diets supplemented with high-protein concentrates) to 100% when urea is the sole source (Salter et al. 1979). In lactating cows fed an 18%-CP alfalfa hay diet, 33% of microbial N is derived from ammonia (Hristov et al. 2005). At typical peptide and AA concentrations in the rumen, ~80% of the microbial N is derived from ammonia (Firkins et al. 2007). In the rumen, 1 mol urea is hydrolyzed by urease to 2 mol $NH_3$ plus 1 mol $CO_2$, with the $NH_3$ being utilized for bacterial protein synthesis or absorbed into blood (Figure 7.8). Intact microbial protein accounts for >50% of total N in the rumen (Bergen and Bates 1984).

The most important initial reaction for microbial assimilation of ammonia is catalyzed by glutamate dehydrogenase to produce Glu, which is then utilized to synthesize Gln, Ala, Asp, and Asn by GS, Glu-pyruvate transaminase, Glu-oxaloacetate transaminase, and Asn synthetase, respectively (Figure 7.10). Glu is also formed from Gln and α-ketoglutarate by Glu synthase. This Glu family of AAs (Glu, Gln, Ala, Asp, and Asn) serves as substrates for the synthesis of all other AAs by microorganisms in the presence of fermentable carbohydrates and sulfur in the rumen. Sulfur is needed for the synthesis of methionine and cysteine, and can be supplied as sulfate or protein. Sulfate $\left(SO_4^{2-}\right)$ is converted to sulfite $\left(SO_3^{2-}\right)$ in ruminal microorganisms via three sequential reactions involving ATP-dependent sulfurylase, ATP-dependent adenosine-5′-phosphosulfate kinase, and NADPH-dependent 3′-phosphoadenosine-5′-phosphosulfate reductase (Wu 2013). Sulfite is reduced to sulfide ($S^{2-}$) by NADPH-dependent sulfite reductase in the microbes, and hydrogen sulfide ($H_2S$) is required for the conversion of serine into cysteine (Figure 7.9). Elemental sulfur (S), two forms of calcium sulfate (hydrated $CaSO_4.2H_2O$ and anhydrous $CaSO_4$), and ammonium sulfate [$(NH_4)_2SO_4$] are effective sources of sulfide for ruminal bacteria. The diets for ruminants should contain N and sulfur at a ratio (g/g) ranging from 12:1 to 16:1, depending on the desired levels of their growth and lactation performance.

### Role of Ruminal Protozoa in Intracellular Protein Degradation

In the rumen, protozoa are active in ruminal protein degradation, and, owing to their large size, can account for about 25% of the total microbial mass in the rumen, depending on the type of rations (Firkins et al. 2007). They engulf and digest, through the use of hydrolytic enzymes (including lysozymes to break down bacterial cell walls), bacteria, fungi, small feed particles, and water-insoluble proteins (Jouany 1996). Protozoa are active in degrading extracellular water-insoluble proteins, but poorly degrade extracellular water-soluble proteins due to their limited engulfment

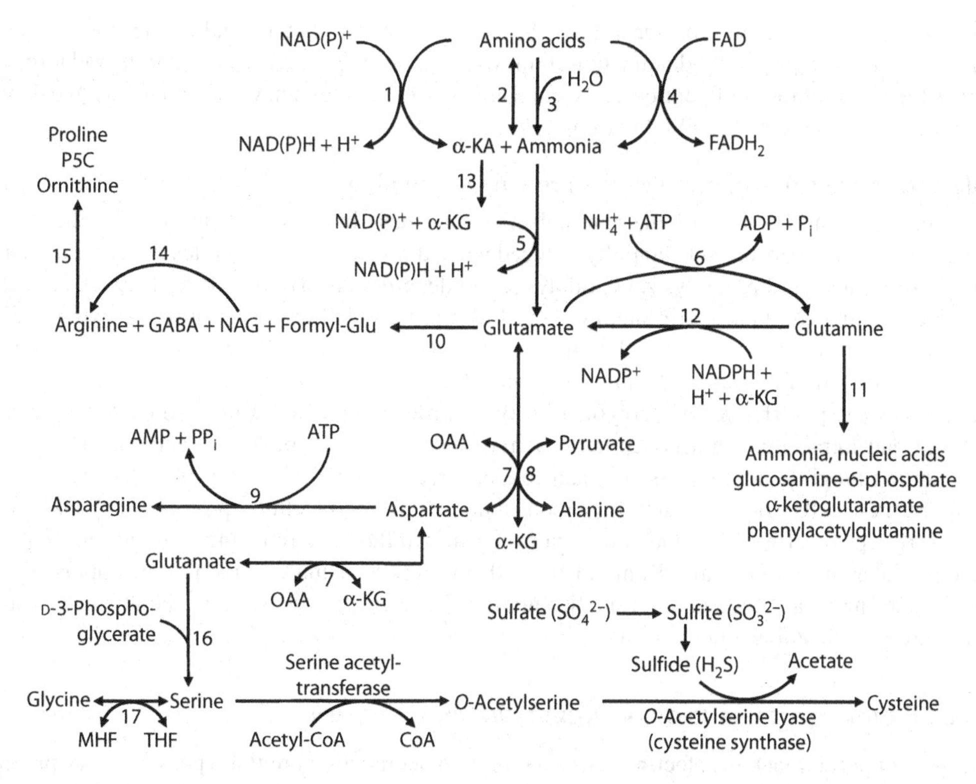


**FIGURE 7.10** Production and utilization of ammonia by microorganisms in the rumen of ruminants. GABA, γ-aminobutyrate; Formyl-Glu, formylglutamate; α-KA, α-ketoacids; α-KG, α-ketoglutarate; NAG, *N*-acetylglutamate; P5C, pyrroline-5-caroxylate. The enzymes that catalyze the indicated reactions are: (1) AA dehydrogenases; (2) AA transaminases; (3) AA deaminases; (4) AA oxidases; (5) glutamate dehydrogenase; (6) glutamine synthetase; (7) glutamate-oxaloacetate transaminase (aspartate transaminase); (8) glutamate-pyruvate transaminase (alanine transaminase); (9) asparagine synthetase; (10) the syntheses of NAG, GABA, P5C, and formyl-Glu from glutamate are catalyzed by NAG synthase, glutamate decarboxylase, γ-glutamyl kinase plus glutamyl semialdehyde dehydrogenase, and complex enzymes, respectively; (11) a series of enzymes required in multiple pathways; (12) glutamate synthase (also known as NADPH-dependent glutamine: α-ketoglutarate amidotransferase; glutamine + 2 α-ketoglutarate + NADPH + H$^+$ → 2 glutamate + NADP$^+$); and (13) the conversion of α-ketoacids to α-ketoglutarate via various reactions; (14) the enzymes for converting NAG into arginine; (15) arginase, ornithine aminotransferase, and P5C reductase; and (16) the enzymes for converting D-3-phosphoglycerate and glutamate into serine; (17) serine hydroxymethyltransferase. MTF, $N^5$-$N^{10}$-methylene tetrahydrofolate; NAG, *N*-acetylglutamate; OAA, oxaloacetate; P5C, pyrroline-5-carboxylate; THF, tetrahydrofolate.

(Firkins and Yu 2015). Like bacteria, protozoa actively deaminate AAs to form ammonia plus their carbon skeletons. However, in contrast to bacteria, protozoa cannot synthesize AAs from ammonia (Jouany 1996) and release large amounts of peptides, AAs, and ammonia (representing ~50% of total ingested protein) into ruminal fluid. Owing to their secretory activity, substantial autolysis, and apoptosis, protozoa are a source of high-activity peptidases in ruminal fluid, which participates in the extracellular hydrolysis of peptides. Thus, through the engulfment of bacteria, extracellular protein, intracellular proteolysis, the release of proteolysis products, and their reuptake, protozoa are key players in the intra-ruminal recycling of N. There is evidence that ≥65% of protozoal protein recycles within the rumen under normal nutritional and physiological conditions (Punia et al. 1992). This extensive N cycle, along with the selective retention of isotrichid protozoa in the rumen, functions to: (1) convert insoluble proteins in the bacterial and fungal membranes and in ruminal fluid into soluble cytosolic proteins; (2) supply a utilizable source of N to generate small peptides, AAs, and ammonia for sustaining bacterial growth; and (3) conserve dietary and endogenous N. This helps to explain, in part, why defaunation (removal of protozoa) decreases protein degradation, as well as the concentrations of peptides, AAs, and ammonia in the rumen, while enhancing N balance in ruminants (Firkins et al. 2007; Males and Purser 1970).

#### Role of Ruminal Fungi in Intracellular Protein Degradation

Fungi can account for ~5% of the ruminal microbial mass in the ruminants fed lignified fiber diets, but their numbers are substantially reduced when diets rich in concentrates are fed. Fungi are capable of intracellular proteolysis, peptidolysis, and deamination (Broderick et al. 1991), but their role in degrading ruminal feed protein (extracellular protein) is limited because the extracellular protease activity of fungal origin is low in the rumen (Brock et al. 1982). In evaluating the seven most common strains of ruminal fungi in culture, Michel et al. (1993) found that only one strain (i.e., *Piromyces* sp.) exhibited proteolytic activity toward extracellular casein. All the seven strains of fungi had intracellular aminopeptidase activity but no carboxypeptidase activity. It is likely that ruminal fungi do not play a significant role in directly degrading feed proteins in the rumen. However, these cells can make an indirect contribution to the extracellular proteolysis by taking up di- and tri-peptides, free AAs, and ammonia from ruminal fluid and reducing the concentrations of these products in ruminal fluid. Ruminal fungi themselves contribute to the protein supply of the host by serving as a source of high-quality microbial protein for digestion in the abomasum and small intestine (Gruninger et al. 2014).

### Major Factors Affecting Protein Degradation in the Rumen

The most important factors affecting microbial protein degradation are the types of dietary protein and carbohydrates, their metabolism to ammonia or lactate, ruminal pH, and microbial number and activity (including the predominant microbial population) in the rumen (Firkins and Yu 2015). Other influential factors include the particle size of the ration, ruminal passage rate, and environmental temperatures. Overall, the microbial ecosystem, including the populations of not only bacteria but also protozoa and fungi, is crucial for the fermentative digestion of protein in the rumen (Nagaraja 2016).

#### Effects of Type of Dietary Protein on Its Degradation in the Rumen

Different dietary proteins have different rates of fermentation in the rumen (Wallace 1994). The rates of ruminal degradation are: 200%–300%/h for soluble proteins (e.g., globulins and some albumins); 5%–15%/h for most albumins and glutelins; 0.1%–1.5%/h for prolamines, extensins, prolamines, plant cell-wall protein, and denatured proteins; and 0.0%/h for Maillard products, lignin-bound proteins, and tannin-bound proteins (Chalupa and Sniffen 1994; Ghorbani 2012). Consistent with the current literature, several definitions on ruminal protein digestion are based on CP content in diets and digestae: (1) RDP, which replaces the earlier term DIP (degraded intake); (2) RUP (rumen-undegraded CP), which replaces the earlier term UIP (undegraded intake CP); (3) MCP (rumen-synthesized microbial CP); and (4) MP (metabolizable protein, defined as the true protein, that is, digested post-rumen), which is calculated as 0.64 × MCP. The rationale for the latter calculation is that microbial CP (as provided by ruminal bacteria and protozoa) contains 80% true protein and the true protein of microbial CP is 80% digestible in the small intestine (NRC 2001).

The proportion of the total dietary protein that is degraded in the rumen varies from 70%–85% for most diets to 30%–40% for less soluble proteins (Table 7.6). Rates of protein degradation in the rumen depend on residence time in the rumen, proteolytic activity of ruminal microorganisms, the type of protein, and the level of feeding. For example, some proteins of animal origin (e.g., feather meal, MBM, and blood meal) are much more resistant to rumen degradation than plant proteins. Much evidence shows that dietary RDP feeds the ruminal bacteria and ensures an adequate supply of microbial protein to the small intestine, whereas dietary RUP (digestible in the abomasum and

**TABLE 7.6**
**Degradation of Dietary Protein and NPN Substances in the Rumen of Cattle**

| Ingredients | CP Content (%) | RDP (%) | RUP (%) |
|---|---|---|---|
| | **(1) Plant-Source Protein Ingredients** | | |
| Alfalfa hay | 22 | 84 | 16 |
| Brewer's grains | 29.2 | 34 | 66 |
| Canola meal | 40.9 | 68 | 32 |
| Corn distiller's grains | 30.4 | 26 | 74 |
| Corn gluten meal | 66.3 | 41 | 59 |
| Soybean meal | 52.9 | 80 | 20 |
| Soypass® | 52.6 | 34 | 66 |
| | **(2) Silage** | | |
| Alfalfa | 19.5 | 92 | 8 |
| Barley | 11.9 | 86 | 14 |
| Corn | 8.6 | 77 | 23 |
| | **(3) Other Plant-Source Ingredients** | | |
| Barley grain | 13.2 | 67 | 33 |
| Barley straw | 4.4 | 30 | 70 |
| Timothy hay | 10.8 | 73 | 27 |
| | **(4) Animal-Source Protein Ingredients** | | |
| Blood meal | 93.8 | 25 | 75 |
| Hydrolyzed feather meal | 85.8 | 30 | 70 |
| Fish meal | 67.9 | 40 | 60 |
| Meat & bone meal | 50 | 47 | 53 |
| | **(3) Nonprotein Nitrogen** | | |
| Urea | 291 | 100 | 0 |

*Sources:* Chalupa, W. and C.J. Sniffen. 1994. In: *Recent Advances in Animal Nutrition*. Edited by P.C. Garnsworthy and D.J.A. Cole. University of Nottingham Press, Nottingham, pp. 265–275; Ghorbani, G.R. 2012. Dynamics of Protein Metabolism in the Ruminant. http://www.freepptdb.com/details-dynamics-of-protein-metabolism-in-the-ruminant.

small intestine) complements the microbial protein for the provision of high-quality protein to the host ruminant (NRC 2001).

## Effects of Type of Carbohydrate on Microbial Protein Synthesis in the Rumen

As the major source of energy for ruminal microbes and an effector of ruminal pH, dietary carbohydrate supply profoundly influences the utilization of ruminal $NH_3$ for microbial protein synthesis (Hristov et al. 2005). Compared with neutral detergent fiber (NDF), intraruminal provision of glucose to lactating cows decreased: (1) ruminal $NH_3$-N flux (including the transfer of blood urea into the rumen); (2) the irreversible disappearance of ruminal ammonia-N from the rumen (including the ammonia absorbed into the blood through the ruminal epithelium plus the ammonia converted into microbial protein); (3) ruminal acetate and ammonia concentrations; and (4) ruminal pH. However, intraruminal administration of glucose increased: (1) ruminal butyrate concentration; (2) microbial N concentration in the rumen; (3) microbial N flow out of the rumen; and (4) the percentage of bacterial N derived from ammonia in lactating cows. Starch had similar effects on the measured variables to those of glucose, except that ruminal ammonia flux or ruminal acetate concentration did not differ between starch and NDF feeding (Table 7.7). Glucose or starch feeding, which decreases ruminal pH, may alter the number and activity of butyrate-, acetate-, and/or ammonia-producing bacteria in the rumen (Firkins et al. 2007). Thus, appropriate amounts of readily fermentable carbohydrates in the diets of ruminants likely inhibit ammonia production from AAs and enhance microbial protein synthesis in the rumen.

### Effects of Dietary Concentrate and Forage Intake on Proteolytic Bacteria in the Rumen

Adequate intake of dietary protein (e.g., 14% CP in the diet of growing beef and 18% CP in the diet of high-producing lactating cows, expressed on the basis of DM content) is essential for the optimal growth and proteolytic activity of ruminal bacteria. Feeding an appropriate amount of concentrates to ruminants increases total microbial population in the rumen, including some active proteolytic bacteria that are also amylolytic bacteria (e.g., *Prevotella ruminicola*, *Ruminobacter amylophilus*, and *Streptococcus bovis*) (Ghorbani 2012). Under these conditions (e.g., in high-producing dairy cows), the ruminal fermentation of dietary protein and the engulfment of bacteria by protozoa are favored, as reported for hay-fed sheep supplemented with or without concentrates (Table 7.8).

**TABLE 7.7**
**Effects of the Type of Dietary Carbohydrate on Ruminal Ammonia N Use in Lactating Dairy Cows**

| Variable | Glucose | Starch | NDF |
|---|---|---|---|
| Dry matter (DM) intake, kg/day | 21.8 | 21.4 | 22.6 |
| Organic matter (OM) intake, kg/day | 19.9 | 19.8 | 20.4 |
| NDF intake, kg/day | 8.3 | 8.3 | 12.4 |
| Nitrogen (N) intake, kg/day | 0.634 | 0.630 | 0.662 |
| Ruminal true digestibility of DM, % | 64.1 | 61.9 | 60.9 |
| Ruminal true digestibility of OM, % | 66.5 | 64.0 | 64.7 |
| Ruminal true digestibility of NDF, % | 57.0 | 59.6 | 56.5 |
| Ruminal true digestibility of N, % | 57.5 | 59.1 | 66.6 |
| $NH_3$-N in ruminal fluid, mM | 8.5[b] | 9.6[b] | 16.4[a] |
| Ruminal $NH_3$-N flux, g/day | 350[b] | 487[a] | 533[a] |
| Microbial N in rumen fluid, g/kg TDOM | 15[a] | 15[a] | 12[b] |
| Irreversible disappearance of ruminal $NH_3$-N, g/day | 230[b] | 343[a] | 320[a] |
| Microbial N flow out of the rumen, g/day | 197[a] | 185[a] | 153[b] |
| Microbial N derived from $NH_3$-N, g/day | 75[b] | 111[a] | 74[b] |
| Bacterial N derived from $NH_3$-N, % | 33[a] | 33[a] | 23[b] |
| Protozoa in rumen, $\log_{10}$/mL | 5.26 | 5.21 | 5.42 |
| Total SCFAs in ruminal fluid, mM | 122 | 139 | 136 |
| Acetate in ruminal fluid, mM | 74.0[b] | 95.4[a] | 94.5[a] |
| Propionate in ruminal fluid, mM | 22.1 | 23.0 | 23.2 |
| Butyrate in ruminal fluid, mM | 22.2[a] | 15.0[b] | 12.4[c] |
| Butyrate/Total SCFAs, mol/100 mol | 18.2[a] | 10.8[b] | 9.1[b] |
| pH in ruminal fluid | 6.00[c] | 6.19[b] | 6.41[a] |

*Source:* Adapted from Hristov, A.N. et al. 2005. *J. Anim. Sci.* 83:408–421.

Late-lactation Holstein cows were fed an all alfalfa-hay (chopped) diet (~18% CP) at 12 h intervals (DM intake = 22.2 kg/d). Glucose, starch, or NDF was introduced intraruminally at 20.6% of DM intake twice daily before each feeding.

[a–c] Within a row, means not sharing the same superscript letters differ ($P < 0.05$).

NDF, neutral detergent fiber (provided from white-oat fiber); SCFAs, short-chain fatty acids.

**TABLE 7.8**
**Effects of Dietary Concentrates on Microbial Protein Synthesis in the Rumen of Hay-Fed Mature Sheep**

| Variable | Hay | 60% Hay + 40% Concentrate[a] |
|---|---|---|
| Organic matter intake, g/day | 804 | 750 |
| Nitrogen intake, g/day | 21.7 | 21.2 |
| Rumen retention time of particles, h | 19.9 | 31.6 |
| Rumen retention time of solutes, h | 11.8 | 10.6 |
| Rumen pH | 6.48 | 6.08 |
| Rumen $NH_3$-N, mg/L fluid | 192 | 225 |
| **Rumen Microbial N, g** | | |
| Total microbial N | 18.3 | 24.0 |
| Bacterial N | 10.9 | 8.54 |
| Protozoal N | 6.93 | 14.9 |
| Fungal N | 0.41 | 0.56 |
| **% of Total Microbial N in Rumen Digesta** | | |
| Fungal N | 2 | 2 |
| Protozoal N | 38 | 62 |
| Bacterial N | 60 | 36 |
| Flow of $NH_3$-N out of the rumen, g/day | 2.80 | 2.2 |
| Duodenal digesta $NH_3$-N, mg/L fluid | 96.5 | 105.5 |
| **Duodenal Digesta Microbial N, g/Day** | | |
| Total microbial N | 14.8 | 15.1 |
| Bacterial N | 13.9 | 13.0 |
| Protozoal N | 0.82 | 1.73 |
| Fungal N | 0.16 | 0.35 |
| **% of Total Microbial N Flow (Duodenal Digesta)** | | |
| Fungi | 1 | 2 |
| Protozoa | 5 | 12 |
| Bacteria | 94 | 86 |
| Flow of $NH_3$-N to duodenum, g/day | 0.98 | 0.99 |

*Source:* Faichney G.J. et al. 1997. *Anim. Feed Sci. Technol.* 64:193–213.

[a] The concentrate mixture contained (g/kg): barley, 825; soybean meal, 110; dried molasses, 47; and mineral-vitamin mix, 18.

Likewise, consumption of fresh forage enhances the proportion of proteolytic bacteria relative to total microbial population in the rumen, which is also beneficial for the ruminal fermentation of low-quality protein (Chalupa et al. 1994). Very high intake of dietary starch rapidly reduces the pH and the number of proteolytic bacteria in the rumen, which in turn adversely affects ruminal protein degradation.

## Nutritional Importance of Protein Digestion in the Rumen

Ruminants are unique in digestive physiology in that they can convert NPN (e.g., urea and ammonia), roughages, and forages into bacterial and protozoal proteins, which are digested terminally in the small intestine into constituent small peptides and AAs. The peptides and AAs are used for the synthesis of high-quality animal proteins in skeletal muscle, the lactating mammary gland, and other tissues. Thus, ruminants can convert low-quality protein and non-protein materials into high-quality products (e.g., meat and milk) for human consumption without a need to compete with monogastric animals or humans for foods or natural resources. This underscores the nutritional and economic significance of the digestion of plant proteins by ruminants. An understanding of these complex processes will aid in: (1) increasing the supply of all AAs to the small intestine for absorption and utilization for tissue protein synthesis; (2) sustaining regional and global animal production; and (3) providing high-quality animal protein to improve human growth, development, and health.

As in all animals, a major loss of dietary protein in ruminants occurs due to inefficiencies of ruminal digestion, extensive catabolism of AAs in the gastrointestinal tract, and suboptimal rates of protein synthesis in tissues (particularly skeletal muscle) (Wu et al. 2014b). For example, only 30%–35% of feed protein is captured in milk and the remaining 65%–70% is lost as nitrogenous compounds in the feces and urine. In ruminant diets, soluble protein should account for 30%–32% of total CP or about half of the RDP level, whereas RUP should be 32%–39% of total CP in the diet (Fellner 2002). Such diets should meet dietary requirements for not only NDF and starches but also total CP, RDP, and RUP. This is because: (1) total CP provides nitrogen sources for microbial protein synthesis in the rumen, which is tightly coupled with ATP production from the glycolysis of glucose and its fermentation to SCFAs in the microbes; (2) RDP is essential for sustaining microbial growth and mass in the rumen; (3) RUP supplies high-quality protein for digestion in the abomasum and small intestine; and (4) dietary NDF helps to maintain a rumen environment that is favorable for fermentation. Consistent with this notion is the finding that, in lactating cows fed diets with CP content between 9% and 17% and without supplemental fats, milk protein yield increases by a 0.02-percentage unit with a 1-percent unit increase in dietary CP (Emery 1978).

## Protecting High-Quality Protein and Supplements of AAs from Rumen Degradation

High-quality dietary protein is required to support maximal growth, reproduction, and lactation performance of beef, dairy cows, sheep, and goats. Degradation of these proteins by ruminal bacteria results in a substantial waste, as not all dietary protein is utilized for microbial protein synthesis. Additionally, microbial protein synthesis requires large amounts of energy and the efficiency of energetic transformations for protein synthesis from AAs is usually less than 75%. Furthermore, supplements of crystalline AAs in the diets of ruminants are not efficacious because of their rapid degradation in the rumen (Tedeschi and Fox 2016). Thus, high-quality protein or supplemental AAs (e.g., Arg, His, Lys, and Met) in the diet should be protected from rumen degradation. Several approaches have been developed to reduce the degradation of protein in the rumen. These methods include the treatment of protein by mild heating, chemical treatment, addition of polyphenolic phytochemicals, and physical encapsulation (e.g., rumen-protected protein). In the small intestine, the coating lipids are readily broken down by lipase to release proteins or AAs. Similarly, nearly all free AAs in diets do not escape the rumen into the abomasum, and supplemental AAs for ruminants should be protected from rumen degradation and generally recognized as safe (GRAS) to ensure both high efficacy and safety. Rumen-protected AAs should be stable, particularly when they are incorporated into silage or forage-based total mixed rations.

### Heating

Heating is one of the earliest methods used to increase the escape of high-quality protein (e.g., casein) from the rumen. The underlying principle is the Maillard reaction, which involves a reaction between certain AAs [particularly the ε-amino groups ($-NH_2$) of lysine residues in protein] and carbonyl compounds ($-HC{=}O$), usually reducing sugars (e.g., glucose) (Chapter 4). The initial reaction is the formation of a Schiff's base, followed by an Amadori rearrangement of Schiff's base to generate an Amadori compound. The formation of Schiff's base is reversible. However, further heating results in the production of melanoidin polymers that are nutritionally unavailable to animals. Heating also helps to denature protease inhibitors in feedstuffs.

### Chemical Treatments

Chemical treatments of dietary protein aid in reducing its solubility and its susceptibility to proteases in the rumen. An example of chemical treatment is the use of formaldehyde (HCHO). An advantage of this method is that most of the formaldehyde-protein reactions are unstable at low pH, such as the pH in the abomasum and the upper part of the small intestine. Therefore, formaldehyde-treated proteins are susceptible to degradation by proteases in the abomasum and the small intestine. However, formaldehyde is a potential carcinogen and is a hazard to animals and humans. Other chemicals and methods used for treating dietary protein (e.g., SBM) include NaOH, ethanol, propionic acid, and calcium lignosulfonate, as well as extrusion and expeller processing (Waltz and Stern 1989). To date, a common method to chemically treat a protein ingredient (e.g., oilseed meal) for manufacturing a rumen-protected product is to mix the feedstuff with calcium lignosulfonate (a by-product of the wool pulp industry containing a variety of sugars, mainly D-xylose), followed by appropriate heating.

### Polyphenolic Phytochemicals

Tannins (natural phytochemicals) are often used to protect protein degradation in the rumen. They spontaneously react with proteins primarily through hydrogen bonding to generate a water-insoluble complex. Such a tannin–protein complex is resistant to ruminal proteases at pH 5.5–6.5. However, in the lumen of the abomasum (pH 2–3), protein is dissociated from the tannins and is available for degradation by proteases. Thus, high-quality proteins can be effectively protected from degradation in the rumen and become available for digestion in the abomasum and then in the small intestine. In practice, tannins may be added directly to feedstuffs for ruminants.

### Physical Encapsulation of Protein or AAs

Early work in the 1970s indicated that certain protein ingredients of animal origin are resistant to rumen degradation (Tamminga 1979). Animal-source protein is more resistant to bacterial proteases than plant-source protein because of its water insolubility resulting from heating during the rendering process to remove any potential pathogens and inactivate any latent proteases from the animal's tissues. To date, the methods for physical encapsulation of proteins or AAs include blood spraying and the use of a hydrogenated lipid layer. Protein supplements are sprayed by blood, followed by heating the mixture to dryness, to effectively coat the surface of proteins. Proteins or AAs can also be coated with hydrogenated lipids (e.g., lecithin or soy oils) to form microcapsules. All these encapsulated proteins and AAs are not colonized to the surface of ruminal bacteria and are less accessible to proteases or AA deaminases in the ruminal fluid.

### Inhibition of AA Degradation

The conversion of AAs to their carbon skeletons and ammonia is catalyzed by AA deaminases. Thus, an inhibition of these enzymes in the rumen can increase the availability of dietary AAs for absorption in the small intestine. In support of this view, dietary supplementation with an inhibitor of AA deaminases (e.g., diphenyliodonium chloride) can enhance the flow of high-quality protein from the rumen into the abomasum and the small intestine, thereby improving growth performance in beef cattle fed diets containing high-quality protein. However, inhibition of AA deaminases can reduce the availability of ammonia for AA synthesis by ruminal bacteria and therefore is not beneficial for ruminants fed diets containing low-quality protein.

## Flow of Microbial Protein from the Rumen into the Abomasum and Duodenum

Ruminal bacteria and protozoa undergo turnover in the rumen to grow new cells and replace the old ones. In addition, microbial lysis occurs within the rumen due to the presence of autolytic enzymes and bacteriocins, as well as bacteriophages and mycoplasmas. Furthermore, ruminal microbes flow out of the rumen into the abomasum and then the duodenum, with the rates for bacteria being greater than those for protozoa. The mean retention times of bacteria and protozoa in the rumen of roughage-fed ruminants are ~20 and 35 h, respectively (Ffoulkes and Leng 1988). Thus, as shown for mature sheep (Table 7.8), protozoal N may account for ~25%–40% of total microbial N in the rumen, but only 1% of total microbial N in the duodenal digesta. Of note, Sok et al. (2017) have estimated that: (1) 40% of the bacteria in the duodenum are present in the fluid phase, which means that they pass with the gastric liquid phase; and (2) 60% of bacteria and most entodiniomorphid protozoa (>90% of protozoa) are found in the particulate phase of the duodenum.

The composition of AAs is similar between rumen bacterial and protozoal proteins, except that the content of Ala, Gly, and Val is higher in rumen bacterial protein than that in rumen protozoal protein, while the opposite is true for Glu plus Gln and Lys (Table 7.9). Much evidence shows that feeding different dietary rations to ruminants can affect the amount of microbial proteins flowing from the rumen into the duodenum, but does not generally influence the AA composition or quality of the microbial proteins (Bergen et al. 1968a; Bergen 2015). In contrast to common belief, the content of only ten AAs is similar between ruminal bacteria protein and casein: His, Leu, Lys, Met, Cys, Phe, Ser, Trp, Tyr, and Val. Since sulfur-containing AAs in casein are known to be inadequate for the maximum growth of young animals (Wu 2013), ruminal microbial protein is not ideal for the growth performance of ruminants. Notably, the content of Ala, Arg, Asp, Asn, Gly, and Thr is

**TABLE 7.9**
**AA Composition (g/100 g Total AAs) of Proteins in Rumen and Small-Intestinal Mixed Bacteria and in Animal Bodies**

| Amino Acid Body[a] | Sheep Rumen Mixed Bacteria[b] | | Sheep Rumen Protozoa[c] | Duodenal Digest[b] | | Casein[c] | Cattle Body[a] | Sheep Body[a] |
|---|---|---|---|---|---|---|---|---|
| | Bergen[b] | Chamberlain[c] | | Sheep[b] | Cows[c] | | | |
| Ala | 6.5 | 7.4 | 4.1 | 7.09 | 5.4 | 2.6 | 7.6 | 6.65 |
| Arg | 5.2 | 4.9 | 4.9 | 4.91 | 5.0 | 3.6 | 7.5 | 6.80 |
| Asp + Asn | 12.1 | 11.7 | 11.6 | 11.3 | 7.7 | 6.5 | 8.7 | 7.95 |
| Cys | 0.54 | – | – | – | – | 0.4 | 1.4 | 1.46 |
| Glu + Gln | 13.4 | 12.9 | 15.1 | 12.1 | 14.4 | 20.9 | 13.8 | 13.4 |
| Gly | 5.0 | 5.3 | 4.1 | 6.48 | 7.4 | 1.8 | 12.1 | 11.3 |
| His | 2.1 | 2.1 | 2.1 | 2.53 | 2.0 | 2.6 | 2.7 | 2.12 |
| Ile | 5.7 | 6.5 | 6.8 | 6.86 | 5.7 | 4.8 | 3.0 | 3.60 |
| Leu | 7.6 | 8.3 | 8.5 | 9.65 | 9.1 | 8.8 | 7.4 | 6.94 |
| Lys | 8.5 | 7.8 | 11.3 | 7.55 | 6.2 | 7.4 | 6.9 | 6.10 |
| Met | 2.4 | 2.4 | 2.1 | 1.23 | 1.8 | 2.6 | 1.8 | 1.90 |
| Phe | 4.9 | 5.5 | 5.8 | 6.24 | 5.4 | 5.0 | 3.9 | 3.46 |
| Pro | 3.5 | 3.8 | 3.7 | 4.63 | 6.9 | 11.7 | 8.7 | 8.55 |
| Ser | 4.5 | 4.6 | 4.5 | 3.11 | 5.2 | 5.4 | 4.7 | 4.52 |
| Thr | 5.4 | 5.8 | 5.2 | 4.78 | 5.8 | 3.8 | 4.3 | 3.68 |
| Trp | 1.4 | – | – | – | – | 1.2 | 1.2 | 1.14 |
| Tyr | 4.4 | 5.0 | 5.4 | 2.71 | 5.1 | 5.3 | 2.7 | 2.70 |
| Val | 6.0 | 6.5 | 5.0 | 7.09 | 6.3 | 5.7 | 4.2 | 4.26 |

[a] Flores, D.A. et al. 1986. *Can. J. Anim. Sci.* 66:1019–1027. Mature sheep were fed fresh alfalfa.
[b] Bergen, W.G. 2015. *Amino Acids.* 47:251–258.
[c] Chamberlain, D.G. et al. 1986. *Grass Forage Sci.* 41:31–38. Mature sheep were fed a diet consisting of hay plus concentrate, whereas non-lactating cows were fed silage plus barley.

much higher, but the content of Glu, Gln, and Pro is much lower, in rumen microbial protein than in casein (Bergen 2015). With a few exceptions (Ala, Glu, Gln, and Lys), the composition of AAs is similar between microbial and protozoal proteins. Interestingly, the percentages of Glu, Gln, and Lys in protozoal protein are 17% and 45% higher than those in bacterial protein. Thus, compared with bacterial protein, protozoal protein may have a better nutritive value for the small intestine and the host, lending additional support for the nutritional importance of the engulfment of bacteria by protozoa in the rumen.

Owing to the addition of endogenous proteins into the abomasum, the composition of all AAs is similar between duodenal digesta and the animal body, except for the following. First, the content of Arg, Gly, and Pro is lower, but that of three branched-chain AAs (BCAAs), Phe, and Thr is higher in the duodenal digesta compared to the animal body. Thus, like nonruminants (Wu 2013), ruminants must synthesize Arg, Gly, and Pro, with endogenous N donors probably being BCAAs, and inadequate synthesis of Arg, Gly, and Pro may limit the maximum growth and production performance of ruminants.

### Digestion of Microbial and Feed Proteins in the Abomasum and Small Intestine

Digestion of protein in the abomasum and small intestine of ruminants is largely similar to that in the stomach and small intestine of nonruminants, with two exceptions for extracellular hydrolysis of bacterial and protozoal proteins. Specifically, in contrast to the stomach of nonruminants, the abomasum of ruminants (e.g., cattle, sheep, and deer) secretes large amounts of gastric lysozymes, which efficiently break down bacterial cell walls by hydrolyzing the β-1,4 glycosidic linkages of membrane polysaccharides (Irwin 1995; Irwin and Wilson 1990). The gastric lysozymes are most active at pH 2–3, in contrast to other lysozymes that exhibit highest activities at pH 7.4 and have broader pH optima. Interestingly, these enzymes are unusually resistant to cleavage by pepsin, thereby prolonging their presence in the lumen of the stomach. Of note, colobine monkeys, which are also foregut fermenters, produce high levels of gastric lysozymes (Irwin 1995). Thus, the diverse foregut fermenters share a digestive strategy to digest bacterial protein. Upon exposure to gastric proteases, proteins of rumen-bacterial origin and feed proteins are hydrolyzed by proteases to large peptides.

The digestion of ruminal protozoa in the abomasum is different from that of ruminal bacteria, due to marked differences in the structures of their cell membranes. The cell membrane of ruminal protozoa and the pellicle (a thin layer outer membrane supporting the cell membrane) of various ruminal protozoa (primarily ciliates) do not consist of β-1,4-linked polysaccharides or lignin. Therefore, no lysozymes are required to break down the protozoal cell membrane. Through the transit of digesta, ruminal protozoa flow to the omasum, where they become inactive and start to disintegrate (Hungate 1966). In the abomasum, protozoa are denatured by HCl, followed by an enzymatic attack by pepsin to form large peptides (Hook et al. 2012). The protozoa that escape proteolysis in the abomasum are further degraded by trypsin in the small intestine to generate large peptides.

In the small intestine of ruminants, the bacteria- and protozoa-derived large peptides are degraded by oligopeptidases to yield di- and tri-peptides and some free AAs, as in nonruminants. These digestion products are absorbed into enterocytes, where the small peptides are hydrolyzed to free AAs. The AAs that are not utilized by the enterocytes are transported through the lamina propria to the intestinal venule, which leads to the portal vein. As in nonruminants, the enterocytes of ruminants, such as mature sheep (Wolff et al. 1972) and growing cattle (Lescoat et al. 1996), take up a large amount of Gln, but no nutritionally significant quantity of other AAs, from the arterial blood during the postabsorptive period.

The true digestibility of microbial protein, which is determined at the terminal ileum after the correction for the flow of endogenous protein, is 85% in mature sheep (Storm and Orskov 1983) and 80% in cows (NRC 2001). Similarly, Larsen et al. (2001) reported that the true digestibility of microbial protein was ~80% in lactating cows fed barley plus concentrate, as measured for most AAs (e.g., Arg, 79.5%; Asp plus Asn, 80.4%; Gly, 79.3%; Ile, 80.4%; Leu, 80.4%; Lys, 81.6%; Met, 78.3%; and Val, 78.9%). The true digestibility of protozoal protein in ruminants is approximately 90% (McDonald et al. 2011), which is about 10%–15% higher than that of bacterial protein (Bergen and Purser 1968; Bergen et al. 1968b).

### Digestion and Absorption of Nucleic Acids in the Small Intestine

The dietary nucleic acids that escape the rumen, as well as the bacterial and protozoal nucleic acids that leave the rumen, are hydrolyzed extracellularly to nucleotides in the small intestine by pancreatic nucleases (e.g., ribonuclease and deoxyribonuclease released from the pancreas) and by intestinal phosphodiesterases (released from the small intestine). Specific pancreatic nucleotidases and nonspecific phosphatases (released from the pancreas) further degrade nucleotides to nucleosides and phosphate (Pi). The digestibility of nucleic acids to nucleosides as well as purine and pyrimidine bases in the small intestine of ruminants is 80%–90% (McDonald et al. 2011; Stentoft et al. 2015).

The nucleosides and phosphate are transported, respectively, into the enterocytes by apical membrane $Na^+$-dependent nucleoside transporters (CNT1, selctive for purine nucleoside; and CNT2, selective for pyrimidine nucleoside) and three $Na^+$-dependent phosphate transporters (NaPi2b, PiT1, and PiT2). The nucleosides that are not absorbed directly are degraded extracellularly by both pancreatic nucleosidases and small-intestinal mucosa-derived nucleoside phosphorylases to form purine or pyrimidine bases. The purine or pyrimidine bases are then transported by $Na^+$-dependent nucleobase transporters into the enterocytes. Like preruminants, the small intestine of ruminants has a high capacity to absorb nucleosides and their bases. In dairy cows, the hepatic removal of purines and pyrimidines is almost the same as their net PDV release (Stentoft et al. 2015).

Nucleic acid + $H_2O$ → Nucleotide (Nuclease; RNAse, or DNAse)
Nucleotide + $H_2O$ → Nucleoside + Pi (Nucleotidase)
Nucleoside + $H_2O$ → Purine or pyrimidine base + Ribose or deoxyribose (Nucleosidase)
Nucleoside + $P_i$ → Purine or pyrimidine base + Ribose-1-phosphate (Nucleoside phosphorylases)

### Nitrogen Recycling in Ruminants and Its Nutritional Implications

Ammonia plays an important role in interorgan AA metabolism in ruminants. The ammonia that is produced in the rumen but is not utilized for synthesis of AAs or polypeptides in microorganisms is absorbed into the blood circulation and converted into urea (Figure 7.11). Ammonia in the rumen fluid may also be utilized by rumen epithelial cells for biosynthetic processes (including the production of urea, Glu, and Gln). Ammonia in the plasma is taken up by the liver for the synthesis of urea via the urea cycle. Some urea is excreted into the urine, and up to 70% of urea undergoes recycling through the blood circulation, depending on dietary CP intake (Wu 2013). About 20% of the circulating urea is taken up by the intestine where it is hydrolyzed by microbial urease to form ammonia plus $CO_2$. Ammonia, which takes up $H^+$ to form $NH_4^+$, can increase the pH of the rumen fluid. Some urea in blood enters the rumen through saliva, and ~15% of the urea recycled to the rumen is via saliva. In the rumen, urea is hydrolyzed by microbial urease to form ammonia plus $CO_2$. The recycled N helps conserve ammonia for biosynthetic processes in the rumen. Since microbial urease hydrolyzes urea into ammonia, urea can be used as a source of N for the diets of ruminants. Urea is well utilized by rumen microorganisms when diets contain <13% CP. Thus, urea has been fed to ruminants as an NPN supplement for more than 100 years. Results of extensive research indicate that urea may represent 15%–25% of CP in diets for beef cattle, cows, and sheep (Kertz 2010).

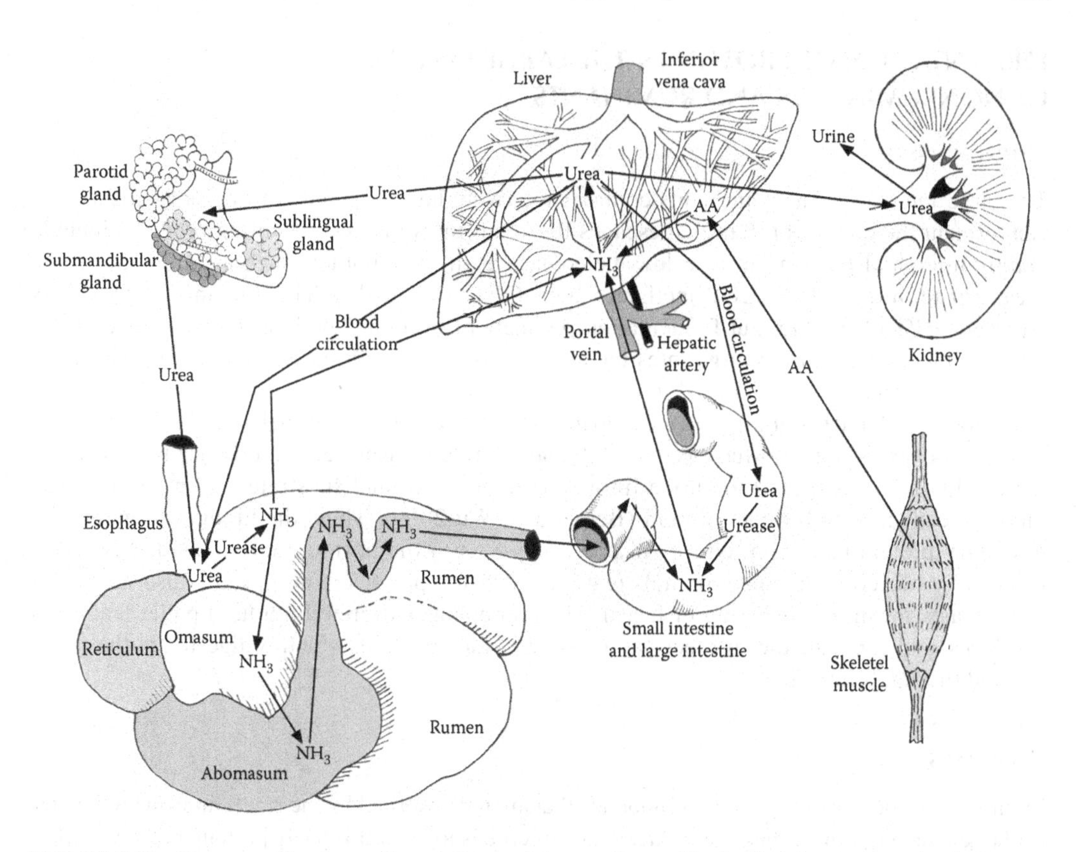


**FIGURE 7.11** Urea recycling in ruminants. Some of the urea formed in the liver from ammonia via the urea cycle enters the saliva, rumen, small intestine, and large intestine through blood circulation. In the rumen and intestinal lumen, urea is hydrolyzed by urease to ammonia, with some of the ammonia being used for synthesis of AAs and proteins by microbes. The remaining ammonia re-enters the liver for the resynthesis of urea, and some of the urea returns to the rumen and intestine, as noted previously. This process, known as urea recycling, helps maximize the efficiency of nitrogen utilization in ruminants.

Urea is a natural substance in forages and is a major form of NPN in conventional ruminant diets. Corn silage and alfalfa may contain up to 50% and 20% of NPN, respectively. Efficacy and safety of dietary supplementation with urea to diets for cattle and sheep depend on many factors, including: (1) the dosage (usually $\leq$1% in a concentrate-containing diet; $\leq$2% in low-CP hay) and frequency, (2) percentages of dietary carbohydrates and CP as well as their digestibilities in the rumen, and (3) adequate supply of phosphorus, sulfur, and trace minerals. It should be borne in mind that the toxicity of ammonia and urea can occur when their concentrations in the rumen are very high. The underlying mechanisms involve: (1) a substantial increase in the rumen pH $\left(\text{urea} \rightarrow 2NH_3 + CO_2; NH_3 + H^+ \rightarrow NH_4^+\right)$, leading to reductions in bacterial growth and synthetic activity in the rumen; (2) removal of α-KG from the Krebs cycle, thereby interfering with ATP production by cells, particularly those in the central nervous system; (3) disturbance of acid–base balance in the circulation; and (4) enhanced synthesis of Gln, which inhibits the synthesis of NO from Arg in endothelial cells and, therefore, blood flow and oxygen supply to vital organs, particularly the brain. It is advantageous to supply urea as a liquid feed supplement with molasses (2.5%–10% of total dietary DM intake) and anhydrous phosphoric acid (orthophosphoric acid, a nontoxic white solid at a temperature <42°C; 0.1%–0.3% of total dietary DM intake) (Broderick and Radloff 2004; Dixon 2013; Kertz 2010). This is because: (1) molasses serves as an energy source for microbial utilization of ammonia and protein synthesis; and (2) phosphoric acid lowers ruminal fluid pH.

## FERMENTATION OF PROTEIN IN THE LARGE INTESTINE OF NONRUMINANTS AND RUMINANTS

### Nonruminants

The large intestine of nonruminants contains relatively large amounts of microorganisms that can ferment the dietary protein that escapes the small intestine. The resulting products include mainly microbial protein but also low-molecular-weight metabolites, such as ammonia, AAs, urea, nitrite, nitrate, $H_2S$, $CO_2$, methane, and SCFAs (Wu 2013). The amounts of free AAs represent <1% of the hindgut fermentation products of protein. The biochemical processes of nitrogen metabolism in the large intestine are similar to those in the rumen of ruminants, but the hindgut fermentation of dietary protein in nonruminants is much less effective than rumen fermentation (Hendriks et al. 2012). Compared to enterocytes, the epithelial cells of the cecum and colon express much lower levels of AA and peptide transporters and, under normal feeding conditions, are exposed to only a limited amount of luminal substrates. Of note, the large intestine cannot absorb intact protein (Bergen and Wu 2009). Thus, the hindgut fermentation of dietary protein has a limited role in providing AAs to the host animals. This disadvantage is partially overcome in some animals (e.g., rabbits) that practice coprophagia (also known as coprophagy, meaning the eating of feces). The coprophages excrete both hard pellet feces and soft feces, and consume the soft feces as a source of food protein, which is digested in the stomach and the small intestine.

### Ruminants

In ruminants, dietary nitrogenous compounds that are not absorbed by the small intestine will enter the large intestine, where they are fermented by microbes to form primarily protein and low-molecular-weight substances (e.g., ammonia, $H_2S$, and SCFAs) (Bergen and Wu 2009). Other sources of N in the large intestine are derived from the recycling of blood urea and ammonia, as well as endogenous protein (e.g., sloughed epithelial cells, enzymes, and mucins). Neither the nitrogenous compounds that are bound to lignin nor the terminal products of the Maillard reaction will be degraded by microbes in the large bowel. The microbial protein synthesis (which helps to remove excessive ammonia from the hindgut) and fecal N excretion increase as the amount of dietary fermentable carbohydrates reaching the cecum and colon increases. As in nonruminants, the microbial protein synthesized in the large intestine is not absorbed into colonocytes and therefore has little nutritive value to the host.

## DIGESTION AND ABSORPTION OF PROTEIN IN FISH

### Developmental Changes of Gastric Proteases in Fish

As noted in Chapter 1, not all fish have a stomach, and agastric fish will not develop a stomach or synthesize gastric proteases even at the adult stage. Precocious fish have a functional stomach at the onset of first exogenous feeding, whereas altricial larvae develop a functional stomach during metamorphosis. In precocious and altricial fish, there are no pepsins at the larval stage, due to the absence of a functional stomach. For example, pepsins are not found in the stomach of larval striped bass or hybrid striped bass until day 16 after hatching, which corresponds to the development of their stomach (Gabaudan 1984). This organ slowly produces pepsin-like enzymes and develops acidification capacity during metamorphosis (Rønnestad et al. 2013). Active pepsins are present in the functional stomach with an acidic environment (e.g., pH 2–3). Although the stomach of most teleosts exhibits similarities in their anatomical and functional ontogeny, there are inter-species variations in the sequence and time of appearance of pepsins.

### Developmental Changes in Extracellular Proteases in the Intestine of Fish

Fish larvae obtain nutrients from the yolk sac for the first several days (e.g., 4–5 days post hatching in striped bass and hybrid striped bass), as they undergo metamorphosis and digestive tract development (García-Gasca et al. 2006; Pedersen et al. 1987). Thereafter (just before the initiation of exogenous feeding), the pancreas of fish synthesizes significant amounts of pancreatic proteases. The abundances of these enzymes increase progressively as the larvae develop. For example, in striped bass and hybrid striped bass, the specific activities of pancreatic trypsin, chymotrypsin, aminopeptidases, elastase, and carboxypeptidases A and B at day 32 post hatching (as larval development nears completion) are 65%–300% greater than those at day 4 (Baragi and Lovell 1986). After the intestine is developed, the pancreas secretes these enzymes into the intestinal lumen, which helps fish to hydrolyze the ingested dietary protein. Depending on fish species and physiological conditions, the quality and quantity of dietary protein, as well as other dietary and environmental factors, the true digestibility of dietary protein in fish generally ranges from 80% to 90% (NRC 2011; Ribeiro et al. 2011). These values are similar to those for land animals. However, rates of protein digestion plus AA absorption may be much lower in fish than in mammals and birds.

## BIOAVAILABILITY OF DIETARY AAS TO EXTRA-DIGESTIVE ORGANS

### Net Entry of Dietary AAs from the Small Intestine into the Portal Vein

Enterocytes release the absorbed, undegraded AAs into the interstitial space of the lamina propria, where they are taken up by the residing capillaries into the intestinal venule. Through the blood circulation, AAs are transported to the small vein and then the portal vein. Since enterocytes, luminal bacteria, and the lamina propria in the mammalian small intestine degrade certain AAs (Burrin and Davis 2004; Wu 1998), not all the AAs released from the hydrolysis of dietary protein enter the portal circulation (Table 7.10). For example, in 30-day-old growing pigs, 96% Glu, 95% Asp, and 67% Gln but only 13% Ala, 13% Asn, 17% Cys, and 18% Gly in the digestible diet are metabolized by the gut during their first pass into the portal circulation (Hou et al. 2016). In 60 kg growing pigs fed every 8 h (3 times daily) a 16%-CP diet (daily feed intake = 3.6% of body weight), hardly any dietary Asp, Gln, and Glu (free or peptide-bound) in the small-intestinal lumen is absorbed to the portal blood (Figure 7.12). On average, ~50% of dietary AAs do not enter the portal vein in postweaning pigs, adult pigs, and adult rats. Thus, in swine fed an adequate-protein diet, except for Arg and Ala, all AAs exhibit a negative balance across the portal vein (i.e., output < input); both Arg and Ala show a positive balance across the portal vein (i.e., output > input) because of their synthesis by enterocytes (Wu 2013). In poultry, whose enterocytes have a limited ability to degrade many AAs (including Arg and Gln) (Wu et al. 1995), it is likely that >50% of dietary AAs can enter the portal vein.

### Extraction of AAs from the Portal Vein by the Liver

AAs from the portal vein are first exposed to the hepatocytes. In growing pigs, the liver has the net uptake of basic and neutral proteinogenic AAs from the portal vein at different proportions of their net portal-vein fluxes, the net release of acidic AAs, and no uptake of Cit (Table 7.10). Generally, the rates of hepatic uptake of AAs in decreasing order are: small neutral AAs > large neutral AAs > BCAAs = basic AAs. On the basis of the portal and hepatic fluxes of AAs, Kristensen and Wu (2012) classified them into three groups. The first group of AAs is those AAs that are absorbed from the small intestine into the portal vein and taken up by the liver at ≥17% of their net portal fluxes: Ala, Asn, Cys, Gly, Met, Phe, Pro, Ser, Trp, and Tyr. The second group of AAs are those AAs that are absorbed from the small intestine into the portal vein and taken up by the liver at ≤10% of their net portal fluxes: Arg, His, Ile, Leu, Lys, Thr, and Val. The third group of AAs is those AAs that exhibit little entry from the small-intestinal lumen into the portal vein: Asp, Gln, and Glu. The

**TABLE 7.10**
**Metabolism of AAs in the Small Intestine and Liver of Growing Pigs and in the Portal-Drained Viscera (PDV) and Liver of Lactating Cows**

| | Growing Pigs | | | Lactating Cows[a] | | |
|---|---|---|---|---|---|---|
| AA | Catabolism in the Small Intestine (SI)[b] | Oral Bioavaila-Bility[c] | Net Uptake or Release by Liver[d] | PDV Recovery of AAs Absorbed from the SI (%) | Net PDV Flux of AAs (g/h)[e] | Net Uptake or Release by Liver[d] |
| Ala | 13 | 87 | +52 | 61 | 7.54 | +11 |
| Arg | 40 | 60 | +8 | 49 | – | +4.9 |
| Asn | 13 | 87 | +56 | – | – | +17 |
| Asp | 95 | 5 | −0.30 g/kg feed[f] | 20 | – | +2.4 |
| Citrulline | 10 | 90 | 0.0 | 85 | – | +0.1 |
| Cys | 17 | 83 | +70 | – | 0.47 | – |
| Gln | 67 | 33 | + 6.4 g/kg feed[f] | – | 0.61 | +5.7 |
| Glu | 96 | 4 | −35 g/kg feed[f] | 12 | 1.38 | –24 |
| Gly | 18 | 82 | +73 | 37 | 3.24 | +15 |
| His | 20 | 80 | +9 | 42 | 1.51 | +4.8 |
| Ile | 35 | 65 | +9 | 38 | 3.73 | +1.9 |
| Leu | 34 | 66 | +9 | 34 | 5.77 | +2.1 |
| Lys | 25 | 75 | +10 | 45 | 5.23 | +2.2 |
| Met | 21 | 79 | +17 | 56 | 2.09 | +9.9 |
| Phe | 22 | 78 | +51 | 45 | 4.20 | +12 |
| Pro | 40 | 60 | +40 | 24 | – | +6.5 |
| Ser | 17 | 83 | +28 | 58 | 4.28 | +19 |
| Thr | 28 | 72 | +10 | 38 | 3.16 | +5.3 |
| Trp | 19 | 81 | +35 | – | 1.51 | +4.2 |
| Tyr | 20 | 80 | +54 | 58 | 3.88 | +11 |
| Val | 35 | 65 | +10 | 29 | 3.82 | +1.3 |

*Source:* Doepel, C.L. et al. 2007. *J. Dairy Sci.* 90:4325–4333; Hou, Y.Q. et al. 2016. *Adv. Nutr.* 7:331–342; Kristensen, N.B. and G. Wu. 2012. In: *Nutritional Physiology of Pigs*. Edited by K.E. Bach, N.J. Knudsen, H.D. Kjeldsen, and B.B. Jensen. Danish Pig Research Center, Copenhagen, Denmark. Chapter 13, pp. 1–17; Lescoat et al. 1996. *Reprod. Nutr. Dev.* 36:137–174; Reynolds, C. K. 2006. In: *Ruminant Physiology*. Edited by K. Sejrsen, T. Hvelplund and M.O. Nielsen.. Wageningen Academic Publishers, The Netherlands, Wageningen, pp. 225–248.

[a] Cows consumed 19.4 kg dry matter/day and produced 16.5 kg milk/day.

[b] % of the AA present in the small-intestinal lumen. AA catabolism occurs in the small-intestinal bacteria plus the small-intestinal mucosa.

[c] % of the AA orally administered to the pig.

[d] % of the portal vein flux, unless specified otherwise. (+) denotes net uptake, and (−) net release.

[e] Net PDV flux in the lactating cow which consumed 18 kg dry matter/day (30.6 Mcal/day net energy and 2,067 g/day metabolizable protein) and produced 40 kg milk/day.

[f] Net uptake or net release per kg feed consumed by growing pigs fed a 16%-CP diet.

60 kg pig liver receives little dietary Asp, Gln, and Glu from the portal vein as noted previously, but takes up 6.4 g Gln/kg feed intake from the portal vein (ultimately the arterial blood), and releases 35 g Glu and 0.3 g Asp per kg feed intake as a result of hepatic AA metabolism. Among all AAs, the percentages of hepatic uptakes of Gly (73%) and Cys (70%) are greatest in growing pigs (Table 7.10).

In growing animals, only a small amount of AAs is degraded in their livers. For example, in 60 kg pigs fed a 16%-CP diet, all the ammonia absorbed into the portal blood is removed during its

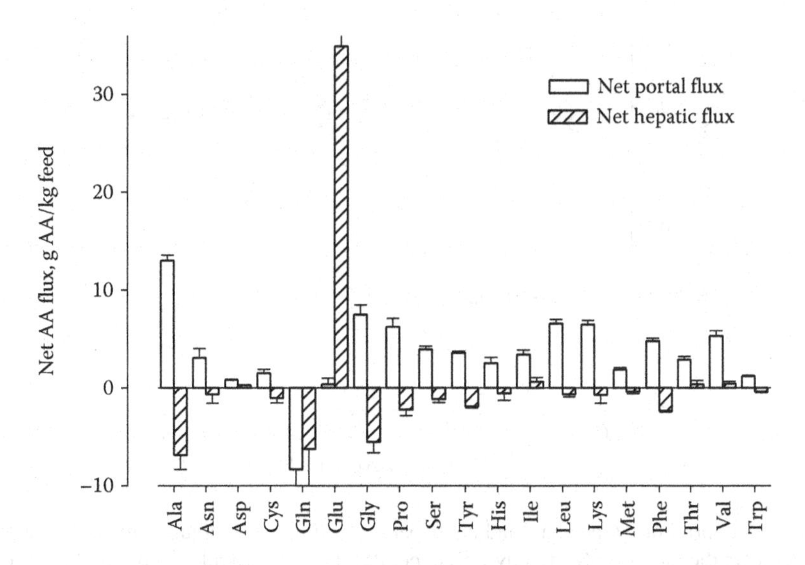


**FIGURE 7.12** Net portal flux (open bar) and net hepatic flux (filled bar) of glucose and AAs in 60 kg growing pigs fed a 16%-CP diet at the rate of 3.6% of body weight per day. Feed was divided into 3 equally sized meals per day at 8 h intervals. A positive flux denotes the net release, and a negative flux the net uptake across the tissues. Hardly any of the dietary Asp, Gln, and Glu (free or peptide-bound) in the small-intestinal lumen is absorbed into the portal blood. The liver takes up Gln from the portal vein, but releases both Asp and Glu. The absolute amount of AA fluxes varies markedly among different AAs. Each data point represents mean ± SEM, $n = 8$. (From Kristensen, N.B. and G. Wu. 2012. In: *Nutritional Physiology of Pigs*. Edited by K.E. Bach, N.J. Knudsen, H.D. Kjeldsen, and B.B. Jensen. Danish Pig Research Center, Copenhagen, Denmark. Chapter 13, pp. 1–17. With permission.)

single passage through the liver, and this organ takes up a small amount of ammonia released from peripheral tissues (Kristensen and Wu 2012). These authors have also reported that 95% of the urea-N released from the liver is accounted for by the hepatic uptake of ammonia from the portal vein and the hepatic artery in 60 kg pigs. In other words, only 5% of the urea-N released by the liver is provided from hepatic AA degradation when the pigs are fed a balanced diet (Figure 7.13). This is consistent with a low rate of hepatic gluconeogenesis in fed pigs (Chapter 5).

## ENDOGENOUS SYNTHESIS OF AAS IN ANIMALS

### Needs for Endogenous Synthesis of AAs in Animals

On the basis of the needs of protein synthesis for "nutritionally essential AAs (EAAs)" (those AAs whose carbon skeletons are not synthesized at all or adequately in animal cells), livestock, poultry, fish, and shrimp are normally fed diets containing minimal levels of CP. This feeding method aims at reducing feed costs and the concentrations of ammonia in the blood circulation. However, recent studies with growing, gestating, and lactating pigs, as well as poultry and fish, indicate that the supply of dietary protein, as currently recommended by the NRC, does not meet their requirements for NEAAs (AAs whose carbon skeletons can be synthesized *de novo* in the body) to achieve maximal growth and production performance (Hou et al. 2016). First, in milk-fed piglets, intake of dietary EAAs greatly exceeds protein accretion in the body, whereas among NEAAs only Asn and Ser in milk exceed the needs for their accretion in the body, and other dietary NEAAs cannot meet the needs for protein accretion in the neonate (Table 7.11). These deficits are particularly severe for Asp, Glu, Gly, and Arg. Accordingly, *de novo* synthesis of these AAs must be active in milk-fed neonates to support weight gains, with the net rates of synthesis of Arg, Gln, and Gly being at least 0.58, 1.15, and 1.20 g/kg body weight per day, respectively. Second, in weanling pigs fed typical

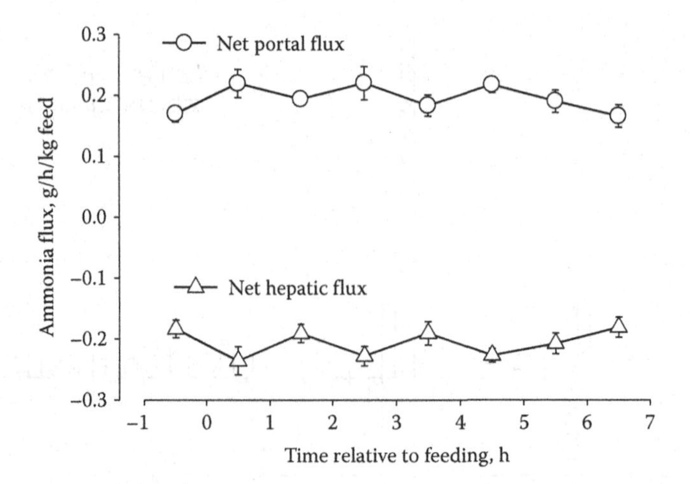


**FIGURE 7.13** Net portal flux (open bar) and net hepatic flux (filled bar) of ammonia in 60 kg growing pigs fed a 16%-CP diet at the rate of 3.6% of body weight per day. Feed was divided into 3 equally sized meals per day at 8 h intervals. A positive flux denotes the net release, and a negative flux the net uptake across the tissues. Each data point represents mean ± SEM, $n = 8$. (From Kristensen, N.B. and G. Wu. 2012. In: *Nutritional Physiology of Pigs*. Edited by K.E. Bach, N.J. Knudsen, H.D. Kjeldsen, and B.B. Jensen. Danish Pig Research Center, Copenhagen, Denmark. Chapter 13, pp. 1–17. With permission.)

corn- and SBM-based diets, dietary EAAs, as well as Asn, Ser, and Ala, exceed the needs for protein synthesis, but dietary Asp, Glu, Gly, Pro, Arg, and Gln cannot meet the needs of the growing piglets and must be synthesized in the body. Third, in gestating gilts typically fed 2 kg of a corn- and SBM-based diet/day containing 12.2% CP, all EAAs except Lys, Trp, and Met exceed their uterine uptake, whereas Ala, Asn, and Ser are the only synthesizable AAs whose supplies in the diet exceed uterine uptake. Other NEAAs (including Arg, Glu, Gln, and Gly) must be synthesized by the gestating dam to support fetal growth and development. Fourth, in lactating sows fed a corn- and soybean meal-based diet containing 18% CP, all dietary EAAs (except for Lys) entering the portal vein exceed their output in sow's milk, whereas dietary Asp, Glu, Gln, and Pro (which are the most abundant AAs in milk protein) cannot meet their output in milk and must be synthesized *de novo* from dietary EAAs. Finally, in growing broiler chickens fed normal protein diets (i.e., an 18%-CP diet between 5 and 21 days of age; a 17%-CP diet between 21 and 35 days of age), Gly, Glu, and Gln must be synthesized from EAAs for muscle growth. In 1- to 42-day-old growing broiler chickens fed a low-protein (16.2% CP) diet, Gly, Pro, Ala, Glu, and Asp must be synthesized from EAAs to sustain protein gains. Thus, since dietary intake cannot meet the needs of animals for NEAAs, their endogenous synthesis and dietary supplementation are necessary for the maximum growth performance of livestock, poultry, and fish (Hou et al. 2016).

## EAAs as Precursors for Synthesis of NEAAs

Four aspects of AA synthesis in animals are noteworthy. Specifically, all animals: (1) cannot synthesize *de novo* the carbon skeletons of the following nine proteinogenic AAs: His, Ile, Leu, Lys, Met, Phe, Thr, Trp, and Val; (2) synthesize *de novo* the following eight proteinogenic AAs: Ala, Asp, Asn, Glu, Gln, Gly, Pro, and Ser (Figure 7.14); (3) hydroxylate Phe into Tyr and convert Met into Cys but not vice versa (Wu 2013); and (4) synthesize Arg in a highly species-specific manner. Many of the synthesized AAs are interconvertible in the animal organisms. In nonruminants, EAAs are ultimately the sources of the amino groups in NEAAs, and provide carbon skeletons for the synthesis of most NEAAs. In ruminants, although there exists a symbiotic relationship

**TABLE 7.11**
**Metabolism of Amino Acids (AAs) in the 14-d-Old Pig (3.9 kg Body Weight) Reared by Sows[a]**

| | AA in Sow's Milk | Dietary AA Entering the Portal Vein | AA Accretion in Extra-Intestina Tissues | Dietary AA Entering the Portal Vein/AA Accretion in Extra-Intestinal Tissues | Extra-Intestinal Metabolism of AA Via Non-Protein Synthesis Pathways | | |
|---|---|---|---|---|---|---|---|
| | | | | | Total Amount | Total Nitrogen (N) | Total Carbon (C) |
| AA | g/L | g/d | g/d | g/g | g/d | mmol N/d | mmol C/d |
| | **Catabolism of AAs Whose Carbon Skeletons Are Not Synthesized by Animal Cells** | | | | | | |
| Cys | 0.72 | 0.50 | 0.40 | 1.25 | 0.10 | 0.83 | 2.48 |
| His | 0.92 | 0.76 | 0.63 | 1.21 | 0.13 | 2.51 | 5.03 |
| Ile | 2.28 | 1.41 | 1.07 | 1.32 | 0.34 | 2.59 | 15.6 |
| Leu | 4.46 | 2.78 | 2.06 | 1.35 | 0.72 | 5.49 | 32.9 |
| Lys | 4.08 | 3.09 | 1.82 | 1.70 | 1.27 | 17.4 | 52.1 |
| Met | 1.04 | 0.85 | 0.57 | 1.49 | 0.28 | 1.88 | 9.38 |
| Phe | 2.03 | 1.50 | 1.05 | 1.43 | 0.45 | 2.72 | 24.5 |
| Thr | 2.29 | 1.32 | 1.03 | 1.28 | 0.29 | 2.43 | 9.74 |
| Trp | 0.66 | 0.52 | 0.33 | 1.58 | 0.19 | 1.86 | 10.2 |
| Tyr | 1.94 | 1.43 | 0.80 | 1.79 | 0.63 | 3.48 | 31.3 |
| Val | 2.54 | 1.51 | 1.28 | 1.18 | 0.23 | 1.96 | 9.82 |
| **Subtotal** | **23.0** | **15.7** | **11.0** | | **4.63** | **43.1** | **203** |
| | **Net Synthesis of AAs Whose Carbon Skeletons Can Be Formed by Animal Cells[b]** | | | | | | |
| Ala | 1.97 | 1.38 | 1.98 | 0.70 | −0.80 | −8.98 | −26.9 |
| Arg | 1.43 | 1.06 | 2.05 | 0.52 | 2.27[6] | 13.0[6] | 0 |
| Asn | 2.53 | 2.00 | 1.07 | 1.87 | −0.93 | −14.1 | −28.2 |
| Asp | 2.59 | 0.11 | 1.29 | 0.085 | 1.18 | 8.87 | 35.5 |
| Glu | 4.57 | 0.21 | 2.36 | 0.089 | 2.15 | 14.6 | 73.1 |
| Gln | 4.87 | 1.42 | 1.52 | 0.93 | 0.10 | 1.37 | 3.40 |
| Gly | 1.12 | 0.82 | 3.41 | 0.24 | 2.59 | 34.5 | 69.0 |
| Pro | 5.59 | 3.12 | 3.66[c] | 0.85 | 0.37 | 3.21 | 16.1 |
| Hydroxyproline | 1.04 | 0.86 | 0.0 | – | −0.86 | −6.56 | −32.8 |
| Ser | 2.35 | 1.72 | 1.34 | 1.28 | −0.38 | −3.62 | −10.8 |
| **Subtotal** | **27.0** | **12.7** | **18.7** | | **5.69** | **42.3** | **98.3** |

*Source:* Hou, Y.Q. et al. 2016. *Adv. Nutr.* 7:331–342.

[a] The milk consumption and body-weight gain of the piglet are 913 mL/day and 235 g/day, respectively.

[b] Rates of AA formation from intestinal catabolism of dietary AAs are estimated to be 1.40, 0.17, and 2.27 g/day for Ala, Pro, and Arg, respectively, and to be negligible for other AAs. The sign "−" denotes the contribution of dietary AA for extraintestinal AA synthesis in a cell- and tissue-specific manner.

[c] Including Pro and hydroxyproline for the calculation of extraintestinal carbon and nitrogen balance.

between the ruminant and its rumen microbes (Hungate 1966), dietary AAs are the major source of N for ruminal AA synthesis. Thus, if a purified diet containing only EAAs is fed to animals, there will be a great shortage of NEAAs for supporting their maximum growth and production performance. Besides developmental changes in the expression of AA-synthetic enzymes, dietary intake of EAAs is by far the single most important factor affecting the *de novo* synthesis of NEAAs in animals.

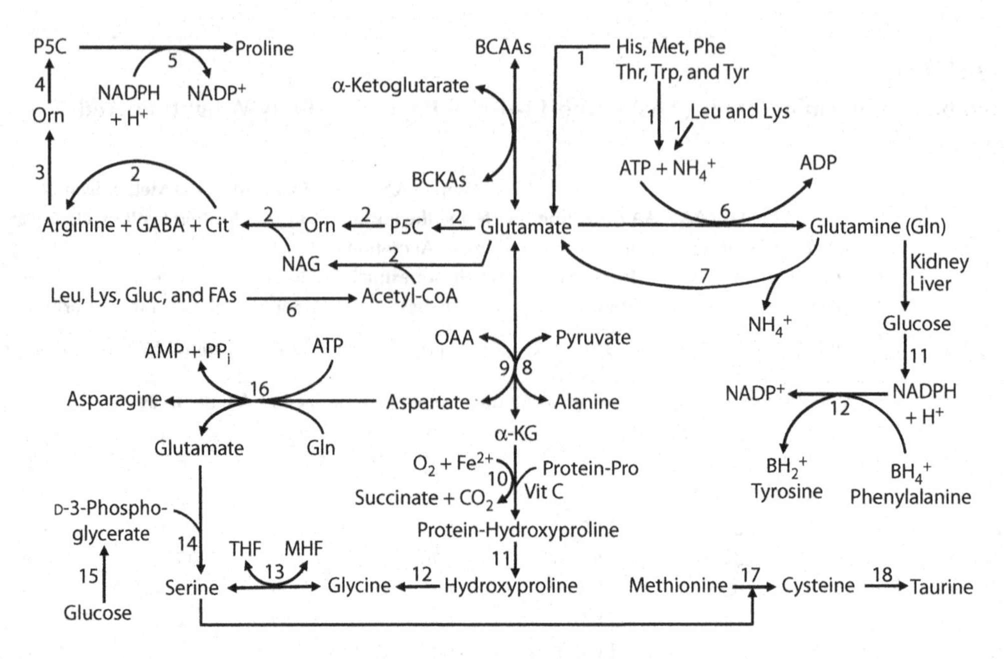


**FIGURE 7.14** Synthesis of AAs in animal cells. BCAAs, branched-chain AAs; BCKAs, branched-chain α-ketoacids. These reactions are cell- and tissue-specific in animals.

## Cell- and Tissue-Specific Syntheses of AAs

It is important to recognize that, within the same animal, the synthesis of AA occurs in a cell- and tissue-specific manner and requires interorgan metabolism of AAs. Some NEAAs can be synthesized in certain tissues but not in others due to the lack of one or more of the required enzymes. Examples are given as follows. First, the livers of mammals can synthesize many NEAAs (e.g., Ala, Glu, Gln, Gly, and Ser) from EAAs, but are not capable of having net synthesis of Cit or Arg under physiological conditions. This is because: (1) Cit is immediately converted into Arg via ASS and ASL; and (2) the Arg is then rapidly hydrolyzed by hepatic arginase to urea plus Orn. The enterocytes of most mammals (including cattle, pigs, rats, and sheep) can synthesize Cit, Arg, and Pro from Gln and Glu, but these pathways are absent from the livers of the same animals due to the lack of P5C synthase.

Second, skeletal muscle, heart, brain, white adipose tissue, mammary tissue, and placenta can synthesize Ala, Asp, Glu, and Gln from BCAAs and α-KG (Harper et al. 1984). Specifically, BCAA transaminase (located in both the cytosol and mitochondria) catalyzes the transamination of BCAAs with α-KG to form BCKAs and Glu. This enzyme is widely expressed in many tissues but its activity is very low in the liver under physiological conditions. Glu-OAA transaminase converts Glu and pyruvate into α-KG and Ala, whereas Gln synthetase synthesizes Gln from Glu and $NH_4^+$ in an ATP-dependent manner. Both Ala and Gln are major vehicles for interorgan transport of nitrogen, and are key substrates for gluconeogenesis. Furthermore, Gln is used for both intestinal Cit synthesis (regulation of NO production and hemodynamics) and renal ammonia production (regulation of acid–base balance).

Third, the small intestine of most mammals can synthesize: (1) Ala, Arg, Asp, Asn, Cit, Orn, and Pro from Glu and Gln; (2) Glu from BCAAs plus glucose, Gln, and Pro; and (3) Tyr from Phe. In many mammalian species, the small intestine releases Ala, Arg, citrulline, ornithine, and Pro in the postabsorptive state, indicating the net synthesis of these AAs by the gut. The pathways for Arg synthesis from Gln, Glu, and Pro in the enterocytes of most mammals are outlined in Figure 7.15. Note that although Arg is formed as an intermediate in mammalian livers via the urea cycle, there is no net synthesis of this AA via this metabolic cycle under physiological conditions. Although Cit is converted into Arg via ASS and ASL, Arg is rapidly hydrolyzed by hepatic arginase to urea plus

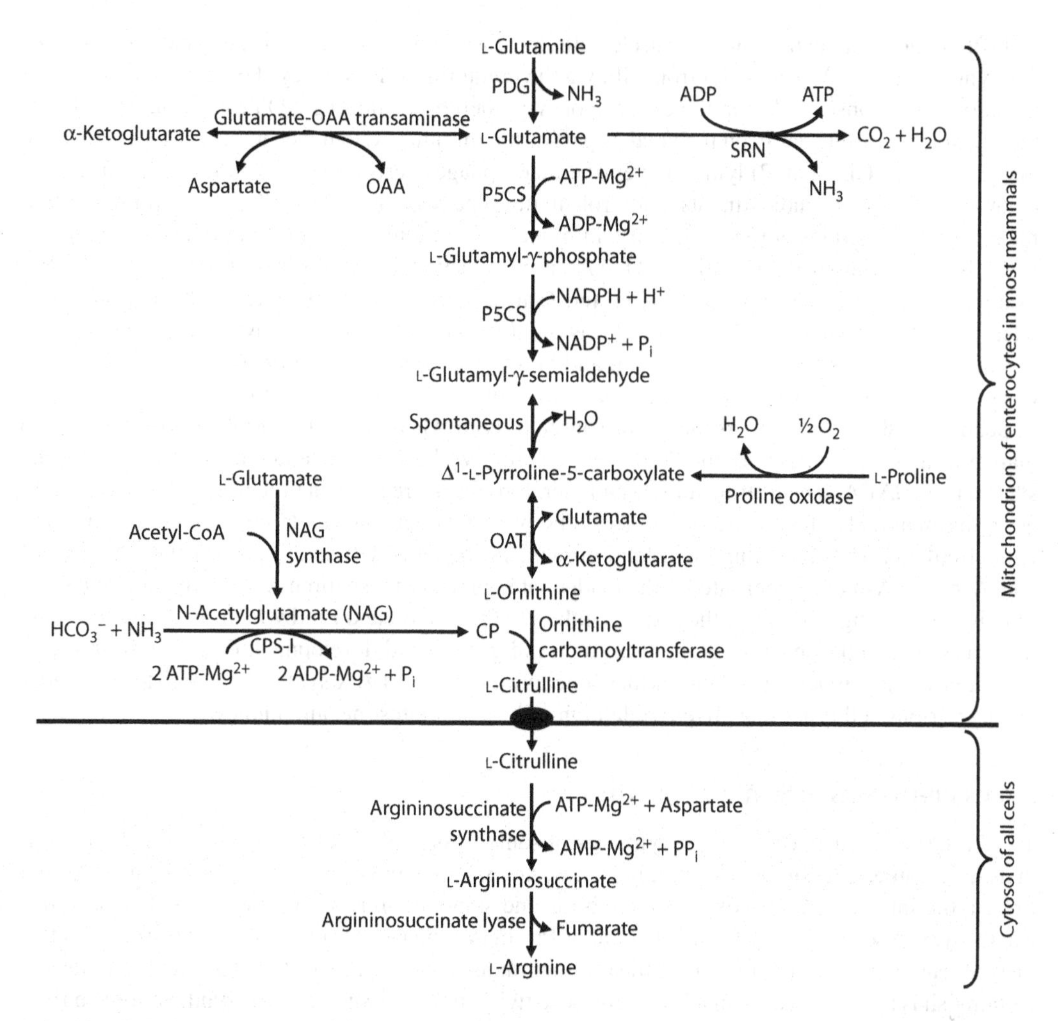


**FIGURE 7.15** Synthesis of citrulline and arginine from glutamine, glutamate, and proline in most mammals (including pigs, ruminants, rats, and humans). Citrulline is synthesized from glutamine, glutamate, and proline almost exclusively in the mitochondria of enterocytes, while all cell types contain cytosolic enzymes for converting citrulline into arginine. The enzymes catalyzing the indicated reactions are: (1) glutaminase (two isoforms: phosphate-independent, and phosphate-activated); (2) γ-glutamyl kinase; (3) glutamyl-γ-phosphate dehydrogenase; (4) nonenzymatic reaction; (5) ornithine aminotransferase; (6) ornithine carbamoyltransferase; (7) argininosuccinate synthase; (8) argininosuccinate lyase; (9) pyrroline-5-carboxylate reductase; (10) carbamoylphosphate synthase II; (11) a series of enzyme-catalyzed reactions involving glutamate dehydrogenase, α-ketoglutarate dehydrogenase, and succinyl-CoA dehydrogenase; (12) *N*-acetylglutamate synthase; (13) acetylglutamate kinase; (14) *N*-acetyl-γ-glutamyl phosphate dehydrogenase; (15) *N*-acetylornithine-δ-aminotransferase; and (16) acetylornithine deacetylase. CP, carbamoyl phosphate.

Orn. Thus, most mammals (e.g., mice, pigs, and rats) have lower requirements for dietary Arg than poultry (e.g., chickens, ducks, and geese) because net Arg synthesis is present in those mammals but absent from birds.

Fourth, the kidneys can synthesize Ala, Asp, Glu, Gly, and Ser, and convert Phe into Tyr. The kidneys also express ASS and ASL for converting the intestine-derived Cit into Arg. These two enzymes are localized within the proximal convoluted tubules with little arginase activity to maximize the release of Arg into the blood circulation. This interorgan-metabolic pathway is known as the intestinal-renal axis for Arg synthesis. Owing to the high rates of blood flow through the kidney, it plays an important role in AA synthesis in animals.

Fifth, endothelial cells, smooth muscle cells, cardiac myocytes, macrophages, and lymphocytes can synthesize Ala, Asp, and Glu from Gln via the glutaminolysis pathway. These cells also convert Cit into Arg to conserve Arg at the expense of Asp, thereby sustaining NO production by NO synthase. Skeletal muscle has been included as part of the immune system, because: (1) this organ is the major source of Gln, and (2) lymphocytes and macrophages derive 35% and 50% of ATP from this pathway, respectively, indicating its major role in immune response. Thus, Gln is a common AA that integrates the functions of the circulatory, immune, and muscular systems in animals.

Cell- and tissue-specific synthesis of AAs is of nutritional and physiological importance. For example, in food-deprived subjects, Ala and Gln account for approximately 50% of total AAs released by the skeletal muscle. The synthesis of Gln from $NH_4^+$ and Glu plays a key role in removing ammonia from skeletal muscle, heart, and brain, with glucose being the primary source of the Glu carbons. Of note, owing to its large mass (40% and 45% of body weight in neonates and adults, respectively), skeletal muscle is the major source of both Ala and Gln in postabsorptive animals to maintain their homeostasis. In the brain, cell-specific synthesis of Glu and Gln is important for the synthesis of GABA (a neurotransmitter) and therefore for the regulation of neurological function. In gestating mammals, the release of Gln from the placenta contributes a large amount of Gln to the fetal circulation for supporting rapid fetal growth. In the fetus, Gln is utilized for the synthesis of Glu, Asp, and Asn to compensate for the inadequate uptake of these three AAs by the gravid uterus. Finally, in lactating mammals, the active synthesis of Glu, Gln, and Pro by mammary tissue results in their high abundances in milk to ensure optimal growth and development of the small intestine and other tissues in neonates. Within the same animal, rates of AA synthesis can differ markedly among various cell types (e.g., liver, skeletal muscle, small intestine, and kidneys).

### Species Differences in Syntheses of AAs

There are species differences in the synthesis of some AAs (Baker 2005). For example, most mammals (e.g., cattle, dogs, humans, mice, pigs, rats, and sheep) can synthesize Arg from Glu, Gln, and Pro via the intestinal-renal axis. However, birds and some mammals (e.g., cats, ferrets, and minks) cannot synthesize Cit or Arg from Glu, Gln, or Pro in the enterocytes of the small intestine, and this may be true in most fish. Also, in contrast to mammals, the synthesis of Pro from Arg in birds and certain fish is limited because of a low arginase activity in their tissues, and the synthesis of Pro from Glu and Gln is absent in birds and perhaps in most fish because of the lack of intestinal P5C synthase. Furthermore, in cats, the conversion of cysteine into taurine is limited due to a low activity of cysteine dioxygenase and of cysteinesulfinate decarboxylase that catalyzes the formation of taurine from cysteinesulfinic acid. Human infants, who have relatively low activities of both cysteine dioxygenase and cysteinesulfinate decarboxylase compared to adults, require the dietary intake of taurine for maintaining normal retinal, cardiac, and skeletal functions. Supplementing taurine to all-plant protein, taurine-free diets enhance growth and feed efficiency in carnivore fish (e.g., the rainbow trout and the Japanese flounder), but not the common carp, suggesting the suboptimal *de novo* synthesis of taurine by certain aquatic species (Li et al. 2009). Finally, the rate of Gly synthesis is much lower than the rate of Gly utilization in poultry, young pigs, and human infants (Graber and Baker 1973; Wu et al. 2014a), but whether this is also true in other species is unknown.

### Synthesis of AAs from Their α-Ketoacids or Analogs in Animal Cells and Bacteria

With the exception of five AAs (L-Arg, L-Cys, L-Lys, L-Thr, and Gly), all proteinogenic AAs can be formed from: (1) their α-ketoacids through L-AA transaminases; and (2) their D-isomers via D-AA oxidases (peroxisomal enzymes containing FAD as a cofactor) and L-AA transaminases (ubiquitously present in both mitochondria and the cytosol) which widely occur in animal tissues. The final steps for the syntheses of L-Arg, L-Cys, and Gly in animal cells or of L-Lys and L-Thr in microbes do not involve transamination, and therefore they do not form from their α-ketoacids in the organisms.

An α-ketoacid ($KA_1$) transaminates with an AA ($AA_2$, usually Glu) to generate a new AA ($AA_1$) and a new α-ketoacid ($KA_2$) (Chapter 1). Since Glu is synthesized from ammonia and α-KG, the conversion of an α-ketoacid into its corresponding L-AA drives the disposal of ammonia for the production of a new L-AA. This is physiologically important for patients with hepatic or renal dysfunction; the formation of a new AA (e.g., Leu) from its α-ketoacid (e.g., α-ketoisocaproate) not only removes ammonia, but also generates a new AA to support protein synthesis and possibly activate anabolic metabolic pathways.

Animal cells lack D-AA transaminases. Therefore, D-AAs do not undergo transamination reactions in mammalian, avian, or other vertebrate cells. However, animal tissues (e.g., liver, kidney, brain, and heart) contain D-AA oxidases (oxidoreductases) to oxidize D-AA (e.g., D-Met) to their corresponding α-ketoacids (e.g., α-keto-γ-methylthiobutyrate, also called 2-keto-4-methylthiobutanoic acid; KMB). Subsequently, L-AA transaminases catalyze the conversion of the α-ketoacid and glutamate into the corresponding L-α-AA (e.g., L-Met) and α-KG. Owing to technical challenges to manufacture L-Met through microbial fermentation, KMB is an effective precursor of L-Met in animals and therefore is a useful additive to the feeds for poultry and swine.

1. D-Methionine + $O_2$ + $H_2O$ + FAD → α-Keto-γ-methylthiobutyrate + $FADH_2$ + $H_2O_2$
2. α-Keto-γ-methylthiobutyrate + L-Glutamate ↔ L-Methionine + α-Ketoglutarate

In recent years, two hydroxy ketoacids of Met, L-2-hydroxy-4-methylthiobutanoic acid, and D-2-hydroxy-4-methylthiobutanoic acid have also been used as the precursors of L-Met through the formation of KMB in farm animals (Figure 7.16). These hydroxyl acids are absorbed mainly by monocarboxylate transporter 1, coupled with the action of the $Na^+/H^+$ exchanger (NHE3). L-2-hydroxy acid oxidase (a $H_2O_2$-producing flavoenzyme in peroxisomes of tissues, mainly the liver and kidneys) oxidizes L-2-hydroxy-4-methylthiobutanoic acid into KMB, whereas D-2-hydroxy acid dehydrogenase (an $H_2O_2$-producing flavoenzyme in the mitochondria of tissues, mainly the liver and kidneys) converts D-2-hydroxy-4-methylthiobutanoic acid into KMB (Zhang et al. 2015). The choice of an L-Met precursor as a feed additive depends on its cost (compared with other sources of L-Met such as MBM, intestinal mucosal protein, and blood meal) and diets.

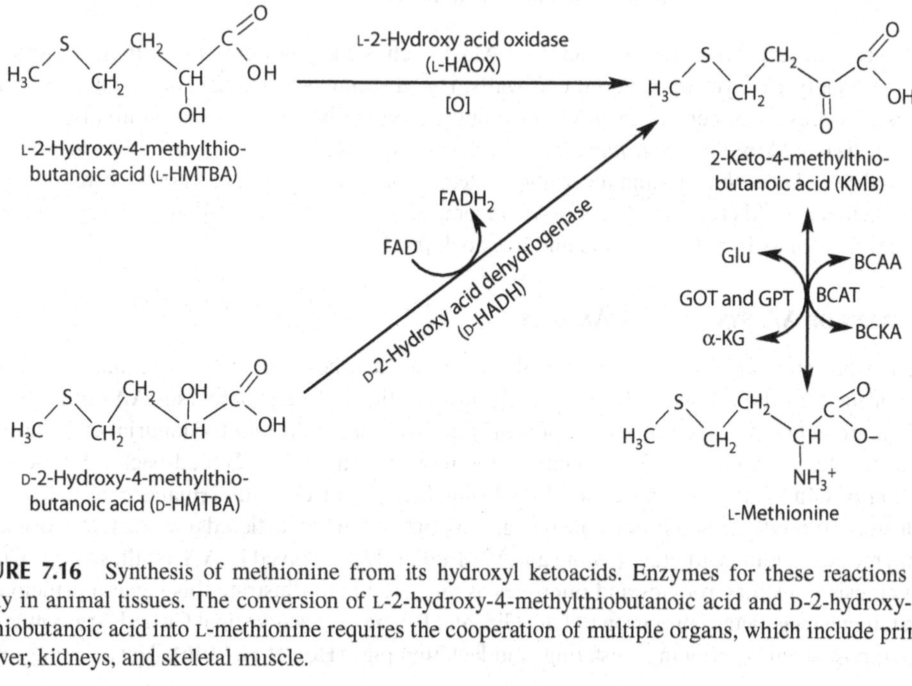

**FIGURE 7.16** Synthesis of methionine from its hydroxyl ketoacids. Enzymes for these reactions occur widely in animal tissues. The conversion of L-2-hydroxy-4-methylthiobutanoic acid and D-2-hydroxy-4-methylthiobutanoic acid into L-methionine requires the cooperation of multiple organs, which include primarily the liver, kidneys, and skeletal muscle.

Bacteria (e.g., those in the intestine) contain D-AA oxidases, as well as D-AA transaminases and L-AA transaminases, and therefore can convert D-AAs to L-AAs. However, the extent of these reactions in the gastrointestinal microbes is unknown. The microbial presence of D-AA transaminases provides an additional route for L-AA synthesis from D-AAs in animals, as shown for D-Trp below. The efficiency of the utilization of D-AAs for the synthesis of L-AAs varies greatly with animal species and D-AAs. For example, the efficiency of L-Leu synthesis from D-Leu is 100%, 50%, and 15% for chicks, rats, and mice, respectively, whereas the efficiency of D-Trp for the synthesis of L-Trp is 20%, 100%, and 30% for chicks, rats, and mice, respectively (Wu 2013).

1. D-Tryptophan + α-Ketoglutarate ↔ Indole-3-pyruvate + L-Glutamate
2. Indole-3-pyruvate + L-Glutamate ↔ L-Tryptophan + α-Ketoglutarate

## Syntheses of D-AAs in Animal Cells and Bacteria

As noted in Chapter 4, D-AAs are present in nature. An AA racemase (also known as D-AA racemase) converts a free L-AA into a free D-AA in animal cells and bacteria. Most AA racemases (including D-aspartate racemase, D-serine racemase, and D-Ala racemase) depend on pyridoxal-5′-phosphate for catalytic activity. These enzymes localize in the cytosol with their respective substrates. Only two AA racemases, D-Asp racemase and D-Ser racemases have been identified in mammals and birds to date. Both D-Asp and D-Asp racemase activity have been identified in: (1) pinealocytes of the pineal gland; (2) pituicytes of the posterior pituitary gland; (3) epinephrine-producing chromaffin cells of the medulla of the adrenal glands; and (4) elongated spermatids of the testes. In the brain, endogenously synthesized D-Asp is important for neurological function, because the entry of D-AA from the peripheral circulation into this organ appears to be limited by the blood–brain barrier. In addition to nervous tissues, D-Asp racemase has been reported in the kidney and liver of mammals, which is in keeping with the presence of D-Asp in these organs. Likewise, all animals (e.g., mammals, birds, and invertebrates) express D-Ser racemase, which converts free L-Ser into D-Ser. This enzyme is enriched in the glial cells of the rat brain that contain high levels of D-Ser.

L-Amino acid (e.g., Ala, Asp, or Ser) ⟷ D-Amino acid (e.g., Ala, Asp, or D-Ser)
D-AA racemase (vitamin $B_6$)

D-Ala racemase converts free L-Ala into D-Ala, which is a key building block in the biosynthesis of the peptidoglycan layer in bacterial cell walls. D-Ala racemases are ubiquitous among microorganisms and present in certain invertebrates, but are typically absent from mammals, birds, and fish. Bacteria (e.g., *Streptococcus faecalis*, *Mycobacterium tuberculosis*, *E. coli*, *Listeria monocytogenes*, and *Bacillus anthracis*) and invertebrates (e.g., *Corbicula japonica*, a brackish-water species; and crayfish) use D-Ala to grow. Thus, D-Ala racemase is an attractive target for the development of novel antimicrobials in both medicine and livestock production.

## Regulation of AA Syntheses in Animals

Under normal nutritional and physiological conditions, syntheses of AAs in animals are limited by one or more of the following factors: (1) the availabilities of their precursor AAs (mainly those AAs that are not synthesized by eukaryotes); (2) intracellular or intramitochondrial concentrations of co-substrates or cofactors; (3) amounts of the required enzymes; (4) feed-back inhibition (e.g., inhibition of Gln synthetase expression by Gln in skeletal muscle cells [Huang et al. 2007]); and (5) allosteric inhibition. Some hormones (e.g., insulin and glucocorticoids) regulate expression of the enzymes (e.g., Gln synthetase [Wang and Watford 2007]) involved in AA synthesis. Use Cit and Arg synthesis in pig enterocytes and microbes as an example to illustrate this general principle.

First, increasing dietary provision of Glu, Gln, and Pro promotes intestinal Cit and Arg synthesis in suckling, postweaning, growing, gestating, and lactating pigs (Hou et al. 2016). Thus, when growing pigs (e.g., 10–20 kg) are fed a low-CP diet (e.g., 14% CP), which supplies all nonsynthesizable AAs at the levels of an intermediate CP-level diet (17% CP) or a normal CP diet (e.g., 20% CP) but does not meet the needs of Arg and all other synthesizable AAs (e.g., Asp and Gly), their growth performance, feed efficiency, and muscle protein gain are suboptimal and their fat deposition in the body is substantially increased. As the dietary CP content decreases from 20% to 17% and to 14% at the same dietary levels of nonsynthesizable AAs but decreasing levels of synthesizable AAs, the daily weight gain of the growing pigs decreases progressively (Li et al. 2016). Similarly, the growth performance of pigs (13–35 kg) decreases progressively as the dietary CP content decreases from 20% to 17.2%, 15.3%, and 13.9% at the same dietary levels of nonsynthesizable AAs but decreasing levels of synthesizable AAs (Peng et al. 2016). These results further support the notion that animals do have dietary requirements of synthesizable AAs for maximal growth and development (Wu et al. 2013a).

Second, intestinal synthesis of Cit and Arg requires *N*-acetylglutamate (NAG, an allosteric activator of carbamoylphosphate synthase-I [CPS-I] in mitochondria). A substantial decrease in the mitochondrial concentration of NAG in the enterocytes of 7- to 21-day-old pigs limits Cit and Arg synthesis, compared with newborn pigs (Wu et al. 2004), as noted previously. Since NAG is actively degraded by deacetylase in the cytosol of cells, *N*-carbamoylglutamate (NCG, a metabolically stable analog of NAG which is not a substrate of deacetylase) can be used as a dietary additive to stimulate intestinal Cit and Arg synthesis in young pigs (Wu et al. 2004). This approach is also effective in enhancing Arg synthesis in gestating pigs and rats.

Third, either a natural surge of cortisol during weaning or intramuscular administration of cortisol increases intestinal Cit and Arg synthesis in 14- to 21-day-old pigs through enhancing: (1) expression of P5C synthase and NAG synthase; and (2) mitochondrial NAG synthesis and concentration in their enterocytes. Fourth, while the purified P5C synthase is inhibited *in vitro* by high concentrations of Orn (a product of P5C transamination by Orn aminotransferase), supplementing the basal diet (containing ~1% Arg) of growing pigs with up to 2% Arg does not reduce Cit plus Arg synthesis from Gln or Pro in their enterocytes (Wu et al. 2016). This is because the Arg-derived Orn is extensively metabolized to Pro in these cells such that their intracellular concentrations of Orn are not sufficiently high to inhibit P5C synthase.

Finally, in many of the metabolic pathways for synthesizing AAs (e.g., Arg, Gln, and Trp) in intestinal bacteria, products are allosteric inhibitors of certain key enzymes (e.g., inhibition of Gln synthetase and anthranilate synthase by Gln and Trp, respectively). Thus, in gastrointestinal (including ruminal) microbes, the rates of incorporation of free AAs into protein can influence the rates of their syntheses from NPN (e.g., ammonia and urea).

## DEGRADATION OF AAS IN ANIMALS

### PARTITION OF AAS INTO PATHWAYS FOR CATABOLISM AND PROTEIN SYNTHESIS

The $K_M$ values of aminoacyl-tRNA synthetases (enzymes initiating protein synthesis) for AAs in cells range from 0.2 to 0.4 mM (Wolfson et al. 1998), which are similar to the intracellular concentrations of most AAs (except for Gln, Glu, Asp, Gly, Pro, and Ala at 2–25 mM; and Arg (nonhepatocytes) and Thr at 1 to 2 mM) but lower than the $K_M$ values of the various enzymes initiating the degradation of AAs (1.5–30 mM) in animal tissues (Krebs 1972). Thus, protein synthesis takes precedence over the degradation of AAs in animals to ensure their survival and to conserve the AAs. However, since AA-degrading enzymes are present in live animals, the catabolism of AAs occurs in the body regardless of their nutritional states, with the rates being the highest immediately after feeding. AAs in excess of their needs for the synthesis of protein and other biologically active substances, as well as their intracellular concentrations in tissues, must be degraded in a cell-specific manner. Although some cell types (e.g., enterocytes in mammals) depend on the oxidation of certain AAs (Gln, Glu, and Asp) as their major metabolic fuels, the use of AAs for ATP production is energetically inefficient when compared with the oxidation of glucose and fatty acids. On average, the efficiencies of energy transfer from protein, fat, and glucose to ATP are 41.5%, 54.8%, and 55.7%, respectively (Wu 2013). In some animals, such as fish and carnivorous mammals, dietary protein may provide the bulk of energy, but knowledge of their utilization of AAs can provide a basis for the development of alternatives (e.g., pyruvate, α-KG, or OAA) in the diets. In mammals, birds and fish, the rates of degradation of AAs generally increase with an increase in their extracellular concentrations. As indicated in Chapter 1, the carbon skeletons of AAs must be eventually converted into acetyl-CoA for net oxidation to $CO_2$ and water. Thus, animals have high capacities to catabolize AAs (e.g., Arg, Gln, Glu, Gly, and Pro) as an adaptive response to their dietary intakes.

## Cell- and Tissue-Specific Degradation of AAs

The degradation of AAs is catalyzed by specific enzymes, whose distribution varies greatly among different cells and tissues of the same species (Wu 2013). This gives rise to cell- and tissue-specific catabolism of AAs (Table 7.12), as indicated by the following examples. First, in pigs and rats, the placenta, mammary gland, and mature red blood cells do not contain the phosphate-activated glutaminase pathway for Gln degradation, but this pathway is highly active in all other cells and tissues (including the small intestine, skeletal muscle, heart, and immunocytes) (Figure 7.17). The

**TABLE 7.12**
**Cell- and Tissue-Specific Catabolism of AAs in Mammals and Birds Under Normal Physiological Conditions**

| | Mammals | | | | | Birds | | | |
|---|---|---|---|---|---|---|---|---|---|
| AA | Entero-Cytes | Liver | Skeletal Muscle | Kidney | Mammary Gland | Entero-Cytes | Liver | Skeletal Muscle | Kidney |
| Ala | Limited | +++ | Limited | ++ | + | Limited | +++ | Limited | ++ |
| Arg | +++ | +++++ | No | +[a] | +++ | No | No | No | +[a] |
| Asn | No | +++ | No | ++ | No | No | +++ | No | ++ |
| Asp | +++++ | +++ | + | ++ | + | ? | +++ | + | ++ |
| Cys | No | +++ | No | ++ | No | No | +++ | No | ++ |
| Gln | +++++ | +++ | ++ | +++ | No | Limited | Limited | ++ | +++ |
| Glu | +++++ | +++ | ++ | +++ | + | ? | +++ | ++ | +++ |
| Gly | Limited | +++ | No | ++ | Limited | Limited | +++ | No | ++ |
| His | No | +++ | No | + | No | No | +++ | No | + |
| Ile | +++ | Limited | +++ | +++ | +++ | +++ | Limited | +++ | +++ |
| Leu | +++ | Limited | +++ | +++ | +++ | +++ | Limited | +++ | +++ |
| Lys | No | +++ | No | + | No | No | +++ | No | + |
| Met | No | +++ | No | + | No | No | +++ | No | + |
| Orn | ++++ | +++ | No | +++ | +++ | + | +++ | No | +++ |
| Phe | No | +++ | No | ++ | No | No | +++ | No | ++ |
| Pro | +++ | ++ | No | ++ | No | ? | ++ | No | ++ |
| Ser | Limited | +++ | No | ++ | Limited | Limited | +++ | No | ++ |
| Thr | No | +++ | No | + | ++ | No | +++ | No | + |
| Tyr | No | +++ | No | + | No | No | +++ | No | + |
| Val | +++ | Limited | +++ | +++ | +++ | +++ | Limited | +++ | +++ |
| D-AA | Limited | + | No | ++ | No | Limited | + | No | ++ |

D-AA, D-mino aacids.
[a] Limited activity in proximal renal tubules where synthesis of arginine from citrulline primarily occurs in kidneys, but is present at high activity in other parts of the renal tissue.

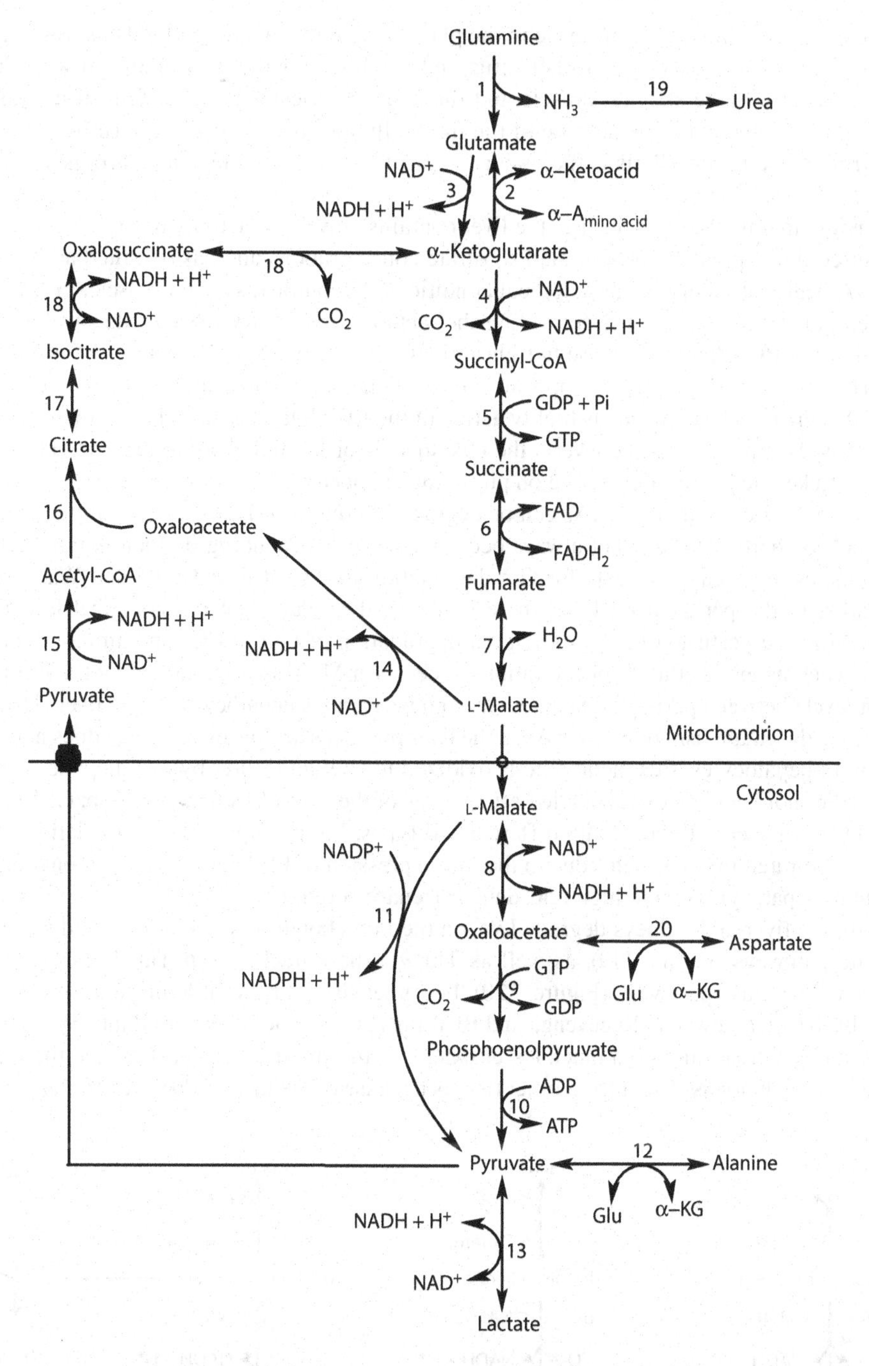


**FIGURE 7.17** Glutamine degradation via the phosphate-activated glutaminase pathway in animals. The enzymes that catalyze the indicated reactions are: (1) phosphate-activated glutaminase; (2) glutamate transaminase; (3) glutamate dehydrogenase; (4) α-ketoglutarate dehydrogenase; (5) succinate thiokinase; (6) succinate dehydrogenase; (7) fumarase; (8) $NAD^+$-linked malate dehydrogenase (cytoplasm); (9) phosphoenolpyruvate carboxykinase; (10) pyruvate kinase; (11) $NADP^+$-linked malate dehydrogenase; (12) glutamate-pyruvate transaminase; (13) lactate dehydrogenase; (14) $NAD^+$-linked malate dehydrogenase (mitochondria); (15) pyruvate dehydrogenase; (16) citrate synthase; (17) aconitase; (18) isocitrate dehydrogenase; (19) conversion of ammonia into urea via the urea cycle. Glutamine degradation to form glutamate, aspartate, and alanine is known as glutaminolysis.

lack of Gln catabolism via glutaminase in the placenta and the lactating gland ensures maximum transfer of Gln from the mother to her fetus and newborn for their optimum growth, development, and health. Since skeletal muscle and the heart synthesize *de novo* Gln from Glu, while degrading this AA to Glu, the net rate of the intracellular Gln–Glu cycle determines the release of Gln from these tissues. This is the major factor affecting the endogenous provision of Gln in animals.

Second, in mammals, birds, or fish, the liver contains only a low activity of BCAA transaminase as measured in the presence of saturated substrate concentrations and has a limited ability to initiate BCAA degradation under physiological conditions. In contrast, skeletal muscle, kidneys, small intestine, and many other tissues (including the lactating mammary tissue) extensively possess a high activity of BCAA transaminase to transaminate BCAAs with α-KG to form BCKAs and glutamate (Figure 7.18). However, the opposite is true for the oxidation of branched-chain α-ketoacids by BCKA dehydrogenase, which is highly active in the liver but only has a low to medium activity in other tissues. The liver also converts the α-ketoacids of Ile and Val into glucose, as well as all BCKAs into ketone bodies, depending on physiological needs.

Third, all AAs other than BCAAs can be degraded in the liver. However, net degradation of the non-branched chain AAs may not always occur in the liver depending on their extracellular concentrations, as reported previously for Gln degradation in the rat liver (Lund and Watford 1976). Specifically, in the perfused rat liver, there is no net degradation of physiological levels of Gln (0.5–1 mM in the perfusion medium), but net degradation of Gln to $CO_2$ and ammonia occurs in the liver when its extracellular concentration exceeds 1 mM. This is explained by the intercellular Gln–Glu cycle between periportal hepatocytes and perivenous hepatocytes in the liver (Haussinger 1990). Since the catabolism of many AAs in the liver produces acetoacetate, which does not undergo oxidation in hepatocytes, this metabolite is oxidized to $CO_2$ and water by extrahepatic tissues and cells. Furthermore, among extrahepatic tissues, rates of the degradation of Ala, Asp, Gln, Glu, Arg, Pro, and Orn vary considerably with different cell types. For example, in pigs, oxidation of Pro to $CO_2$ is very limited in enterocytes due to the low expression of P5C dehydrogenase, but occurs at a high rate in hepatocytes due to high P5C dehydrogenase activity.

Fourth, the liver and kidneys degrade Lys via the mitochondrial saccharopine and peroxisomal pipecolate pathways (Figure 7.19), as well as Thr via the mitochondrial Thr dehydrogenase and cytosolic dehydratase pathways (Figure 7.20), but other tissues have little or no ability to oxidize Lys or Thr to $CO_2$ and water (Benevenga and Blemings 2007). Phe is converted into Tyr in the liver, kidneys, and pancreas, and, to a much lesser extent, in the small intestine, skin, and the brain, but this Phe hydroxylation is absent from other tissues because of the lack of Phe hydroxylase. Note that

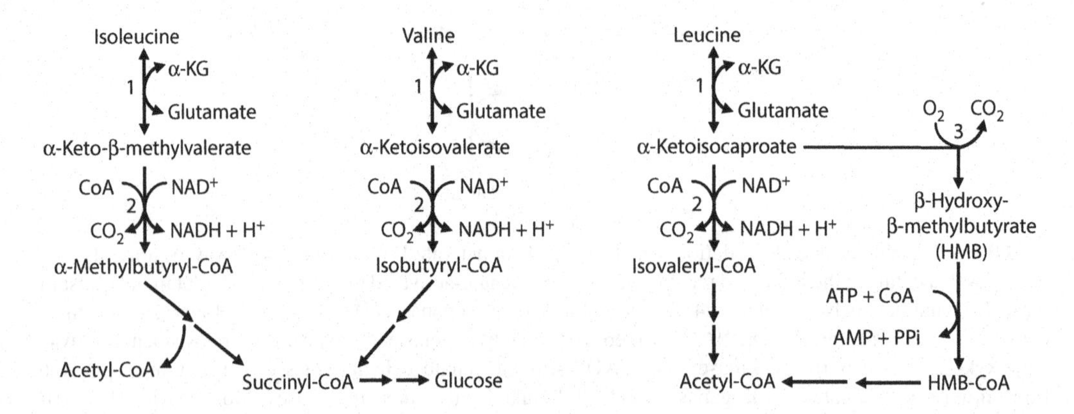


**FIGURE 7.18** Degradation of BCAAs in animals. The enzymes that catalyze the indicated reactions are: (1) BCAA transaminase; (2) branched-chain α-ketoacid dehydrogenase; (3) α-ketoisocaproate dioxygenase; and (4) HMB-CoA synthase.

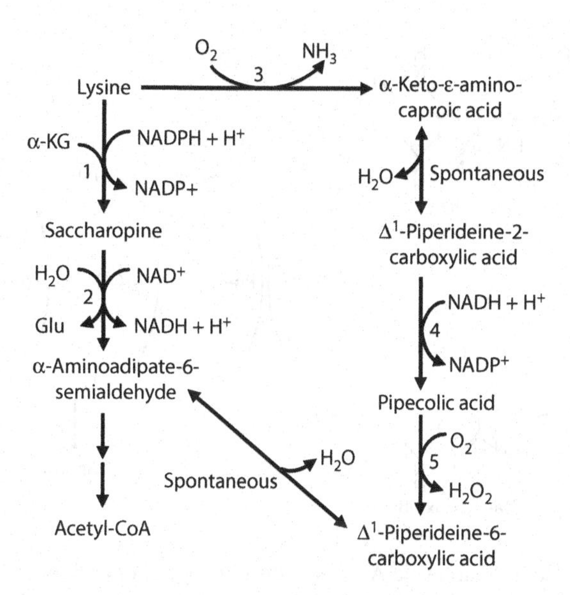


**FIGURE 7.19** Lysine degradation in the liver of animals. Lysine is degraded via the mitochondrial saccharopine pathway and the peroxisomal pipecolate pathway. The enzymes that catalyze the indicated reactions are: (1) lysine: α-ketoglutarate reductase; (2) saccharopine dehydrogenase ($NAD^+$, glutamate-forming); (3) lysine oxidase (a peroxisomal protein); (4) peperideine-2-carboxylic acid reductase; and (5) pipecolate oxidase (a peroxisomal protein). α-KG, α-ketoglutarate.

the hydroxylation of Phe, as well as other aromatic AAs and Arg, requires tetrahydrobiopterin ($BH_4$) as an essential factor (Figure 7.21).

Finally, although Met is converted into SAM by SAM synthase in many cell types to provide SAM for the synthesis of spermidine and spermine from putrescine, the liver is the only organ that can degrade Met into Cys, taurine, $CO_2$, and water in animals (Stipanuk 2004). The pathway for Met catabolism via the transsulfuration pathway is outlined in Figure 7.22. Like Met, Trp degradation can be initiated in multiple tissues (Figure 7.23), but the liver is the only organ to oxidize Trp to $CO_2$ and water. In animals, Trp is catabolized via the kynurenine, serotonin, and transamination pathways. The kynurenine pathway involves the deamination and decarboxylation of tryptophan to form

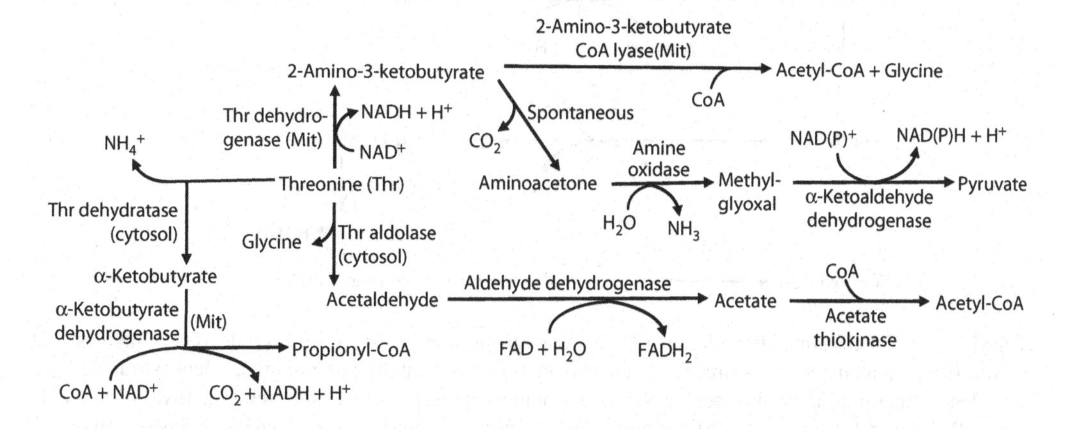


**FIGURE 7.20** Threonine degradation in the liver of animals. Threonine degradation in the liver is initiated primarily by threonine dehydrogenase (a mitochondrial enzyme) and, to a much lesser extent, threonine dehydratase and threonine aldolase (cytosolic enzymes). Products of threonine catabolism include glycine, pyruvate, and propionyl-CoA.

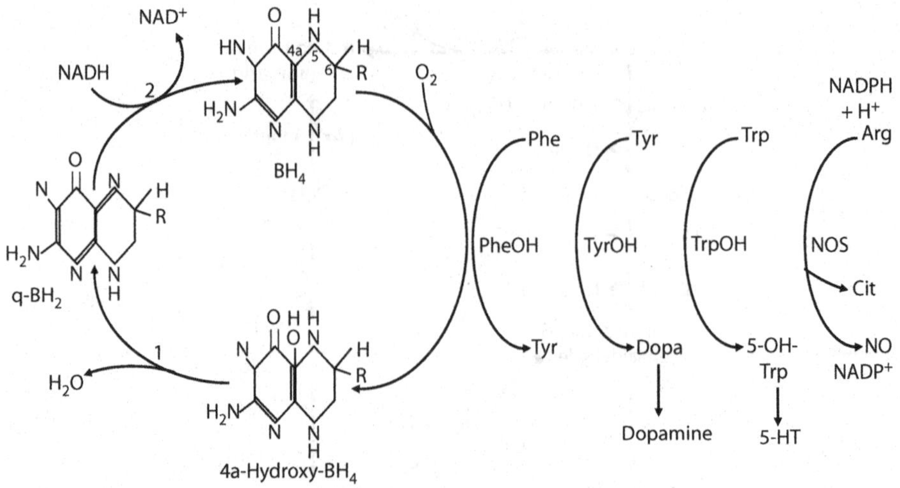

**FIGURE 7.21** Hydroxylation of aromatic AAs by hydroxylases and of arginine by NO synthase in animal tissues. These reactions require tetrahydrobiopterin as an essential cofactor. NOS, NO synthase; PheOH, phenylalanine hydroxylase; TrpOH, tryptophan hydroxylase; TyrOH, tyrosine hydroxylase.

kynurenine, and occurs primarily in the liver and brain (Le Floc'h et al. 2011). The further catabolism of kynurenine produces indoleacetic acid, niacin, pyruvate, and acetyl-CoA. Quantitatively, the kynurenine pathway accounts for the degradation of over 95% of the available peripheral Trp. The serotonin pathway depends on the $BH_4$-dependent hydroxylation and vitamin $B_6$-dependent decarboxylation of Trp to generate serotonin (5-hydroxytryptamine), and takes place mainly in the

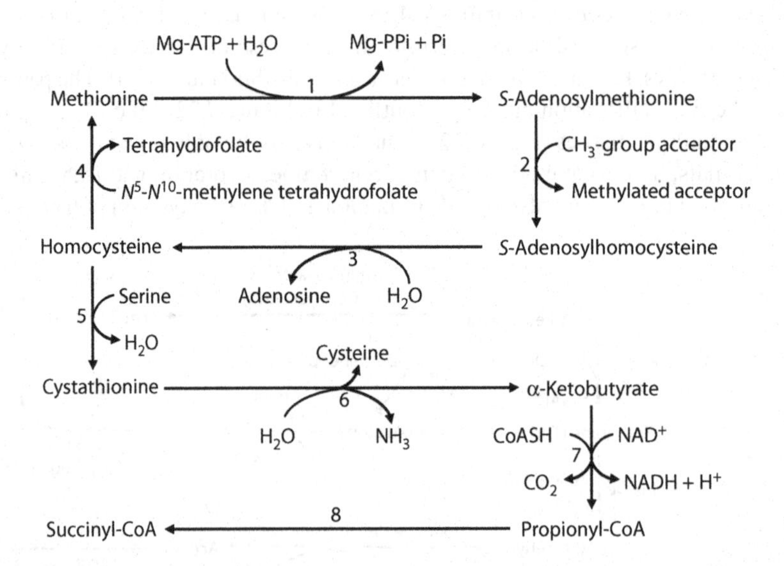


**FIGURE 7.22** Methionine degradation via the transsulfuration pathway in animals. The enzymes that catalyze the indicated reactions are: (1) *S*-adenosylmethionine synthase (methionine adenosyltransferase); (2) *S*-adenosylmethionine methylase; (3) *S*-adenosylhomocysteinase; (4) homocysteine methyltransferase (a vitamin B12-dependent enzyme); (5) cystathionine β-synthase (a pyridoxal phosphate-dependent enzyme); (6) cystathionine γ-lyase (a pyridoxal phosphate-dependent enzyme); (7) α-ketobutyrate dehydrogenase; (8) and a series of enzymes (propionyl-CoA carboxylase, methylmalonyl-CoA racemase, and methylmalonyl-CoA mutase [a vitamin B12-dependent enzyme]). All the carbons of cysteine are derived from serine. Many tissues can convert Met into SAM, but the liver is the only organ to oxidize Met into Cys, Tau, $CO_2$, and water.

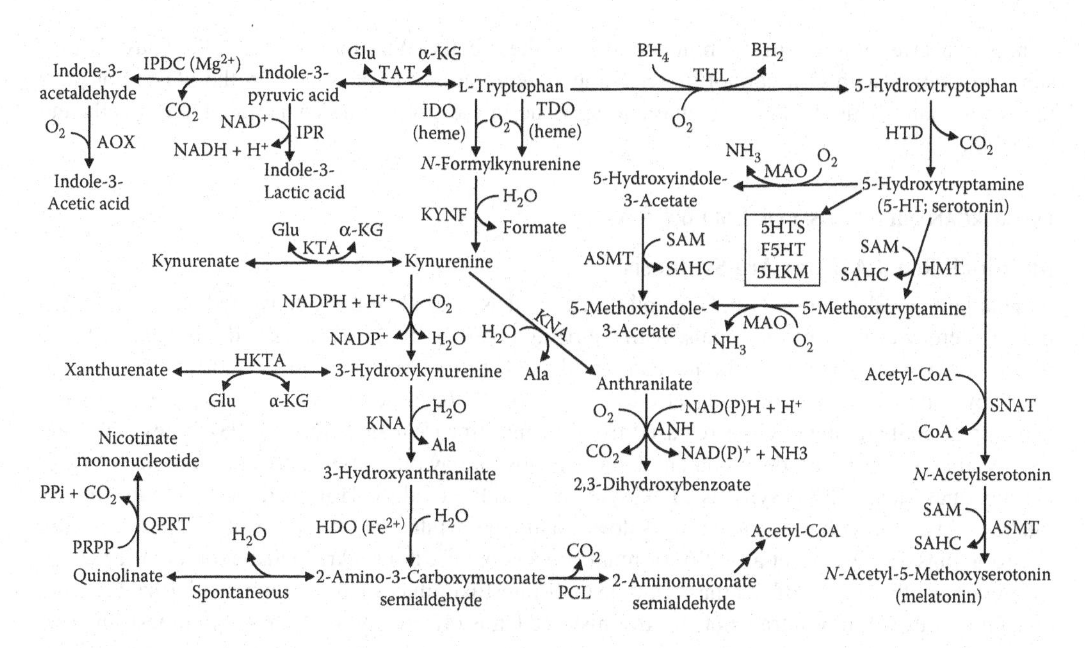


**FIGURE 7.23** Tryptophan degradation in animals. Degradation of L-tryptophan is initiated by indoleamine 2,3-dioxygenase (IDO), tryptophan 2, 3-dioxygenase (TDO), and tryptophan hydroxylase (THL). These pathways are cell- and tissue-specific. Serotonin, melatonin, and their metabolites can form sulfate and glucuronide conjugates for excretion in urine and feces. Products of tryptophan catabolism include NAD, serotonin, melatonin, kynurenine, indoles, and acetyl-CoA. Many tissues can initiate Trp catabolism, but the liver is the only organ to oxidize Met into Cys, Tau, $CO_2$, and water. AMSR, 2-aminomuconate semialdehyde reductase; ANH, anthranilate hydroxylase [also known as Anthranilate 3-monooxygenase (deaminating)]; AOC, aldehyde oxidase; ASMT, *N*-acetylserotonin *O*-methyltransferase; F5HT, formyl 5-hydroxytryptamine; HDO, 3-hydroxyanthranilate dioxygenase; 5HKM, 5-hydroxykynuremine; HKTA, 3-hydroxykynurenine transaminase; HMT, 5-hydroxyindole-*O*-methyltransferase; 5-HT, 5-hydroxytryptamine; HTD, 5-hydroxytryptophan decarboxylase; 5HTS, 5-hydroxytryptamine sulfate; 5-HTP, 5-hydroxy-l-tryptophan; IPDC, indole-3-pyruvate decarboxylase (a thiamine diphosphate-dependent enzyme); IPR, indole-3-pyruvate reductase; KAD, α-ketoadipate dehydrogenase; KHL, kynurenine hydroxylase; KNA, kynureninase; KTA, kynurenine transaminase; KYN, kynurenine; KYNF, kynurenine formamidase; MAO, monoamine oxidase; NADS, NAD synthase; NER, nonenzymatic reaction; NGH, NAD glycohydrolase; OCR, oxalocrotonate reductase; PCL, picolinate carboxylase; PLP, pyridoxal phosphate; PRPP, 5-phosphoribosyl-1-pyrophosphate; QPRT, quinolinate phosphoribosyl transferase; SNAT, serotonin-*N*-acetyltransferase; SAM, *S*-adenosylmethionine; SAHC, *S*-adenosylhomocyteine; SR, a series of reactions for conversion of glutaryl-CoA to acetyl-CoA; and TAT, tryptophan aminotransferase; The following enzymes require pyridoxal phosphate for catalytic activities: HTD, HKTA, KNA, KTA, and TAT. QPRT is inhibited by high concentrations of leucine.

neuronal cells of the gastrointestinal tract and brain. Serotonin is a biogenic amine that functions as a neurotransmitter and gastrointestinal hormone. Thus, like AA synthesis, the catabolism of most AAs takes place in a tissue- and cell-specific manner.

## Compartmentalization of AA Degradation in Cells

An interesting characteristic of AA degradation in animals is complex compartmentalization (Haüssinger 1990). This means that: (1) the metabolic pathways for AA catabolism are specific to certain organelles; and (2) extracellularly and intracellularly derived AAs may have very different metabolic fates. For example, in pig enterocytes, Pro oxidation to P5C by Pro oxidase occurs only in mitochondria, whereas Orn decarboxylase is expressed in the cytosol but not in the mitochondria. Also, the Orn generated from Gln in the mitochondria of pig enterocytes, but not extracellular

Orn, is converted into Cit in the mitochondria of these cells (Wu and Morris 1998). Thus, dietary supplementation with Orn cannot increase the concentration of Cit or Arg in the plasma of pigs, rats, or humans. This illustrates a challenging issue in the studies of AA metabolism in cells and the whole body.

## Interorgan Metabolism of Dietary AAs

### Intestinal–Renal Axis for Arg Synthesis

As noted previously, dietary Gln, Glu, and Pro, as well as arterial Gln, are converted into Cit and Arg in the enterocytes of most mammals, with Cit being taken up by the kidneys and other extrahepatic tissues for Arg production. In the neonates of those Cit-producing mammals, most of the Cit produced by enterocytes is further converted into Arg locally because of high ASS and ASL activities, and only a small amount of Cit is released from the intestine (Wu and Morris 1998). Rates of Cit and Arg syntheses depend on developmental stages, substrate availabilities, and intestinal activities of key enzymes, such as NAG synthase, P5C synthase, and Pro oxidase. However, increasing the dietary intake of Arg within physiological ranges does not affect the intestinal synthesis of Cit from Glu, Gln, or Pro in pigs or rats (Wu et al. 2016) or renal conversion of Cit into Arg (Dhanakoti et al. 1992). In the mammals that lack P5C synthase in the small-intestinal mucosa and do not synthesize Cit from Glu, Gln, or Pro, oral or intravenously administered Cit is effectively used for Arg synthesis *in vivo*.

### Renal Gln Utilization for Regulation of Acid–Base Balance

Through renal ammoniagenesis, Gln plays an important role in regulating acid–base balance by producing $NH_3$ (ammonia), which then combines with $H^+$ (proton) to form $NH_4^+$ for excretion in the urine (Xue et al. 2010). Under acidotic conditions, which occur during intensive exercise, early lactation, and late pregnancy and in animals with type-I diabetes mellitus, renal utilization of Gln is markedly increased to meet the need of ammonia production for the removal of $H^+$. The sources of the Gln for renal uptake are mainly the skeletal muscle, WAT, and liver. In acidotic animals, suppression of Gln degradation in the small intestine and immunocytes also increases the availability of Gln in the blood for extraction by the kidneys.

### Gln and Ala Synthesis from BCAAs

In mammals, most dietary Gln does not enter the portal vein. Therefore, the circulating Gln must be derived primarily from *de novo* synthesis. Dietary BCAAs absorbed from the small intestine enter the portal vein and largely bypass the liver due to the near absence of hepatic BCAA catabolism. BCAAs in the blood are taken up by extrahepatic tissues, where these AAs are transaminated with α-KG by cytosolic and mitochondrial BCAA transaminases to form Glu and BCKAs. Thus, BCAAs donate the amino group to Glu. Glu is either amidated with ammonia by Gln synthetase to form Gln, or transaminated with pyruvate and α-KG to yield Ala and Asp, respectively (Figure 7.24). Glucose is the major source of the carbon skeletons of Gln, Glu, Ala, and Asp. The $NH_4^+$ for Gln synthesis is supplied from the blood. In skeletal muscle, an additional source of ammonia for Gln synthesis is inosine monophosphate through the purine nucleotide cycle, particularly during exercise (Figure 7.25). During fasting, both Ala and Gln are major precursors for the renal synthesis of glucose (Watford et al. 1980).

In mammals and birds, skeletal muscle, heart, adipose tissue, and lungs, as well as the placenta in gestating dams and the mammary gland in lactating mothers, have high BCAA transaminase activities and therefore play an important role in initiating BCAA catabolism in the body (Harper et al. 1984). However, these extrahepatic tissues only partially decarboxylate BCKAs due to the relatively low activity of BCKA dehydrogenase, releasing most of the BCKAs into the blood. The BCKAs are taken up primarily by the liver for: (1) oxidation to $CO_2$ and water; (2) gluconeogenesis (except for the ketoacid of Leu); (3) ketogenesis; and (4) synthesis of lipids. At present, little is known about BCAA metabolism in various tissues of fish and shrimp.

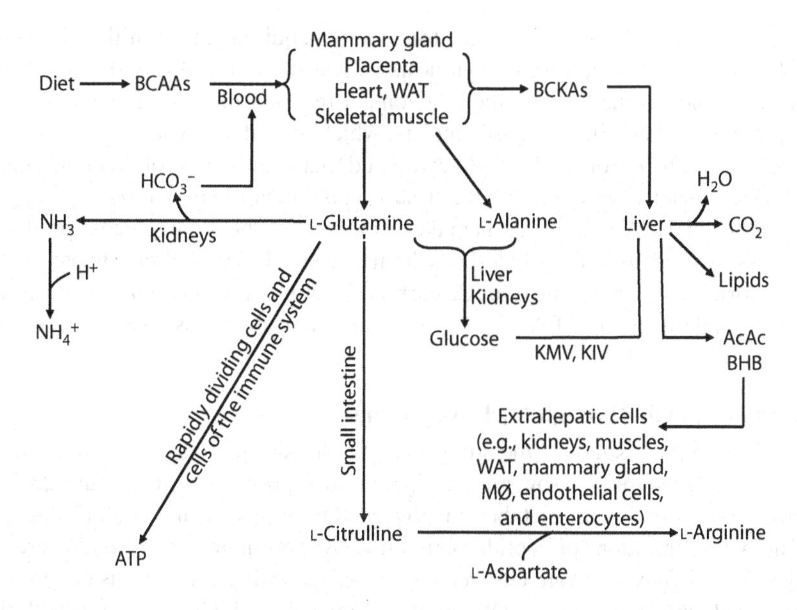


**FIGURE 7.24** Interorgan metabolism of BCAAs in animals. Dietary BCAAs are absorbed into the blood, largely bypass the liver, and are catabolized in skeletal muscle to synthesize glutamine and alanine. The transamination of BCAAs in the muscle also results in the release of branched-chain α-ketoacids (BCKAs). Glutamine and alanine are taken up by the liver and kidneys for glucose synthesis. Glutamine is a major metabolic fuel in enterocytes and immunocytes, a major substrate for citrulline synthesis in the small intestine of most mammals, and a major regulator of acid-base balance through renal ammoniagenesis and $HCO_3^-$ absorption. Arginine is synthesized from citrulline in all cell types. BCKAs released from the skeletal muscle are taken up by the liver where they are either oxidized or converted into glucose, ketone bodies, and lipids. AcAc, acetoacetate; BHB, β-hydroxybutyrate; KIV, α-ketoisovalerate; KMV, α-keto-β-methylvalerate; MØ, macrophages.

Endogenous synthesis of Gln plays an important role in animal growth and development. This is because: (1) Gln is essential for the synthesis of protein (including glycoproteins), nucleic acids, aminosugars, and NAD(P), and (2) these roles of Gln cannot be replaced by any other AA. For example, both glycoproteins and nucleic acids are critical for the growth and development of embryos and fetuses. This is consistent with the fact that Gln is the most abundant AA in the plasma of most postnatal animals (including ruminants, rats and chickens) and is one of the two most abundant AAs in the plasma of pigs and sheep (with the other AA being Gly) (Wu 2013).

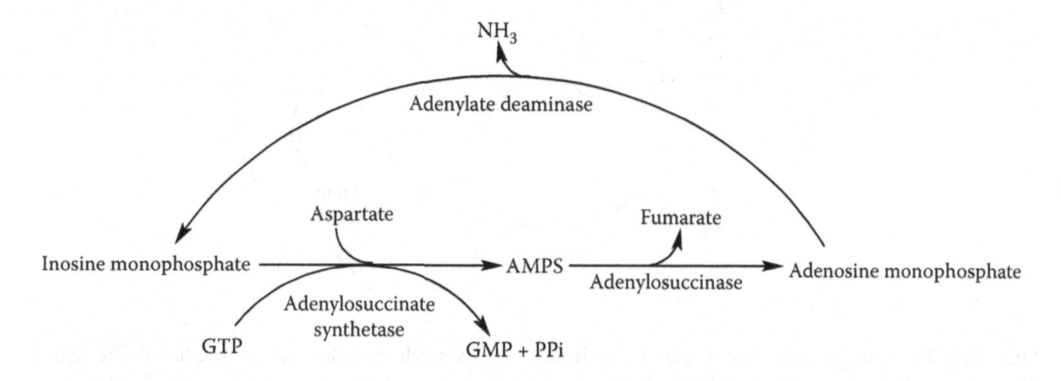


**FIGURE 7.25** The purine nucleotide cycle for ammonia production in skeletal muscle. AMP, adenosine monophosphate; AMPS, adenosine monophosphate succinate; GTP, guanosine triphosphate; GMP, guanosine monophosphate; IMP, inosine monophosphate.

The supply of Ala from diets is inadequate to meet the requirements of milk-fed mammals, such as piglets. This necessitates endogenous synthesis of Ala from BCAAs by the skeletal muscle of neonates. For example, on the basis of the Ala content in sow's milk, milk meets at most 66% of the need for protein synthesis in 14-day-old piglets, which must daily synthesize at least 0.18 g Ala/kg body weight (Wu 2010). Hou et al. (2016) estimated that at least 30% of Ala in tissue proteins is provided from endogenous synthesis. In all animals, under conditions of food deprivation or when food intake is reduced, BCAA-derived Ala makes a major contribution to glucose production by the liver and kidneys and therefore the whole-body homeostasis of glucose (see Chapter 5). The use of glucose for the formation of pyruvate (the Ala carbon skeleton) in skeletal muscle, the release of Ala from the muscle, and the uptake of Ala by the liver for gluconeogenesis constitute the glucose–Ala cycle in animals (Figure 7.26).

## Conversion of Pro to Gly through Hydroxyproline

The milk of all mammals studied (including pigs, cattle, sheep, goats, and humans) is severely deficient in Gly. For example, in sow-reared piglets, milk provides at most only 23% of Gly for tissue protein synthesis and other metabolic pathways. Of interest, Wang et al. (2013) reported the presence of high concentrations of peptide-bound hydroxyproline in sow's milk. There is evidence that hydroxyproline is converted into Gly in the kidneys, providing endogenous Gly to support neonatal growth, development, and health (Wu et al. 2013a). Through Gly synthesis, both the carbons and nitrogen of the Pro molecule are effectively spared in milk-fed neonates. This pathway likely plays an important role in maintaining Gly homeostasis in animals, particularly in milk-fed young mammals.

## NO-Dependent Blood Flow

Utilization of dietary AAs requires cooperation among many different organs, and therefore, blood flow through them. Rates of blood flow, which affect the transport of AAs and other nutrients across tissues, are regulated by NO. This free radical is synthesized from Arg by $BH_4$- and NADPH-dependent NO synthase in virtually all cell types (Blachier et al. 2011). In endothelial cells and

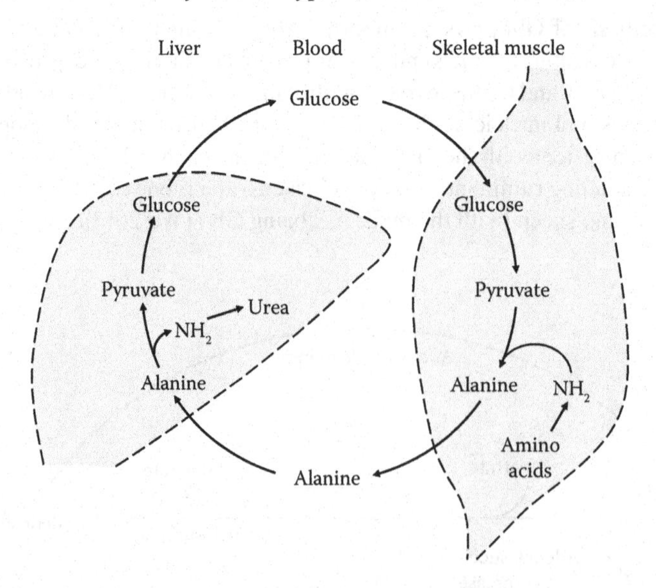


**FIGURE 7.26** The glucose-alanine cycle in animals. The liver releases glucose into the blood circulation. Skeletal muscle takes up arterial glucose for generation of pyruvate, which is used for alanine synthesis via transamination. Skeletal muscle releases alanine, which is converted into urea and glucose in the liver. There is no net synthesis of glucose by the glucose-alanine cycle, when the source of pyruvate in the muscle is glucose.

placentae, Arg stimulates $BH_4$ synthesis by enhancing the expression of GTP cyclohydrolase I (Wu et al. 2009). NO is a major vasodilator released by endothelial cells of blood vessels to control blood flow to tissues, such as the small intestine, utero-placental unit, liver, skeletal muscle, and mammary gland. Without dietary Arg or Glu- Gln- and Pro-derived endogenous Arg, there is insufficient blood flow and insufficient interorgan metabolism of AAs in animals (Wu 2013).

## Regulation of AA Oxidation to Ammonia and $CO_2$

In animals, the oxidation of AAs to ammonia and $CO_2$ is regulated by many factors: (1) allosteric activators or inhibitors; (2) reversible phosphorylation and dephosphorylation of enzymes; (3) concentrations of substrates and cofactors; (4) concentrations of activators and inhibitors of enzymes; (5) signal transduction; (6) changes in cell volume; and (7) other forms of regulation of enzyme activity (Wu 2013). Some of these factors related to the oxidation of AA-derived pyruvate and α-KG have been discussed in Chapter 5. The following well-documented examples substantiate these principles.

First, GDH, which is a protein in the inner mitochondrial matrix, catalyzes the interconversion of Glu $\leftrightarrow$ α-KG + $NH_4^+$. In the liver and possibly other tissues, the chemical equilibrium of this enzyme favors the production of ammonia from Glu under physiological conditions. GDH is allosterically activated by ADP and Leu but inhibited by GTP and ATP (Li et al. 2012). This has nutritional and physiological importance. For example, when extracellular concentrations of Leu are elevated through high protein intake or Leu supplementation, GDH in pancreatic β-cells is activated to enhance energy metabolism, the ATP-sensitive $K^+$ channel, and membrane depolarization, leading to an increase in insulin release. Likewise, mutations in GDH that abrogate allosteric GTP inhibition result in high levels of insulin and ammonia in plasma (Li et al. 2012). Therefore, allosteric regulation of GDH plays an important role in insulin homeostasis and whole-body nutrient metabolism.

Second, some enzymes in AA metabolism are known to be modified by phosphorylation and dephosphorylation. Whether phosphorylation of an enzyme increases or decreases its catalytic activity varies with individual enzymes. For example, BCKA dehydrogenase is inactivated by phosphorylation and activated by dephosphorylation. This enzyme is present mainly in the phosphorylated (inactive) form in the heart and skeletal muscle but in the dephosphorylated (active) form in the liver and kidneys (Brosnan and Brosnan 2006). Consumption of a high-protein diet by animals increases BCKA dehydrogenase activity in the heart and kidneys by increasing the conversion of the enzyme from the phosphorylated into the dephosphorylated form. Similarly, cortisol and glucagon enhance BCAA degradation in bovine mammary epithelial cells, whereas insulin and growth hormone stimulate the phosphorylation of BCKA dehydrogenase in the cells to reduce BCAA oxidative decarboxylation (Flynn et al. 2009; Lei et al. 2013). In contrast to BCKA dehydrogenase, the activities of Phe hydroxylase, Trp hydroxylase, Tyr hydroxylase, and Tyr aminotransferase are enhanced by protein phosphorylation but inhibited by protein dephosphorylation. This kind of metabolic control does not involve a change in the amount of the enzyme protein, but allows for rapid changes in product formation in a tissue- and substrate-specific manner.

Third, concentrations of substrates and cofactors play an important role in regulating AA metabolism, as illustrated by BCAA catabolism in skeletal muscle exposed to ketone bodies. Both acetoacetate and β-hydroxybutyrate inhibit the transamination of BCAAs by suppressing the conversion of glucose into pyruvate and then α-KG (Wu and Thompson 1988). Conversely, the inhibitory effect of ketone bodies on BCAA transamination is prevented by the addition of pyruvate, which generates α-KG. Ketone bodies also inhibit the oxidative decarboxylation of BCKA in extrahepatic tissues (including skeletal muscle, mammary tissue, kidneys, and the small intestine) in the absence or presence of pyruvate. The oxidation of acetoacetate and β-hydroxybutyrate to $CO_2$ and water in these tissues requires both CoA-SH and $NAD^+$, thereby decreasing the availability of these cofactors for BCKA dehydrogenase. Thus, competition for the cofactors of enzymes is a major mechanism responsible for the effect of ketone bodies on inhibiting BCAA catabolism in skeletal muscle.

Fourth, the availability of activators and inhibitors can affect metabolic fluxes, respectively. For example, chronic high concentrations of lactate (e.g., 10–20 mM) in plasma are associated with severe hypocitrullinemia and hypoargininemia but hyperprolinemia in infants. Kinetics analysis of enzymatic activity revealed noncompetitive inhibition of enterocyte Pro oxidase by lactate (decreased maximal velocity and unaltered $K_M$) (Dillon et al. 1999). This provides a biochemical basis for the treatment of lactate-induced hyperammonemia in neonates. Another example of enzyme inhibition is the competitive inhibition ($K_i = 1.0–1.6\ \mu M$) of all NOS isoforms by $N^G$-monomethy-L-arginine (NMMA) and asymmetric dimethylarginine (ADMA). The concentrations of these methylarginines in plasma are elevated in patients with obesity, diabetes, cardiovascular disease, and renal dysfunction. Reductions in NMMA and ADMA can improve their metabolic profiles and health.

Fifth, signal transduction in cells, which is brought about by their responses to extracellular chemicals (including nutrients, hormones, cytokines, drugs, toxins, or phytochemicals), can regulate AA catabolism in animals. For example, glucagon stimulates glycine oxidation in the mitochondria of hepatocytes (Jois et al. 1989), whereas cortisol promotes the catabolism of Arg, Gln, Orn, and Pro in enterocytes (Flynn et al. 2009). The responses of AA degradation to cell signaling may be cell-specific, as cAMP increases the synthesis of tyrosine aminotransferase in the liver and kidneys but not in the small intestine or skeletal muscle. Defects in signal transduction can cause: (1) impairments in growth, development, and homeostasis; (2) increased susceptibility to infectious diseases; and (3) obesity, diabetes, cardiovascular disorders, DNA mutation, cancer, and other diseases.

Sixth, changes in cell volume occur in response to alterations in uptake of AAs or extracellular osmolarity. For example, upon ingestion of a meal and fluids, AAs, glucose, ions, and water are transported into the cell, leading to cell swelling (Haüssinger 1990). Conversely, loss of cellular water in dehydration leads to cell shrinkage. The maintenance of adequate cell volume is a major prerequisite for cell survival, growth, and development. Cell swelling induced by AAs or hypotonicity stimulates Gln degradation, but cell shrinkage increases net synthesis of AAs in the perfused rat liver. Furthermore, cell swelling decreases, but cell shrinkage increases, BCAA catabolism and the release of Gln and Ala from the rat skeletal muscle. Finally, an increase in cell volume promotes Gln catabolism in both lymphocytes and macrophages. This may have physiological and immunological importance, as the volume of immunocytes increases in response to mitogenic stimulation and immunological activation.

## Detoxification of Ammonia as Urea via the Urea Cycle in Mammals

### The Urea Cycle for Disposal of Ammonia in Mammals

Oxidation of AAs in all animals produces ammonia. In aqueous solution, free ammonia is at equilibrium with ammonium ion ($NH_3 + H^+ \leftrightarrow NH_4^+$). At pH 7.4°C and 37°C, approximately 1.6% and 98.4% of ammonia exist as free $NH_3$ and $NH_4^+$, respectively. Here, free $NH_3$ and $NH_4^+$ are collectively referred to as ammonia. Physiological concentrations of ammonia are essential to life because it participates in many reactions to: (1) synthesize carbamoylphosphate in the cytosol by CPS-II; (2) bridge AA metabolism with glucose metabolism; and (3) regulate acid–base balance in the kidneys. However, excess ammonia in blood is particularly toxic to the brain, as well as embryos and fetuses, and therefore must be removed through the formation of urea primarily via the hepatic urea cycle (Figure 7.27). The liver converts extracellular (blood) and intracellularly generated ammonia into urea. In growing pigs, nearly all (95%) of the urea-N released from the liver is derived from the hepatic uptake of ammonia from the portal vein and the hepatic artery, as noted previously. This indicates a low rate of AA degradation in the liver under physiological conditions. It is now known that enterocytes of postnatal mammals can also synthesize urea from extracellular and mitochondrially generated ammonia (Wu 1995).

Urea, which is highly water-soluble and nontoxic, is a desirable form to dispose of ammonia in mammals which periodically excrete water as the major component of urine. Urea elimination via the kidneys involves: (1) glomerular filtration; (2) reabsorption in the proximal renal tubules into

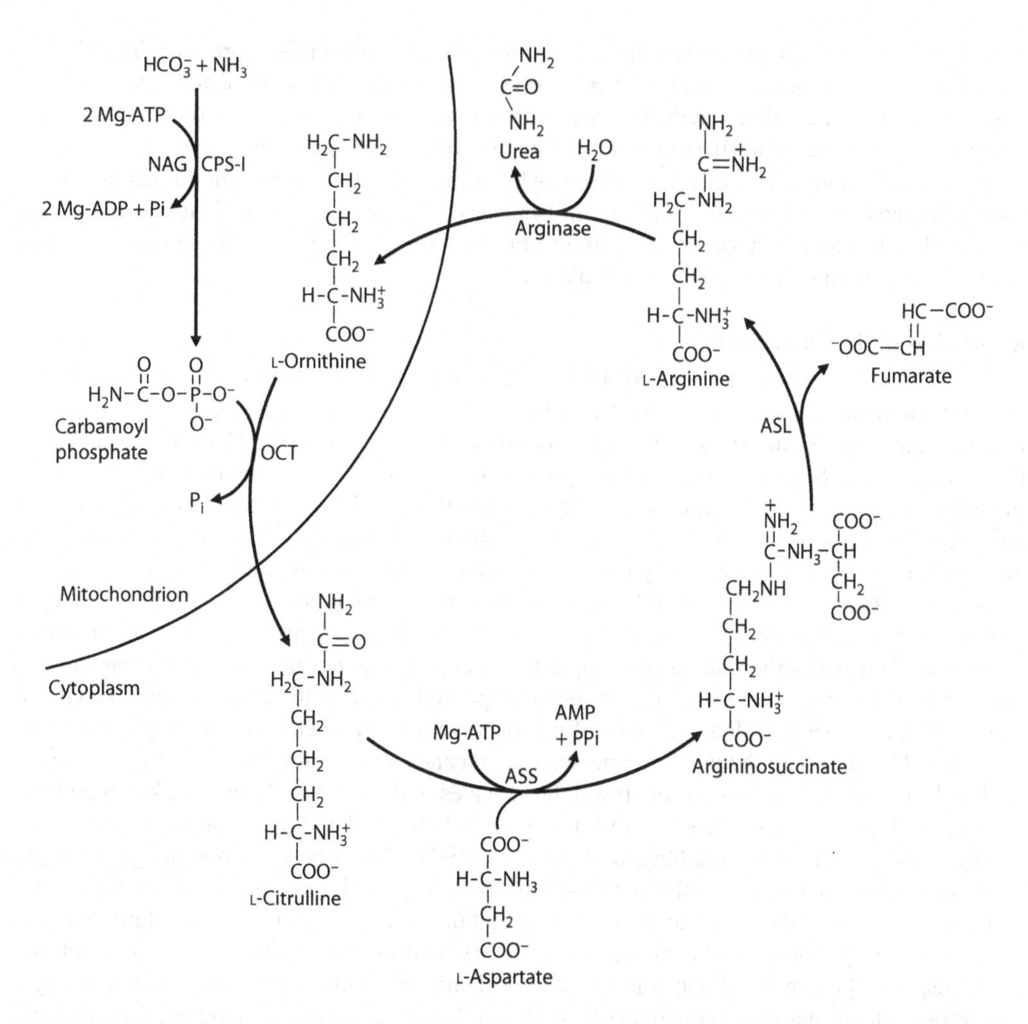


**FIGURE 7.27** Synthesis of urea from ammonia and bicarbonate in mammals. This is the major metabolic pathway for ammonia detoxification in mammalian species. The synthesis of urea from ammonia and bicarbonate involves both the mitochondrion and the cytoplasm. Citrulline exits the mitochondrion into the cytoplasm where it is converted into arginine, which is rapidly hydrolyzed by arginase into urea plus ornithine. Ornithine is then reused for another turnover of the cycle. ASL, argininosuccinate lyase; ASS, argininosuccinate synthase; CPS-I, carbamoylphosphate synthase-I; NAG, *N*-acetylglutamate.

blood through facilitated or carrier-mediated transporters; and (3) the movement of the remaining urea through the collecting duct as part of urine.

## Energy Requirement of Urea Synthesis

Urea synthesis: (1) starts with $NH_3$ (rather than $NH_4^+$) and $HCO_3^-$ (rather than $CO_2$) as the substrates for CPS-I; (2) involves the cytosol and mitochondria, as well as substrate channeling in both compartments; and (3) requires 6.5 mol ATP per 2 mol ammonia. The formation of 1 mol urea from 1 mol each of ammonia, Asp, and $HCO_3^-$ requires 4 mol ATP for urea-cycle reactions and 2.5 mol ATP for the incorporation of 1 mol ammonia into 1 mol Asp. The latter reaction is expressed as follows:

$$NH_4^+ + \alpha\text{-Ketoglutarate} + NADH + H^+ \rightarrow \text{Glutamate} + NAD^+ \text{(equivalent to 2.5 mol ATP)}$$

$$\text{Glutamate} + \text{Oxaloacetate} \leftrightarrow \alpha\text{-Ketoglutarate} + \text{Aspartate}$$

Since the detoxification of protein-derived ammonia as urea consumes approximately 10%–15% of ATP produced from the oxidation of AAs, optimizing the quality and quantity of dietary AA requirements by mammals can reduce urea production, thereby improving the efficiency of protein and energy utilization. When the rate of formation of carbamoylphosphate from ammonia, $CO_2$, and ATP exceeds the rate of conversion of carbamoylphosphate plus Orn into Cit in mitochondria, carbamoylphosphate exits into the cytoplasm for synthesis of orotate (Wu 2013). This can occur when there is: (1) a deficiency of Orn carbamoyltransferase or Arg; (2) an excess intake of dietary protein; or (3) a high concentration of ammonia in plasma.

### Regulation of the Urea Cycle

The activity of the urea cycle is controlled primarily by the availability of substrates (e.g., AA and ammonia) and cofactors (e.g., $Mn^{2+}$ and $Mg^{2+}$) in plasma. Thus, in animals with low protein intake, hepatic urea synthesis is depressed to conserve both energy and N. Conversely, increasing the dietary intake of protein beyond the optimal AA requirements of the animal progressively increases ureagenesis in the mammalian liver. Second, changes in the activities of urea cycle enzymes also influence hepatic ureagenesis. For example, the expression and activities of hepatic urea cycle enzymes are enhanced by the high intake of dietary protein and AAs to facilitate the removal of AA-derived ammonia from the body. In contrast, the hepatic expression of urea cycle enzymes is markedly reduced in response to the low intake of dietary protein or AAs as an adaptation mechanism. Thus, the sudden consumption of a large amount of dietary protein immediately after chronic protein malnutrition can result in hyperammonemia and even death. Likewise, in mammalian neonates with low activities of one or more urea cycle enzymes, high-protein intake may exceed the ability of the liver to remove ammonia and cause deaths. This may be more severe for low-birth-weight than normal-birth-weight neonates. CPS-I and ASS are two key regulatory enzymes in hepatic urea synthesis. Third, the urea cycle is regulated by allosteric activators Arg (activator of NAG synthase) and NAG (activator of CPS-I). Thus, when Arg is deficient, ammonia exits mitochondria into the cytoplasm, where ammonia is utilized for the synthesis of purines and then orotate and uric acid. High levels of orotate and uric acid potentially result in fatty liver and gout, respectively. Fourth, reducing extracellular pH reduces hepatic ureagenesis by inhibiting AA transport. Thus, in metabolic acidosis, Gln is channeled to the kidneys for ammoniagenesis. In contrast, increasing extracellular pH from 7.4 to 7.6 enhances glutaminase activity and urea synthesis in the liver.

Finally, urea synthesis is also regulated by some hormones (Morris 2002). For example, growth hormone reduces the expression and activities of CPS-I, ASS, ASL, arginase, and glutaminase in the liver, thereby contributing to the conservation of AAs for protein synthesis. Growth hormone and insulin reduce the concentrations of AAs in the plasma by increasing net protein synthesis in skeletal muscle, thereby reducing the availability of the AA substrates for urea synthesis (Bush et al. 2002). In contrast, high levels of glucocorticoids upregulate the expressions of AA-degrading enzymes and of urea cycle enzymes through a cAMP-dependent mechanism, thereby promoting the production of ammonia and urea under catabolic conditions. At present, little is known about the hormonal regulation of the urea cycle in enterocytes of the small intestine.

## Detoxification of Ammonia as Uric Acid in Birds

### Uric Acid Synthesis for Disposal of Ammonia in Birds

Uric acid is a weak organic acid with a $pK_a$ of 5.75. At physiological pH values, uric acid is present primarily as monosodium urate (the chemically stable form of uric acid). In birds, uric acid is synthesized from ammonia as the major product of AA catabolism, with the liver being the most active site, followed by the kidneys and pancreas (Figure 7.28). This is true for some animals (e.g., lizards and snakes) and perhaps most species of fish which lack the urea cycle (Singer 2003). Uric

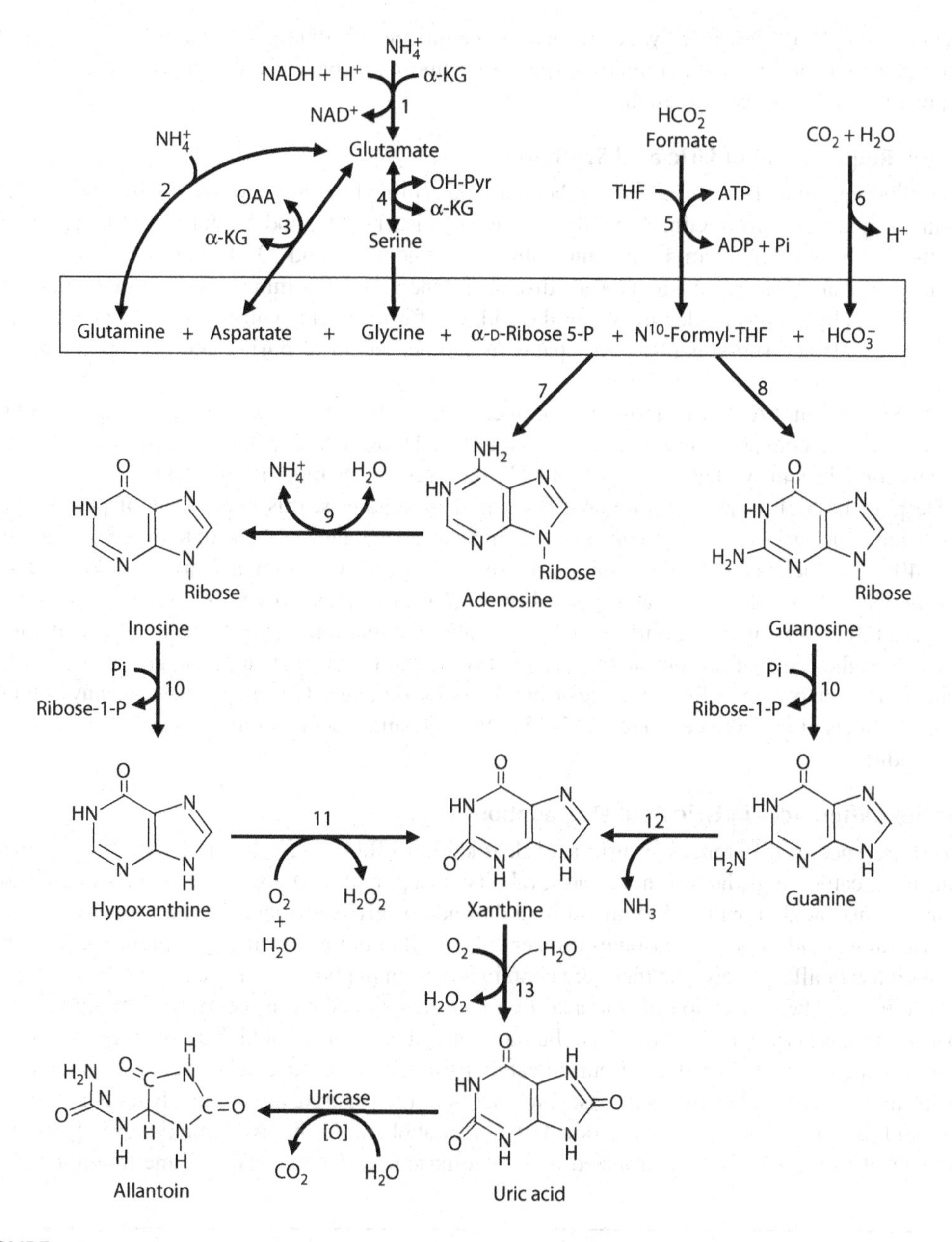


**FIGURE 7.28** Synthesis of uric acid from ammonia and bicarbonate in birds and mammals. This is the major metabolic pathway for ammonia detoxification in birds. The enzymes that catalyze the indicated pathways are: (1) glutamate dehydrogenase; (2) glutamine synthetase; (3) glutamate-oxaloacetate transaminase; (4) glutamate-hydroxypyruvate transaminase; (5) $N^{10}$-formyl-tetrahydrofolate synthetase; (6) carbonic anhydrase; (7) a series of enzymes for adenosine synthesis; (8) a series of enzymes for guanosine synthesis; (9) adenosine deaminase; (10) purine nucleoside phosphorylase; (11) xanthine oxidase; (12) guanine deaminase (guanase); and (13) xanthine oxidase.

acid synthesis also exists in the livers and other tissues of mammals. Like the urea cycle in mammals, the synthesis of uric acid also starts with ammonia and $HCO_3^-$ and requires mitochondria and cytosol. Specifically, ammonia is first incorporated into Gln (mitochondria), Asp (mitochondria and cytosol), and Gly (mitochondria and cytosol). These AAs then react with $HCO_3^-$ and $N^{10}$-formyl-tetrahydrofolate in the cytosol to form purines (adenosine and guanosine) via a series of enzyme-catalyzed steps. Finally, adenosine and guanosine are oxidized to xanthine and then uric acid in the cytosol. In many mammalian species (excluding primates) and various insects, uric acid can be oxidized by uricase to allantoin.

### Energy Requirement of Uric acid Synthesis

The ATP requirements for uric acid synthesis are determined by three events: (1) formation of adenosine or guanosine from Gln, Asp, Gly, ribose-5-P, bicarbonate, and $N^{10}$-formyl-tetrahydrofolate; (2) the incorporation of ammonia into Gln, Asp, and Gly; and (3) formation of $N^{10}$-formyl-tetrahydrofolate from formate and tetrahydrofolate. One mole of ammonia is generated from 1 mol of adenosine by adenosine deaminase in the pathway for uric acid synthesis from adenosine. This ammonia molecule subsequently participates in another round of purine and uric acid synthesis. The incorporation of 4 mol $NH_4^+$ into 1 mol uric acid requires 19.5 mol ATP if adenosine is an intermediate or 18.5 mol ATP if guanosine is an intermediate (Wu 2013). Assuming that equal amounts of ammonia are converted into uric acid through the adenosine and guanosine pathways, the entire process for uric acid synthesis from 4 mol $NH_4^+$ requires, on average, 19 mol ATP.

Despite the high energy requirement for uric acid synthesis, this pathway is of physiological importance for birds. First, uric acid synthesis in birds contributes to their higher body temperature (e.g., 40°C in chickens and ducks) than in mammals (e.g., 37°C in humans and pigs). Second, uric acid is relatively insoluble in water (solubility = 0.2 mM in plasma) and is excreted as a concentrated salt, therefore allowing birds to conserve water and maintain a low body weight during long-distance flights. Second, at physiological concentrations, uric acid is a scavenger of oxygen free radicals and can protect cells and tissues from oxidative damage. This may counteract any potential adverse effects of hyperglycemia (e.g., 12–15 mM in plasma) occurring in birds under normal feeding conditions.

### Species Differences in Uric Acid Degradation

There are species differences in uric acid degradation (Table 7.13). In the livers of most mammals (e.g., cattle, dogs, horses, mice, pigs, rabbits, sheep, and rats), except for humans and higher primates, uric acid is oxidized to allantoin (a diureide of glyoxylic acid) by the copper-containing uricase (urate oxidase) in peroxisomes (Singer 2003). Allantoin-producing mammals do not express allantoinase or allantoicase and therefore contain allantoin in plasma and release this purine metabolite in urine. The conversion of uric acid to allantoin also occurs in the kidneys of amphibia. In contrast, uricase is absent from tissues of humans and other primates, and therefore they excrete uric acid in urine as the end product of purine catabolism. Likewise, uricotelic species (e.g., chickens, ducks, and geese) do not express uricase, and therefore they excrete quantitatively large amounts of uric acid in urine as the major end product of AA catabolism. In the liver and kidneys of amphibia and teleost fish, allantoin is hydrolyzed by allantoinase (a mitochondrial enzyme in amphibia but

**TABLE 7.13**
**Species Differences in Excretion of Major Nitrogenous Metabolites by Animals**

| Metabolite | Animal Species |
|---|---|
| Urea | Mammals, terrestrial amphibians, teleost fish, elasmobranchii (sharks, rays, and skates), some aquatic reptiles, and some aquatic turtles (chelonians; but absent in most of them) |
| Uric acid | Birds, land reptiles (including squamate reptiles, such as lizards and snakes; lacking the hepatic urea cycle), Dalmation dogs, molluscs, some terrestrial crustaceans, and various insects |
| Allantoin | Most mammals except for primates, earthworms, lizards, aquatic turtles (chelonians), and various insects |
| Allantoic acids | Various insects |
| Ammonia | Aquatic amphibians, most fish, aquatic turtles (chelonians), earthworms, crustaceans, dipnoans, and some insects |

a cytosolic and peroxisomal enzyme in fish) to form allantoic acid, which is further hydrolyzed by allantoicase (a peroxisomal enzyme) to urea and glyoxylic acid. Uric acid and its metabolites are excreted by the kidneys through urate/anion exchangers.

### Regulation of Uric Acid Synthesis

Uric acid synthesis is regulated by the same nutritional and hormonal factors as noted for urea synthesis. In addition, the conversion of ammonia and bicarbonate is affected by the concentration of tetrahydrofolate as well as the activities of adenosine deaminase, purine nucleoside phosphorylase, and xanthine oxidase/xanthine dehydrogenase in cells. Thus, one-carbon-unit metabolism modulates the production of uric acid via the synthesis of purine nucleosides. Of note, $N^{10}$-formyl-tetrahydrofolate synthetase is a folate enzyme that catalyzes the formylation of tetrahydrofolate in an ATP-dependent manner. This enzyme is part of a trifunctional protein called $C_1$-tetrahydrofolate synthase. Besides its $N^{10}$-formyl-tetrahydrofolate synthetase activity, $C_1$-tetrahydrofolate synthase also contains $N^{5,10}$-methenyltetrahydrofolate cyclohydrolase and $N^{5,10}$-methylenetetrahydrofolate dehydrogenase activities. Cytokines (e.g., tumor necrosis factor-$\alpha$, interferon-$\gamma$, interleukin-1, and interleukin-6) and glucocorticoids all increase expression of xanthine dehydrogenase/xanthine oxidase in many cell types, thereby stimulating uric acid production under inflammatory and stressful conditions.

## Comparison between Urea and Uric Acid Synthesis

Urea and uric acid syntheses share some common features, namely: (1) the use of the same raw materials (ammonia, Asp, bicarbonate, and ATP); (2) the formation of a neutral AA (Cit vs Gln) in the mitochondria and a basic substance (Arg vs. xanthine) in the cytosol as intermediates; and (3) the production of a neutral end product (urea vs. sodium urate at physiological pH) (Figure 7.29). However, there are many differences between uric acid and urea syntheses: (1) the requirement of 46% more ATP to detoxify 1 mol ammonia via uric acid synthesis than through urea synthesis; (2) AAs and purines, respectively, as intermediates in urea and uric acid syntheses; (3) the participation of bicarbonate in mitochondrial and cytosolic reactions, respectively, for urea and uric acid syntheses; (4) the need of tetrahydrofolate in uric acid, but not urea, synthesis; (5) the use of Gly as

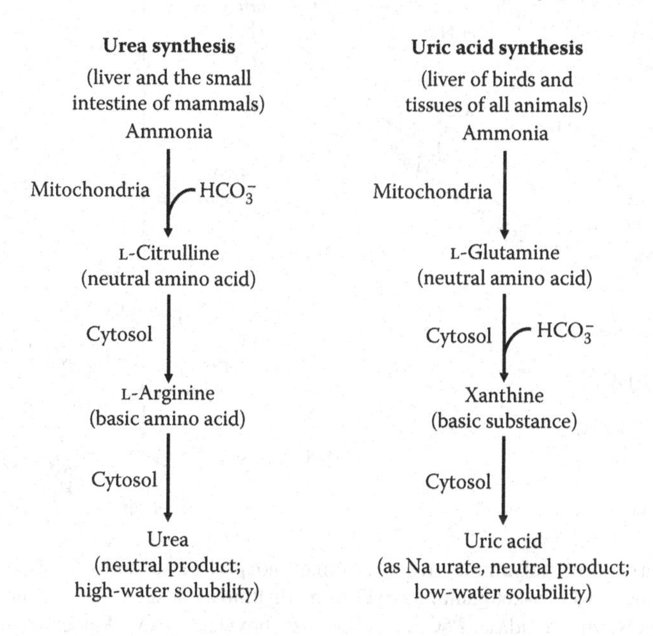


**FIGURE 7.29** Comparison between urea and uric acid syntheses in animals.

a direct substrate for uric acid synthesis, but only as a source of ammonia in urea synthesis; (6) the occurrence of urea synthesis from ammonia only in mammals and a limited species of fish, but the presence of uric acid synthesis in all animal species; and (7) ureagenesis being cell-specific but uric acid synthesis taking place in virtually all cells. Thus, different species develop different strategies for ammonia disposal to meet their metabolic and physiological needs.

## Species-Specific Degradation of AAs

Different animal species exhibit different pathways for the metabolism of some AAs possibly as an adaptation to diets and living environments, as well as physiological and anatomical changes during evolution (Davis and Austic 1997; Wright 1995). Let us use the Arg metabolism to illustrate this notion. For example, ovine placentomes express high arginase activity to degrade Arg to Orn and urea, so that Orn is utilized for the synthesis of Pro (present at relatively low content in forages) and polyamines (Kwon et al. 2003). In ruminants, urea can be recycled for AA and protein syntheses by ruminal bacteria. Thus, the presence of arginase in the placentomes of ruminants would not result in an irreversible loss of Arg nitrogen. Sheep can also utilize agmatine (a product of Arg decarboxylation by Arg decarboxylase in microbes and ovine conceptuses) to form polyamines via agmatinase (Figure 7.30). To further spare Arg, gestating sheep store a large amount of Cit (e.g., 10 mM on day 60 of gestation) and a smaller quantity of Arg (e.g., 2 mM on day 60 of gestation) in allantoic fluid.

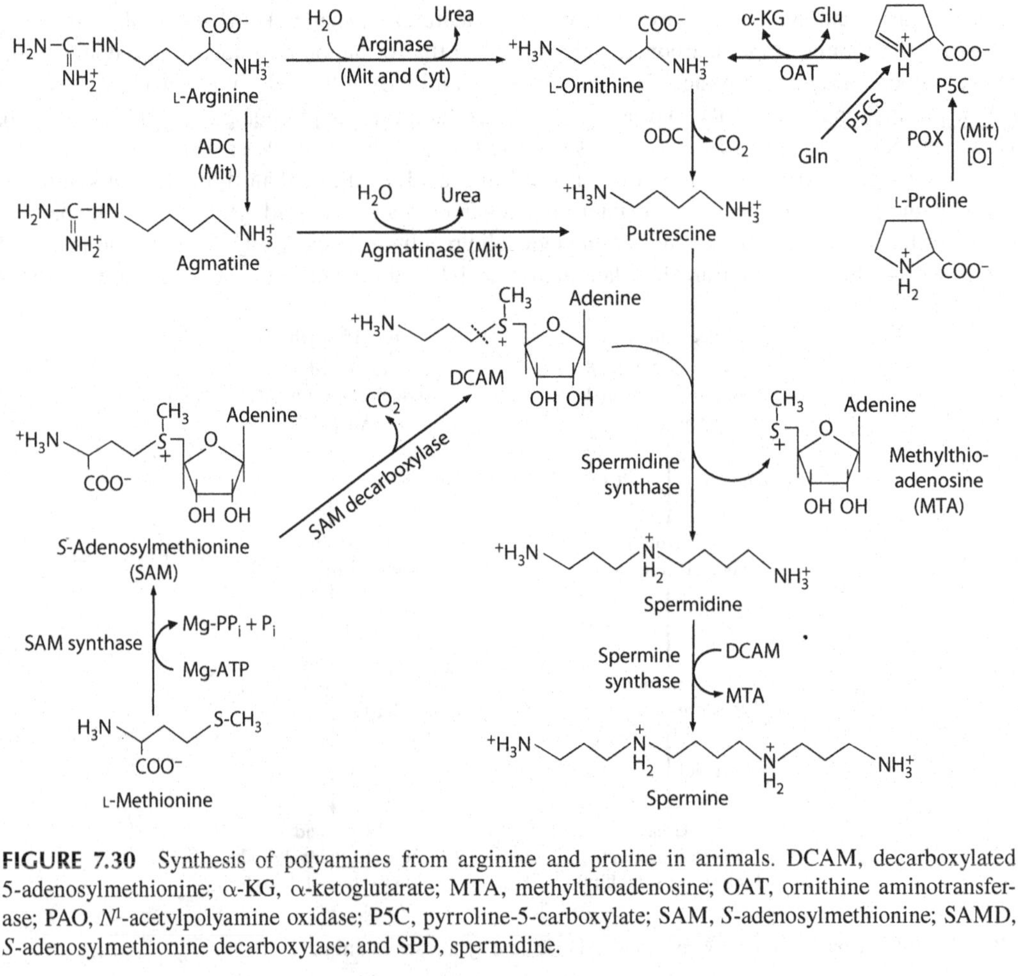

**FIGURE 7.30** Synthesis of polyamines from arginine and proline in animals. DCAM, decarboxylated 5-adenosylmethionine; α-KG, α-ketoglutarate; MTA, methylthioadenosine; OAT, ornithine aminotransferase; PAO, $N^1$-acetylpolyamine oxidase; P5C, pyrroline-5-carboxylate; SAM, *S*-adenosylmethionine; SAMD, *S*-adenosylmethionine decarboxylase; and SPD, spermidine.

Since Cit is readily converted into Arg in fetal extrahepatic tissues, Cit in the allantoic fluid serves as a reservoir of Arg in ovine fetuses. In contrast, pigs exhibit a very different picture of Cit and Arg metabolism than sheep during the entire pregnancy (Wu et al. 2013a,b). Specifically, the porcine placenta does not contain arginase activity and therefore effectively transfers Arg from the mother to the fetus. Thus, gestating pigs have an unusually high concentration of Arg (e.g., 4–6 mM on day 40 of gestation) but only a low concentration of Cit (e.g., 0.06–0.07 mM on day 40 of gestation) in allantoic fluid. To overcome the lack of arginase for polyamine synthesis from Arg in the pig placenta, this tissue expresses both Pro oxidase and Orn aminotransferase to convert Pro into Orn, which then serves as the substrate for Orn decarboxylase to form putrescine (Figure 7.30). Since the extraintestinal tissues of the pig do not use urea for AA synthesis due to the lack of urease, the absence of arginase from its placenta helps to conserve Arg, while allowing Pro (a product of the catabolism of Glu and Gln, abundant AAs in swine diets) to serve as the carbon skeleton for polyamine synthesis. To date, there is no evidence for polyamine synthesis from Arg via Arg decarboxylase and agmatinase in pigs, which is in sharp contrast to sheep (Wang et al. 2014). Thus, different animals utilize different mechanisms to regulate AA homeostasis in the body.

While enzymes for degrading AAs share functional activities among animal species, tissue-specific expression of these enzymes differ markedly between mammals and birds. This conclusion is supported by the following lines of evidence. First, Gln is extensively degraded in enterocytes of mammals, but occurs at a very low rate in enterocytes of chickens (Wu et al. 1995). This helps explain why the concentration of Gln (~1 mM) in the plasma of chickens is twice that (~0.5 mM) in postnatal mammals. Second, in the liver of chickens, Gln synthetase is a mitochondrial enzyme and traps the mitochondrion-derived ammonia for the synthesis of Gln, which is then used for uric acid production in the cytosol. In birds, net synthesis of Gln can occur in the mitochondrion, because this organelle has a very low activity of phosphate-activated glutaminase. In contrast, the liver of mammals contains a very high activity of phosphate-activated glutaminase, which would prevent net Gln synthesis if Gln synthetase was localized in the mitochondrion (Haüssinger 1990). Thus, the presence of Gln synthetase in the cytosol of the mammalian liver makes it possible for hepatocytes to synthesize Gln and aids in detoxifying blood-borne ammonia as a neutral AA. Third, as noted previously, arginase is absent from the hepatocytes of birds but is present at an exceedingly high activity in the liver of mammals to initiate Arg catabolism (Figure 7.31). Also, intestinal Orn aminotransferase is very abundant in pigs but is weakly expressed in chickens (Wu et al. 1995). Differences in AA catabolism among animal species are a metabolic basis for their different requirements of dietary AAs (Baker 2005).

## Major Products of AA Catabolism in Animals

As alluded to previously, different AAs have different catabolic pathways but share several common steps to generate some common intermediates: pyruvate, oxaloacetate, α-KG, fumarate, succinyl-CoA, and acetyl-CoA (Chapter 1). Transamination is an important step to initiate the degradation of AAs in animal cells, but the catabolism of many AAs also starts with other reactions, such as cleavage, deamination, decarboxylation, dioxygenation, hydrolysis, and hydroxylation. However, the catabolism of some AAs (e.g., Arg [Figure 7.31] and Lys) is not initiated by transamination. Complete oxidation of many AAs to $CO_2$, water, and ammonia requires interorgan cooperation, as noted previously for BCAA catabolism. The major end products of AA catabolism in animals are $CO_2$, ammonia, urea, uric acid, and sulfate (Table 7.14). Other metabolites of AAs with nutritional and physiological importance include: (1) glucose; (2) short-, medium-, and long-chain fatty acids, cholesterol, and ketone bodies; (3) signaling gases (NO, CO, and $H_2S$); (4) aminosugars, nucleotides, and heme; (5) antioxidants (e.g., glutathione, creatine, carnitine, taurine, melanin, melatonin, indoles, urocanate, and anthranilic acid; as well as carnosine, anserine, and balenine); (6) non-gaseous neurotransmitters (e.g., GABA, *N*-acetylcholine, serotonin, and dopamine); (7) hormones (e.g., thyroid hormones, epinephrine, and norepinephrine); (8) ethanolamine, histamine, polyamines,

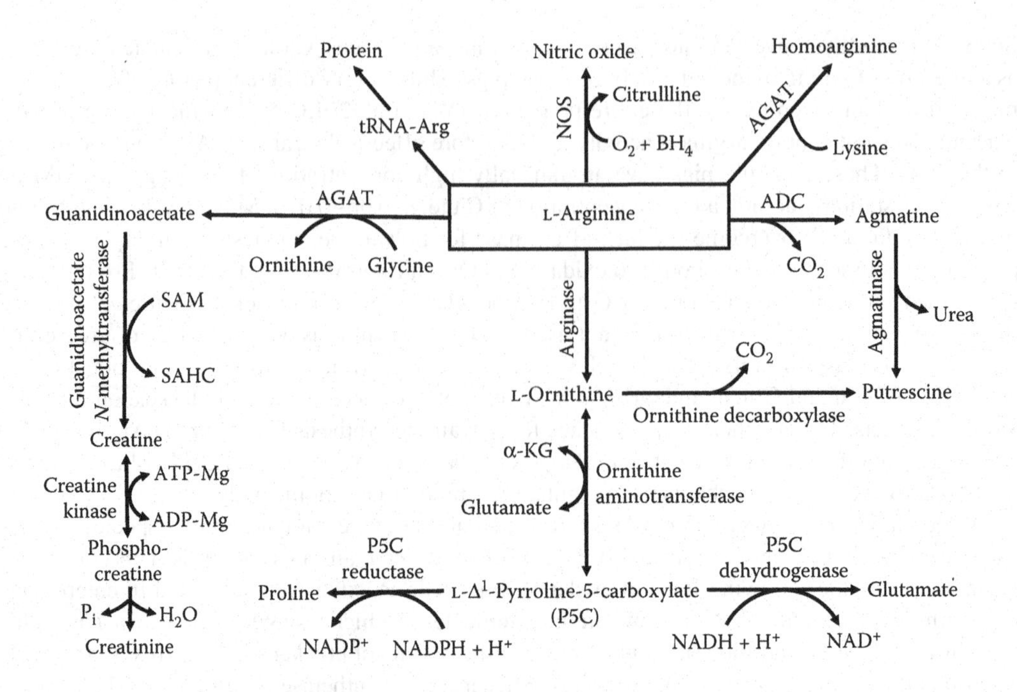


**FIGURE 7.31** Arginine catabolism via multiple pathways in animals. Arginase is the major pathway to initiate arginine degradation in mammals, birds, and fish. Large amounts of creatine are synthesized in all animals. In some tissues (e.g., skeletal muscle and brain) of mammals and birds, phosphocreatine serves to store ATP. The spontaneous loss of creatine as creatinine is 1.7% per day. ADC, arginine decarboxylase; AGAT, arginine:glycine amidinotransferase; BH4, (6R)-5,6,7,8-tetrahydro-L-biopterin; α-KG, α-ketoglutarate; NOS, nitric oxide synthase; SAM, *S*-adenosylmethionine; SAHC, *S*-adenosylhomocysteine.

homoarginine, and agmatine; (9) D-AAs (e.g., D-Ser and D-Asp); and (10) others (e.g., SAM, bilirubin, niacin, and betaine). Thus, many AAs not only serve as the precursors of protein but also regulate key metabolic pathways to improve health, survival, growth, development, lactation, and reproduction of animals. Those AAs are called functional AAs (Wu 2013).

## INTRACELLULAR PROTEIN TURNOVER

Dietary protein is converted into tissue protein in animals through a series of complex digestive and metabolic processes. The tissue protein is not static, but undergoes continuous degradation and synthesis, which is collectively called intracellular protein turnover (Figure 7.32). The balance between the rates of these two processes is the determinant of protein accretion in cells and tissue (e.g., skeletal muscle) growth in animals (Bergen et al. 1987; Buttery 1983). A protein gain in animals results from a greater rate of protein synthesis than protein degradation, whereas a protein loss in stressed animals under catabolic or disease conditions is caused by a greater rate of protein degradation than protein synthesis. When the rate of protein synthesis is equal to that of proteolysis, there will be no net change in protein mass, which occurs in healthy adults. However, protein balance in tissues is not zero postprandially. Thus, studies of intracellular protein turnover in tissues, particularly skeletal muscle (the major reservoir of protein in the body), have important implications for improving the growth performance and feed efficiency of livestock, poultry, and fish (Wu 2009).

### INTRACELLULAR PROTEIN SYNTHESIS

The process of cytosolic protein synthesis in eukaryotic organisms includes five steps: (1) gene transcription to form mRNA; (2) initiation of mRNA translation to generate peptides at ribosomes;

**TABLE 7.14**
**Major Metabolites and Functions of AAs in Animals[a]**

| Amino Acid | Metabolites | Major Functions |
|---|---|---|
| Amino acids | Ammonia | Bridge AA and glucose metabolism; regulation of acid-base balance |
| | Urea | Removal of excess nitrogen from mammals |
| | Glucose | A major energy source for brain and red blood cells |
| | Ketone bodies | Energy substrates for extrahepatic tissues; signaling molecules |
| | Fatty acids | Membrane components; components of TAGs for energy storage |
| Alanine | D-Alanine | A component of the peptidoglycan layer in bacterial cell walls |
| β-Alanine | Coenzyme A | Numerous metabolic reactions (e.g., pyruvate dehydrogenase) |
| | Pantothenic acid | Metabolic reactions (e.g., fatty acid synthesis) |
| | Antioxidant dipeptides | Carnosine (β-alanyl-L-histidine), carcinine (β-alanyl-histamine), anserine (β-alanyl-1-methyl-L-histidine), and balenine (β-alanyl-3-methylhistidine) |
| Arginine | Nitric oxide | A signaling molecule; a major vasodilator; a neurotransmitter |
| | Agmatine | Inhibition of NOS; synthesis of putrescine in ruminant conceptuses |
| | Ornithine | Urea cycle; syntheses of proline, glutamate, and polyamines (PA) |
| | Methylarginines | Competitive inhibition of NOS |
| Aspartate | Arginine | See above (Cit + Asp → Arginine) |
| | D-Aspartate | Activation of NMDA receptors in brain |
| Cysteine | Taurine | Antioxidant; regulation of cellular redox state; osmolyte |
| | $H_2S$ | A signaling molecule; a major vasodilator; a neurotransmitter |
| Glutamate | NAG | Urea cycle; intestinal arginine synthesis |
| | γ-Aminobutyrate | Inhibitory or excitatory neurotransmitter, depending on the region of brain |
| Glutamine | Glu and Asp | Excitatory neurotransmitters; the malate shuttle; cell metabolism |
| | Glucosamine-6-P | Synthesis of aminosugars and glycoproteins; cell growth and development |
| | Ammonia | Renal regulation of acid-base balance |
| Glycine | Heme | Hemoproteins (e.g., hemoglobin, myoglobin, catalase, and cytochrome c) |
| | Bilirubin | Natural ligand of aryl hydrocarbon receptor in the cytoplasm |
| Histidine | Histamine | Allergic reaction; vasodilator; gastrointestinal tract function |
| | Imidazoleacetate | Analgesic and narcotic actions |
| | Urocanate | Modulation of skin immunity; protecting the skin against ultraviolet radiation |
| Ile, Leu, and Val | Gln and Ala | See above for "Glutamine" and "Alanine" |
| Leucine | HMB | Regulation of immune response and skeletal muscle protein synthesis |
| Lysine | Hydroxylysine | Structure and function of collagen |
| Methionine | Homocysteine | Oxidant; inhibition of nitric oxide synthesis |
| | Betaine | Methylation of homocysteine to methionine; one-carbon-unit metabolism |
| | Cysteine | Cellular metabolism and nutrition |
| | SAM | Methylation of proteins and DNA; creatine, epinephrine, and PA synthesis |
| | Taurine | Antioxidant; osmolytes; conjugation with bile acids |
| | Phospholipids | Synthesis of lecithin and phosphatidylcholine cell signaling |
| Phenylalanine | Tyrosine | See below for "Tyrosine" |
| Proline | $H_2O_2$ | Killing pathogens; a signaling molecule; an oxidant |
| | P5C | Cellular redox state; ornithine, citrulline, arginine, and PA synthesis |
| Serine | Glycine | See above for "Glycine" |
| | D-Serine | Activation of NMDA receptors in brain |
| Threonine | Mucins | Maintaining intestinal integrity and function |
| Tryptophan | Serotonin | Neurotransmitter; regulation of food intake |
| | *N*-Acetylserotonin | Antioxidant |
| | Melatonin | Antioxidant; circadian rhythms |
| | Anthranilic acid | Inhibiting production of proinflammatory T-helper-1 cytokines |
| | Niacin | A component of NAD(H) and NADP(H) |
| | Indoles | Natural ligands of the aryl hydrocarbon receptor; regulation of immunity |

(*Continued*)

**TABLE 7.14 (*Continued*)**
**Major Metabolites and Functions of AAs in Animals[a]**

| Amino Acid | Metabolites | Major Functions |
|---|---|---|
| Tyrosine | Dopamine | Neurotransmitter; regulation of immune response |
| | EPN & NEPN | Neurotransmitters; cell metabolism |
| | Melanin | Antioxidant; pigmentation of skin and hair |
| | $T_3$ and $T_4$ | Regulation of energy and protein metabolism |
| Arg & Met | Polyamines | Gene expression; DNA and protein synthesis; cell function |
| Arg, Met, & Gly | Creatine | Antioxidant; antiviral; antitumor; energy metabolism in muscle and brain |
| Cys, Glu, & Gly | Glutathione | Free radical scavenger; antioxidant; cell metabolism; gene expression |
| Gln, Asp, & Gly | Nucleic acids | Components of RNA and DNA; protein synthesis |
| | Uric acid | Antioxidant; detoxification of ammonia in birds |
| Lys & Met | Carnitine | Transport of long-chain fatty acids into mitochondria for oxidation |
| Ser & Met | Choline | A component of acetylcholine and phosphatidylcholine; betaine synthesis |

*Source:* Wu, G. 2013. *Amino Acids: Biochemistry and Nutrition*. CRC Press, Boca Raton, Florida.

[a] Unless indicated, the AAs mentioned herein are L-amino acids. BCAA, branched-chain AAs; SAM, *S*-adenosylmethionine; EPN, epinephrine; HMB, β-hydroxy-β-methylbutyrate; NMDA, *N*-methyl-D-aspartate receptor (a glutamate receptor and ion channel protein found in nerve cells); NEPN, norepinephrine; NOS, nitric oxide synthase; PA, polyamines; TAGs, triacylglycerols; $T_3$, triiodothyronine; $T_4$, thyroxine.

(3) peptide elongation to produce protein; (4) termination as recognized by a terminating codon on the mRNA; and (5) posttranslational modifications of the newly synthesized protein (Figure 7.33). In bacteria, transcription in the nucleus is closely coupled with the subsequent translation in the rough endoplasmic reticulum. tRNA is necessary for translation, because mRNA does not directly recognize any AA but can bind to a tRNA that carries a corresponding AA (Manning and Cooper 2017). In essence, the mRNA synthesized from DNA encodes the polypeptide with each AA designated by a specific codon (three nucleotides). Thus, tRNAs serve as the adaptors to translate genetic information from nucleic acids (e.g., DNAs) into proteins

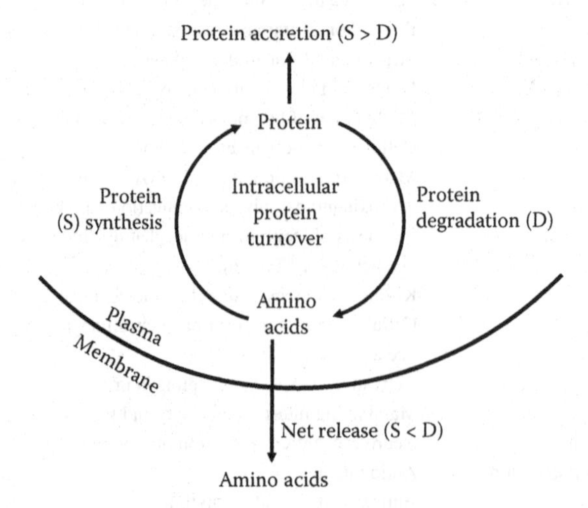


**FIGURE 7.32** Intracellular protein turnover in animals. The balance between protein synthesis and protein degradation in the cell determines its protein accretion and release of AAs.

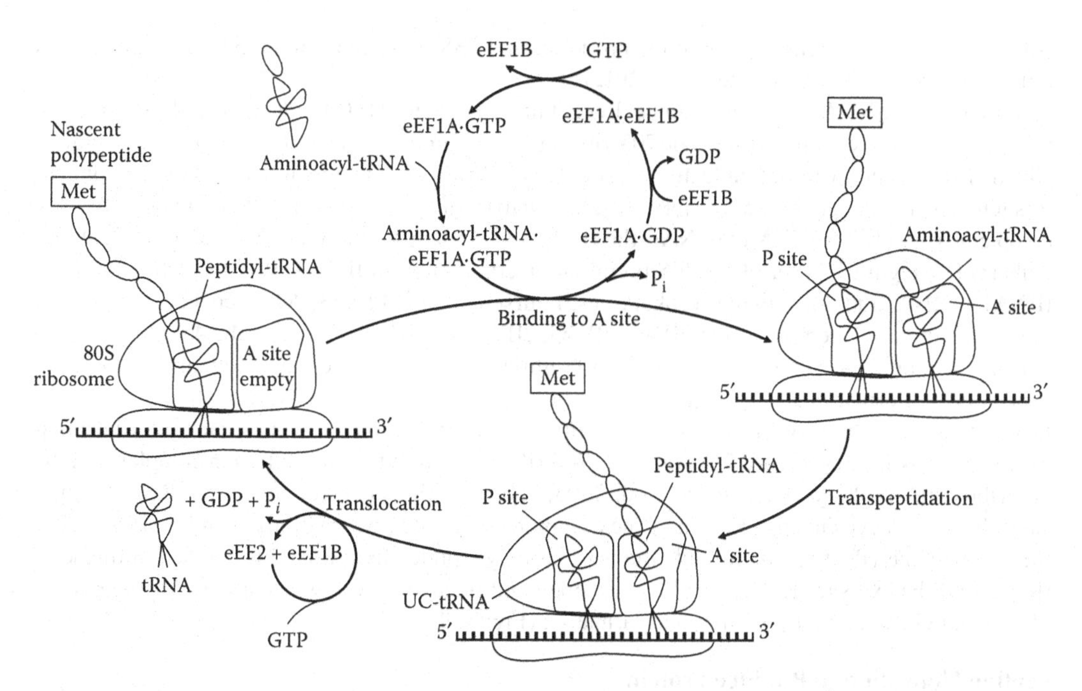


**FIGURE 7.33** The pathway of protein synthesis in animal cells. The 80S ribosome is the functional site for the translation of mRNA into protein. These processes require: enzymes (aminoacyl-tRNA synthetase and peptidyltransferase), eukaryotic initiation factors (eIF), elongation factors (eEF), and release factors (eRF). eEF1A·GTP is required for the binding of an incoming aminoacyl-tRNA to the A site, and eEF1A·GDP is recycled into eEF1A·GTP under the action of eEF1B. Polypeptide elongation is terminated by a terminating codon on the mRNA template. Peptidyltransferase, together with eRF1, hydrolyzes peptidyl-tRNA to release the newly synthesized peptide. UC-tRNA, uncharged tRNA.

## Gene Transcription to form mRNA

The first step in protein synthesis is the transcription of a DNA gene to form rRNA, mRNA, and tRNA in the nucleus by RNA polymerases I, II, and III, respectively. These processes are similar between eukaryotic and prokaryotic cells (Lackner and Bähler 2008). Each tRNA contains a tri-nucleotide sequence (collectively known as an anticodon), which is complementary to a codon on mRNA for a specific AA. The mRNA has a 5′-cap (methyl-guanosyl triphosphate), which is critical for protection from RNases in the nucleus. In eukaryotic organisms, most mRNA molecules are polyadenylated at the 3′ end via the covalent linkage of a polyadenylyl moiety. The poly(A) tail and its associated proteins protect mRNA from degradation by exonucleases. Eukaryotic precursor mRNA requires extensive processing (including the methylation of guanosine by SAM-dependent guanine-$N^7$-methyltransferase, and the removal of introns [splicing] by the spliceosome [a ribozyme]) to become mature mRNA before transport through the nuclear pore to ribosomes in the cytoplasm (Manning and Cooper 2017).

## Initiation of mRNA Translation to Generate Peptides at Ribosomes

Before protein synthesis is initiated, the 80S ribosome is formed from 60S and 40S subunits in eukaryotic cells. In prokaryotic cells, the 70S ribosome is formed from 50S and 30S subunits. The steps of this process are similar between eukaryotic and prokaryotic cells, but more initiation factors are required by eukaryotes than prokaryotes and the sizes of the ribosomes differ. For example, the 40S subunit in eukaryotic cells contains an 18S RNA that is homologous to the prokaryotic 16S RNA, whereas the 60S subunit in eukaryotic cells contains three RNAs: the 5S and 28S RNAs (which are the counterparts of the prokaryotic 5S and 23S molecules) and a 5.8S RNA (which is unique to eukaryotes) (Kong and Lasko 2012).

Initiation of mRNA translation can be divided into four steps: (1) GTP-dependent dissociation of the 80S ribosome (e.g., in animals) or 70S ribosome (e.g., in bacteria) into its constituent subunits, which is controlled by initiation factors (e.g., eukaryotic initiation factors [eIF]) and elongation factors (eukaryotic elongation factors [eEF]); (2) formation of the 43S preinitiation complex (ternary complex) from eIF2, GTP, Met-tRNAi (the tRNA for binding to the initial Met), and 40S subunit (eukaryotes; Figure 7.34) or of the 30S preinitiation complex from IF2, GTP, *N*-formylmethionine-tRNAi, mRNA, and 30S subunit (prokaryotes; Laursen et al. 2005); (3) ATP-dependent formation of the 48S initiation complex from eIF4E, eIF4G, eIF4A, eIF4G, mRNA, and the 43S preinitiation complex (eukaryotes; Figure 7.32) or of the 30S initiation complex through codon–anticodon interaction and conformational change (prokaryotes; Laursen et al. 2005); and (4) formation of the translationally active 80S ribosome from the 48S initiation complex, the 60S ribosome, and ribosomal protein S6 (eukaryotes; Figure 7.32) or of the 70S ribosome from the 30S initiation complex and the 50S ribosome (prokaryotes; Laursen et al. 2005). The 80S ribosome contains three RNA-binding sites: the aminoacyl site (also known as the acceptor site; A site), which binds an aminoacyl-tRNA; the peptidyl site (P site), which binds the nascent polypeptide chain linked to the last aminoacyl-tRNA; and the exit site (E site, usually not recognized in eukaryotes), which allows for the release of deacylated tRNA after peptide-bond formation (Figure 7.35).

### Peptide Elongation to Produce Protein

Active translation occurs on the functional 80S ribosome complex where the ribosome reads mRNA in the 5′–3′ direction. During this process, each tRNA that carries the corresponding AA moves through the 80S ribosome from the A site to the P site and then exits the ribosome via the E site. Elongation factors are crucial for addition of an AA to a polypeptide and for peptide elongation. Protein synthesis occurs at a high speed and accuracy. Eukaryotic and prokaryotic ribosomes can incorporate 6 and 18 AA per second, respectively. This rapid process of peptide elongation starts with the ATP-dependent activation of AA to form aminoacyl-tRNA, which is catalyzed by each of 20 different aminoacyl-tRNA synthetases, in addition to Met-tRNAi. During elongation, AAs are continually added to the peptide, eventually forming a polypeptide or protein chain bound together through peptide bonds.

Amino acid + tRNA + ATP → Amino acyl-tRNA + AMP + PPi (aminoacyl-tRNA synthetase)

### Termination of Peptide Chain Elongation

After multiple cycles of elongation to polymerize AAs into a protein molecule, the completion of the polypeptide chain elongation is recognized in the A site by the terminating signal known as the nonsense or terminating codon (e.g., UGA, UAG, or UAA) on the mRNA. Except for the special Sec-$tRNA_{(Sec)}$, tRNA normally does not have an anticodon that can recognize such a termination codon. Rather, the recognition of a termination codon residing in the A site of the 80S ribosome is performed by eukaryotic protein release factors (eRF) (e.g., eRF1, eRF2, and eRF3). The stop codon induces the binding of a release factor that prompts the disassembly of the entire ribosome–mRNA complex. eRF1 recognizes UAA and UAG, whereas eRF2 recognizes UAA and UGA. In complexes with GTP, eRF3 promotes the binding of eRF1 and eRF2 to the 80S ribosome, and the eRF then hydrolyzes the bond between the peptide and the terminal tRNA. GTP hydrolysis triggers the dissociation of the eRF from the ribosome, which dissociates into the 40S and 60S subunits for another cycle of protein synthesis.

### Posttranslational Modifications of Newly Synthesized Proteins

Most of the newly synthesized proteins have no biological activities when released from the ribosome. The polypeptides must undergo appropriate modifications in the cytoplasm and/or on the

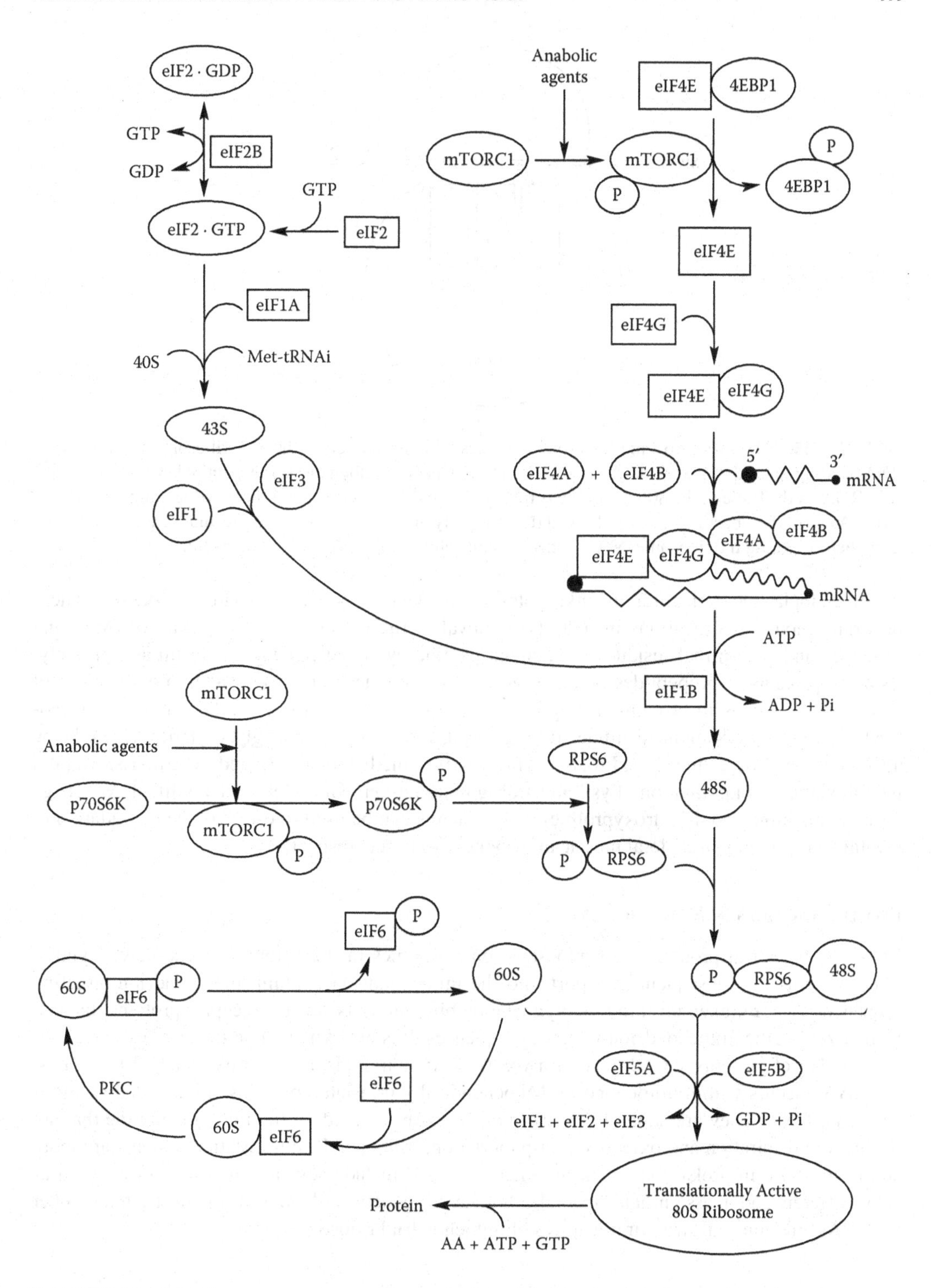


**FIGURE 7.34** Initiation processes for protein synthesis in animal cells. In the presence of various initiation factors and the mRNA template, 40S and 60S ribosomes combine to form the translationally active 80S ribosome where protein synthesis in the cytoplasm and mitochondria takes place. eIF, eukaryotic initiation factor; 4EBP1, eIF4E-binding protein 1; mTORC1, complex 1 of mammalian or mechanistic target of rapamycin; p70S6K, ribosomal protein S6 kinase 1 (a 70 kDa protein); PKC, protein kinase C; RPS6, ribosomal protein S6; S, Svedberg unit of flotation.

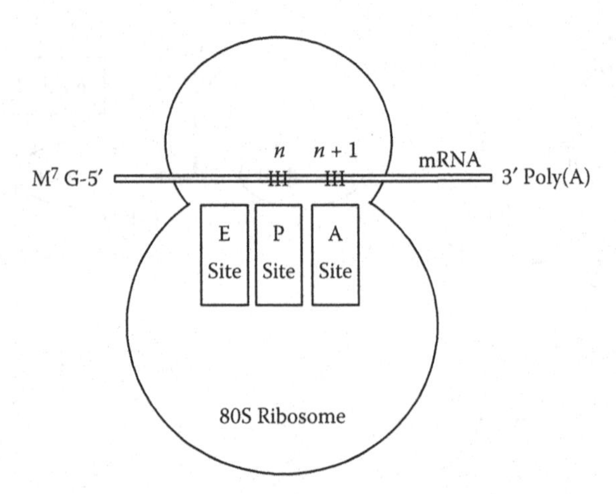


**FIGURE 7.35** The 80S ribosome for protein synthesis in animal cells. The 80S ribosome contains three RNA-binding sites designated as A, P, and E. During peptide elongation, the peptidyl moiety from the AA-tRNA on the P site of the 80S ribosome is transferred to the acceptor end of the existing aminoacyl-tRNA on the A site of the ribosome. The discharged tRNA rapidly dissociates from the P site and is transferred to the E site before exiting the ribosome. $M^7G$, 7-methylguanylate cap; Poly(A), polyadenylyl tail.

rough endoplasmic reticulum in eukaryotes (equivalent to becoming mature proteins). These posttranslational modifications include: (1) removal of the initiating AA (e.g., Met or fMet) and of the C- and N-terminal residues (e.g., signal peptide by signal peptidase); (2) limited proteolysis of proproteins or propeptides (inactive proteins or peptides); and (3) covalent modifications of certain AA residues in proteins or peptides, including acetylation (Lys), ADP-ribosylation, biotinylation, γ-carboxylation, disulfide linkage (Cys), flavin attachment, glycosylation (Lys), heme attachment, hydroxylation (Lys, Pro, Ser, Thr, and Tyr), methylation (Arg and Lys), myristoylation, palmitoylation, ubiquitination (Lys), and transglutamination. The release of modified AAs (e.g., 3-methylhistidine and 4-hydroxyproline) from proteins can be used to estimate the degradation of myofibrillar proteins in skeletal muscle and connective tissue, respectively.

### Protein Synthesis in Mitochondria

Most mitochondrial proteins are synthesized on ribosomes in the cytoplasm. The newly synthesized proteins for subsequent transport into the mitochondrion contain mitochondrion-targeting sequences and are taken up into this organelle by binding to its surface receptor proteins that can recognize specific mitochondrion-targeting sequences. It is now known that the synthesis of a limited number of proteins (e.g., 8 in certain yeasts, 13 in mammals, and approximately 20 in plants) from AAs occurs within mitochondria. Mitochondrially translated proteins are encoded by mitochondrial DNA. They are subunits of enzyme complexes located on the inner membrane that are involved in respiration and oxidative phosphorylation. Mitochondrial translation systems are more similar to those in prokaryotes than in eukaryotes, and include several unusual features, such as some different codon assignments from the "universal" genetic code, the use of a restricted number of tRNAs, and unusual structural features of mitochondrial ribosomes.

### Energy Requirement of Protein Synthesis

One mole of protein consist of various quantities of different AAs that amount to the sum of 1 mol of AA. Intracellular protein synthesis requires substantial amounts of energy, primarily in the forms of ATP and GTP. The energy-dependent reactions include: (1) AA activation to form tRNA-AA; (2) the entry of tRNA-AA into the A site on the ribosome (initiation of peptide chain formation) that requires the cleavage of GTP to GDP; and (3) the translocation of the newly formed peptidyl-tRNA from the A site to the P site on the ribosome (chain elongation); and (4) termination of polypetide synthesis.

1. AA activation: ATP → AMP + PPi (2 high energy phosphate bonds)
2. Initiation of peptide chain formation: GTP → GDP + Pi (1 high energy phosphate bond)
3. Peptide chain elongation: GTP → GDP + Pi (1 high energy phosphate bond)
4. Termination of polypeptide synthesis: GTP → GDP + Pi (1 high energy phosphate bond)

Thus, an equivalent of 5 mol ATP (5 ATP → 5 ADP + 5 $P_i$) is required to synthesize 1 mol protein. In addition, the transport of some AAs into cells requires ATP (e.g., 0.5 mol ATP/mol AA on average). This consideration is nutritionally relevant because dietary (exogenous) AAs are required for protein maintenance and accretion in animals. Thus, 5.5 mol ATP are needed to synthesize 1 mol or 100 g protein from extracellular AAs, which amount to 118 g AAs based on the composition of AAs in the pig body (Wu 2013). When AAs are derived within the cell through synthesis or intracellular protein degradation, the energetic cost of protein synthesis is 5 mol ATP per 1 mol or 100 g protein. The energy released during protein synthesis contributes to "heat increment" after an animal eats a meal containing protein.

### Measurement of Protein Synthesis

Labeled AA tracers (nonmetabolizable AAs; e.g., Leu for liver and Phe for skeletal muscle) are used to measure protein synthesis in isolated tissues or incubated cells (Bergen et al. 1987; Klasing et al. 1987; Wu and Thompson 1990). For example, with the use of $^{14}$C-Phe as a tracer plus 1 mM Phe in a medium to study protein synthesis in skeletal muscle, the rate of protein synthesis (measured by the incorporation of $^{14}$C-Phe into protein) within a 2 h period is calculated as:

Amount of $^{14}$C-Phe radioactivity in protein (dpm)/Specific radioactivity of $^{14}$C-Phe in the precursor pool (dpm/nmol) = nmol Phe/2 h

The fractional rate of protein synthesis is calculated as:

Specific activity of $^{14}$C-Phe radioactivity in protein (dpm/nmol)/Specific radioactivity of $^{14}$C-Phe in the precursor pool (dpm/nmol) × 100 = %/2 h

The absolute amount of protein synthesis is calculated as:

Amount of protein in tissue (mg) × fractional rate of protein synthesis [%/(2 h × 100)] = mg/2 h

In all these calculations, the amount of tissue used for incubation should be taken into consideration.

Many methods involving tracers have also been developed to measure *in vivo* protein synthesis in tissues of the animal, which include: (1) single administration of a tracer AA; (2) flooding dose technique (e.g., young animals; 10–30 min labeling of protein); and (3) constant infusion of a tracer AA (larger animals; 4–6 h labeling of protein) (Davis and Reeds 2001; Southorn et al. 1992; Watford and Wu 2005). Measurement of whole-body protein synthesis based on two- or more-compartment models has also been validated for use in animals (Waterlow et al. 1978). The most common methods are the flooding dose technique and the constant infusion of a tracer. However, the experimental approach chosen for measuring tissue protein synthesis *in vivo* should be dictated by the scientific question being addressed. For example, the short-term flooding dose technique is useful for tissues (e.g., liver and small intestine) with high rates of protein synthesis to minimize the recycling of the tracer, and for tissues (skeletal muscle and heart in young animals) with lower rates of protein synthesis. In contrast, the long-term constant infusion technique is appropriate for tissues with lower rates of protein synthesis in large animals to reduce the cost of tracer and achieve a steady state of precursor specific radioactivity or isotope enrichment (Bergen et al. 1987).

## Intracellular Protein Degradation

### Proteases for Intracellular Protein Degradation

Protein degradation is catalyzed by proteases, with the resultant peptides being hydrolyzed by oligo-, tri-, and di-peptidases (Baracos et al. 1986; Wu 2013). Most proteases are hydrolases (also known as peptidases), but some (e.g., Asn peptide lyases) are not. Therefore, the terms "proteases" and "peptidases" should not be treated as synonymous. Proteases are classified according to: (1) reaction type (e.g., exopeptidases and endopeptidases); (2) the chemical nature of the enzyme's catalytic site (e.g., Ser, Cys, Asp, Thr, Glu, Asn, and metallo proteases); and (3) their evolutionary relationship (e.g., families, and families with related structures are grouped into clans) (Rawlings et al. 2012). The classification and naming of enzymes based on the type of reaction is the primary principle of the enzyme nomenclature of the International Union of Biochemistry and Molecular Biology.

### Intracellular Proteolytic Pathways

Intracellular proteins are degraded via highly selective pathways to maintain a dynamic state of protein turnover (Bergen 2008). Proteases are present in the cytoplasm, plasma membrane, and many organelles of the cell (Goldberg 2003). Besides the cytoplasm and the lysosome, peptidases are present in the plasma membrane, mitochondria, nucleus, and rough endoplasmic reticulum. Thus, intracellular proteolytic pathways are classified according to the location of proteases: lysosomal and nonlysosomal systems (Figure 7.36).

1. *The lysosomal proteolytic pathway*. Proteins are delivered from the cytoplasm to the lysosome via the endocytic pathway mediated by endocytosis or autophagy (self-eating). Once cytosolic proteins are inside the lysosome, they are denatured due to the low pH and then hydrolyzed by proteases to release AAs. These proteases include: (1) cathepsin B (cysteine protease) with both endopeptidase and exopeptidase (C-terminus) activities; (2) cathepsin H (cysteine protease; a glycoprotein) with both endopeptidase and exopeptidase (N-terminus) activities; (3) cathepsin L (a major lysosomal cysteine protease; endopeptidase); (4) cathepsin D (aspartate protease; endopeptidase); (5) cathepsin K (cysteine protease in osteoclasts and bronchial

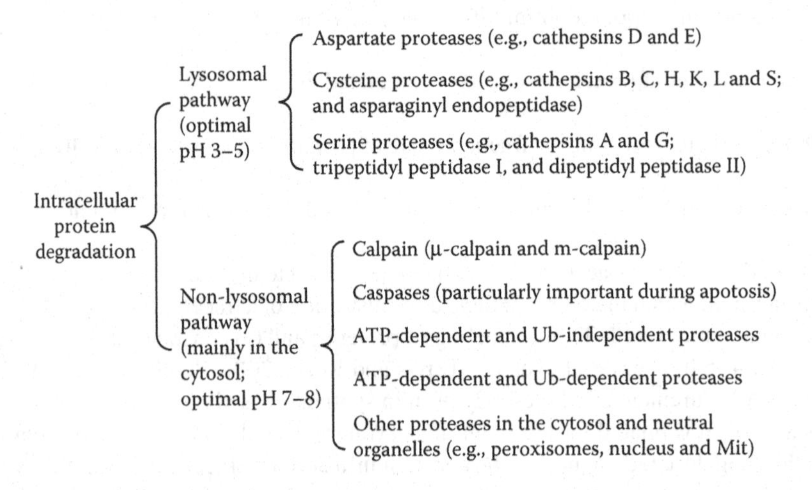


**FIGURE 7.36** Intracellular pathways for protein degradation in animal cells. Proteins enter the lysosome from the cytosol via autophagy, endocytosis, and crinophagy. The lysosomal pathway is responsible for the degradation of endocytosed proteins and nonmyofibrillar proteins under conditions of nutritional deprivation (20%–30% of total cellular proteins). The nonlysosomal pathway is responsible for the degradation of normal short-lived proteins; abnormal, denatured, and aged proteins under basal metabolic conditions; and myofibrillar and nonmyofibrillar proteins under conditions of nutritional deprivation (70%–80% of total cellular proteins). Mit, mitochondria; Ub, ubiquitin.

epithelium); and (6) other proteases, such as cathepsins C (myeloid cells), F (macrophages), O (widespread), V (thymic epithelium), W ($CD8^+$ T-cells), and Z (widespread) (Ciechanover 2012; Goldberg 2003). The optimal pH for lysosomal proteases is 3–5. Thus, some weak bases (e.g., ammonia, methylamine, chloroquine, or monensin [an ionophore]) inhibit lysosomal protein degradation by increasing intralysosomal pH above 5.0. The lysosomal proteolytic system participates in the intracellular degradation of (1) endocytosed proteins and (2) nonmyofibrillar proteins under conditions of nutritional deprivation. Studies involving the use of inhibitors of lysosomal enzymes indicate that, in the presence of physiological concentrations of insulin, glucose, and AAs, the lysosomal proteolytic system contributes to the degradation of 30%–35% and 20%–25% of intracellular proteins in enterocytes and skeletal muscle, respectively (Wu 2013). The lysosomal system is not involved to a significant extent in the degradation of myofibrillar proteins in skeletal, cardiac, or smooth muscles.

2. *The nonlysosomal proteolytic pathways.* A variety of low- and high-molecular-mass proteases are found outside the lysosome. Based on catalytic mechanisms, the nonlysosomal pathway for proteolysis can be divided into: (1) the $Ca^{2+}$-dependent proteolytic system (calpain); (2) the caspases (e.g., caspases 1, 3, and 9; cysteine proteases); (3) the ATP-dependent, ubiquitin-independent proteolytic system (e.g., the 20S proteasome); and (4) the ATP- and ubiquitin-dependent proteolytic system (e.g., the 26S proteasome) (Goll et al. 2008). All of these protein degradation pathways are present in the cytoplasm and may also be expressed in certain organelles (e.g., peroxisomes, nucleus, and mitochondria). The optimal pH for nonlysosomal proteases is 7–8. The nonlysosomal system is responsible for the degradation of (1) normal short-lived proteins; (2) abnormal, denatured, and aged proteins under basal metabolic conditions; and (3) both myofibrillar and nonmyofibrillar proteins under conditions of nutritional deprivation (Wu 2013). Depending on cell type, the nonlysosomal system can contribute to the degradation of 70%–80% of intracellular proteins in the presence of physiological concentrations of insulin, glucose, and AA.

### Biological Half-Lives of Proteins

Owing to their different AA sequences and structures, different proteins are degraded in animal cells at different rates. Thus, the half-lives of intracellular proteins range from several minutes for short-lived proteins to days for long-lived proteins and to months for very long-lived proteins (Wu 2013). Abnormal proteins are more rapidly degraded than normal proteins. The rates of degradation of normal proteins vary widely with their functions. Enzymes at key metabolic control points usually have a much shorter half-life than those that catalyze near-equilibrium reactions. For example, Orn decarboxylase (which catalyzes a rate-controlling step of polyamine synthesis) has a half-life of 11 min, whereas actin and myosin (cytoskeletal proteins) in skeletal muscle have a half-life of $\geq$30 days.

### Energy Requirement for Intracellular Protein Degradation

The energy requirement for peptide-bond cleavage cannot be explained by thermodynamic considerations, since the hydrolysis of peptide bonds is an exergonic process (Goll et al. 2008). However, experimental evidence shows that ATP is required for protein breakdown by: (1) ATP-dependent but ubiquitin-independent proteases (2 ATP molecules per peptide bond); and (2) the ATP- and ubiquitin-dependent 26S proteasome (equivalent to 3 ATP molecules per peptide bond). Combining all proteolytic pathways in cells, approximately 2 ATP molecules are used for the cleavage of one peptide bond in proteins.

### Measurements of Intracellular Protein Degradation

Intracellular protein degradation releases free AAs. Thus, the rate of protein degradation is also measured by the release of a nonmetabolizable AA (labeled or nonlabeled AA) from intracellular proteins by cells or tissues (Bergen 2008). Such a measurement is affected by the reincorporation of AAs into newly synthesized proteins. In incubated cells or tissues whose pathway of protein synthesis is not inhibited, the release of an AA is an indicator of only net protein degradation, and protein synthesis should be determined simultaneously to calculate the rate of protein degradation. In contrast, when an inhibitor of protein synthesis (e.g., 0.5 mM cycloheximide) is included in the incubation medium, the release of an AA is an indicator of total protein degradation (which can simply be called protein degradation) in cells or tissues (Wu and Thompson 1990). In studies involving the release of a labeled AA from labeled proteins, inclusion of a high concentration of the unlabeled AA in the incubation medium (e.g., 1 mM Phe in medium for skeletal muscle and intestinal cells) is sufficient to minimize the reincorporation of the labeled tracer AA into the protein pool.

Net protein degradation = Protein degradation − Protein synthesis
Protein degradation = Net protein degradation + Protein synthesis

Measurements of intracellular protein degradation *in vivo* also involve a labeled AA (Waterlow et al. 1978). Stable isotope tracers are often used in humans and large farm animals, because they are ethically acceptable and safe for studies. In contrast, radioactive tracers are good choices for studying *in vivo* protein degradation in rodents and small farm animals because of high sensitivity, easy analysis, and low costs. In rapidly growing animals, assessment of intracellular protein degradation can be based on fractional rates of protein synthesis and protein growth, as follows:

$$K_d = K_s - K_g$$

$K_d$ (%/day) is the fractional rate of protein degradation
$K_s$ (%/day) is the fractional rate of protein synthesis
$K_g$ (%/day) is the fractional rate of protein growth

Urinary excretion of 3-methylhistidine is often used as a noninvasive method to estimate whole-body muscle proteolysis in certain species of animals (Young and Munro 1978). As noted previously, posttranslational methylation of some His residues in actin and myosin proteins generates 3-methylhistidine residues. After these proteins are hydrolyzed by intracellular proteases, 3-methylhistidine is produced by skeletal, smooth, and cardiac muscles and is not reincorporated into proteins (Bergen et al. 1987). 3-Methylhistidine is quantitatively excreted in the urine in some species (including cats, cattle, chickens, deer, frogs, humans, rats, and rabbits), and therefore can be a useful noninvasive technique for measuring *in vivo* protein degradation in these animals. In some species (e.g., dogs, goats, mice, pigs, and sheep), 3-methylhistidine cannot be quantitatively excreted in the urine, and thus is not a useful indicator of muscle protein degradation. In pigs, sheep, and goats, 3-methylhistidine reacts with β-alanine to form β-alanyl-L-3-methylhistidine. In dogs, 3-methylhistidine undergoes decarboxylation to form 3-methylhistamine and a large amount of 3-methylhistidine is excreted in the feces. In mice, 3-methylhistidine is also decarboxylated to form 3-methylhistamine, followed by oxidative deamination to yield 1-methylimidazole-4-acetic acid, whereas 3-methylhistidine can be acetylated to *N*-acetyl-3-methylhistidine.

## Nutritional and Physiological Significance of Protein Turnover

Both protein synthesis and protein degradation require significant amounts of energy. In maintenance, the intracellular protein turnover requires a total of 7 mol ATP per 1 mol of protein (5 mol ATP for protein synthesis and 2 mol ATP for protein degradation). This does not appear to have an advantage of efficient utilization of dietary energy. Then the question is why do cells continuously degrade the proteins that have been synthesized? Also, during fasting in animals, including humans, a decrease in protein loss would be advantageous to their survival. Why does protein breakdown continue even under catabolic conditions? These questions can be answered in light of the nutritional and physiological significance of protein turnover.

1. Protein turnover regulates cellular levels of proteins (including enzymes) and cell growth.

   Cellular protein = Protein synthesis − Protein degradation

   Growth of animals depends on the balance between the rates of protein synthesis and protein degradation in their tissues, particularly skeletal muscle (Table 7.15). The rate of protein synthesis is much greater than the rate of protein deposition in growing animals (Davis et al. 2004). For example, in 30-kg pigs, an increase in the deposition of 1 g protein in the body requires the synthesis of 1.5–2 g protein coinciding with the degradation of 0.5–1 g protein (Reeds 1989). In general, the deposition of 1 g protein in tissues is associated with the retention of 3 g water. Thus, protein accretion is the major determinant of BW gain in animals. The efficiency of protein gain in the body decreases with age, primarily because the fractional rate of protein synthesis is reduced with advanced age, while the fractional rate of protein degradation remains largely unchanged, as reported for 30 to 90 kg pigs (Davis et al. 2004; Reeds et al. 1980).

   Changes in cellular protein concentrations are also important for the metabolic control of enzymes in various pathways, such as AA oxidation, the urea cycle, gluconeogenesis, ketogenesis, and the Krebs cycle. Maintenance of intracellular and extracellular homeostasis of proteins is consistent with their essential functions in: (1) cell structure (integral and peripheral membrane proteins); (2) extracellular matrix (collagen, elastin, and proteoglycans); (3) enzyme-catalyzed reactions; (4) gene expression (e.g., histones and methylases); (5) hormone-mediated effects (e.g., insulin and growth hormone, and placental lactogen); (6) muscle contraction (actin, myosin, tubulin, tropomyosin, and troponin); (7) osmotic regulation (e.g., proteins in plasma); (8) protection (e.g., blood clotting factors, antibodies, and interferons); (9) regulation of metabolism (e.g., calmodulin, leptin, and osteopontin); (10) storage of nutrients and $O_2$ (e.g., ferritin, metallothionein, and myoglobin); and (11) transport of nutrients and $O_2$ (e.g., albumin, hemoglobin, and plasma lipoproteins). Thus, a loss of more than 50% of the protein from the body is not compatible with the survival of animals.
2. Protein turnover is required for the ongoing production of rapidly growing cells (e.g., epithelial cells of the gastrointestinal tract, mammary glands, skin, and placental cells); reticulocytes; lymphocytes, macrophages, and other immunocytes; and eggs and sperm of female and male reproductive systems, respectively. For example, the rapid growth of neonatal enterocytes requires high rates of net protein synthesis. In addition, when an

**TABLE 7.15**
**Effects of Dietary Protein Quality and Energy Intake on Protein Deposition in Growing Pigs (30–40 kg Body Weight)**

| | Change (g Protein/Day) in | | |
|---|---|---|---|
| Diet | Protein Deposition | Protein Synthesis | Protein Degradation |
| Feed intake (3 times vs. 2 times Maintenance intake)[a] | +62 | +97 | +35 |
| Protein quantity (29% vs. 15% CP in diet) | +23 | +127 | 104 |
| Protein quality (sufficient vs. insufficient lysine) | +75 | +40 | −35 |
| Dietary energy (with or without added carbohydrate) | +43 | +20 | −23 |
| Dietary energy (with or without added fats) | +60 | +20 | −40 |

*Source:* Reeds, P.J. 1989. In: *Animal Growth Regulation*. Edited by D.R. Campion, G.J. Hausman, and R.J. Martin. Plenum Publishing Corporation, pp. 183–210.

[a] Maintenance requirements were 7.4 MJ metabolizable energy/day and 8.1 g digestible CP/day per kg body-weight$^{0.75}$.

animal is immunologically challenged, T-cells and B-cells rapidly proliferate so that large amounts of lymphokines and antibodies are generated to mount a successful response. Furthermore, successful wound healing, which is critical to the recovery of patients from injury, requires proliferation of endothelial cells, angiogenesis, collagen synthesis, granulation tissue formation, epithelialization, and wound contraction by the action of myofibroblasts. Increased provision of AAs, particularly Arg, Pro, and Gly, can promote protein synthesis and accelerate wound healing in injured animals.

3. Protein degradation is required to remove aged, abnormal, and denatured proteins due to changes in extracellular and intracellular environments (e.g., pollution, heat stress, and the oxidative stress induced by free radicals and other oxidants). The presence of abnormal proteins within cells may interfere with the normal cellular metabolism, or result in changes in cell volume and osmolarity. In addition, protein degradation plays an important role in adaptation to nutritional deprivation (e.g., such as fasting and lack of dietary protein intake) and pathological conditions (e.g., burn, cancer, infection, inflammation, and injury) by supplying AAs (e.g., Ala, Gln, and Arg) for gluconeogenesis, ammoniagenesis, ATP production, synthesis of essential proteins, production of neurotransmitters, generation of gaseous signaling molecules, and immunity.

## Nutritional and Hormonal Regulation of Intracellular Protein Turnover

### Dietary Provision of AAs and Energy

The synthesis of proteins, including potent anabolic hormones (e.g., insulin, growth hormone, and insulin-like growth factor-I), requires all of its building blocks (i.e., AAs), as well as sufficient energy, enzymes, and cofactors (Wu 2013). In addition, AAs stimulate the release of these hormones from the endocrine organs. Thus, the availability of the AAs, which are provided ultimately in diets, is crucial for protein synthesis in all animals (Buttery 1983). For example, in 30 kg pigs, the rate of whole-body protein synthesis is 270 g/day at energy equilibrium, and is increased to 406 and 512 g/day, respectively, when their ration supplies twice and three times their maintenance (7.4 MJ metabolizable energy/day and 8.1 g digestible CP/day per kg body-weight$^{0.75}$) requirements (Reeds et al. 1980). Compared with carbohydrate supplementation, adding an isocaloric amount of fats to the diet of growing pigs does not affect protein synthesis but reduces protein degradation, resulting in greater protein deposition in the whole body (Table 7.15). It is likely that the metabolism of fats is more effective at sparing AAs for tissue protein synthesis than carbohydrates.

All proteinogenic AAs must be present in the cytosol at the same time and in the proper ratios to ensure optimal synthesis of proteins in cells. This nutritional principle is the basis for feeding animals with diets containing adequate amounts of high-quality protein, which provides optimal ratios and sufficient concentrations of AAs in the plasma for protein synthesis in the whole body. Thus, as reported for young pigs (Reeds 1989), an improvement in dietary protein quality can result in greater protein deposition in the body than a simple increase in the amount of low-quality protein intake (Table 7.15).

### MTOR Cell Signaling

Initiation of polypeptide formation is upregulated by the activation of MTOR (a highly conserved serine/threonine protein kinase), which integrates diverse signals from nutrients, hormones, and growth factors to upregulate protein synthesis in tissues, including skeletal muscle and placenta (Bazer et al. 2014; Suryawan et al. 2011). The MTOR system consists of two structurally and functionally distinct components: MTOR complex 1 (MTORC1) and MTOR complex 2 (MTORC2) (Figure 7.37). The enzymatic activity of MTOR depends on its phosphorylation by an upstream kinase, which is activated by growth hormone, insulin, insulin-like growth factor-1, and a variety of growth factors, glucose, or an AA (e.g., Arg, Gln, Leu, Gly, Pro, and Trp) (Columbus et al. 2015; Sun et al. 2016; Xi et al. 2012). The activated MTOR phosphorylates two downstream target proteins:

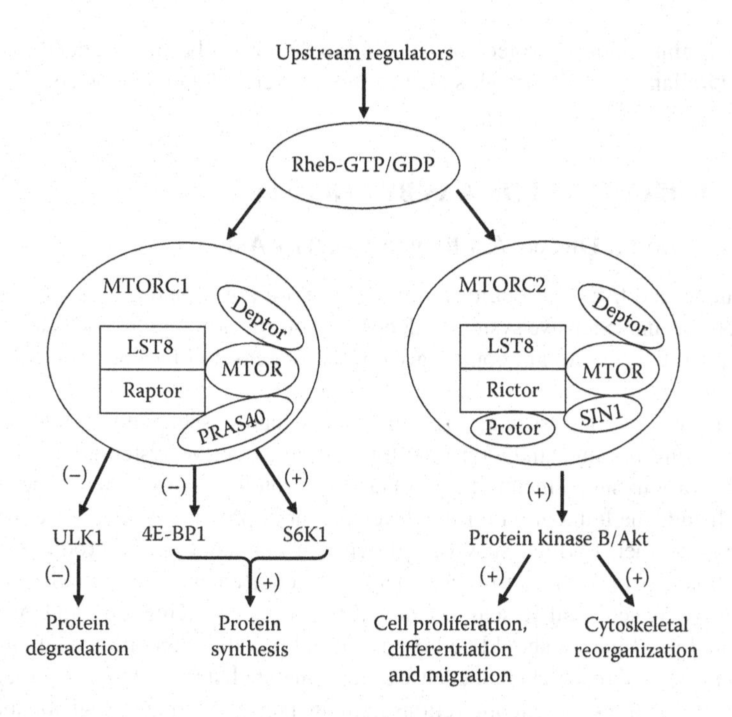


**FIGURE 7.37** The MTOR complexes in animal cells to regulate intracellular protein turnover. eIF4E-BP1, eukaryotic initiation factor 4E-binding protein-1; LST8, lethal with SEC13 protein 8 (also known as GβL); MTORC1, mechanistic target of rapamycin complex 1; MTORC2, mechanistic target of rapamycin complex 2; PRAS40, proline-rich Akt substrate of 40 kDa; SIN1, stress-activated MAP kinase interacting protein 1; ULK1, unc 51-like kinase 1.

eIF4E–BP1 (eIF4E-binding protein-1, a translational repressor protein) and ribosomal protein S6 kinase-1 (S6K1). In a non-phosphorylated state, eIF4E–BP1 binds tightly to eIF4E (an initiation factor) with high affinity, such that free eIF4E is not available to bind eIF4G (another initiation factor) to form a translationally active complex. When eIF4E–BP1 is phosphorylated, eIF4E is dissociated from eIF4E–BP1 to bind with eIF4G, generating the eIF4F–eIF4G complex. In contrast, S6K1 phosphorylation results in the phosphorylation of ribosomal protein S6 (RPS6) to yield the RPS6–48S complex and finally the translationally active 80S ribosome for the initiation of polypeptide synthesis. Besides the regulation of protein synthesis, activation of MTORC1 also inhibits ULK1 (unc 51-like autophagy activating kinase) to suppress autophagy and lysosomal protein degradation in cells. Activation of MTORC2 stimulates cell proliferation, differentiation, and migration, as well as cytoskeletal reorganization (Figure 7.35). Thus, the combined actions of MTORC1 and MTORC2 play an important role in the growth and development of cells, particularly at fetal and neonatal stages (Bazer et al. 2015).

### Physiological and Pathological Stresses

Under stress conditions (e.g., heat, cold, transportation, weaning, and social mixing stresses) where the circulating levels of glucocorticoids are markedly elevated, muscle protein synthesis is depressed and muscle proteolysis is augmented to cause no or even negative weight gain in animals (including mammals, birds, and fish) (McAllister et al. 2000; Samuels and Baracos 1995; Southorn et al. 1990). An effective approach to ameliorate the stress-induced negative protein balance may be dietary supplementation with Yucca extracts (120–180 ppm), a structural analogue of glucocorticoids (Chapter 3). By antagonizing glucocorticoids, *Yucca Schidigera* extracts can improve protein deposition and growth performance in animals (e.g., chickens reared at high ambient temperatures) (Rezaei et al. 2017). Likewise, in diseases (including sepsis), inflammatory cytokines stimulate muscle protein degradation and inhibit muscle proteolysis, leading to the loss of body protein (Baracos et al. 1987; Bergen 2008; Orellana et al. 2011). This is even more severe when the subjects cannot eat or they eat very little.

## DIETARY REQUIREMENTS FOR AAS BY ANIMALS

### Needs for Formulating Dietary AA Requirements of Animals

Livestock, poultry, and fish of agricultural importance are raised under various production conditions (e.g., intensive and extensive systems), depending on species, region, and season. For example, pigs, chickens, and dairy cows are commonly housed in pens and fed their formulated rations (an intensive system), whereas waterfowl (e.g., ducks and geese) often graze pasture and watersheds in developing countries. In contrast, many ruminants (e.g., cattle, sheep, goats, and deer) and horses usually graze pasture in rangeland, consume forages (an extensive system), and/or receive feedlot diets containing various supplemental levels of energy, protein, vitamins, and minerals. Knowledge of AA metabolism is the foundation for the development of protein or AA supplements to the diets of farm animals for their optimal survival, growth, development, and reproduction. Many countries have established committees to recommend AA requirements for animals (e.g., the NRC in the United States, Agricultural Research Council in the United Kingdom, and Animal Nutrition Research Council in China). It should be borne in mind that these recommendations serve only as guides for producers and researchers, because animal metabolism is a dynamic process and its rate can change markedly in response to alterations in many nutritional, physiological, and environmental factors.

### General Considerations of Dietary Requirements of AAs

In determining dietary requirements of AAs by animals, oxidation of AAs in the body should be taken into consideration (Figure 7.38). First, regardless of AA balance in the diet, when the dietary intake of a given AA is augmented, its oxidation is increased according to the substrate–enzyme relationship of Michaelis–Menton kinetics. Thus, when the dietary intake of a given AA (e.g., Lys)

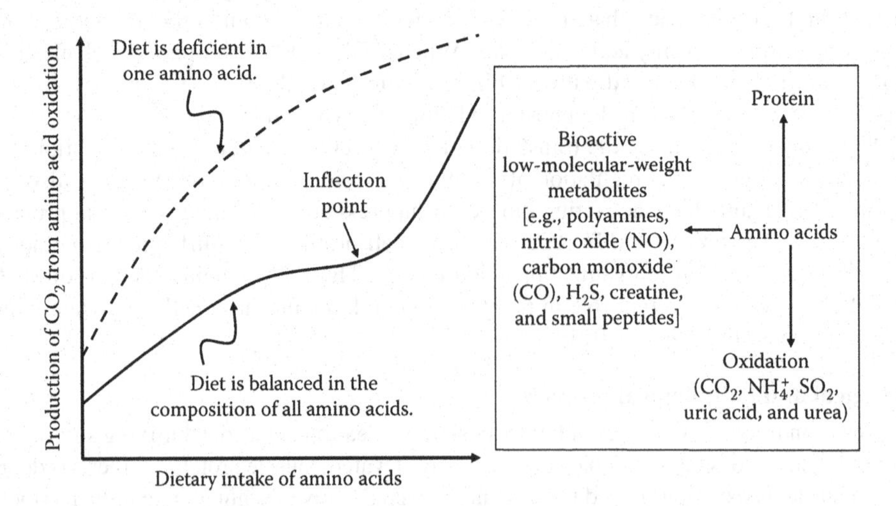


**FIGURE 7.38** The relationship between the oxidation of AAs and protein synthesis in animals. The interrelationships between AA oxidation and the dietary intake of AAs in animals. In animals fed an AA-adequate diet, an excess of a specific AA (indicated by the inflection point) results in an increase in its oxidation but not necessarily the oxidation of other AAs. In contrast, when an AA (particularly an AA not synthesized by animals) is deficient in a diet, protein synthesis is impaired and the oxidation of other AAs is increased with increasing dietary intake of AAs.

is below the animal's requirement, its oxidation is reduced to spare it for protein synthesis. As noted previously, the tRNA-AA synthases have much lower $K_M$ values for AA substrates than the enzymes that degrade AAs. Only a small fraction of dietary AAs is available for oxidation in animals fed an AA-balanced diet. Excessive AAs are usually not stored in tissues and must be oxidized to $CO_2$, water, ammonia, and urea. Second, when the dietary intake of a given AA is optimal for protein synthesis, its oxidation is at a minimum level, in comparison with its excess. In an AA-balanced diet, an excess of an AA would increase its oxidation, but not necessarily the oxidation of other AAs. In contrast, in an AA-imbalanced diet, when one of the AAs whose carbon skeleton is not synthesized by animal cells (e.g., Lys) is deficient in the diet, the oxidation of other AAs (e.g., Phe) is increased gradually with increasing dietary intake of other AAs. This is because the short supply of the limiting AA limits the utilization of other AAs for protein synthesis and all the non-limiting AAs are degraded in a tissue-specific manner.

Dietary requirements of AAs can be classified as qualitative and quantitative. Qualitative requirements refer to the question of "what is needed by animals for maintenance and production (e.g., growth, lactation, reproduction, and sports competition)?" Quantitative requirements refer to the question of "how much is required by animals for maintenance and production?" Both terms are practically important in animal feeding practices. Traditionally, growth or N balance experiments are employed to determine both qualitative and quantitative requirements of dietary AAs by animals.

## Qualitative Requirements of Dietary AAs

As noted preciously, AAs were traditionally classified as EAAs, conditionally essential AAs (CEAAs), and NEAAs. The term "EAAs" was coined in 1912 and these AAs must be provided to animals to maintain their growth and nitrogen balance. The EAAs are His, Ile, Leu, Lys, Met, Phe, Thr, Trp, and Val in all animals, and this list also includes Arg in birds and most fish species. CEAAs are AAs that which normally can be synthesized in adequate amounts by animals but must be provided in the diet to meet optimal needs under certain conditions (e.g., weaning and infection [Ewaschuk et al. 2011; Wu 2010]) wherein rates of utilization are greater than rates of synthesis. The CEAAs are Arg, Gln, Glu, Gly, and Pro for most mammals, and are Gln, Glu, Gly, and Pro for birds and most fish. In contrast, NEAAs were considered to be dispensable in diets. In most mammals (e.g., humans, rats, and pigs), the traditionally classified NEAAs are Ala, Arg, Asn, Asp, Cys, Glu, Gln, Gly, Pro, Ser, and Tyr. Although the concepts of EAAs and NEAAs have been used for over a century, growing evidence from studies with pigs, poultry, and fish has shown that animals do have dietary requirements of NEAAs to fulfill their genetic potential for maximum growth, reproduction, lactation, and production performance, as well as optimal health and well-being (Hou et al. 2015; Yoshida et al. 2016). Thus, the term "NEAAs" should no longer be used in nutritional sciences. Hou and Wu (2017) recommended that "NEAAs" be replaced by a new term "AASAs," that is, AAs that are synthesizable *de novo* in animal cells. Since an animal has dietary requirements for all proteinogenic AAs, they should not be classified as EAAs or NEAAs.

The ability of animals to synthesize AASAs *de novo* has nutritional and physiological significance in ensuring their constant provision to the cell for maintaining its homeostasis. One can argue that the selective conservation of pathways for the syntheses of AASAs indicates that they are indispensable for the metabolic needs and survival of animals (Wu 2013). Conversely, the lack of EAA synthesis can help to: (1) spare phosphoenolpyruvate, D-erythrose-4-phosphate, and acetyl-CoA for the formation of glucose, nucleotides, and fatty acids, respectively; (2) reduce energy expenditure; and (3) minimize the numbers of proteins and intermediary metabolites, as well as metabolic complexity and cell size in animals. While protein biosynthesis requires all proteinogenic AAs, AASAs confer many functions that cannot be fulfilled by EAAs. In addition, AASAs are more abundant in the body than EAAs, and the needs for AASAs for growth, lactation, and egg production are greater than those for EAAs (Hou et al. 2016).

Another concept often used in protein nutrition is "limiting AA," which is defined as an AA that is in the shortest supply from the diet relative to its requirements by an animal for maintenance, growth, and health. Limiting AAs are usually EAAs. The first limiting AA is often an EAA that is present in the diet in the least amount, as compared to the animal's daily requirement (Kim et al. 2005; Liao et al. 2015; Trottier et al. 1997). For example, Lys and Met are normally the first limiting AAs for swine and poultry diets, respectively, and are most often the limiting AAs for ruminants fed corn- and forage-based diets (Baker and Han 1994; Benevenga and Blemings 2007; Hanigan et al. 1998; Le Floc'h et al. 2011). Results from nutritional studies indicate that, in conventional swine diets, the second, third, and fourth limiting AA are usually methionine, tryptophan, and threonine, respectively.

### Quantitative Requirements of Dietary AAs

The classic method to assess AA requirements of animals involves growth or N balance studies during a period of time (e.g., days or weeks). Minimal requirements of AAs can also be estimated by so-called factorial analysis, namely, the loss of N in animals fed a protein-free diet (maintenance) + N deposited in animals + N excreted as animal products (e.g., milk, eggs, wool, and fetuses). Modern tracer techniques for assessing dietary AA requirements by animals have been developed. Recommended requirements of dietary EAAs are available for domestic and laboratory animals (NRC 2017), and those for dietary AASAs for pigs and chickens have recently been published (Wu 2014). Generally, the requirements of dietary AAs by animals decrease with advanced age. Of note, dietary requirements of AAs are much greater in growing fish (e.g., 30%–60% CP) than in growing (5–100 kg BW) pigs (20%–14% CP) and growing (0.05–3 kg BW) broilers (20%–16% CP). Since the composition of AAs in the carcass is similar among different animal species and the relative rates of growth in fish are not necessarily greater than those for mammals and birds, fish may have low rates of syntheses of AASAs and require sufficient provision of these AAs in diets to compensate for their inadequate endogenous synthesis.

1. *Growth or N balance studies for determining dietary requirements of AAs.* Young animals (e.g., piglets, chicks, and rats) are very sensitive to dietary provision of AAs, and therefore their growth performance is a useful indicator of their needs for dietary AAs (Baker 2005; Kim and Wu 2004). To further assess protein deposition in the body, N balance studies are often conducted with growing animals that require dietary AAs for maintenance and growth. When there is no N accumulation in the body (zero N equilibrium), N intake from the diet should be equal to N excretion in various forms including: (a) urea, ammonia, nitrite, nitrate, AAs, and other nitrogenous substances in urine; (b) NO gas; (c) fecal nitrogenous substances (N output); and (d) N losses through the hair and skin (Young and Borgonha 2000). When dietary provision of an AA is deficient, N balance in animals is not optimal and can even be negative. To date, with the availability of improved techniques for rapid and accurate AA analysis, AA but not N balance should be measured in animal research or production.
2. *Factorial method for determining AA requirements.* Dietary requirements for AAs by the whole body or a tissue of interest (e.g., the small intestine) can be estimated based on factorial analysis, namely, the sum of fecal and urinary N in response to a protein-free diet (maintenance), AA deposited in the body, and AA excreted as important products (e.g., milk and fetal growth). For certain AAs, the factorial method can also be based on the sum of the needs for the AA for metabolic pathways and obligatory losses of the AA via secretions from the body. The obligatory loss of AA occurs through hair, sweat, nasal secretions, and seminal fluid (males), when an animal is fed an essentially N-free diet that meets energy requirements (Wu 2014). The factorial method is particularly useful for determining dietary requirements of AAs that are synthesized in mammalian cells.
3. *Tracer studies for determining dietary requirements of AAs and protein.* The rate of oxidation of an AA depends on its concentration in the free pools (e.g., plasma and intracellular fluids), the nutritional status, and the physiological needs of the subject. As noted

previously, excessive amounts of AAs are generally not stored in the body and will be disposed of primarily via oxidation. A marked increase in the oxidation of an AA is usually an indicator of its excessive availability in the body, provided there are no significant changes in the concentrations of regulatory hormones, coenzymes, cofactors, or metabolites. In other words, if the supply of an AA exceeds its needs by the animal, this AA is oxidized to $CO_2$, water, ammonia, and urea (Figure 7.15). In the direct AA oxidation method, the production of $CO_2$ from a test AA (e.g., L–[1–$^{13}$C]Lys) is measured to estimate its dietary requirement by the animal. In the indicator (indirect) AA oxidation method, the production of $CO_2$ from an AA (e.g., L–[1–$^{13}$C]Phe) other than the test AA (e.g., Pro) is determined to estimate the dietary requirement of the test AA (Ball et al. 1986). Since the early 1980s, the direct and indirect AA oxidation techniques have been used to determine dietary requirements of many EAAs by swine and poultry (Elango et al. 2012).

Each method for determining dietary requirements of AAs has its own strengths and weaknesses. The N balance study is a simple and relatively inexpensive approach to estimate dietary requirements of AAs by animals, but is insensitive to the metabolic needs of AAs within a short period and is beset with large variations among animals (Table 7.16). The common advantages of both the direct and the indicator AA oxidation methods over the N balance technique are that (a) dietary requirements of AAs can be estimated within a few hours after several days of adaptation to experimental diets; and (b) changes in whole-body oxidation of a specific AA in response to different intakes of dietary AA can be assessed. However, both N balance and isotope studies do not take into consideration functional needs of AAs beyond protein synthesis in animals.

1. *Physiological, metabolic, and anatomical criteria for assessing dietary requirements of AAs.* Determination of dietary requirements of EAAs for animals is simpler than that of AASAs because the organisms respond more sensitively and more rapidly to a deficiency of an EAA in the diet. The end points for determining dietary EAA requirements by animals (e.g., mortality, morbidity, food intake, growth, lactation, and reproductive performance) can be used to estimate their dietary requirements of AASAs. Additional criteria can also be helpful and include assessments of physiological parameters (e.g., concentrations of hormones, hemoglobins, ammonia, urea, AAs, nitrogenous metabolites, lipids,

**TABLE 7.16**
**Limitations of Nitrogen Balance Studies in Assessing Dietary Requirements of AAs by Animals**

(1) Failure to account for all the losses of N from the body, resulting in underestimation of AA requirements;
(2) High variability in daily N balance, as small changes in N deposition may not be detected;
(3) Failure to detect functional changes in cells and organs or to fully evaluate dietary requirements of AAs;
(4) Not being sufficiently sensitive to dietary intake of certain AAs (e.g., Arg and His) particularly within a short experimental period;
(5) An inability to provide information about the cellular processes of the intermediary metabolism of AAs or protein;
(6) Difficulty in interpreting the experimental data either when dietary protein intake is high or when dietary protein intake is low, because enzyme systems adapt and AA oxidation can be altered;
(7) N balance being strongly influenced by dietary energy intake, environmental conditions, and changes in endocrine status;
(8) Requirement of a relatively long period of adaptation to an experimental diet (e.g., 5–7 days for rats and pigs);
(9) Possible inconsistency between animal growth and N balance, as an animal can lose weight and still be in a positive nitrogen balance; and
(10) Like all bioassays, the response per increment of intake declines as the maximum attainable response is approached.

*Source:* Wu, G. 2013. *Amino Acids: Biochemistry and Nutrition.* CRC Press, Boca Raton, Florida.

and glucose in plasma, as well as concentrations of neurotransmitters, glutathione, creatine, and polyamines in tissues) (Wu et al. 2014a). Furthermore, dietary requirements of AASAs can be based on any abnormal values for anatomical, physiological, biochemical, and immunological indices, including (a) abnormalities in small-intestinal morphology, mass, absorptive capacity, and integrity; (b) imbalances among AAs and high concentrations of ammonia in plasma and urine; (c) dysfunctional regulation of nutrient metabolism to reduce muscle protein gain, promote white-fat accretion, and cause metabolic syndrome in the body; (d) impaired response of peripheral lymphocytes to stimulation by mitogens; (e) abnormal blood chemistry; and (f) abnormal organ function (e.g., impaired vision, skin lesions, and skeletal muscular weakness). Thus, multiple variables can be used to define dietary requirements of AASAs by animals, and the choices should depend on species and goals.

### Factors Affecting Dietary Requirements of AAs

Dietary requirements of AAs by animals are highly dynamic and are affected by a variety of factors (Field et al. 2002; Wu 2013). These factors include: (a) dietary composition (e.g., AA content and proportions, energy intake, presence or absence of other substances, and food processing); (b) physiological characteristics of animals (e.g., age, sex, genetic backgrounds, circadian clock, hormones, pregnancy, lactation, and physical activity); (c) pathological states (e.g., injury, infection, trauma, neoplasia, diabetes, obesity, cardiovascular disease, and fetal growth restriction); and (d) the living environment (e.g., hot or cold ambient temperatures, toxic agents, air pollution, sanitation, noise, and social grouping). Thus, caution should be exercised when one uses any recommended values of dietary AA requirements for animals. Feeding practice should be the best way to test a nutritional theory.

### The "Ideal Protein" Concept

The "ideal protein" concept, which was conceptualized for diets of chickens in the late 1950s, refers to optimal proportions and amounts of EAAs (Arg, His, Ile, Leu, Lys, Met, Phe, Thr, Trp, and Val) without the consideration of any "NEAAs" (Fisher and Scott 1954). It was thought that the composition of EAAs in diets should be the same as that in eggs or casein. However, approaches based on this proposition were largely unsuccessful. An improvement in chicken growth performance was achieved when the profile of EAAs in the chick carcass was used to formulate dietary EAAs, but the result remained unsatisfactory (Klain et al. 1960). Subsequent studies showed that inclusion of both EAAs and several "NEAAs" (cystine, Gly, Pro, and Glu) in diets yielded better results on chicken growth performance than EAAs alone (Baker et al. 1968; Graber and Baker 1973). This extensive research culminated in several versions of the "chick AA requirement standard" for the first three weeks post-hatching (e.g., Baker and Han 1994; Sasse and Baker 1973), possibly because of the concerns that: (1) the published data on the composition of glycine, proline, and hydroxyproline in the chicken carcass were highly inconsistent, and (2) inclusion of a large amount of Glu (e.g., 13 times the lysine value) in diets as an isonitrogenous control might interfere with the transport, metabolism, and utilization of other dietary AAs. The NRC (1994) and Baker (1997) did not include Glu, Gly, or Pro in an ideal protein for diets of 0- to 56-day-old chickens. Omission of these three and other proteinogenic AASAs from the "ideal protein" is not desirable due to their important nutritional and physiological roles in poultry (Wu et al. 2014a).

Research on the dietary ideal protein for chickens laid a foundation for studies with growing pigs. Cole (1980) suggested that swine diets could be formulated to contain ideal ratios of Ile, Leu, Lys, Met, Phe, Thr, Trp, and Val (with Lys as the reference value) based on their content in the pig carcass. This idea was adopted by the Agricultural Research Council (ARC, 1981) and NRC (1998). Of note, His and all AASAs (including Arg) were not included in the ideal protein concept of the ARC for growing pigs or by Wang and Fuller (1989) for 25 to 50 kg gilts. This oversight was partially corrected by Chung and Baker (1992) in their work involving 10–20 kg swine through the addition of Arg, Gly, His, and Pro (42%, 100%, 32%, and 33% of Lys, respectively) to the basal diet containing 1.2% true digestible Lys. However, owing to incomplete knowledge of AA biochemistry and nutrition, the NRC (1998) did not recognize the needs of pigs for dietary Pro or Gly. Consequently, Pro and Gly were removed from the ideal protein in swine diets (Baker 2000; Kim et al. 2005). This conceptual foundation is flawed because: (1) the pattern of AAs in the diet does not match that in the animal body due to their extensive catabolism at different rates in the small intestine (Wu et al. 2014a); and (2) with the exception of Arg, all AASAs were not included in the ideal protein (Kim et al. 2001). Much evidence shows that animals have dietary requirements for all proteinogenic AAs in proper proportions and adequate amounts (Hou et al. 2015; Hou and Wu 2017).

## EVALUATION OF THE QUALITY OF DIETARY PROTEIN AND AAS

The quality of any dietary protein depends on the following factors: (1) the amounts and profile of its AAs; and (2) the digestibility and availability of its AAs to the animal relative to requirements for all AAs. A protein that has a balanced composition of all AAs but cannot be hydrolyzed by proteases in the gastrointestinal tract cannot be a high-quality protein for animals. Thus, although the analysis of the AA content in feedstuffs is necessary to predict which AA is deficient or excessive in the diet, this chemical method should not be used as the sole means of evaluating the nutritive quality of feed proteins. Therefore, biological studies to determine protein digestibility *in vivo* and the animal's growth performance must be carried out concurrently with the determination of dietary AA composition (Chapter 4). In human nutrition, various AA scoring systems have been used over the past three decades, including the protein digestibility corrected AA score (PDCAAS, recommended in 1989) and the digestible indispensable AA score (DIAAS, recommended in 2011) (FAO 2013).

In the PDCAAS system, a single value of apparent (e.g., fecal) CP digestibility is used as the digestibility of each EAA in the dietary protein, and the ratio of the amount (mg) of an apparently digestible EAA in 1 g of the dietary protein to the amount (mg) of the same EAA in 1 g of the reference protein is calculated for each EAA, and the lowest value is designated as the PDCAAS. In the DIAAS system, the ratio of the amount (mg) of a truly digestible EAA in 1 g of the dietary protein to the amount (mg) of the same EAA in 1 g of the reference protein is calculated for each EAA, and the lowest value is designated as the DIAAS.

$$\text{PDCAAS}(\%) = \frac{\begin{matrix}\text{Amount (mg) of a nutritionally essential} \\ \text{amino acid (EAA) in 1 g of the dietary protein}\end{matrix} \times \begin{matrix}\text{Apparent digestibility of} \\ \text{the dietary crude protein}\end{matrix}}{\text{Amount (mg) of the same EAA in 1 g of the reference protein}} \times 100$$

$$\text{DIAAS}(\%) = \frac{\begin{matrix}\text{Amount (mg) of a nutritionally essential amino} \\ \text{acid (EAA) in 1 g of the dietary protein}\end{matrix} \times \begin{matrix}\text{True digestibility of the amino} \\ \text{acid in the dietary protein}\end{matrix}}{\text{Amount (mg) of the same EAA in 1 g of the reference protein}} \times 100$$

### Analysis of AAs in Diets and Feed Ingredients

Proteins in complete diets or feed ingredients must be hydrolyzed to individual AAs before AA analysis. This is usually done by both acid and alkaline hydrolyses (Chapter 4). When feedstuffs are finely ground, their proteins can be hydrolyzed with known proteases of microbial, plant, and animal origin. Alternatively, feed can be incubated with fluids obtained from the stomach and small intestine of postabsorptive animals to mimic the *in vivo* digestion process. Free AAs can be measured by HPLC, gas chromatography, or enzymic methods. Owing to its accuracy, speed, and low costs, HPLC is by far the most powerful technique for AA analysis. Values from AA analysis can tell us which AA in dietary proteins might be deficient, adequate, or excessive, but give little information on their availability to the animal. A good quality protein contains high percentages of Cys, Lys, Met, Thr, and Trp. Glu, Gln, Asn, Asp, plus BCAAs represent most of the AA content in both plant and animal proteins. Certain plant (e.g., peanut meal and cottonseed meal) and animal (e.g., fish meal and gelatin) products provide high levels of arginine. However, feedstuffs of animal origin usually contain higher percentages of Cys, Lys, Met, Thr, and Trp than feedstuffs of plant origin. Unlike other animal products, Ile content is relatively low in red blood cells or blood meal (only 22% of Leu). Overall, feedstuffs of animal origin (except for gelatin which is abundant in Pro and OH-Pro but deficient in most EAAs) are excellent sources of all AAs for livestock, avian, and aquatic species.

## Determination of Protein Digestibility

### Apparent vs. True Digestibility of Dietary Protein

Since the ileum is the last segment of the small intestine, the content of AAs in dietary protein and in the lumen of the distal ileum is used to determine the digestibility of dietary protein (Moughan and Rutherfurd 2012). However, such values should only be considered as "apparent digestibility." This is due to the large flow of endogenous AAs into the lumen of the small intestine, as shown in growing pigs (Table 7.17) and lactating cows (Table 7.18). The sources of the endogenous AAs include saliva, bile, gastric plus pancreatic plus intestinal secretions, epithelial cells sloughed off the digestive tract, and possibly intestinal bacteria. Sauer and de Lange (1992) reported that endogenous CP in the small intestine of growing pigs fed soybean meal-, canola meal-, wheat-, and barley-based diets was 25.5, 30.5, 27.4, and 27.7 g/kg DM intake, respectively. In all animals, there is usually

**TABLE 7.17**
**Dietary and Endogenous Sources of Nitrogen in the Lumen of The Pig Intestine**[a]

| Source | Amount of N (mg/kg Body Weight) |
|---|---|
| Sources of N in the Small Intestine | |
| Diet | 1530 |
| Endogenous source | 500 |
| Saliva | 14 |
| Stomach | 180 |
| Bile | 50 |
| Pancreatic secretions | 56 |
| Small-intestinal secretions | 100 |
| Microorganisms in the lumen | 100 |
| Absorption of N in the small intestine | 1600 |
| Secretions of N into the lumen of the large intestine | 65 |
| Absorption of N in the large intestine | 320 |
| Fecal N excretion | 175 |

*Source:* Data are adapted from Fuller, M.F. and P.J. Reeds. 1998. Nitrogen cycling in the gut. *Annu. Rev. Nutr.* 18:385–411 and Bergen and Wu (2009).

[a] Estimated from the 30–50 kg growing pig consuming an 18%-CP diet.
Dry matter intake is 5.3% of body weight per day.

**TABLE 7.18**
**Dietary and Endogenous Sources of CP in the Lumen of the Small Intestine of The Lactating Cows**

| Source | Amount (kg/Day per Cow) |
|---|---|
| Dietary CP | 2.26 |
| Duodenal CP | 2.58 |
| Endogenous source | 0.41 |
| Net duodenal | 2.17 |
| Apparent ileal digestible CP | 1.84 |
| Endogenous ileal CP | 0.21 |
| (from the undigested endogenous duodenal CP) | (0.105) |
| (from the nonreabsorbed endogenous small intestine) | (0.105) |
| True ileal digestible CP | 1.94 |

*Source:* Lapierre, H. et al. 2006. *J. Dairy Sci.* 89(E. Suppl.):E1–E14.

a net flow of endogenous AAs into the lumen of the ileum, leading to substantial underestimation (up to 30%) of the true digestibility of dietary protein in the small intestine (Reynolds and Kristensen 2008; Sauer et al. 2000). A cornstarch-based nitrogen-free diet is often used to estimate basal endogenous AA flow ($AA_{EIb}$) in the small intestine of nonruminants, but such a technique is not applicable to ruminants because ruminal fermentation capacity would be greatly inhibited. Rather, labeled AAs (e.g., $^{15}$N-Phe and $^{15}$N-Lys) are often used to determine endogenous AA flow in the small intestine of ruminants (e.g., sheep and cattle).

1. When all digesta are collected at the terminal ileum, the apparent or true ileal digestibility of an AA can be calculated as follows (Knabe et al. 1989; Liao et al. 2005):

$$\text{Apparent ileal digestibility of AA} = \frac{\text{AA intake (g)} - \text{AA in ileal digesta (g)}}{\text{AA intake (g)}}$$

$$= 1 - \frac{\text{AA in ileal digesta (g)}}{\text{AA intake (g)}}$$

$$\text{True ileal digestibility of AA} = \frac{\text{AA intake (g)} - [\text{AA in ileal digesta (g)} - \text{AA}_{\text{EI}}\text{ (g)}]}{\text{AA intake (g)}}$$

$$= \text{Apparent ileal digestibility of AA} + \frac{\text{AA}_{\text{EI}}\text{ (g)}}{\text{AA intake (g)}}$$

$AA_{EI}$ is the total flow of the endogenous AA into the lumen of the ileum (i.e., total amount of the endogenous AA present in ileal digesta), expressed as g. $AA_{EI}$ can be measured using an $^{15}$N-labeled AA (e.g., $^{15}$N-Leu) or homoarginine (Yin et al. 2015). When $AA_{EIb}$ is measured, instead of $AA_{EI}$, the value is called standardized ileal digestibility (SID).

2. When an indigestible marker (e.g., 0.3% $Cr_2O_3$) is added to the diet to eliminate the need for total collection of ileal digesta (Mavromichalis et al. 2001), the apparent or true ileal digestibility of an AA can be calculated as follows, with all the measured variables being expressed as g/kg DM. Note that the term "Indicator content in diet/Indicator content in ileal digesta" is used to correct for the rate of recovery of $Cr_2O_3$ from the ileal digesta.

$$\text{Apparent ileal digestibility of AA} = \frac{\text{AA content in diet} - \text{AA content in ileal digesta} \times \dfrac{\text{Indicator content in diet}}{\text{Indicator content in ileal digesta}}}{\text{AA content in diet}}$$

$$= 1 - \frac{\text{AA content in ileal digesta}}{\text{AA content in diet}} \times \frac{\text{Indicator content in diet}}{\text{Indicator content in ileal digesta}}$$

$$\text{True ileal digestibility of AA} = \frac{\text{AA content in diet} - \left(\text{AA content in ileal digesta} - AA_{EI}\right)}{\text{AA content in diet}} \times \frac{\text{Indicator content in diet}}{\text{Indicator content in ileal digesta}}$$

$$= \text{Apparent ileal digestibility of AA} + \frac{AA_{EI}}{\text{AA content in diet}} \times \frac{\text{Indicator content in diet}}{\text{Indicator content in ileal digesta}}$$

$AA_{EI}$ is the total flow of the endogenous AA into the lumen of the ileum (i.e., total amount of the endogenous AA present in ileal digesta), expressed as g/kg diet DM.

### Measurement of $AA_{EIb}$ in the Small Intestine with the Use of an Indicator Technique

When an indigestible marker (e.g., 0.3% $Cr_2O_3$) is added to a cornstarch-based N-free diet, $AA_{EIb}$ in the small intestine of an animal can be measured. All the measured variables are expressed as g/kg DM. Accordingly, the unit of $AA_{EIb}$ is g/kg DM.

$$AA_{EIb} = \text{Endogenous AA in ileal digesta} \times \frac{\text{Indicator content in diet}}{\text{Indicator content in ileal digesta}}$$

### Measurement of Protein Digestibility of a Feed Ingredient Added to a Basal Diet

If it is desirable to measure protein digestibility of a feed ingredient added to a basal diet, the principles of the calculations of protein digestibility are the same as those for the basal diet, except that changes in ileal AA content due to the added test ingredient should be accounted for.

1. When all digesta are collected at the terminal ileum, the formula for calculating the apparent or true digestibility of a protein-bound AA in the test ingredient is as follows:

$$\text{Apparent ileal digestibility of AA} = \frac{\text{AA intake from test ingredient (g)} - [\text{AA in ileal digesta}_{\text{Basal+Test}} \text{ minus AA in ileal digesta}_{\text{Basal}} \text{(g)}]}{\text{AA intake from test ingredient (g)}}$$

$$\text{True ileal digestibility of AA} = \text{Apparent ileal digestibility of AA} + \frac{AA_{EI} \text{ resulting from test ingredient (g)}}{\text{AA intake from test ingredient (g)}}$$

AA in ileal $\text{digesta}_{\text{Basal+Test}}$ is the amount of AA in the ileal digesta of the animal fed the basal diet plus test ingredient, and AA in ileal $\text{digesta}_{\text{Basal}}$ is the amount of AA in the ileal digesta of the animal fed the basal diet.

2. When an indigestible marker (e.g., 0.3% $Cr_2O_3$) is added to the diet to eliminate the need for total collection of ileal digesta, the apparent or true ileal digestibility of an AA can be calculated as follows, with all the measured variables being expressed as g/kg DM.

$$\text{Apparent ileal digestibility of AA} = 1 - \frac{[\text{AA content in ileal digesta}_{\text{Basal+Test}} \text{ minus AA content in ileal digesta}_{\text{Basal}}]}{\text{AA content in test ingredient}} \times \frac{\text{Indicator content in diet}}{\text{Indicator content in ileal digesta}}$$

$$\text{True ileal digestibility of AA} = \begin{matrix}\text{Apparent ileal} \\ \text{digestibility of AA}\end{matrix} + \frac{\text{AA}_{\text{EI}} \text{ resulting from test ingredient}}{\text{AA intake from test ingredient}} \times \frac{\text{Indicator content in diet}}{\text{Indicator content in ileal digesta}}$$

AA in ileal $\text{digesta}_{\text{Basal + Test}}$ is AA content in the ileal digesta of the animal fed the basal diet plus test ingredient, whereas AA in ileal $\text{digesta}_{\text{Basal}}$ is AA content in the ileal digesta of the animal fed the basal diet.

### Animal Feeding Experiments to Determine the Quality of Dietary Protein

The quality of dietary protein is best evaluated by determining its bioavailability to animals (Table 7.19). The test animals are usually chicks and rats based on practical convenience and low costs. Ideally, this is performed using multiple levels of a test protein in the diet that provides adequate caloric intake. Traditional concepts for protein utilization include: (1) protein digestibility, which is

**TABLE 7.19**
**Evaluation of Dietary Protein Quality for Animals**

| Method | Equation |
|---|---|
| | **Chemical Analysis** |
| Chemical score | For example, Lys/$\text{Lys}_{\text{egg}}$ or Met/$\text{Met}_{\text{egg}}$, with the lowest ratio being the chemical score |
| EAA index | Geometric mean of ratios of EAAs in a test protein to those in a reference protein |
| Dye-binding | Reaction of Lys ε-$NH_2$ in protein with fluoro-2,4-dinitrobenzene |
| Mutual AA ratios | Retaining EAAs whose ratios in the test protein are similar to those in a reference protein |
| | **Animal Experiments** |
| Biological value | = [NI − (FN − MFN) − (UN − EUN)] ÷ [NI − (FN − MFN)] × 100 |
| Protein efficiency ratio | = weight gain/total protein intake |
| Net protein ratio | = (weight gain [test diet] + weight loss [N-free diet])÷total protein intake (test diet) |
| Relative N utilization | = (weight gain [test diet] + 0.1 [initial + final weight])÷total N intake |
| Net protein utilization | = [NI − (FN − MFN) − (UN − EUN)]÷NI × 100 |
| Nitrogen growth index | = slope of the regression of weight gain (Y-axis) on N intake (X-axis) |

EUN, Endogenous urinary N; FN, Fecal N; MFN, Metabolic fecal N; NI, Dietary N intake; FN − MFN, Amount of N from the diet that is excreted in the feces; UN − EUN, Amount of N from the diet that is excreted in the urine; NI − (FN − MFN) − (UN − EUN), Amount of dietary N retained by a test animal; NI − (FN − MFN), Amount of dietary N that is absorbed by a test animal.

a measure of the dietary AA that is made available to the animal after digestion and absorption; and (2) biological value, which is a measure of how efficiently the absorbed AA is utilized to synthesize proteins in the animal. Overall protein utilization, as indicated by net protein utilization, reflects both protein digestibility and biological value. This method has been most widely used in animal growth studies involving the utilization of dietary protein that can be either in a fixed amount or at varying levels in the diet. Thus, feeding experiments can give meaningful information on the availability of dietary AAs to animals. Such studies normally involve small animals such as rats and chicks because of both practical convenience and low costs.

The methods to evaluate the quality of dietary protein include: (a) biological value (the fraction of absorbed N retained in the body for maintenance and growth of the animal); (b) protein efficiency ratio (the gain in body weight per gram of dietary protein or N consumed); (c) net protein ratio (similar to the protein efficiency ratio method but with the consideration of maintenance requirement by the animal); (d) net protein utilization (similar to the biological value method but with the use of dietary N absorbed by the test animal rather than total N intake); (e) slope ratio (also called the nitrogen growth index), (i.e., the slope of the regression of weight gain [Y-axis] on dietary N intake [X-axis]); and (f) relative nitrogen utilization (inclusion of a factor for the protein utilized for maintenance) (Table 7.19). The common weaknesses of these methods are that: (a) the components of weight gains in animals are not known and weight gains may not necessarily result from protein deposition; (b) fecal N and urinary N in animals fed a protein-free diet may not reflect their true endogenous values under normal feeding conditions; and (c) factors that impair the function of the gastrointestinal tract will reduce the utilization of dietary protein independent of its quality (Wu 2013). Thus, test feed-ingredients should be free of anti-nutritional factors, the digestive physiology of animals considered, and protein accretion in test animals measured during the experimental period.

## SUMMARY

AAs are building blocks of protein in feedstuffs and animals. In the stomach of nonruminants, dietary protein is denatured by HCl and then broken down by proteases (e.g., pepsins). The stimulatory or inhibitory factors for the control of gastric acid secretion act primarily through affecting the production of gastrin (stimulatory) or somatostatin (inhibitory) in the mucosa of the stomach and duodenum. In ruminants, dietary protein is degraded by microbial proteases, peptidases, and deaminases to generate ammonia and free AAs for microbial protein synthesis in the rumen. Ruminal microbes flow into the abomasum (the true stomach), where their membranes are lyzed by lysozymes to release protein, which then undergoes hydrolysis by proteases. The most common strategy to increase the escape of high-quality dietary protein from the rumen aims at minimizing proteolysis, peptidolysis, and deamination, while maximizing the digestibility of the escaped protein. Optimal protein supply to the host ruminant requires adequate RDP and energy to maximize the capture of dietary OM in microbial protein. In both nonruminants and ruminants, the gastric digesta enters the duodenum, where it is neutralized by pancreatic and duodenal secretions. The terminal digestion of protein and polypeptides occurs primarily in the jejunum under the combined actions of pancreas- and small intestine-derived proteases, as well as oligo-, tri-, and di-peptidases, to release tripeptides and dipeptides (~80%) and free AAs (~20%). Bacteria present in the lumen of the small intestine can degrade large amounts of the protein digestion products. The remaining small peptides and AAs are absorbed into enterocytes of the small intestine by PepT1 and AA transporters, respectively, with the rate of peptide transport being greater than that of free AAs. More than one AA transporter can transport a certain AA, and a group of AAs with similar chemical structures compete for the same transporter. Within the enterocytes of all animals, peptides are hydrolyzed into AAs. Of note, Asp, Glu, and Gln are extensively oxidized as metabolic fuels in the intestinal mucosa of mammals and serve as substrates for Cit and Arg syntheses in the enterocytes of most mammals (e.g., pigs and ruminants). The AAs which are not degraded by the enterocytes are transported through the basolateral membrane into the lamina propria of the small intestine.

The AAs that enter the portal vein participate in interorgan metabolism. BCAAs largely bypass the liver, and are taken up by the skeletal muscle, heart, adipose tissue, mammary gland, and placenta. In the extrahepatic tissues, BCAAs are transaminated to form Glu, which is either amidated with $NH_4^+$ to yield Gln or transaminated with pyruvate (or OAA) to generate Ala (or Asp). Ala and Gln are substrates for hepatic and renal gluconeogenesis, whereas Gln is extracted by the small intestine and kidneys to produce Cit and ammonia, respectively. Cit is also converted into Arg by the kidneys. In animals, AAs are used for the production of peptides, proteins, and low-molecular-weight metabolites (e.g., gaseous signaling molecules, neurotransmitters, and antioxidant small peptides). Intracellular protein undergoes continuous synthesis and degradation in an energy-dependent manner to constitute protein turnover, which regulates protein deposition, cell growth, removal of oxidized protein, and whole-body homeostasis. As components of this metabolic cycle, AAs are catabolized and synthesized via compartment-, cell-, and tissue-specific reactions. Some AAs or their metabolites activate cell signaling pathways to regulate nutrient metabolism and, therefore, the accretion of protein, fat, and glycogen in the body; these AAs are called functional AAs. The ammonia generated from AA catabolism is detoxified primarily as urea in the liver of mammals and as uric acid in birds, and is directly released by most fish into their living environment. In post-weaning mammals, enterocytes are also capable of ureagenesis as the first line of defense against dietary and gut-derived ammonia. Although animals can synthesize many AAs from the traditionally classified EAAs, these pathways cannot provide sufficient AASAs for maximal survival, growth, fertility, or lactation in farm animals. Thus, livestock, poultry, and fish have dietary requirements for both EAAs and AASAs, namely, all proteinogenic AAs. It is not optimal to consider only EAAs or the "ideal protein concept" in formulating animal diets. This is a new paradigm shift in our knowledge of AA nutrition. To meet animal needs, diets must provide adequate amounts of AAs in proper proportions. The quality of dietary protein is assessed by both quantifying its AA composition and determining its ability to support the growth of young animals (e.g., chicks, rats, and piglets). Optimizing AA nutrition through dietary supplementation with high-quality protein or AAs is an efficient and feasible way to enhance the yields and efficiency of livestock, poultry, and fish production, while ensuring the optimal health of animals and reducing the generation of animal wastes on farms.

## REFERENCES


Agricultural Research Council (United Kingdom) 1981. *The Nutrient Requirements of Pigs: Technical Review. Commonwealth Agricultural Bureaux*, Slough, U.K.

Austic, R.E. 1985. Development and adaptation of protein digestion. *J. Nutr.* 115:5686–5697.

Averill, B.A. 1996. Dissimilatory nitrite and nitric oxide reductases. *Chem. Rev.* 96:2951–2964.

Baracos, V.E., W.T. Whitmore, and R. Gale. 1987. The metabolic cost of fever. *Can. J. Physiol. Pharmacol.* 65:1248–1254.

Baragi, V. and R.T. Lovell. 1986. Digestive enzyme activities in striped bass from first feeding through larva development. *Trans. Am. Fish. Soc.* 115:478–484.

Baker, D.H. 1997. Ideal amino acid profiles for swine and poultry and their applications in feed formulation. *BioKyowa Tech. Rev.* 9:1–24.

Baker, D.H. 2000. Recent advances in use of the ideal protein concept for swine feed formulation. *Asian-Aust. J. Anim. Sci.* 13:294–301.

Baker, D.H. 2005. Comparative nutrition and metabolism: Explication of open questions with emphasis on protein and amino acids. *Proc. Natl. Acad. Sci. USA.* 102:17897–17902.

Baker, D.H. 2009. Advances in protein-amino acid nutrition of poultry. *Amino Acids* 37:29–41.

Baker, D.H. and Y. Han. 1994. Ideal amino acid profile for broiler chicks during the first three weeks post-hatching. *Poult. Sci.* 73:1441–1447.

Baker, D.H., M. Sugahara, and H.M. Scott. 1968. The glycine-serine interrelationship in chick nutrition. *Poult. Sci.* 47:1376–1377.

Ball, R.O., J.L. Atkinson, and H.S. Bayley. 1986. Proline as an essential amino acid for the young pig. *Br. J. Nutr.* 55:659–668.

Baracos, V., R.E. Greenberg, and A.L. Goldberg. 1986. Influence of calcium and other divalent cations on protein turnover in rat skeletal muscle. *Am. J. Physiol.* 250:E702–710.

Barrett, K.E. 2014. *Gastrointestinal Physiology*. McGraw Hill, New York.

Bazer, F.W., G. Wu, G.A. Johnson, and X.Q. Wang. 2014. Environmental factors affecting pregnancy: Endocrine disrupters, nutrients and metabolic pathways. *Mol. Cell. Endocrinol.* 398:53–68.

Bazer, F.W., W. Ying, X.Q. Wang, K.A. Dunlap, B.Y. Zhou, G.A. Johnson, and G. Wu. 2015. The many faces of interferon tau. *Amino Acids* 47:449–460.

Benevenga, N.J. and K.P. Blemings. 2007. Unique aspects of lysine nutrition and metabolism. *J. Nutr.* 137:1610S–1615S.

Bergen, W.G. 2008. Measuring in vivo intracellular protein degradation rates in animal systems. *J. Anim. Sci.* 86 (Suppl. 14):E3–E12.

Bergen, W.G. 2015. Small-intestinal or colonic microbiota as a potential amino acid source in animals. *Amino Acids* 47:251–258.

Bergen, W.G. and D.B. Bates. 1984. Ionophores: Their effect on production efficiency and mode of action. *J. Anim. Sci* 58:1465–1483.

Bergen, W.G., D.R. Mulvaney, D.M. Skjaerlund, S.E. Johnson, and R.A. Merkel. 1987. In vivo and *in vitro* measurements of protein turnover. *J. Anim. Sci.* 65(Suppl. 2):88–106.

Bergen, W.G. and D.B. Purser. 1968. Effect of feeding different protein sources on plasma and gut amino acids in the growing rat. *J Nutr.* 95:333–340.

Bergen, W.G. and G. Wu. 2009. Intestinal nitrogen recycling and utilization in health and disease. *J. Nutr.* 139:821–825.

Bergen, W.G., D.B. Purser, and J.H. Cline. 1968a. Effect of ration on the nutritive quality of rumen microbial protein. *J. Anim. Sci.* 27:1497–1501.

Bergen, W.G., D.B. Purser, and J.H. Cline. 1968b. Determination of limiting amino acids of rumen-isolated microbial proteins fed to rat. *J. Dairy Sci.* 51:1698–1700.

Blachier, F., A.M. Davila, R. Benamouzig, and D. Tome. 2011. Channelling of arginine in NO and polyamine pathways in colonocytes and consequences. *Front. Biosci.* 16:1331–1343.

Brinkhuis, J. and T.A. Payens. 1985. The rennet-induced clotting of para-kappa-casein revisited: Inhibition experiments with pepstatin A. *Biochim. Biophys. Acta* 832:331–336.

Brock, F.M., C.W. Forsberg, and J.G. Buchanan-Smith. 1982. Proteolytic activity of rumen microorganisms and effects of proteinase inhibitors. *Appl. Environ. Microbiol.* 44:561–569.

Broderick, G.A. and W.J. Radloff. 2004. Effect of molasses supplementation on the production of lactating dairy cows fed diets based on alfalfa and corn silage. *J. Dairy Sci.* 87:2997–3009.

Broderick, G.A., R.J. Wallace, and E.R. Ørskov. 1991. Control of rate and extent of protein degradation. In: *Physiological Aspects of Digestion and Metabolism in Ruminants.* Edited by T. Tsuda and Y. Sasaki. Academic Press, Orlando, Florida, pp. 541–592.

Bröer, S. and M. Palacín. 2011. The role of amino acid transporters in inherited and acquired diseases. *Biochem. J.* 436:193–211.

Brosnan, J.T. and M.E. Brosnan. 2006. Branched-chain amino acids: Enzyme and substrate regulation. *J. Nutr.* 136:207S–211S.

Burrin, D.G. and T.A. Davis. 2004. Proteins and amino acids in enteral nutrition. *Curr. Opin. Clin. Nutr. Metab. Care* 7:79–87.

Bush, J.A., G. Wu, A. Suryawan, H.V. Nguyen, and T.A. Davis. 2002. Somatotropin-induced amino acid conservation in pigs involves differential regulation of liver and gut urea cycle enzyme activity. *J. Nutr.* 132:59–67.

Buttery, P.J. 1983. Hormonal control of protein deposition in animals. *Proc. Nutr. Soc.* 42:137–148.

Chalupa, W. and C.J. Sniffen. 1994. Carbohydrate, protein and amino acid nutrition of dairy cows. In: *Recent Advances in Animal Nutrition.* Edited by P.C. Garnsworthy and D.J.A. Cole. University of Nottingham Press, Nottingham, pp. 265–275.

Chamberlain, D.G., P.C. Thomas, and J. Quig. 1986. Utilization of silage nitrogen in sheep and cows: Amino acid composition of duodenal digesta and rumen microbes. *Grass Forage Sci.* 41:31–38.

Chelikani, P.K., D.R. Glimm, D.H. Keisler, and J.J. Kennelly. 2004. Effects of feeding or abomasal infusion of canola oil in Holstein cows. 2. Gene expression and plasma concentrations of cholecystokinin and leptin. *J. Dairy Res.* 71:288–296.

Chen, L.X., P. Li, J.J. Wang, X.L. Li, H.J. Gao, Y.L. Yin, Y.Q. Hou, and G. Wu. 2009. Catabolism of nutritionally essential amino acids in developing porcine enterocytes. *Amino Acids* 37:143–152.

Chen, L.X., Y.L. Yin, W.S. Jobgen, S.C. Jobgen, D.A. Knabe, W.X. Hu, and G. Wu. 2007. In vitro oxidation of essential amino acids by intestinal mucosal cells of growing pigs. *Livest. Sci.* 109:19–23.

Chiba, L.I., A.J. Lewis, and E.R. Peo Jr. 1991. Amino acid and energy interrelationships in pigs weighing 20 to 50 kilograms: I. Rate and efficiency of weight gain. *J. Anim. Sci.* 69:694–707.

Chung, T.K. and D.H. Baker. 1992. Ideal amino acid pattern for ten kilogram pigs. *J. Anim. Sci.* 70:3102–3111.

Ciechanover, A. 2012. Intracellular protein degradation: From a vague idea thru the lysosome and the ubiquitin-proteasome system and onto human diseases and drug targeting. *Biochim. Biophys. Acta* 1824:3–13.

Cole, D.J.A. 1980. The amino acid requirements of pigs: The concept of an ideal protein. *Pig News Info.* 1:201–205.

Columbus, D.A., J. Steinhoff-Wagner, A. Suryawan, H.V. Nguyen, A. Hernandez-Garcia, M.L. Fiorotto, and T.A. Davis. 2015. Impact of prolonged leucine supplementation on protein synthesis and lean growth in neonatal pigs. *Am. J. Physiol.* 309:E601–E610.

Colvin, B.M. and H.A. Ramsey. 1968. Soy flour in milk replacers for young calves. *J. Dairy Sci.* 51:898–904.

Cranwell, P.D. 1995. Development of the neonatal gut and enzyme systems. In: *The Neonatal Pig: Development and Survival.* Edited by M.A. Varley. CAB International, Wallingford, Oxon, U.K, pp. 99–154.

Daenzer, M., K.J. Petzke, B.J. Bequette, and C.C. Metges. 2001. Whole-body nitrogen and splanchnic amino acid metabolism differ in rats fed mixed diets containing casein or its corresponding amino acid mixture. *J. Nutr.* 131:1965–1972.

Dai, Z.L., Z.L. Wu, S.Q. Hang, W.Y. Zhu, and G. Wu. 2015. Amino acid metabolism in intestinal bacteria and its potential implications for mammalian reproduction. *Mol. Hum. Reprod.* 21:389–409.

Dai, Z.L., G. Wu, and W.Y. Zhu. 2011. Amino acid metabolism in intestinal bacteria: Links between gut ecology and host health. *Front. Biosci.* 16:1768–1786.

Dai, Z.L., J. Zhang, G. Wu, and W.Y. Zhu. 2010. Utilization of amino acids by bacteria from the pig small intestine. *Amino Acids* 39:1201–1215.

Davis, A.J. and R.E. Austic. 1997. Dietary protein and amino acid levels alter threonine dehydrogenase activity in hepatic mitochondria of Gallus domesticus. *J. Nutr.* 127:738–744.

Davis, T.A., J.A. Bush, R.C. Vann, A. Suryawan, S.R. Kimball, and D.G. Burrin. 2004. Somatotropin regulation of protein metabolism in pigs. *J. Anim. Sci.* 82(E-Suppl.):E207–E213.

Davis, T.A. and P.J. Reeds. 2001. Of flux and flooding: The advantages and problems of different isotopic methods for quantifying protein turnover *in vivo*: II. Methods based on the incorporation of a tracer. *Curr. Opin. Clin. Nutr. Metab. Care.* 4:51–56.

Debray, L., I. Le Huerou-Luron, T. Gidenne, and L. Fortun-Lamothe. 2003. Digestive tract development in rabbit according to the dietary energetic source: Correlation between whole tract digestion, pancreatic and intestinal enzymatic activities. *Comp. Biochem. Physiol. A* 135:443–455.

Dhanakoti, S.N., J.T. Brosnan, M.E. Brosnan, and G.R. Herzberg. 1992. Net renal arginine flux in rats is not affected by dietary arginine or dietary protein intake. *J. Nutr.* 122:1127–1134.

Dillon, E.L., D.A. Knabe, and G. Wu. 1999. Lactate inhibits citrulline and arginine synthesis from proline in pig enterocytes. *Am. J. Physiol. Gastrointest. Liver Physiol.* 276:G1079–G1086.

Dixon, R.M. 2013. Controlling voluntary intake of molasses-based supplements in grazing cattle. *Anim. Prod. Sci.* 53:217–225.

Doepel, C.L., G.E. Lobley, J.F. Bernier, P. Dubreuil, and H. Lapierre. 2007. Effect of glutamine supplementation on splanchnic metabolism in lactating dairy cows. *J. Dairy Sci.* 90:4325–4333.

Dorward, D.A., C.D. Lucas, G.B. Chapman, C. Haslett, K. Dhaliwal, and A.G. Rossi. 2015. The role of formylated peptides and formyl peptide receptor 1 in gverning neutrophil function during acute inflammation. *Am. J. Pathol.* 185:1172–1184.

Elango, R., R.O. Ball, and P.B. Pencharz. 2012. Recent advances in determining protein and amino acid requirements in humans. *Br. J. Nutr.* 108(Suppl. 2):S22–S30.

Emery, R.S. 1978. Feeding for increased milk protein. *J. Dairy Sci.* 61:825–828.

Ewaschuk, J.B., G.K. Murdoch, I.R. Johnson, K.L. Madsen, and C.J. Field. 2011. Glutamine supplementation improves intestinal barrier function in a weaned piglet model of *Escherichia coli* infection. *Br. J. Nutr.* 106:870–877.

Faichney G.J., C. Poncet, B. Lassalas, J.P. Jouany, L. Millet, J. Doré, and A.G. Brownlee. 1997. Effect of concentrates in a hay diet on the contribution of anaerobic fungi, protozoa and bacteria to nitrogen in rumen and duodenal digesta in sheep. *Anim. Feed Sci. Technol.* 64:193–213.

FAO (Food and Agriculture Organizations of the United Nations) 2013. *Dietary Protein Quality Evaluation in Human Nutrition.* Rome, Italy.

Fellner, V. 2002. Rumen microbes and nutrient management. *Proceedings of American Registry of Professional Animal Scientists—California Chapter Conference*, October, 2002, Coalinga, CA.

Ffoulkes, D. and R.A. Leng. 1988. Dynamics of protozoa in the rumen of cattle. *Br. J. Nutr.* 59:429–436.

Field, C.J., I.R. Johnson, and P.D. Schley. 2002. Nutrients and their role in host resistance to infection. *J. Leukoc. Biol.* 71:16–32.
Firkins, J.L. and Z. Yu. 2015. How to use data on the rumen microbiome to improve our understanding of ruminant nutrition. *J. Anim. Sci.* 93:1450–1470.
Firkins, J.L., Z. Yu, and M. Morrison. 2007. Ruminal nitrogen metabolism: Perspectives for integration of microbiology and nutrition for dairy. *J. Dairy Sci.* 90(E. Suppl.):E1–E16.
Fisher, H. and H.M. Scott. 1954. The essential amino acid requirements of chicks as related to their proportional occurrence in the fat-free carcass. *Arch. Biochem. Biophys.* 51:517–519.
Flores, D.A., L.E. Phillip, D.M. Veira, and M. Ivan. 1986. Digestion in the rumen and amino acid supply to the duodenum of sheep fed ensiled and fresh alfalfa. *Can. J. Anim. Sci.* 66:1019–1027.
Flynn, N.E., J.G. Bird, and A.S. Guthrie. 2009. Glucocorticoid regulation of amino acid and polyamine metabolism in the small intestine. *Amino Acids* 37:123–129.
Fuller, M.F. and P.J. Reeds. 1998. Nitrogen cycling in the gut. *Annu. Rev. Nutr.* 18:385–411.
Gabaudan, J. 1984. Posthatching morphogenesis of the digestive system of striped bass. *Ph.D. Dissertation*, Auburn University, Auburn, Alabama.
García-Gasca, A., M.A. Galaviz, J.N. Gutiérrez, and A. García-Ortega. 2006. Development of the digestive tract, trypsin activity and gene expression in eggs and larvae of the bullseye puffer fish *Sphoeroides annulatus*. *Aquaculture* 251:366–376.
Gerrits, W.J.J., J. Dijkstra, and J. France. 1997. Description of a model integrating protein and energy metabolism in preruminant calves. *J. Nutr.* 127:1229–1242.
Ghorbani, G.R. 2012. *Dynamics of Protein Metabolism in the Ruminant.* http://www.freepptdb.com/details-dynamics-of-protein-metabolism-in-the-ruminant. Accessed on January 16, 2017.
Gilbert, E.R., E.A. Wong, and K.E. Webb, Jr. 2008. Peptide absorption and utilization: Implications for animal nutrition and health. *J. Anim Sci.* 86:2135–2155.
Giuffrida, P., P. Biancheri, and T.T. MacDonald. 2014. Proteases and small intestinal barrier function in health and disease. *Curr. Opin. Gastroenterol.* 30:147–153.
Goldberg, A.L. 2003. Protein degradation and protection against misfolded or damaged proteins. *Nature* 426:895–899.
Goll, D.E., G. Neti, S.W. Mares, and V.F. Thompson. 2008. Myofibrillar protein turnover: The proteasome and the calpains. *J. Anim. Sci.* 86(14 Suppl.):E19–E35.
Graber, G. and D.H. Baker. 1973. The essential nature of glycine and proline for growing chickens. *Poul. Sci.* 52:892–896.
Gruninger, R.J., A.K. Puniya, T.M. Callaghan, J.E. Edwards, N. Youssef, S.S. Dagar, K. Fliegerova et al. 2014. Anaerobic fungi (phylum Neocallimastigomycota): Advances in understanding their taxonomy, life cycle, ecology, role and biotechnological potential. *FEMS Microbiol. Ecol.* 90:1–17.
Hanigan, M.D., J.P. Cant, D.C. Weakley, and J.L. Beckett. 1998. An evaluation of postabsorptive protein and amino acid metabolism in the lactating dairy cow. *J. Dairy Sci.* 81:3385–3401.
Harper, A.E., R.H. Miller, and K.P. Block. 1984. Branched-chain amino acid metabolism. *Annu. Rev. Nutr.* 4:409–454.
Haüssinger, D. 1990. Nitrogen metabolism in liver: Structural and functional organization and physiological significance. *Biochem. J.* 267:281–290.
Hendriks, W.H., J. van Baal, and G. Bosch. 2012. Ileal and faecal protein digestibility measurement in humans and other non-ruminants—A comparative species view. *Br. J. Nutr.* 108(Suppl. 2):S247–S257.
Higgins, C.F. and M.M. Gibson. 1986. Peptide transport in bacteria. *Methods Enzymol.* 125:365–377.
Hook, S.E., J. Dijkstra, A.D.G. Wright, B.W. McBride, and J. France. 2012. Modeling the distribution of ciliate protozoa in the reticulo-rumen using linear programming. *J. Dairy Sci.* 95, 255–265.
Hou, Y.Q. and G. Wu. 2017. Nutritionally nonessential amino acids: A misnomer in nutritional sciences. *Adv. Nutr.* 8:137–139.
Hou, Y.Q., K. Yao, Y.L. Yin, and G. Wu. 2016. Endogenous synthesis of amino acids limits growth, lactation and reproduction of animals. *Adv. Nutr.* 7:331–342.
Hou, Y.Q., Y.L. Yin, and G. Wu. 2015. Dietary essentiality of "nutritionally nonessential amino acids" for animals and humans. *Exp. Biol. Med.* 240:997–1007.
Hristov, A.N., J.K. Ropp, K.L. Grandeen, S. Abedi, R.P. Etter, A. Melgar, and A.E. Foley. 2005. Effect of carbohydrate source on ammonia utilization in lactating dairy cows. *J. Anim. Sci.* 83:408–421.
Huang, Y.F., Y. Wang, and M. Watford. 2007. Glutamine directly downregulates glutamine synthetase protein levels in mouse $C_2C_{12}$ skeletal muscle myotubes. *J. Nutr.* 137:1357–1361.
Hungate, R.E. 1966. *The Rumen and Its Microbes.* Academic Press, New York.

Hyde, R., P.M. Taylor, and H.S. Hundal. 2003. Amino acid transporters: Roles in amino acid sensing and signalling in animal cells. *Biochem. J.* 373:1–18.

Irie, M., T. Terada, M. Okuda, and K. Inui. 2004. Efflux properties of basolateral peptide transporter in human intestinal cell line Caco-2. *Pflugers Arch.* 449:186–194.

Irwin, D.M. 1995. Evolution of the bovine lysozyme gene family: Changes in gene expression and reversion of function. *J. Mol. Evol.* 41:299–312.

Irwin, D.M. and A.C. Wilson. 1990. Concerted evolution of ruminant stomach lysozymes. Characterization of lysozyme cDNA clones from sheep and deer. *J. Biol. Chem.* 265:4944–4952.

Jois, M., B. Hall, K. Fewer, and J.T. Brosnan. 1989. Regulation of hepatic glycine catabolism by glucagon. *J. Biol. Chem.* 264:3347–3351.

Jouany, J.P. 1996. Effect of rumen protozoa on nitrogen utilization by ruminants. *J. Nutr.* 126:1335S–1346S.

Kertz, A.F. 2010. Urea feeding to dairy cattle: A historical perspective and review. *Prof. Anim. Sci.* 26:257–272.

Kim, S.W., D.H. Baker, and R.A. Easter. 2001. Dynamic ideal protein and limiting amino acids for lactating sows: The impact of amino acid mobilization. *J. Anim. Sci.* 79:2356–2366.

Kim, S.W. and G. Wu. 2004. Dietary arginine supplementation enhances the growth of milk-fed young pigs. *J. Nutr.* 134:625–630.

Kim, S.W., G. Wu, and D.H. Baker. 2005. Ideal protein and amino acid requirements by gestating and lactating sows. *Pig News Inform.* 26:89N–99N.

Klain, G.J., H.M. Scott, and B.C. Johnson. 1960. The amino acid requirements of the growing chick fed a crystalline amino acid diet. *Poult. Sci.* 39:39–44.

Klasing, K.C., C.C. Calvert, and V.L. Jarrell. 1987. Growth characteristics, protein synthesis, and protein degradation in muscles from fast and slow-growing chickens. *Poult. Sci.* 66:1189–1196.

Knabe, D.A., D.C. LaRue, E.J. Gregg, G.M. Martinez, and T.D. Tanksley, Jr. 1989. Apparent digestibility of nitrogen and amino acids in protein feedstuffs by growing pigs. *J. Anim. Sci.* 67:441–458.

Koeln, L.L., T.G. Schlagheck, and K.E. Webb Jr. 1993. Amino acid flux across the gastrointestinal tract and liver of calves. *J. Dairy Sci.* 76:2275–2285.

Kong, J. and P. Lasko. 2012. Translational control in cellular and developmental processes. *Nature Rev. Genet.* 13:383–394.

Krebs, H. 1972. Some aspects of the regulation of fuel supply in omnivorous animals. *Adv. Enzyme Regul.* 10:397–420.

Kristensen, N.B. and G. Wu. 2012. Metabolic functions of the porcine liver. In: *Nutritional Physiology of Pigs*. Edited by K.E. Bach, N.J. Knudsen, H.D. Kjeldsen, and B.B. Jensen. Danish Pig Research Center, Copenhagen, Denmark, Chapter 13, pp. 1–17.

Kwon, H., G. Wu, F.W. Bazer, and T.E. Spencer. 2003. Developmental changes in polyamine levels and synthesis in the ovine conceptus. *Biol. Reprod.* 69:1626–1634.

Lackner, D.H. and J. Bähler 2008. Translational control of gene expression from transcripts to transcriptomes. *Int. Rev. Cell Mol. Biol.* 271:199–251.

Lam, P. and M.M.M. Kuypers. 2011. Microbial nitrogen cycling processes in oxygen minimum zones. *Annu. Rev. Mar. Sci.* 3:317–345.

Lapierre, H., D. Pacheco, R. Berthiaume, D.R. Ouellet, C.G. Schwab, P. Dubreuil, G. Holtrop, and G.E. Lobley. 2006. What is the true supply of amino acids for a dairy cow? *J. Dairy Sci.* 89(E. Suppl.):E1–E14.

Larsen, M., T.G. Madsen, M.R. Weisbjerg, T. Hvelplund, and J. Madsen. 2001. Small intestinal digestibility of microbial and endogenous amino acids in dairy cows. *J. Anim. Physiol. Anim. Nutr.* 85:9–21.

Laursen, B.S., H.P. Sørensen, K.K. Mortensen, and H.U. Sperling-Petersen. 2005. Initiation of protein synthesis in bacteria. *Microbiol. Mol. Biol. Rev.* 69:101–123.

Lee, C. and K.A. Beauchemin. 2014. A review of feeding supplementary nitrate to ruminant animals: Nitrate toxicity, methane emissions, and production performance. *Can. J. Anim. Sci.* 94:557–570.

Le Floc'h, N., W. Otten, and E. Merlot. 2011. Tryptophan metabolism, from nutrition to potential therapeutic applications. *Amino Acids* 41:1195–1205.

Lei, J., D.Y. Feng, Y.L. Zhang, S. Dahanayaka, X.L. Li, K. Yao, J.J. Wang, Z.L. Wu, Z.L. Dai, and G. Wu. 2013. Hormonal regulation of leucine catabolism in mammary epithelial cells. *Amino Acids* 45:531–541.

Lescoat, P., D. Sauvant, and A. Danfær. 1996. Quantitative aspects of blood and amino acid flows in cattle. *Reprod. Nutr. Dev.* 36:137–174.

Li, M., C. Li, A. Allen, C.A. Stanley, and T.J. Smith. 2012. The structure and allosteric regulation of mammalian glutamate dehydrogenase. *Arch. Biochem. Biophys.* 519:69–80.

Li, P., K.S. Mai, J. Trushenski, and G. Wu. 2009. New developments in fish amino acid nutrition: Towards functional and environmentally oriented aquafeeds. *Amino Acids* 37:43–53.

Li, Y.H., H.K. Wei, F.N. Li, S.W. Kim, C.Y. Wen, Y.H. Duan, Q.P. Guo, W.L. Wang, H.N. Liu, and Y.L. Yin. 2016. Regulation in free amino acid profile and protein synthesis pathway of growing pig skeletal muscles by low-protein diets for different time periods. *J. Anim. Sci.* 94:5192–5205.

Liao, S.F., W.C. Sauer, A.K. Kies, Y.C. Zhang, M. Cervantes, and J.M. He. 2005. Effect of phytase supplementation to diets for weanling pigs on the digestibilities of crude protein, amino acids, and energy. *J. Anim. Sci.* 83:625–633.

Liao, S.F., T. Wang, and N. Regmi. 2015. Lysine nutrition in swine and the related monogastric animals: Muscle protein biosynthesis and beyond. *SpringerPlus* 4:147.

Lin, C., D.C. Mahan, G. Wu and S.W. Kim. 2009. Protein digestibility of porcine colostrum by neonatal pigs. *Livest. Sci.* 121:182–186.

Lund, P. and M. Watford. 1976. Glutamine as a precursor of urea. In: *The Urea Cycle.* Edited by S. Grisolia, R. Baguena, and F. Mayor. John Wiley & Sons, New York, pp. 479–488.

Males, J.R. and D.B. Purser. 1970. Relationship between rumen ammonia levels and the microbial population and volatile fatty acid proportions in faunated and defaunated sheep. *Appl. Microbiol.* 19:483–490.

Manning, K.S. and T.A. Cooper. 2017. The roles of RNA processing in translating genotype to phenotype. *Nat. Rev. Mol. Cell Biol.* 18:102–114.

Matthews, J.C. 2000. Amino acid and peptide transport system. In: *Farm Animal Metabolism and Nutrition.* Edited by J.P.F. D'Mello. CAPI Publishing, Wallingford, Oxon, UK, pp. 3–23.

Mavromichalis, I., T.M. Parr, V.M. Gabert, and D.H. Baker. 2001. True ileal digestibility of amino acids in sow's milk for 17-day-old pigs. *J. Anim. Sci.* 79:707–713.

McAllister, T.A., J.R. Thompson, and S.E. Samuels. 2000. Skeletal and cardiac muscle protein turnover during cold acclimation in young rats. *Am. J. Physiol.* 278:R705–R711.

McDonald, P., R.A. Edwards, J.F.D. Greenhalgh, J.F.D. Greenhalgh, C.A. Morgan, and L.A. Sinclair. 2011. *Animal Nutrition*, 7th ed. Prentice Hall, New York.

McKnight, J.R., M.C. Satterfield, W.S. Jobgen, S.B. Smith, T.E. Spencer, C.J. Meininger, C.J. McNeal, and G. Wu. 2010. Beneficial effects of L-arginine on reducing obesity: Potential mechanisms and important implications for human health. *Amino Acids* 39:349–357.

McLaughlin, J.T., R.B. Lomax, L. Hall, G.J. Dockray, D.G. Thompson, and G. Warhurst. 1998. Fatty acids stimulate cholecystokinin secretion via an acyl chain length-specific, $Ca^{2+}$-dependent mechanism in the enteroendocrine cell line STC-1. *J. Physiol.* 513:11–18.

Michel, V., G. Fonty, L. Millet, F. Bonnemoy, and P. Gouet. 1993. In vitro study of the proteolytic activity of rumen anaerobic fungi. *FEMS Microbiol. Lett.* 110:5–10.

Morris, S.M. Jr. 2002. Regulation of enzymes of the urea cycle and arginine metabolism. *Annu. Rev. Nutr.* 22:87–105.

Moss, A.R., J.-P. Jouany, and J. Newbold. 2000. Methane production by ruminants: Its contribution to global warming. *Ann. Zootech.* 49:231–253.

Moughan, P.J. and S.M. Rutherfurd. 2012. Gut luminal endogenous protein: implications for the determination of ileal amino acid digestibility in humans. *Br. J .Nutr.* 108 (Suppl. 2):S258–263.

Moughan, P.J., V. Ravindran, and J.O.B. Sorbara. 2014. Dietary protein and amino acids—Consideration of the undigestible fraction. *Poult. Sci.* 93:2400–2410.

Nagaraja, T.G. 2016. Microbiology of the rumen. In: *Rumenology.* Edited by D.D. Millen, M.D.B. Arrigoni, and R.D.L. Pacheco, Springer, New York, NY, pp. 39–61.

National Research Council (NRC) 1994. *Nutrient Requirements of Poultry.* National Academy Press, Washington, DC.

National Research Council (NRC) 1998. *Nutrient Requirements of Swine.* National Academy Press, Washington, DC.

National Research Council (NRC) 2001. *Nutrient Requirements of Dairy Cattle.* National Academy Press, Washington, DC.

National Research Council (NRC) 2011. *Nutrient Requirements of Fish and Shrimp.* National Academy Press, Washington, D.C.

National Research Council (NRC) 2017. http://www.nationalacademies.org/nrc/. Accessed on June 1, 2017.

Naylor, J.M., T. Leibel, and D.M. Middleton. 1997. Effect of glutamine or glycine containing oral electrolyte solutions on mucosal morphology, clinical and biochemical findings, in calves with viral induced diarrhea. *Can. J.Vet. Res.* 61:43–48.

Nir, I., Z. Nitsan, and M. Mahagna, 1993. Comparative growth and development of the digestive organs and of some enzymes in broiler and egg type chicks after hatching. *Br. Poult. Sci.* 34:523–532.

Nitzan, Z., E.A. Dunnington, and P.B. Siegel. 1991. Organ growth and digestive enzyme levels to fifteen days of age in lines of chickens differing in body weight. *Poult. Sci.* 70:2040–2048.

Noy, Y. and D. Sklan. 1995. Digestion and absorption in the young chick. *Poult. Sci.* 74:366–373.

Officer, D.I., E.S., Batterham, and D.J. Farrel. 1997. Comparison of growth performance and nutrient retention of weaner pigs given diets based on casein, free amino acids or conventional proteins. *Br. J. Nutr.* 77:731–744.

Orellana, R.A., F.A. Wilson, M.C. Gazzaneo, A. Suryawan, T.A. Davis, and H.V. Nguyen. 2011. Sepsis and development impede muscle protein synthesis in neonatal pigs by different ribosomal mechanisms. *Pediatr. Res.* 69:473–478.

Owsley, W.F., D.E. Orr, Jr., and L.F. Tribble. 1986. Effects of age and diet on the development of the pancreas and the synthesis and secretion of pancreatic enzymes in the young pig. *J. Anim. Sci.* 63:497–504.

Pedersen, B.H., E.M. Nilssen, and K. Hjelmeland. 1987. Variations in the content of trypsin and trypsinogen in larval herring (*Clupea harengus*) digesting copepod nauplii. *Mar. Biol.* 94:171–181.

Peng, X., L. Hu, Y. Liu, C. Yan, Z.F. Fang, Y. Lin, S.Y. Xu et al. 2016. Effects of low-protein diets supplemented with indispensable amino acids on growth performance, intestinal morphology and immunological parameters in 13–35 kg pigs. *Animal* 10:1812–1820.

Porter, J.W.G. 1969. Digestion in the pre-ruminant animal. *Proc. Nutr. Soc.* 28:115–121.

Pun, H.H.L. and L.D. Satter. 1975. Nitrogen fixation in ruminants. *J. Anim. Sci.* 41:1161–1163.

Punia, B.S., J. Leibholz., and G.J. Faichney. 1992. Rate of production of protozoa in the rumen and the flow of protozoal nitrogen to the duodenum in sheep and cattle given a pelleted diet of lucerne hay and barley. *J. Agric. Sci.* 118:229–236.

Rampilli, M., R. Larsen, and M. Harboe. 2004. Natural heterogeneity of chymosin and pepsin in extracts of bovine stomachs. *Int. Dairy J.* 15:1130–1137.

Raufman, J.-P. 1992. Gastric chief cells: Receptors and signal-transduction mechanisms. *Gastroenterology* 102:699–710.

Rawlings, N.D., A.J. Barrett, and A. Bateman. 2012. MEROPS: The database of proteolytic enzymes, their substrates and inhibitors. *Nucleic Acids Res.* 40:D343–D350.

Reeds, P.J. 1989. Reguation of protein turnover. In: *Animal Growth Regulation.* Edited by D.R. Campion, G.J. Hausman, and R.J. Martin. Plenum Publishing Corporation, New York, NY, pp. 183–210.

Reeds, P.J., D.G. Burrin, T.A. Davis, and M.L. Fiorotto. 1993. Postnatal growth of gut and muscle: Competitors or collaborators. *Proc. Nutr. Soc.* 52:57–67.

Reeds, P.J., D.G. Burrin, B. Stoll, and J.B. van Goudoever. 2000. Role of the gut in the amino acid economy of the host. *Nestle Nutr. Workshop Ser. Clin. Perform Programme.* 3:25–40.

Reeds, P.J., A. Cadenhead, M.F. Fuller, G.E. Lobley, and J.D. McDonald. 1980. Protein turnover in growing pigs. Effects of age and food intake. *Br. J. Nutr.* 43:445–455.

Reynolds, C.K. 2006. Splanchnic metabolism of amino acids in ruminants. In: *Ruminant Physiology.* Edited by K. Sejrsen, T. Hvelplund, and M.O. Nielsen. Wageningen Academic Publishers, The Netherlands, Wageningen, pp. 225–248.

Reynolds, C.K. and N.B. Kristensen. 2008. Nitrogen recycling through the gut and the nitrogen economy of ruminants: An asynchronous symbiosis. *J. Anim. Sci.* 86(14 Suppl.):E293–E305.

Rezaei, R., J. Lei, and G. Wu. 2017. Dietary supplementation with *Yucca schidigera* extract alleviates heat stress-induced growth restriction in chickens. *J. Anim. Sci.* 95 (Suppl. 4):370–371.

Ribeiro, F.B., E.A.T. Lanna, M.A.D. Bomfim, J.L. Donzele, M. Quadros, and P.D.S.L. Cunha. 2011. True and apparent digestibility of protein and amino acids of feed in Nile tilapia. *R. Bras. Zootec.* 40:939–946.

Rojas, O.J. and H.H. Stein. 2017. Processing of ingredients and diets and effects on nutritional value for pigs. *J. Anim. Sci. Biotechnol.* 8:48.

Rønnestad, I., M. Yúfera, B. Ueberschär, L. Ribeiro, Ø. Sæle, and C. Boglione. 2013. Feeding behaviour and digestive physiology in larval fish: Current knowledge, and gaps and bottlenecks in research. *Rev. Aquaculture* 5(Suppl. 1):S59–S98.

Russell, J.B., J.D. O'Connor, D.G. Fox, P.J. Van Soest, and C.J. Sniffen. 1992. A net carbohydrate and protein system for evaluating cattle diets: I. Ruminal fermentation. *J. Anim. Sci.* 70:3551–3561.

Salter, D.N., K. Daneshaver, and R.H. Smith. 1979. The origin of nitrogen incorporated into compounds in the rumen bacteria of steers given protein- and urea-containing diets. *Br. J. Nutr.* 41:197–209.

Samuels, S.E. and V.E. Baracos. 1995. Tissue protein turnover is altered during catch-up growth following *Escherichia coli* infection in weanling rats. *J. Nutr.* 125:520–530.

San Gabriel, A. and H. Uneyama. 2013. Amino acid sensing in the gastrointestinal tract. *Amino Acids* 45:451–461.

Sasse, C.E. and D.H. Baker. 1973. Modification of the Illinois reference standard amino acid mixture. *Poult. Sci.* 52:1970–1972.

Sauer, W.C. and K. de Lange. 1992. Novel methods for determining protein and amino acid digestibility values in feedstuffs. In: *Modern Methods in Protein Nutrition and Metabolism.* Edited by S. Nissen. Academic Press, London.

Sauer, W.C., M.Z. Fan, R. Mosenthin, and W. Drochner. 2000. Methods for measuring ileal amino acid digestibility in pigs. In: *Farm Animal Metabolism and Nutrition.* Edited by J.P.F. D'Mello. CAPI Publishing, Wallingford, Oxon, UK, pp. 279–307.

Sauer, W.C. and L. Ozimek. 1986. Digestibility of amino acids in swine—Results and their practical applications—A review. *Livest. Sci. Prod.* 15:367–388.

Shah, B.P., P. Liu, T. Yu, D.R. Hansen, and T.A. Gilbertson. 2012. TRPM5 is critical for linoleic acid-induced CCK secretion from the enteroendocrine cell line, STC-1. *Am. J. Physiol. Cell Physiol.* 302:C210–C219.

Shepherd, E.J., N. Lister, J.A. Affleck, J.R. Bronk, G.L. Kellett, I.D. Collier, P.D. Bailey, and C.A. Boyd. 2002. Identification of a candidate membrane protein for the basolateral peptide transporter of rat small intestine. *Biochem. Biophys. Res. Commun.* 296:918–922.

Sherriff, R.M., M.F. Broom, and V.S. Chadwick. 1992. Isolation and purification of N-formylmethionine aminopeptidase from rat intestine. *Biochim. Biophys. Acta* 1119:275–280.

Singer, M.A. 2003. Do mammals, birds, reptiles and fish have similar nitrogen conserving systems? *Comp. Biochem. Physiol. B.* 134:543–558.

Sok, M., D.R. Ouellet, J.L. Firkins, D. Pellerin, and H. Lapierre. 2017. Amino acid composition of rumen bacteria and protozoa in cattle. *J. Dairy Sci.* 100:1–9.

Southorn, B.G., J.M. Kelly, and B.W. McBride. 1992. Phenylalanine flooding dose procedure is effective in measuring intestinal and liver protein synthesis in sheep. *J. Nutr.* 122:2398–2407.

Southorn, B.G., R.M. Palmer, and P.J. Garlick. 1990. Acute effects of corticosterone on tissue protein synthesis and insulin-sensitivity in rats *in vivo*. *Biochem. J.* 272:187–191.

Spooner, H. 2012. *Protein: An Important Nutrient. Horse Extension Program.* Michigan State University, East Lansing, MI.

Stentoft, C., B.A. Røjen, S.K. Jensen, N.B. Kristensen, M. Vestergaard, and M. Larsen. 2015. Absorption and intermediary metabolism of purines and pyrimidines in lactating dairy cows. *Br. J. Nutr.* 113:560–573.

Stipanuk, MH. 2004. Sulfur amino acid metabolism: Pathways for production and removal of homocysteine and cysteine. *Annu. Rev. Nutr.* 24:539–577.

Stoll, B. and D.G. Burrin. 2006. Measuring splanchnic amino acid metabolism *in vivo* using stable isotopic tracers. *J. Anim. Sci.* 84(Suppl.):E60–E72.

Storm, E. and E.R. Orskov. 1983. The nutritive value of rumen microorganisms in ruminants. *Br. J. Nutr.* 50:463–470.

Sun, K.J., Z.L. Wu, Y. Ji, and G. Wu. 2016. Glycine regulates protein turnover by activating Akt/mTOR and inhibiting expression of genes involved in protein degradation in C2C12 myoblasts. *J. Nutr.* 146:2461–2467.

Suryawan, A., R.A. Orellana, M.L. Fiorotto, and T.A. Davis. 2011. Leucine acts as a nutrient signal to stimulate protein synthesis in neonatal pigs. *J. Anim. Sci.* 89:2004–2016.

Tamminga, S. 1979. Protein degradation in the forestomachs of ruminants. *J. Anim. Sci.* 49:1615–1625.

Tarvid, I.L. 1991. Early postnatal development of peptide hydrolysis in chicks and guinea pigs. *Comp. Biochem. Physiol.* 99A:441–447.

Tarvid, I.L. 1992. Effect of early postnatal long-term fasting on the development of peptide hydrolysis in chicks. *Comp. Biochem. Physiol.* 101A:161–166.

Tedeschi, L.O. and D.G. Fox. 2016. *The Ruminant Nutrition System.* XanEdu, Acton, MA.

Trottier, N.L., C.F. Shipley, and R.A. Easter. 1997. Plasma amino acid uptake by the mammary gland of the lactating sow. *J. Anim. Sci.* 75:1266–1278.

Van Dijk, S., A.J. Lobsteyn, T. Wensing, and H.J. Breukink. 1983. Treatment of nitrate intoxication in a cow. *Vet. Rec.* 112:272–274.

Vogels, G.D. and C. Van der Driet. 1976. Degradation of purines and pyrimidines by microorganisms. *Bacteriol. Rev.* 40:403–468.

Wallace, R.J. 1994. Amino acid and protein synthesis, turnover, and breakdown by rumen microorganisms. In: *Principles of Protein Metabolism in Ruminants.* Edited by J.M. Asplund. CRC Press, Boca Raton, Florida, pp. 71–111.

Waltz, D.M. and M.D. Stern. 1989. Evaluation of various methods for protecting soya-bean protein from degradation by rumen bacteria. *Anim. Feed Sci. Technol.* 25:111–122.

Wang, T., J.M. Feugang, M.A. Crenshaw, N. Regmi, J.R. Blanton, Jr., and S.F. Liao. 2017. A systems biology approach using transcriptomic data reveals genes and pathways in porcine skeletal muscle affected by dietary lysine. *Int. J. Mol. Sci.* 18:885.

Wang, T.C. and M.F. Fuller. 1989. The optimum dietary amino acid patterns for growing pigs. 1. Experiments by amino acid deletion. *Br. J. Nutr.* 62:77–89.

Wang, W.W., R. Rezaei, Z.L. Wu, Z.L. Dai, J.J. Wang, and G. Wu. 2013. Concentrations of free and peptide-bound hydroxyproline in the sow's milk and piglet plasma. *Amino Acids* 45:595.

Wang, X.Q., J.W. Frank, D.R. Little, K.A Dunlap, M.C. Satterfiled, R.C. Burghardt, T.R. Hansen, G. Wu, and F.W. Bazer. 2014. Functional role of arginine during the peri-implantation period of pregnancy. I. Consequences of loss of function of arginine transporter *SLC7A1* mRNA in ovine conceptus trophectoderm. *FASEB J.* 28:2852–2863.

Wang, Y. and M. Watford. 2007. Glutamine, insulin and glucocorticoids regulate glutamine synthetase expression in C2C12 myotubes, Hep G2 hepatoma cells and 3T3 L1 adipocytes. *Biochim. Biophys. Acta* 1770:594–600.

Waterlow, J.C. 1995. Whole-body protein turnover in humans—Past, present, and future. *Annu. Rev. Nutr.* 15:57–92.

Waterlow, J.C., D.J. Millward, and P.J. Garlick. 1978. *Protein Turnover in Mammalian Tissues and in the Whole Body*. Amsterdam, The Netherlands.

Watford, M., P. Vinay, G. Lemieux, and A. Gougoux. 1980. The regulation of glucose and pyruvate formation from glutamine and citric-acid-cycle intermediates in the kidney cortex of rats, dogs, rabbits and guinea pigs. *Biochem. J.* 188:741–748.

Watford, M., and G. Wu. 2005. Glutamine metabolism in uricotelic species: Variation in skeletal muscle glutamine synthetase, glutaminase, glutamine levels and rates of protein synthesis. *Comp. Biochem. Physiol. B.* 140:607–614.

Wilson, R.H. and J. Leibholz. 1981. Digestion in the pigs between 7 and 35 d of age. 4. The digestion of amino acids in pigs given milk and soya-bean proteins. *Br. J. Nutr.* 45:347–357.

Wolff, J.E., E.N. Bergman, and H.H. Williams. 1972. Net metabolism of plasma amino acids by liver and portal-drained viscera. *Am. J. Physiol.* 223:438–446.

Wolfson, A.D., J.A. Pleiss, and O.C. Uhlenbeck. 1998. A new assay for tRNA aminoacylation kinetics. *RNA* 4:1019–1023.

Wright, P.A. 1995. Nitrogen excretion: Three end products, many physiological roles. *J. Exp. Biol.* 198:273–281.

Wu, G. 1995. Urea synthesis in enterocytes of developing pigs. *Biochem. J.* 312:717–723.

Wu, G. 1997. Synthesis of citrulline and arginine from proline in enterocytes of postnatal pigs. *Am. J. Physiol.* 272:G1382–G1390.

Wu, G. 1998. Intestinal mucosal amino acid catabolism. *J. Nutr.* 128:1249–1252.

Wu, G. 2009. Amino acids: Metabolism, functions, and nutrition. *Amino Acids* 37:1–17.

Wu, G. 2010. Functional amino acids in growth, reproduction and health. *Adv. Nutr.* 1:31–37.

Wu, G. 2013. *Amino Acids: Biochemistry and Nutrition*. CRC Press, Boca Raton, Florida.

Wu, G. 2014. Dietary requirements of synthesizable amino acids by animals: A paradigm shift in protein nutrition. *J. Anim. Sci. Biotechnol.* 5:34.

Wu, G., F.W. Bazer, Z.L. Dai, D.F. Li, J.J. Wang, and Z.L. Wu. 2014a. Amino acid nutrition in animals: Protein synthesis and beyond. *Annu. Rev. Anim. Biosci.* 2:387–417.

Wu, G., A.G. Borbolla, and D.A. Knabe. 1994b. The uptake of glutamine and release of arginine, citrulline and proline by the small intestine of developing pigs. *J. Nutr.* 124:2437–2444.

Wu, G., J. Fanzo, D.D. Miller, P. Pingali, M. Post, J.L. Steiner, and A.E. Thalacker-Mercer. 2014b. Production and supply of high-quality food protein for human consumption: Sustainability, challenges and innovations. *Ann. N.Y. Acad. Sci.* 1321:1–19.

Wu, G., N.E. Flynn, W. Yan, and D.G. Barstow, Jr. 1995. Glutamine metabolism in chick enterocytes: Absence of pyrroline-5-carboxylate synthase and citrulline synthesis. *Biochem. J.* 306:717–721.

Wu, G., D.A. Knabe, and N.E. Flynn. 1994a. Synthesis of citrulline from glutamine in pig enterocytes. *Biochem. J.* 299:115–121.

Wu, G., D.A. Knabe, and N.E. Flynn. 2005. Amino acid metabolism in the small intestine: biochemical bases and nutritional significance. In: *Biology of Metabolism of Growing Animals*. Edited by D.G. Burrin and H.J. Mersmann. Elsevier, New York, pp. 107–126.

Wu, G., D.A. Knabe, and S.W. Kim. 2004. Arginine nutrition in neonatal pigs. *J. Nutr.* 134:2783S–2390S.

Wu, G. and S.M. Morris, Jr. 1998. Arginine metabolism: Nitric oxide and beyond. *Biochem. J.* 336:1–17.

Wu, G. and J.R. Thompson. 1988. The effect of ketone bodies on alanine and glutamine metabolism in isolated skeletal muscle from the fasted chick. *Biochem. J.* 255:139–144.

Wu, G. and J.R. Thompson. 1990. The effect of glutamine on protein turnover in chick skeletal muscle. *Biochem. J.* 265:593–598.

Wu, G., Z.L. Wu, Z.L. Dai, Y. Yang, W.W. Wang, C. Liu, B. Wang, J.J. Wang and Y.L. Yin. 2013a. Dietary requirements of "nutritionally nonessential amino acids" by animals and humans. *Amino Acids* 44:1107–1113.

Wu, G., F.W. Bazer, T.A. Davis, S.W. Kim, P. Li, J.M. Rhoads, M.C. Satterfield, S.B. Smith, T.E. Spencer, and Y.L. Yin. 2009. Arginine metabolism and nutrition in growth, health and disease. *Amino Acids* 37:153–168.

Wu, G., F.W. Bazer, G.A. Johnson, R.C. Burghardt, X.L. Li, Z.L. Dai, J.J. Wang, and Z.L. Wu. 2013b. Maternal and fetal amino acid metabolism in gestating sows. *Soc. Reprod. Fertil. Suppl.* 68:185–198.

Wu, Z.L., Y.Q. Hou, S.D. Hu, F.W. Bazer, C.J. Meininger, C.J. McNeal, and G. Wu. 2016. Catabolism and safety of supplemental L-arginine in animals. *Amino Acids* 48:1541–1552.

Xi, P.B., Z.Y. Jiang, Z.L. Dai, X.L. Li, K. Yao, C.T. Zheng, Y.C. Lin, J.J. Wang, and G. Wu. 2012. Regulation of protein turnover by L-glutamine in porcine intestinal epithelial cells. *J. Nutr. Biochem.* 23:1012–1017.

Xue, Y., S.F. Liao, K.W. Son, S.L. Greenwood, B.W. McBride, J.A. Boling, and J.C. Matthews. 2010. Metabolic acidosis in sheep alters expression of renal and skeletal muscle amino acid enzymes and transporters. *J. Anim. Sci.* 88:707–717.

Yang, C., J.A. Rooke, I. Cabeza, and R.J. Wallace. 2016. Nitrate and inhibition of ruminal methanogenesis: Microbial ecology, obstacles, and opportunities for lowering methane emissions from ruminant livestock. *Front. Microbiol.* 7:132.

Yang, Y.X., Z.L. Dai, and W.Y. Zhu. 2014. Important impacts of intestinal bacteria on utilization of dietary amino acids in pigs. *Amino Acids* 46:2489–2501.

Yasugi, S. and T. Mizuno. 1981. Developmental changes in acid proteases of the avian proventriculus. *J. Exp. Zool. A* 216:331–335.

Yen, J.T. 2001. Digestive system. In: *Biology of the Domestic Pig*. Edietd by W.G. Pond and H.J. Mersmann. Cornell University Press, Ithaca, NY, pp. 390–453.

Yen, J.T., B.J. Kerr, R.A. Easter, and A.M. Parkhurst. 2004. Difference in rates of net portal absorption between crystalline and protein-bound lysine and threonine in growing pigs fed once daily. *J. Anim. Sci.* 82:1079–1090.

Yin, J., W.K. Ren, Y.Q. Hou, M.M. Wu, H. Xiao, J.L. Duan, Y.R. Zhao et al. 2015. Use of homoarginine for measuring true ileal digestibility of amino acids in food protein. *Amino Acids* 47:1795–1803.

Yoshida, C., M. Maekawa, M. Bannai, and T. Yamamoto. 2016. Glutamate promotes nucleotide synthesis in the gut and improves availability of soybean meal feed in rainbow trout. *Springerplus* 5:1021.

Young, V.R. and S. Borgonha. 2000. Nitrogen and amino acid requirements: The Massachusetts Institute of Technology amino acid requirement pattern. *J. Nutr.* 130:1841S–1849S.

Young, V.R. and H.N. Munro. 1978. Nτ-Methylhistidine (3-methylhistidine) and muscle protein turnover: An overview. *Fed. Proc.* 37:2291–2300.

Zhang, S., E.A. Wong, and E.R. Gilbert. 2015. Bioavailability of different dietary supplemental methionine sources in animals. *Front. Biosci.* E7, 478–490.

Zhanghi, B.M. and J.C. Matthews. 2010. Physiological importance and mechanisms of protein hydrolysate absorption. In: *Protein Hydrolysates in Biotechnology*. Edited by V.K. Pasupuleki and A.L. Demain. Springer Science, New York, pp. 135–177.

# 8 Energy Metabolism

Energy is not matter but is contained in matter. Carbohydrates, lipids, protein, and amino acids (AAs) are the primary sources of dietary energy for animals (Jobgen et al. 2006; van Milgen et al. 2000), with the proportions of these nutrients in diets differing among carnivores, herbivores, and omnivores (Stevens and Hume 2004). An animal must survive before it can grow and produce food (e.g., muscle, milk, or eggs) for human consumption (Pond et al. 1995). Animals will not grow and will lose body weight (BW) if their dietary intake of energy is insufficient because metabolic processes and tissue accretions require adequate energy (Milligan 1970; Verstegen and Henken 1987). A major cost of animal production is maintaining the basal energy requirement of the body (e.g., maintaining a stable body temperature in mammals and birds, muscular activity, and essential physiological function) (Kleiber 1961). The animal requires additional energy for the purpose of production, including tissue growth (and wool growth), fattening, lactation, draught power, transport, pregnancy, or egg formation, depending on the living environment, species, breeds, sex and age (McDonald et al. 2011). Thus, the efficiency of the utilization of dietary energy is of great importance for productivity, economic returns, and sustainability in animal agriculture.

Adenosine triphosphate (ATP) is the major currency of energy in organisms, because it is used by all cells for biochemical reactions and physiological processes (Dai et al. 2013; Newsholme and Leech 2009). All animals obtain their biological energy from the cell-specific oxidation of fatty acids, glucose, and AAs that are derived, respectively, from fats, starch/glycogen, and protein/free AAs in diets (Jobgen et al. 2006). In general, small endothermic animals have a higher basal metabolic rate (BMR) per kg BW than larger ones because the former have a larger surface area, lose heat faster, and require more energy to maintain a constant internal temperature (Blaxter 1989; Speakman 2005). Results from 138 studies involving 69 species of teleost fish (representing 28 families and 12 orders) indicate that the rates of resting oxygen consumption (mmol/h) are positively correlated with body mass and environmental temperature (Clarke and Johnston 1999). In the same animal species, different tissues have different rates of energy metabolism to meet their physiological needs, and the type of energy substrate varies with tissue and developmental stage (Milligan and Summers 1986). For example, in growing pigs and rats, the small intestine utilizes glutamate, glutamine, and aspartate as its major metabolic fuels, whereas fatty acids provide the bulk of ATP to the liver and skeletal muscle (Jobgen et al. 2006). The conversion of food energy to biological energy requires complex pathways for metabolism of the macronutrients to $CO_2$ and water, as discussed in Chapters 5–7. Since all forms of energy are convertible into heat, heat production is measured by direct or indirect calorimetry studies of animal energy metabolism (Blaxter 1971). The objective of this chapter is to highlight the partitioning of food energy in animals, as well as the energy systems used in feedstuff evaluation and feeding.

## BASIC CONCEPTS OF ENERGY

### Definition of Energy

Energy may be defined as the capacity to do work (Newsholme and Leech 2009). There are various forms of energy, including chemical, thermal, electrical, and radiant energy, all of which can be interconvertible by suitable means. Chemical energy is the energy stored in bonds between atoms within a molecule. Energy can be added or released from a molecule by rearranging its chemical bonds (Brown et al. 2003). Both in foods and animals, energy is stored primarily in carbohydrates, fats, fatty acids, proteins, and AAs. The energy released from the oxidation of fatty acids, glucose,

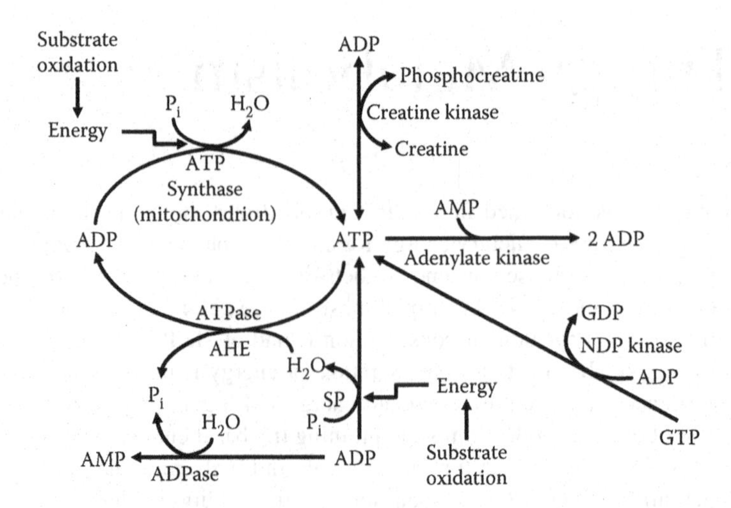


**FIGURE 8.1** ATP synthesis in animals. Energy is released from substrates (glucose, glycerol, lactate, fatty acids, and AAs) during their oxidation in animal cells. This energy is subsequently used to drive the synthesis of ATP from ADP through: (1) substrate level phosphorylation and (2) mitochondrial oxidative phosphorylation. In skeletal muscle and the brain, ATP is stored as phosphocreatine. The rate of ATP utilization is matched by the rate of ATP production. GTP is converted into ATP by nucleoside-diphosphate (NDP) kinase. AHE, transmembrane ATPase (e.g., $Na^+/K^+$-ATPase and $H^+/K^+$-ATPase); SP, substrate-level phosphorylation.

and AAs is used for the synthesis of ATP, guanosine triphosphate (GTP), cytidine triphosphate (CTP), and uridine triphosphate (UTP) (Newsholme and Leech 2009). Among these nucleotides, ATP is the most abundant and important for energy metabolism in animal cells, but GTP, UTP, and CTP participate in some special reactions (e.g., G-protein signaling mechanisms, as well as the synthesis of protein, lactose, and glycogen) (Lodish et al. 2000). The metabolism of energy in the whole body may lead to anabolism (energy storage) or catabolism (energy mobilization) (Verstegen and Henken 1987).

According to the first law of thermodynamics, energy can neither be created nor destroyed, and can only be converted from one form into another (Brown et al. 2003). Thus, there is no energy production in organisms, and inadequate intake of dietary energy will always result in energy deficits (Blaxter 1989). In the ecosystem, the radiant energy of the sun is converted into chemical energy in green plants. The latter are consumed by animals for conversion into biological energy (mainly in the form of ATP) plus heat (Figure 8.1). In all organisms, when chemical reactions release energy, it goes into the surroundings (Lodish et al. 2000). Energy metabolism in cells or animals can be defined as biochemical reactions involved in the transformation of various forms of chemical energy. Since the efficiency of trapping energy released from substrate oxidation is <60% (Chapter 1), these processes generate heat.

## Unit of Energy in Animal Nutrition

The thermochemical calorie (cal), which is based on the caloric value of benzoic acid as the reference standard, has been used as the basic energy unit in animal nutrition (McDonald et al. 2011). Traditionally, 1 cal is defined as the heat required to increase the temperature of 1 g water in an insulated tank by 1°C (usually from 14.5°C to 15.5°C) at a pressure of 1 atmosphere. Since the calorie is inconveniently small, the kilocalorie (kcal; 1 kcal = 1000 cal) or the megacalorie (mcal; 1 mcal = $10^3$ kcal = $10^6$ cal) is often used. The term "large calorie", written as Calorie (Cal), sometimes appears in literature (1 Cal = 1 kcal). However, the international unit of energy is the joule (J) (The International Bureau of Weights and Measures [IBWM] 2006), which is named after the English physicist James Prescott Joule (1818–1889). The International Union of Nutritional Sciences and the International Union of Physiological Sciences have recommended the joule (J) as the energy unit for use in nutritional and physiological studies. This suggestion has been almost universally adopted (Hargrove 2007). In physics, one joule is defined as the energy transferred to (or work done on) an object when a force of one newton acts on that object in the direction of its motion through a distance of one meter (i.e., 1 newton meter or N · m) (IBWM 2006). One joule is also equivalent to the energy dissipated as heat when an electric current of one ampere passes through a resistance of one ohm for one second. The work of moving 1 kg by 1 m against gravitational acceleration at the sea level equals 9.807 (IBWM 2006); namely, 1 kg · m = 9.807 J (1 kg · km = 9.807 kJ). For unit conversion, 1 cal = 4.1842 J. However, owing to convenience, the unit of calories is still used to formulate diets on farms.

## Gibbs Free Energy

The second law of thermodynamics states that energy transfers increase the entropy or disorder of the system (e.g., an insulated tank, a test tube, a cell, a tissue, or an animal) (Brown et al. 2003). Thus, the natural direction of change is always toward greater entropy (more disorder). An example is the oxidation of glucose (a highly organized molecule) into $H_2O$ and $CO_2$ (less organized molecules). Animals use biological energy to counteract the increasing disorder of the system through growth (e.g., building skeletal muscle or bones, deposition of white adipose tissue to store energy, and increased accumulation of collagen; that is, toward a more organized system in the animal body) (Newsholme and Leech 2009). As the organisms grow via energy-dependent reactions, the release of heat (expressed as kcal per animal) increases, and the entropy of the surroundings (the overall system) increases (Lodish et al. 2000). Thus, the thermodynamically open system of an animal, which involves energy exchanges with its surrounding environment, does not defy the laws of thermodynamics. In the animal body, a portion of the energy that is available to do work (e.g., carrying out a biochemical reaction, nutrient absorption, skeletal muscle contraction, and urinary excretion of metabolites) is termed Gibbs free energy (Lodish et al. 2000). It is named after the American mathematician Josiah Willard Gibbs (1839–1903). Thus, Gibbs free energy, which is a measure of the useful energy of a system, takes into consideration the changes in the enthalpy (heat) and entropy (degree of disorder) of a reaction (Brown et al. 2003).

$$\Delta G = \Delta H - T\,\Delta S$$

$\Delta G$ = change in Gibbs free energy; $\Delta S$ = change in entropy (disorder); $\Delta H$ = change in enthalpy (heat); T = absolute temperature (in Kelvin).

Note that $\Delta H$ is independent of the pathway, but depends on only the substrates and products (Lodish et al. 2000). When an organic substrate (e.g., glucose) is oxidized to $CO_2$ and $H_2O$ in either an animal or a bomb calorimeter, the $\Delta H$ is the same. However, when the oxidation of an organic substrate (e.g., protein) in an animal generates products (e.g., $CO_2$, $H_2O$, ammonia, and urea) that are different from those in a bomb calorimeter (e.g., $CO_2$, $H_2O$, and $N_2$), the resulting $\Delta H$ values are not the same (Wu 2013). This becomes important when heat production is calculated according to data on $O_2$ consumption and $CO_2$ production generated from studies involving indirect calorimetry.

Whether a chemical reaction can occur spontaneously depends on changes in Gibbs free energy ($\Delta G$). When $\Delta G < 0$, the reaction takes place spontaneously (exergonic) (Lodish et al. 2000). There is a positive flow of energy from the system to the surroundings, for example, heat production. An exergonic (exothermic) reaction results in products which have stronger bonds (lower energy) and are more stable than the reactants. When $\Delta G = 0$, the reaction is said to be at equilibrium (no net production of products); an example of this reaction is the transamination of an AA (Wu 2013). When $\Delta G > 0$, the reaction does not take place spontaneously, and energy must be fed into the system in order for the reaction to occur (endergonic). An endothermic reaction absorbs free energy (usually, but not always, heat) from its surroundings to break bonds in reactants and generate products with higher energy (Newsholme and Leech 2009). Examples of this reaction include photosynthesis in plants, the solubilization of salts (e.g., NaCl and KCl) in water for intestinal absorption of ions, and the phosphorylation of glucose to form glucose-6-phosphate. Evaporation of water from animals is also an endothermic process that requires the input of heat into the system.

Constant interconversions of energy occur in animals. For example, in live cells, a reaction (including a spontaneous reaction) releases free energy, which can be used to power another reaction (including a nonspontaneous reaction) (Newsholme and Leech 2009). Therefore, metabolic pathways, which can be defined as a consecutive series of chemical reactions where the product of one reaction is the reactant of the next reaction (Chapter 1), always produce heat. This means that energy metabolism is a highly active physiological process.

The $\Delta G$ of a biochemical reaction can be calculated using the following equation:

$$\Delta G = \Delta G^\circ + 2.3\ RT\ \log X$$

$\Delta G^\circ$: Standard free energy change

$$X = [B]/[A] \text{ for } A \rightarrow B, \text{ or } X = ([B_1] \times [B_2])/([A_1] \times [A_2]) \text{ for } A_1 + A_2 \rightarrow B_1 + B_2$$

R: Gas constant (1.987 cal/(K × mol) or 8.314 J/(K × mol))
T: Kelvin temperature (K). (37°C = 310 K; 25°C = 298 K; 0°C = 273 K)

As noted previously, a chemical reaction either absorbs or releases energy, and always involves breaking the bonds of reactants and making bonds in products (Brown et al. 2003). Under physiological conditions, ATP, GTP, and UTP are hydrolyzed to provide energy for driving energy-dependent biochemical reactions, nutrient transport, and muscular contractions (Chapters 5–7), with the heat being released into the surroundings. Thus, energy metabolism is the foundation of life.

## ATP Synthesis in Cells

There are two mechanisms for the synthesis of ATP from ADP in animals: (1) substrate level phosphorylation, and (2) oxidative phosphorylation (Chapter 1). Substrate-level phosphorylation refers to the synthesis of ATP from ADP and inorganic phosphate (Pi) directly during a biochemical reaction. Examples can be seen in glycolysis and the mitochondrial Krebs cycle. Substrate-level phosphorylation via glycolysis is the only mechanism for ATP production by anaerobic microorganisms (e.g., those present in the rumen) (Newsholme and Leech 2009). This indicates the importance of dietary carbohydrates for ATP supply to ruminal microorganisms. Indeed, glycolysis plays a more important role in ATP synthesis by animal cells under anaerobic rather than aerobic conditions, and is the only pathway to generate ATP in cells containing no mitochondria (e.g., mammalian red blood cells) (Chapter 5). Oxidative phosphorylation refers to the synthesis of ATP from ADP and Pi when the reducing equivalents (NADH, NADPH, and $FADH_2$) are oxidized via the mitochondrial electron transport system (Chapter 1). In the presence of an adequate supply of oxygen, oxidative phosphorylation is the major mechanism for ATP production in most animal cells (Figure 8.1). The amount of energy required to synthesize either 1 mol ATP from 1 mol ADP plus 1 mol Pi or 1 mol GTP from 1 mol GDP plus 1 mol Pi is 85.4 kJ/mol (McDonald et al. 2002).

Phosphocreatine plays a critical role in storing energy by forming: (1) phosphocreatine from ATP and creatine via creatine kinase in the nerves and skeletal muscle of mammals and birds; and (2) phosphoarginine from ATP and Arg via Arg kinase in aquatic invertebrates (Clark et al. 2012). In both phosphocreatine and phosphoarginine, chemical bonds form after the valence electrons of two or more atoms interact to make them more stable. In response to physiological needs, phosphocreatine and phosphoarginine are hydrolyzed by enzymes to provide energy, which is used for biochemical reactions and physiological events (Newsholme and Leech 2009).

## PARTITION OF FOOD ENERGY IN ANIMALS

Food energy is partitioned into various fractions on the basis of nutrient digestion and metabolism in animals (Baldwin and Bywater 1984). The scheme is shown in Figure 8.2. Different energy systems are used to formulate the diets of different animal species because of differences in their digestive physiology and anatomy (Wu et al. 2007). Factors that affect digestion, absorption, and metabolism of dietary nutrients can also influence the efficiency of their utilization by animals (Moughan et al. 2000; Noblet et al. 1994).

### GROSS ENERGY

Gross energy (GE) is defined as the energy released as heat (called heat of combustion) when a substance is fully oxidized in a bomb calorimeter, which contains a strong metal chamber resting in an insulated tank of water (a thermodynamically closed system) (McDonald et al. 2011). The heat produced from substrate oxidation is calculated from the rise in temperature of the surrounding water. Heat of combustion is often referred to as the change in the enthalpy of the reaction ($\Delta H$). $\Delta H$ is independent of the chemical pathway by which a process is carried out, and depends only on the differences in chemical energy before and after the process has occurred (i.e., the substrates and products) (Newsholme and Leech 2009). For example, the $\Delta H$ of fat is the same when it is completely oxidized to $CO_2$ and $H_2O$ in a bomb calorimeter or an animal. This is also true for starch and glucose. In contrast, protein is completely oxidized to $CO_2$, $H_2O$, and nitrogen oxides ($NO_x$) in

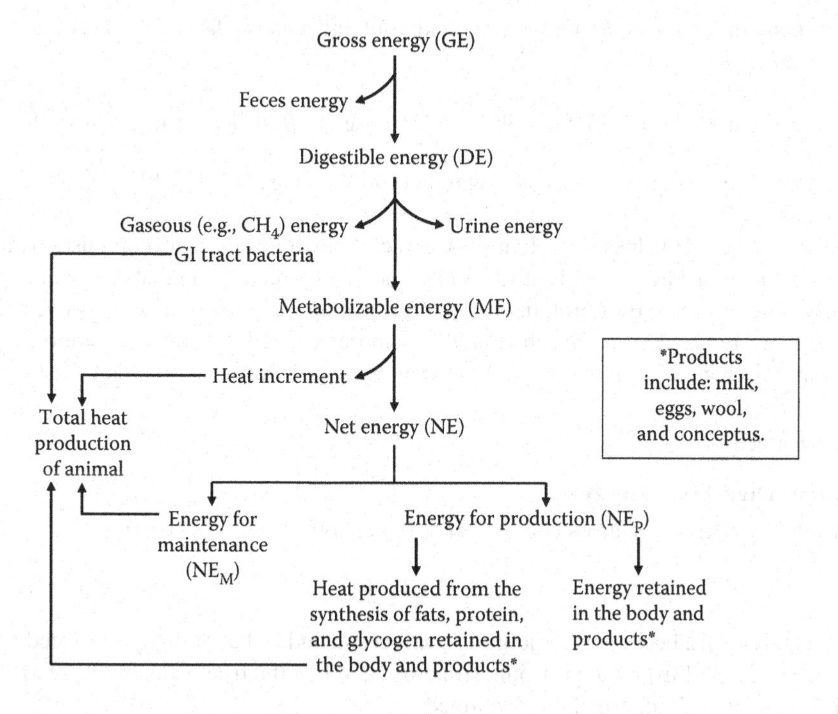


**FIGURE 8.2** Partitioning of food energy into various fractions in animals. When feces energy is determined, apparent DE is obtained. True DE can be calculated on the basis of the true digestibility of macronutrients in diets. Metabolizable energy (ME) values of feedstuffs may vary greatly within the same animal and among animal species, depending on the dietary content of fiber, fat, carbohydrate, and protein. Heat is produced by an animal via: (1) basal metabolism (maintenance); (2) gastrointestinal (GI) tract bacteria; (3) heat increment of feeding; and (4) the synthesis of fats, protein, and glycogen retained in the body of the animal and its products (e.g., milk, eggs, and wool). Net energy (NE) can better predict the efficiency of dietary energy for maintenance and production than gross energy, DE, and ME. NE can be partitioned into NE for maintenance ($NE_m$) and production ($NE_p$).

a bomb calorimeter, but incompletely oxidized to $CO_2$, $H_2O$, ammonia, urea, uric acid, nitrate, creatinine, and other nitrogenous metabolites in an animal. Thus, the biological ΔH of protein is lower than its value of the heat of combustion (i.e., GE) obtained from a bomb calorimeter.

Oxidation of fat and starch in a bomb calorimeter and an animal:

$$\text{Fat} + O_2 \dashrightarrow CO_2 + H_2O$$

$$\text{Starch} + O_2 \dashrightarrow CO_2 + H_2O$$

Oxidation of protein in a bomb calorimeter:

$$\text{Protein} + O_2 \dashrightarrow CO_2 + H_2O + NO_x$$

Oxidation of protein in an animal:

$$\text{Protein} + O_2 \dashrightarrow CO_2 + H_2O + \text{ammonia, urea, uric acid, nitrate, creatinine, and other metabolites}$$

GE of a diet can be calculated according to the content of dietary carbohydrate, fat, and protein (i.e., 4.1 kcal/g starch, 3.7 kcal/g glucose or simple sugar, 9.4 kcal/g fat, and 5.4 kcal/g protein).

$$\text{GE (kcal/kg diet)} = (\%\ \text{fat} \times 9.4 + \%\ \text{starch} \times 4.1 + \%\ \text{protein} \times 5.4) \times 10$$

(for a diet containing fat, starch/glycogen, and protein; e.g., % fat = 10, % starch = 65, and % protein = 20)

$$\text{GE (kcal/kg diet)} = (\%\ \text{fat} \times 9.4 + \%\ \text{glucose} \times 3.7 + \%\ \text{protein} \times 5.4) \times 10$$

(for a diet containing fat, glucose/simple sugar, and protein; e.g., % fat = 10, % glucose = 65, and % protein = 20)

Table 8.1 lists the ΔH values of protein, fats, and carbohydrates in bomb combustion and animal oxidation. On the gram basis, the GE of fat is 74% and 129% greater than that of protein and starch, respectively, whereas the GE of protein is 32% greater than that of starch. This is because fat and protein are more reduced than carbohydrate. The more reduced an organic compound (i.e., the higher the hydrogen atom content), the more oxygen is required for its oxidation to $H_2O$.

## Digestible Energy

### Definition of Digestible Energy

Digestible energy (DE) is the gross energy minus the energy of the feces (FE).

$$\text{DE} = \text{GE} - \text{FE}$$

This is apparent DE, because the energy of the feces includes that of undigested feed and that of the substances secreted from the gastrointestinal tract. When the true digestibility of organic matters (OM) is determined, the true DE is obtained.

### Losses of Fecal Energy in Various Animals

The energy in the feces represents the single largest loss of the ingested energy. In ruminants, the heat produced during digestive fermentation is positively correlated with the fiber content of the diet; the higher the fiber intake, the more the heat generated from the gastrointestinal tract. In these animals, fecal energy accounts for 20%–30% and 40%–50% of GE, respectively, when concentrates and roughage are fed. Fecal energy represents ~ 40%, 20%, 20%, and 25% of the GE in horses, pigs, poultry, and fish, respectively (Pond et al. 2005). The higher fecal energy value found

**TABLE 8.1**
**ΔH Values of Organic Substances in Bomb Combustion and Animal Oxidation[a]**

| | Bomb Calorimeter | | | Animal Oxidation | | | | |
|---|---|---|---|---|---|---|---|---|
| **Nutrient** | **kcal/g** | **kJ/g** | **kJ/mol** | **kcal/g** | **kJ/g** | **kJ/mol** | **ATP Yield (mol/mol)** | **Efficiency (%) of ATP Production from Substrate Oxidation** |
| Fat[b] (mw 806) | 9.39 | 39.3 | 31,676 | 9.39 | 39.3 | 31,676 | 336.5 | 54.8 |
| Palmitate (mw 256) | 9.35 | 39.1 | 10,031 | 9.35 | 39.1 | 10,031 | 106 | 54.5 |
| Protein (mw 100) | 5.40 | 22.6 | 2260 | 4.10 | 17.2 | 1720 | 20 | 45.7 (mammal) |
| Protein (mw 100) | 5.40 | 22.6 | 2260 | 3.74 | 15.7 | 1566 | 18.2 | 41.6 (bird) |
| Protein (mw 100) | 5.40 | 22.6 | 2260 | 4.91 | 20.5 | 2054 | 23.9 | 54.6 (fish) |
| Starch (residue mw 162) | 4.11 | 17.2 | 2786 | 4.11 | 17.2 | 2786 | 30 | 55.7 |
| Lactose (mw 342) | 3.92 | 16.4 | 5630 | 3.92 | 16.4 | 5630 | 60 | 55.0 |
| Sucrose (mw 342) | 3.94 | 16.5 | 5640 | 3.94 | 16.5 | 5640 | 60 | 55.0 |
| Glucose (mw 180) | 3.73 | 15.6 | 2803 | 3.73 | 15.6 | 2803 | 30 | 55.3 |
| Galactose (mw 180) | 3.73 | 15.6 | 2803 | 3.73 | 15.6 | 2803 | 30 | 55.3 |
| Glycerol (mw 92) | 4.30 | 18.0 | 1655 | 4.30 | 18.0 | 1655 | 18.5 | 57.7 |
| Lactic acid (mw 90) | 3.56 | 14.9 | 1344 | 3.56 | 14.9 | 1344 | 15 | 57.6 |
| Ethanol (mw 46) | 7.10 | 29.7 | 1366 | 7.10 | 29.7 | 1366 | 15 | 56.7 |
| Acetic acid (mw 60) | 3.25 | 13.6 | 816 | 3.25 | 13.6 | 816 | 8 | 50.6 |
| Propionic acid (mw 74) | 4.97 | 20.8 | 1536 | 4.97 | 20.8 | 1536 | 17.5 | 58.8 |
| Butyric acid (mw 88) | 5.95 | 24.9 | 2193 | 5.95 | 24.9 | 2193 | 22 | 51.8 |
| Glutamate (mw 147) | 3.66 | 15.3 | 2244 | 1.72 | 7.21 | 1060 | 20.5 | 47.2 (mammal) |
| Glutamate (mw 147) | 3.66 | 15.3 | 2244 | 1.60 | 6.69 | 984 | 18.7 | 43.1 (bird) |
| Glutamate (mw 147) | 3.66 | 15.3 | 2244 | 1.85 | 7.75 | 1139 | 24.4 | 56.2 (fish) |
| Creatine (mw 131) | 4.23 | 17.7 | 2323 | 0.0[c] | 0.0 | 0.0 | – | – |
| Creatinine (mw 113) | 4.94 | 20.7 | 2336 | 0.0[c] | 0.0 | 0.0 | – | – |
| Urea (mw 60) | 2.51 | 10.5 | 632 | 0.0[c] | 0.0 | 0.0 | – | – |
| Uric acid (mw 168) | 2.73 | 11.4 | 1920 | 0.0[c] | 0.0 | 0.0 | – | – |
| Ammonia ($NH_3$, mw 17) | 5.37 | 22.5 | 382 | 0.0[c] | 0.0 | 0.0 | – | – |
| Allantoin (mw 158) | 2.59 | 10.8 | 1714 | 0.0[c] | 0.0 | 0.0 | – | – |
| Methane (mw 16) | 13.3 | 55.6 | 891 | 0.0[c] | 0.0 | 0.0 | – | – |

*Source:* Cox, J.D. and G. Pilcher. 1970. *Thermochemistry of Organic and Organometallic Compounds*. Academic Press: New York. pp. 1–643; and Wu, G. 2013. *Amino Acids: Biochemistry and Nutrition*. CRC Press, Boca Raton.

[a] The calculation does not involve substrate oxidation via the formation of glucose or ketone bodies. If propionate is first converted into glucose, which is subsequently oxidized into $CO_2$ and $H_2O$, the net production of ATP is 11.5 mol per 1 mol propionate. If butyrate is first converted into D-β-hydroxybutyrate, which is subsequently oxidized into $CO_2$ and $H_2O$, the net production of ATP is 20 mol per 1 mol butyrate.

[b] Tripalmitoylglycerol (tripalmitin).

[c] For nonruminants.

MW = molecular weight.

in horses (herbivores) consuming their habitual fibrous diets compared to that in non-herbivorous nonruminants ingesting little forage can be explained by the fact that plant cell-wall material in the diets of the former is not digested in the foregut and enters the large intestine, where it is fermented. The enlarged colon and cecum of an adult horse have the capacity of 60 and 25–35 L, respectively; the combined fermentation in the large intestine contributes to the digestion of 30% protein, 15%–30% soluble non-starch polysaccharides, and 75%–85% of plant cell-wall polysaccharides in diets (Ralston 1984). When fed a mixture of hay and concentrates, the digestibility of organic matter in horses is 85% of that in ruminants, indicating a high ability of horses to utilize forages among

**TABLE 8.2**
**Calculation of Gross Energy and DE of Diets for Animals[a]**

| | Starch | | Lipids | | Protein | | Gross Energy[b] (GE) | Digestible Energy[c] | |
|---|---|---|---|---|---|---|---|---|---|
| Animal | Content in Diet (%) | True Digestibility | Content in Diet (%) | True Digestibility | Content in Diet (%) | True Digestibility | (kcal/kg Diet) | Amount (kcal/kg Diet) | % of GE |
| Pigs[d] | 50 | 0.95 | 10 | 0.92 | 18 | 0.87 | 3967 | 3663 | 92.3 |
| Chickens[e] | 50 | 0.95 | 6 | 0.92 | 20 | 0.90 | 3699 | 3443 | 93.1 |
| Ruminants | 65 | 0.40–0.95 (0.675) | 5 (2–8) | 0.72 | 14 (10–18) | 0.65 | 3898 | 2633 | 67.5 |
| Horses | 10 | 0.95 | 6 | 0.92 | 14 | 0.85 | 1731 | 1552 | 89.7 |
| Fish | 20 | 0.85 | 10 | 0.90 | 40 | 0.85 | 3922 | 3381 | 86.2 |

[a] Dietary dry matter content is 90%. Within the same species, optimal nutrient contents in diets vary with productive purposes and ages. In this table, averaged values are used for calculation.

[b] Gross energy (kcal/kg diet) = (% starch × 10 × 4.11 kcal/g) + (% lipids × 10 × 9.4 kcal/g) + (% protein × 10 × 5.4 kcal/g). Using the diet for pigs as an example, gross energy (kcal/kg diet) = (50×10×4.11) + (10×10×9.4) + (18×10×5.4) = 3967 kcal/kg diet.

[c] DE (kcal/kg diet) = (% starch × digestibility × 10 × 4.11 kcal/g) + (% lipids × digestibility × 10 × 9.4 kcal/g) + (% protein × digestibility × 10 × 5.4 kcal/g). Using the diet for pigs as an example, gross energy (kcal/kg diet) = (50 × 0.95 × 10 × 4.11) + (10 × 0.92 × 10 × 9.4) + (18 × 0.87 × 10 × 5.4) = 3663 kcal/kg diet.

[d] Pigs (2 months of age) are fed cereal grains.

[e] Chickens (4 weeks of age) are fed cereal grains.

nonruminants (Hintz 1975). Owing to the complexity of hind-gut fermentation in horses, dietary DE values vary greatly among their feedstuffs. When pigs are fed a diet containing 5% fiber, their large intestine can ferment as much as 50% of cellulose and hemicellulose in cereal grains and their products (McDonald et al. 2011). In contrast, the rates of hind-gut fermentation in poultry (Qaisrani et al. 2015), fish, and shrimp (Stevens and Hume 2004) are much lower than those for horses. Since dogs and cats have a small hind-gut where fermentation is limited (Stevens and Hume 2004), dietary DE values will be low if these carnivores are fed a fibrous diet. In all animals, the true DE values should be calculated by adding, to the apparent DE, the amount of energy of endogenous (gastrointestinal) secretions that are present in the feces. In other words, the true DE is always greater than apparent DE. Like the apparent DE, the true DE can be calculated on the basis of the content and true digestibility of macronutrients in diets (Table 8.2).

## Measurements of the Digestibility of Feeds

A digestion experiment involves the collection of ileal digesta or feces from an animal which is kept in a specially designed crate (for facilitating the separation of feces from urine) and fed a constant amount of a test diet. The time required for feed to pass through the gastrointestinal tract differs markedly between ruminants and nonruminants (Chapter 1). A pretest period (e.g., 4–6 days for pigs and horses; 8–10 days for ruminants) is necessary for the digestive tract to be free of residues from previous feeds and for an animal to adapt to the test diet. The period of ileal digesta or feces collection varies with animal species (e.g., 4–6 days for pigs and horses or 8–10 days for ruminants). The digestibility of a concentrate feed for ruminants is generally determined as the difference in the digestibility of roughage (the basal diet) and that of the roughage plus concentrate to ensure sufficient provision of dietary fiber to the rumen. In poultry, which normally excrete both feces and urine from a single orifice, the determination of fecal digestibility requires that urinary flow be diverted from the cloaca to a collecting device. However, this procedure is not needed when the ileal digesta is obtained.

## Metabolizable Energy

Metabolizable energy (ME) is DE minus the energy in urine (UE) and the energy in combustible gases ($E_{gases}$) leaving the digestive tract. Feces and urine must be collected from individual animals placed in metabolism cages, whereas a respiratory chamber is required to measure methane production in ruminants.

$$ME = DE - UE - E_{gases}$$

The gases are mainly methane (which contains 13.3 kcal/g; Cox and Pilcher 1970) and, to a lesser extent, ammonia, $H_2$, $H_2S$, and $CO_2$. Loss of combustible gases through intestinal digestion is negligible in monogastric animals, but is nutritionally and quantitatively significant in ruminants and hind gut fermenters (Stevens and Hume 2004). Fermentation in the rumen and the hindgut produces large amounts of gases, which can represent 7%–8% of dietary ME intake (McDonald et al. 2011). In addition, when dietary carbohydrates, proteins, and fats are fermented to short-chain fatty acids (SCFAs) in the rumen, the energy released from the reactions is not fully trapped in the products or by the bacteria (Chapter 5). Thus, enhancing the fermentation of fiber to SCFAs in the rumen and the subsequent utilization of the SCFAs by the host tissue will substantially reduce the gaseous energy of the ration and improve feed efficiency.

Methane can account for 6%–12% and 1%–4% of the dietary GE intake in cattle and horses, respectively. In pigs, the $E_{gas}$ represents only a small fraction (ranging from 0.1% to 3%) of DE, depending on the diet and environmental temperature (Velayudhan et al. 2015). Owing to the different rates of fermentation in the digestive tract of animal species, the ME values of feedstuffs may differ widely among nonruminants and ruminants, particularly when they are fed diets containing high percentages of fibrous by-products or nonstarch polysaccharides (Table 8.3). Of note, the use of these ingredients for animal feeding is growing globally. Thus, owing to large variations in their ME values, the National Research Council (NRC 2012) no longer recommends ME as the energy system for formulating swine diets.

Urine energy results primarily from the excretion of incompletely oxidized nitrogenous compounds (e.g., urea, uric acid, ammonia, creatinine, and nitrate) under normal conditions (Wu 2013). However, products of the oxidation of fatty acids and ketogenic AAs (e.g., ketone bodies) are also present in the urine of most animals, and the amounts are substantially increased in animals with type-I diabetes mellitus. Urine energy accounts for 2%–3%, 4%–5%, and 4%–4.5% of dietary GE intake in pigs, cattle, and horses, respectively (Bondi 1987; Velayudhan et al. 2015). Urea, uric acid, creatinine, and ammonia contain 2.51, 2.73, 4.94, and 5.37 kcal/g, respectively (Cox and Pilcher 1970). Since they are the major end products of AA oxidation in animals, the physiological energy of protein is much lower than its GE, as noted previously. Thus, the high intake of dietary protein is associated with low ME in all animals, when compared with the isocaloric intake of fats and starch (Verstegen and Henken 1987).

ME is the portion of the food energy that is available for metabolic processes in an animal (Blaxter 1989). The efficiency of ME utilization is affected by energy substrates, their metabolic pathways, physiological states of the animal, and the ambient environment. Dietary ME is utilized more efficiently when animals are fed diets below maintenance requirements, compared to diets above maintenance requirements (i.e., fat and protein deposition) (Table 8.4). This is because the metabolic transformation for the synthesis of fat and protein in all animals is always less than 100% (see the sections below). The dietary ME from fat is utilized more efficiently when animals are fed diets either below or above maintenance requirements in comparison with the dietary ME from protein, because the energetic efficiency of the synthesis of fat is higher than that of protein (Verstegen and Henken 1987). Owing to differences in digestion and metabolism, the values of dietary ME (Table 8.5) and the efficiency of its utilization differ greatly among animals. For example, ME is 80%–86% (average 83%) of DE in ruminants (beef cattle, sheep, and goats), 94%–97% (average of 95.5%) of DE in pigs, and 60%–65% of GE in horses, depending on diets. In chickens, ME is 75%–80% of GE, depending on diets (McDonald et al. 2011; Pond et al. 1995).

**TABLE 8.3**
**Metabolizable Energy Values of Feed Ingredients for Animals**

| Animal | Feed | Gross Energy (GE) | Energy Present in | | | Metabolizable Energy | |
|---|---|---|---|---|---|---|---|
| | | | Feces | Urine | Methane | Amount | % of GE |
| Fowl | Corn | 18.4 | 2.2[a] | – | – | 16.2 | 88.0 |
| | Wheat | 18.1 | 2.8[a] | – | – | 15.3 | 84.5 |
| | Barley | 18.2 | 4.9[a] | – | – | 13.3 | 73.1 |
| Pig | Corn | 18.9 | 1.6 | 0.4 | – | 16.9 | 89.4 |
| | Oats | 19.4 | 5.5 | 0.6 | – | 13.3 | 68.6 |
| | Barley | 17.5 | 2.8 | 0.5 | – | 14.2 | 81.1 |
| | Coconut cake meal | 19.0 | 6.4 | 2.6 | – | 10.0 | 52.6 |
| Sheep | Barley | 18.5 | 3.0 | 0.6 | 2.0 | 12.9 | 69.7 |
| | Dried ryegrass (young) | 19.5 | 3.4 | 1.5 | 1.6 | 13.0 | 66.7 |
| | Dried ryegrass (mature) | 19.0 | 7.1 | 0.6 | 1.4 | 9.9 | 52.1 |
| | Grass hay (young) | 18.0 | 5.4 | 0.9 | 1.5 | 10.2 | 56.7 |
| | Grass hay (mature) | 17.9 | 7.6 | 0.5 | 1.4 | 8.4 | 46.9 |
| | Grass silage | 19.0 | 5.0 | 0.9 | 1.5 | 11.6 | 61.1 |
| Cattle | Corn | 18.9 | 2.8 | 0.8 | 1.3 | 14.0 | 74.1 |
| | Barley | 18.3 | 4.1 | 0.8 | 1.1 | 12.3 | 67.2 |
| | Wheat bran | 19.0 | 6.0 | 1.0 | 1.4 | 10.6 | 55.8 |
| | Lucerne hay | 18.3 | 8.2 | 1.0 | 1.3 | 7.8 | 42.6 |

*Source:* Adapted from McDonald, P. et al. 2011. *Animal Nutrition*, 7th ed. Prentice Hall, New York.

*Note:* Values are MJ/kg dry matter, except for the % of GE. The GE values were determined in the laboratory. Different sources of corn and barley were used for different studies.

[a] Energy in feces plus urine.

Over the past 25 years, the ME system has been used widely in the swine and poultry industries (de Lange and Birkett 2005). Thus, data on the dietary ME values of conventional feedstuffs for nonruminants are available in the literature (de Lange and Birkett 2005; Le Goff and Noblet 2001). Of note, the use of the ME system is unique for poultry feeding, because poultry void both urine and feces into the same opening and are conveniently collected together (Sibbald 1982). The ME values of swine and poultry diets can be readily determined through standard metabolism and digestion experiments (McDonald et al. 2011).

## Net Energy and Heat Increment

Net energy (NE) is ME minus the heat increment (HI) associated with feeding. HI is part of the whole-body heat production in animals that results from the activity of feeding, food digestion, and nutrient metabolism (Bondi 1987). NE consists of the energy for maintenance ($NE_m$) and the energy for production ($NE_p$), such as growth, lactation, and gestation. NE is a better indicator of the energy value of feedstuffs than ME if the efficiency of their ME utilization for maintenance and production differs substantially. This situation likely arises from the feeding of fibrous diets, which stimulate the activities of gastrointestinal tract bacteria and mucosal cells, as well as intestinal motility (Chapter 5). Of note, NE is much more difficult to determine and more complex than ME (Blaxter 1989).

$$NE = ME - HI$$

### *Definition of HI*

HI is also called the specific dynamic effect of foods. The major causes of HI include: (1) nutrient digestion and absorption (e.g., chewing and mastication of feeds, fermentation in the rumen, active

**TABLE 8.4**
**Efficiency of Utilization of Metabolizable Energy (ME) Below Maintenance and for Fat and Protein Deposition above Maintenance in Animals[a]**

| Nutrient | Animal | Efficiency (% of ME) | | Heat Increment (% of ME) | |
|---|---|---|---|---|---|
| | | Below Maintenance | Above Maintenance[b] | Below Maintenance | Above Maintenance[b] |
| Carbohydrate | Nonruminants | 94 | 78 | 6 | 22 |
| | Ruminants | 80 | 54 | 20 | 46 |
| | Other herbivores | 90 | 64 | 10 | 36 |
| | Birds | 95 | 77 | 5 | 23 |
| Fat | Nonruminants | 98 | 85 | 2 | 15 |
| | Ruminants | 92[c] | 79 | 8[c] | 21 |
| | Other herbivores | 92[c] | 79 | 8[c] | 21 |
| | Birds | 95 | 78 | 5 | 22 |
| Protein | Nonruminants | 77 | 64 | 23 | 36 |
| | Ruminants | 70 | 45 | 30 | 55 |
| | Other herbivores | 76 | 50 | 24 | 50 |
| | Birds | 80 | 55 | 20 | 45 |
| Regular diets | Man | 90 | 75 | 10 | 25 |
| | Rat | 90 | 75 | 10 | 25 |
| | Dog | 85 | 70 | 15 | 30 |
| | Pig | 85 | 70 | 15 | 30 |
| | Rabbit | 80 | 65 | 20 | 35 |
| | Horse | 75 | 60 | 25 | 40 |
| | Cattle | 70 | 50 | 30 | 50 |
| | Sheep | 70 | 50 | 30 | 50 |
| | Chicken | 90 | 75 | 10 | 25 |

*Source:* Blaxter, K.L. 1989. *Energy Metabolism in Animals and Man*. Cambridge University Press, New York, NY.

[a] Different animals consume their habitual diets. The corresponding heat increment for utilization of dietary ME increases as the amount of energy for maintenance or production decreases.

[b] Used for deposition of fat and protein.

[c] Tedeschi, L.O. and D.G. Fox. 2016. *The Ruminant Nutrition System: An Applied Model for Predicting Nutrient Requirements and Feed Utilization in Ruminants*. XanEdu, Acton, MA.

**TABLE 8.5**
**Energy Values of Feedstuffs for Animals[a]**

| Animal | Gross Energy (GE) | Digestible Energy (DE, % of GE) | Metabolizable Energy (ME, % of DE) | Net Energy (NE, % of ME) |
|---|---|---|---|---|
| Pigs | 100 | 90–92 | 96 | 82 |
| Chickens | 100 | 92–93 | 96 | 80 |
| Ruminants | 100 | 66–68 | 82 | 80 |
| Horses | 100 | 80–90 | 90–95 for cereals<br>84–88 for forages | 80 |
| Fish | 100 | 85–88 | 97 | 90–95 |

[a] These are estimated values, depending on a variety of dietary, animal, and environmental factors.

**TABLE 8.6**
**Heat Increment of Feeding (% of ME)**

| Nutrient | Pig | Sheep | Cattle | Chickens | Salmonids | Rainbow Trout |
|---|---|---|---|---|---|---|
| Fat | 9 | 29 | 35 | 10 | – | 1.4 |
| Starch | 17 | 32 | 37 | 18 | – | 3.5 |
| Protein | 26 | 54 | 52 | 44 | – | 3.3 |
| Mixed rations | 10–40 | 35–70 | 35–70 | 25–30 | 2.5 | 1.6 |

*Source:* Adapted from Bondi, A.A. 1987. *Animal Nutrition*. John Wiley & Sons, New York, NY for pigs, ruminants and chickens; and from Smith, R.R. et al. 1978. *J. Nutr.* 108:1025–1032 for salmonids (Atlantic salmon) and rainbow trout.

transport of nutrients by enterocytes and other cell types, and fermentation in the hindgut); (2) gastrointestinal movement; (3) non-production metabolism in an animal (e.g., synthesis of urea and uric acid); and (4) the physiological activities of various organs (e.g., kidneys, skeletal muscle, and heart) associated with feeding (Johnson et al. 1990; Lobley 1990; Noblet and Etienne 1987). The values of HI in pigs, sheep, cattle, chickens, and salmons are summarized in Table 8.6. The HI increases when the intake of food or dietary fiber is enhanced (Blaxter 1989).

### *Differences in HI Among Energy Substrates*

The HI of energy substrates fed to mammals and birds is: protein > carbohydrates > fat. The greater HI value for protein than that of carbohydrates or fats can be explained by the following biochemical reactions (Wu 2013). First, intracellular protein turnover requires large amounts of energy. Second, disposal of ammonia as urea in mammals and as uric acid in birds requires large amounts of energy. Third, energy is required to concentrate and excrete nitrogenous compounds by the kidneys. Finally, the oxidation of the carbon skeletons and nitrogen of AAs produces heat, particularly in cases of AA imbalance. Protein has a lower HI when used for protein synthesis than when used for oxidation to provide energy, because the latter is always associated with the conversion of AA-derived ammonia into urea or uric acid.

Intestinal absorption of lipids requires virtually no ATP, and the transport of fatty acids through the plasma and organelle (e.g., mitochondria) membranes of all cells is largely energy-independent (Chapter 6). In contrast, intestinal and renal absorption of glucose requires ATP, and the transport of the carboxylic acids (e.g., pyruvate) of glucose by all cell types is energy-dependent (Chapter 5). All these factors explain why the HI associated with the feeding of fat is much lower than that for glucose or protein in nonruminants. Among all macronutrients, protein has the highest HI in mammals and birds, as noted previously. Thus, during heat stress, protein is not an ideal source of energy for the whole bodies of land animals. However, certain cell types in mammals as well as possibly birds and fish have specific requirements for some AAs as major metabolic fuels (e.g., glutamate, glutamine, and aspartate for enterocytes in pigs, and glutamine for lymphocytes in pigs and rats) (Jobgen et al. 2006).

In nonruminant mammals and birds, although the HI of starch is greater than that of fat, starch/glucose should be provided in diets as a major source of energy, particularly under stress (e.g., heat stress) and disease conditions. This is because: (1) the oxidation of fatty acids in animals produces more oxidants (e.g., $H_2O_2$ and superoxide anion) than that of equal molar glucose (Chapters 5 and 6); (2) saturated fatty acids increase the risk for insulin resistance and metabolic syndrome, whereas under physiological conditions the concentration of glucose in the plasma is constant and not elevated; and (3) fatty acids, particularly polyunsaturated fatty acids, are more prone to chemical oxidation than glucose at high ambient temperatures.

### *Species Differences in HI*

The HI value is greater in ruminants than in monogastric animals (Blaxter 1989), because of the following reasons. First, greater amounts of energy are required for eating (including chewing and swallowing) and ruminating in ruminants, with the energy costs being 3%–6% and 0.3% of dietary ME intake, respectively. Second, greater movement of the gastrointestinal tract (including the rumen and the hind gut) in ruminants produces a larger amount of heat than nonruminants. The rates of the conversion of ME into NE in ruminants under various physiological conditions are as follows: maintenance, 70%–80%; lactation, 60%–70%; growth, 40%–60%; and pregnancy, 10%–25% (Bondi 1987; McDonald et al. 2011). These values are lower than those for nonruminants, as noted previously.

The disposal of nitrogenous wastes and the pathways of fat utilization in fish differ from those of mammals and birds (Chapter 7). For example, most fish lack the hepatic urea cycle and directly excrete ammonia into the surrounding water. In addition, most fish have a lower capacity to oxidize glucose and fatty acids than AAs. Smith et al. (1978) measured the HI in salmonids fed a complete diet or a purified macronutrient (fat, protein, or carbohydrate). These authors observed that heat production increased about 30 min after feeding and the increases remained elevated for 1–5 h, depending on the amount and type of the ingested material. Of interest, the HI of protein in the fish was 3%–10% of the dietary ME (depending on species) and was much lower than the HI for mammals or birds (Smith et al. 1978). This further supports the notion that high rates of urea and uric acid syntheses are the major cause of the HI associated with protein feeding to mammals and birds, respectively. Moreover, the HI of starch in fish did not differ from that of protein, but was higher than the HI of fat, as in land animals. Overall, the HI of complete diets in salmonids was <3% of the dietary ME, which is 10% of that in nonruminants and 5%–10% of the HI in ruminants. Thus, the net energy of protein is higher for fish than for mammals or birds.

NE is the portion of the food energy that is available to the animal for maintenance (e.g., sustaining the life processes; $NE_m$) and productive purposes (e.g., growth and fattening, as well as the production of milk, eggs, and wool; $NE_p$). In other words, the NE value of a food is used to sustain the BMR of an animal and to support production (e.g., tissue gain or secretions) (Baldwin and Bywater 1984). The $NE_m$ is fully converted into heat. Note that some of $NE_p$ is also converted into heat during the synthesis of fats, protein, and glycogen retained in the body and products (e.g., milk, eggs, and wool) because the efficiencies of the conversion of dietary fat into body fat and of dietary protein or AAs into body protein are always less than 100% (Table 8.7). NE represents ~80% of the ME (or ~30%–32% of the GE) in ruminants fed high-quality concentrates and in horses; ~82% of the ME (or 60%–62% of GE) in pigs; 80% of the ME (or 58%–60% of GE) in laying hens; and 90%–95% of the ME in fish (Table 8.2). In animals, lean tissue growth generally increases with increasing dietary intake of NE up to a point where the rate of protein deposition in skeletal muscle reaches a maximum as determined by the genetic capacity and environment (including nutrition) (Campbell 1988; van Milgen et al. 2001). Any additional provision of energy beyond this point will result in a marked increase in lipid deposition with only a modest increase in lean tissue gain (Campbell 1988).

#### *Factors Affecting the Dietary NE*

Factors that affect the ME value of a diet also affect its NE. In addition, NE is also influenced by the heat increment. Thus, the NE value of a feedstuff is not fixed, but varies with diets, ages, or phases of animal production and the environment (Kil et al. 2013; Tedeschi and Fox 2016). For example, for all animals, feeds with high percentages of protein and nonstarch polysaccharides usually have lower NE values than feeds with high percentages of starch and fats (Baldwin and Bywater 1984). The NE of diets for swine and ruminants is generally in the following order: growth > lactation > gestation (Bondi 1987; Pond et al. 2005). Owing to a higher energetic efficiency of fat synthesis than protein synthesis, NE is used more efficiently for fat deposition than for protein accretion in mammals, birds, fish, and shrimp.

#### *Measurement of HI*

HI, like total whole-body heat production, is often measured using direct or indirect calorimetry methods (Blaxter 1971). Direct calorimetry is simple in theory but difficult in practice. In direct

**TABLE 8.7**
**The Energetic Efficiencies of Biosynthetic Processes in Animals**

| Substrate | Product in Animal | Efficiency of Energy Transfer (%) |
|---|---|---|
| | **Fat (Tripalmitin) Synthesis** | |
| 3 mol palmitate plus 1/2 mol glucose | Fat[a] | 98.1 |
| 8 mol acetate plus 1/2 mol glucose | Fat[a] | 86.4 |
| Glucose | Fat[a] | 81.4 |
| Protein | Fat[a] | 59.0 |
| Dietary fat | Fat[a] | 98.9 |
| | **Carbohydrate Synthesis** | |
| Lactate | Glucose | 87.8 |
| Protein | Glucose | 62.3 |
| Glucose | Lactose | 97.5 |
| Glucose | Glycogen | 93.7 |
| | **Protein Synthesis** | |
| Amino acids | Protein | 80.8 |

[a] Tripalmitoylglycerol (tripalmitin).

calorimetry, the animal calorimeter is an airtight insulated chamber, in which oxygen is supplied by the flow of air, and the heat produced by the animal increases the temperature of a surrounding medium. Sensible heat is lost from the body surface to the environment by radiation, conduction, and convection (Verstegen and Henken 1987). Evaporative heat is lost from the surface of the skin and the respiratory tract. In indirect calorimetry, the magnitude of energy metabolism is estimated on the basis of the volume of $O_2$ consumed by an animal, the volume of $CO_2$ produced by the animal, and a respiratory quotient ($RQ = CO_2/O_2$) (Table 8.8). Calculation of heat production from the measurement of gaseous exchange is based on the principle that $\Delta H$ is independent of the pathway but depends only on the difference in energy between substrates and products, as explained later in this chapter.

## ENERGETIC EFFICIENCY OF METABOLIC TRANSFORMATIONS IN ANIMALS

Each of the two terminal phosphate bonds of ATP contains 51.6 kJ/mol, but a greater amount of energy (i.e., 85.4 kJ/phosphate bond) is required to form the high-energy bond (Newsholme and Leech 2009). In other words, the energy conserved through the synthesis of ATP from ADP plus Pi is 51.6 kJ/mol, and the efficiency of ATP synthesis is only 60%. Owing to these values, the energetic efficiency of substrate oxidation in cells and animals can be calculated. Examples are given for the oxidation of nutrients in mammals (Table 8.4). In general, the efficiency of metabolic transformation can be calculated as energy trapped in the product/energy value of the precursor (Bottje and Carstens 2009). Of note, the efficiency of energy transfer from the oxidation of protein to ATP in mammals and birds is about 16% and 24%, respectively, lower than that of glucose, starch, palmitate, and fat. As noted in Chapter 7, there is a greater requirement of ATP for uric acid synthesis than urea synthesis, and most fish directly release almost exclusively ammonia into the surrounding water. Thus, the energetic efficiency of the oxidation of AAs is: fish > mammals > birds.

$$\text{Efficiency of energy transfer (\%)} = \frac{\text{Energy trapped in product}}{\text{Energy value of precursor}} \times 100\%$$

**TABLE 8.8**
**Measurement of Heat Production by Animals Based on Respiratory Quotients (RQ)**

| Substrate | RQ ($CO_2/O_2$, vol/vol) | Heat of Combustion | | Heat Produced from Substrate Oxidation per L of $O_2$ Consumed | | Percentage (%) of Total Heat Produced by the Oxidation of Substrate | |
|---|---|---|---|---|---|---|---|
| | | kJ/g | kcal/g | kJ/L | kcal/L | $CH_2O$[a] | Fat[b] |
| Carbohydrate | 1.00 | 16.74 | 4.0 | 21.12 | 5.047 | 100 | 0 |
| Fat | 0.707 | 37.66 | 9.0 | 19.61 | 4.686 | 0 | 100 |
| Protein | 0.831 | 22.59 | 5.4 | 18.62 | 4.450 | – | – |
| **Mixture of Carbohydrate:Fat (g/g)** | | | | | | | |
| 15:85 | 0.751[c] | 34.52[d] | 8.25 | 19.84[e] | 4.742[f] | 16.0[a] | 84.3[b] |
| 30:70 | 0.795 | 31.38 | 7.50 | 20.06 | 4.794 | 31.6 | 68.4 |
| 40:60 | 0.824 | 29.29 | 7.00 | 20.21 | 4.830 | 47.7 | 58.3 |
| 50:50 | 0.854 | 27.20 | 6.50 | 20.36 | 4.866 | 52.0 | 48.0 |
| 60:40 | 0.883 | 25.11 | 6.00 | 20.52 | 4.904 | 61.8 | 38.2 |
| 70:30 | 0.912 | 23.02 | 5.50 | 20.67 | 4.940 | 71.5 | 28.5 |
| 85:15 | 0.956 | 19.88 | 4.75 | 20.89 | 4.993 | 85.9 | 14.1 |

*Sources:* Adapted from Kleiber, M. 1961. *The Fire of Life*. John Wiley, New York, NY; Lusk, G. 1924. *J. Biol. Chem.* 59:41–42.

*Note:* Carbohydrate ($CH_2O$) consists of 35.7% starch and 64.3% sucrose. Fat is 1-palmitoleoyl-2-oleoyl3-stearoyl-glycerol. Heat production from protein oxidation is not included in the calculations.

[a] Calculated as follows: [504.7 × (RQ – 0.707)]/[5.047 × (RQ – 0.707) + 4.686 × (1 – RQ)].

[b] Calculated as follows: [468.6 × (1 – RQ)]/[5.047 × (RQ – 0.707) + 4.686 × (1 – RQ)].

[c] Calculated as follows: (0.15×1.00) + (0.85 × 0.707) = 0.751. Values of RQ for other mixtures of carbohydrate:fat were calculated in the same manner [(i.e., proportion of carbohydrate × 1.00) + (proportion of fat × 0.707)].

[d] Calculated as follows: (0.15 × 16.74) + (0.85 × 37.66) = 34.52. Values of the heat of combustion for other mixtures of carbohydrate:fat were calculated in the same manner [i.e., proportion of carbohydrate × 16.74) + (proportion of fat × 37.66)].

[e] Calculated as follows: (0.15 × 21.12) + (0.85 × 19.61) = 19.84. Values of the heat produced from substrate oxidation per L of $O_2$ consumed for other mixtures of carbohydrate:fat were calculated in the same manner [i.e., proportion of carbohydrate × 21.12) + (proportion of fat × 19.61)].

[f] 1 kJ = 4.1842 kcal. The value (kcal/L) can also be calculated as follows: 4.686 + 0.361 × (RQ – 0.707)/0.293.

$$\text{Efficiency of energy transfer from substrate to ATP via oxidation (\%)}$$
$$= \frac{\text{Mole of net ATP produced per mole of substrate oxidize} \times 51.6\,\text{kJ/mol}}{\text{Combustion energy of substrate (kJ/mole)}} \times 100\%$$

$$\text{Efficiency of energy transfer from amino acids to protein (\%)}$$
$$= \frac{\text{Energy of protein}}{\text{Energy of amino acids + Energy of ATP or GTP needed for protein synthesis}} \times 100\%$$

As noted previously, the amount of energy required for the production of ATP from ADP and Pi is 85.4 kJ/mol ATP (McDonald et al. 2011). This constant is required for the calculation of energetic efficiencies of biosynthetic processes, which differ among different metabolic pathways (Wester 1979). The values of energetic efficiencies for the syntheses of fats, glucose, lactose, glycogen, and protein from their respective precursors are summarized in Table 8.7. The details of the calculations are provided in the following sections. Note that based on the composition of AAs in the piglet body, the average molecular weight of protein is 100 (Wu 2013). This value can be used to calculate the energetic efficiency of protein synthesis from AAs.

1. 8 mol acetate plus 1/2 mol glucose to 1 mol fat (tripalmitin) in the cytosol

| | |
|---|---|
| 8 mol acetate | 6,528 kJ |
| 8 mol acetate ---> 8 acetyl-CoA | 1,366 kJ (16 mol ATP) |
| 7 mol acetyl-CoA ---> 7 mol malonyl-CoA | 598 kJ (7 mol ATP) |
| 7 mol malonyl-CoA to 1 mol palmitate | 2,989 kJ (14 NADPH or 35 ATP) |
| 1 mol palmitate ---> 1 mol palmitoyl-CoA | 171 kJ (2 ATP) |
| Energy for the synthesis of 1 mol palmitoyl-CoA | 11,652 kJ |
| Energy for the synthesis of 3 mol palmitoyl-CoA | 34,956 kJ |
| 1/2 mol glucose | 1,402 kJ |
| 1/2 mol glucose ---> 1 mol dihydroxyacetone-P | 85.4 kJ (1 mol ATP) |
| 1 mol dihydroxyacetone ---> 1 mol glycerol-3-P | 214 kJ (1 NADH or 2.5 ATP) |
| Energy for the synthesis of 1 mol glycerol-3-P | 1,701 kJ (=1,402 + 85 + 214) |
| Total energy for the synthesis of 1 mol tripalmitin | 36,657 kJ (= 34,956 + 1,701) |
| Energy in 1 mol tripalmitin | 31,676 kJ |
| Efficiency of synthesis = | (31,676/36,657) × 100% = 86.4% |

2. 3 mol palmitate plus 1/2 mol glucose to 1 mol fat (tripalmitin) in the cytosol

| | |
|---|---|
| 3 mol palmitate | 30,093 kJ (10,031 kJ/mol) |
| 3 mol palmitate ---> 3 mol palmitoyl-CoA | 512 kJ (6 ATP) |
| Energy for the synthesis of 3 mol palmitoyl-CoA | 30,605 kJ |
| 1/2 mol glucose | 1,402 kJ |
| 1/2 mol glucose ---> 1 mol dihydroxyacetone-P | 85.4 kJ (1 mol ATP) |
| 1 mol dihydroxyacetone ---> 1 mol glycerol-3-P | 214 kJ (1 NADH or 2.5 ATP) |
| Energy for the synthesis of 1 mol glycerol-3-P | 1,701 kJ (= 1,402 + 85.4 + 214) |
| Total energy for the synthesis of 1 mol tripalmitin | 32,306 kJ (= 30,605 + 1,701) |
| Energy in 1 mol tripalmitin | 31,676 kJ |
| Efficiency of synthesis = | (31,676/32,306) × 100% = 98.1% |

3. Glucose to fat (tripalmitin) [involving both the cytosol and mitochondria (Mit)]

| | |
|---|---|
| 4 mol glucose | 11,212 kJ |
| 4 mol glucose ---> 8 pyruvate | (−8 mol ATP and −4 mol NADH) |
| 8 mol pyruvate ---> 8 mol acetyl-CoA (Mit) | (−8 mol NADH) |
| 8 mol acetyl-CoA (Mit) ---> cytosolic 8 mol acetyl-CoA | (+8 mol ATP) |
| 7 mol acetyl-CoA ---> 7 mol malonyl-CoA (cytosol) | (+7 mol ATP) |
| 7 mol malonyl-CoA to 1 mol palmitate | (+14 mol NADPH) |
| 1 mol palmitate ---> palmitoyl-CoA | (+2 mol ATP) |
| Net ATP required (9 ATP) | 769 kJ (9 ATP) |
| Net NAD(P)H required (2 mol) | 427 kJ (2 mol NAD(P)H or 5 mol ATP) |
| Energy for the synthesis of 1 mol palmitoyl-CoA | 12,408 kJ (= 11,212 + 769 + 427) |
| Energy for the synthesis of 3 mol palmitoyl-CoA | 37,224 kJ |
| 1/2 mol glucose | 1,402 kJ |

| | |
|---|---|
| 1/2 mol glucose ---> 1 mol dihydroxyacetone-P | 85.4 kJ (1 mol ATP) |
| 1 mol dihydroxyacetone ---> 1 mol glycerol-3-P | 214 kJ (1 NADH or 2.5 ATP) |
| Energy for the synthesis of 1 mol glycerol-3-P | 1,701 kJ |
| Total energy for the synthesis of 1 mol tripalmitin | 38,925 kJ (= 37,224 + 1,701) |
| Energy in 1 mol tripalmitin | 31,676 kJ |
| Efficiency of synthesis = | (31,676/38,925) × 100% = 81.4% |

4. Protein (AAs) to fat (tripalmitin) [involving both the cytosol and mitochondria (Mit)]

$C_{4.3}H_7O_{1.4}N_{1.2}$ (protein without the sulfur atom) – $C_{0.6}H_{2.4}O_{0.6}N_{1.2}$ (0.6 urea) ---> $C_{3.7}H_{4.6}O_{0.8}$

To form 8 mol pyruvate ($C_{24}$), 6.5 mol protein is required. (1 mol protein ---> 3.7 mol C or 1.23 mol pyruvate)

| | |
|---|---|
| 6.5 mol protein | 14,690 kJ (2,260 kJ/mol protein) |
| 6.5 mol protein ---> 3.9 mol urea (= 0.6×6.5) | (+25.4 mol ATP; 6.5 mol ATP/mol urea) |
| 6.5 mol protein ---> 8 mol pyruvate | (−30 mol ATP) |
| 8 mol pyruvate ---> 8 mol acetyl-CoA (Mit) | (−20 mol ATP) |
| 8 mol acetyl-CoA (Mit) ---> cytosolic 8 mol acetyl-CoA | (+8 mol ATP) |
| 7 mol acetyl-CoA ---> 7 mol malonyl-CoA (cytosol) | (+7 mol ATP) |
| 7 mol malonyl-CoA to 1 mol palmitate | (+14 mol NADPH) |
| 1 mol palmitate ---> palmitoyl-CoA | (+2 mol ATP) |
| Net ATP requirement (−7.6 mol ATP) | −649 kJ (−7.6 mol ATP) |
| NADPH required (14 mol) | 2,989 kJ (14 mol NADPH or 35 mol ATP) |
| Energy for the synthesis of 1 mol palmitoyl-CoA | 17,030 kJ (= 14,690 – 649 + 2,989) |
| Energy for the synthesis of 3 mol palmitoyl-CoA | 51,090 kJ |
| 0.811 mol protein ($C_3/C_{3.7}$ = 0.811) | 1,833 kJ |
| 0.811 mol protein ---> 0.49 mol urea | (+3.2 mol ATP; 6.5 mol ATP/mol urea) |
| 0.811 mol protein ---> 1 mol pyruvate | (−3.7 mol ATP; 4.6 mol ATP/mol protein) |
| 1 mol pyruvate ---> 1/2 glucose | (+5.5 mol ATP) |
| 1/2 mol glucose ---> 1 mol dihydroxyacetone-P | (+1 mol ATP) |
| 1 mol dihydroxyacetone ---> 1 mol glycerol-3-P | (+1 mol NADH) |
| Net ATP requirement (6 mol ATP) | 512 kJ (6 mol ATP) |
| Net NADH required (1 mol) | 214 kJ (1 mol NADH or 2.5 mol ATP) |
| Energy for the synthesis of 1 mol glycerol-3-P | 2,559 kJ (= 1,833 + 512 + 214) |
| Total energy for the synthesis of 1 mol tripalmitin | 53,649 kJ (= 51,090 + 2,559) |
| Energy in 1 mol tripalmitin | 31,676 kJ |
| Efficiency of synthesis = | (31,676/53,649) × 100% = 59.0% |

5. Dietary fat to body fat (tripalmitin)

| | |
|---|---|
| 1 mol fat (tripalmitin) | 31,676 kJ |
| 1 mol fat ---> 2 mol palmitate + 1 mol MAG | 0 kJ |
| 2 mol palmitate ---> 2 mol palmitoyl-CoA | 342 kJ (4 ATP) |
| 2 mol palmitoyl-CoA + 1 mol MAG --> tripalmitin | 0 kJ |
| Energy for the synthesis of 1 mol tripalmitin | 32,018 kJ |
| Energy in 1 mol tripalmitin | 31,676 kJ |
| Efficiency of synthesis = | (31,676/32,018) × 100% = 98.9% |

MAG = monoacylglycerol.

## 6. Lactate to glucose

| | |
|---|---|
| 2 mol lactate | 2,688 kJ |
| 2 mol pyruvate ---> 2 mol oxaloacetate | 171 kJ (2 mol ATP) |
| 2 oxaloacetate ---> 2 mol phosphoenolpyruvate | 171 kJ (2 mol GTP) |
| 2 mol 3-phosphoglycerate ---> 2 mol BPG | 171 kJ (2 mol ATP) |
| Energy for the synthesis of 1 mol glucose | 3,201 kJ |
| Energy in 1 mol glucose | 2,803 kJ |
| Efficiency of synthesis = | (2,803/3,201) × 100% = 87.8% |

BPG = 1,3-bisphosphoglycerate.

## 7. Protein to glucose

$C_{4.3}H_7O_{1.4}N_{1.2}$ (protein without the sulfur atom) – $C_{0.6}H_{2.4}O_{0.6}N_{1.2}$ (0.6 urea) ---> $C_{3.7}H_{4.6}O_{0.8}$

To form 2 mol pyruvate ($C_{24}$), 1.62 mol protein is required. (1 mol protein ---> 3.7 mol C)

| | |
|---|---|
| 1.62 mol protein | 3661 kJ (2,260 kJ/mol protein) |
| 1.62 mol protein ---> 0.97 mol urea (= 0.6×1.62) | (+6.3 mol ATP; 6.5 mol ATP/mol urea) |
| 1.62 mol protein ---> 2 mol pyruvate | (−7.5 mol ATP) |
| 2 mol pyruvate ---> 2 mol oxaloacetate | (+2 mol ATP) |
| 2 oxaloacetate ---> 2 mol phosphoenolpyruvate | (+2 mol GTP) |
| 2 mol 3-phosphoglycerate ---> 2 mol BPG | (+2 mol ATP) |
| 2 mol BPG ---> 2 mol Glyceraldehyde 3-P | (+2 mol NADH) |
| Net ATP requirement (4.8 mol ATP) | 410 kJ (4.8 mol ATP) |
| Net NADH required (2 mol) | 427 kJ (2 mol NADH or 5 mol ATP) |
| Energy for the synthesis of 1 mol glucose | 4,498 kJ (= 3,661 + 410 + 427) |
| Energy in 1 mol glucose | 2,803 kJ |
| Efficiency of synthesis = | (2,803/4,498) × 100% = 62.3% |

BPG = 1,3-bisphosphoglycerate.

## 8. Glucose to lactose

| | |
|---|---|
| 2 mol glucose | 5,606 kJ |
| 1 mol glucose ----> 1 mol glucose-1-P | 85.4 kJ (1 mol ATP) |
| 1 mol glucose-1-P ----> 1 mol UDP-Glucose | 85.4 kJ (1 mol ATP) |
| Energy for the synthesis of 1 mol lactose | 5,777 kJ |
| Energy in 1 mol lactose | 5,630 kJ |
| Efficiency of synthesis = | (5,630/5,777) × 100% = 97.5% |

## 9. Glucose to glycogen

| | |
|---|---|
| 1 mol glucose | 2,803 kJ |
| 1 mol glucose ---> 1 mol glucose-1-P | 85.4 kJ (1 mol ATP) |
| 1 mol glucose-1-P ---> 1 mol UDP-Glucose | 85.4 kJ (1 mol ATP) |
| Energy for the incorporation of 1 mol glucose | 2,974 kJ |
| Energy in 1 mol glycogen | 2,786 kJ |
| Efficiency of synthesis = | (2,786/2,974) × 100% = 93.7% |

10. AAs to protein

| | |
|---|---|
| 118 g AAs (based on AA composition in pigs) | 2,326 kJ |
| 0.5 mol ATP needed for transport of 1 mol AAs | 43 kJ (0.5 mol ATP) |
| 5 mol ATP/mol AAs (synthesis of 1 mol protein) | 427 (5 mol ATP; 85.4 kJ/mol) |
| Energy for the synthesis of 1 mol protein | 2,796 kJ (= 2,326 + 43 + 427) |
| Energy in 1 mol protein (100 g protein) | 2,260 kJ |
| Efficiency of protein synthesis = | (2,260/2,796) × 100% = 80.8% |

Energetic efficiency in the utilization of food energy by animals varies among species, physiological state, the type of production, physical activity, health status, the living environment (e.g., temperature, humidity, noise, toxins, and air pollution), and dietary composition. For example, pigs are always more efficient in utilizing dietary energy for both maintenance and production than cattle, because of lower HI in pigs than in cattle (Table 8.4). In the same species, food energy is utilized more efficiently for maintenance or lactation than for growth or fattening, and milk production is almost as efficient as maintenance in terms of energetic efficiency. This phenomenon can be explained by the following reasons. First, the rates of ATP-dependent processes (e.g., the turnover of proteins, triacylglycerols [TAGs], and glucose) at maintenance are lower than those for production, and the heat generated from nutrient oxidation by animals is used to maintain their body temperatures. Second, for production, heat is always produced when proteins, fats, and carbohydrates are synthesized from their precursors and is lost to the surroundings, and the efficiencies of these metabolic transformations are always <100%. As shown in Table 8.7, energetic efficiencies in the conversion of glucose and protein into fats are only 81% and 59%, respectively. Third, immediately after being synthesized and processed, proteins, fats, and lactose are excreted from the mammary epithelial cells into the lumen of the lactiferous duct without being subject to intracellular or extracellular degradation under normal physiological conditions. In contrast, intracellular constituent proteins in tissues (e.g., skeletal muscle, intestine, and liver), which are major DM components of animal growth, undergo continuous synthesis and degradation that require a large amount of ATP (Chapter 7). In addition, the maintenance of TAGs in white adipose tissue requires energy. Animals with exposure to air pollution inhale toxins and oxidants from the surrounding environment and also generate endogenous oxidants from metabolism; all these harmful substances can inhibit nutrient absorption, digestion, and utilization, including the oxidation of NADH and $FADH_2$ via the mitochondrial electron transport system for ATP production. Finally, fever and infection result in increased whole-body heat production (maintenance energy requirement) and, therefore, a decreased efficiency in the utilization of dietary energy for production (Baracos et al. 1987). This catabolic response, along with reduced food intake, contributes to negative energy balance in the affected host and constitutes a large metabolic cost.

It should be understood that all animals can adjust to the sub-maintenance dietary energy levels with a higher energetic efficiency than the above-maintenance requirements (Table 8.4). It is also noteworthy that some animals can adapt well to elevated environmental temperatures by lowering metabolic needs to stabilize their body weight and physiological conditions, as reported for Hereford × Boran steers in Kenya (Ledger and Sayers 1977) and Brahman (*Bos indicus*) cattle in South Asia, the United States, and Australia (Butterworth, 1985). The physiological adaptation of animals to nutrient availability and other environmental factors has important implications for livestock (e.g., cattle) and poultry (e.g., chickens) production in tropical and subtropical regions of the world.

## DETERMINATION OF HEAT PRODUCTION AS AN INDICATOR OF ENERGY EXPENDITURE BY ANIMALS

### Total Heat Production by Animals

Heat is produced by an animal via: (1) basal metabolism (maintenance); (2) gastrointestinal (GI) tract bacteria; (3) heat increment of feeding; and (4) the synthesis of fats, protein, and glycogen retained in the body and products. Fasting heat production by a food-deprived animal is a measure of its basal metabolism. In a fed animal, heat is produced from basal metabolism plus feeding-associated activities, including the digestion, absorption, and metabolism of dietary nutrients.

Small animals not only have a larger surface area than larger ones and a higher metabolic rate but also produce more heat than larger animals per kg BW. Expressed per metabolic body weight (body weigh$^{0.75}$), the rate of heat production is relatively constant throughout the animal kingdom (Baldwin 1995; Blaxter 1989). Within the same animal, different tissues have different metabolic rates and therefore exhibit different rates of heat production. This notion is exemplified by studies with rats (Table 8.9) and ruminants (Table 8.10). The percentage contribution of skeletal muscle to the whole-body fasting heat production is similar between rats and ruminants. In contrast, the percentage contribution of the digestive tract to the whole-body fasting heat production is much greater in ruminants than in rats, because of greater mass and more active fermentation in the former than in the latter (Stevens and Hume 2004). Since blood circulation provides oxygen and nutrients to tissues, the rate of blood flow is positively correlated to heat production by the tissues.

Energy needs of animals are met through the oxidation of fatty acids, glucose, and AAs in a cell- and tissue-specific manner (Jobgen et al. 2006). The oxidation of 1 mol NADH and 1 mol $FADH_2$ yields 2.5 and 2 mol ATP in mitochondria-containing cells, respectively. Thus, in all animals,

**TABLE 8.9**
**Rates of Resting Oxygen Consumption by Major Tissues of Fasted Adult Rats**

| | | $O_2$ Consumption in the Fasting State | | | Heat Production in the Fasting State | | |
|---|---|---|---|---|---|---|---|
| Whole-Body or Specific Tissue | Body Weight or Tissue Weight in a 300-g Adult Rat (g) | Rate (mL/100 g per min) | Total Amount (mL/300 g Rat per min) | % of Whole Body Fasting $O_2$ Consumption | Rate (kcal/100 g per h) | Total Amount (kcal/300 g Rat per h) | % of Whole Body Fasting Heat Production |
| Whole body | 300 | 2.0 | 6.0 | 100 | 0.576 | 1.73 | 100 |
| BAT | 0.61 | 48 | 0.293 | 4.9 | 13.8 | 0.084 | 4.9 |
| Heart | 1.53 | 19.4 | 0.297 | 5.0 | 5.59 | 0.086 | 5.0 |
| Kidneys | 2.63 | 19.1 | 0.502 | 8.3 | 5.50 | 0.145 | 8.4 |
| Liver | 10.8 | 15.9 | 1.72 | 28.7 | 4.58 | 0.495 | 28.6 |
| Brain | 1.61 | 10.3 | 0.166 | 2.8 | 2.97 | 0.048 | 2.8 |
| Small intestine | 6.10 | 6.4 | 0.390 | 6.5 | 1.84 | 0.112 | 6.5 |
| Spleen | 0.77 | 2.2 | 0.017 | 0.28 | 0.63 | 0.0049 | 0.28 |
| Testes | 3.58 | 1.7 | 0.061 | 1.0 | 0.49 | 0.018 | 1.0 |
| Lungs | 1.63 | 1.0 | 0.016 | 0.27 | 0.29 | 0.0047 | 0.27 |
| Skeletal muscle | 135 | 0.92 | 1.24 | 20.7 | 0.27 | 0.358 | 20.7 |
| WAT | 33.9 | 0.18 | 0.061 | 1.01 | 0.052 | 0.018 | 1.01 |

*Source:* Adapted from Assaad, H. et al. 2014. *Front. Biosci.* 19:967–985.

*Note:* The mean body weight of male Sprague–Dawley rats was 300 g (275–325 g). Rats were fasted for 16 h before rates of oxygen consumption by the whole body, kidneys, liver, and other tissues were measured.

BAT, brown adipose tissue; WAT, white adipose tissue.

**TABLE 8.10**
**Contributions of Tissues to Fasting Heat Production by Ruminants**

| Tissue | Percentage of Empty Body Weight (%) | Percentage of Cardiac Blood Output (%) | Percentage of Fasting Heat Production (%) |
|---|---|---|---|
| Skeletal muscle | 41 | 18 | 23.0 |
| White adipose tissue | 15 | 9.6 | 8.0 |
| Gastrointestinal tract | 6.5 | 23.0 | 9.0 |
| Skin | 6.3 | 8.0 | 2.7 |
| Nervous tissue | 2.0 | 10 | 12 |
| Liver | 1.6 | 27 | 22.5 |
| Heart | 0.6 | 4.1 | 10 |
| Kidneys | 0.3 | 13.4 | 7.0 |
| Other | 27.7 | 9.9 | 5.8 |

*Source:* Adapted from Baldwin, R.L. 1995. *Modeling Ruminant Digestion and Metabolism*. Chapman & Hall, New York, NY.

approximately 55% of the chemical energy in glucose and fatty acids is conserved in energy-rich phosphate bonds (primarily ATP), with the remaining being converted into heat (Chapters 5 and 6). The yields of ATP production from protein oxidation are ~ 46%, 42%, and 55%, respectively, in mammals, birds, and fish, with the remaining energy being converted into heat (Chapter 1). This is because of the different metabolic fates of the ammonia generated from AA oxidation in these animal species. Energy-dependent biochemical reactions and physiological processes include intracellular protein turnover, the urea cycle, gluconeogenesis, nutrient transport, various "futile cycles," Na/K-ATPase activity and ion pumping (which may account for 10% of whole-body heat production in animals), renal resorption, gut motility, as well as cardiac and skeletal muscle contractions. These processes utilize approximately one-third of the energy released from ATP hydrolysis, with the remaining chemical energy being converted into heat (Wester 1979). In cells, rates of ATP utilization are precisely matched by rates of ATP production (Dai et al. 2013). In mammals (e.g., rats and humans) possessing brown adipose tissue, its unique uncoupling protein-1 inhibits ATP synthesis from ADP and Pi, thereby dissipating all the chemical energy from mitochondrial substrate oxidation into heat (Chapter 1). Thus, the energy released from the oxidation of macronutrients is ultimately transformed into heat in animals. In other words, heat production is a useful indicator of energy expenditure by animals.

## Direct Calorimetry for Measurement of Heat Production

Direct calorimetry is used to measure the amount of heat produced by an animal enclosed within an airtight and insulated chamber (known as a calorimeter) (McDonald et al. 2011). Such a technique was first used by Antoine Lavoisier and coworkers in the late 1700s for measuring metabolic rates in animals. Specifically, this pioneer determined the heat production of a guinea pig through observing the amount of ice melted in an insulated chamber that contained both ice and the test animal. Direct calorimetry can accurately quantify the rate of heat production as an indicator of the metabolic rate in both metabolically normal and abnormal states (Kaiyala and Ramsay 2011). Heat is lost from an animal through four avenues: (1) conduction (heat transfer from the warmer animal to a cooler surface by direct contact); (2) convection (heat transfer by the bulk flow of a liquid or gas away from the animal); (3) radiation (heat transfer via long wave [3–100 μm] electromagnetic wave energy emitted by the animal) and (4) evaporation (heat transfer via the transformation of body water from the liquid to the gas phase in the respiratory passages and on the skin) (Bondi 1987). The first three types of heat loss are collectively known as sensitive heat loss.

There are four types of direct calorimeters: isothermal, heat-sink, convection, and differential (Blaxter 1989). In an isothermal direct calorimeter, its wall temperature is kept constant through the use of constant-temperature water in a jacket or bath surrounding the animal chamber. The sensitive heat loss is taken up by the water circulated through coils within the chamber, and is computed on the basis of a difference in temperatures between entry and exit water, as well as the rate of water flow. Evaporative heat loss is calculated according to a difference in moisture content between entry and exit air, as well as the volume of the air drawn through the chamber (Kaiyala and Ramsay 2011). In heat-sink direct calorimetry, the sensible heat released into the calorimeter chamber is removed via a water-cooled heat exchanger, within which water circulates through a jacket in the calorimeter walls surrounding the test animal. The transfer of dry heat from the animal is calculated on the basis of water's specific heat, flow rate, and temperature increase, but evaporative heat loss is estimated by a different method (Mclean and Tobin 1987). In direct convection calorimetry, the sensitive heat loss from an animal is determined by measuring the differences in both temperature and enthalpy between the entry and exit air, whereas evaporative heat loss is computed from the rate of gas flow and the change in the concentration of water vapor. Finally, in direct differential calorimetry, two identical chambers are used to separately house an animal and an electric heater adjusted to yield identical temperature increases in both chambers, with the heat supplied to the heater equating to heat loss from the animal (Blaxter 1989). Since it is expensive to build direct calorimetry instruments, heat production by animals is now often measured with the use of the indirect calorimetry methods described below.

## Indirect Calorimetry for Measurement of Heat Production

Indirect calorimetry is a technique that provides accurate estimates of heat production from measurements of $CO_2$ production and $O_2$ consumption by an animal, thereby eliminating the need for using a complex, delicate, and costly instrument to directly determine heat production by direct calorimetry (Blaxter 1989; Carstens et al. 1987; Lusk 1924). Advances in gas exchange measurement have made indirect calorimetry readily available for animal research. This technique is based on the principles that: (1) there are no considerable reserves of $O_2$ in animals and their uptake of $O_2$ reflects the oxidation of organic nutrients; (2) chemical energy in the body is derived from the oxidation of carbohydrates, fats, and proteins to $CO_2$ and $H_2O$; (3) the ratios of $O_2$ consumption to $CO_2$ production resulting from the oxidation of these macronutrients are constant in animals; (4) the oxidation of fatty acids, glucose, and non-nitrogenous substances to $CO_2$ and $H_2O$ in animals yields the same amounts of heat as those from combustion in a bomb calorimeter; and (5) the oxidation of protein in animals generates urea (as the major nitrogenous end-product), $CO_2$, and $H_2O$. Requirements of $O_2$ for heat production differ among macronutrients (Mclean and Tobin 1987). In mammals and birds, the consumption of 1 mol $O_2$ by the animal produces 5.00, 4.61, and 4.49 mol ATP, respectively, from the complete oxidation of 1 mol glucose, fatty acid (palmitate), and protein; in other words, the amount of $O_2$ required for the synthesis of the same amount of ATP from energy substrates is protein > fats > glucose. In fish, which release ammonia into the surrounding water, the energetic efficiency of ATP production from protein oxidation is ~ 55% (Table 8.1), which is essentially the same as that for fats and glucose.

### Closed-Circuit Indirect Calorimetry

In the closed-circuit system, the animal breathes the same air from the chamber or prefilled container (spirometer), and $CO_2$ in expired air is absorbed by a canister of soda lime (potassium hydroxide) in the breathing circuit for measurement (Mclean and Tobin 1987). An oxygen analyzer attached to the chamber or spirometer records $O_2$ uptake from changes in the system's volume. Since $O_2$ is continuously used by the animal, the chamber or environment may eventually become hypoxic in a closed-circuit system, thus limiting the period of the RQ measurement.

### Open-Circuit Indirect Calorimetry

In the open-circuit system, the animal inhales ambient air with a constant composition of $O_2$ (e.g., 20.93%), $CO_2$ (e.g., 0.04%), and $N_2$ (e.g., 79.04%), and expired gases are then analyzed (Assaad et al. 2014). The changes in $O_2$ and $CO_2$ percentages in expired air, compared with those in inspired ambient air, indirectly reflect rates of energy metabolism in the body. Additionally, in the open-circuit system, air flows through the chamber at a rate that constantly replenishes the $O_2$ depleted by the animal while simultaneously removing the $CO_2$ and water vapor produced by the animal (Mclean and Tobin 1987). Owing to its convenience, computer-controlled open-circuit indirect calorimetry is now widely used for measuring energy expenditure in animals for hours or days (Assaad et al. 2014).

RQ is defined as the ratio of the volume of $CO_2$ produced (L/kg BW per h) to the volume of $O_2$ consumed (L/kg BW per h).

Respiratory Quotient (RQ) = moles of $CO_2$ produced/moles of $O_2$ consumed

$$1 \text{ mole of gas} = 22.41 \text{ L}$$

The function of the lungs should be normal to obtain accurate values of $O_2$ consumption and $CO_2$ production by animals. HP is then calculated from the values of $O_2$ consumption and $CO_2$ production according to the Brouwer (1965) equation:

$$\text{HP (kcal)} = 3.82 \times VO_2 \text{ (in L)} + 1.15 \times VCO_2 \text{ (in L)}$$

If the unit of $VO_2$ and $VCO_2$ is L/kg BW per h, the unit of heat production should be kcal/kg BW per h.

When AA oxidation and the urinary excretion of nitrogen are considered, $\Delta H$ (kJ/mol) = 16.34 $VO_2$ (L) + 4.50 $VCO_2$ (L) – 3.92 N (g). The calculations are shown in Table 8.11. The coefficients for calculating heat production based on the metabolic data on $O_2$ consumption, $CO_2$ production, urinary nitrogen excretion, and methane production in different animals are summarized in Table 8.12. Note that the production of large amounts of methane by ruminants and horses should be taken into consideration in estimating whole-body heat production.

## COMPARATIVE SLAUGHTER TECHNIQUE FOR ESTIMATING HEAT PRODUCTION

The comparative slaughter technique can be used to estimate whole-body heat production by animals, as well as their energy requirement for maintenance and growth (Tedeschi et al. 2002). Let

**TABLE 8.11**
**$\Delta H$, $O_2$ Consumption, and $CO_2$ Production by Animals**

| Compound | $\Delta H$ (Animal) (kJ/mol) | $O_2$ Consumed (mol, a) | $CO_2$ Produced (mol, b) | N Excreted (mol, c) | Equation |
|---|---|---|---|---|---|
| Glucose | 2803 | 6 | 6 | 0 | 2803 = 6a + 6b + 0c |
| Palmitic acid | 10,039 | 23 | 16 | 0 | 10,039 = 23a + 16b + 0c |
| Alanine | 1296 | 3 | 2.5 | 1 | 1296 = 3a + 2.5b – 1c |

*Source:* Blaxter, K.L. 1989. *Energy Metabolism in Animals and Man.* Cambridge University Press, Cambridge, UK.

*Note:* Solving the three equations gives: a = 366.3 kJ/mol $O_2$ (or 16.34 kJ/L $O_2$), b = 100.8 kJ/mol $CO_2$ (or 4.50 kJ/L $CO_2$), and c = −54.9 kJ/mol N (or −3.92 kJ/g N). Thus, $\Delta H$ (kJ/mol) = 16.34 $VO_2$ (L) + 4.50 $VCO_2$ (L) – 3.92 N (g).

Note that when the oxidation of sucrose, oleic acid, and glutamate is considered, a = 355.7 kJ/mol $O_2$ (or 15.87 kJ/L $O_2$), b = 114.8 kJ/mol $CO_2$ (or 5.12 kJ/L $CO_2$), and c = 107.3 kJ/mol N (or 7.66 kJ/g N). $\Delta H$ (kJ/mol) = 15.87 $VO_2$ (L) + 5.12 $VCO_2$ (L) – 7.66 N (g).

**TABLE 8.12**
**Coefficients for Estimating Heat Production Based on Metabolic Data in Animals**[a]

| Authors | $O_2$ Consumption (kJ/L) | $CO_2$ Production (kJ/L) | Urinary N Excretion (kJ/g) | Methane Production (kJ/L) | Heat Production (MJ/day) |
|---|---|---|---|---|---|
| | | | **Nonruminant Mammals (Including Man)** | | |
| Blaxter (1989)[b] | 16.20 | 4.94 | −5.80 | – | 9.99 |
| Weir (1949) | 16.50 | 4.63 | −9.08 | – | 9.96 |
| Ben-Porat et al. (1983) | 16.37 | 4.57 | −13.98 | – | 9.80 |
| Brockway (1987) | 16.57 | 4.50 | −5.90 | – | 10.00 |
| | | | **Ruminants (Cattle and Sheep)** | | |
| Blaxter (1989) | 16.07 | 5.23 | −5.26 | −2.40 | 10.04 |
| Brouwer (1965) | 16.18 | 5.16 | −5.93 | −2.42 | 10.01 |
| | | | **Birds** | | |
| Farrell (1974) | 16.20 | 5.00 | −1.20 | – | 10.08 |

*Source:* Ben-Porat, M. S. et al. 1983. *Am. J. Physiol.* 244:R764–769; Blaxter, K.L. 1989. *Energy Metabolism in Animals and Man.* Cambridge University Press, New York, NY; Brockway, J.M. 1987. *Human Nutrition: Clinical Nutrition.* 41C:463–471; Brouwer, E. 1965. *Energy Metabolism.* edited by K.L. Blaxter, Academic Press, London. pp. 441–443; Farrell, D.J. 1974. *Energy Requirements of Poultry*, edited by T.R. Morris, and B.M. Freeman, British Poultry Science Ltd., Edinburgh, U.K., pp. 1–24; Weir, J.B. 1949. *J. Physiol. (London)* 109:1–9.

[a] The coefficients for the whole bodies of different animal species are derived from the equations in Table 8.11.

[b] The heat production was calculated for an $O_2$ consumption of 500 L/day, a $CO_2$ production of 400 L/day, and a urinary nitrogen (N) excretion of 15 g/day.

us use cockerels (male chickens) as an example (Fuller et al. 1983). When the birds were fed a diet providing an ME of 2255 kJ over a period of 4 days, they gained 68 g body weight (final body weight of 2823 g – initial body weight of 2755 g), which is equivalent to 679 kJ (i.e., NE for growth). Assuming that methane production is negligible, heat production (including heat increment, maintenance energy requirement, and intermediary metabolism) by the birds is calculated to be 1576 kJ (2255–679 = 1567) during 4 days. Analysis of gaseous exchange data from open-circuit indirect calorimetry indicated the heat production of 1548 kJ by the same animals. Thus, the efficiency of ME for growth in the 2.8 kg cockerels is 30%. Owing to its ability to directly measure net tissue gains over an experimental period, the comparative slaughter method is considered as the gold standard for determining the NE content of feeds for animals (Kil et al. 2011; McDonald et al. 2011).

### Lean Tissues and Energy Expenditure

The metabolic rate of an animal is not linearly proportional to its body weight or tissue mass (Campbell 1988). Additionally, relationships between metabolic rate and body weight differ between small and large mammals (Blaxter 1971). This complex picture is further complicated by the fact that different tissues have different rates of metabolism, heat production, or $O_2$ consumption per kg tissue weight (e.g., heart > kidney > liver > small intestine > skeletal muscle > white adipose tissue) (Table 8.9). Interestingly, the brain, liver, heart, kidneys, and small intestine account for 7.6% of the body weight but 51.4% of whole-body $O_2$ consumption in nonruminants. In ruminants, the digestive tract and liver, which are highly active in fermentation and metabolism, can contribute to as much as 50% of total heat production of the whole body (Table 8.10). Although the rate of $O_2$ consumption or energy expenditure per kg tissue in resting skeletal muscle is much lower than that for internal organs, this tissue contributes to 20.7% of the whole-body $O_2$ consumption due to its large mass. In contrast, white adipose tissue accounts for 12.4% of the body weight but only 1% of the whole-body $O_2$ consumption or heat production due to its low metabolic rate. Thus, there is considerable debate about an appropriate way to express data on $O_2$ consumption, $CO_2$ production, and energy expenditure by animals (Even and Nadkarni 2012).

The weights of internal organs (other than white adipose tissues) and skeletal muscle are relatively constant per kg BW, but the weight of white adipose tissue is substantially increased in obese animals compared with lean animals (Jobgen et al. 2006). Thus, expression of whole-body $O_2$ consumption or heat production data per kg BW or metabolic weight (the BW raised to the power of 0.75) may lead to an underestimation of metabolic activities (including energy expenditure) in the fat-free tissues or lean body mass of obese animals (Assaad et al. 2014). Therefore, the simple division of metabolism variables by BW or metabolic weight does not provide accurate information to compare true metabolic rates between normal-weight and obese animals. A solution to overcoming this problem is to determine body composition, including the weights of white adipose tissue, brown adipose tissue, and other major $O_2$-consuming tissues in each animal. Then, data on rates of energy metabolism in animals fed the low fat or high fat diet can be more accurately expressed per kg non-fat mass. If the weights of non-white fat tissues (e.g., skeletal muscle, liver, heart, kidneys, small intestine, and brown adipose tissue) do not differ between low fat- and high fat-fed animals, data on energy metabolism (i.e., rates of $O_2$ consumption, $CO_2$ production, and heat production) can be expressed per animal to indicate its metabolic activity (Assaad et al. 2014). However, this is not the case, because the non-fat masses of some tissues (e.g., skeletal muscle, heart, liver, and kidneys) are increased in high fat-fed animals than in low fat-fed animals. When the rates of whole-body $O_2$ consumption or energy expenditure are expressed per kg body weight, data should be interpreted as such.

## Usefulness of RQ Values in Assessing Substrate Oxidation in Animals

Owing to the different composition of C, O, and H in glucose, fatty acids, and protein, the oxidation or synthesis of these nutrients gives different RQ values (Kleiber 1961). Thus, RQ can reveal information on the nature of oxidation of energy substrates or about anabolic pathways in animals (Table 8.13). For example, RQ is 1.00 and 0.70 for the oxidation of glucose and fatty acids, respectively. In addition, RQ values between 0.80 and 0.85 implicate oxidation of fatty acids, glucose, and AAs to $CO_2$ and water. Furthermore, RQ values between 0.67 and 0.70 suggest that animals mobilize fat stores, providing fatty acids for oxidation and glycerol for gluconeogenesis. In animals, oxidation of glucose, fatty acids, and AAs occurs simultaneously in a cell- and tissue-specific manner. The

**TABLE 8.13**
**Respiratory Quotients (RQ) for Substrate Oxidation and for Synthetic Pathways in Animals**

| Oxidation to $CO_2$ and $H_2O$ | RQ Value | Synthetic Pathways | RQ Value |
|---|---|---|---|
| Glucose | 1.00 | Glucose to fatty acids[c] | 8.00 |
| Glycerol | 0.857 | Glucose to fat[b] | 2.05 |
| Protein[a] | 0.831 | Protein to fat[b] | 1.26 |
| Fat[b] | 0.703–0.710 | Protein to fatty acids[c] | 1.22 |
| Fatty acids[c] | 0.696 | Glycerol to glucose | 0.667 |
| Ethanol | 0.667 | Protein or AAs to glucose | 0.333 |

[a] Protein ($C_{4.3}H_7O_{1.4}N_{1.2}$).
[b] RQ = 1 for tripalmitoylglycerol ($C_{51}O_6H_{98}$), and RQ = 0.710 for trioleoylglycerol.
[c] Palmitate.

contribution of each substrate to the whole-body $O_2$ consumption can be calculated on the basis of RQ values (Table 10.6).

RQ values for oxidation of glucose, fatty acids, fat, and protein can be calculated based on the established biochemical reactions. Examples are given as follows:

1. For glucose oxidation:
   $C_6H_{12}O_6 + 6\ O_2$ -----> $6\ CO_2 + 6\ H_2O$
   $RQ = 6\ CO_2/6\ O_2 = 1.00$
2. For fatty acid oxidation (e.g., palmitate):
   $C_{16}H_{32}O_2 + 23\ O_2$ -----> $16\ CO_2 + 16\ H_2O$
   $RQ = 16\ CO_2/23\ O_2 = 0.696$
3. For fat (tripalmitoylglycerol) oxidation:
   Oxidation of tripalmitoylglycerol (tripalmitin, Chapter 3):
   $C_{51}H_{98}O_6 + 72.5\ O_2$ -----> $51\ CO_2 + 49\ H_2O$
   $RQ = 51\ CO_2/72.5\ O_2 = 0.703$
   Oxidation of 1-palmitoleoyl-2-oleoyl3-stearoyl-glycerol (Chapter 3)
   $C_{55}H_{103}O_6 + 77.75\ O_2$ -----> $55\ CO_2 + 51.5\ H_2O$
   $RQ = 55\ CO_2/77.75\ O_2 = 0.707$
   Oxidation of trioleoylglycerol (triolein, Chapter 3):
   $C_{57}H_{105}O_6 + 80.25\ O_2$ -----> $57\ CO_2 + 52.5\ H_2O$
   $RQ = 57\ CO_2/80.25\ O_2 = 0.710$
4. For protein oxidation:
   $C_{4.3}H_7O_{1.4}N_{1.2}$ (protein)
   Oxidation of 1.2 mole of N to 0.6 mole of urea ($CH_4ON_2$)
   $C_{4.3}H_7O_{1.4}N_{1.2}$ (protein) – $C_{0.6}H_{2.4}O_{0.6}N_{1.2}$ (0.6 mole of urea) ----> $C_{3.7}H_{4.6}O_{0.8}$
   $C_{3.7}H_{4.6}O_{0.8} + 4.45\ O_2$ ---------> $3.7\ CO_2 + 2.3\ H_2O$
   $RQ = 3.7\ CO_2/4.45\ O_2 = 0.831$

RQ values for the syntheses of fatty acids, fat, glucose, and protein can also be calculated based on the established biochemical reactions (Table 8.8). Examples are given as follows:

1. Fatty acid synthesis from glucose:
   $4\ C_6H_{12}O_6 + O_2$ -----> $C_{16}H_{32}O_2 + 8\ CO_2 + 8\ H_2O$
   $RQ = 8\ CO_2/1\ O_2 = 8$
   Fat (e.g., tripalmitoylglycerol; $C_{51}O_6H_{98}$) synthesis from glucose:
   $31\ C_6H_{12}O_6 + 41\ O_2$ ------> $2\ C_{51}O_6H_{98} + 84\ CO_2 + 88\ H_2O$
   $RQ = 84\ CO_2/41\ O_2 = 2.05$
2. Glucose synthesis from protein:
   After oxidation of protein nitrogen to urea, $C_{3.7}H_{4.6}O_{0.8}$ is available for glucose synthesis.
   $C_{3.7}H_{4.6}O_{0.8} + 2.1\ O_2 + 2\ H^+$ ------> $0.5\ C_6H_{12}O_6 + 0.7\ CO_2 + 0.6\ H_2O$
   $RQ = 0.7\ CO_2/2.1\ O_2 = 0.333$
3. Glucose synthesis from glycerol:
   $3\ C_3H_8O_3 + 4.5\ O_2$ ------> $C_6H_{12}O_6 + 3\ CO_2 + 6\ H_2O$
   $RQ = 3\ CO_2/4.5\ O_2 = 0.667$

### Caution in the Interpretation of RQ Values

In order for an RQ value to accurately indicate the metabolism of animals, they must have a healthy respiratory system to inhale $O_2$ and exhale $CO_2$ (Blaxter 1989; Kleiber 1961). The following issues should be borne in mind in using indirect calorimetry to determine heat production by animals. First, there may be differences in $CO_2$ produced and $CO_2$ exhaled by the animal during a period of time due

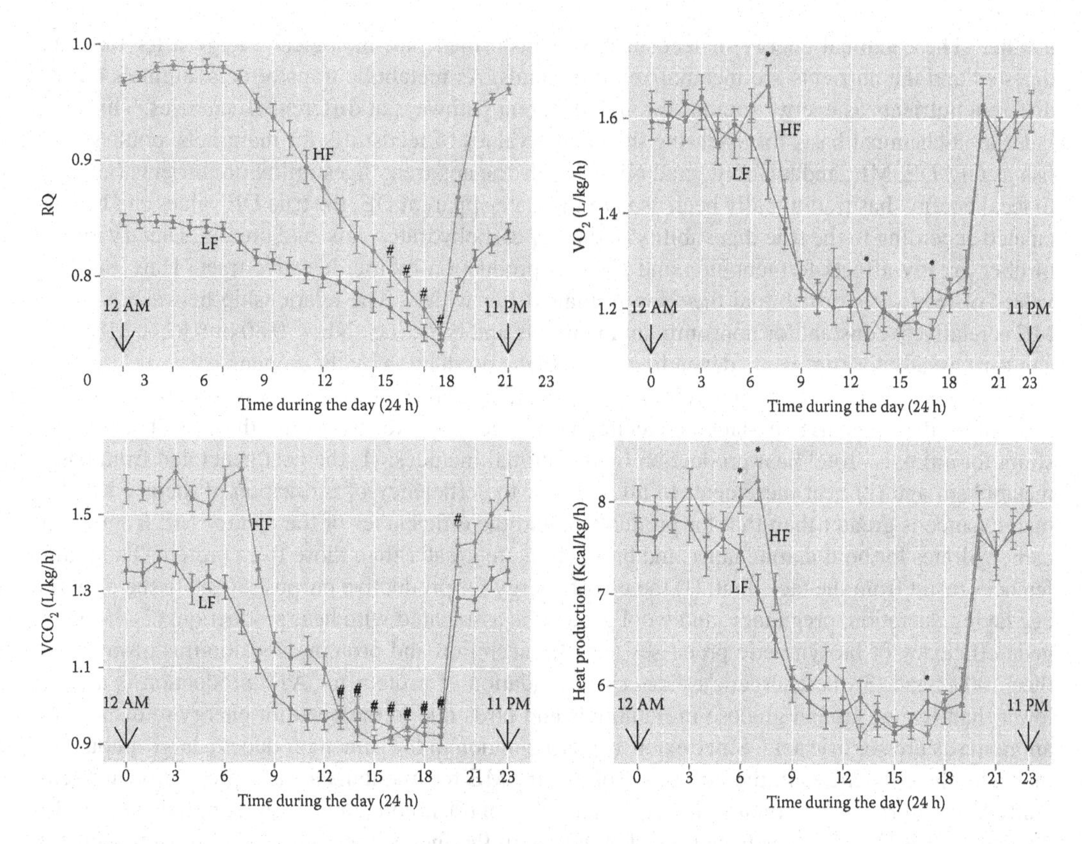


**FIGURE 8.3** Energy metabolism of male Sprague–Dawley rats (Charles River Laboratories) fed a low-fat (LF) or high-fat (HF) diet. Rats were fed an LF or HF diet between 4 and 13 weeks of age. At 13 weeks of age, rats were placed in a computer-controlled Oxymax instrument (an open circuit calorimeter; Columbus Instruments, OH) to measure 24-h $O_2$ consumption, $CO_2$ production, RQ, and heat production. Values are mean ± SEM during the day (24 h) at the end of the study. There were 16 rats per diet group, which consumed food at night. The feeding time was between 7:00 p.m. and 6:00 a.m. The sign "*" denotes a significant effect of diet at the indicated time point ($P < 0.05$). The sign "#" denotes no significant effect of diet at the indicated time point. (Adapted from Assaad, H. et al. 2014. *Front. Biosci.* 19:967–985. Copyright 2014, with permission from Frontiers in Bioscience.)

to pulmonary dysfunction (i.e., respiratory acidosis) or metabolic alkalosis. Second, in ruminants, the $CO_2$ and methane produced through anaerobic fermentation by the rumen cannot be distinguished from those produced through oxidative metabolism by the body tissues. This may also be a problem for obese animals which may have a greater population of anaerobes in the gastrointestinal tract than their nonobese counterparts (Zhao 2013). Third, when large amounts of ketone bodies are synthesized from acetyl-CoA, $O_2$ is consumed but no $CO_2$ is produced (RQ = 0 for fatty acid oxidation through ketogenesis). Finally, there are diurnal changes in RQ among animals due to different metabolic activities at different times, as shown for rats (Figure 8.3). Thus, a short-term measurement of RQ may not be valid, depending on the time relative to the last feeding (Assaad et al. 2014).

## SUMMARY

Energy is an important concept in nutrition and may be defined as the capacity for doing work. Energy itself is not a nutrient but is contained within nutrients, primarily carbohydrates, lipids, protein, and AAs. According to the first law of thermodynamics, energy is conserved in any system. Specifically, energy is neither created nor destroyed, but is interconverted from one form into another. The chemical energy of feedstuffs is transformed into biological energy after they are digested and the nutrients are metabolized in animals. As metabolic transformers, animals utilize different nutrients as energy sources through different pathways at different efficiencies. This provides a biochemical basis for assessing the energy values of feedstuffs for mammals, poultry, and fish as GE, DE, ME, and NE ($NE_m$ and $NE_g$). While the apparent digestibility of nutrients (leading to fecal energy) has traditionally been used to estimate apparent DE, the true DE values can be calculated according to the true digestibility of dietary carbohydrates, fats, and protein. Dietary intake of fiber greatly affects fermentation and gaseous production by the digestive tract. Thus, the ME values of feedstuffs or habitual diets for animals differ widely. The relationship between NE and ME is relatively constant for nonruminant mammals and birds (i.e., NE = 0.80 or 0.82 × ME), but can vary greatly for ruminants depending on methane production by the rumen.

The measurement of heat production by direct calorimetry, indirect calorimetry (based on RQ values), or the comparative slaughter technique is necessary to determine the NE of any feedstuffs for animals. Total heat production by the animal includes: (1) the heat generated from basal metabolism and (2) heat increment. In all animals, the efficiency of utilization of dietary ME for maintenance is greater than that for production, and the efficiencies of the dietary ME from fat or carbohydrates for both maintenance and production are greater than those from protein. These differences result from the facts that: (1) the use of energy for productive purposes (e.g., tissue growth, egg laying, lactation, pregnancy, and wool growth) is associated with heat production; (2) the energetic efficiency of biosynthetic processes (e.g., fat accretion and protein deposition) is always less than 100%; and (3) the energetic efficiency of oxidation of protein for ATP production is always lower than that of fat and glucose in mammals and birds due to the need for energy to dispose of ammonia as urea or uric acid. Since extensive fermentation in the rumen produces a large amount of methane, the efficiencies in the utilization of dietary ME for maintenance and production are generally lower in ruminants than in nonruminants. In contrast, compared with mammals and birds, fish have a greater NE value because of low HI. With the increasing inclusion of nonconventional feedstuffs in animal diets, the use of NE will better predict the efficiency of dietary energy for both maintenance and production and therefore precise formulation of diets. Improving the efficiency of utilization of dietary energy is essential to reduce the costs of animal production and resource use, thereby sustaining the global livestock, poultry, and aquaculture industries.

## REFERENCES

Assaad, H., K. Yao, C.D. Tekwe, S. Feng, F.W. Bazer, L. Zhou, R.J. Carroll, C.J. Meininger, and G. Wu. 2014. Analysis of energy expenditure in diet-induced obese rats. *Front. Biosci.* 19:967–985.

Baldwin, R.L. 1995. *Modeling Ruminant Digestion and Metabolism.* Chapman & Hall, New York, NY.

Baldwin, R.L. and A.C. Bywater. 1984. Nutritional energetics of animals. *Annu. Rev. Nutr.* 4:101–114.

Baracos, V.E., W.T. Whitmore, and R. Gale. 1987. The metabolic cost of fever. *Can. J. Physiol. Pharmacol.* 65:1248–1254.

Ben-Porat, M., S. Sideman, and S. Bursztein. 1983. Energy metabolism rate equations for fasting and post-absorptive subjects. *Am. J. Physiol.* 244:R764–769.

Blaxter, K.L. 1971. Methods of measuring the energy metabolism and interpretation of results obtained. *Fed. Proc.* 30:1436–1443.

Blaxter, K.L. 1989. *Energy Metabolism in Animals and Man.* Cambridge University Press, Cambridge, U.K.

Bondi, A.A. 1987. *Animal Nutrition.* John Wiley & Sons, New York, NY.

Bottje, W.G. and G.E. Carstens. 2009. Association of mitochondrial function and feed efficiency in poultry and livestock species. *J. Anim. Sci.* 87 (Suppl. 14):E48–63.

Brockway, J.M. 1987. Derivation of formulae used to calculate energy expenditure in man. *Hum. Nutr.: Clin. Nutr.* 41C:463–471.

Brown, T.L., H.E. LeMay Jr, B.E. Bursten, and J.R. Burdge. 2003. *Chemistry: The Central Science.* Prentice Hall, Upper Saddle River, New Jersey.

Brouwer, E. 1965. Report of sub-committee on constants and factors. *Energy Metabolism.* In: Edited by K.L. Blaxter, Academic Press, London, UK., pp. 441–443.

Butterworth M.H. 1985. *Beef Cattle Nutrition and Tropical Pastures.* Longman Inc., New York,

Campbell, R.G. 1988. Nutritional constraints to lean tissue accretion in farm animals. *Nutr. Res. Rev.* 1:233–253.

Carstens, G.E., D.E. Johnson, M.D. Holland, and K.G. Odde. 1987. Effects of prepartum protein nutrition and birth weight on basal metabolism in bovine neonates. *J. Anim. Sci.* 65:745–751.

Clark, S.A., O. Davulcu, and M.S. Chapman. 2012. Crystal structures of arginine kinase in complex with ADP, nitrate, and various phosphagen analogs. *Biochem. Biophys. Res. Commun.* 427:212–217.

Clarke, A. and N.M. Johnston. 1999. Scaling of metabolic rate with body mass and temperature in teleost fish. *J. Anim. Ecol.* 68:893–905.

Cox, J.D. and G. Pilcher. 1970. *Thermochemistry of Organic and Organometallic Compounds.* Academic Press, New York. pp. 1–643.

Dai, Z.L., Z.L. Wu, Y. Yang, J.J. Wang, M.C. Satterfield, C.J. Meininger, F.W. Bazer, and G. Wu. 2013. Nitric oxide and energy metabolism in mammals. *BioFactors* 39:383–391.

de Lange, C.F.M. and S.H. Birkett. 2005. Characterization of useful energy content in swine and poultry feed ingredients. *Can. J. Anim. Sci.* 85:269–280.

Even, P.C. and N.A. Nadkarni. 2012. Indirect calorimetry in laboratory mice and rats: Principles, practical considerations, interpretation and perspectives. *Am. J. Physiol. Regul. Integr. Comp. Physiol.* 303:R459–476.

Farrell, D.J. 1974. General principles and assumptions of calorimetry. In: *Energy Requirements of Poultry.* Edited by T.R. Morris, and B.M. Freeman, British Poultry Science Ltd., Edinburgh, U.K., pp. 1–24.

Fuller, H.L., N.M. Dale, and C.F. Smith. 1983. Comparison of heat production of chickens measured by energy balance and by gaseous exchange. *J. Nutr.* 113:1403–1408.

Hargrove, J.L. 2007. Does the history of food energy units suggest a solution to "Calorie confusion"? *Nutr. J.* 6:44.

Hintz, H.F. 1975. Digestive physiology of the horse. *J. S. Afr. Vet. Assoc.* 46:13–7.

International Bureau of Weights and Measures (IBWM), 2006. *The International System of Units (SI).* Stedi Media, Paris, France.

Jobgen, W.S., S.K. Fried, W.J. Fu, C.J. Meininger, and G. Wu. 2006. Regulatory role for the arginine-nitric oxide pathway in metabolism of energy substrates. *J. Nutr. Biochem.* 17:571–588.

Johnson, D.E., K.A. Johnson, and R.L. Baldwin. 1990. Changes in liver and gastrointestinal tract energy demands in response to physiological workload in ruminants. *J. Nutr.* 120:649–655.

Kaiyala, K.J. and D.S. Ramsay. 2011. Direct animal calorimetry, the underused gold standard for quantifying the fire of life. *Comp. Biochem. Physiol. A* 158:252–264.

Kil, D.Y., F. Ji, L.L. Stewart, R.B. Hinson, A.D. Beaulieu, G.L. Allee, J.F. Patience, J.E. Pettigrew, and H.H. Stein. 2011. Net energy of soybean oil and choice white grease in diets fed to growing and finishing pigs. *J. Anim. Sci.* 89:448–459.

Kil, D.Y., B.G. Kim, and H.H. Stein. 2013. Feed energy evaluation for growing pigs. *Asian-Australas. J. Anim. Sci.* 26:1205–1217.

Kleiber, M. 1961. *The Fire of Life.* John Wiley, New York, NY.

Le Goff, G. and J. Noblet. 2001. Comparative total tract digestibility of dietary energy and nutrients in growing pigs and adult sows. *J. Anim. Sci.* 79:2418–2427.

Ledger, H.P. and A.R. Sayers. 1977. The utilization of dietary energy by steers during periods of restricted food intake and subsequent re-alimentation. 1. The effect of time on the maintenance requirements of steers held at constant five weights. *J. Agric. Sci.* 88:11–26.

Lobley, G.E. 1990. Energy metabolism reactions in ruminant muscle: Responses to age, nutrition and hormonal status. *Reprod. Nutr. Dev.* 30:13–34.

Lodish, H., A. Berk, S.L. Zipursky, P. Matsudaira, D. Baltimore, and J. Darnell. 2000. *Molecular Cell Biology*, 4th ed. W. H. Freeman, New York, NY.

Lusk, G. 1924. Animal calorimetry. Analysis of the oxidation of the mixture of carbohydrate and fat. *J. Biol. Chem.* 59:41–42.

McDonald, P., R.A. Edwards, J.F.D. Greenhalgh, C.A. Morgan, and L.A. Sinclair. 2011. *Animal Nutrition*, 7th ed. Prentice Hall, New York.

McDonald, P., R.A. Edwards, J.F.D. Greenhalgh, and C.A. Morgan. 2002. *Animal Nutrition*, 6th ed. Prentice Hall, New York.

Mclean, J. and G. Tobin. 1987. *Animal and Human Calorimetry.* Cambridge University Press, Cambridge, UK.

Milligan, L.P. 1970. Energy efficiency and metabolic transformations. *Fed. Proc.* 30:1454–1458.

Milligan, L.P. and M. Summers. 1986. The biological basis of maintenance and its relevance to assessing responses to nutrients. *Proc. Nutr. Soc.* 45:185–193.

Moughan, P. J., Verstegen, M. W. A. and Visser-Reyneveld, M. 2000. *Feed Evaluation—Principles and Practice.* Wageningen Academic Publishing, Wageningen, the Netherlands.

National Research Council (NRC). 2012. *Nutrient Requirements of Swine.* National Academy Press, Washington, DC.

Newsholme, E.A. and T.R. Leech. 2009. *Functional Biochemistry in Health and Disease.* John Wiley & Sons, West Sussex, UK.

Noblet, J. and M. Etienne. 1987. Metabolic utilization of energy and maintenance requirements in lactating sows. *J. Anim. Sci.* 64:774–781.

Noblet, J., X.S. Shi, and S. Dubois. 1994. Effect of body weight on net energy value of feeds for growing pigs. *J. Anim. Sci.* 72:648–657.

Pond, W.G., D.B. Church, K.R. Pond, and P.A. Schoknecht. 2005. *Basic Animal Nutrition and Feeding*, 5th ed. Wiley, New York.

Pond, W.G., K.R. Pond, and D.B. Church. 1995. *Basic Animal Nutrition and Feeding*, 4th Ed. Wiley, New York.

Qaisrani, S.N., M.M. van Krimpen, R.P. Kwakkel, M.W.A. Verstegen, and W.H. Hendriks. 2015. Dietary factors affecting hindgut protein fermentation in broilers: A review. *World Poult. Sci. J.* 71:139–160.

Ralston, S.L. 1984. Controls of feeding in horses. *J. Anim. Sci.* 59:1354–1361.

Sibbald, I.R. 1982. Measurement of bioavailable energy in poultry feeding stuffs. *Can. J. Anim. Sci.* 62:983–1048.

Smith, R.R., G.L. Rumsey, and M.L. Scott. 1978. Heat increment associated with dietary protein, fat, carbohydrate and complete diets in salmonids: Comparative energetic efficiency. *J. Nutr.* 108:1025–1032.

Speakman, J.R. 2005. Body size, energy metabolism and lifespan. *J. Exp. Biol.* 208:1717–1730.

Stevens, C.E. and I.D. Hume. 2004. *Comparative Physiology of the Vertebrate Digestive System.* Cambridge University Press, New York, NY.

Tedeschi, L.O. and D.G. Fox. 2016. *The Ruminant Nutrition System: An Applied Model for Predicting Nutrient Requirements and Feed Utilization in Ruminants.* XanEdu, Acton, MA.

Tedeschi, L.O., C. Boin, D.G. Fox, P.R. Leme, G.F. Alleoni, and D.P. Lanna. 2002. Energy requirement for maintenance and growth of Nellore bulls and steers fed high-forage diets. *J. Anim. Sci.* 80:1671–1682.

van Milgen, J., N. Quiniou, and J. Noblet. 2000. Modelling the relation between energy intake and protein and lipid deposition in growing pigs. *Anim. Sci.* 71:119–130.

van Milgen, J., J. Noblet, and S. Dubois. 2001. Energetic efficiency of starch, protein and lipid utilization in growing pigs. *J. Nutr.* 131:1309–1318.

Verstegen, M.W.A. and A.M. Henken. 1987. *Energy Metabolism in Farm Animals.* Springer, New York, NY.

Velayudhan, D.E., I.H. Kim, and C.M. Nyachoti. 2015. Characterization of dietary energy in swine feed and feed ingredients: A review of recent research results. *Asian-Australas J. Anim. Sci.* 28:1–13.

Weir, J.B. 1949. New methods of calculating metabolic rate with special references to protein metabolism. *J. Physiol. (London)* 109:1–9.

Wester, A.J.F. 1979. The energetic efficiency of metabolism. *Proc. Nutr. Soc.* 40:121–128.

Wu, G. 2013. *Amino Acids: Biochemistry and Nutrition.* CRC Press, Boca Raton.

Wu, Z., D. Li, Y. Ma, Y. Yu, and J. Noblet. 2007. Evaluation of energy systems in determining the energy cost of gain of growing-finishing pigs fed diets containing different levels of dietary fat. *Arch. Anim, Nutr.* 61:1–9.

Zhao, L.P. 2013. The gut microbiota and obesity: From correlation to causality. *Nat. Rev. Microbiol.* 11:639–647.

# 9 Nutrition and Metabolism of Vitamins

Vitamins are organic compounds required in small amounts for normal metabolism and growth of animals and humans. Hopkins (1912) demonstrated that a synthetic diet containing purified casein, lard, sucrose, starch, and inorganic salts was inadequate for the growth of young rats, but adding a small quantity of milk (4.7 calories/g diet) to this synthetic diet helped the animals grow normally. The term "accessory factors," which were thought to contain amino nitrogen and be essential for animal growth, were named "vitamines" (meaning vital amines) by Casimir Funk in the same year. It is now known that only a few vitamins contain amino nitrogen (Berdanier 1998). The seminal finding of Hopkins challenged the dogma held at the time that only four nutritional factors were essential for animals: proteins, carbohydrates, fats, and minerals.

Although the discovery of vitamins dates back to the beginning of the twentieth century, the association between certain diseases and vitamin deficiencies was recognized much earlier (Semba 2012). For example, at the beginning of the seventeenth century, the beneficial effect of lemon in preventing and curing scurvy in humans was known. In 1753, Lind, a British naval physician, reported that scurvy in humans could be prevented by inclusion of salads and fruits in the diet. At the end of the nineteenth century, Eijkmann found that the disease beriberi in humans could be cured by giving the patients brown rice grain rather than polished rice. However, only after the discovery of vitamins, it was recognized that their specific deficiencies result in characteristic diseases, such as scurvy, beriberi, rickets, pellagra, and xerophthalmia (Zempleni et al. 2013).

The system of naming vitamins by letters of the alphabet was convenient and was generally accepted before the discovery of their chemical nature. However, chemical names are increasingly used to describe vitamins of the B complex ($B_1$, $B_2$, $B_3$, $B_5$, $B_6$, $B_{12}$, biotin, and folic acid). Vitamins are classified as water or lipid soluble based on their solubility in water or fat (Table 9.1). The absorption and transport of dietary lipid-soluble vitamins are closely linked to the metabolism of lipids, low-density lipoproteins (LDLs), very low-density lipoproteins (VLDLs), and high-density lipoproteins (HDLs). Although some substances such as *p*-aminobenzoic acid, carnitine, choline, flavonoids, lipoic acid, *myo*-inositol, pyrroloquinoline quinone (PQQ), and ubiquinones have been called vitamins at various times, such classifications have not generally been accepted. These factors can be classified as quasi-vitamins, namely, vitamin-like compounds (Combs 2012). Some vitamins are single substances (e.g., riboflavin and pantothenic acid), and others are members of the families of chemically related compounds—vitamers (e.g., nicotinic acid and nicotinamide for niacin; retinol, retinal, and retinoic acid for vitamin A). In animal nutrition, requirements for vitamins are expressed as mg or international units (UI) per kg body weight or percentages of complete diets (McDonald et al. 2011). The main objective of this chapter is to highlight the sources, metabolism, and functions of vitamins.

## CHEMICAL AND BIOCHEMICAL CHARACTERISTICS OF VITAMINS

### General Characteristics of Vitamins

Vitamins have various structures, but have some common biochemical characteristics (Combs 2012). These features are that (1) vitamins are organic nutrients that are required in small amounts for biochemical reactions; (2) many vitamins (especially lipid-soluble vitamins, as well as vitamins $B_1$, $B_3$, $B_6$, and $B_{12}$) are destroyed by oxidation, heat, light, or certain metals, and, therefore, conditions of storage and processing of feeds can influence their biological values; (3) most vitamins, except niacin and

**TABLE 9.1**
**Vitamins Important in Animal Nutrition**

| Water-Soluble Vitamins | | Water-Insoluble Vitamins | |
|---|---|---|---|
| **Conventional Name** | **Chemical Name** | **Conventional Name** | **Chemical Name** |
| Vitamin $B_1$ | Thiamin | Vitamin A | Retinol |
| Vitamin $B_2$ | Riboflavin | Vitamin $D_2$ (plant) | Ergocalciferol |
| Vitamin $B_3$ | Niacin (nicotinamide) | Vitamin $D_3$ | Cholecalciferol |
| Vitamin $B_5$ | Pantothenic acid | Vitamin E | Tocopherol |
| Vitamin $B_6$ | Pyridoxine | Vitamin $K_1$ (plant) | Phylloquinone |
| Vitamin $B_{12}$ | Cyanocobalamin | Vitamin $K_2$ (bacteria) | Menaquinone |
| Biotin | Biotin | Vitamin $K_3$ (synthetic) | Menadione* |
| Folate ($B_9$) | Pteroylglutamic acid | | |
| Vitamin C | Ascorbic acid | | |

* Chemically, menadione is a water-soluble substance. However, it is metabolized to lipid-soluble, bioactive menaquinone in animals.

vitamin D, cannot be synthesized by animal cells, making almost all vitamins essential nutrients for nonruminant animals; (4) vitamins are neither degraded to provide energy nor used for cell structural purposes; (5) many vitamins (including B complex vitamins, folate, and vitamin C) serve as coenzymes for enzymes, while lipid-soluble vitamins fulfill specific functions in the body, such as the maintenance of vision (vitamin A), the utilization of dietary calcium (vitamin D), blood clotting (vitamin K), and regulation of gene expression; (6) some vitamins (e.g., vitamins C and E) are potent antioxidants; (7) most vitamins are not utilized in the form in which they are absorbed from the intestine, and are converted or modified to their active forms; (8) some vitamins are covalently attached to enzymes or tightly associated with enzymes via a noncovalent linkage; (9) small-intestinal absorption of water-soluble vitamins occurs via specific carrier proteins, whose expression is regulated at transcriptional and/or posttranscriptional levels; and (10) the absence or relative deficiency of vitamins in the diet results in characteristic deficiency states and diseases. Like any other nutrients, excess vitamins are toxic to animals (DiPalma and Ritchie 1977). The chemical properties of vitamins are summarized in Table 9.2.

## General Sources of Vitamins for Animals

Many plants are capable of synthesizing vitamins (Berdanier 1998). Thus, most feedstuffs contain vitamins, but the content of vitamins varies widely. For example, concentrate feeds contain B vitamins, while forages are good sources of carotenes. In contrast, dried feedstuffs of plant sources provide vitamin $D_2$, but it is virtually absent from typical corn- and soybean meal-based diets for poultry and swine. Furthermore, animal products are rich in most vitamins (including lipid-soluble vitamins) but are deficient in vitamin C and pantothenic acid, whereas plants are good sources of many water-soluble vitamins, vitamin E, and vitamin K (Table 9.3). Finally, microbial synthesis of the B complex vitamins and vitamin K occurs in the rumen of ruminants and in the large intestine of animals (Combs 2012). With the exceptions of vitamin $B_{12}$, vitamin K, and biotin, intestinal bacteria do not contribute a nutritionally significant quantity of vitamins to the animal hosts. The jejunum portion of the small intestine is the major site for the absorption of all dietary vitamins but vitamin $B_{12}$. The latter is absorbed primarily by the ileum. Although the epithelial cells of the large intestine express vitamin transporters, the rates of vitamin transport by colonocytes of the large intestine are much lower than those for enterocytes of the small intestine (Said 2011). Intestinal transport of water- and lipid-soluble vitamins is summarized in Table 9.4.

Provitamins are the compounds that are not vitamins themselves but function as vitamins after a chemical change (Zempleni et al. 2013). The best examples are the carotenes (precursors of vitamin A), subcutaneous provitamin D (precursor of vitamin $D_3$), and tryptophan (precursor of niacin).

**TABLE 9.2**
**Discovery and Chemical Properties of Vitamins**

| Vitamin | Vitamers | MW (g/mol) | Absorption Maximum (nm) | Melting Point (°C) | Color at 25°C | Form at 25°C |
|---|---|---|---|---|---|---|
| | | | **Lipid-Soluble Vitamins** | | | |
| Vitamin A (1915)[a] | Retinol | 286.4 | 325 | 62–64 | Yellow | Crystal |
| | Retinal | 284.4 | 373 | 61–64 | Orange | Crystal |
| | Retinoic acid | 300.4 | 351 | 180–182 | Yellow | Crystal |
| Vitamin D (1919) | Vitamin $D_2$ | 396.6 | 265 | 115–118 | White | Crystal |
| | Vitamin $D_3$ | 384.6 | 265 | 84–85 | White | Crystal |
| Vitamin E (1922) | α-Tocopherol | 430.7 | 294 | 2.5 | Yellow | Oil |
| | γ-Tocopherol | 416.7 | 298 | −2.4 | Yellow | Oil |
| Vitamin K (1929) | Vitamin $K_1$ | 450.7 | 242, 248, 260 | −20 | Yellow | Oil |
| | Vitamin $K_2$ | 649.2 | 269, 325 | 54 | Yellow | Crystal |
| | Vitamin $K_3$* | 172.2 | 243, 248, 261<br>270, 325–328<br>246, 262, 333 | 105–107 | Yellow | Crystal |
| | | | **Water-Soluble Vitamins** | | | |
| Vitamin C (1907) | Free acid | 176.1 | 245 | 190–192 | White | Crystal |
| | Sodium salt | 198.1 | 245 | 218 | White | Crystal |
| Thiamin (1906) | Free form | 265.4 | 243 (pH 2.3) | 164 | White | Crystal |
| | Disulfide form | 562.7 | 235, 265 (pH 7.4) | 177 | Yellow | Crystal |
| | Hydrochloride | 337.3 | – | 164 | White | Crystal |
| | Mononitrate | 327.4 | – | 196–200 | White | Crystal |
| Riboflavin (1933) | Free form | 376.4 | 220–225, 266<br>371, 444, 475 | 278 | Orange to yellow | Crystal |
| Niacin (1926) | Nicotinic acid | 123.1 | 263 | 237 | White | Crystal |
| | Nicotinamide | 122.1 | 263 | 128–131 | White | Crystal |
| Vitamin $B_6$ (1934) | Pyridoxal | 167.2 | 293 | 165 | White | Crystal |
| | Pyridoxine-HCl | 205.6 | 255, 326 | 160 | White | Crystal |
| Biotin (1926) | Free form | 244.3 | – | 167 | White | Crystal |
| Pantothenic acid (1931) | Free form | 219.2 | – | – | Yellow | Oil |
| | Calcium salt | 476.5 | – | 195 | White | Crystal |
| Folate (1931) | Monoglutamate | 441.1 | 256, 283, 368 | 250 | Orange to yellow | Crystal |
| Vitamin $B_{12}$ (1926) | Cyanobalamin | 1355.4 | 278, 361, 550 | >300 | Red | Crystal |

*Source:* Combs, G.F. 2012. *The Vitamins: Fundamental Aspects in Nutrition and Health*. Academic Press. New York, NY; and Open Chemistry Database, https://pubchem.ncbi.nlm.nih.gov.

[a] The number in parentheses refers to the year when the specific vitamin was discovered.

* Chemically, menadione is a water-soluble substance. However, it is metabolized to lipid-soluble, bioactive menaquinone in animals.

The efficiency of conversion of provitamins into vitamins varies with the substrates, as well as the species and developmental stage of animals (Combs 2012).

## WATER-SOLUBLE VITAMINS

Apart from their solubility properties, water-soluble vitamins have little in common from the chemical point of view. They are present in plant- and animal-source foods at various concentrations

**TABLE 9.3**
**Vitamins from Major Plant- and Animal-Source Foods**

| Micronutrient | Plant-Source Foods | Animal-Source Foods |
|---|---|---|
| Thiamin (vitamin $B_1$) | Peas and other legumes, nuts, whole grains, and wheat germ | Meat, liver, milk, eggs, and other animal products |
| Riboflavin (vitamin $B_2$) | Wheat germ, whole grains, nuts, legumes, and green vegetables | Meat, liver, milk, eggs, and other animal products |
| Niacin (vitamin $B_3$) | Whole grains, wheat germ, nuts, legumes, and vegetables | Meat, liver, milk, eggs, and other animal products |
| Vitamin $B_6$ | Nuts, legumes, whole grains, vegetables, and bananas | Meat, liver, milk, eggs, and other animal products |
| Pantothenic acid | Whole grains, legumes, nuts, and vegetables | Meat, liver, milk, eggs, and other animal products |
| Biotin | Whole grains, legumes, nuts, and vegetables | Meat, liver, milk, eggs, and other animal products |
| Folic acid (vitamin $B_9$) | Peas and other legumes, nuts, juice whole grains, and leafy vegetables | Liver, milk, eggs, meat, and other animal products |
| Vitamin $B_{12}$ | Absent from plants | Meat, liver, milk, eggs, and other animal products |
| Vitamin C | Abundant in fresh vegetables, juice tomatoes, green tea, and potatoes, but virtually absent from whole grains | Liver, milk, eggs, meat, and other animal products |
| Vitamin A | Absent from plants; however, dark, green, orange, or yellow vegetables are good sources of provitamin A | Liver, milk, eggs, meat, and butter |
| Vitamin D | Absent from plants; however, sun-dried vegetables contain vitamin $D_2$ | Milk, eggs, and liver are good sources of vitamin $D_3$ |
| Vitamin E | Vegetable oils and wheat germ oil | Meat, liver, milk, eggs, fat, and other animal products |
| Vitamin K | Alfalfa, pepper, whole grains, vegetables, and bananas | Meat, liver, milk, eggs, and other animal products |

*Source:* Wu, G. et al. 2014. *Ann. N.Y. Acad. Sci.* 1321:1–19.

(Table 9.5). As noted previously, most of these nutrients are not synthesized in animal cells and must be supplied in nonruminant diets (Pond et al. 1995). Their synthesis in the rumen may not be sufficient for maximal growth and production performance of ruminants (McDonald et al. 2011). Water-soluble vitamins are absorbed in the small intestine (primarily in the jejunum for all vitamins but vitamin $B_{12}$) via specific transporters into the portal vein (Halsted 2003). Most of the water-soluble vitamins are transported in the blood in their free forms but some are carried in their protein-bound forms. Except for vitamin $B_{12}$, these nutrients are excreted from the body primarily in the urine (Zempleni et al. 2013). The storage of water-soluble vitamins in tissues is limited and they rarely accumulate at toxic concentrations (DiPalma and Ritchie 1977).

## Thiamin (Vitamin $B_1$)

### *Structure*

Thiamin, which consists of a substituted pyrimidine joined by a methylene bridge to a substituted thiazole (Figure 9.1), is the first member of the family of water-soluble vitamins to be discovered. This vitamin has maximum absorption wavelengths of 235 and 265 nm, which correspond to its pyrimidine and thiazole moieties, respectively. The active form of vitamin $B_1$ is thiamin diphosphate (pyrophosphate), which is synthesized from thiamin by ATP-dependent thiamin

**TABLE 9.4**
**Transport of Vitamins from the Intestinal Lumen across Enterocytes and Colonocytes in Animals**

| | Apical Membrane Transporter (Intestinal Lumen into Enterocyte) | | Basolateral Membrane Transport (Enterocyte into Lamina Propria) |
|---|---|---|---|
| **Vitamin** | **Conventional Name** | **Gene Name** | |
| Thiamin | Thiamin transporter 1 (ThTr1; $Na^+$-independent) | SLC19A2 | Transmembrane protein carrier |
| | Thiamin transporter 2 (ThTr2; $Na^+$-independent) | SLC19A3 | |
| | Thiamin pyrophosphate transporter in colonocytes (energy-dependent but $Na^+$-independent) | SLC44A4 | |
| Riboflavin | Riboflavin transporter-1 (RF-1; $Na^+$-independent) | SLC52A1 | Transmembrane protein carrier |
| | Riboflavin transporter-2 (RF-2; $Na^+$-independent) | SLC52A3 | |
| Niacin | Niacin carrier (H-dependent, $Na^+$-independent) | ??? | Transmembrane protein carrier |
| | Sodium-coupled monocarboxylate transporter | SLC5A8 | |
| Pantothenate | Multivitamin transporter ($Na^+$-dependent) | SLC19A6, 5A6 | $Na^+$-independent transporter |
| Vitamin $B_6$ | Vitamin $B_6$ carrier ($H^+$-dependent, $Na^+$-independent) | ??? | Transmembrane protein carrier |
| Biotin | Multivitamin transporter ($Na^+$-dependent) | SLC19A6, 5A6 | $Na^+$-independent transporter |
| Vitamin $B_{12}$[a] | Receptor-mediated endocytosis | ??? | Multidrug resistance protein-1 |
| Folate | Reduced-folate carrier-1 (RFC-1, $Na^+$-independent) | SLC19A1 | Multidrug resistance proteins |
| | Reduced-folate carrier-1 (RFC-2, $Na^+$-independent) | ??? | |
| | $H^+$-coupled folate transporter | SLC46A1 | |
| Vitamin C | Vitamin C transporter-1 ($Na^+$-dependent) | SLC23A1 | Transmembrane protein carrier |
| | Vitamin C transporter-2 ($Na^+$-dependent) | SLC23A2 | |
| DHAA | GLUT2 (facilitative, $Na^+$-independent) | SLC2A2 | Transmembrane protein carrier |
| | GLUT8 (facilitative, $Na^+$-independent) | SLC2A8 | |
| Vitamins A, D, E, K | Passive diffusion via lipid micelles | – | Passive diffusion via chylomicrons and VLDLs |

[a] Cubilin for the intrinsic factor–vitamin $B_{12}$ complex, and the asialoglycoprotein receptor for the haptocorrin–vitamin $B_{12}$ complex.
"???" indicates the lack of information.
DHAA, dehydroascorbic acid.

diphosphotransferase (Manzetti et al. 2014). Thiamin is unstable particularly under alkaline conditions because of its quaternary nitrogen, cleaved to the thiol form in water, and easily oxidized to thiamin disulfide and other derivatives (e.g., thiochrome).

### *Sources*

Thiamin is present in a variety of foods of plant (particularly cereal grains) and animal origin, as well as in yeast. However, most manufactured foods contain only low concentrations of this vitamin (Combs 2012). Thiamin is concentrated in the outer layers of seeds, in the germ, and in the growing areas of roots, leaves, and shoots. Yeasts (e.g., dried brewer's and baker's yeasts), fermentation products, unrefined cereal grains, and animal products (e.g., egg yolk, liver, kidney, and pork muscle) are good sources of thiamin. The synthetic vitamin is sold in the form of thiamin-HCl, because it is more stable.

### *Absorption and Transport*

Thiamin pyrophosphate is released from dietary proteins during hydrolysis in the gastrointestinal tract and then hydrolyzed to thiamin. Thiamin is absorbed into enterocytes mainly through thiamin transporters 1 and 2 (ThTrl and ThTr 2), which are pH-dependent and $Na^+$-independent carriers (Said 2011). The rate of thiamin transport is greatest in the jejunum and ileum. There are

**TABLE 9.5**
**Content of Water-Soluble Vitamins and Choline in Feedstuffs**

| Feedstuff | Biotin | Choline | Folate | Niacin | Pantothenic Acid | Riboflavin | Thiamin | Vitamin $B_6$ | Vitamin $B_{12}$ |
|---|---|---|---|---|---|---|---|---|---|
| Alfalfa, 17% CP | 0.54 | 1.40 | 4.36 | 38 | 29 | 13.6 | 3.4 | 6.5 | 0.00 |
| Barley grain | 0.14 | 1.03 | 0.31 | 55 | 8.0 | 1.8 | 4.5 | 5.0 | 0.00 |
| Blood meal[a] | 0.03 | 852 | 0.10 | 31 | 2.0 | 2.4 | 0.4 | 4.4 | 44 |
| Blood meal[b] | 0.28 | 485 | 0.40 | 23 | 3.7 | 3.2 | 0.3 | 4.4 | – |
| Canola meal | 0.98 | 6700 | 0.83 | 160 | 9.5 | 5.8 | 5.2 | 7.2 | 0.00 |
| Casein, dried | 0.04 | 205 | 0.51 | 1 | 2.7 | 1.5 | 0.4 | 0.4 | – |
| Corn grain | 0.06 | 620 | 0.15 | 24 | 6.0 | 1.2 | 3.5 | 5.0 | 0.00 |
| CSM[c] | 0.30 | 2933 | 1.65 | 40 | 12 | 5.9 | 7.0 | 5.1 | 0.00 |
| Feather meal | 0.13 | 891 | 0.20 | 21 | 10 | 2.1 | 0.1 | 3.0 | 78 |
| Fish meal, Menhaden | 0.13 | 3056 | 0.37 | 55 | 9.0 | 4.9 | 0.5 | 4.0 | 143 |
| Flax meal | 0.41 | 1512 | 1.30 | 33 | 14.7 | 2.9 | 7.5 | 6.0 | 0.00 |
| MBM[d] | 0.08 | 1996 | 0.41 | 49 | 4.1 | 4.7 | 0.4 | 4.6 | 90 |
| Milk powder[e] | 0.25 | 1393 | 0.47 | 12 | 36.4 | 19.1 | 3.7 | 4.1 | 36 |
| Oat grain | 0.24 | 946 | 0.30 | 19 | 13 | 1.7 | 6.0 | 2.0 | 0.00 |
| Peanut meal, sol. extr. | 0.39 | 1854 | 0.50 | 170 | 53 | 7.0 | 5.7 | 6.0 | 0.00 |
| PBM[f] | 0.09 | 6029 | 0.50 | 47 | 11.1 | 10.5 | 0.2 | 4.4 | – |
| Rice bran | 0.35 | 1135 | 2.20 | 293 | 23 | 2.5 | 22.5 | 26 | 0.00 |
| Rice grain[g] | 0.08 | 1003 | 0.20 | 25 | 3.3 | 0.4 | 1.4 | 28 | 0.00 |
| Safflower meal, sol. extr. | 1.03 | 820 | 0.50 | 11 | 33.9 | 2.3 | 4.6 | 12 | 0.00 |
| Sorghum grain | 0.26 | 668 | 0.17 | 41 | 12.4 | 1.3 | 3.0 | 5.2 | 0.00 |
| SBM[h] | 0.27 | 2794 | 1.37 | 34 | 16 | 2.9 | 4.5 | 6.0 | 0.00 |
| Sunflower meal, sol. extr. | 1.40 | 3791 | 1.14 | 264 | 29.9 | 3.0 | 3.0 | 11.1 | 0.00 |
| Wheat bran | 0.36 | 1232 | 0.63 | 186 | 31 | 4.6 | 8.0 | 12 | 0.00 |
| Wheat grain[i] | 0.11 | 778 | 0.22 | 48 | 9.9 | 1.4 | 4.5 | 3.4 | 0.00 |
| Yeast (brewer's dried) | 0.63 | 3984 | 9.90 | 448 | 109 | 37.0 | 91.8 | 42.8 | 1 |

*Source:* National Research Council (NRC). 1998. *Nutrient Requirements of Swine*, National Academy Press, Washington, DC.

*Note:* Values are mg/kg (on the as-fed basis), except for vitamin $B_{12}$ (μg/kg). sol. extr., solvent extraction.

[a] Conventional blood meal.

[b] Blood meal, spray or ring dried (93% dry matter).

[c] Cottonseed meal (solvent extract, 41% CP).

[d] Meat and bone meal (93% dry matter).

[e] Bovine milk (skim, dried; 96% dry matter).

[f] Poultry by-product meal (93% dry matter).

[g] Polished, broken.

[h] Soybean meal (solvent extracted, 89% dry matter).

[i] Hard red, winter.

reports that thiamin pyrophosphate itself can be directly transported by colonocytes via an energy-dependent, $Na^+$-independent transporter (SLC44A4) (Nabokina et al. 2014). Thiamin exits the intestinal epithelial cell through its basolateral membrane via a specific transporter. After entering the portal vein, thiamin is transported in the protein-bound form into various tissues (e.g., the liver) where it is converted back into thiamin pyrophosphate by the action of thiaminokinase (Brown 2014). A specific thiamin-binding protein has been identified in rat serum and liver, as well as hens' eggs (Combs 2012). A small amount of the body's thiamin also exists as thiamin monophosphate and thiamin triphosphate.

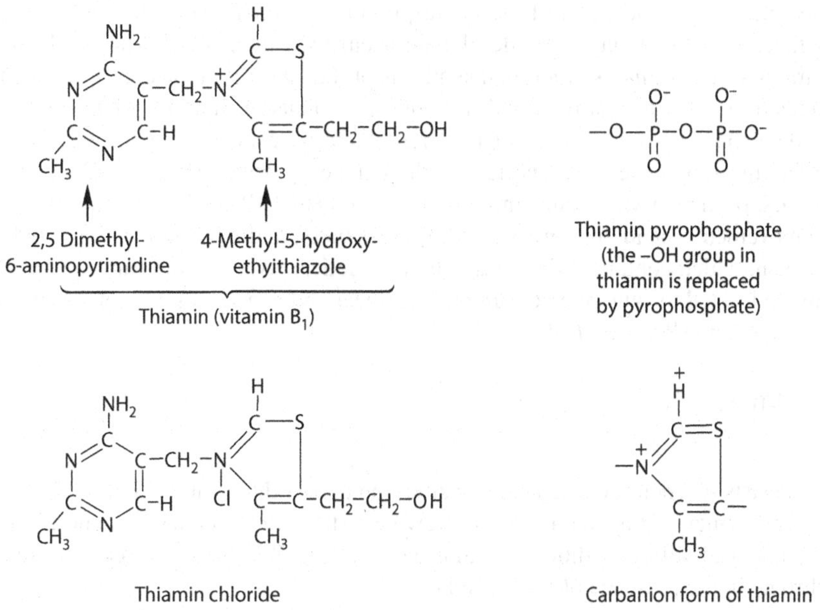

2,5 Dimethyl-6-aminopyrimidine

4-Methyl-5-hydroxy-ethyithiazole

Thiamin (vitamin $B_1$)

Thiamin pyrophosphate (the -OH group in thiamin is replaced by pyrophosphate)

Thiamin chloride

Carbanion form of thiamin

**FIGURE 9.1** The chemical structure of thiamin (vitamin $B_1$). This vitamin consists of a substituted pyrimidine joined by a methylene bridge to a substituted thiazole. Thiamin is chemically unstable in aqueous solutions.

### *Functions*

Thiamin diphosphate is a coenzyme in enzymatic reactions involving the transfer of an aldehyde unit: (1) oxidative decarboxylation of α-ketoacids for ATP production and (2) transketolase reactions in the pentose phosphate pathway and for valine synthesis in microorganisms, plants, and yeasts (Bettendorff et al. 2014). In these reactions, thiamin diphosphate provides a reactive carbon on the thiazole that forms a carbanion, which is then free to add to the carbonyl group of α-ketoacids. Examples for the oxidative decarboxylation of α-ketoacids are catalyzed by pyruvate, α-ketoglutarate, or branched-chain α-ketoacid dehydrogenase complex. Their reactions are outlined as follows:

Pyruvate→Acetyl-CoA + $CO_2$ (pyruvate dehydrogenase complex)
α-Ketoglutarate→Succinyl-CoA + $CO_2$ (α-ketoglutarate dehydrogenase complex)
α-Ketoacids of branched-chain amino acids→R-CO-CoA + $CO_2$ (branched-chain ketoacid dehydrogenase complex)

### *Deficiency and Diseases*

Thiamin deficiency produces poor appetite, anorexia, weight loss, edema, heart problems, muscular and nerve degeneration, and progressive dysfunction of the neurological system. These deficiency syndromes are collectively called the disease of beriberi (Jones and Hunt 1983), a term originally used by the natives of Indonesia for "leg disorders, including weakness, edema, pain, and paralysis". In humans, the populations most at risk of developing thiamin deficiency are chronic alcoholics, those overly dependent on polished rice as a staple, and those consuming large amounts of raw seafood due to the activity of thiaminase (Vedder et al. 2015). Thiaminase activity is destroyed by high temperatures or cooking. The ataxia and ocular symptoms associated with thiamin deficiency in alcoholics are known as Wernicke's disease, which is caused by decreased intake of nutrients, reduced absorption, and impaired ability to utilize the absorbed vitamin.

In addition to the general symptoms of beriberi, some characteristics of thiamin deficiency occur in farm animals. For example, pigs have inflammatory lesions of the gastrointestinal tract, diarrhea, occasional vomiting, dermatitis, hair loss, and respiratory dysfunction (Roche 1991). In chicks fed a thiamin-deficient diet for 10 days, they develop polyneuritis, which is characterized by head retraction and paralysis. In ruminants, microbial synthesis of the vitamin in the digestive tract plus exogenous sources in the diet normally provides adequate amounts of thiamin (McDonald et al. 2011). However, when there is high activity of bacterial thiaminase in the rumen (e.g., lactic acidosis caused by feeding rapidly fermentable feeds), the deficiency condition known as cerebrocortical necrosis occurs, particularly in young animals (Jones and Hunt 1983). This disease is characterized by circling movements, head pressing, stargazing, blindness, and muscular tremors. In horses consuming bracken, which contains thiaminase, thiamin deficiency symptoms appear. In all animals, beriberi can be treated through the consumption of meat and vegetables, as well as dietary supplementation with niacin (Pond et al. 1995).

## Riboflavin (Vitamin $B_2$)

### *Structure*

Riboflavin consists of a heterocyclic isoalloxazine ring attached to ribitol (Figure 9.2). It is a yellow and fluorescent pigment. This vitamin is relatively heat-stable in either acid or neutral solutions, but is destroyed under alkaline conditions (Thakur et al. 2016). Riboflavin decomposes to lumiflavin and lumichrome in the presence of visible light.

### *Sources*

Riboflavin is synthesized by plants and microorganisms but not by animal cells (García-Angulo 2017). Animals obtain riboflavin by consuming foods of plant and animal origins. The liver is an excellent source of riboflavin, and considerable amounts are present in kidneys, meat, and dairy products. Dark green leafy vegetables are good sources of riboflavin, but cereal grains are poor

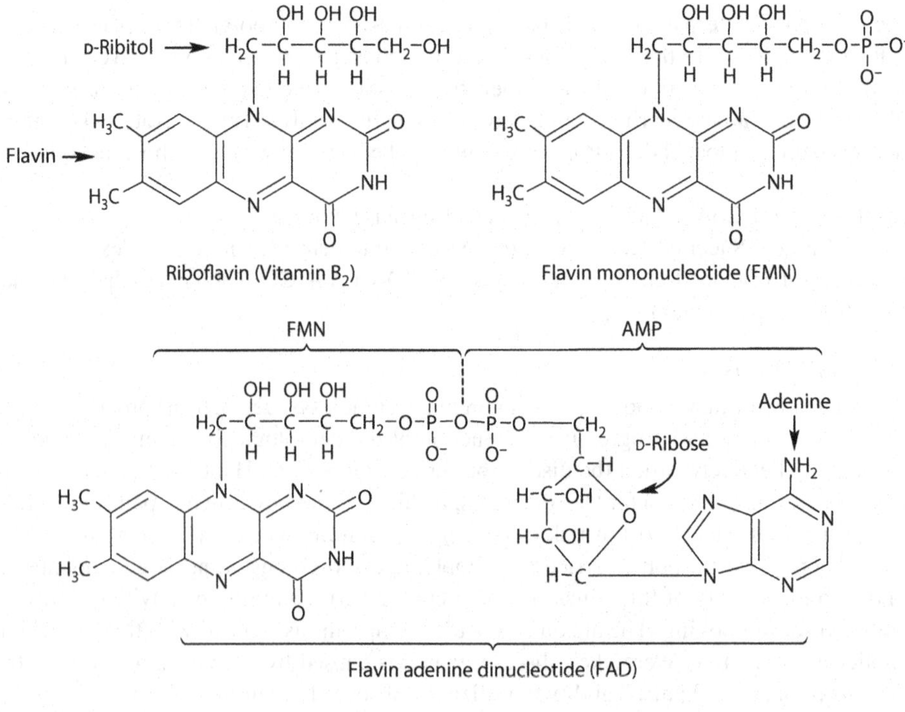

**FIGURE 9.2** The chemical structure of riboflavin (vitamin $B_2$). This vitamin consists of a heterocyclic isoalloxazine ring attached to ribitol. It is destroyed under alkaline conditions or by visible light.

sources of riboflavin. Thus, riboflavin is widely present in foods (Thakur et al. 2016). In plant- and animal-source feedstuffs, this vitamin is almost exclusively bound to proteins in the form of flavin mononucleotide (FMN) and flavin adenine dinucleotide (FAD).

### *Absorption and Transport*

Dietary FMN and FAD are hydrolyzed by intestinal phosphatases (alkaline phosphatase, FAD pyrophosphatase [which converts FAD into FMN], and FMN phosphatase) to generate free riboflavin prior to absorption by enterocytes. The major site of digestion is the jejunum. The digestibility of riboflavin from animal products is greater than that from plant products (Bates 1997). The apical membrane of the enterocytes contains riboflavin transporters (RF-1 and RF-2), which are $Na^+$-independent but moderately sensitive to pH (Said 2011). These cells can convert most of the absorbed riboflavin into FMN by ATP-dependent flavokinase, with FMN being further metabolized into FAD. The remaining free riboflavin exits the enterocyte across its basolateral membrane into the lamina propria through a specific transporter, enters the venous blood circulation, and is transported in the plasma in both free and protein-bound forms (~50% in either form). About 80% of FMN in the plasma (which is derived primarily from the lysis of cells) is bound to proteins. The proteins that weakly bind, through hydrogen bonding, both riboflavin and FMN in the plasma are globulins and fibrinogen, with albumin being the major one.

### *Functions*

Riboflavin is a major component of FMN and FAD. FMN is formed by ATP-dependent phosphorylation of riboflavin. FAD is synthesized from FMN with ATP by FAD synthase; in this reaction, the AMP moiety of ATP is transferred to FMN. FMN and FAD are cofactors of oxidoreductase enzymes known as flavoproteins. FMN and FAD are usually bound to their apoproteins via a non-covalent linkage. Many flavoprotein enzymes contain one or more metals as essential cofactors and are known as metalloflavoproteins (Powers 2003). About 10% of FAD in the cell is covalently bound to enzymes such as succinate dehydrogenase and monoamine oxidase. In reactions catalyzed by flavoprotein enzymes, $FMNH_2$ and $FADH_2$ are produced from FMN and FAD, respectively. The flavoprotein enzymes are widespread in animals, and participate in many biochemical reactions, including the synthesis of cholesterols, steroids, and vitamin D (Pinto and Cooper 2014). Examples of flavoproteins are given in Table 9.6.

### *Deficiency and Diseases*

The signs of riboflavin deficiency in animals include low appetite, reduced growth, reduced feed efficiency, lesions of the mouth known as cheilosis (cracks and fissures at the corners of the mouth) and angular stomatitis (inflammation of the oral mucosa), and reduced glutathione reductase activity in erythrocytes. Other symptoms include dermatitis, a rash on the scrotum or vulva, photophobia, degenerative changes in the nervous system, endocrine dysfunction, and anemia (Jones and Hunt 1983). A severe deficiency, which can be induced experimentally in animals, results in failure to grow and reproduce, dermatitis, and nerve degeneration. In view of the many metabolic functions of riboflavin, it is surprising that dietary riboflavin deficiency does not lead to major life-threatening conditions. This is perhaps because riboflavin is tightly bound to proteins in animals. The turnover rate of riboflavin may be very slow and thus it may take a very long time to deplete this vitamin in cells. In addition to these general symptoms, some characteristics of riboflavin deficiency occur in farm animals (Pond et al. 1995). For example, in pigs, deficiency symptoms include poor appetite, growth restriction, vomiting, skin eruptions, and eye abnormalities. For sows, dietary riboflavin is essential to maintain normal estrus activity and prevent premature birth. In chicks, riboflavin-deficient chicks grow poorly and develop "curled toe paralysis" in which chicks walk on their hocks with the toes curled inward (Baker et al. 1999). This is a specific symptom caused by peripheral nerve degeneration. In breeding hens, a deficiency of riboflavin causes decreased hatchability. Embryonic abnormalities occur,

**TABLE 9.6**
**Flavoprotein Enzymes in Animals**

| Enzyme | Cofactor | Function |
|---|---|---|
| L-Amino acid oxidase | FMN | L-Amino acids → Ketoacids + $NH_3$ |
| NADH dehydrogenase[a] | FMN | Mitochondrial electron transport |
| Pyridoxine phosphate oxidase | FMN | Vitamin $B_6$ metabolism |
| D-Amino acid oxidase | FAD | D-Amino acids → Ketoacids + $NH_3$ |
| Choline dehydrogenase | FAD | Choline degradation |
| Dihydrolipoyl dehydrogenase | FAD | Oxidative decarboxylation of α-ketoacids |
| Dimethylglycine dehydrogenase | FAD | Choline degradation |
| Fatty acyl-CoA dehydrogenase | FAD | Fatty acid oxidation |
| Glutathione reductase | FAD | Reduction of GSSG to 2 GSH |
| Methylene-$H_4$ folate reductase | FAD | Production of 5-methyl-$H_4$ folate |
| Mitochondrial glycerol-3-P dehydrogenase | FAD | Transfer of cytosolic reducing equivalents into mitochondria |
| Monoamine oxidase | FAD | Metabolism of neurotransmitters |
| Monomethylglycine dehydrogenase | FAD | Choline degradation |
| Nitric oxide synthase | FAD/FMN | Arginine + $O_2$ → Citrulline + NO |
| Sphinganine oxidase | FAD | Sphingosine synthesis |
| Succinate dehydrogenase[b] | FAD | Krebs cycle |
| Xanthine oxidase | FAD | Purine degradation |

[a] Also known as NADH-ubiquinone reductase: NADH + $H^+$ + UQ ↔ $NAD^+$ + $UQH_2$ (ubiquinol).
[b] Also known as succinate-ubiquinone reductase: Succinate + UQ ↔ Fumarate + $UQH_2$.

including the characteristic "clubbed down" symptom in which the down feather continues to grow inside the follicle, forming a coiled feather (Wyatt et al. 1973). In ruminants, riboflavin is synthesized by the ruminal microorganisms. Thus, deficiencies of riboflavin are rare in ruminants with a functional rumen. However, riboflavin deficiencies have been reported for young calves and lambs, and symptoms include loss of appetite, diarrhea, and lesions in the corners of the mouth.

## NIACIN (VITAMIN $B_3$)

### *Structure*

Niacin is the generic name for nicotinic acid and nicotinamide (Figure 9.3), which are colorless and have an optical absorption maximum at 262 nm (Kamanna et al. 2013). Nicotinic acid is a monocarboxylic acid derivative of pyridine. Nicotinamide is a relatively stable vitamin, and is not easily destroyed by heat, acids, alkalis, or oxidation.

### *Sources*

Niacin is found widely as nicotinamide in animal tissues and as protein-bound nicotinic acid in plants (Table 9.3). In cereal grains, much of niacin is present in a bound form that is not readily available to humans, pigs, and poultry. In corn, niacin is in a bound unavailable form, niacytin, from which niacin can be released by pretreatment with hot alkali (calcium oxide). In Central America, soaking corn in lime water before the preparation of tortillas can effectively protect against pellagra (Carpenter 1983). Tryptophan can be converted to nicotinate mononucleotide in all animal species (Figure 9.3), but the efficiency of the conversion is low, especially in cats, fish, and poultry (e.g., 45:1 on a weight basis in chicks) (Yao et al. 2011). Rich sources of niacin are liver, meats, yeasts (brewer's and baker's yeasts), groundnut, and sunflower meals.

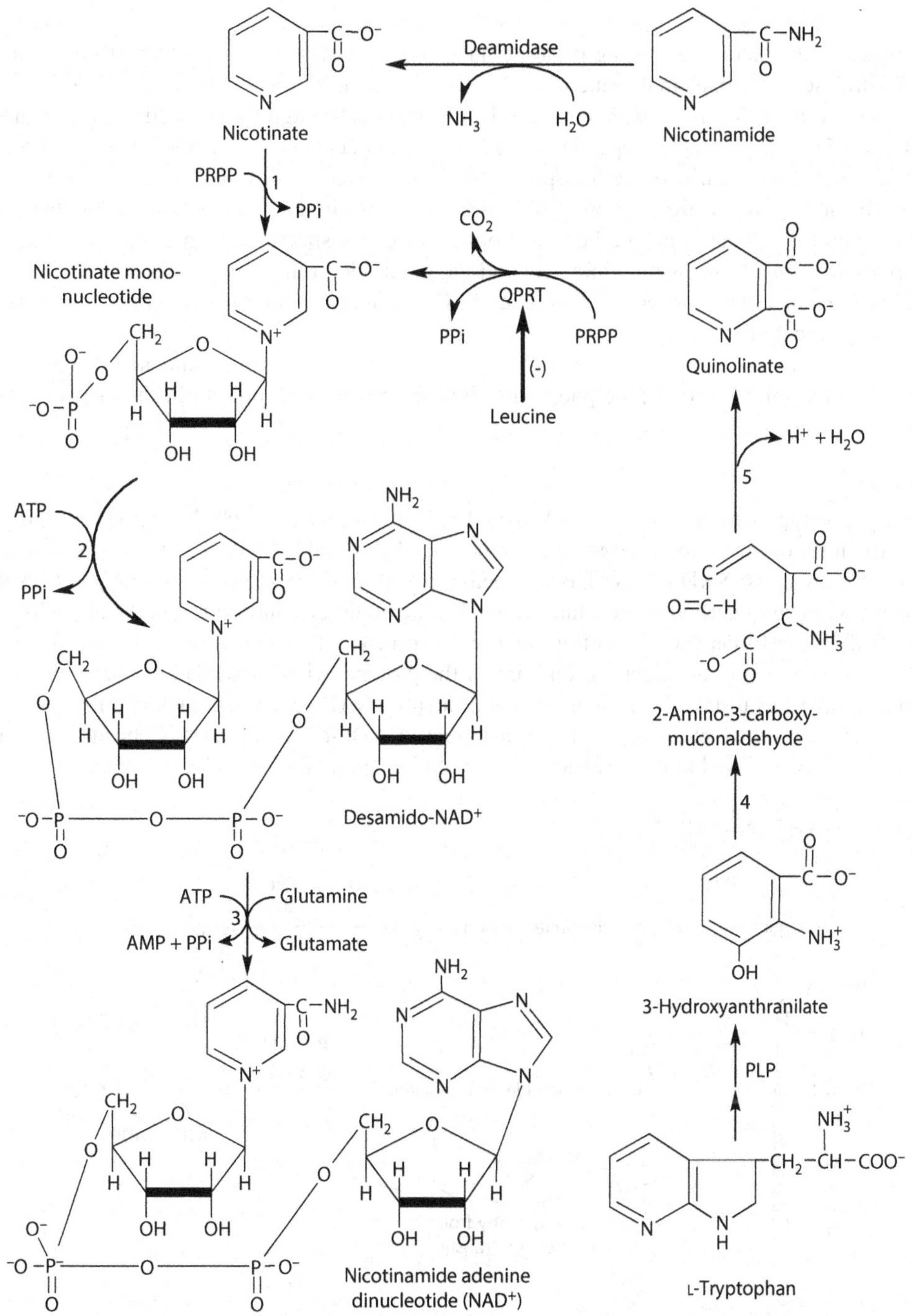

**FIGURE 9.3** The chemical structure of niacin (vitamin $B_3$) and its synthesis from tryptophan in animals. Niacin is the generic name for nicotinic acid (a monocarboxylic acid derivative of pyridine) and its derivative, nicotinamide. Nicotinic acid is synthesized from tryptophan via a series of reactions in animals. PLP, pyridoxal phosphate; PRPP, 5-phosphoribosyl-1-pyrophosphate; QPRT, quinolinate phosphoribosyl transferase.

### *Absorption and Transport*

Hydrolysis of the niacin-containing pyridine nucleotides ([NAD(H) and NADP(H)]) by NAD(P)-glycohydrolase (an intestinal mucosal enzyme) generates nicotinamide and ADP-ribose. Nicotinamide and nicotinic acid are absorbed by enterocytes through a specific high-affinity (apparent $K_m$ of 0.53 μM), acidic-pH-dependent, and $Na^+$-independent carrier (Nabokina et al. 2005). The sodium-coupled monocarboxylate transporter SLC5A8 (apparent $K_m$ of 0.23–0.3 mM) may play a role in the absorption of high pharmacological doses of niacin. Niacin exits the enterocyte across its basolateral membrane into the lamina propria through a specific transporter. This vitamin is transported in the plasma as nicotinic acid and nicotinamide in the unbound form and is taken up by tissues via the anion transport system (e.g., SLC5A8 in erythrocytes), $Na^+$-dependent transport system (e.g., renal tubules), and energy-dependent system (e.g., brain) (Kamanna et al. 2013). Inside the cells, nicotinic acid (nicotinate) is converted to nicotinamide adenine dinucleotide (NAD) and nicotinamide adenine dinucleotide phosphate (NADP) by enzymes present in the cytosol of most cells (Figure 9.4).

### *Functions*

Niacin is a component of NAD and NADP) (Bogan and Brenner 2008). Nicotinic acid (nicotinate) is the form of niacin required for the synthesis of NAD and NADP by enzymes present in the cytosol of most cells. NAD and NADP are coenzymes for many oxidoreductase enzymes involved in the metabolism of carbohydrates, fatty acids, ketone bodies, amino acids, and alcohol (MacKay et al. 2012). NAD(P)-dependent reactions involve the transfer of two electrons and two protons, and NAD(P) accepts two of the electrons and one of the protons, with the second proton remaining in solution. Besides its usual role as an oxidant or reductant, NAD serves as a substrate for poly(ADP-ribose) polymerase, which catalyzes the attachment of ADP-ribose to various chromosomal proteins. Thus, NAD is used in the posttranslational modification of a variety of proteins.

$$NAD(P)^+ + AH_2 \leftrightarrow NAD(P)H + H^+ + A$$

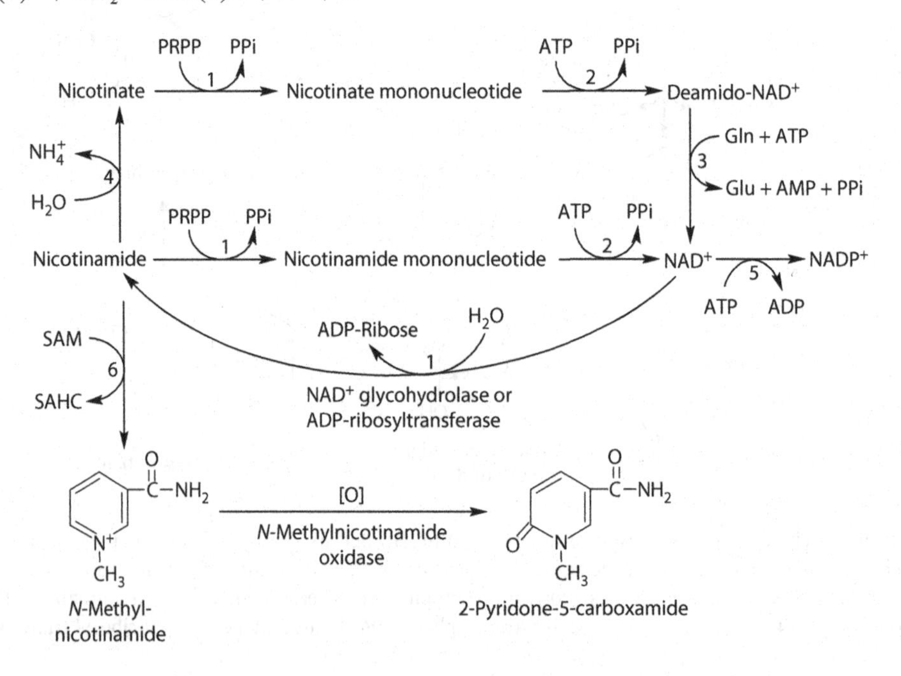


**FIGURE 9.4** Nicotinate metabolism in animals. Nicotinate is converted into $NAD^+$ and $NADP^+$ via ATP-dependent reactions. Nicotinic acid and nicotinamide are interconvertible in animals. PRPP, 5-phosphoribosyl-1-pyrophosphate; SAHC, *S*-adenosylhomocysteine; SAM, *S*-adenosylmethionine.

### *Deficiency and Diseases*

Severe niacin deficiency results in a disease known as pellagra, first noted in the 1760s in Spain and Italy where corn was popular. Given the roles of ATP and redox signaling in cellular metabolism, it is not surprising that pellagra is characterized by severe dermatitis and fissured scabs, diarrhea, and mental depression. The disease is also associated with the four D's: dermatitis, diarrhea, dementia, and death (Carpenter 1983). Dependence on sorghum is also pellagragenic, not because of low tryptophan but because of sorghum's high leucine content (Gopalan and Jaya Rao 1975). Excess dietary leucine can bring about niacin deficiency by inhibiting quinolinate phosphoribosyl transferase (QPRT), a key enzyme in the conversion of tryptophan to NAD. Because vitamin $B_6$ is involved as a cofactor in the synthesis of niacin from tryptophan, vitamin $B_6$ deficiency can potentiate a deficiency in niacin. Other conditions leading to symptoms of pellagra include administration of some drugs, such as isoniazid (an antituberculosis drug) (in which tryptophan metabolism is directed to serotonin), and Hartnup disease (in which tryptophan absorption by the small intestine is impaired) (Bogan and Brenner 2008). In pigs, deficiency symptoms include poor growth, anorexia, enteritis, vomiting, and dermatitis (Roche 1991). In poultry, niacin deficiency causes bone disorders, feathering abnormalities, and inflammation of the mouth and upper part of the esophagus (Jones and Hunt 1983). When pigs and poultry are fed diets with a high maize content, niacin deficiency may occur, but niacin deficiency rarely occurs in ruminants with a functional rumen (Niehoff et al. 2009). Pellagra in nonruminants can be cured by dietary supplementation with niacin.

## PANTOTHENIC ACID (PANTOTHENATE)

### *Structure*

Pantothenic acid (vitamin $B_5$) is an amide of pantoic acid and ß-alanine (Figure 9.5).

The anion form of this vitamin is called pantothenate, and its more stable form (commercially available) is D-calcium pantothenate. Thus, vitamin $B_5$ can be considered as a peptide consisting of ß-alanine and a butyrate derivative. Pantothenic acid is a yellow, viscous oil, but its salts (with

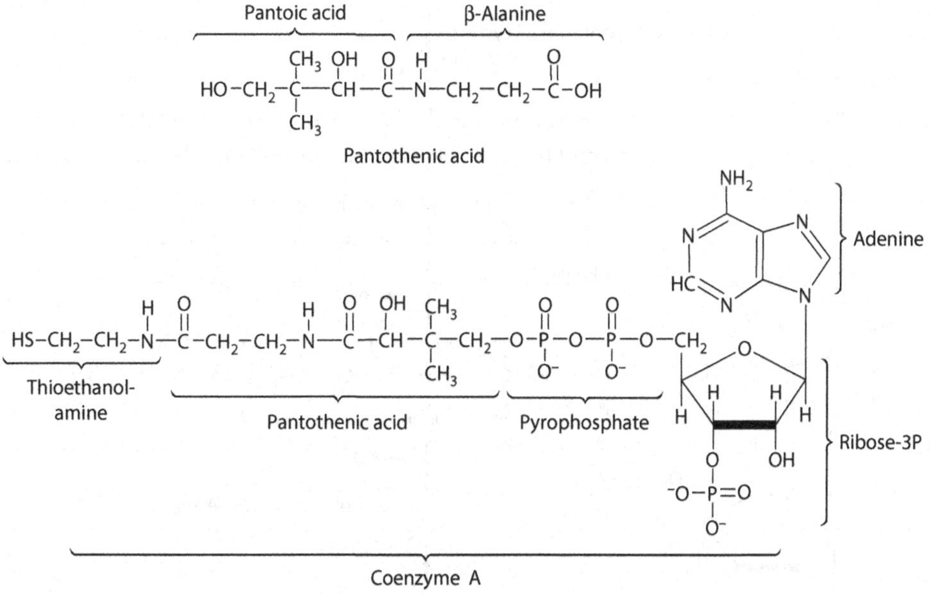

**FIGURE 9.5** The chemical structure of pantothenic acid (vitamin $B_5$). This vitamin is an amide of pantoic acid and ß-alanine.

calcium and other minerals) are white crystalline substances. In the dry form, the salts of pantothenic acid are stable at 25°C but are hygroscopic.

*Sources*

Pantothenic acid is widely distributed in nature, and thus its name was derived from the Greek *pantothen*, meaning "present everywhere." This vitamin is synthesized by plants and microorganisms (Figure 9.6), but not by animal cells (Coxon et al. 2005). Pantothenic acid is present in foods primarily as coenzyme A (CoA) and, to a lesser extent, protein-bound 4′-phosphopantetheine. In the latter, a 4-phosphopantetheine moiety is linked via its phosphate group to the hydroxyl group of serine in protein. Pantothenic acid is particularly abundant in animal products (e.g., liver, egg yolk), yeast, groundnuts, whole-grain cereals, alfalfa, and legumes.

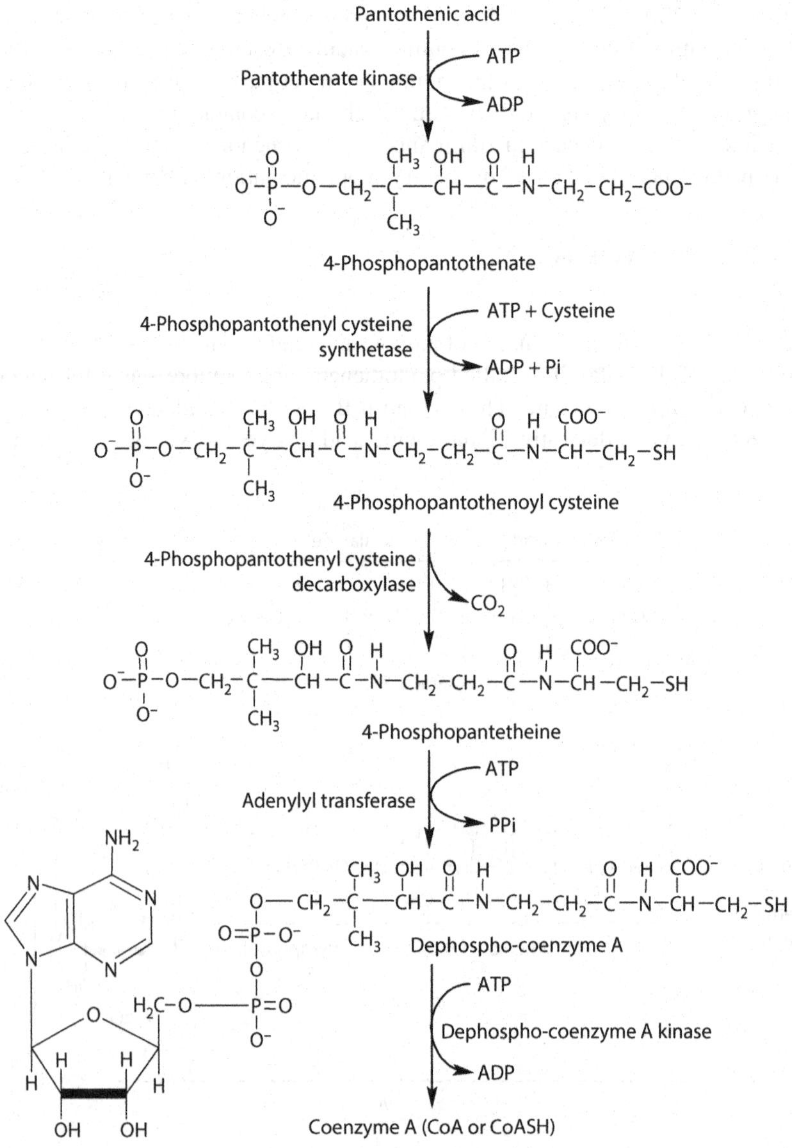

Pantothenic acid
Pantothenate kinase
ATP
ADP
4-Phosphopantothenate
4-Phosphopantothenyl cysteine synthetase
ATP + Cysteine
ADP + Pi
4-Phosphopantothenoyl cysteine
4-Phosphopantothenyl cysteine decarboxylase
$CO_2$
4-Phosphopantetheine
Adenylyl transferase
ATP
PPi
Dephospho-coenzyme A
Dephospho-coenzyme A kinase
ATP
ADP
Coenzyme A (CoA or CoASH)

**FIGURE 9.6** Conversion of pantothenic acid into CoA in animal cells.

### *Absorption and Transport*

CoA and protein-bound 4′-phosphopantetheine in diets do not readily cross cell membranes (including those of the intestine), and must be hydrolyzed to pantothenic acid prior to its intestinal absorption. Specifically, in the lumen of the small intestine, dietary CoA is hydrolyzed to dephospho-CoA, 4′-phosphopantetheine, and pantetheine (Shibata et al. 1983). The two responsible phosphatases are (1) pyrophosphatase, which acts on diphosphate bonds, and (2) orthophosphatase (also known as orthophosphoric monoester phosphohydrolase), which acts on orthophosphoric monoesters. The protein-bound 4′-phosphopantetheine in the diet is hydrolyzed by orthophosphatase to release 4′-phosphopantetheine. The 4′-phosphopantetheine is then dephosphorylated by pyrophosphatase or phosphatase to yield pantetheine, which is hydrolyzed by the intestinal pantetheinase into pantothenic acid and cysteine. Ultimately, pantothenic acid is readily absorbed into the enterocytes through the sodium-dependent multivitamin transporter (Vadlapudi et al. 2012). The exit of this vitamin across the basolateral membrane of the enterocyte into the lamina propria is mediated by a $Na^+$-independent carrier. In the plasma, pantothenic acid is transported in the free form. Interestingly, erythrocytes carry most of this vitamin in the blood.

### *Functions*

In animal cells, pantothenic acid is converted to 4′-phosphopantetheine, which is the prosthetic group of (1) CoA; (2) acyl carrier protein (ACP) of the fatty acid synthase complex (Figure 9.7); and (3) $N^{10}$-formyltetrahydrofolate dehydrogenase, which catalyzes the conversion of $N^{10}$-formyltetrahydrofolate to tetrahydrofolate, an essential cofactor in the metabolism of nucleic acids and AAs (Smith and Song 1996). CoA is involved in many reactions: the Krebs cycle, fatty acid synthesis and oxidation, AA metabolism, ketone body metabolism, cholesterol synthesis, acetylcholine synthesis, heme synthesis, and conjugation of bile salts (Zempleni et al. 2013). ACP plays an important role in fatty acid synthesis. Dietary pantothenic acid is essential for all mammalian species studied (including humans, pigs, dogs, rodents, and cats) as well as for poultry and fish (Combs 2012).

### *Deficiencies and Diseases*

Deficiency of pantothenic acid is rare because the substance is widely distributed in foods. Deficiency of pantothenic acid can be induced experimentally, which results in a loss of appetite, slow growth, skin lesions, loss of hair, depression, fatigue, ulceration of the intestine, weakness, and eventually death (Zempleni et al. 2013). Interestingly, the "burning foot syndrome" has been ascribed to pantothenic acid deficiency in prisoners of war (Berdanier 1998). In pigs, a deficiency of pantothenic acid results in poor growth, diarrhea, loss of hair, scaliness of the skin, and a characteristic "goose-stepping" gait. In severe cases, pigs cannot stand (Roche 1991). Deficiency of this vitamin has been reported for commercial herds of pigs. In poultry, deficiency of this vitamin results in growth

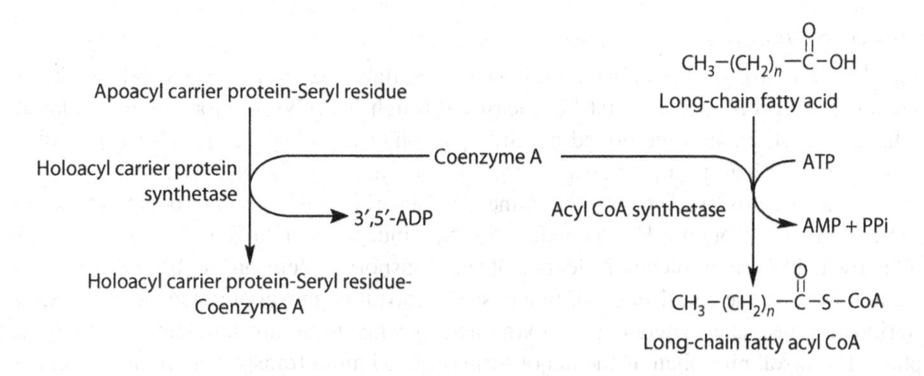


**FIGURE 9.7** Role of CoA as a coenzyme for holoacyl carrier protein synthetase and acyl-CoA synthetase in animal cells.

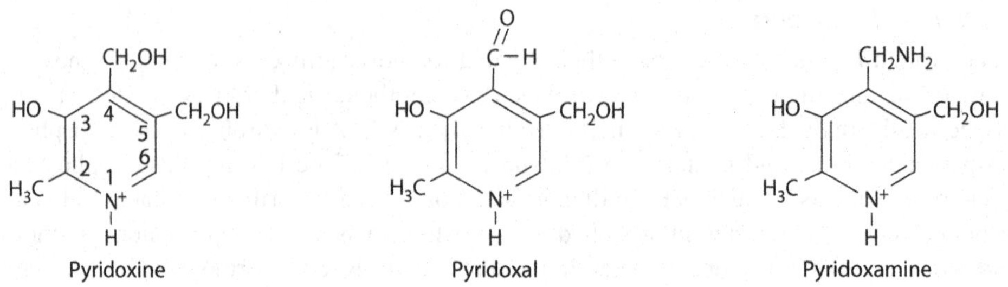

**FIGURE 9.8** The chemical structure of $B_6$ as a pyridine derivative. The three biologically active forms of vitamin $B_6$ are pyridoxal, pyridoxine, and pyridoxamine.

restriction, dermatitis, and reduced hatchability (Jones and Hunt 1983). Deficiency of pantothenic acid is rare in ruminants because rumen microorganisms can synthesize all B complex vitamins (Ragaller et al. 2011).

## Pyridoxal, Pyridoxine, and Pyridoxamine (Vitamin $B_6$)

### *Structure*

The name pyridoxine given to vitamin $B_6$ reflects its structure as a pyridine derivative. Three biologically active forms of vitamin $B_6$ are now recognized: pyridoxal, pyridoxine, and pyridoxamine (Figure 9.8). These three forms are interconvertible in animals, with the parent substance of vitamin $B_6$ being pyridoxine (Hayashi 1995). Active vitamin $B_6$ is mainly pyridoxal phosphate. Pyridoxine, pyridoxal phosphate, and pyridoxamine phosphate are the main representatives of vitamin $B_6$ in the diet, and all three have equal vitamin activity because they can be interconverted in the body (Figure 9.9). The amine and aldehyde derivatives of pyridoxine are less stable than pyridoxine. Vitamin $B_6$ is destroyed by heat.

### *Sources*

The vitamin is present in plants mainly as pyridoxine glycoside, whereas animal products contain pyridoxine, pyridoxal, and pyridoxamine (Ueland et al. 2015). Poultry, fish, liver, eggs, meat, milk, yeast, bananas, vegetables, cereal grains, and nuts are good sources of vitamin $B_6$. A large proportion of vitamin $B_6$ in foods is bound to protein via the ε-amino groups of lysine residues and the sulfhydryl groups of cysteine residues. In plants, this vitamin is also present in glycosylated forms (e.g., 5′-*O*-(β-D-glucopyranosyl) pyridoxine). Pyridoxine is the major vitamin $B_6$ in plant-source foods, whereas pyridoxal and pyridoxamine are the primary forms of the vitamin in animal-source foods. Pyridoxine-HCl is stable at 25°C and used for dietary supplementation.

### *Absorption and Transport*

Much of the vitamin $B_6$ in foods is not biologically available due to low digestibility. The vitamin in glycosides and proteins must first be released through hydrolysis before its intestinal absorption. The enterocyte membrane-bound alkaline phosphatase hydrolyzes pyridoxal phosphate and pyridoxamine phosphate into pyridoxal and pyridoxamine, respectively. All forms of vitamin $B_6$ (i.e., pyridoxal, pyridoxine, and pyridoxamine) are absorbed into the enterocytes (mainly of the jejunum and ileum) through a $H^+$-dependent but $Na^+$-independent carrier (Said 2011). At present, little is known about the molecular identity of the transport protein on the basolateral membrane of the enterocyte. In the small-intestinal mucosa, pyridoxal is phosphorylated by pyridoxal kinase into pyridoxal phosphate, whereas pyridoxine and pyridoxamine are metabolized into pyridoxal phosphate. Pyridoxal phosphate is the major form of the vitamin transported in blood and is tightly bound to proteins (primarily albumin in the plasma, and hemoglobin in erythrocytes) via the Schiff base linkage. A smaller amount of pyridoxal, pyridoxine, and pyridoxamine is also transported in

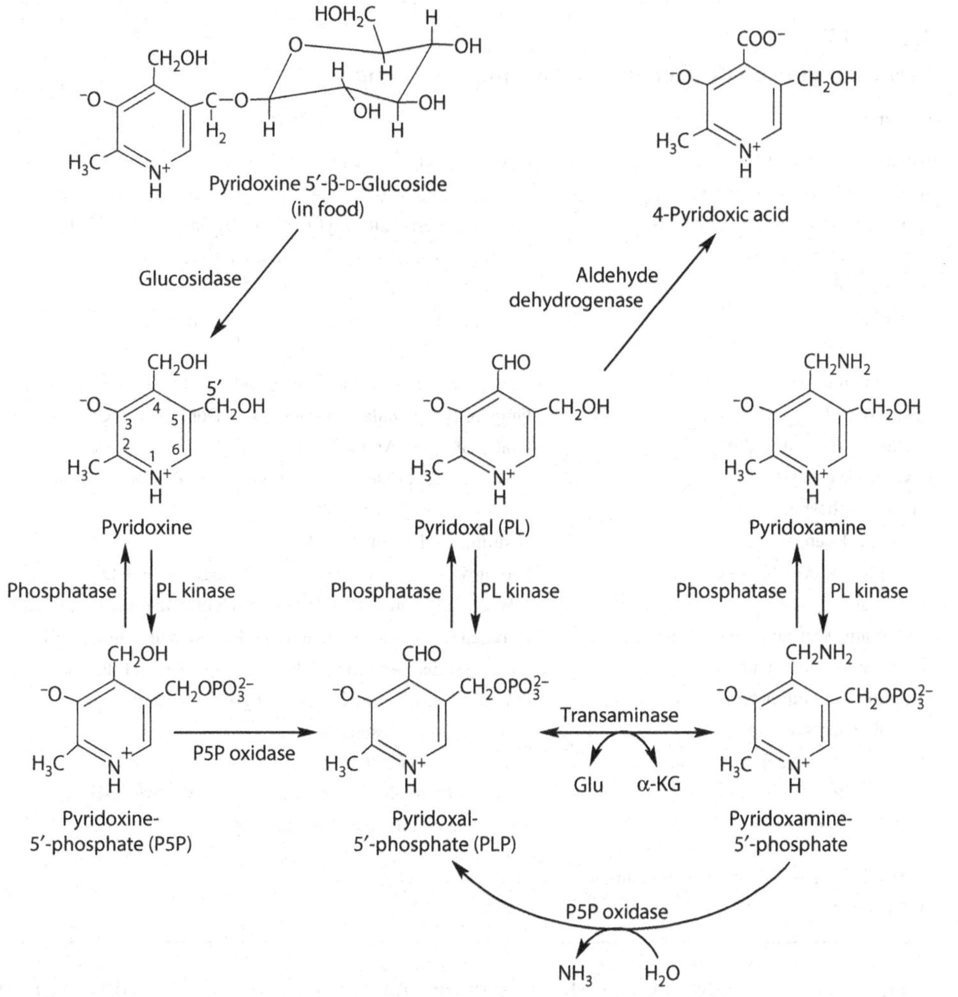

**FIGURE 9.9** Interconversion of pyridoxal, pyridoxine, and pyridoxamine in animal cells.

the plasma in the protein-bound forms. Phosphorylation of the absorbed pyridoxine, pyridoxal, and pyridoxamine, and their binding to proteins, which occur in both the small-intestinal mucosa and blood, play an important role in the intestinal absorption of vitamin $B_6$.

Extraintestinal cells take up vitamin $B_6$ through a specific membrane transporter. The rate of uptake of pyridoxal by animal cells is greater than that of pyridoxal phosphate (Combs 2012). Most tissues contain pyridoxal kinase, which catalyzes the phosphorylation by ATP of the unphosphorylated forms of the vitamin to their respective phosphate esters. Pyridoxic acid is the end product of vitamin $B_6$ degradation, and is excreted in urine.

### *Functions*

Pyridoxal phosphate is the coenzyme of several enzymes involved in amino acid metabolism (Table 9.7). By entering into a Schiff base combination between its aldehyde group and the amino group of an $\alpha$-amino acid, pyridoxal phosphate can facilitate changes in the three remaining bonds of the $\alpha$-amino carbon to allow (1) transamination, (2) decarboxylation, or (3) threonine aldolase activity (Figure 9.10). The mechanism whereby vitamin $B_6$ participates in AA transamination is outlined in Figure 9.11. In addition, pyridoxal phosphate is covalently bound to glycogen phosphorylase via an initial Schiff base with the $\varepsilon$-amino group of a lysine residue of the enzyme and plays an important

**TABLE 9.7**
**Pyridoxal Phosphate-Dependent Enzymes in Animals**

| Enzyme | Function |
|---|---|
| Amino acid racemase | L-Amino acid ↔ D-Amino acid |
| Amino acid (AA) transaminase | $AA_1$ + α-Ketoacid$_1$ ↔ $AA_2$ + α-Ketoacid$_2$ |
| Aminolevulinic acid (AL) synthase | Heme synthesis; Succinyl-CoA + Glycine → AL + $CO_2$ |
| Arginine decarboxylase | Arginine → Agmatine (Argamine) + $CO_2$ |
| Aspartate decarboxylase | Aspartate → ß-Alanine + $CO_2$ |
| Cystathionase | Cystathionine → Cysteine + α-Ketobutyrate |
| Cysteine sulfinate decarboxylase | Cysteine sulfinate → Taurine |
| Cystathionine synthase | Homocysteine + Serine → Cystathionine |
| DOPA decarboxylase | Dihydroxyphenylalanine (DOPA) → Dopamine + $CO_2$ |
| Glutamate (Glu) decarboxylase | Glutamate → γ-Aminobutyrate + $CO_2$ |
| Glycine cleave system | Glycine + $H_4$ folate → $CO_2$ + $NH_3$ + $N^5N^{10}$-$CH_2$-$H_4$ folate |
| Glycogen phosphorylase | Glycogen → Glucose 1-P |
| Histidine decarboxylase | Histidine → Histamine + $CO_2$ |
| Ketosphinganine synthase[a] | Palmitoyl-CoA + Serine → Ketosphinganine + $CO_2$ |
| Kynureninase | 3-Hydroxykynurenine + $H_2O$ → 3-Hydroxyanthranilate + Ala |
| Kynurenine transaminase | Kynurenine + α-Ketoglutarate → Kynurenate + Glutamate |
| Methionine (Met) synthase | Homocysteine + 5-Methyl-$H_4$ folate → Met + $H_4$ folate |
| Ornithine aminotransferase | Ornithine + α-Ketoglutarate ↔ Pyrroline-5-carboxylate + Glu |
| Ornithine decarboxylase | Ornithine → Putrescine + $CO_2$ |
| Phosphatidylserine decarboxylase | Synthesis of phosphatidylethanolamine |
| Serine hydroxymethyltransferase | Serine + $H_4$ folate → Glycine + $N^5$,$N^{10}$-Methylene-$H_4$ folate |
| Threonine aldolase | Threonine → Glycine + Acetaldehyde |

[a] Also known as 3-dehydrosphinganine-L-serine synthetase.
Ala, alanine.

role in stabilizing the conformational structure of the enzyme (Helmreich 1992). Muscle glycogen phosphorylase accounts for 70%–80% of the total body vitamin $B_6$.

### *Deficiencies and Diseases*

AA metabolism is impaired in animals with vitamin $B_6$ deficiency. The symptoms of vitamin $B_6$ deficiency are generally similar among animal species: hyperammonemia, hyperhomocysteinemia,

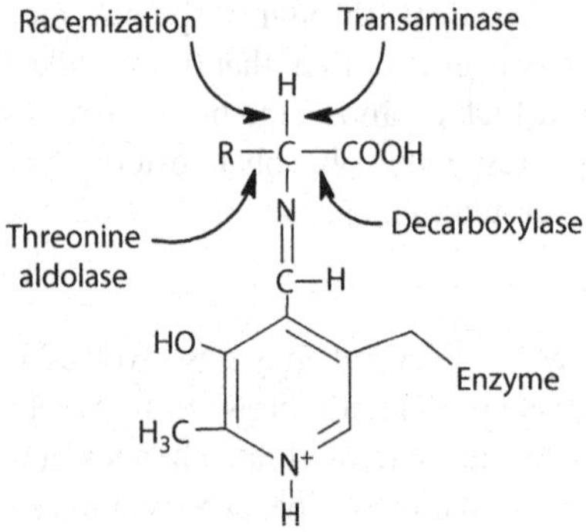

**FIGURE 9.10** Roles of vitamin $B_6$ in amino acid transamination and decarboxylation, as well as threonine degradation. Pyridoxal phosphate is the major form of vitamin $B_6$ for these reactions.

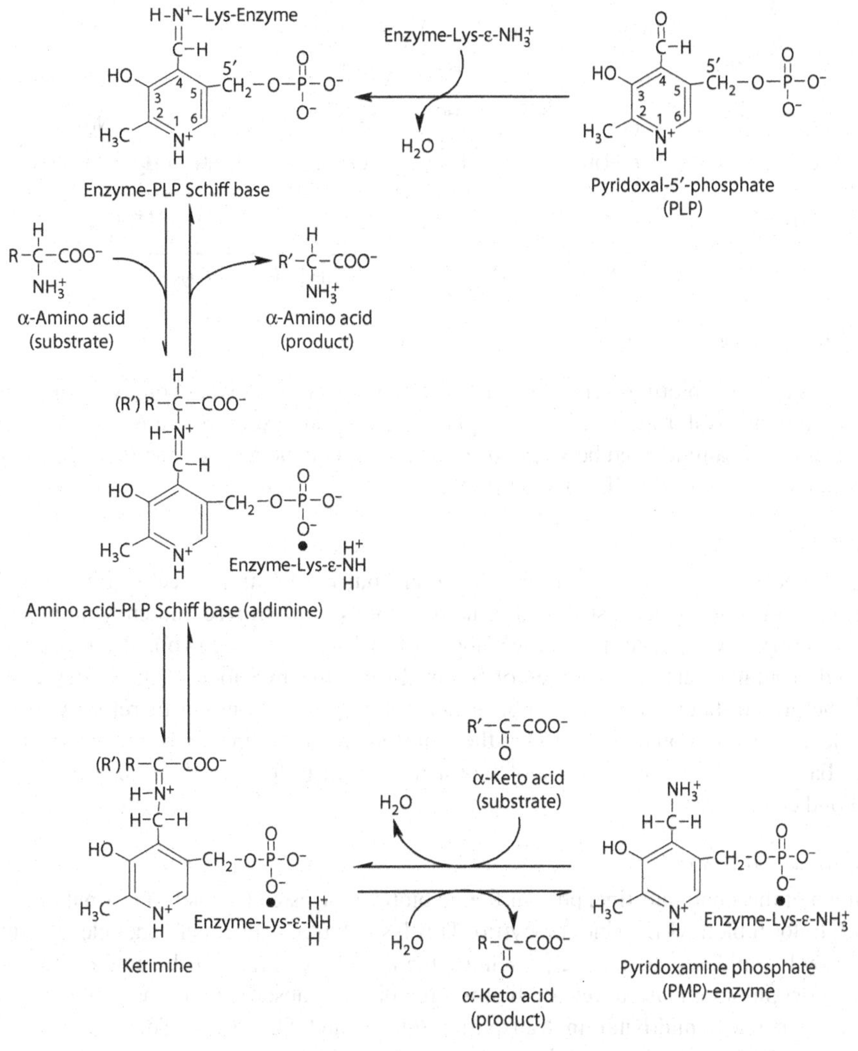

**FIGURE 9.11** The mechanism whereby vitamin $B_6$ participates in amino acid transamination. In this reaction, a new amino acid is formed from an α-ketoacid and an amino acid.

oxidative stress, cardiovascular dysfunction, alterations in the skin and nervous tissues, anemia, growth restriction, depression, confusion, seizure (a neurological problem), skin lesions, and sometimes convulsion (Ahmad et al. 2013). Vitamin $B_6$ deficiency is often found in chronic alcoholics, because of (1) a low intake of the vitamin, (2) alcohol-induced impairments in the metabolism of the vitamin, and (3) reduced hydrolysis of the phosphate bond of pyridoxal phosphate (Halsted and Medici 2011). Vitamin $B_6$ deficiency can occur in nursing infants whose mothers are depleted of the vitamin due to its inadequate intake. A widely used antituberculosis drug, isoniazid, can induce vitamin $B_6$ deficiency by forming a hydrazone with pyridoxal. In pigs, deficiency of vitamin $B_6$ results in poor growth, convulsions, impaired immune function, and anemia with high levels of iron in the spleen (Roche 1991).

## Biotin

### *Structure*

Biotin is an imidazole derivative widely distributed in foods of animal and plant origin. It is a sulfur-containing vitamin (Figure 9.12). In the crystalline form, this vitamin is stable at 25°C.

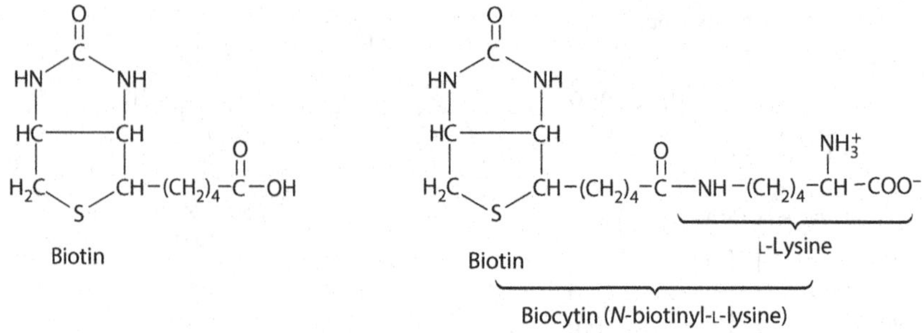

Biotin

L-Lysine

Biotin

Biocytin (*N*-biotinyl-L-lysine)

**FIGURE 9.12** The chemical structure of biotin. This sulfur-containing vitamin is an imidazole derivative.

In an aqueous solution, biotin is sensitive to degradation under oxidative, strongly acidic, or strongly alkaline conditions (Waldrop et al. 2012). In plant and animal tissues, biotin is usually bound to its enzymes through an amide bond between the C-2 of its thiophane nucleus and the ε-amino group of a protein-bound lysine residue (Berdanier 1998).

### *Sources*

Biotin is synthesized by plants, bacteria, and fungi, but not by animal cells (Fugate and Jarrett 2012). This vitamin is widely distributed in natural foods, in both free and enzyme-bound forms, but mostly in very low concentrations (McMahon 2002). Liver, milk, egg yolk, dried yeast, oilseeds, alfalfa, and vegetables are rich sources of biotin. In plant-source foods (e.g., barley and wheat), much of the protein-bound vitamin is not released during digestion and therefore is biologically unavailable. A large portion (about 50%) of the requirement for biotin may be met by synthesis from intestinal bacteria. The bioavailability of biotin in feedstuffs for intestinal absorption is usually $<50\%$ (Pond et al. 1995).

### *Absorption and Transport*

In the lumen of the small intestine, protein-bound biotin is digested by gastrointestinal proteases and peptidases to form biotinyl-L-lysine (biocytin). This lysyl–biotin adduct is further cleaved into lysine and biotin by biotinidase, an enzyme present on the apical membrane of the enterocytes. Milk and blood also contain biotinidase to release biotin. Free biotin is absorbed into the enterocytes through the sodium-dependent multivitamin transporter (Quick and Shi 2015). This transporter is also expressed on the apical membrane of the epithelial cells of the large intestine. Biotin exits the enterocytes and colonocytes through their basolateral membranes into the lamina propria via a specialized $Na^+$-independent transporter. Intestinal biotin uptake is upregulated by a dietary deficiency of biotin, but downregulated by a dietary excess of biotin (Said 2011). This adaptive regulation may be mediated via changes in the number (and/or activity) of the biotin transporters, but not in their affinity.

Biotin is transported in the plasma in the free form. About 12% of the total biotin in the plasma is covalently bound and another 7% is reversibly bound to proteins (Zempleni et al. 2013). Extraintestinal tissues take up biotin through specific transporters, including the $Na^+$-dependent multivitamin transporter (SLC5A6) (Uchida et al. 2015). Inside the cells, biotin is attached to its apoenzymes through the formation of an amide linkage with the ε-amino group of a specific lysine residue. This biochemical reaction, which is called protein biotinylation, is catalyzed by biotin protein ligase.

### *Functions*

In mammals, birds, fish, and microbes, biotin is a coenzyme of four ATP-dependent carboxylases: pyruvate carboxylase, acetyl-CoA carboxylase, propionyl-CoA carboxylase, and ß-methylcrotonyl-CoA carboxylase (Table 9.8). Biotin is covalently bound to the enzymes via the terminal amino group of a lysine residue (Figure 9.13). Two additional biotin-dependent carboxylases are present in microbes, but not in animal cells: urea amidolyase (which enables microbes to hydrolyze urea to

**TABLE 9.8**
**Biotin-Dependent Enzymes in Animal and Microbes**

| Enzyme | Function |
|---|---|
| | **Animals and Microbes** |
| Pyruvate carboxylase | Pyruvate + $CO_2$→Oxaloacetate (gluconeogenesis, provision of OAA for Krebs cycle) |
| Acetyl-CoA carboxylase | Acetyl-CoA + $CO_2$→Malonyl-CoA (fatty acid synthesis, regulation of CPT I activity in outer mitochondria membrane, fuel sensing mechanism) |
| Propionyl-CoA carboxylase | Propionyl-CoA + $CO_2$→D-Methylmalonyl-CoA (gluconeogenesis from propionate) |
| ß-Methylcrotonyl-CoA carboxylase | ß-Methylcrotonyl-CoA + $CO_2$→ß-Methylglutaconyl-CoA (catabolism of leucine and certain isoprenoid compounds) |
| | **Microbes** |
| Urea amidolyase (urea carboxylase) | ATP + Urea + $HCO_3^-$→ADP + Phosphate + Urea-1-carboxylate (providing a source of nitrogen in microbial metabolism) |
| Geranyl-CoA carboxylase | ATP + Geranoyl-CoA + $HCO_3^-$→ADP + Phosphate + 3-(4-Methylpent-3-en-1-yl)pent-2-enedioyl-CoA |

ammonia and $CO_2$) and geranyl-CoA carboxylase (which participates in isoprenoid catabolism in microbes) (Waldrop et al. 2012).

*Deficiencies and Diseases*

Biotin deficiency is rare, but can occur in humans consuming raw eggs (Zempleni et al. 2013). This is because egg white contains a heat-labile protein (avidin), which binds very tightly with biotin via a noncovalent linkage, thereby preventing the absorption of biotin by the intestine. Avidin is destroyed during cooking. The absence of carboxylate synthase, which attaches biotin to the lysine residue of the biotin carrier protein, results in multiple carboxylase deficiencies and causes biotin deficiency syndromes (Tong 2013). A rare genetic deficiency of biotinidase also causes biotin deficiency in 1/40,000 infants. The syndromes of biotin deficiency include growth restriction, depression, muscle

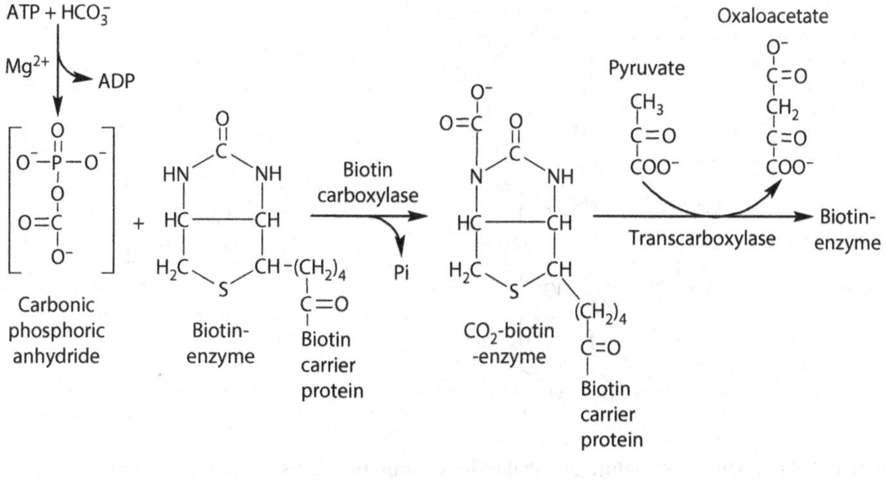

**FIGURE 9.13** The mechanism whereby biotin participates in the carboxylation of monocarboxylic acids.

pain, dermatitis, neurological disorders, anorexia, and extreme tiredness. In pigs, biotin deficiency results in poor growth, foot lesions, hair loss, a dry scaly skin, and impaired reproductive function (Roche 1991). In poultry, biotin deficiency causes reduced growth, dermatitis, leg bone abnormalities, cracked feet, poor feathering, and fatty liver and kidney syndrome (Jones and Hunt 1983). The fatty liver and kidney syndrome, which occurs mainly in 2- to 5-week-old chicks, is a fatal condition, in which the liver and kidneys are pale and swollen, and contain abnormal lipid depositions. In rats, a deficiency of biotin suppresses the expression and activity of ornithine carbamoyltransferase (a urea-cycle enzyme), leading to hyperammonemia (Maeda et al. 1996).

## VITAMIN $B_{12}$ (COBALAMIN)

### *Structure*

Vitamin $B_{12}$ (cobalamin) is an octahedral cobalt complex consisting of a porphyrin-like ring and a cobalt ion at its center (Figure 9.14). Cobalt occurs in three oxidation states: $Co^+$, $Co^{2+}$, and $Co^{3+}$ (Stadtman 2002). For example, in the liver, vitamin $B_{12}$ exists as methylcobalamin ($Co^+$), 5-deoxyadenosylcobalamin ($Co^{2+}$), and hydroxocobalamin. The commercial preparation of vitamin $B_{12}$ is cyanocobalamin ($Co^{3+}$), and is the most stable form of the vitamin. Vitamin $B_{12}$ has the most complex structure of all the vitamins. The free form of this vitamin is sensitive to acidic conditions and is stabilized after its binding to specific proteins.

### *Sources*

Vitamin $B_{12}$ is synthesized exclusively by microorganisms, but not animal cells (Raux et al. 2000). Thus, this vitamin is not needed in ruminant diets, if they provide sufficient cobalt, and inorganic

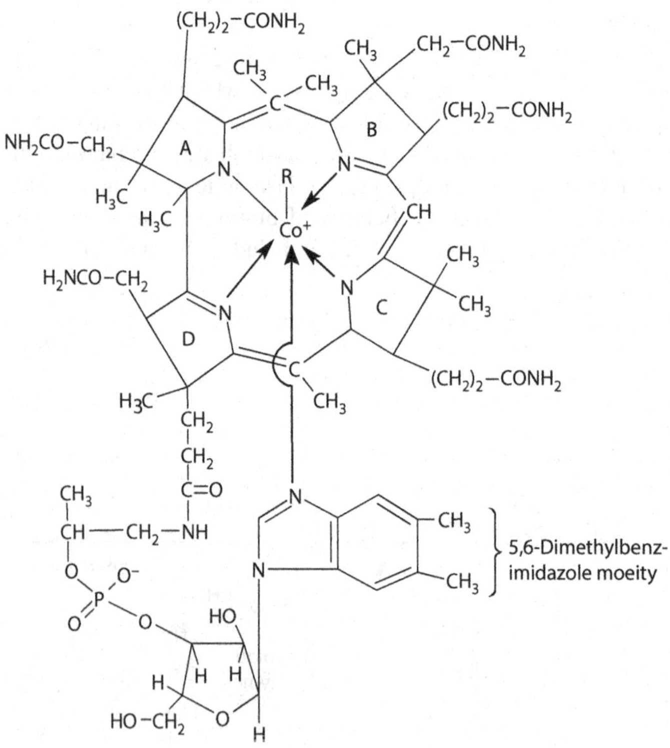

**FIGURE 9.14** The chemical structure of cobalamin (vitamin $B_{12}$). This vitamin is an octahedral cobalt complex consisting of a porphyrin-like ring and a cobalt ion at its center.

cobalt salts (Georgievskii 1982). Vitamin $B_{12}$ is absent from plants and plant-derived cereals, unless they are contaminated by microorganisms. All animal tissues contain vitamin $B_{12}$, which is derived from their diets and intestinal bacteria synthesis. This vitamin is conserved in the liver. Good sources of vitamin $B_{12}$ are the liver, meats (particularly beef), poultry, milk (e.g., 0.4 μg/L in human breast milk and 4.0 μg/L in cow's milk), and fish (Gille and Schmid 2015). All vitamin $B_{12}$ found in animals and our environment originated from $B_{12}$ synthesis in microorganisms. The naturally occurring vitamin $B_{12}$ in foods is bound to its enzyme proteins in the coenzyme form (Gruber et al. 2011). Preformed vitamin $B_{12}$ must be supplied to preruminants and nonruminants.

*Absorption and Transport*

Intestinal absorption of vitamin $B_{12}$ occurs primarily in the ileum, but also occurs in the jejunum and large intestine. This is a complex physiological and biochemical process (Alpers and Russell-Jones 2013). Within the lumen of the stomach, vitamin $B_{12}$ is released from foods through gastric acidification and proteolysis (particularly the action of pepsin). This vitamin then binds to the intrinsic factor (IF, a secreted glycoprotein) and haptocorrin (HC, also known as the R-protein) in the stomach. The major sources of IF vary with species: parietal cells of the gastric mucosa (the fundic glands) in humans, ruminants (e.g., cattle and sheep), guinea pigs, and rabbits; parietal cells of the abomasum mucosa (the fundic glands) in ruminants (e.g., cattle and sheep); abomasum chief cells of the gastric mucosa (the fundic glands) in rats and mice; pyloric glands of the gastric mucosa and mucosal cells of the duodenum in pigs; and pancreatic ductal cells in dogs (Alpers and Russell-Jones 2013; McKay and McLeay 1981). Of interest, like the dogs, stomach preparations from black slugs, cats, chickens, edible snails, eels, frogs, lobsters, plaice, sea trout, and toads do not contain the IF (Hippe and Schwartz 1971); the major source of the IF in these species may be the pancreas. The IF binds the four cobalamins (methylcobalamin, adenosylcobalamin, cyanocobalamin, and aquacobalamin) with equal affinity. HC is produced from the salivary glands and gastric gland, but their proportions differ among different species. The third vitamin $B_{12}$-binding protein is transcobalamin, which is produced by enterocytes of the small intestine. Additionally, mammalian milk contains another vitamin $B_{12}$-binding protein (cobalophilin). These cobalamin-bonding proteins share the same overall structural scaffold and each of them carries a single vitamin $B_{12}$ molecule (Nielsen et al. 2012).

The IF is resistant, but HC is sensitive, to degradation by proteases (trypsin>chymotrypsin> elastase) in the small-intestinal lumen. In neonatal mammals, as demonstrated for 1- to 28-day-old pigs (Ford et al. 1975; Trugo et al. 1985), when IF production is low, HC and cobalophilin play an important role in the intestinal absorption of vitamin $B_{12}$. In adults, vitamin $B_{12}$ absorption is primarily dependent on its binding to the IF. In all animals, the ileum of the small intestine is the primary site for the absorption of dietary vitamin $B_{12}$ as noted previously. The trafficking of this vitamin from the intestinal lumen into the intestinal epithelial cell is mediated by a specific receptor protein on the apical membrane of the enterocyte. This receptor (e.g., cubilin for the IF–vitamin $B_{12}$ complex, and the asialoglycoprotein receptor for the HC–vitamin $B_{12}$ complex) is most abundant in the ileum among the intestinal segments. The vitamin $B_{12}$-binding protein–vitamin $B_{12}$ complex enters the enterocyte via endocytosis and is subsequently transported into its lysosomes. After the lysosomal proteases hydrolyze the vitamin $B_{12}$-binding protein, vitamin $B_{12}$ is released. Cobalamin F transports vitamin $B_{12}$ from the lysosome into the cytosol, where the free vitamin $B_{12}$ binds to a cytosolic protein called cobalamin C, which is involved in the decyanation of cyanocobalamin and dealkylation of alkylcobalamins. Vitamin $B_{12}$ is then passed on to another cytosolic protein called cobalamin D, and exits the enterocyte across its basolateral membrane into the lamina propria through the multidrug resistance protein 1 (MRP1) (Beedholm-Ebsen et al. 2010). MRP1 is a member of the ATP-binding cassette (ABC) transporter family of proteins that couples ATP hydrolysis to the transport of substances against a concentration gradient.

After entering the venous blood circulation, vitamin $B_{12}$ binds to proteins in the plasma known as transcobalamins, which are needed for the transport of the vitamin to the tissues (Hall 1977).

Transcobalamin II, which is synthesized and released by several tissues (including the liver and small intestine) like transcobalamins I and III, is the chief transporter of vitamin $B_{12}$ in the plasma. The vitamin $B_{12}$–transcobalamin complex is taken up by extraintestinal cells through an endocytic receptor called the transmembrane CD320 protein (Nielsen et al. 2012). This protein is heavily glycosylated and belongs to the low-density lipoprotein receptor family. Upon endocytosis, transcobalamin is degraded in the lysosomes to release vitamin $B_{12}$ (hydroxocobalamin), which is converted to methylcobalamin in the cytosol or enters the mitochondria for conversion into 5′-deoxyadenosylcobalamin. Like other water-soluble vitamins, vitamin $B_{12}$ is not stored in the tissues (e.g., the liver and kidneys) of livestock species (Suttle 2010), poultry, and fish.

Unlike other water-soluble vitamins, vitamin $B_{12}$ is excreted from animals mainly via biliary secretion in the feces and, to a much lesser extent, the urine. In nonruminants (particularly patients with pernicious anemia), urinary excretion of the vitamin after its oral administration is often used to determine whether the animal can absorb vitamin $B_{12}$ properly; this is called the Schilling test. In ruminants, vitamin $B_{12}$ exits the rumen via microbes or bound to the salivary HC, and is released during digestion in the abomasum (Smith and Marston 1970). Lactating cows fed normal diets excrete approximately 87% of all excreted cobalt in the feces, 1.0% in urine, and 12% in milk, whereas nonlactating cows excrete approximately 98% of all excreted cobalt in the feces and 2.0% in urine (Georgievskii 1982). Because of the high efficiency of the enterohepatic circulation in reabsorbing vitamin $B_{12}$ in the ileum via the IF-mediated transport, most of the bile-derived vitamin $B_{12}$ is retained in the body. The total daily excretion of this vitamin via the feces and urine represents <1% of the total body reserves in animals.

### *Functions*

The active vitamin $B_{12}$ coenzymes are methylcobalamin and 5′-deoxy- adenosylcobalamin (Gruber et al. 2011). Methylcobalamin is the coenzyme required for the synthesis of (1) methionine from homocysteine and (2) tetrahydrofolate from $N^5$-methyltetrahydrofolate by methionine synthase (Figure 9.15). The metabolic significance of this reaction is to detoxify homocysteine and maintain intracellular stores of methionine, while regenerating $H_4$ folate from $N^5$-methyltetrahydrofolate available for the synthesis of purine, pyrimidine, and nucleic acid. 5′-Deoxyadenosylcobalamin is the coenzyme required for the synthesis of succinyl-CoA from L-methylmalonyl-CoA by methylmalonyl-CoA mutase (Nielsen et al. 2012). This is a key reaction in the conversion pathway of propionate to an intermediate of the Krebs cycle and therefore to glucose. The synthesis of glucose from propionate is particularly for ruminants, because propionate is a major product of microbial fermentation in the rumen and because little glucose is absorbed from the small intestine of ruminants.

### *Deficiencies and Diseases*

Without supplementation, a deficiency of vitamin $B_{12}$ is common among nonruminants fed plant-source ingredients, ruminants with inadequate intake of cobalt, and farm-raised fish (Pond et al. 1995). In most animals, gastric bypass surgery and gastric atrophy (typically caused by persistent infection with *Helicobacter pylori*), which leads to reduced production of the IF, result in vitamin $B_{12}$ deficiency (Jones and Hunt 1983). In humans, vegans are at risk of actual dietary deficiency of vitamin $B_{12}$, because the vitamin is found only in foods of animal origin or in microorganisms, but not in plants. In addition, the lack of a bioavailable IF due to its binding with self-antibodies results in a deficiency of vitamin $B_{12}$ (pernicious anemia, an autoimmune disease). Furthermore, an inherited defect in the synthesis of methylcobalamin or 5′-deoxyadenosylcobalamin causes vitamin $B_{12}$ deficiency (Gruber et al. 2011). Likewise, vitamin $B_{12}$ deficiency may occur as a result of a parasitic infection by tapeworms, which can arise from the consumption of infected raw fish and be passed to the consumer's gut, thereby limiting the availability of vitamin $B_{12}$ to the animal host.

Numerous metabolic disorders are caused by inadequate intake of dietary vitamin $B_{12}$. For example, a deficiency of this vitamin results in decreased activity of methionine synthase and methylmalonyl-CoA mutase, impaired DNA (purine and thymidylate) synthesis, reduced cell division,

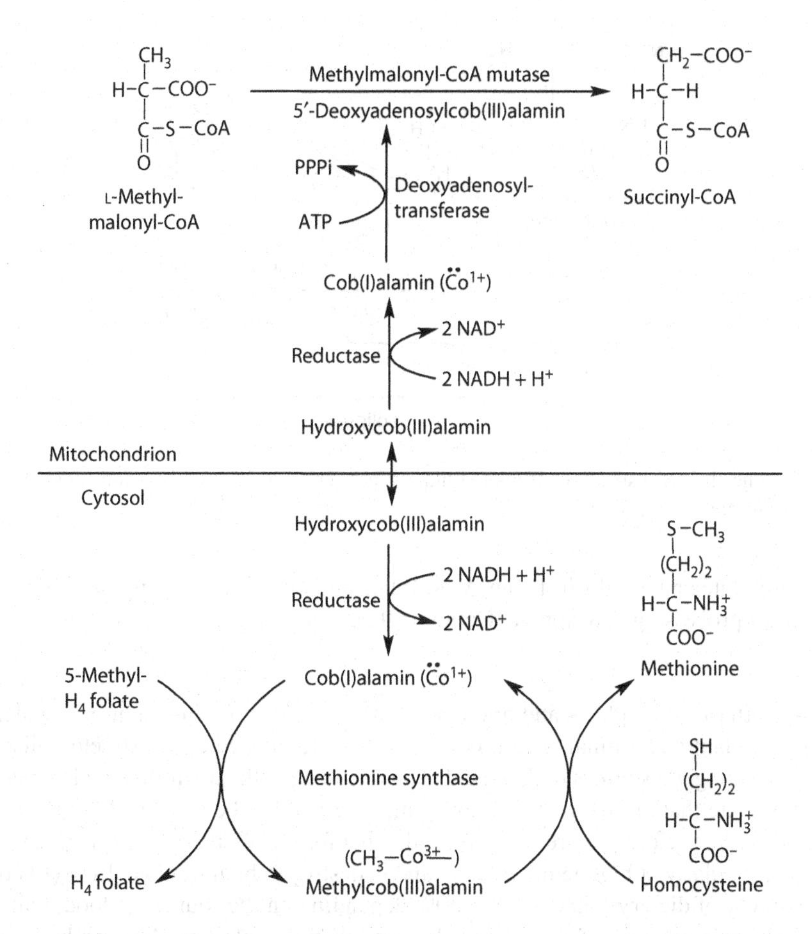


**FIGURE 9.15** Role of vitamin $B_{12}$ as a coenzyme for methylmalonyl-CoA mutase and methionine synthase. These reactions occur in hepatocytes.

impaired formation of the nucleus of new red blood cells with consequent accumulation in the bone marrow of megaloblasts. Homocystinuria (accumulation of homocysteine) and methylmalonic aciduria (accumulation of methylmalonic acid) also occur in animals and humans with vitamin $B_{12}$ deficiency. Neurological disorders associated with vitamin $B_{12}$ deficiency may be secondary to a relative deficiency of methionine.

## Folate

### *Structure*

Folate (vitamin $B_9$) refers to folic acid (also known as pteroylglutamic acid) and its derivatives, which act as coenzymes for one-carbon metabolism (Shane 2008). Folic acid consists of a pteridine base, *p*-aminobenzoic acid, and glutamic acid (Figure 9.16), and is the parent structure of the large family of pteridine derivatives. Folates may contain one or more glutamate residues as a γ-linked polypeptide chain. For example, in plants, folate exists as a polyglutamate conjugate consisting of seven glutamate residues (Butterworth and Bendich 1996). In animal tissues, the major form of folate is a pentaglutamyl conjugate containing five glutamate residues (Zhao and Goldman 2013). Essentially, all cellular folates occur in the polyglutamyl form. Folates that carry one-carbon units at varying oxidation states and bound to one or two nitrogen atoms (e.g., $N^5$,$N^{10}$-methylenetetrahydrofolate) are named according to the specific carbon moiety bound. The reduced folates

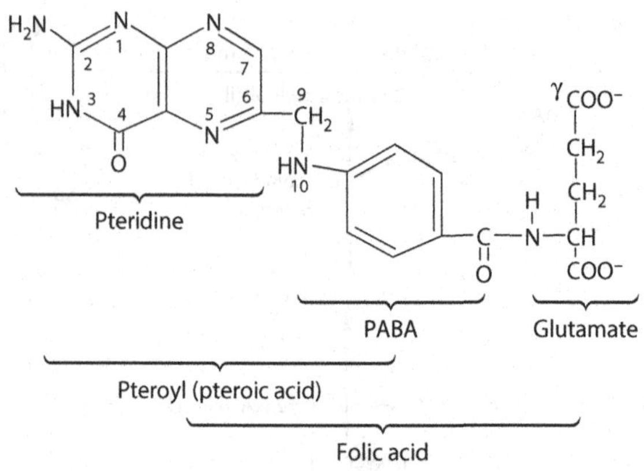

Pteridine
PABA
Glutamate
Pteroyl (pteroic acid)
Folic acid

**FIGURE 9.16** The chemical structure of folate (vitamin $B_9$). This vitamin refers to folic acid (also known as pteroylglutamic acid) and its derivatives.

include dihydrofolate and tetrahydrofolate. Most folates in foods can be easily oxidized under aerobic conditions of processing and storage (Combs 2012).

### *Sources*

Folic acid is synthesized by plants and microbes (Sahr et al. 2005). This vitamin is widely distributed in foods of plant and animal origin. Green leafy materials, cereals, extracted oilseed meals, and orange juice are good sources of folic acid. The liver, egg yolk, and milk are also major sources of the vitamin. Note that animal cells cannot synthesize *p*-aminobenzoic acid or attach glutamate to pteroic acid, and therefore require folate from the diet for metabolism. Folate is readily degraded by moisture, particularly at high temperatures, and is destroyed by ultraviolet light (Lucock 2000). The bioavailability of dietary folate is 30%–80% depending on the sources of food, with the folate in animal products being better digested and absorbed than the folate in plant products.

### *Absorption and Transport*

As noted previously, dietary folate exists in the form of mono- and polyglutamates, which are called folymonoglutamates and folypolyglutamates, respectively. Folymonoglutamates, but not folypolyglutamates, are absorbed by enterocytes and colonocytes. Thus, folypolyglutamates must be hydrolyzed into folymonoglutamates prior to their absorption. This digestion process occurs mainly in the proximal part of the small intestine and involves the enzyme folylpoly-$\gamma$-glutamate carboxypeptidase (also known as $\gamma$-glutamyl hydrolase or conjugase) that is localized on the apical membrane of the enterocyte. The intestinal activity of folylpoly-$\gamma$-glutamate carboxypeptidase is increased by folate deficiency but decreased by folate excess (Said et al. 2000). Both the proton-coupled folate transporter (PCFT, SLC46A1) and two reduced-folate carriers (RFC-1, SLC19A1; RFC-2), which are expressed in the apical membrane of intestinal epithelial cells, are responsible for intestinal absorption of folymonoglutamate (Said 2011). RFCs, which are $H^+$-dependent but $Na^+$-independent, are the major transporters for folates in mammalian cells. Upon entering the enterocytes, most folymonoglutamate is reduced to tetrahydrofolate ($H_4$ folate) by folate reductase, which uses NADPH as a donor of reducing equivalents (Figure 9.17). $N^5$-methyl-$H_4$ folate is also formed in these cells, which is the major form of folate in the plasma. Little is known about the molecular identity of the folate transport system on the basolateral membrane of intestinal epithelial cells. However, members of the multidrug resistance proteins may play an important role in transporting intracellular folate across the basolateral membrane of the enterocyte into the lamina propria (Zhao and Goldman 2013).

In most animal species, free folate is transported in the plasma as folymonoglutamate derivatives (mainly $N^5$-methyl-$H_4$ folate) (Zempleni et al. 2013). They are taken up by extraintestinal

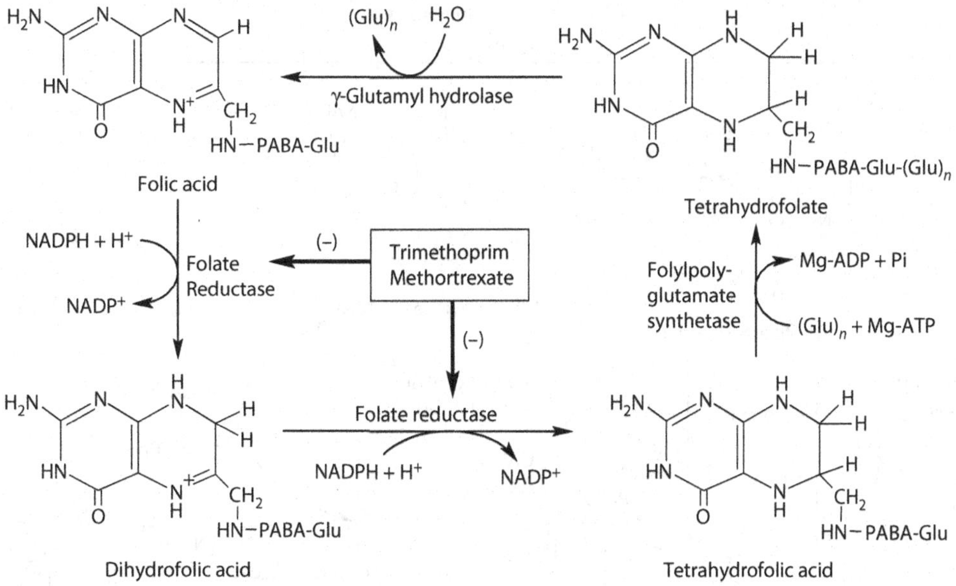

FIGURE 9.17 Conversion of folate into tetrahydrofolate in animal cells.

cells through PCFT, RFCs, and high-affinity folate receptors (FRs). Except for RCF, which is ubiquitously expressed in animal tissues, the distribution of PCFT and the high-affinity FRs is tissue-specific. In particular, PCFT is highly expressed in the small intestine as noted previously and also in the kidneys, liver, placenta, and spleen, but to a lesser extent, in the brain, testes, and lung. Much lower levels of PCFT are expressed in the terminal ileum and colon. Likewise, three FRs are expressed at the cell membrane in a tissue-specific manner (Zhao et al. 2011). For example, FRα is expressed on the membrane of epithelial tissues (e.g., the placenta, the apical brush-border membrane of proximal renal tubular cells, retinal pigment epithelium, and the choroid plexus). FRβ is present in hematopoietic tissues (e.g., spleen, thymus, and $CD34^+$ monocytes) and macrophages. FRδ is highly abundant in natural and TGFβ-induced regulatory T cells, whereas FRγ is a secreted protein. The kidneys play an important role in folate homeostasis. In particular, folates are filtered via the glomerulus and reabsorbed via the apical FRα-mediated endocytosis from the lumen of the renal tubule into the tubular epithelial cell. The reabsorbed folate will then be transported across the tubular epithelial cell into the bloodstream by its basolateral folate transporters.

### *Functions*

Active folate in cell metabolism is tetrahydrofolate ($H_4$ folate) in the form of tetrahydrofolate polyglutamates. $H_4$ folates are the carriers of activated one-carbon units and are used as cofactors in reactions that comprise one-carbon metabolism. The one-carbon units carried by $H_4$ folates represent methyl ($CH_3$–), methylene (–$CH_2$–), methenyl (–CH=), formyl (O=CH–), and formimino (HN=CH–), which are all metabolically interconvertable (Figure 9.18). $N^{10}$-formyl-$H_4$ folate contributes to the C-2 and C-8 of the purine ring structure. $N^5$-$N^{10}$-methylene-$H_4$ folate provides the methyl group for the synthesis of thymidylate, an event that is essential to DNA synthesis (Figure 9.19) and the formation of red blood cells. Thus, folate is required for the following processes: (1) interconversion of serine and glycine; (2) synthesis of purines; (3) histidine degradation; and (4) provision of methyl groups essential for methylation reactions, such as choline and methionine synthesis (Ducker and Rabinowitz 2017). Note that serine is the major source of one-carbon units carried by folate, whereas formiminoglutamate (a metabolite of L-histidine) can also

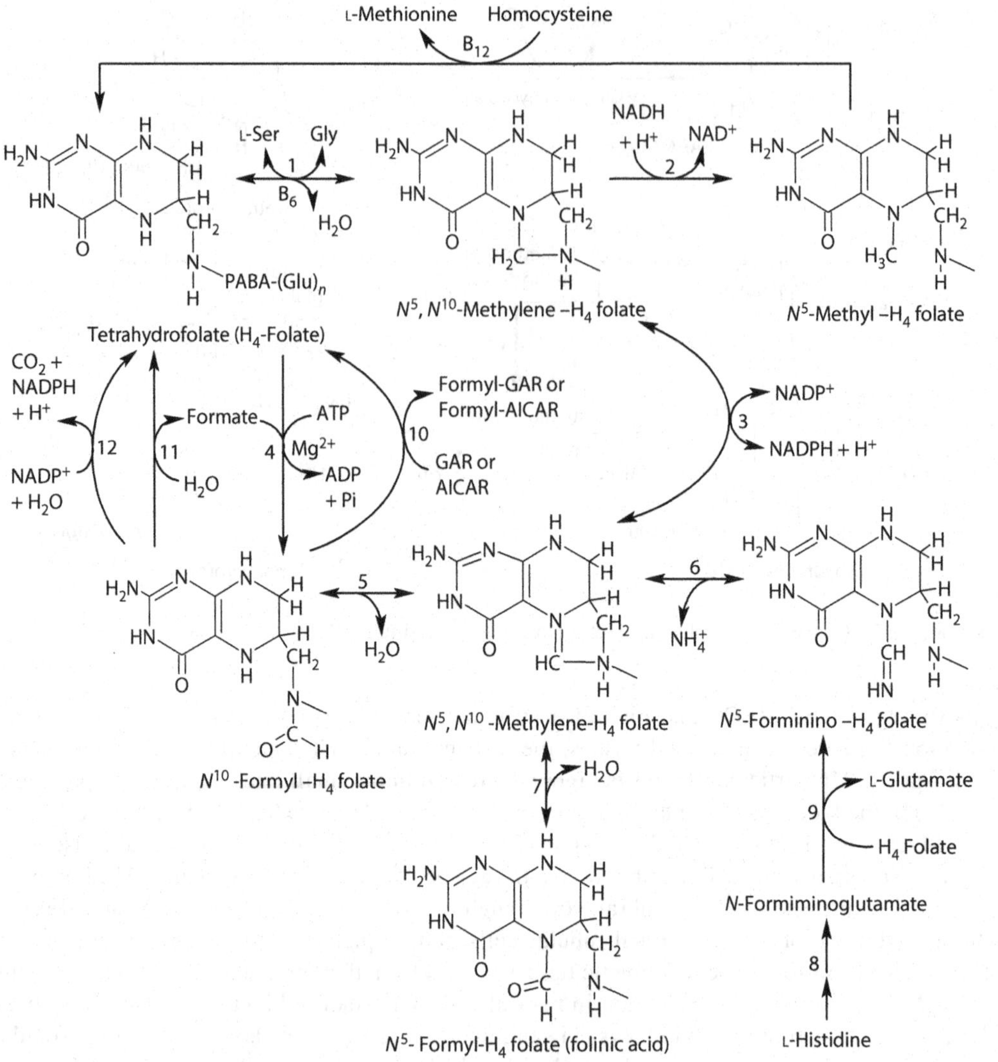

**FIGURE 9.18** One-carbon metabolism in animal cells. The one-carbon units carried by $H_4$ folates represent methyl ($CH_3$–), methylene (–$CH_2$–), methenyl (–CH=), formyl (O=CH–), and formimino (HN=CH–), which are all metabolically interconverted in animal cells. AICAR, 5-amino-4-imidazolecarboxamide riboside; GAR, glycinamide ribonucleotide.

transfer its formimino group to $H_4$ folate to form $N^5$-formimino-$H_4$ folate (Wang et al. 2012). Finally, folate is required for the microbial production of methane from formate or $CO_2$ plus $H_2$ (Chapter 5).

### *Deficiencies and Diseases*

Risk factors in folate deficiency include (1) inadequate intake of folate; (2) chronic consumption of alcohol in place of food; (3) heating of foods and dilution in cooking water; (4) increased requirement due to pregnancy and lactation in mammals or egg laying in birds; (5) treatment with methotrexate (an inhibitor of folate reductase); and (6) vitamin $B_{12}$ deficiency. The reason why vitamin $B_{12}$ deficiency induces folate deficiency is that vitamin $B_{12}$ is required for the conversion of folate from a form ($N^5$-methyl-$H_4$ folate) with a limited use into a form ($H_4$ folate) that participates in a variety of reactions. Severe metabolic disorders occur in folate-deficient animals, particularly during embryonic, fetal,

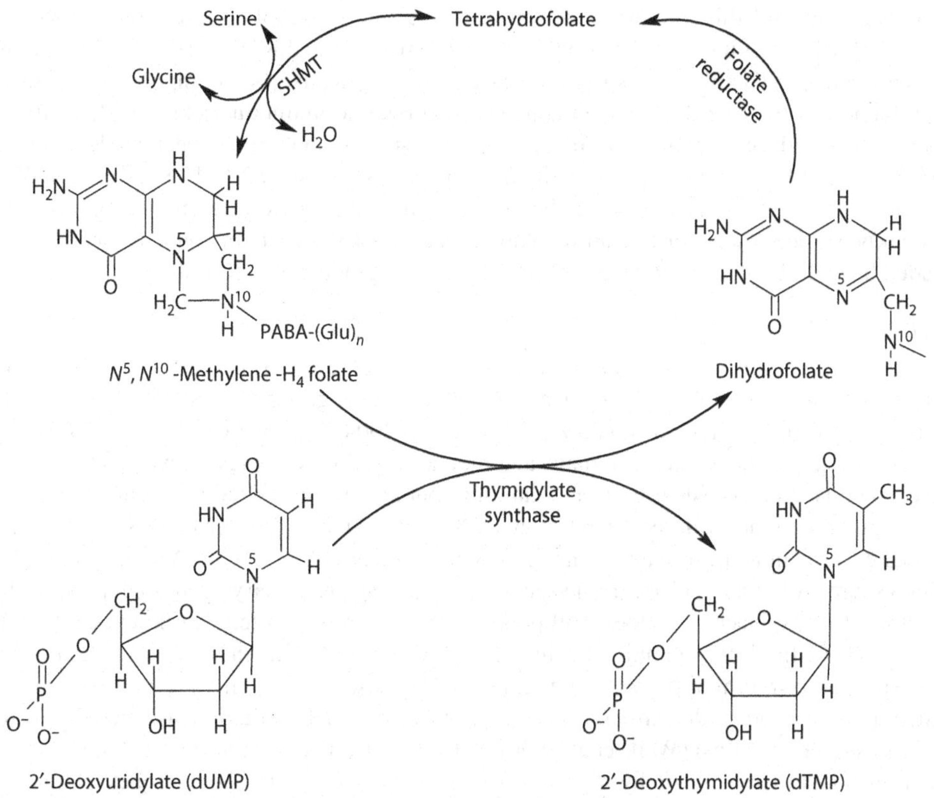

**FIGURE 9.19** Role of tetrahydrofolate in the formation of 2′-deoxythymidylate (dTMP), a precursor of DNA. $N^5,N^{10}$-Methylene-$H_4$ folate, which is generated from tetrahydrofolate, is a coenzyme for thymidylate synthase.

and neonatal development (Ducker and Rabinowitz 2017). For example, folate deficiency causes megaloblastic anemia, because one-carbon metabolism is necessary for the formation of red blood cells. Folate deficiency during pregnancy can cause neural tube defects such as spina bifida in infants (Fleming and Copp 1998). The complexities of the interaction between vitamin $B_{12}$ and folate are a consequence of their common participation in the methionine synthase reaction. Folate deficiency can occur in chickens and turkeys fed diets containing practical ingredients, with symptoms including poor growth, reduced feed efficiency, anemia, poor bone development, and poor egg hatchability (Pesti et al. 1991; Sherwood et al. 1993). This may be due to a low ability of poultry to synthesize folate in their intestinal bacteria and a low ability of folate absorption by their hindguts. Folate deficiency rarely occurs in other farm animals because of the presence of the vitamin in commonly used ingredients and the synthesis of the vitamin by intestinal bacteria. However, under conditions (e.g., gestation and lactation) when the requirements of folic acid are increased, dietary supplementation of folic acid is necessary. Note that folinic acid (5-formyl tetrahydrofolic acid) is a metabolically active analog of tetrahydrofolate. It can be used to treat folate deficiency in animals. For example, folinic acid is often administered to methotrexate-treated cancer patients at the appropriate time to alleviate damage to their bone marrow and gastrointestinal mucosa cells (Zempleni et al. 2013).

## Ascorbic Acid (Vitamin C)

### *Structure*

Vitamin C (also known as ascorbic acid) is a glucose derivative with the chemical name of 2,3-didehydro-L-threo-hexano-1,4-lactone. It is a white, crystalline, and water-soluble substance.

The oxidized form of this vitamin is dehydroascorbic acid (also called L-dehydroascorbic acid) (Wells and Xu 1994). Vitamin C has weak acidic and strong reducing properties, and can stabilize unpaired electrons. Therefore, it is used to scavenge free radicals, protect biomolecules (e.g., tetrahydrobiopterin) from oxidation in an aqueous solution, and maintain metal ions (e.g., iron and copper) in their reduced forms (Englard and Seifter 1986). This vitamin is heat-stable in an acidic solution and readily decomposed under alkaline conditions (Figure 9.20). The destruction of vitamin C at high temperatures is enhanced by exposure to light. Dehydroascorbic acid is not ionized in a weakly acidic solution or a neutral solution, and is not stable in an aqueous solution as it is degraded by hydrolytic ring opening to form 2,3-dioxo-L-gulonic acid (Combs 2012).

*Sources*

Vitamin C is essentially absent from grains (McDonald et al. 2011). It is synthesized from glucose via the uronic acid pathway in the liver of most mammals (e.g., pigs, dogs, cats, and ruminants) and in the liver and kidneys of poultry (Mahan et al. 2004; Maurice et al. 2004; Ranjan et al. 2012). However, in primates (e.g., humans and monkeys) and guinea pigs, as well as some species of insects, birds, fish, and invertebrates, vitamin C cannot be synthesized from glucose due to the lack of L-gulonolactone oxidase (Zempleni et al. 2013). In contrast to other water-soluble vitamins, intestinal bacteria in nonruminants do not have a net synthesis of vitamin C (Wrong et al. 1981).

Good sources of vitamin C are fresh vegetables, including green leafy plants, bell peppers, broccoli, citrus fruits, spinach, tomatoes, and potatoes. Animal products (e.g., milk and eggs) contain some vitamin C. In plant- and animal-source foods, vitamin C exists in the reduced and oxidized forms. The oxidized form of the vitamin is converted into ascorbic acid in intestinal epithelial cells by glutathione-dependent dehydroascorbic acid reductase, which is the intrinsic activity of thioltransferases (glutaredoxins) (Wells et al. 1990). In ruminants, dietary vitamin C is totally degraded in the rumen and there is virtually no net synthesis of this vitamin by the microbes (Ranjan et al.

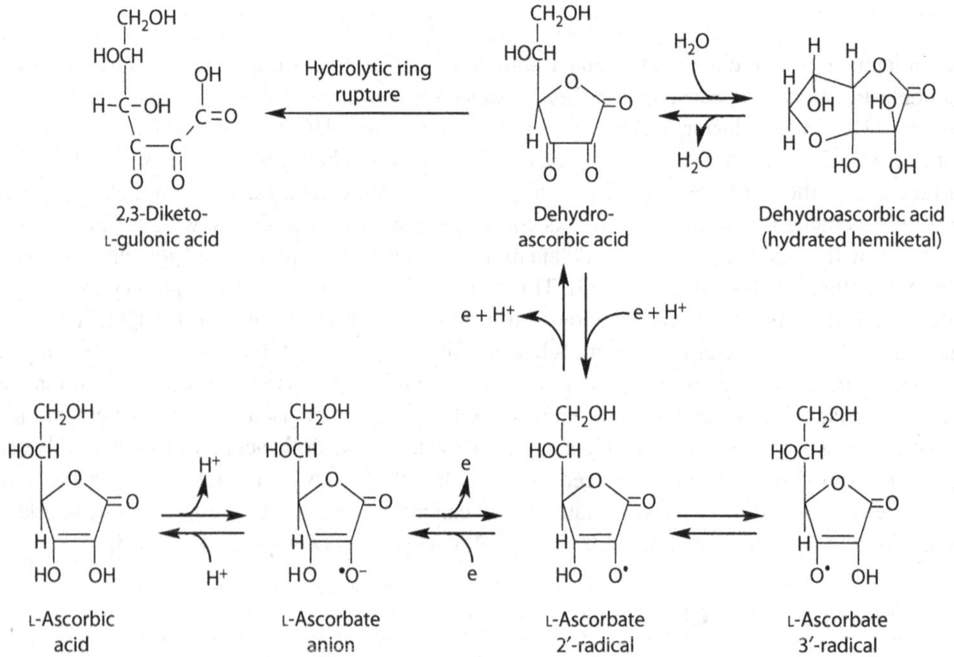

**FIGURE 9.20** The chemical structure of vitamin C and its oxidation to L-ascorbate 2′-radical and dehydroascorbic acid in animal cells.

2012). Thus, it is difficult to increase milk's vitamin C content through dietary supplementation of the unprotected vitamin.

*Absorption and Transport*

Vitamin C is absorbed by the small intestine into the blood circulation. The apical membrane of the enterocyte contains sodium-dependent vitamin C transporters (SVCT) 1 and 2 (the products of the SLC23A1 and SLC23A2 genes, respectively) to take up dietary vitamin C (Bürzle et al. 2013). SVCT1 is expressed in the intestine, liver, and kidney, but SVCT2 is widely distributed in animal tissues. In contrast, dehydroascorbic acid is absorbed into the enterocyte via facilitative ($Na^+$-independent) glucose transporters GLUT2 and GLUT8 that are competitively inhibited by hexoses (e.g., glucose and fructose) and flavonoids (e.g., phloretin and quercetin) (Corpe et al. 2013). Vitamin C exits the enterocyte across its basolateral membrane into the lamina propria via a specific protein carrier. Thus, dietary sugars and flavonoids (e.g., derived from fruits and vegetables) may modulate vitamin C bioavailability in animals. In addition, intestinal absorption of vitamin C is upregulated by its dietary deficiency but downregulated by its dietary excess (Said 2011).

In animals, vitamin C is transported in the plasma in the free form, which usually has no detectable dehydroascorbic acid. Vitamin C is taken up by extraintestinal tissues via SVCT2 and participates in many biochemical reactions (see the section below). In cells, this vitamin may be oxidized to ascorbyl free radical and then to dehydroascorbic acid by losing one electron in each step (Figure 9.20). Dehydroascorbic acid undergoes irreversible hydrolysis to 2,3-diketo-L-gulonic acid, which is oxidized to $C_5$ fragments (xylose, xylonic acid, and lyxonic acid), $C_4$ fragments (L-erythrulose and L-threonate), oxalate, $H_2O$, and $CO_2$ (Figure 9.21). The proportions of these products vary with animal species (e.g., almost completely as $H_2O$ and $CO_2$ in rats and guinea pigs, but primarily as oxalate in humans) (Combs 2012). Vitamin C can be regenerated from (1) ascorbyl free radical by NADPH-dependent semidehydroascorbyl reductase and (2) dehydroascorbic acid through its reduction by the reduced form of glutathione (GSH) or lipoic acid nonenzymatically or by GSH-dependent dehydroascorbic acid reductase. All these reactions help to conserve vitamin C.

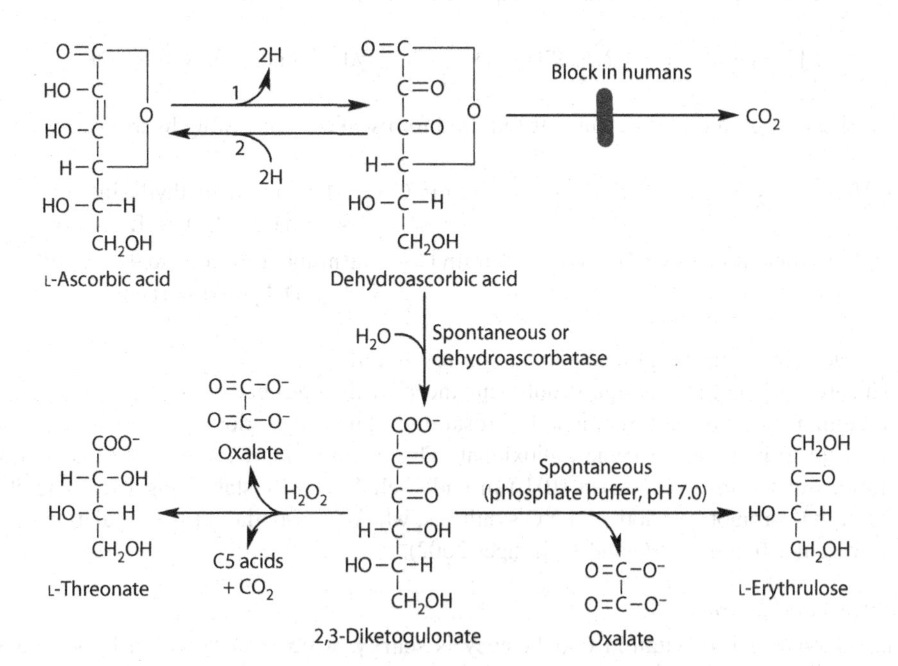


**FIGURE 9.21** Vitamin C catabolism in animals. The degradation products of this vitamin include $CO_2$, L-threonate, oxalate, and L-erythrulose in a species-dependent manner.

### *Functions*

Vitamin C is a donor of reducing equivalents, and can reduce compounds such as $O_2$, nitrate, and cytochromes a and c (Englard and Seifter 1986; Padayatty and Levine 2016). Vitamin C can help to maintain a metal cofactor of some enzymes in the reduced state (e.g., $Cu^+$ in monooxygenase and $Fe^{2+}$ in dioxygenases, including α-ketoglutarate- and $O_2$-dependent histone demethylases). The following reactions depend on vitamin C and, in some cases, one or more additional cofactors:

1. Synthesis of hydroxyproline by prolyl hydroxylase ($Fe^{2+}$) in collagen (posttranslational reaction) that requires vitamin C and α-ketoglutarate (α-KG).

$$\text{–Pro– (peptide)} + {}^{18}O_2 + \alpha\text{-KG} \rightarrow \text{–}{}^{18}\text{OH–Pro–} + [{}^{18}\text{O}]\text{Succinate} + CO_2$$

2. Synthesis of hydroxylysine by lysyl hydroxylase ($Fe^{2+}$) in collagen (posttranslational reaction).

$$\text{–Lys– (peptide)} + {}^{18}O_2 + \alpha\text{-KG} \rightarrow \text{–}{}^{18}\text{OH–Lys–} + [{}^{18}\text{O}]\text{Succinate} + CO_2$$

3. Oxidation of tyrosine at the steps catalyzed by *p*-hydroxyphenylpyruvate hydroxylase ($Fe^{2+}$) and homogentisate oxidase ($Fe^{2+}$)

$$p\text{-Hydroxyphenylpyruvate} + O_2 \rightarrow \text{Homogentisate} + CO_2$$
$$\text{Homogentisate} + O_2 \rightarrow \text{Maleylacetoacetate}$$

4. Synthesis of catecholamines from tyrosine by dopamine ß-hydroxylase.

$$\text{Dopamine} + O_2 \rightarrow \text{Norepinephrine}$$

5. Synthesis of bile acid (vitamin C is required at the initial 7α-hydroxylase step).

$$\text{Cholesterol} + O_2 + \text{NADPH} + H^+ \rightarrow 7\alpha\text{-Hydroxycholesterol} + \text{NADP}^+$$

6. Synthesis of carnitine (vitamin C is required for two $Fe^{2+}$-containing hydroxylases).

$$\varepsilon\text{-}N\text{-Trimethyllysine} + \alpha\text{-KG} + O_2 + \text{Vitamin C} \rightarrow \beta\text{-Hydroxytrimethyllysine} + \text{Succinate} + CO_2 + \text{Dehydroascorbate}$$
$$\gamma\text{-Butyrobetaine} + \alpha\text{-KG} + O_2 + \text{Vitamin C} \rightarrow \text{Carnitine} + \text{Succinate} + CO_2 + \text{Dehydroascorbate}$$

7. Steroidogenesis in the adrenal cortex requires vitamin C.
8. The absorption of iron is significantly enhanced by the presence of vitamin C.
9. Vitamin C inhibits the formation of nitrosamines during digestion.
10. Vitamin C is a water-soluble antioxidant. This vitamin increases intracellular concentrations of tetrahydrobiopterin ($BH_4$) in endothelial cells by stabilizing $BH_4$. Therefore, vitamin C promotes endothelial NO synthesis, which is essential for the regulation of cardiovascular function (Wu and Meininger 2002).

### *Deficiencies and Diseases*

The classic syndrome of vitamin C deficiency is scurvy, which can be cured by the consumption of fruits and fresh vegetables (Padayatty and Levine 2016). The disease is related to defective collagen synthesis in the connective tissue (e.g., blood vessels). In addition to connective tissue abnormalities (including subcutaneous and other hemorrhages [bleeding], soft swollen gums, loose teeth, and capillary fragility), impaired wound healing, muscle weakness, fatigue, depression, poor growth, reduced feed intake, and increased risk for infectious diseases can also occur in animals with vitamin C deficiency (Jones and Hunt 1983). Because farm animals can synthesize vitamin C, its severe deficiency normally does not occur. However, under certain conditions (e.g., heat stress), the demand for vitamin C may be greater than its endogenous synthesis and, therefore, a dietary supplement may be beneficial for improving animal health and productivity (Ranjan et al. 2012; Roche 1991).

## LIPID-SOLUBLE VITAMINS

Lipid-soluble vitamins are all isoprene derivatives. Concentrations of vitamin E and β-carotene in plant- and animal-source foods are shown in Table 9.9. Except for vitamin $D_3$, they are not synthesized in animal cells and must be supplied in ruminant diets (Pond et al. 1995). Their synthesis in the rumen may not be sufficient for maximal growth and production performance of ruminants (McDonald et al. 2011). Lipid-soluble vitamins are absorbed efficiently by the small intestine (primarily in the jejunum) when diets contain lipids (Meydani and Martin 2001). The absorbed vitamins are assembled into chylomicrons (vitamins A, D, E, and K) and VLDLs (vitamin E) in the

**TABLE 9.9**
**Content of Lipid-Soluble Vitamins and β-Carotene in Feedstuffs**

| Feedstuff | Vitamin E | β-Carotene | Feedstuff | Vitamin E | β-Carotene |
|---|---|---|---|---|---|
| Alfalfa | 49.8 | 94.6 | Oat grain | 7.8 | 3.7 |
| Barley grain | 7.4 | 4.1 | Peanut meal | 2.7 | 0.00 |
| Blood meal[a] | 1.0 | 0.00 | Pea seeds | 0.2 | 1.0 |
| Blood meal[b] | 1.0 | 0.00 | Rice bran | 9.7 | 0.0 |
| Canola meal | 13.4 | – | Rice grain[g] | 2.0 | 0.0 |
| Corn grain | 8.3 | 0.8 | Safflower meal | 16.0 | 0.00 |
| CSM[c] | 14.0 | 0.2 | Sorghum grain | 5.0 | 0.00 |
| Feather meal | 7.3 | 0.0 | SBM[h] | 2.3 | 0.2 |
| Fish meal | 5.0 | 0.0 | Sunflower meal | 9.1 | 0.00 |
| Flax meal | 2.0 | 0.2 | Wheat bran | 16.5 | 1.0 |
| Flax meal | 2.0 | 0.2 | Wheat bran | 16.5 | 1.0 |
| MBM[d] | 1.6 | 0.00 | Wheat grain[i] | 11.6 | 0.4 |
| Milk[e] | 4.1 | 0.00 | Yeast[j] | 10.0 | 0.0 |
| PBM[f] | trace | – | | | |

*Source:* National Research Council (NRC). 1998. *Nutrient Requirements of Swine*, National Academy Press, Washington, D.C.

*Note:* Values are mg/kg (on the as-fed basis).

[a] Conventional blood meal.
[b] Blood meal, spray or ring dried.
[c] Cottonseed meal (solvent extract, 41% CP).
[d] Meat and bone meal (93% dry matter).
[e] Bovine milk (skim, dried; 96% dry matter).
[f] Poultry by-product meal (93% dry matter).
[g] Polished, broken.
[h] Soybean meal (solvent extracted, 89% dry matter).
[i] Hard red, winter.
[j] Yeast, brewer's dried.

enterocyte for export across its basolateral membrane into either the intestinal lymphatics (mammals and fish) or the portal vein (birds and reptiles) (Chapter 6). Like any other hydrophobic lipid, lipid-soluble vitamins are transported in the blood in their protein-bound forms, and are excreted from the body primarily in the feces via the bile (Zempleni et al. 2013). Because of the body's ability to store surplus lipid-soluble vitamins, toxicity can result from their excessive intake, with risk being vitamin A > vitamin D > vitamin K > vitamin E (Zempleni et al. 2013).

## VITAMIN A

### *Structure*

Vitamin A is chemically known as all-*trans*-retinol (the alcohol form). The term "retinoids" has been used to describe both the natural forms and the synthetic analogs of retinol. Vitamin A is a polyisoprenoid compound containing a cyclohexenyl ring (Figure 9.22). It is present in animal tissues and stored in the liver mainly as retinol esters. Retinol derivatives are retinal (the aldehyde form) and retinoic acid (the acid form), which are called retinoids (Cascella et al. 2013). Most of the preformed vitamin A in animal-source foods is in the form of retinyl esters. Vitamin A is a pale yellow crystalline solid, insoluble in water but soluble in fat and various fat solvents. It is readily destroyed by oxidation on exposure to air and light. A related compound with the formula $C_{20}H_{27}OH$, originally found in fish, has been designated dehydroretinol or vitamin $A_2$. A group of compounds that are similar to vitamin A are pro-vitamin A carotenoids, such as α-carotene, β-carotene, and γ-carotene.

Retinol and retinal are interconverted by NAD(P)H-dependent retinaldehyde reductase. However, once formed from retinal, retinoic acid cannot be converted back to retinal or to retinol (Blomhoff et al. 1992). ß-Carotene is converted to vitamin A by ß-carotene dioxygenase and retinaldehyde reductase mainly in enterocytes (Figure 9.23), but this reaction is absent from the cat. Because ß-carotene is not efficiently metabolized to vitamin A, the biological activities of ß-carotene and vitamin A are not equivalent on a per weight basis. In humans, 6.0 mg of ß-carotene is equivalent to 1.0 mg of retinol (Combs 2012).

### *Sources*

Foods of animal origin (e.g., liver, eggs, milk, and butter) contain vitamin A largely in the form of retinyl esters (retinol esterified with a molecule of long-chain fatty acid, such as palmitic acid). The liver is a good source of vitamin A. For example, concentrations of vitamin A in the livers of various animals (μg/g liver) are as follows: pig, 30; cow, 45; rat, 75; man, 90; sheep, 180; horse, 180; hen, 270; codfish, 600; halibut, 3,000; polar bear, 6,000; and soup-fin-shark, 15,000 (McDonald

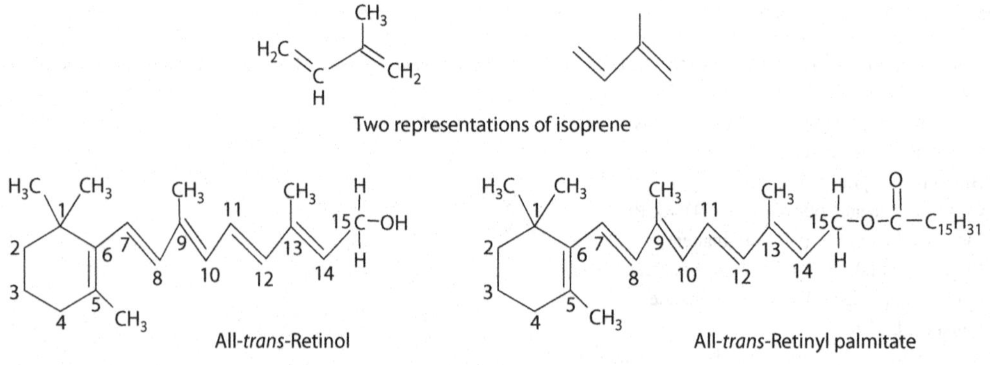

Two representations of isoprene

All-*trans*-Retinol

All-*trans*-Retinyl palmitate

**FIGURE 9.22** The chemical structure of vitamin A. This vitamin is an isoprene derivative containing a cyclohexenyl ring. The term "retinoids" has been used to describe both the natural forms and the synthetic analogs of retinol.

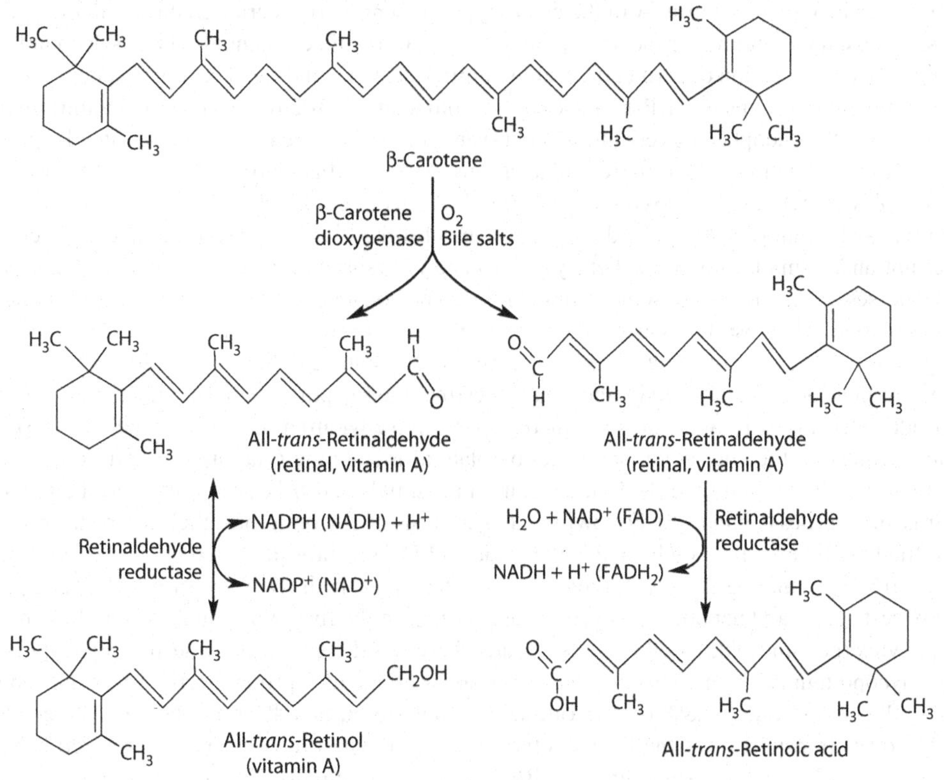

**FIGURE 9.23** Conversion of β-carotene into vitamin A. This NADPH-dependent reaction occurs in enterocytes.

et al. 2011). Plants do not contain vitamin A. However, some plants are rich sources of provitamin A, which takes the form of a family of compounds called carotenoids. Vegetables that are dark green, orange, and yellow are good sources of carotenoids. The efficiencies (%) of the conversion of carotene to vitamin A in animals are rats, 100; chickens, 100; pig, 30; cattle, 24; sheep, 30; horse, 33; man, 33; and dogs, 67 (Berdanier 1998). An international unit (IU) is used to standardize the biological activity of vitamin A and provitamin A carotenoids in various forms (Combs 2012).

1 IU of vitamin A = 0.30 μg crystalline all-*trans*-retinol
= 0.344 μg retinyl acetate
= 0.55 μg retinyl palmitate
= 0.6 μg β-carotene
= 1.2 μg other provitamin A carotenoids

*Absorption and Transport*

In the lumen of the small intestine, dietary retinol esters are dispersed in bile droplets and hydrolyzed by pancreatic enzymes (triglyceride lipase and lipase-related protein 2, as well as intestinal phospholipase B) to yield retinol (Reboul et al. 2006). The latter is solubilized with lipids and bile salts to form micelles, which are taken up by the enterocyte (primarily in the jejunum) through its apical membrane via passive diffusion. In contrast to retinol, carotenoids are taken up by enterocytes through their binding to a scavenger receptor class B, type I, which is also a receptor for high-density lipoproteins and other lipophilic compounds, including tocopherols (Van Bennekum et al.

2005). Esterification of vitamin A in the enterocyte is essential to generate a concentration gradient across its apical membrane for the absorption of the vitamin and carotenoids. This is accomplished through (1) the conversion of carotenoids into vitamin A; (2) the binding of retinol to specific cellular retinoid-binding proteins (CRBPs), including the abundant CRBP2 that transports vitamin A from the cytosol to the endoplasmic reticulum; and (3) enzymatic esterification with saturated long-chain fatty acids by the action of lecithin:retinol acyltransferase and diacylglycerol *O*-acyltransferase 1 in the endoplasmic reticulum (O'Byrne et al. 2005; Wongsiriroj et al. 2008).

In rats and poultry, most of the dietary carotene absorbed into the intestinal mucosa is cleaved to retinol and a small amount of dietary β-carotene is absorbed into the circulation. In humans, cattle, horses, pigs, and sheep, some carotenoids escape conversion in the small intestine and enter the circulation. The absorbed carotenoids are transported in the blood, carried to tissues (see the paragraphs below), and contribute to the pigmentation of meat, eggs, and milk. Being water soluble, dietary retinoic acid is absorbed by the small intestine into the portal vein (Arnhold et al. 2002).

Inside enterocytes, retinol esters are incorporated into chylomicrons (O'Byrne et al. 2005). The chylomicrons exit the enterocyte across its basolateral membrane (via passive diffusion) into the intestinal lymphatics and then the bloodstream in mammals and fish, or into the portal circulation in birds and reptiles (Chapter 6). Following the hydrolysis of chylomicrons, their remnants (containing retinyl esters) are taken up by hepatocytes via an LDL receptor-mediated process (Chelstowska et al. 2016). The internalized REs then undergo enzymatic hydrolysis by carboxyl ester lipases, carboxylesterases, and hepatic lipases to release retinol. In the liver, vitamin A is stored as an ester in lipocytes (perisinusoidal stellate cells, located between the capillaries and the hepatocytes) as a lipoglycoprotein complex. This complex consists of about 13% protein (retinol-binding protein, RBP), 42% retinyl esters, 28% triglycerides, 13% cholesterol, and 4% phospholipids (Vogel et al. 1999). For its transport from the liver to other tissues, the vitamin A ester is hydrolyzed intracellularly to retinol, which is then bound to RBP. The resulting retinol–RBP is processed in the Golgi apparatus and secreted into the plasma. The processed retinol–RBP complex exits the liver into the blood and is taken up into extrahepatic cells via plasma-membrane receptors. Thus, after its mobilization from the liver, vitamin A is transported in the plasma in the RBP-bound form. In extrahepatic cells, retinol is bound to a specific CRBP (Kono and Arai 2015). The lactating mammary glands secrete most vitamin A as retinyl esters. Interestingly, in the eggs of reptiles, retinal is the major retinoid and retinol is present at much lower levels, whereas significant amounts of both retinol and retinal are stored in the eggs of birds (Irie et al. 2010).

Concentrations of retinoic acid in the plasma and tissues are much lower than those of retinol. For example, in mice, the concentrations of all-*trans*-retinoic acid in the plasma (6 pmol/mL) and tissues (e.g., 15 and 20 pmol/g in the liver and kidney, respectively) are 2–3 orders of magnitudes less than total retinol (Vogel et al. 1999). Unlike vitamin A, retinoic acid is transported in the plasma primarily in an albumin-bound form. Carotenoids that are not converted into vitamin A in enterocytes are incorporated into chylomicrons, which exit the cells into the lymphatic circulation. Through lipoprotein metabolism in the blood, carotenoids retained in the chylomicron remnants are internalized by the liver. This organ assembles vitamin A into VLDLs for secretion into the blood circulation.

#### *Functions*

Vitamin A has multiple functions in animals (Figures 9.24 and 9.25). Except for vision, most physiological actions of vitamin A are mediated by its bioactive metabolite retinoic acid (Cascella et al. 2013). For proper vision, retinol is converted into retinal, which is a component of the visual pigment known as rhodopsin (Figure 9.24). Rhodopsin occurs in the rod cells of the retina, cells that are responsible for vision under low-light conditions. When rhodopsin is exposed to light, it dissociates to form all-*trans*-retinal and opsin; this reaction is coupled with the opening of a calcium ion channel in the membrane of the rod cell. The rapid flux of calcium ion triggers a nerve impulse, allowing light to be perceived by the brain.

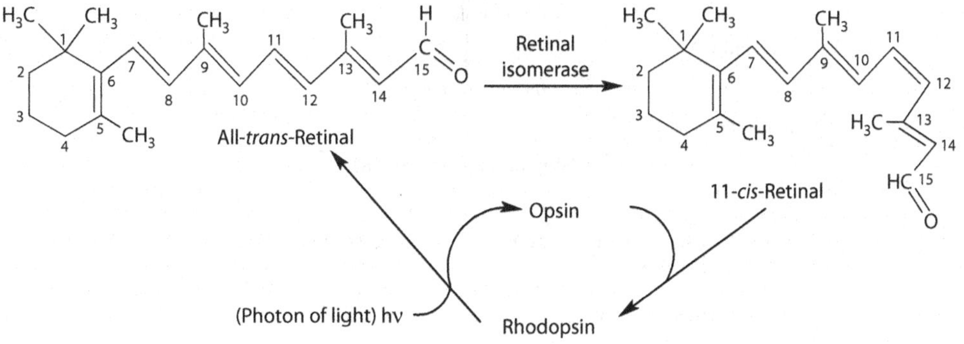

FIGURE 9.24 The mechanism whereby vitamin A is essential for vision. Retinol is converted into retinal, which is a component of the visual pigment known as rhodopsin (a component of the rod cells of the retina). When rhodopsin is exposed to light, it dissociates to form all-*trans*-retinal and opsin; this reaction is coupled with the opening of a calcium ion channel in the membrane of the rod cell. The rapid flux of calcium ion triggers a nerve impulse, allowing light to be perceived by the brain.

Both retinol and retinoic acid play an important role in regulating gene expression by binding to the nuclear retinoid X receptor, RXR (Figure 9.26), as steroid hormones do. Retinoic acid can also alter the activities of transcription factors to promote the transcription of downstream target genes into mRNAs and eventually proteins (Chelstowska et al. 2016). There are reports that retinol and 9-*cis*-retinoic acid upregulate the expression of ornithine aminotransferase in intestinal epithelial cells (Dekaney et al. 2008) and inducible NO synthase (Zou et al. 2007). In addition, retinoic acid participates in the synthesis of glycoproteins. This may account for, in part, the effect of retinoic acid in promoting cell growth and differentiation. Compelling evidence shows that retinol or retinoic acid is required for (1) maintenance of the integrity of normal epithelial tissues (e.g., the skin, small intestine, kidneys, blood vessels, uterus, placenta, and male reproductive tract); (2) spermatogenesis, embryonic survival, and fetal growth and development; (3) synthesis of glycoaminoglycans and growth of osteoclasts; (4) hematopoiesis; and (5) lymphoid organ development, antibody production

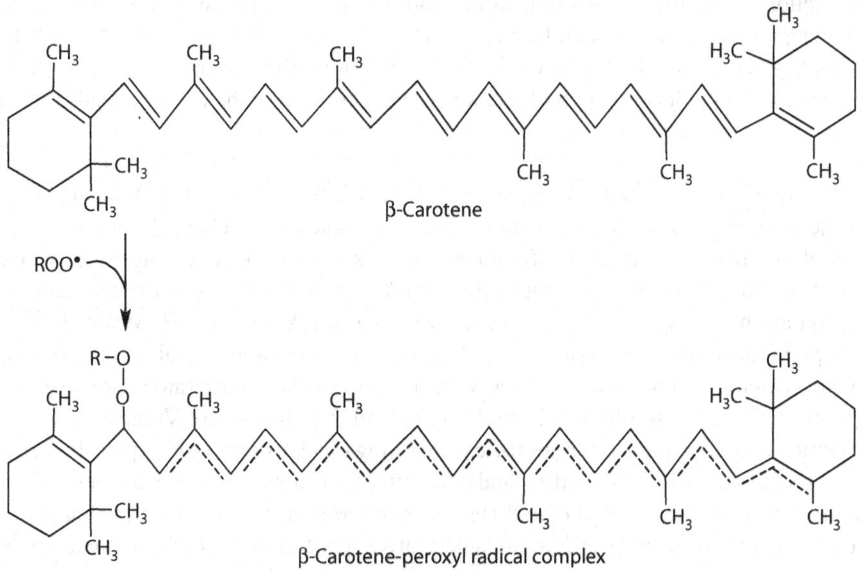

FIGURE 9.25 The formation of a resonance-stabilized carbon-centered radical from a peroxyl radical (ROO•) and β-carotene. Carotene-like substances (shown in Figure 9.27) also have anti-oxidative functions.

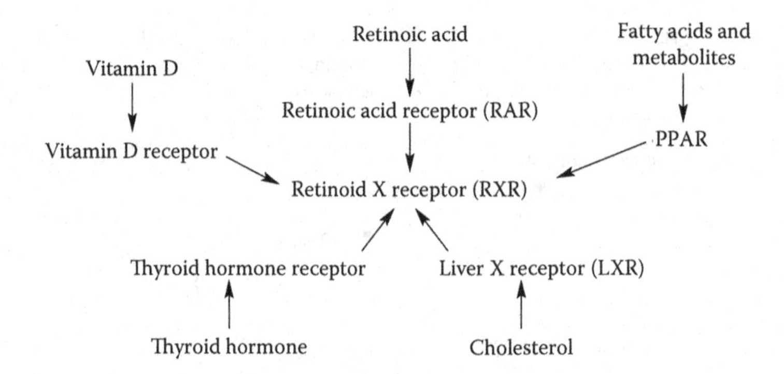


**FIGURE 9.26** Retinoic acid regulates gene expression by binding to the nuclear *retinoid X receptor*, RXR, thereby altering the activities of transcription factors to promote the *transcription* of downstream target genes into mRNAs.

by B-lymphocytes, and immune responses to pathogens. Finally, ß-carotene can stabilize organic peroxide free radicals within its conjugated alkyl structure (Figure 9.26) and is an antioxidant at low oxygen concentration. A group of carotene-like compounds with an antioxidative activity are shown in Figure 9.27, but lycopene, lutein and zeaxanthin have no vitamin A activity (Yeum and Russell 2002). Collectively, vitamin A is essential for vision, growth and development of cells (particularly epithelial cells), embryonic survival, and immunocompetence.

### *Deficiencies and Diseases*

Vitamin A deficiency occurs in animals consuming poor diets, such as those with low contents of vitamin and provitamin A. Vitamin A deficiency restricts animal growth, impairs the function of many tissues and cells, increases risk for infectious diseases, induces testicular damage, and causes embryonic death/fetal resorption (Clagett-Dame and DeLuca 2002; Stephensen 2001). The initial symptom of vitamin A deficiency is defective night vision (night blindness, a defect in the retina). This disorder occurs when liver stores of the vitamin are nearly exhausted (Collins and Mao 1999). Further depletion of vitamin A leads to keratinization of epithelial tissues of the eyes, lungs, gastrointestinal and genitourinary tracts, and decreased mucous secretion. Finally, the deterioration of the eye's tissues (e.g., cornea), which is known as xerophthalmia (the extreme dryness of the conjunctiva) and keratomalacia (dryness with ulceration and perforation of the cornea), leads to blindness.

### *Excesses*

Vitamin A toxicity occurs when the capacity of RBP for binding vitamin A has been exceeded such that the cells are exposed to unbound retinol or retinoic acids. Thus, chronic consumption of high levels of vitamin A is dangerous (Soprano and Soprano 1995). Assessing vitamin A status in animals with subclinical toxicity is complicated by the fact that this range of retinol concentrations in the plasma are not sensitive indicators of hepatic vitamin A reserves. However, the syndromes of overt hypervitaminosis A include severe liver fibrosis, bone and eye abnormalities, hair loss, neurological symptoms, irritability, nausea, vomiting, headache, and teratogenicity, such as birth defects (Penniston and Tanumihardjo 2006; Soprano and Soprano 1995). Vitamin A as a teratogen has been demonstrated in many animal species, including chicks, dogs, guinea pigs, hamsters, mice, monkeys, rabbits, rats, and pigs (Collins and Mao 1999). Of note, there are species differences in sensitivity to hypervitaminosis A due to differences in vitamin A metabolism, as indicated by the toxicity of 13-*cis*-retinoic acid (isotretinoin, a derivative of vitamin A) that is mediated by its isomerization to the all-*trans*-retinoic acid (Nau 2001). Specifically, the sensitive species (primates and rabbits) metabolize 13-*cis*-retinoic acid to the active 13-*cis*-4-ketoretinoic acid, and their placental transfer of 13-*cis*-retinoic acid is extensive, whereas the insensitive species (rats and mice) eliminate

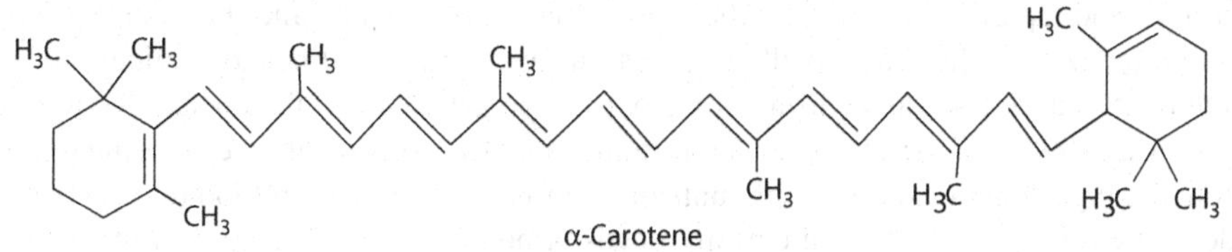

α-Carotene

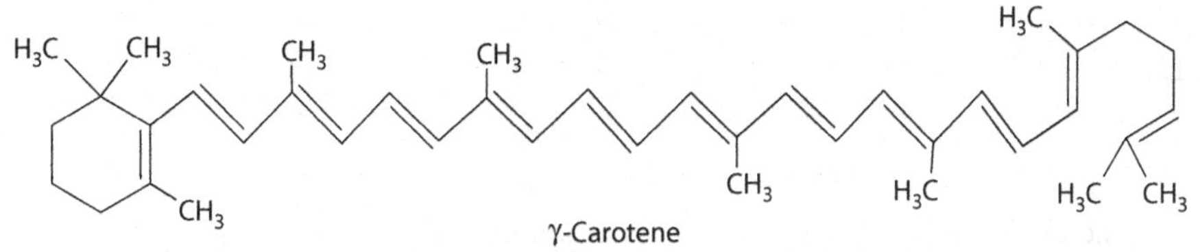

γ-Carotene

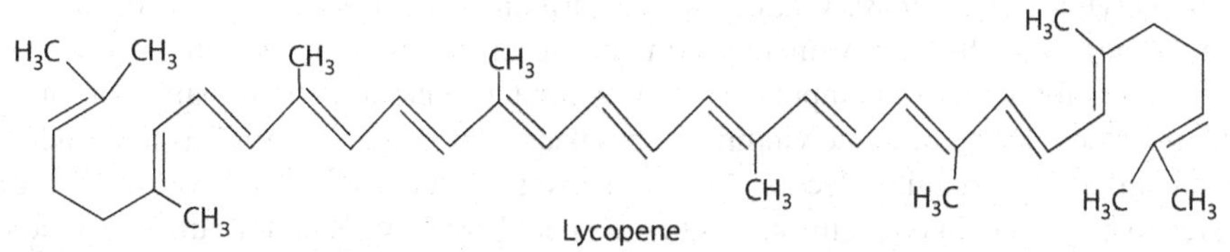

Lycopene

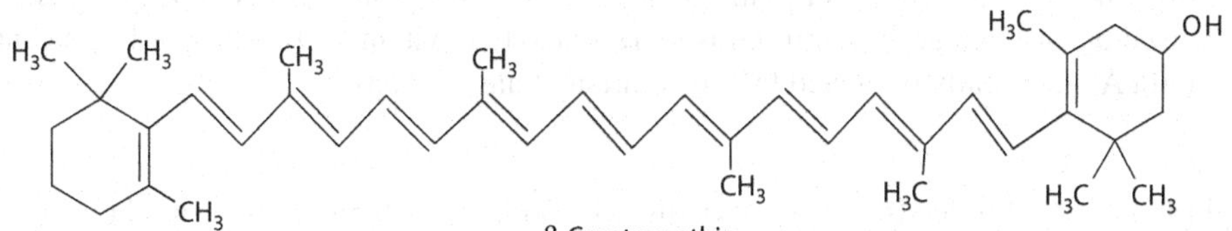

β-Cryptoxanthin

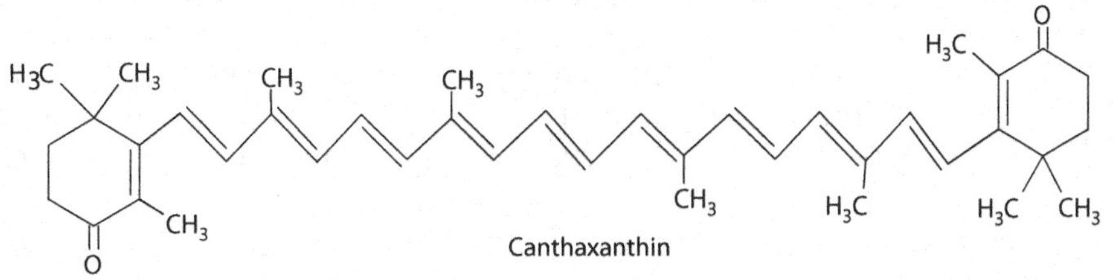

Canthaxanthin

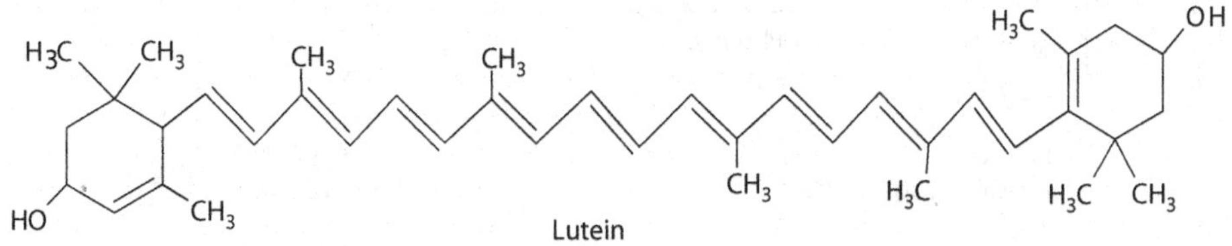

Lutein

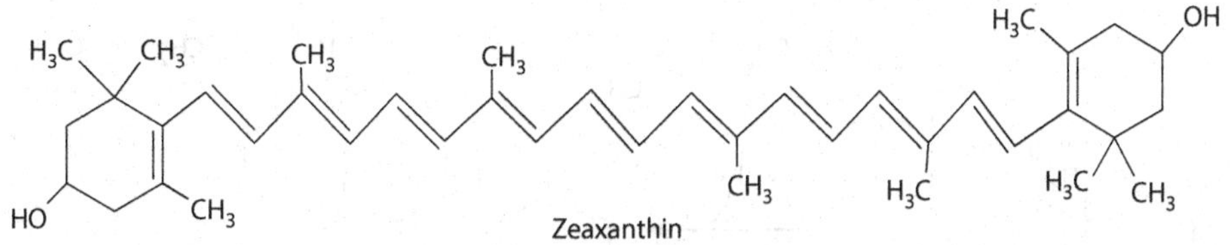

Zeaxanthin

**FIGURE 9.27** Carotene-like substances with anti-oxidative capacities in animal cells. α-Carotene, γ-carotene, β-cryptoxanthin, and canthaxanthin can be converted into vitamin A in the small-intestinal enterocytes and gastrointestinal bacteria of most animals, including ruminants, swine, dogs, poultry, and fish, but the efficiency of conversion is very low as compared to β-carotene (Gross and Budowski 1966; McDonald et al. 2011; Yeum and Russell 2002). Cats cannot synthesize vitamin A from any carotenoids. Lycopene, lutein and zeaxanthin are not precursors of vitamin A in mammals, birds or fish.

13-*cis*-retinoic acid rapidly through detoxification to the β-glucuronide, and their placental transfer of 13-*cis*-retinoic acid is limited. Results of research involving gene-knockout mice indicate that excess vitamin A causes acute and chronic toxicity by hyperactivation of the nuclear RAR and RXR (Collins and Mao 1999). Carotenemia, which is manifested by a yellow-orange coloring of the skin, results from the ingestion of excessive amounts of vitamin A precursors in food (e.g., carrots). This may be desirable for the production of certain breeds of poultry in some regions of the world.

## VITAMIN D

### *Structure*

Vitamin D is a steroid prohormone (Figure 9.28). The two most important forms are ergocalciferol (vitamin $D_2$) and cholecalciferol (vitamin $D_3$). In animals, vitamin D is metabolized to 1,25-dihydroxyvitamin D (Jones et al. 1998). Vitamin $D_3$ is a hormone known as calcitriol, which plays a central role in calcium and phosphorus metabolism. The term "vitamin $D_1$" was originally suggested by earlier workers for an active component, but it was later found to consist mainly of vitamin $D_2$ and some impurities. Thus, the name vitamin $D_1$ has been abolished. Vitamin D is not water soluble but is soluble in fat and organic solvents. Although a water-soluble sulfate derivative of vitamin D was reported to be present in cow's milk, this finding could not be verified for human breast milk or cow's milk (Okano et al. 1986). Both vitamin $D_2$ and vitamin $D_3$ are unstable upon overirradiation and oxidized during storage. Vitamin $D_3$ is more stable than vitamin $D_2$. Vitamin D concentrates, like vitamin A, are usually protected by the addition of antioxidants.

### *Sources*

Vitamin D is limited in feedstuffs for animals. This vitamin is rarely present in plants, except in sun-dried roughages (Peterlik 2012). An unfortified, typical corn- and soybean meal-based diet

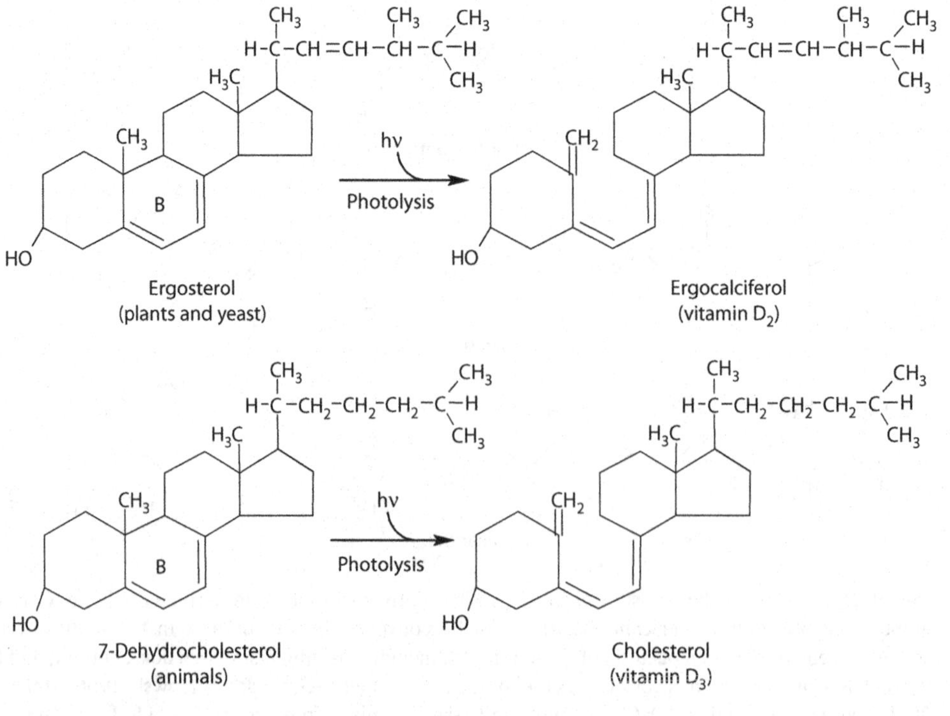

Ergosterol (plants and yeast) → hν Photolysis → Ergocalciferol (vitamin $D_2$)

7-Dehydrocholesterol (animals) → hν Photolysis → Cholesterol (vitamin $D_3$)

**FIGURE 9.28** The chemical structure of vitamin A and its synthesis from ergosterol (a component of plants and yeast) and 7-dehydrocholesterol (a subcutaneous component of the skin) in animals.

contains no vitamin D (Pond et al. 1995). In animals, this vitamin is present in small amounts in certain tissues and is abundant only in some fish. Halibut liver and cod liver oils are rich sources of vitamin $D_3$ (Egaas and Lambertsen 1979). The content of this vitamin in muscle meat is generally much lower than that in the liver, and the content of vitamin D in egg yolks ranges between the values for meat and offal. Unfortified cow's milk and dairy products are generally low in vitamin D, but butter has a high content of this vitamin (Schmid and Walther 2013).

Most animals (e.g., cattle, poultry, pigs, sheep, and rats) can synthesize vitamin $D_3$. Specifically, when the skin is exposed to sunlight (ultraviolet irradiation), the B-ring of 7-dehydrocholesterol is cleaved to yield cholecalciferol (vitamin $D_3$) (DeLuca 2016). This conversion is most active with the light of wavelengths between 280 and 310 nm. Therefore, vitamin D is called the "sunshine vitamin." The rates of vitamin $D_3$ synthesis in animals vary with their living environments, because (1) the amount of ultraviolet radiation that reaches the earth's surface depends on latitude and atmospheric conditions; (2) ultraviolet radiation is greater in the tropics than in the temperate regions; and (3) the presence of clouds, smoke, and dust will reduce ultraviolet radiation (Christakos et al. 2016). Thus, air pollution impairs vitamin $D_3$ synthesis in grazing animals, including lactating cows (Weir et al. 2017). Because ultraviolet radiation cannot pass through ordinary window glass, animals housed indoors lack a subcutaneous synthesis of vitamin $D_3$. Ultraviolet radiation is more effective in animals with light-colored skins than those with dark skins. There are reports that cats and dogs, when exposed to appropriate ultraviolet irradiation, do not synthesize vitamin $D_3$ from 7-dehydrocholesterol in their skins (How et al. 1994). This may also be true for other carnivores.

In plants, the ultraviolet radiation of sunlight also cleaves the B-ring of ergosterol to generate ergocalciferol (vitamin $D_2$). There are reports that 1 kg of hay contains between 800 and 1700 IU of vitamin $D_2$ (McDonald et al. 2011). Like plants, yeast is also rich in ergosterol and its radiation results in the formation of vitamin $D_2$.

Vitamin $D_2$ is almost as effective as vitamin $D_3$ in stimulating intestinal absorption of calcium and phosphate for most mammals (e.g., cattle, sheep, pigs, and humans) (Christakos et al. 2016). However, vitamin $D_2$ has a very low biological activity in chickens and other birds (only ~10% of the potency of vitamin $D_3$) (Proszkowiec-Weglarz and Angel 2013). Thus, poultry feeds must be fortified with vitamin $D_3$. For a few of the mammalian species (e.g., New World monkeys), vitamin $D_3$ is much more potent than vitamin $D_2$ on a weight basis (DeLuca 2016). In practice, with exceptions for poultry and certain monkeys, safe levels of vitamin $D_2$ can prevent abnormal bone development, as can vitamin $D_3$. Thus, the equivalency of vitamin $D_3$ to vitamin $D_2$ varies due to the factors mentioned previously.

$$1 \text{ IU of vitamin D} = 0.025\,\mu\text{g of crystalline vitamin } D_3.$$

### *Absorption and Transport*

In the lumen of the small intestine, dietary vitamin $D_3$ and vitamin $D_2$ are solubilized with lipids and bile salts, and absorbed from the micelles by enterocytes via passive diffusion (Reboul 2015). Following absorption (primarily in the jejunum), vitamin $D_3$ and $D_2$ are assembled into chylomicrons in enterocytes. The vitamin D-containing chylomicrons exit the enterocyte across its basolateral membrane (via passive diffusion) into the intestinal lymphatics and then the bloodstream in mammals and fish, or into the portal circulation in birds and reptiles (Chapter 6). Through the metabolism of lipoproteins in the blood, the vitamin D-containing chylomicrons are converted into chylomicron remnants, which are subsequently taken up by the liver through receptor-mediated mechanisms (Chapter 6). Unlike other lipid-soluble vitamins, vitamin D is not stored in the liver but is distributed almost evenly among various tissues (Combs 2012). Transport of vitamin $D_3$ from the sites of its cutaneous synthesis into the liver via the blood is mediated by a specific protein, called vitamin D-binding protein (also known as transcalciferin, an α-globulin). This binding protein has a higher affinity toward 1,25-dihydroxyvitamin $D_3$ than the vitamin $D_2$ derivative. In the liver, vitamin D is hydroxylated into 25-hydroxyvitamin $D_3$ or 25-hydroxyvitamin $D_2$, which is subsequently exported into the blood. The hepatocyte-derived 25-hydroxyvitamin D is transported in the plasma bound to the vitamin D-binding protein. Vitamin D, if used externally, can also be absorbed effectively across the lipid bilayers of the skin.

*Functions*

Interorgan metabolism of vitamin D (Figure 9.29) is required for exerting its potent biological activity (DeLuca 2016). Specifically, in the liver of mammals as well as both the liver and the kidneys of birds, vitamin $D_3$ is converted to 25-hydroxyvitamin $D_3$ by vitamin $D_3$-25-hydroxylase. This enzymatic activity involves cytochrome P-450-dependent mixed-function oxygenase. The 25-hydroxyvitamin $D_3$ is the major form of vitamin $D_3$ in the blood circulation and the major storage form in the liver. In the renal tubules of the kidneys, bone, and placenta, the 25-hydroxyvitamin $D_3$ is further converted to 1,25-dihydroxyvitamin $D_3$ (calcitriol) by 25-hydroxyvitamin $D_3$-1-hydroxylase. Hypocalcemia, hypophosphatemia, and parathyroid hormone increase the activity of 1-hydroxylase, while 1,25-dihydroxyvitamin $D_3$ decreases the enzyme's activity. Vitamin $D_3$-25-hydroxylase and 25-hydroxyvitamin $D_3$-1-hydroxylase are mitochondrial enzymes. Vitamin $D_2$ undergoes the same transformations as vitamin $D_3$ in animals. The 1,25-dihydroxyvitamin $D_3$ is transported in the plasma bound to the vitamin D-binding protein.

The vitamin D hormone (1,25-dihydroxyvitamin $D_3$ or 1,25-dihydroxyvitamin $D_2$) binds the calcitriol receptor in the nucleus, thereby stimulating gene transcription and the formation of specific mRNAs that code for calcium- and phosphate-binding proteins (Christakos et al. 2016).

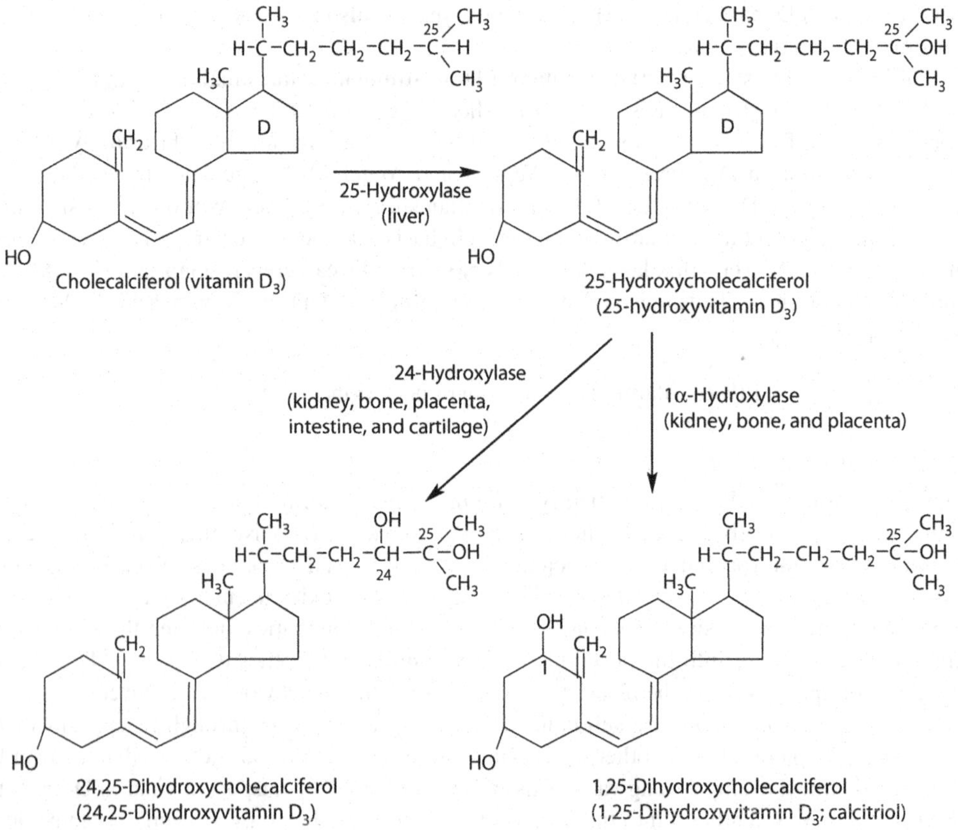

Cholecalciferol (vitamin $D_3$)

25-Hydroxylase (liver)

25-Hydroxycholecalciferol (25-hydroxyvitamin $D_3$)

24-Hydroxylase (kidney, bone, placenta, intestine, and cartilage)

1α-Hydroxylase (kidney, bone, and placenta)

24,25-Dihydroxycholecalciferol (24,25-Dihydroxyvitamin $D_3$)

1,25-Dihydroxycholecalciferol (1,25-Dihydroxyvitamin $D_3$; calcitriol)

**FIGURE 9.29** Conversion of vitamin $D_3$ into 1,25-dihydroxyvitamin $D_3$ (calcitriol) through interorgan cooperation. The latter is a hormone in animals.

1,25-Dihydroxyvitamin $D_3$ has three important physiological effects: (1) activation of the vitamin D-dependent calcium and phosphate transport systems of the enterocyte; (2) stimulation of the osteoclasts for the release of calcium and phosphate from bone; and (3) enhancement of calcium and phosphate resorption by the kidney (DeLuca 2016). Approximately 65% and 80% of the filtered calcium and phosphate are reabsorbed primarily within the proximal tubule under normal dietary intakes of the minerals (Christakos et al. 2016). Thus, vitamin D is essential for the regulation of calcium and phosphorus metabolism and consequently for the calcification and growth of bones.

Let us use "milk fever" to highlight the function of vitamin D. Milk fever is a disease in cows whose plasma calcium levels drop below 5 mg/100 mL (DeGaris and Lean 2008). The disease occurs when a cow has been fed an alfalfa diet high in calcium before giving birth to a calf (calving) and lactation. When calving, the cow has a low appetite, and the intake of calcium from the diet becomes inadequate. The body requires a period of adjustment to activate the calcium-mobilizing mechanisms. Because the prior consumption of high-calcium diets leaves these mechanisms in the nonactivated state, the sudden decrease in feed intake by the lactating cow does not allow the animal to adjust and mobilize bone calcium at an adequate rate. The consequence is a rapid drop in plasma calcium concentration, which can lead to coma, and sometimes death. Milk fever can be treated by intravenous administration of calcium or 1,25-dihydroxyvitamin $D_3$ into the sick lactating cow.

*Deficiencies and Diseases*

There is no need for a dietary source of vitamin D if animals (except for cats and dogs) are exposed to sunlight for at least a short period of time during the day. However, vitamin D (preferably vitamin $D_3$) must be supplemented to plant-based diets of the livestock and poultry housed entirely indoors. Also, because the content of vitamin $D_2$ in dried hay varies considerably, vitamin D supplementation is desirable, especially for young ruminants and pregnant animals on winter diets. When animals and humans are not exposed to sunlight or do not receive adequate amounts of vitamin $D_3$ in their diets, a deficiency of vitamin D occurs. Animals with vitamin D deficiency exhibit abnormal growth and development (DeLuca 2016). Specifically, vitamin D deficiency causes rickets in young animals and children, and this disease is characterized by the low deposition of calcium and phosphate in bones. Vitamin D deficiency also results in osteomalacia in adults, in which there is reabsorption of deposited bone tissue. Note that rickets and osteomalacia can also be caused by a dietary deficiency of calcium or phosphorus or by an imbalance between these two minerals. In young cattle, vitamin D deficiency syndromes include swollen knees. In pigs, deficiency syndromes are usually enlarged joints, broken bones, stiffness of the joints, and occasionally paralysis (Roche 1991). In poultry, a deficiency of vitamin D causes weak legs as in all other animals, as well as reduced egg production and poor eggshell quality (Proszkowiec-Weglarz and Angel 2013). In all young animals, vitamin D deficiency restricts their skeletal growth and development, leading to short stature.

*Excesses*

Excess vitamin D or 25-hydroxyvitamin D is toxic to animals (DeLuca 2016). The symptoms of vitamin D intoxication are thirst, itchiness, diarrhea, malaise, weight loss, polyuria, diminished appetite, neurological deterioration, hypertension, irritability, nausea, vomiting, and headache. In addition, severe hypercalcemia, hyperphosphatemia, and hypermineralization occur in many tissues to cause excessive calcification, particularly the kidneys, aorta, heart, lung, and subcutaneous tissue. Bone pain is common in hypervitaminosis D. Different animals may have different sensitivity to excess vitamin D in diets. There are reports that 1,25-dihydroxyvitamin D is not responsible for toxicity caused by vitamin D or 25-hydroxyvitamin D (DeLuca et al. 2011). Of note, the elevated plasma concentration of calcium in hypervitaminosis D can be reduced by treatment with adrenal cortical steroids (Dipalma and Ritchie 1977).

## Vitamin E

### *Structure*

Vitamin E was discovered nearly 100 years ago in vegetable oils as a factor required for reproduction in rats. This nutrient was required to prevent fetal resorption in gestating rats fed lard-containing diets that were easily oxidizable (Niki and Traber 2012). It was given the name tocopherol (*tokos* = childbirth, *phero* = bear, *ol* = an alcohol or phenol). Vitamin E refers to a group of tocol and tocotrienol derivatives that exhibit the biological activity of D-α-tocopherol.

Tocopherols and tocotrienols are called chromanols, which protect cells from lipid peroxidation. Tocopherols are all isoprenoid-substituted 6-hydroxychromanes (tocols), namely, side-chain derivatives of a methylated 6-chromanol nucleus. The most active form of tocopherol is D-α-tocopherol (Figure 9.30), and other tocopherols with a much weaker biological activity include D-β-tocopherol, D-γ-tocopherol, and D-δ-tocopherol (Traber 2007). These four naturally occurring tocol compounds differ in the number of methyl groups (3, 2, or 1 "$-CH_3$" groups) present in their aromatic ring, but have the same three chiral centers (2*R*, 4′*R*, and 8′*R*) in the phytol (side) chain. Thus, tocopherol has eight possible stereoisomers. D-α-Tocopherol has the widest natural distribution and the greatest biological activity of the vitamin E group (Table 9.10). The β, γ, and δ forms of D-tocopherol have only about 8.1%, 3.4%, and 0.4% of the activity of D-α-tocopherol (Combs 2012). Like tocopherol, tocotrienol also has α, β, γ, and δ isomers, but has only one chiral center (2*R* in naturally occurring tocotrienols or 2*S* in synthetic tocotrienols). Tocotrienols differ from tocopherols by possessing three double bonds in the phytol (side) chain, as these bonds are absent from tocopherols (Figure 9.30).

DL-α-Tocopherol was chemically synthesized in the early 1970s and its acetate ester was then adopted as the international standard for assessing the biological activities of all other forms of the vitamin. To date, the synthetic preparations of vitamin E (the acetate ester form) for animal feeding include all eight possible stereoisomers and are designated with the prefix all-*rac*-.

### *Sources*

Vitamin E is widely distributed in feedstuffs. Vegetable oils (e.g., corn, soybean, sunflower seed, safflower seed, and peanut oil) are good sources of this vitamin. Animal fats (e.g., butter and lard) and products (e.g., fish, eggs, and beef) also provide some vitamin E. However, corn and wheat grains are poor sources of this vitamin. For example, concentrations of total tocopherols in feedstuffs (mg/kg DM) are as follows: corn grain, 4–10; fish meal, 21; lucerne meal, 190–250;

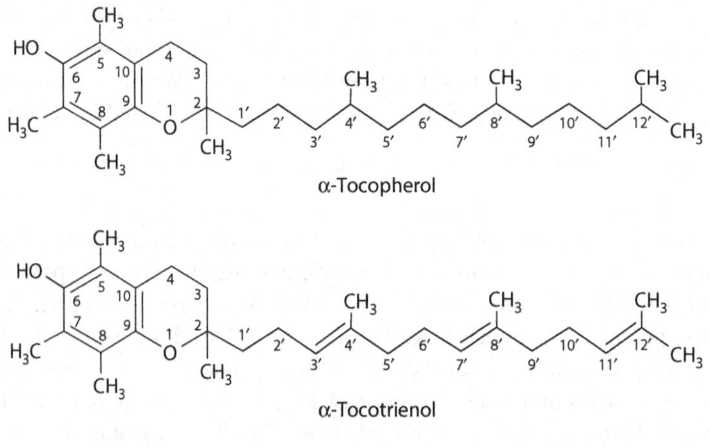

α-Tocopherol

α-Tocotrienol

**FIGURE 9.30** The chemical structures of α-tocopherol and α-tocotrienol. They are called chromanols. Tocopherols are all isoprenoid-substituted 6-hydroxychromanes (tocols). Tocotrienols differ from tocopherols by possessing three double bonds in the phytol (side) chain, as these bonds are absent from tocopherols.

**TABLE 9.10**
**Synthetic and Naturally Occurring Compounds with Vitamin E Activity[a]**

| Compound | Systematic Name | Biopotency (IU/mg Material) |
|---|---|---|
| | **Synthetic Tocopherol** | |
| All-*rac*-α-Tocopheryl acetate[b] | 2*RS*,4′*RS*,8′*RS*-5,7,8-Trimethyltocylacetate | 1.0 |
| All-*rac*-α-Tocopherol[b] | 2*RS*,4′*RS*,8′*RS*-5,7,8-Trimethyltocol | 1.1 |
| | **Naturally Occurring Tocopherol** | |
| *R,R,R*-α-Tocopherol[b] | 2*R*,4′*R*,8′*R*-5,7,8-Trimethyltocol | 1.49 |
| *R,R,R*-ß-Tocopherol | 2*R*,4′*R*,8′*R*-5,8-Dimethyltocol | 0.12 |
| *R,R,R*-γ-Tocopherol | 2*R*,4′*R*,8′*R*-5,7-Dimethyltocol | 0.05 |
| *R,R,R*-δ-Tocopherol | 2*R*,4′*R*,8′*R*-8-Monomethyltocol | 0.006 |
| | **Derivative of Tocopherol** | |
| *R,R,R*-α-Tocopheryl acetate | 2*R*,4′*R*,8′*R*-5,7,8-Trimethyltocyl acetate | 1.36 |
| | **Naturally Occurring Tocotrienol** | |
| *R*-α-Tocotrienol | *trans*-2*R*-5,7,8-trimethyltocotrienol | 0.32 |
| *R*-β-Tocotrienol | *trans*-2*R*-5,8-dimethyltocotrienol | 0.05 |
| *R*-γ-Tocotrienol | *trans*-2*R*-5,7-dimethyltocotrienol | 0.0 |
| *R*-δ-Tocotrienol | *trans*-2*R*-8-momomethyltocotrienol | 0.0 |

*Source:* Combs, G.F. 2012. *The Vitamins: Fundamental Aspects in Nutrition and Health.* Academic Press, New York, NY.

[a] The four naturally occurring tocopherols differ in the number of methyl groups present in their aromatic ring, but have the same three chiral centers (2*R*, 4′*R*, and 8′*R*) in the phytol (side) chain. In contrast, tocotrienol has only one chiral center (2*R* in naturally occurring tocotrienols). Both tocopherols and tocotrienols have α, β, γ, and δ isomers, and they are all antioxidants.

[b] Recognized as having vitamin E activity.

safflower oil, 500; soybean oil, 1,000; soybean meal, 3–6; various green forages, 200–400; wheat germ oil, 1,700–5,000; and wheat grain, 30–35 (McDonald et al. 2011). Accordingly, concentrations of α-tocopherol in feedstuffs (mg/kg DM) are as follows: corn grain, 0.5–3; fish meal, 21; lucerne meal, 180–240; safflower oil, 350; soybean oil, 100; soybean meal, 1; various green forages, 200–400; wheat germ oil, 800–1,200; and wheat grain, 15–18 (McDonald et al. 2011). Thus, α-tocopherol accounts for nearly 100% of total tocopherols in fish meal and lucerne meal, but only 10% of total tocopherols in corn grain and soybean meal. Vitamin E is not very stable in storage, and its stability can be greatly improved by esterifying its hydroxyl group with acetic acid to form α-tocopheryl acetate (Byers and Perry 1992). Although fish liver oils are good sources of vitamin A and D, they have insignificant amounts of vitamin E. Vitamin E is destroyed by cooking and food processing, including deep-freezing.

$$\begin{aligned}1\text{ IU of vitamin E} &= 0.67\text{ mg D-}\alpha\text{-tocopherol (natural)}\\ &= 0.90\text{ mg DL-}\alpha\text{-tocopherol (synthetic)}\end{aligned}$$

### *Absorption and Transport*

In the lumen of the small intestine, dietary vitamin E (in the acetate ester or free alcohol form) is solubilized with lipids and bile salts. The esterified forms of the vitamin are hydrolyzed by pancreatic and duodenal-mucosal esterases to release its free alcohol form. The vitamin E-containing micelle is absorbed by enterocytes (primarily in the jejunum) via passive diffusion (Niki and Traber 2012). The efficiency of absorption of the acetate ester form of vitamin E is similar to that of its free alcohol form. Active fat absorption promotes the absorption of vitamin E by the small intestine. Impaired fat absorption leads to vitamin E deficiency because tocopherol is found dissolved in the fat of the diet and is liberated and absorbed during fat digestion (Zingg 2015).

Inside the enterocyte, vitamin E is assembled into chylomicrons and VLDLs. These vitamin E-containing lipoproteins exit the enterocyte across its basolateral membrane (via passive diffusion) into the intestinal lymphatics and then the bloodstream in mammals and fish, or into the portal circulation in birds and reptiles (Chapter 6). Through the metabolism of lipoproteins in the blood, vitamin E-rich chylomicrons and VLDLs are converted into chylomicron remnants and LDLs, respectively. Unlike vitamins A and D, there is no specific carrier protein for vitamin E in the plasma.

The vitamin E-containing lipoproteins in the plasma are taken up by the liver through receptor-mediated mechanisms (Chapter 5). Inside hepatocytes, a protein (called α-tocopherol transfer protein) stimulates the movement of vitamin E between membrane vesicles and carries this vitamin to the nascent VLDLs (Ulatowski and Manor 2013). The vitamin E-containing VLDLs are then released from the hepatocytes into the blood. In the circulation, some of the VLDLs are converted into LDLs by lipoprotein lipases, and some vitamin E is transferred to HDLs. The presence of vitamin E in lipoproteins helps to protect both proteins and polyunsaturated fatty acids in plasma. In the blood, vitamin E exchanges rapidly between lipoproteins and erythrocytes, which have a high rate of vitamin E turnover (25%/h), to protect these cells. Thus, vitamin E is transported in the plasma via lipoproteins. The vitamin E-containing LDLs are taken up into cells through the LDL receptor, and the intracellular degradation of the endocytosed LDLs (Chapter 5) releases vitamin E. The intracellular transport of vitamin E requires specific tocopherol-binding proteins (Kono and Arai 2015). In white adipose tissue, vitamin E is stored mainly in the triacylglycerol fraction. In contrast, in most nonadipose cells, this vitamin is present almost exclusively in plasma and organelle membranes. In animals, vitamin E is stored primarily in white adipose tissue and liver.

*Functions*

Vitamin E is an antioxidant against peroxidation of polyunsaturated fatty acids in cellular and subcellular membrane phospholipids (Fang et al. 2002). Tocopherols act as antioxidants by breaking free radical chain reactions because of their ability to transfer a phenolic hydrogen to a peroxyl free radical of a peroxidized polyunsaturated fatty acid (Figure 9.31).

ROO· + Tocopherol-OH → ROOH + Tocopherol-O·
ROO· + Tocopherol-O· → ROOH + Non-free radical product
Tocopherol-O· + Vitamin C (red) + 2 GSH → Tocopherol-OH + Vitamin C (oxi) + GSSG

The non-free radical oxidation product is conjugated with glucuronic acid via the 2-hydroxy group and excreted in bile acid. In this reaction, tocopherol is not recycled after carrying out its functions and must be replenished from the diet. The antioxidant action of tocopherol is effective in solutions with high oxygen concentrations and in tissues exposed to high $O_2$ partial pressures, for example, the erythrocyte membrane, the membranes of the respiratory tree, the retina, and nerve tissues (Traber 2007). By keeping the cell membrane intact, vitamin E α-tocopherol is necessary for the structure of lipid bilayers, cell adhesion, nutrient transport, and gene expression. Furthermore, by affecting protein–membrane and lipid–membrane interactions, vitamin E can alter the trafficking of intracellular proteins and lipids, as well as cell signaling (Zingg 2015). Because reactive oxygen species may initiate diseases, antioxidant nutrients (including vitamin E) may prevent infertility, muscular and neurological degeneration, cardiac dysfunction, skin lesions, and aging.

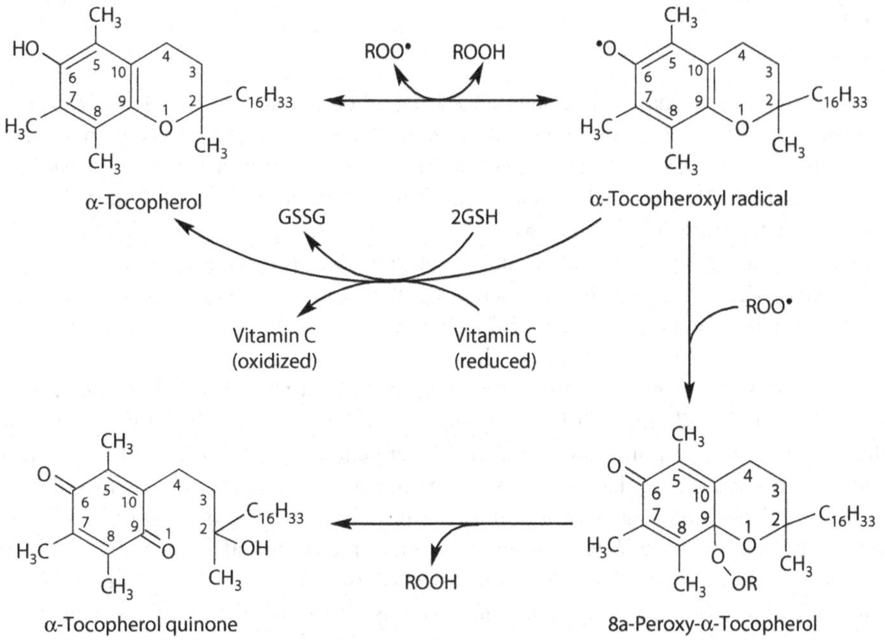

**FIGURE 9.31** Role of α-tocopherol in protecting cells against oxidants. α-Tocopheroxyl radical, a product of vitamin E oxidation, is converted into α-tocopherol via glutathione- and vitamin-dependent reactions.

### *Deficiencies and Diseases*

Deficiency of vitamin E may cause anemia in newborns and adults, due to the decreased production of hemoglobin and a shortened erythrocyte life span (Niki and Traber 2012). In all females and males, vitamin E deficiency results in impaired reproduction (e.g., a decrease in sperm production and dead fetuses, spontaneous abortion, and fetal resorption), muscle weakness and muscular dystrophy, skin and ocular lesions, and edema (Jones and Hunt 1983). Hepatic damage and muscular degeneration (myopathy) are the most frequent manifestations of vitamin E deficiency in laboratory and farm animals, and is a useful sign for diagnosis. These diseases include liver necrosis in rats and pigs, exudative diathesis in chicks due to increased capillary permeability, white muscle disease in lambs and calves. Diets for animals (e.g., gestating and lactating sows, cows in lactating and dry periods, growing broilers, and growing fish) must contain vitamin E to maintain optimal health, growth, and feed efficiency (Politis 2012; Pond et al. 1995). Of particular note, D-α-tocopherol, but not its isomers or tocotrienols, can prevent neural damage or fetal resorption in vitamin E-deficient animals (Zempleni et al. 2013).

### *Excesses*

When tocopherol is oxidized, it becomes a free radical species (Fang et al. 2002). Thus, high levels of dietary vitamin E can be toxic to animals. The syndromes of hypervitaminosis E include hepatic injuries and excess white-fat accumulation in rats, testicular atrophy in hamsters, slow development of secondary sex characteristics in roosters, and a teratogenic effect in mice (Dipalma and Ritchie 1977). Chicks with vitamin E toxicity exhibit reductions in growth rate, thyroid function, mitochondrial respiration, bone calcification, and hematocrit, but increases in reticulocytosis (March et al. 1968, 1973) and lethality of chick embryos (Bencze et al. 1974). Finally, dietary supplementation with excess vitamin E enhances the risk of developing heart failure after myocardial infarction (Marchioli et al. 2006) and all-cause mortality (Miller et al. 2005) in human subjects. Thus, excess vitamin E should be avoided in animal diets.

## Vitamin K

### *Structure*

Vitamin K is the generic name for 2-methyl-1,4-naphthoquinone and all of its derivatives with the biological activity of phylloquinone. Vitamins of the K group are polyisoprenoid-substituted napthoquinones (Figure 9.32). Phylloquinone ($K_1$) is the major form of vitamin K found in plants. Menaquinone (vitamin $K_2$) is synthesized by intestinal bacteria and found in animal tissues. The letter "K" originates from the German word "koagulation" (coagulation, blood clotting). Vitamin $K_3$ (menadione) is a synthetic vitamin K, and is not found naturally. The catabolism of vitamin $K_1$ in the intestine can generate vitamin $K_3$, whereas the metabolism of vitamin $K_3$ in animals can lead to vitamin $K_2$ (menaquinone) (Hirota et al. 2013). Dihydrovitamin K is the active form of vitamin K. Vitamins $K_1$ and $K_2$ are lipid soluble, while vitamin $K_3$ is water soluble.

The discovery of vitamin K had three independent beginnings with toxicological, nutritional, and biochemical studies (Ferland 2012). In toxicology, a hemorrhagic (bleeding) disease arose in cattle that had been eating spoiled sweet clover. Clover generally contained a bitter chemical called coumarin. During spoilage, microbes convert coumarin into dicumarol (4-hydroxydicoumarin), which inhibits 2,3-epoxide reductase and thus inhibits the recycling of vitamin K (Figure 9.33). The dicoumarol in the spoiled clover caused the death of many animals, especially after dehorning and castration procedures. Similarly, the administration of Warfarin, which is structurally similar to dicoumarol (Figure 9.34), is now commonly used as a drug to (1) induce experimental anticoagulation in animals; (2) treat blood clotting (e.g., deep vein thrombosis and pulmonary embolism); and (3) prevent stroke in certain patients with blood-thickening conditions (Clark et al. 2015). In nutrition, rats fed a lipid-deficient diet suffered from a bleeding disease. However, this disease could be cured by treatment with (1) an extract of alfalfa that contained vitamin $K_1$ and (2) spoiled fishmeal that contained vitamin $K_2$. The finding that phthocol was effective in treating the bleeding disease provided an early clue to the structure of vitamin K. In biochemistry, as noted previously, vitamin K was found to be required for the biological activities of blood clotting factors and vitamin K-dependent proteins. This work helped to elucidate the mechanisms whereby vitamin K is an essential nutrient in all animals.

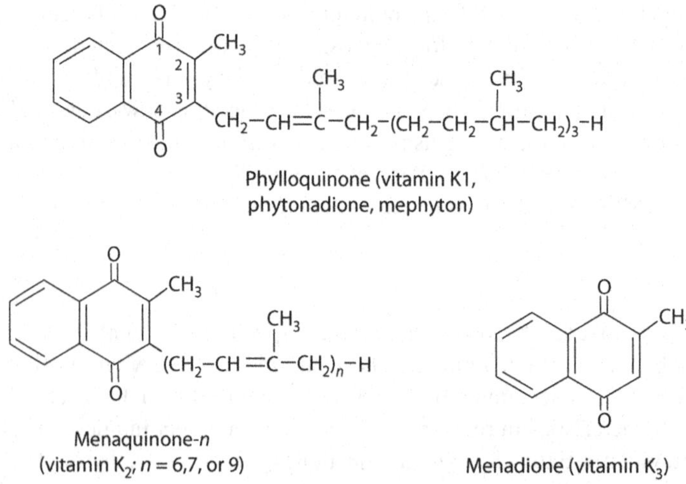

Phylloquinone (vitamin K1, phytonadione, mephyton)

Menaquinone-*n* (vitamin $K_2$; $n$ = 6,7, or 9)

Menadione (vitamin $K_3$)

**FIGURE 9.32** The chemical structure of vitamin K. Vitamins of the K group are polyisoprenoid-substituted napthoquinones. Phylloquinone ($K_1$) is the major form of vitamin K found in plants, whereas menaquinone (vitamin $K_2$) is synthesized by intestinal bacteria. Vitamin $K_3$ (menadione) is a synthetic, water-soluble vitamin K.

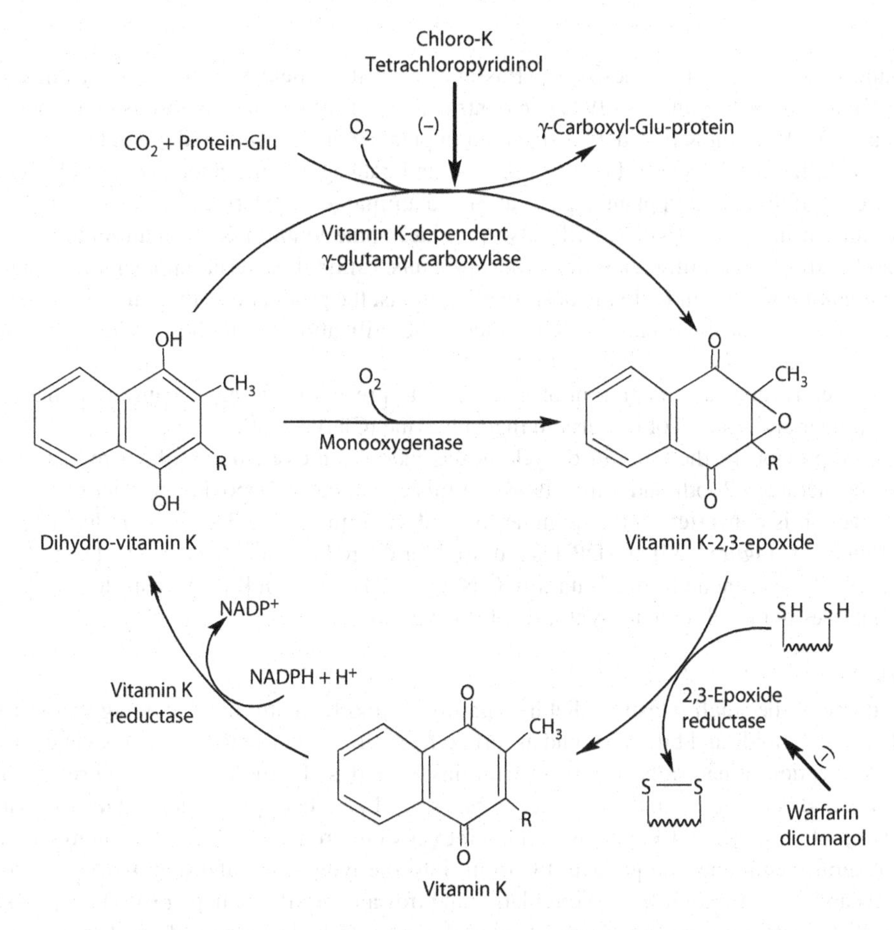


**FIGURE 9.33** Vitamin K recycling in animal cells. Vitamin K-2,3-epoxide is converted into vitamin K by 2,3-epoxide reductase. This enzyme is inhibited by Warfarin and dicumarol.

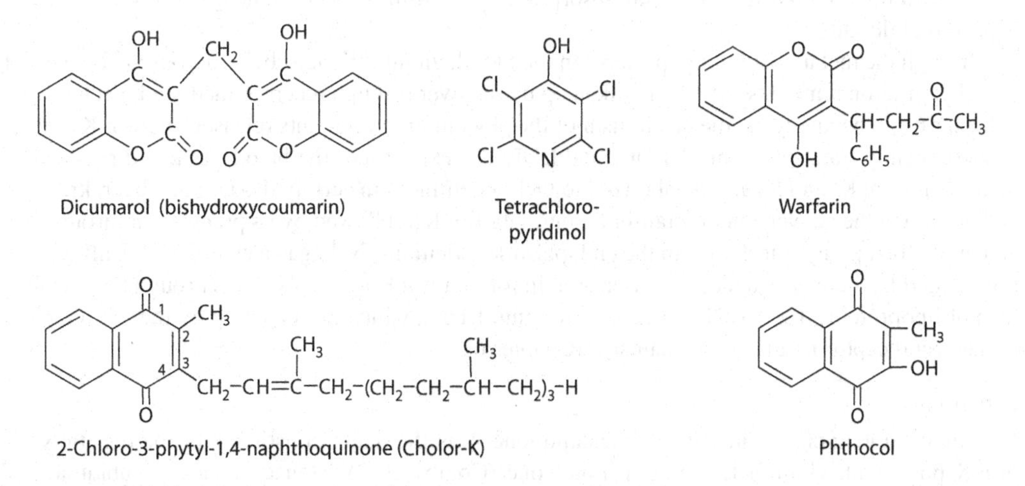


**FIGURE 9.34** The chemical structures of vitamin K antagonists.

### *Sources*

Plants and green algae can synthesize $K_1$ (Basset et al. 2016), whereas bacteria can synthesize vitamin $K_2$ (Bentley and Meganathan 1982). In contrast, there is no *de novo* synthesis of any vitamin K in animal cells. Vitamin K is widely distributed in plants, with bananas and green leafy vegetables (e.g., spinach, lettuce, broccoli, brussels sprouts, and cabbage) being good sources of vitamin K (Shearer et al. 1996). Certain plant (e.g., alfalfa) and animal (e.g., meat) feedstuffs are good sources of this vitamin in animal tissues. Milk also provides some vitamin K for mammalian neonates. Fruits and grains contain little vitamin K. In ruminants, ruminal bacteria supply a nutritionally significant quantity of vitamin $K_2$ to the host. In all animals, the production of vitamin $K_2$ by intestinal bacteria can also contribute vitamin K for metabolic utilization by the hosts. However, bacterial synthesis of vitamin $K_2$ is insufficient to meet the needs of the animals for this vitamin. Preterm neonates often receive administration of vitamin K to prevent bleeding, because they have only a limited number and species of bacteria in their intestine (Clarke 2010).

As noted previously, the vitamin K cycle in the endoplasmic reticulum allows reduced vitamin K to be regenerated (Booth and Suttie 1998). In this cycle, the 2,3-epoxide product of the carboxylation reaction is converted to the quinone form of vitamin K by 2,3-epoxide reductase, using a dithiol reductant (Figure 9.33). NADPH is required for the reduction of the quinone form of vitamin K to the dihydroxyquinone form of vitamin K. Note that the vitamin K cycle helps to conserve vitamin K but does not result in a net synthesis of this vitamin.

### *Absorption and Transport*

In the lumen of the small intestine, dietary vitamin $K_1$ and $K_2$ (naturally occurring vitamin K) are solubilized with lipids and bile salts, and absorbed from the micelles by enterocytes via passive diffusion. Absorption of naturally occurring vitamins $K_1$ and $K_2$ by the intestine requires normal fat absorption, and occurs only in the presence of bile salts, like other lipid-soluble vitamins. Inside the enterocyte, vitamins $K_1$ and $K_2$ are assembled into chylomicrons, which exit the enterocyte across its basolateral membrane (via passive diffusion) into the lymphatics and then the bloodstream in mammals and fish, or into the portal circulation in birds and reptiles (Chapter 6). The water-soluble vitamin $K_3$ and its naturally occurring structural analog (5-hydroxy-menadione [plumbagin]) are absorbed into enterocytes and colonocytes via their apical membrane multidrug resistance-linked ABC drug transporter-2 (ABCG2) (Shukla et al. 2007). Both vitamin $K_3$ and plumbagin exit the intestinal epithelial cells across their basolateral membranes via MRP1 (also known as ABC drug transporter-1 [ABCC1]). Absorbed vitamin $K_3$ and plumbagin enter the portal circulation. In contrast to vitamins $K_1$ and $K_2$, intestinal absorption of vitamin $K_3$ and plumbagin does not directly depend on bile salts.

Through the metabolism of lipoproteins in the blood, vitamin K-rich chylomicrons are converted into chylomicron remnants, which are taken up by the liver through receptor-mediated mechanisms (Chapter 6). In hepatocytes, the catabolism of the chylomicron remnants releases vitamin K, which is subsequently transferred into VLDLs and LDLs for export into the blood. As noted previously, dietary vitamin $K_1$ and $K_3$ are metabolized to yield vitamin $K_2$ in certain tissues (e.g., liver, kidneys, and brain) via the conversion of vitamin $K_1$ into vitamin $K_3$, followed by its prenylation through the action of UbiA prenyltransferase in the endoplasmic reticulum (Nakagawa et al. 2010). Unlike vitamins A and D, there is no specific carrier protein for vitamin K in the plasma. Through the metabolism of lipoproteins, the VLDLs are converted into LDLs, which are taken up by the extrahepatic tissues via receptor-mediated mechanisms (Chapter 6).

### *Functions*

In animals, a long-chain vitamin $K_2$ (menaquinone-4) is the major constituent of the hepatic vitamin K pool, with vitamin $K_1$ being a minor one (Combs 2012). Menaquinone-4 is ubiquitously present in extrahepatic tissues, with high concentrations in the brain, kidney, and pancreas. Vitamin K is a coenzyme of procoagulation factors (II, VII, IX, and X) via contact-activation (intrinsic)

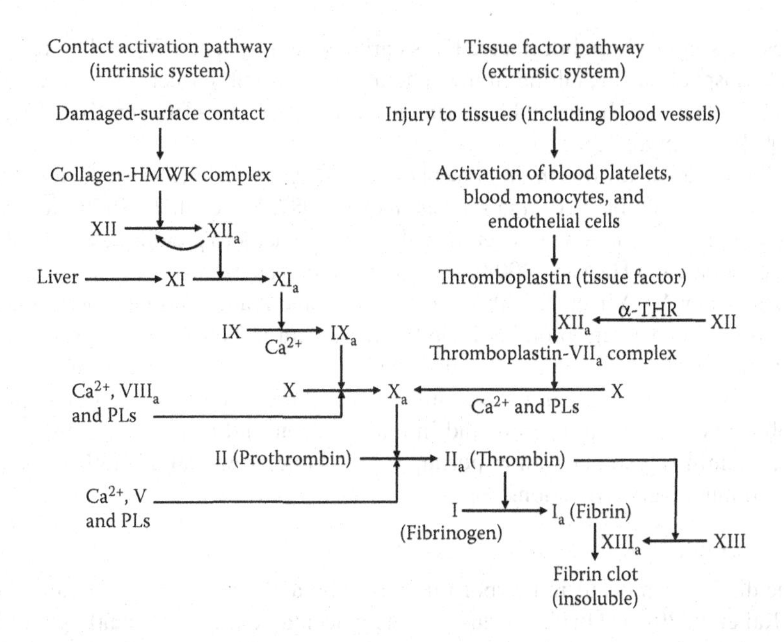


**FIGURE 9.35** Contact activation (intrinsic) and tissue factor (extrinsic) pathways for blood clotting. Coagulation requires many proteins, which are synthesized by the liver and circulate as zymogens (inactive forms) in the blood. Most of these proteins are serine proteases, but factors VIII and V are glycoproteins and factor XIII is a transglutaminase. Procoagulants (factors II, VII, IX, and X) depend on vitamin K for activity. An active form of coagulants is indicated by a subscript letter "a." In the intrinsic pathway, all factors are present in the plasma, and the formation of a collagen/high-molecular-weight kininogen complex due to contact with the damaged surface of tissues triggers a cascade of reactions to form an insoluble fibrin clot. In the extrinsic pathway, some cell types (e.g., blood platelets and monocytes, as well as endothelial cells) of the injured tissues release thromboplastin (tissue factor plus phospholipids), which triggers a cascade of reactions to form an insoluble fibrin clot. The extrinsic pathway is the primary pathway for coagulation in animals. PLs, phospholipids; α-THR, α-thrombin.

and tissue-factor (extrinsic) pathways (Figure 9.35). Specifically, procoagulation factors (including II, VII, IX, and X) are synthesized by the liver and circulate in the blood as zymogens (inactive forms) in the blood. Many of them are serine proteases. Activation of these zymogens requires a cascade of vitamin K-dependent reactions, which include the carboxylation of some glutamate residues in the zymogens to form γ-carboxyglutamates (Figure 9.36). The γ-carboxyglutamates of zymogens chelate $Ca^{2+}$ to form biologically active enzymes (proteins). For example, 10 of the

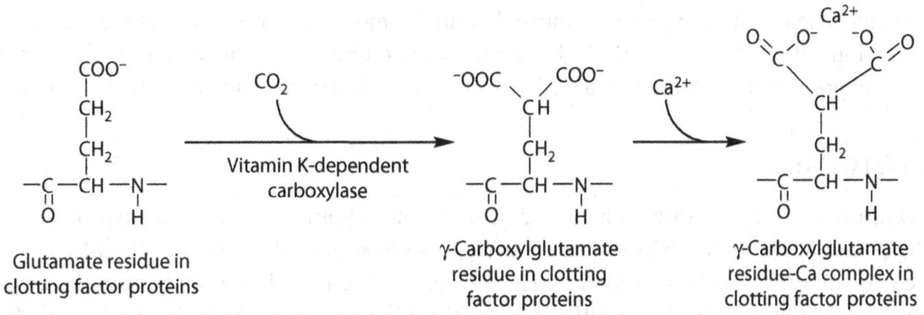

$CO_2$

Vitamin K-dependent carboxylase

$Ca^{2+}$

Glutamate residue in clotting factor proteins

γ-Carboxylglutamate residue in clotting factor proteins

γ-Carboxylglutamate residue-Ca complex in clotting factor proteins

**FIGURE 9.36** Vitamin K-dependent carboxylation of coagulating protein factors. This posttranslational modification of glutamate residues to form γ-carboxyglutamate (Gla) is catalyzed by a vitamin K-dependent carboxylase.

glutamate residues in prothrombin (factor II) is carboxylated by factor $X_a$ in the presence of $Ca^{2+}$, factor V, and phospholipids, resulting in the generation of thrombin (factor $II_a$). The latter converts the soluble fibrinogen into the insoluble fibrin clot in the presence of factor $XIII_a$ (Figure 9.35) to stop bleeding (Basset et al. 2016).

Vitamin K also plays a key role in the control of hemostasis by serving as a cofactor of anticoagulation proteins, namely, proteins S, C, and Z (Esmon et al. 1987; Yin et al. 2000). Protein S (named for Seattle, Washington, where it was discovered in 1979) is a cofactor to protein C, which inhibits factors $V_a$ and $VIII_a$ (Castoldi and Hackeng 2008). Protein Z is a cofactor of a serpin (serine protease inhibitor) that inhibits factor $X_a$ (Yin et al. 2000). Proteins S, C, and Z are important for normal blood flow.

Other vitamin K-dependent proteins include osteocalcin (a bone-specific protein), matrix Gla protein (an inhibitor of soft tissue calcification), and growth arrest-specific gene 6 (Gas-6) protein (which plays a role in platelet aggregation; migration and proliferation of vascular smooth muscle cells; thromboembolism, inflammation, and immune response) (Shearer et al. 1996; Shiraki et al. 2015). Thus, vitamin K also plays an important role in bone growth and health, as well as cardiovascular and immunological functions.

#### *Deficiencies and Diseases*

Hemorrhagic disease can occur in newborn infants, who are particularly vulnerable to vitamin K deficiency (Rai et al. 2017). This is because (1) the placenta does not efficiently pass vitamin K to the fetus and (2) the gut is essentially sterile immediately after birth. If prothrombin (factor II) concentrations in the plasma drop too low because of vitamin K deficiency, the hemorrhagic (bleeding) syndrome may appear. Both subcutaneous and internal hemorrhages are manifested in the young and adults when vitamin K is grossly inadequate, leading to the loss of blood and anemia. In all animals, vitamin K deficiency can be caused by fat malabsorption, which may be associated with pancreatic dysfunction, biliary disease, atrophy of the intestinal mucosa, or any cause of steatorrhea (excess fat in fecal discharges) (Ferland 2012; Jones and Hunt 1983). In addition, sterilization of the large intestine by antibiotics can result in vitamin K deficiency when its dietary intake is limited. Diseases of vitamin K deficiency can be cured through oral (nonruminants) or intravenous (ruminants) administration of this vitamin.

#### *Excesses*

Vitamin $K_3$ is an oxidant and also undergoes monovalent reduction to the semiquinone radical, which can be further oxidized by $O_2$ to the quinone, with the formation of superoxide anion (Basset et al. 2016). This form of vitamin K has been reported to oxidize hemoglobin into methemoglobin (Broberger et al. 1960). Thus, high concentrations of vitamin $K_3$ in the blood cause erythrocyte instability, hemolysis, and fatal anemia (Finkel, M.J. 1961), as well as jaundice, hyperbilirubinemia, and kernicterus in infants (Owens et al. 1971). In addition, intramuscular injection of $K_1$ into the buttock may result in sciatic nerve paralysis (Dipalma and Ritchie 1977). Irritability, nausea, vomiting, and headache also occur in hypervitaminosis K. Furthermore, administration of high doses of vitamin $K_3$ can induce renal toxicosis in the horse, as indicated by renal colic, hematuria, azotemia, and electrolyte abnormalities (Rebhun et al. 1984). This is likely due to oxidative stress in the kidneys.

## QUASI-VITAMINS

Quasi-vitamins include *p*-aminobenzoic acid, carnitine, choline, flavonoids, *myo*-inositol, lipoic acid, PQQ, and ubiquinones. Most of them are soluble in water. They are absorbed by enterocytes via apical membrane carrier mediators and enter either the portal vein or lymphatics depending on their chemical structures (Figure 9.37). Except for *p*-aminobenzoic acid and flavonoids, these nutrients are known to be essential for metabolism and physiology in animals. Some of them act like vitamins but have not been generally recognized as vitamins because of (1) historical reasons, (2) much higher amounts of dietary requirements than most vitamins, and (3) the lack of evidence for

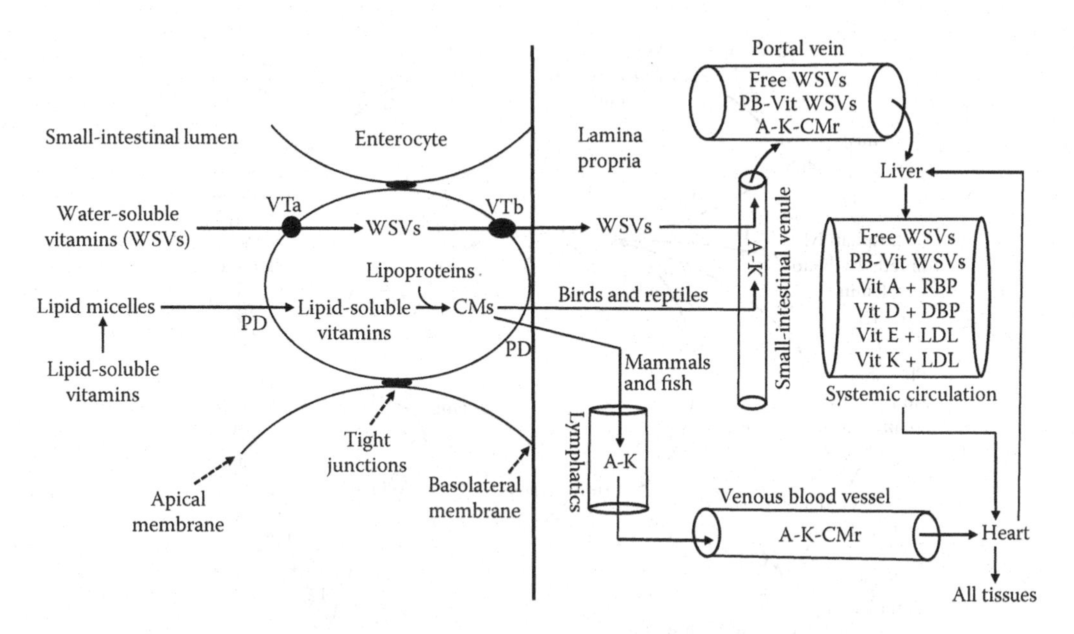


**FIGURE 9.37** Absorption and transport of water- and lipid-soluble vitamins in animals. Water- and lipid-soluble vitamins are absorbed by enterocytes into the lamia propria via specific transporters and passive diffusion, respectively. These vitamins enter the portal vein and lymphatics, respectively, in mammals and fish, but all the vitamins are absorbed into the portal vein in birds and reptiles. The vitamins are transported in the blood in their free or protein-bound forms, and are ultimately taken up by the liver and other cells of the body via specific transporters (water-soluble vitamins except for vitamin $B_{12}$) and receptor-mediated endocytosis (vitamin $B_{12}$ and all lipid-vitamin vitamins). A-K, chylomicrons (CM) containing vitamins A, D, E, and K; A-K-CMr, chylomicron remnants (CM) containing vitamins A, D, E, and K; BDP, vitamin D-binding protein; free WSVs, vitamins (niacin, pantothenic acid, biotin, folate, vitamin C, and 50% riboflavin) are transported in the plasma in their free (unbound) forms; PB-Vit-WSVs, vitamins (thiamin, vitamin $B_6$, vitamin $B_{12}$, and 50% riboflavin) are transported in the plasma in their protein-bound forms; PD, passive diffusion; RBP, retinol-binding protein; VTa, apical membrane transporters for water-soluble vitamins; VTb, basolateral membrane transporters for water-soluble vitamins.

the occurrence of diseases resulting from their dietary deficiencies in diets. Excess quasi-vitamins are rare but can occur after high doses of oral, subcutaneous, or intravenous administration to cause toxicity (e.g., reduced feed intake, growth depression, dizziness, nausea, vomiting, and diarrhea) (Combs 2012).

## Choline

### *Structure*

Choline was first isolated by Adolph Strecker from pig and cattle bile in 1862 and first chemically synthesized by Oscar Liebreich in 1865. The chemical structure of choline is 2-hydroxy-*N*,*N*,*N*,-trimethylethanaminium (also known as (β-hydroxyethyl)trimethylammonium) (Chapter 4). As a quaternary saturated amine, choline is a strong organic base and is soluble in water. When heated in an alkaline solution, choline decomposes to trimethylamine $^+N\text{–}(CH_3)_3$ (a compound with a fishy odor) and glycol ($HO\text{–}CH_2\text{–}CH_2\text{–}OH$). Slow degradation of choline occurs during storage.

### *Sources*

Choline is widely present in feedstuffs, mostly in the form of phosphatidylcholine (PC). Less than 10% of choline occurs as the free base or sphingomyelin (Chapter 3). Animal liver, brain, and kidney, as well as egg yolk, wheat germ, and soybeans, are rich sources of choline. Corn contains a

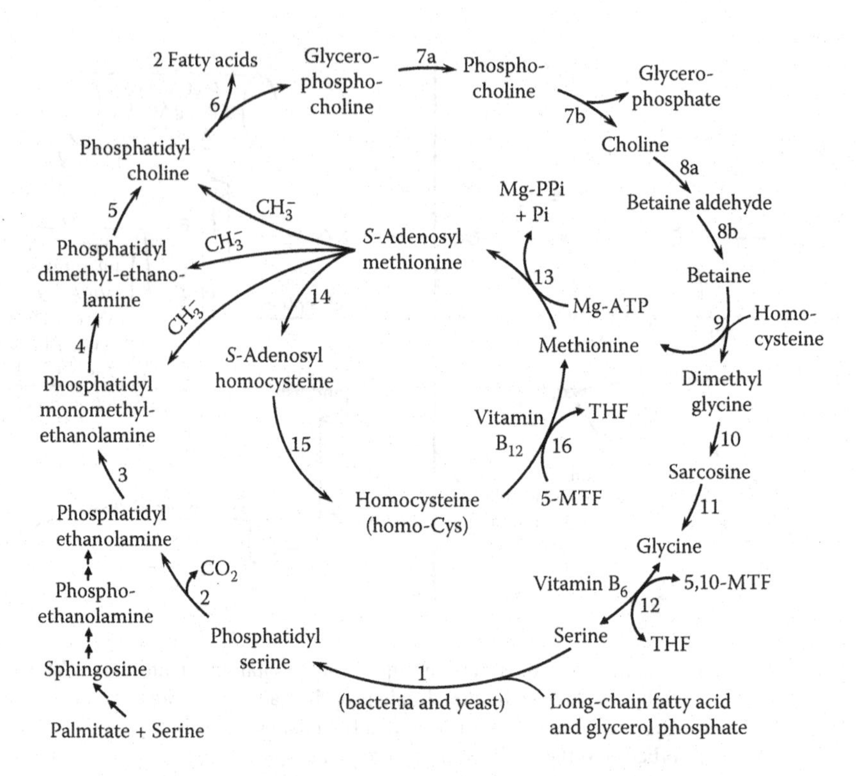


**FIGURE 9.38** *De novo* synthesis of choline from methionine, serine, and palmitate in the liver of animals. Rats have a limited capacity for choline synthesis. In chickens, this pathway is not developed until after 13 weeks of age. Reaction 1 occurs only in bacteria, while all other reactions are present in animal cells and bacteria. The enzymes that catalyze the indicated reactions are (1) a series of enzymes for phosphatidylserine synthesis (Chapter 6); (2) phosphatidylserine decarboxylase; (3) phosphatidyl aminoethanol (phosphatidylethanolamine) *N*-methyltransferase; (4) phosphatidyl *N*-monomethylaminoethanol (phosphatidyl *N*-monomethylethanolamine) *N*-methyltransferase; (5) phosphatidyl *N*-dimethylaminoethanol (phosphatidyl *N*-dimethylethanolamine) *N*-methyltransferase; (6) phospholipases $A_1$ and $A_2$; (7a) glycerophosphocholine phosphodiesterase; (7b) phosphocholine phosphatase; (8a) choline dehydrogenase; (8b) betaine aldehyde dehydrogenase; (9) betaine:homocysteine methyltransferase; (10) dimethylglycine dehydrogenase (a flavoprotein), which catalyzes the oxidative demethylation of dimethylglycine to sarcosine; (11) sarcosine dehydrogenase (a flavoprotein), which catalyzes the oxidative demethylation of sarcosine to glycine; (12) serine hydroxymethyltransferase; (13) *S*-adenosylmethionine synthetase (methionine adenosyltransferase); sarcosine (*N*-methylglycine); (14) *S*-adenosylmethionine-dependent enzymes; (15) *S*-adenosylhomocysteine hydrolase; and (16) $N^5$-methyltetrahydrofolate:homocysteine methyltransferase. SAM, *S*-adenosylmethionine; 5,10-MTF, $N^5$-$N^{10}$-methylene-tetrahydrofolate; 5-MTF, $N^5$-methyltetrahydrofolate; THF, tetrahydrofolate.

low content of both choline (only half the levels found in barley, oats, and wheat) and nondetectable betaine (<0.1% of the value found in whole wheat grain) (Bruce et al. 2010). Because betaine has a choline-sparing effect (Combs 2012), dietary requirements for choline by animals fed a wheat-based diet are much lower than animals fed a corn-based diet.

Most animal species synthesize *de novo* choline from methionine, serine, and palmitate via phosphatidylserine (PS) as an immediate in the liver (Figure 9.38). The chemical structures of some metabolites are illustrated in Figure 9.39. In this metabolic pathway, SAM is used as the methyl donor to sequentially convert PS into phosphatidylethanolamine (PE) via PS *N*-methyltransferase and then into phosphatidyl methylethanolamine and phosphatidyl dimethylethanolamine via PE *N*-methyltransferase. Rat tissues possess a low activity of PS *N*-methyltransferase and, therefore, have a limited capacity to *de novo* synthesize choline (Zempleni et al. 2013). In chicken tissues, PS *N*-methyltransferase activity is absent until after 13 weeks of age (Combs 2012). In mammals, birds,

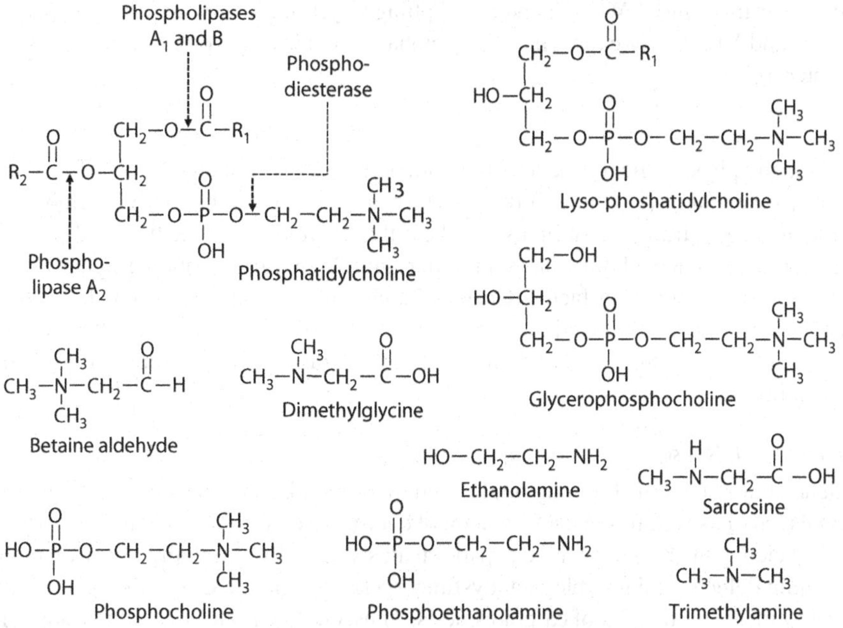

**FIGURE 9.39** The chemical structures of some metabolites in the pathway of choline synthesis.

and most fish, the synthesis of choline cannot meet their requirements, and, therefore, choline (as choline chloride or choline bitartrate, or PC) must be supplied in diets.

### *Absorption and Transport*

Depending on the form of dietary choline, it is absorbed by the small intestine into the lymphatic or portal circulation. In the lumen of the small intestine, dietary PC is hydrolyzed by a high activity of phospholipase $A_2$ (from the pancreas; cleaving the β-ester bond) to generate lyso-PC and one molecule of fatty acid. Some PC is hydrolyzed by phospholipase $A_2$, as well as phospholipases $A_1$ and B (from the intestinal mucosa; cleaving the α-ester bond), to yield glycerolphosphorylcholine (GPC) and two molecules of fatty acids. GPC is further hydrolyzed by GPC diesterase (from the pancreas) to form choline and glycerol phosphate. Because the activity of phospholipase $A_2$ is much greater than that of phospholipases $A_1$ and B, lyso-PC is the major product of PC digestion in the small intestine. Lyso-PC is absorbed into enterocytes primarily via simple diffusion (Chapter 6). About one-third of free choline in the lumen of the small intestine is taken up into enterocytes via choline transporter-1 (an apical membrane $Na^+$-dependent, high-affinity transporter, $K_M < 10$ μM), as well as organic cation transporters (OCTs) 1 and 2 (Kato et al. 2006). Once inside the enterocytes, lyso-PC and free choline are re-esterified into PC. The PC is then packaged into chylomicrons and VLDLs for export into the lymphatics (mammals) or the portal vein (birds, fish, and reptiles) and is transported in the blood as lipoproteins (Chapter 6). The choline that is not esterified in the enterocyte exits the cell through its basolateral membrane into the lamina propria via a choline/$H^+$ antiport (Zempleni et al. 2013). About two-thirds of free choline in the lumen of the small intestine is degraded by intestinal bacteria to form trimethylamine, which is readily absorbed into the portal vein.

In the lumen of the small intestine, some sphingomyelin is hydrolyzed by intestinal alkaline sphingomyelinase and neutral ceramidase to sphingosine, phosphoethanolamine, and LCFA (Nilsson and Duan 2006). Sphingosine is absorbed into enterocytes primarily via simple diffusion. In these cells, most sphingosine is acylated into sphingomyelin, while some sphingosine is converted to palmitate and ethanolamine via a series of enzyme-catalyzed reactions, and the resultant palmitate is esterified into TAGs (Chapter 6). Sphingomyelin, along with TAGs, is packaged into chylomicrons and VLDLs for export into the lymphatics and is transported in the blood as lipoproteins (Chapter 6).

### *Functions*

Choline has many physiological functions in animals (Ennis and Blakely 2016). As a component of PC, choline is essential to (1) maintain the structure and function of biological membranes and (2) promote the interorgan transport of lipids and the efflux of lipids from the liver and small intestine. As a precursor of ceramide, choline plays an important role in transmembrane signaling. As a component of the platelet-activating factor (Chapter 3), choline participates in blood clotting, inflammation, conceptus implantation, and uterine contraction. Finally, as a substrate for the synthesis of acetylcholine (a neurotransmitter) by choline acetyltransferase, choline is required for neurological function in animals.

### *Deficiencies and Diseases*

Choline deficiency occurs in (1) young poultry fed diets containing a low content of choline and (2) other animals fed diets containing a low content of choline or methionine (Combs 2012). Syndromes of choline deficiency in animals include hepatic steatosis, fatty liver, impaired growth, reduced feed efficiency, brain defects, and neurological dysfunction (Zeisel and da Costa 2009). In addition, choline deficiency increases the risk of carcinogenesis. Thus, choline is an essential nutrient for animals that cannot synthesize sufficient amounts to meet their metabolic requirements.

## Carnitine

### *Structure*

Carnitine was found to be a constituent of vertebrate skeletal muscle in 1905. It is now known to be present in nearly all animal tissues, especially the skeletal muscle, heart, and liver, where the rates of LCFA oxidation are high. Carnitine is a quaternary amine and its chemical structure (β-hydroxy-γ-*N*-trimethylaminobutyrate [Chapter 4]) was established in 1927. Carnitine is a strong organic base and is soluble in water.

### *Sources*

Carnitine is abundant in meats and dairy products (Combs 2012), but is low or absent in plants (Panter and Mudd 1969). The liver of animals can synthesize carnitine from peptide-bound lysine, methionine, α-KG, vitamin C, and iron via a series of enzyme-catalyzed reactions (Vaz and Wanders 2002). However, the synthesis of carnitine in insects is limited. *De novo* synthesis of carnitine has not been demonstrated in any bacterial species (Meadows and Wargo 2015). A dietary supplemental form of carnitine is acetylcarnitine, which is also a physiological metabolite of carnitine in animal tissues.

### *Absorption and Transport*

In the lumen of the small intestine, acylcarnitine is cleaved by pancreatic carboxylester lipase to form carnitine and LCFA. Carnitine is absorbed into enterocytes primarily via (1) OCT2, which is a $Na^+$-dependent, high-affinity transporter localized in the apical membrane and (2) AA transporter $B^{0,+}$. In these cells, some carnitine is acetylated by carnitine acetyltransferase to form acetylcarnitine (Gross et al. 1986). Carnitine exits the enterocyte into the lamina propria via OCT3, which is a $Na^+$-independent transporter localized in the basolateral membrane (Durán et al. 2005). Absorbed carnitine enters the portal circulation and becomes available for utilization by extraintestinal tissues. Unabsorbed carnitine is degraded to trimethylamine, malic acid, and betaine by microbes in the small and large intestines (Meadows and Wargo 2015). These metabolites are absorbed into the portal circulation via transmembrane transporters. Carnitine is transported in the blood in both free and acetylated forms, and is taken up by extraintestinal tissues via OCT2 against concentration gradients. Like AAs and glucose, carnitine is reabsorbed by the renal glomerulus into the blood circulation.

Acetyl-CoA + Carnitine ↔CoA + Acetylcarnitine (Carnitine acetyltransferase)

Dietary acetylcarnitine is absorbed into enterocytes via AA transporter $B^{0,+}$ (Wu 2013). Inside these cells, some acetylcarnitine is deacetylated into carnitine, which is transported as noted previously. The transporter $B^{0,+}$ and OCT3 mediate the efflux of acetylcarnitine from the enterocyte across its basolateral membrane into the lamina propria. The rate of intestinal acetylcarnitine transport is faster than that of carnitine (Gross et al. 1986). Absorbed acetylcarnitine enters the portal circulation and becomes available for utilization by extraintestinal tissues to form carnitine.

#### *Functions*

Carnitine is required for the transport of LCFAs from the cytosol into mitochondria for oxidation to $CO_2$ and $H_2O$ and ATP production (Chapter 6). This is the major source of energy for the skeletal muscle, heart, and liver in (1) nonruminants and preruminants under fed or fasting conditions and (2) ruminants when the ruminal production of SCFAs is low or under food-deprivation conditions.

#### *Deficiencies and Diseases*

Animals exhibit carnitine deficiency when its dietary intake, intestinal absorption, or *de novo* synthesis is inadequate. Syndromes include (1) skeletal myopathy, muscle necrosis, cardiomyopathy, and fatigue because of insufficient energy provision to muscle fibers and cardiomyocytes; (2) reduced protein synthesis, increased proteolysis, and increased AA oxidation to ammonia in skeletal muscle due to excess fat-induced insulin resistance; (3) fatty liver and hypoglycemia due to insufficient oxidation of LCFAs (resulting in their accumulation) and insufficient energy supply for gluconeogenesis in hepatocytes; (4) hyperammonemia due to impaired ammonia detoxification via the urea cycle that results from an inhibition of carbamoylphosphate synthase-I by LCFA-CoA (e.g., palmitoyl-CoA) in hepatocytes; (5) neurological dysfunction as a result of hypoglycemia and hyperammonemia; and (6) hyperlipidemia because of impaired oxidation of LCFAs to $CO_2$ and $H_2O$ in the whole body (Zempleni et al. 2013).

### *MYO*-INOSITOL

#### *Structure*

*myo*-Inositol is a water-soluble 6-carbon sugar related to D-glucose and occurs naturally in nine possible isomeric forms. However, only *myo*-inositol (*cis*-1,2,3,5 *trans*-4,6-cyclohexane-hexanol) is biologically important as a nutrient (Figure 9.40).

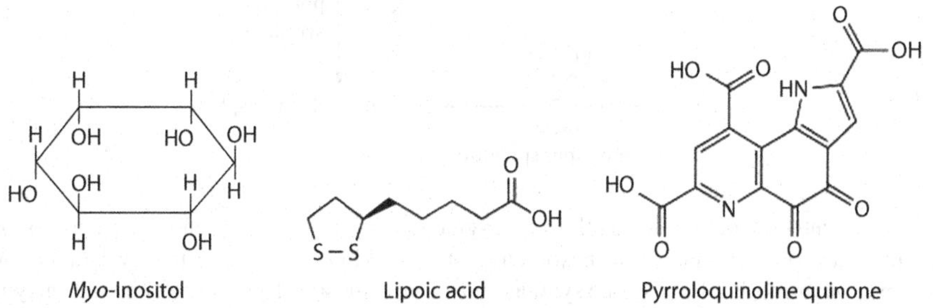

*Myo*-Inositol    Lipoic acid    Pyrroloquinoline quinone

**FIGURE 9.40** Chemical structures of *myo*-inositol, lipoic acid, and pyrroloquinoline quinone. These substances are present in mammals, birds, fish, and microorganisms.

### *Sources*

*myo*-Inositol is widely distributed in plants and animal products, as part of phosphatidylinositol in cell membranes, as free inositol, and as a component of phytic acid. The latter is present in many grain products. Phytate and phytic acid can bind calcium, magnesium, iron, zinc, and other divalent ions, thereby reducing their absorption by the small intestine. Animal tissues (e.g., liver, kidney, brain, and testes) and bacteria can synthesize *myo*-inositol from D-glucose (Geiger and Jin 2006), and this metabolic pathway is outlined in Figure 9.41.

### *Absorption and Transport*

Depending on the form of *myo*-inositol, it is absorbed from the small intestine into the lymphatics (phosphatidylinositol) or portal circulation (free inositol) with a high efficiency. In the rumen of ruminants and in the lumen of the small intestine of all animals, phytic acid can be converted into *myo*-inositol by microbial phytase with the removal of the phosphate groups (Chapter 10). The efficiency of this conversion in the digestive tract depends on animal species. Ruminants and horses have a greater capacity for utilizing dietary phytate than swine and poultry.

*myo*-Inositol is absorbed into the enterocyte via $Na^+$-coupled *myo*-inositol transporter-2 (SMIT2), which is a secondary active transporter (Aouameur et al. 2007). This sugar exits the enterocyte across its basolateral membrane via a diffusive ($Na^+$-independent) carrier-mediated mechanism (Reshkin et al. 1989). Glucose transport systems in the apical membrane of the enterocyte, such as SGLT1 or GLUT5, do not contribute to *myo*-inositol uptake. Likewise, GLUT2 does not mediate *myo*-inositol efflux from the enterocyte across its basolateral membrane. Depending on the form of *myo*-inositol, it is transported in the blood as lipoproteins (phosphatidylinositol) or a predominantly free form (free inositol). *myo*-Inositol in the blood is taken up by the liver via carrier-mediated diffusion, by the brain via SMIT1 and SMIT2, by the renal medulla via SMIT1, and by proximal tubule cells in the kidney cortex via SMIT2 (Aouameur et al. 2007). SMIT2 is responsible for the reabsorption of *myo*-inositol from the glomerular filtrate. A major difference between SMIT1 and SMIT2 is that D-chiro-inositol (an epimer of *myo*-inositol) is transported by SMIT2 with high affinity but is not transported by SMIT1, whereas L-fucose is transported by SMIT1 but not by SMIT2.

### *Functions*

*myo*-Inositol is incorporated into phosphatidylinositol in animal cells. Phosphatidylinositol plays an important role in cell metabolism and signaling by serving as (1) a constituent of cell membranes and (2) a mediator of cellular responses to external stimuli. For example, inositol-1,4,5-triphosphate

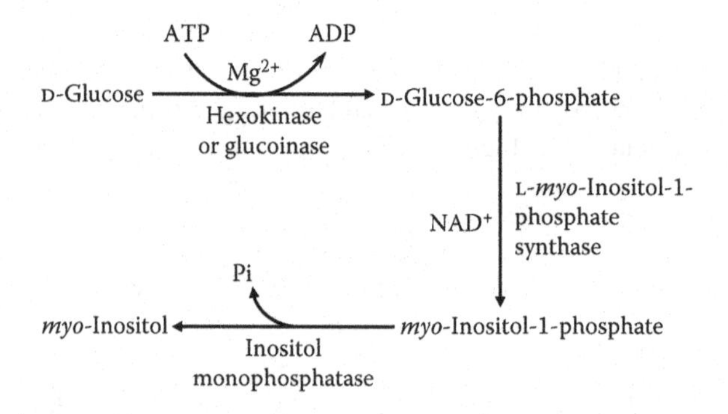


**FIGURE 9.41** Synthesis of *myo*-inositol from D-glucose in animal cells and microbes. D-Glucose is converted into glucose-6-phosphate by hexokinase or glucokinase. The internal cyclization of glucose 6-phosphate by L-*myo*-inositol-l-phosphate synthase forms *myo*-inositol-1-phosphate, and this enzyme has the absolute requirement for $NAD^+$ with no net gain in NADH. Thus, the overall reaction for the generation of *myo*-inositol-1-phosphate is tightly coupled with oxidation and reduction. Finally, inositol monophosphatase catalyzes the dephosphorylation of *myo*-inositol-1-phosphate to yield *myo*-inositol.

($IP_3$) is an intracellular second messenger that stimulates the release of $Ca^{2+}$ from the endoplasmic reticulum to the cytosol, which in turn activates a variety of $Ca^{2+}$-dependent protein kinases (including protein kinase C) and pathways (Gill et al. 1989).

### *Deficiencies and Diseases*

Most animal species (including the fish species abalone and channel catfish) can synthesize sufficient *myo*-inositol, and therefore it is not considered to be a dietary essential nutrient (Burtle and Lovell 1989; Mai et al. 2001; Zempleni et al. 2013). However, a lack of *myo*-inositol in diets results in feed intake depression, impaired growth, reduced feed efficiency, and skin lesions in some aquatic animals, including common carp, red sea bream, Japanese eel, rainbow trout, chinook salmon, and shrimp (Mai et al. 2001). Of interest, male gerbils can sufficiently synthesize *myo*-inositol, but female gerbils cannot (Chu and Hegsted 1980). The absence of *myo*-inositol from the diet causes intestinal lipodystrophy and reduced survival in female gerbils. Under some conditions such as diabetes (with large amounts of *myo*-inositol being excreted in urine), infections, and heat stress (impaired *myo*-inositol synthesis), *myo*-inositol may be a conditionally essential nutrient in diets for animals (Combs 2012).

## Lipoic Acid

### *Structure*

Lipoic acid (a yellow solid compound) is also known as α-lipoic acid and thioctic acid (Figure 9.40). This water-soluble organosulfur compound consists of two sulfur atoms (at $C_6$ and $C_8$) connected by a disulfide bond (the oxidized form). The $C_6$ atom is chiral and the molecule exists as two enantiomers ((*R*)-(+)-lipoic acid and (*S*)-(−)-lipoic acid) and as a racemic mixture (*R*/*S*)-lipoic acid. The reduced form of lipoic acid is known as dihydrolipoic acid.

### *Sources*

Lipoic acid is present in plant and animal products. Exogenous free lipoic acid from the diet is activated by ATP-dependent lipoate-activating enzyme, and the product is then transferred by lipoyltransferase to lipoic acid-dependent enzymes (Figure 9.42). Gastrointestinal bacteria and the mitochondria of animal cells can synthesize a small amount of lipoic acid from octanoic acid (Cronan 2016). In the presence of *S*-adenosylmethionine, lipoyl synthase inserts two sulfur atoms from the iron–sulfur centers of the enzyme to form lipoyl-ACP. The latter is transferred to lipoic acid-dependent enzymes (e.g., pyruvate dehydrogenase). Thus, either the exogenous or the endogenously synthesized lipoic acid (the *R*-isomer) can be bound to the ε-$NH_2$ group of a lysine residue

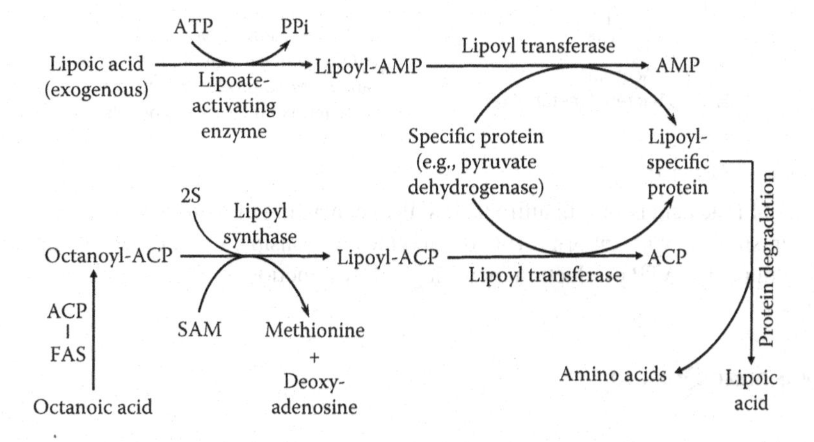


**FIGURE 9.42** Synthesis of specific protein-bound lipoic acid from octanoic acid in the mitochondria of animal cells and in bacteria. ACP, acyl carrier protein; FAS, fatty acid synthase; SAM, *S*-adenosylmethionine.

in a lipoyl-specific protein. In animal cells, oxidized lipoic acid can be converted by an NADPH-dependent enzyme (e.g., glutathione reductase) into dihydrolipoate.

### *Absorption and Transport*

In the lumen of the small intestine, protein-bound lipoic acid is degraded by proteases to release lipoic acid. The latter is absorbed into enterocytes via the $Na^+$-dependent monocarboxylic acid transporter and the sodium-dependent multivitamin transporter (Quick and Shi 2015). In the cells, some lipoic acid is reduced to dihydrolipoate. Both lipoic acid and dihydrolipoate exit enterocytes through their basolateral membranes into the lamina propria via a specialized $Na^+$-independent transporter. Absorbed lipoic acid and dihydrolipoate enter the portal circulation and are transported in the blood primarily as free acids.

### *Functions*

Lipoic acid is a component of lipoamide (Chapter 5), which is a coenzyme for α-ketoacid dehydrogenase complexes, including pyruvate dehydrogenase, α-KG dehydrogenase, and branched-chain α-ketoacid dehydrogenase complexes, in animal cells and microbes. These enzymes play important roles in pyruvate decarboxylation to acetyl-CoA, the activity of the Krebs cycle, and branched-chain AA catabolism, respectively. Therefore, lipoic acid is essential for ATP production from the oxidation of glucose, AAs, and fatty acids in a tissue-specific manner. In addition, lipoic acid is a cofactor for the acetoin dehydrogenase complex (also known as acetyl-CoA:acetoin *O*-acetyltransferase), which degrades acetoin (a product of the decarboxylation of α-acetolactate in bacteria that gives butter its characteristic flavor) (Cronan 2016). Like α-ketoacid dehydrogenase complexes, the acetoin dehydrogenase complex requires thiamin diphosphate as a cofactor. Furthermore, the H-protein (one of the four proteins in the glycine cleavage system [also known as the glycine decarboxylase complex]) contains lipoamide; therefore, lipoic acid is essential for glycine degradation in the liver and kidneys of animals, and in microbes. Finally, high concentrations of dihydrolipoate can scavenge reactive oxygen and nitrogen species (Moura et al. 2015).

α-Ketoacid + CoA + $NAD^+$→Acyl-CoA + NADH + $H^+$ (α-ketoacid dehydrogenase complex, animal cells and bacteria)
Acetoin + CoA + $NAD^+$→Acetaldehyde + Acetyl-CoA + NADH + $H^+$ (acetoin dehydrogenase complex, bacteria)

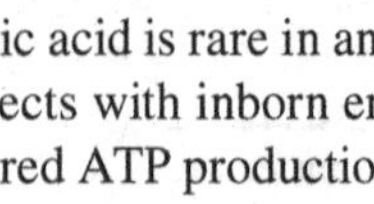

O, $CH_3$, $H_3C$, OH

Acetoin
($C_4H_8O_2$, a bacterial metabolite)

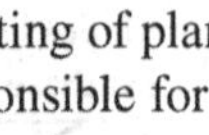

O, $H_3C$, H

Acetaldehyde
($C_2H_4O$, a natural metabolite in bacteria and plants; a product of ethanol oxidation in the liver of animals)

### *Deficiencies and Diseases*

A deficiency of lipoic acid is rare in animals fed diets consisting of plant- or animal-source ingredients. However, subjects with inborn errors of enzymes responsible for endogenous lipoic acid synthesis exhibit impaired ATP production, neurological dysfunction, muscle weakness, and abnormal AA catabolism.

## Pyrroloquinoline Quinone

### *Structure*

PQQ (4,5-dihydro-4,5-dioxo-1*H*-pyrrolo-[2,3-*f*]quinoline-2,7,9-tricarboxylic acid) or methoxatin (Figure 9.40) was discovered in the late 1970s as a water-soluble cofactor of bacterial oxidoreductases.

This aromatic tricarboxylic acid with a fused heterocyclic (*o*-quinone) ring system is now known to be present in yeast, plants, and animals. It is a stable substance in physiological solutions, although its C-5 carbonyl group is reactive toward nucleophiles (e.g., thiol groups). Enzymes containing PQQ are called quinoproteins. In bacteria, PQQ is a member of *ortho*-quinone cofactors that include tryptophan tryptophylquinone, trihydroxyphenylalanyl quinone, lysine tyrosylquinone, and the copper-complexed cysteinyltyrosyl radical (Stites et al. 2000).

#### *Sources*

PQQ is present in plant (e.g., vegetables, fruits, and legumes) and animal (e.g., milk, meats, and eggs) products (Stites et al. 2000). It can be synthesized from glutamate and tyrosine residues of a PqqA polypeptide (e.g., 24 AAs in *Methylobacillus flagellatum*) by gastrointestinal bacteria as an endogenous source for their hosts (Puehringer et al. 2008). Animal cells do not contain enzymes for PQQ synthesis.

#### *Absorption and Transport*

Little is known about the transporters of PQQ absorption by the small intestine. However, a study with mice showed that orally administered PQQ was readily absorbed (62%, range 19%–89%) in the lower intestine into the portal circulation (Smidt et al. 1991). It is possible that ABCG2 mediates the uptake of PQQ into the enterocyte across its apical membrane and that MRP1 is responsible for the efflux of PQQ from the cell across its basolateral membrane. Absorbed PQQ enters the portal circulation. Greater than 95% of PQQ in the blood is associated with the cell fraction, with the remaining in the plasma (Smidt et al. 1991). PQQ is taken up from the blood primarily by the kidneys and skin and, to a lesser extent, other tissues. Most (81%) of absorbed PQQ is excreted by the kidneys within 24 h.

#### *Functions*

PQQ is a redox cofactor in cells. In certain (e.g., methane-generating) bacteria, it acts as a coenzyme for oxidoreductases, including methanol dehydrogenase, ethanol dehydrogenase, and membrane-bound glucose dehydrogenase. It is unknown whether PQQ is essential for enzymes in animal cells. However, there is evidence that PQQ catalyzes the nonspecific oxidation of (1) pyridoxamine phosphate to pyridoxal phosphate and (2) peptidyl lysine residues in elastin and collagen to aldehyde products (known as allysines). These reactive aldehydes undergo spontaneous chemical reactions with other aldehyde residues or unmodified lysine residues to form cross-linking, which is essential for the stabilization of collagen fibrils and for the elasticity of elastin in animals. Furthermore, the radical-scavenging activity of the reduced form of PQQ is 7.4-fold greater than that of vitamin C (Ouchi et al. 2009). As an antioxidant, PQQ has cardio- and neuro-protective effects, while improving mitochondrial biogenesis and function. Therefore, dietary supplementation of 0.2 mg/kg PQQ · $Na_2$ can enhance the antioxidative status, growth performance, and carcass yield of broiler chicks (Samuel et al. 2015; Wang et al. 2015).

#### *Deficiencies and Diseases*

PQQ deficiency is rare in animals fed diets consisting of plant- and animal-source ingredients. There are reports that mice fed a PQQ-free diet exhibited suboptimal embryonic survival, neonatal growth, skin lesions, and impaired immunity (Killgore 1989; Steinberg et al. 1994). Of interest, maximal animal growth could be achieved when the basal diet contained as little as 1 nmol or 300 ng of PQQ per g of diet (Steinberg et al. 1994).

### Ubiquinones

#### *Structure*

Ubiquinones are a group of lipid-soluble 1,4-benzoquinone derivatives with isoprenoid side chains of different lengths. A physiologically important ubiquinone is ubiquinone $Q_{10}$ (also known as ubiquinone Q or coenzyme Q), where Q refers to the quinone group and the subscript "10" is the number of isoprenyl subunits. The structure of the 6-chromanol of coenzyme Q is similar to that of the oxidized form of vitamin E or vitamin K.

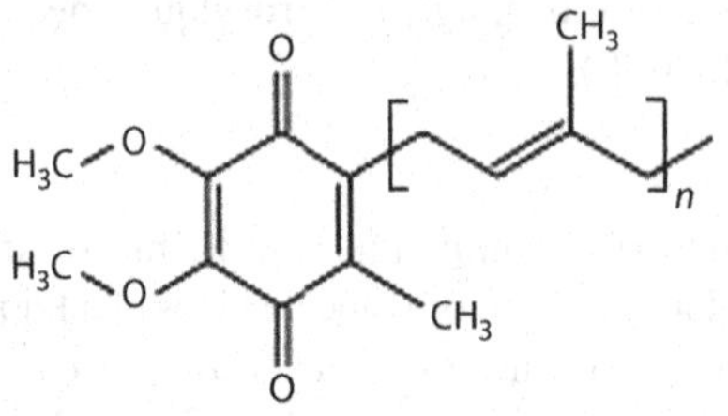

Ubiquinone

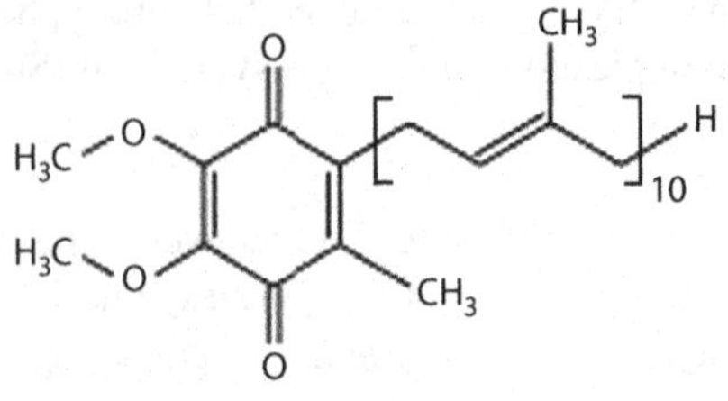

Coenzyme $Q_{10}$ (coenzyme Q)

*Sources*

Ubiquinones occur in plant- and animal-source ingredients. Gastrointestinal bacteria and the hepatocytes of animals can synthesize coenzyme Q from (1) tyrosine (the precursor of the benzoquinone structure) and (2) acetyl-CoA (the substrate of the isoprene side chain), with mevalonate as an intermediate (Bentinger et al. 2010). In the hepatocytes of mammals, birds, and fish, coenzyme Q synthesis involves mitochondria, the endoplasmic reticulum, and peroxisomes (Figure 9.43).

*Absorption and Transport*

In the lumen of the small intestine, dietary ubiquinones are solubilized with lipids and bile salts and absorbed from the micelles by enterocytes via passive diffusion. Upon entering the enterocyte, ubiquinones are assembled into chylomicrons, which exit the enterocyte across its basolateral membrane (via passive diffusion) into the lymphatics and then the bloodstream in mammals and fish, or into the portal circulation in birds and reptiles (Chapter 6). Ubiquinones in the blood are taken up by extraintestinal cells as a component of VLDLs or LDLs via specific receptors (Chapter 6). Dietary ubiquinones (e.g., coenzyme Q) have a low bioavailability to animals (Acosta et al. 2016).

*Functions*

There are three redox states of $CoQ_{10}$: fully oxidized (ubiquinone), semiquinone (ubisemiquinone), and fully reduced (ubiquinol) (Chapter 1). The capacity of ubiquinone as a two-electron carrier (moving between the quinone and quinol forms) and as a one-electron carrier (moving between semiquinone and one of the other forms) is essential for its role in the mitochondrial electron transport chain (complexes I and II). This is because the iron–sulfur clusters of cytochromes can only accept one electron at a time. In addition, like vitamin E, ascorbic acid, and β-carotene, coenzyme Q has a potent antioxidant property and can scavenge free radical species. Thus, coenzyme Q can alleviate syndromes in vitamin E-deficient animals (e.g., mice and rats) (Combs 2012).

*Deficiencies and Diseases*

There is little evidence for impaired metabolism or physiological function due to a lack of dietary coenzyme Q in animals, indicating a sufficient synthesis of this quasi-vitamin. However, because coenzyme Q shares a biosynthetic pathway with cholesterol, interference of lipid metabolism can cause a deficiency of coenzyme Q when the conversion of acetyl-CoA into mevalonate is inhibited by some β-blockers, blood pressure-lowering drugs, and statins (inhibitors of HMG-CoA synthase) (Acosta et al. 2016).

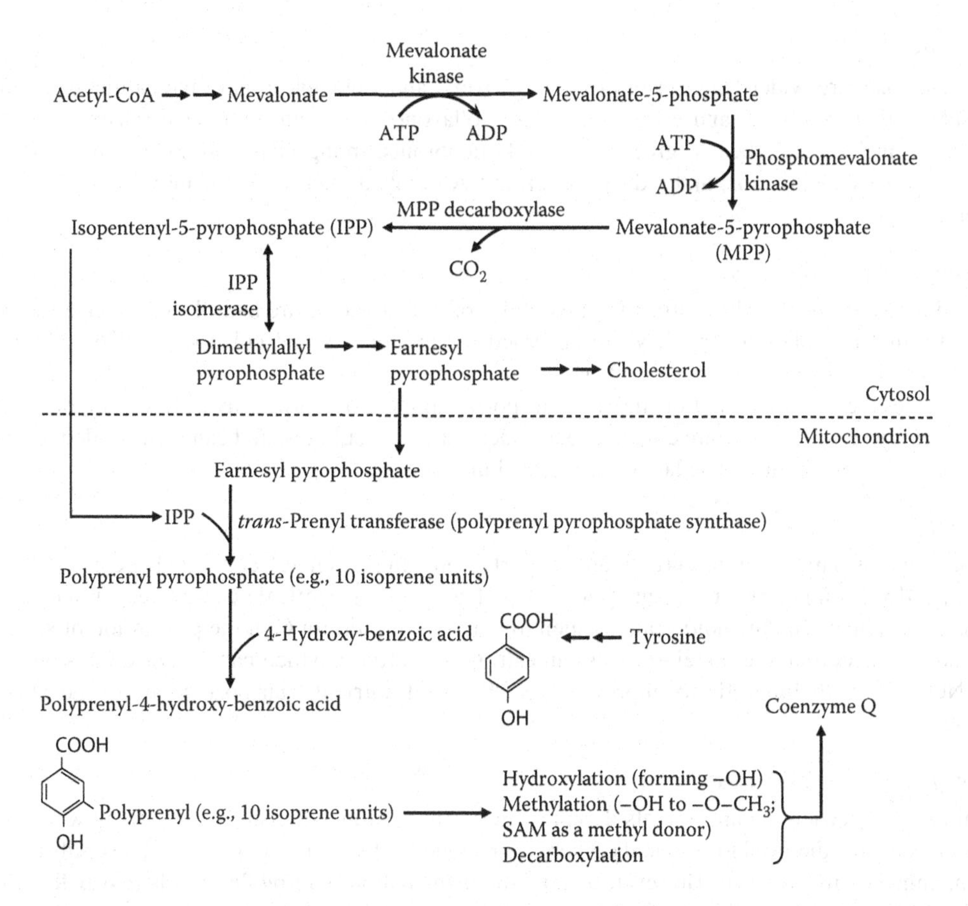


**FIGURE 9.43** Synthesis of coenzyme Q in the hepatocytes of mammals, birds, and fish. Tyrosine is converted into the benzoquinone structure in mitochondria, and acetyl-CoA is the substrate for the formation of the isoprene side chain in the endoplasmic reticulum and peroxisomes. Hydroxymethylglutaryl-CoA (HMG-CoA) reductase, which is a rate-controlling enzyme in the generation of mevalonate from acetyl-CoA, is an integral protein of the endoplasmic reticulum membrane. The enzymes that convert mevalonate into farnesyl pyrophosphate are localized in peroxisomes. The last reactions involving the hydroxylation, methylation, and decarboxylation of polyprenyl-4-hydroxy-benzoic acid occur in mitochondria.

## Bioflavonoids

### *Structure*

Bioflavonoids are a mixture of water-soluble polyphenolic derivatives of 2-phenyl-1,4-benzopyrone that consist of two phenyl rings (A and B) and one heterocyclic ring (C). They occur naturally as glycosides. Examples are flavan-3-ol, quercetin, and isoflavone (Schmitt and Dirsch 2009).

2-Phenyl-1,4-benzopyrone

Flavan-3-ol (flavanol)

Quercetin

Isoflavone [eg., genistein (5-OH, 7-OH, 4′-OH); and daidzein (7-OH, 4′-OH)]

### *Sources*

Bioflavonoids are widely present in plants (e.g., fruits and vegetables) and, like carotenoids, contribute to their red, blue, and yellow pigments. Isoflavones (e.g., genistein and daidzein) occur in legumes, including soybeans, green beans, alfalfa sprouts, mung bean sprouts, cowpeas, kudzu roots, red clover blossoms, and red clover sprouts. Animals do not have enzymes for synthesizing bioflavonoids.

### *Absorption and Transport*

In the lumen of the small intestine, the glycosides of bioflavonoids are hydrolyzed by glycosidases of intestinal microbes before they are absorbed by enterocytes and colonocytes (Combs 2012). However, the molecular properties of bioflavonoid transporters are unknown. Absorbed bioflavonoids enter the portal circulation and are transported in the blood primarily as free compounds. In the liver, these compounds are conjugated as glucuronides or sulfates, and can be degraded to various phenolic metabolites. The latter are excreted in the urine.

### *Functions*

Bioflavonoids have a potent antioxidant property and can scavenge free radical species (Panche et al. 2016; Rahman and Hongsprabhas 2016). These phytochemicals can protect tissues from oxidative injury. Bioflavonoids can augment the action of vitamin C in the prevention of scurvy. Of note, genistein and daidzein possess an estrogenic activity, which can enhance the synthesis of NO by endothelial cells to improve blood flow and nutrient transport (Schmitt and Dirsch 2009).

### *Deficiencies and Diseases*

Animals fed nutrient-balanced diets do not exhibit abnormal metabolism or physiology when they do not consume dietary bioflavonoids. There is no evidence for nutritional roles of these substances in mammals, birds, or fish. However, dietary supplementation with bioflavonoids is beneficial for animal health under conditions of oxidative stress.

## *PARA*-AMINOBENZOIC ACID

### *Structure*

*para*-Aminobenzoic acid (also known as 4-aminobenzoic acid) consists of a benzene ring substituted with an amino group and a carboxyl group. It is a white solid that is soluble in water.

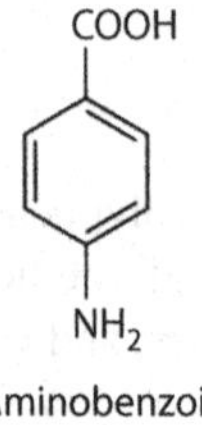

COOH

$NH_2$

*para*-Aminobenzoic acid

### *Sources*

*para*-Aminobenzoic acid occurs in plants, brewer's yeast, bacteria, and whole grains (Combs 2012). It is synthesized from chorismic acid (a product of phosphoenolpyruvate and erythrose-4-phosphate) by gastrointestinal bacteria, but not animal cells. The contribution of these bacteria to folate in animal tissues is limited. Thus, mammals, birds, and fish must ingest folate or its rich sources (e.g., green leafy vegetables). Primarily as a component of diets, *para*-aminobenzoic acid is found in animal products, such as the liver, kidneys, and skeletal muscle.

### *Absorption and Transport*

In the lumen of the small intestine, *para*-aminobenzoic acid is absorbed rapidly by enterocytes via a $Na^+$-independent transporter (passive diffusion) (Imai et al. 2017). Upon entering the enterocyte, some of this substance is acetylated into *N*-acetyl-*para*-aminobenzoic acid by arylamine *N*-acetyltransferase. Absorbed *para*-aminobenzoic acid enters the portal circulation. In the liver, *para*-aminobenzoic acid is metabolized to *N*-acetyl-*para*-aminobenzoic acid. Both *para*-aminobenzoic acid and *N*-acetyl-*para*-aminobenzoic acid are excreted in the urine.

### *Functions*

*para*-Aminobenzoic acid is a precursor for the synthesis of folate in bacteria (Combs 2012). Thus, this substance may play a role in the metabolism and growth of intestinal bacteria. *para*-Aminobenzoic acid antagonizes the bacteriostatic effect of sulfonamide drugs and can be used as a UV-screening agent due to its high absorbance in the UV range (Zempleni et al. 2013).

### *Deficiencies and Diseases*

Animals fed nutrient-balanced diets do not exhibit abnormal metabolism or physiology when they do not consume dietary *para*-aminobenzoic acid. There is no evidence for nutritional roles of this compound in mammals, birds, or fish. Synthesis of this compound by intestinal bacteria appears to meet their needs for folate, but such a microbial source of folate is inadequate for the host (Zempleni et al. 2013).

## SUMMARY

Vitamins are organic substances needed in small amounts by animals. These nutrients are important for (1) nutrient metabolism by serving as coenzymes for a wide array of enzymes (e.g., pyruvate dehydrogenase complex, acetyl-CoA carboxylase, and ornithine decarboxylase); (2) antioxidative reactions (e.g., vitamins C and E); and (3) regulating gene expression and biological activities of proteins (e.g., nuclear retinoid X receptor, intestinal and renal calcium transporters, and coagulation factors). Based on their solubility in water, vitamins are classified as water soluble (vitamins $B_1$, $B_2$, $B_3$, $B_5$, $B_6$, and $B_{12}$, as well as biotin and folate) or lipid soluble (vitamins A, D, E, and K). All vitamins are sensitive to destruction by oxidation and high temperatures. Other than these chemical properties, vitamins have little in common in their structures. Although requirements of animals for these nutrients are quantitatively low, almost all of them must be supplied in nonruminant diets, with an exception of vitamin D in those animals which are regularly exposed to sunlight. Compared with nonruminants, dietary requirements of ruminants for vitamins are much lower because a functional rumen can synthesize all these nutrients when protein, carbohydrates, and cobalt are adequate in diets. Some compounds with vitamin-like roles (e.g., carnitine, choline, *myo*-inositol, ubiquinones, PPQ, and bioflavonoids) are called quasi-vitamins. Most of them are soluble in water and nutritionally dispensable, but may provide health benefits to animals.

Vitamins are absorbed primarily by the small intestine and transported in the blood through different mechanisms (Figure 9.37). Specifically, water-soluble vitamins are absorbed into the enterocyte (primarily in the jejunum for most of them, but in the ileum for vitamin $B_{12}$) through its apical membrane via specific transporters. Some transporters are $Na^+$-dependent, while others are $Na^+$-independent. These vitamins exit the intestinal epithelial cell across its basolateral membrane into the lamina propria via specific transporters, and then enter the portal circulation. Most vitamins (niacin, pantothenic acid, biotin, folate, vitamin C, and 50% riboflavin) are transported in plasma in their free (unbound) forms, but several vitamins (thiamin, vitamin $B_6$, vitamin $B_{12}$, and 50% riboflavin) are transported in the plasma in their protein-bound forms. Water-soluble vitamins in the blood are taken up by all cells of the body via specific transporters and, in the case of vitamin $B_{12}$, via receptor-mediated endocytosis. In contrast, all dietary lipid-soluble vitamins are solubilized with lipids and bile salts as micelles in the lumen of the small intestine, and the micelles are subsequently taken up by enterocytes via passive diffusion. In the enterocytes, the absorbed lipid-soluble vitamins are assembled into chylomicrons and, in the case of vitamin E, also into VLDLs. The intestine-derived lipoproteins exit the enterocyte across its basolateral membrane (via passive diffusion) into the intestinal lymphatics and then the bloodstream in mammals and fish, or into the portal circulation in birds and reptiles. Through the metabolism of lipoproteins in the blood, the lipid-soluble vitamins-containing chylomicrons and VLDLs are converted into chylomicron remnants and LDLs, respectively, which are subsequently taken up by the liver through receptor-mediated mechanisms. Lipid-soluble vitamins are transported in the plasma in their protein-bound forms.

**TABLE 9.11**
**Dietary and Metabolically Active Forms of Vitamins and Quasi-Vitamins**

| Vitamin | Major Dietary Forms | Metabolically Active Forms | Major Function |
|---|---|---|---|
| | | **Lipid-Soluble Vitamins** | |
| Vitamin A | Retinyl palmitate and acetate; Provitamin A (β-carotene) | Retinol, retinal, retinoic acid | Vision, epithelial cell function, and gene expression |
| Vitamin D | Cholecalciferol (D3), ergocalciferol ($D_2$) | 1,25-Dihydroxy-vitamin D | Skeletal growth and development |
| Vitamin E | All-*rac*-α-tocopherol acetate | α-, β-, γ-, and δ-Tocopherols | Antioxidative function |
| Vitamin K | Phylloquinones, menaquinones, and menadione sodium bisulfite* | Phylloquinones, menaquinones | Blood clotting in response to bleeding |
| | | **Water-Soluble Vitamins** | |
| Vitamin C | L-Ascorbate | L-Ascorbate, dehydroascorbate | Hydroxylation of Pro and Lys residues in collagen; antioxidant |
| Thiamin | Thiamin, thiamin pyrophosphate | Thiamin pyrophosphate | Oxidative decarboxylation of KA |
| Riboflavin | FMN, FAD, flavoproteins, riboflavin | FMN, FAD | Cofactors of flavoproteins |
| Niacin | NAD(P), nicotinamide, nicotinic acid | NAD(P) | Coenzymes of oxidoreductases |
| Vitamin $B_6$ | Pyridoxal and pyridoxamine 5′-phosphate | Pyridoxal 5′-phosphate | Coenzyme for AA transaminase |
| Biotin | Biocytin, D-biotin | D-Biotin | ATP-dependent carboxylation |
| Pantothenate | CoA, acyl-CoA, Ca pentothenate | CoA | A component of CoA and ACP |
| Folate | Mono-, poly-, and pteroylglutamates | THF, 5-MTF, 5-10-MTF | One-carbon metabolism |
| Vitamin $B_{12}$ | Cyano-, methyl-, DA-cobalamins | Methyl- or DA-cobalamin | Removal of homocysteine |
| | | **Quasi-Vitamins** | |
| Choline | Phosphatidylcholine, choline chloride | Acetylcholine | Neurotransmission |
| Carnitine | Carnitine (meat), acetylcarnitine | | Oxidation of LCFAs |
| *myo*-Inositol | Phosphatidylinositol, phytate | Phosphatidylinositol | Cell signaling |
| PQQ | Pyrroloquinoline quinone (PQQ) | PQQ | A redox cofactor |
| Lipoic acid | Protein-bound lipoic acid, free lipoic acid | Protein-bound lipoic acid | Oxidative decarboxylation of KA |
| Ubiquinones | Ubiquinones | Coenzyme Q (in animals) | Mitochondrial electron transport |
| Bioflavonoids | Glycosides of bioflavonoids | Bioflavonoids | Antioxidants, pigments |
| PABA | *para*-Aminobenzoic acid (PABA) | PABA | Synthesis of folate in bacteria |

*Source:* Combs, G.F. 2012. *The Vitamins: Fundamental Aspects in Nutrition and Health.* Academic Press, New York, NW; and Open Chemistry Database, https://pubchem.ncbi.nlm.nih.gov

AA, amino acid; ACP, acyl carrier protein; DA, 5′-deoxyadenosyl; KA, α-ketoacids; 5,10-MTF, $N^5$-$N^{10}$-methylene-tetrahydrofolate; 5-MTF, $N^5$-methyltetrahydrofolate; THF, tetrahydrofolate.

* Chemically, menadione is a water-soluble substance. However, it is metabolized to lipid-soluble, bioactive menaquinone in animals.

Most vitamins are not utilized in the form in which they are absorbed from the intestine, and are converted or modified to their active forms (Table 9.11). Dietary requirements of mammals, birds, fish, and other animals for vitamins are affected by physiological states (e.g., pregnancy, lactation, physical activity, egg laying, and hatching), environment (e.g., low or high temperatures), and disease (e.g., bacterial, parasite, and viral infections). Deficiencies of vitamins can greatly reduce animal growth, development, fertility, immunity, production, and feed efficiency, and can also be lethal in severe cases, due to the impairments of ATP production, antioxidative responses, protein synthesis, and cellular signal transduction. Young animals are more sensitive to vitamin deficiencies than adults. The specific syndromes of deficiencies are usually characteristic of each vitamin (e.g., head retraction in niacin-deficient chicks, connective tissue dysfunction in vitamin C-deficient animals, and xerophthalmia in vitamin A-deficient subjects). Most diseases of vitamin deficiencies, particularly at their early stages, can be cured by dietary supplementation or intravenous/intramuscular administration. Like any other nutrients, dietary intake or parenteral provision of excessive vitamins (particularly lipid-soluble vitamins) are toxic to animals, particularly during embryonic and fetal development. Therefore, the status of vitamins must be monitored regularly and their supply (including dietary supplementation) carefully controlled.

## REFERENCES


Acosta, M.J., L. Vazquez Fonseca, M.A. Desbats, C. Cerqua, R. Zordan, E. Trevisson, and L. Salviati. 2016. Coenzyme Q biosynthesis in health and disease. *Biochim. Biophys. Acta* 1857:1079–1085.

Ahmad, I., T. Mirzal, K. Qadeer, U. Nazim, and F.H.M. Vaid. 2013. Vitamin B6: Deficiency diseases and methods of analysis. *Pak. J. Pharm. Sci.* 26:1057–1069.

Alpers, D.H. and G. Russell-Jones. 2013. Gastric intrinsic factor: The gastric and small intestinal stages of cobalamin absorption. A personal journey. *Biochimie* 95:989–994.

Aouameur, R., S. Da Cal, P. Bissonnette, M.J. Coady, and J.-Y. Lapointe. 2007. SMIT2 mediates all *myo*-inositol uptake in apical membranes of rat small intestine. *Am. J. Physiol.* 293:G1300–G1307.

Arnhold, T., H. Nau, S. Meyer, H.J. Rothkoetter, and A.D. Lampen. 2002. Porcine intestinal metabolism of excess vitamin A differs following vitamin A supplementation and liver consumption. *J. Nutr.* 132:197–203.

Baker, D.H., H.M. Edwards 3rd, C.S. Strunk, J.L. Emmert, C.M. Peter, I. Mavromichalis, and T.M. Parr. 1999. Single versus multiple deficiencies of methionine, zinc, riboflavin, vitamin B-6 and choline elicit surprising growth responses in young chicks. *J. Nutr.* 129:2239–2245.

Basset, G.J., S. Latimer, A. Fatihi, E. Soubeyrand, and A. Block. 2016. Phylloquinone (vitamin K1): Occurrence, biosynthesis and functions. *Mini-Rev. Med. Chem.* 16.

Bates, C.J. 1997. Bioavailability of riboflavin. *Eur. J. Clin. Nutr.* 51 (Suppl. 1):S38–42.

Beedholm-Ebsen, R., K. van de Wetering, T. Hardlei, E. Nexø, P. Borst, and S.K. Moestrup. 2010. Identification of multidrug resistance protein 1 (MRP1/ABCC1) as a molecular gate for cellular export of cobalamin. *Blood* 115:1632–1639.

Bencze, B., E. Ugrai, F. Gerloczy, and I. Juvancz. 1974. The effect of tocopherol on the embryonal development. *Int. J. Vitam. Nutr. Res.* 44:180–183.

Bentinger, M., M. Tekle, and G. Dallner. 2010. Coenzyme Q: Biosynthesis and functions. *Biochem. Biophys. Res. Commun.* 396:74–79.

Bentley, R. and R. Meganathan. 1982. Biosynthesis of vitamin K (menaquinone) in bacteria. *Microbiol. Rev.* 46:241–280.

Berdanier, C.D. 1998. *Advanced Nutrition: Micronutrients.* CRC Press, Boca Raton, FL.

Bettendorff, L., B. Lakaye, G. Kohn, and P. Wins. 2014. Thiamine triphosphate: A ubiquitous molecule in search of a physiological role. *Metab. Brain Dis.* 29:1069–1082.

Blomhoff, R., M.H. Green, and K.R. Norum. 1992. Vitamin A: Physiological and biochemical processing. *Annu. Rev. Nutr.* 12:37–57.

Bogan, K.L. and C. Brenner. 2008. Nicotinic acid, nicotinamide, and nicotinamide riboside: A molecular evaluation of $NAD^+$ precursor vitamins in human nutrition. *Annu. Rev. Nutr.* 28:115–130.

Booth, S.L. and J.W. Suttie. 1998. Dietary intake and adequacy of vitamin K. *J. Nutr.* 128:785–788.

Broberger, O., L. Ernster, and R. Zetterstrom. 1960. Oxidation of human hemoglobin by vitamin K3. *Nature* 188:316–317.

Brown, G. 2014. Defects of thiamine transport and metabolism. *J. Inherit. Metab. Dis.* 37:577–585.
Bruce, S.J., PA. Guy, S. Rezzi, and A.B. Ross. 2010. Quantitative measurement of betaine and free choline in plasma, cereals and cereal products by isotope dilution LC-MS/MS. *J. Agric. Food Chem.* 58:2055–2061.
Burtle, G.J. and R.T. Lovell. 1989. Lack of response of channel catfish (*Ictalurus punctatus*) to dietary *myo*-inositol. *Can. J. Fish. Aquat. Sci.* 46:218–221.
Bürzle, M., Y. Suzuki, D. Ackermann, H. Miyazaki, N. Maeda, B. Clémençon, R. Burrier, and M.A. Hediger. 2013. The sodium-dependent ascorbic acid transporter family SLC23. *Mol. Aspects Med.* 34:436–454.
Butterworth, C.E. Jr. and A. Bendich. 1996. Folic acid and the prevention of birth defects. *Annu. Rev. Nutr.* 16:73–97.
Byers, T. and G. Perry. 1992. Dietary carotenes, vitamin C, and vitamin E as protective antioxidants in human cancers. *Annu. Rev. Nutr.* 12:139–159.
Carpenter, K.J. 1983. The relationship of pellagra to corn and the low availability of niacin in cereals. *Experientia Suppl.* 44:197–222.
Cascella, M., S. Bärfuss, and A. Stocker. 2013. *Cis*-retinoids and the chemistry of vision. *Arch. Biochem. Biophys.* 539:187–195.
Castoldi, E. and T.M. Hackeng. 2008. Regulation of coagulation by protein S. *Curr. Opin. Hematol.* 15:529–536.
Chelstowska, S., M.A.K. Widjaja-Adhi, J.A. Silvaroli, and M. Golczak. 2016. Molecular basis for vitamin A uptake and storage in vertebrates. *Nutrients* 8:676.
Christakos, S., P. Dhawan, A. Verstuyf, L. Verlinden, and G. Carmeliet. 2016. Vitamin D: Metabolism, molecular mechanism of action, and pleiotropic effects. *Physiol. Rev.* 96:365–408.
Chu, S.H. and D.M. Hegsted. 1980. *Myo*-inositol deficiency in gerbils: Comparative study of the intestinal lipodystrophy in *Meriones unguiculatus* and *Meriones libycus*. *J. Nutr.* 110:1209–1216.
Clagett-Dame, M. and H.F. DeLuca. 2002. The role of vitamin A in mammalian reproduction and embryonic development. *Annu. Rev. Nutr.* 22:347–381.
Clarke, P. 2010. Vitamin K prophylaxis for preterm infants. *Early Hum. Dev.* 86 (Suppl. 1):17–20.
Clark, N.P., D.M. Witt, L.E. Davies, E.M. Saito, K.H. McCool, J.D. Douketis, K.R. Metz, and T. Delate. 2015. Bleeding, recurrent venous thromboembolism, and mortality risks during Warfarin interruption for invasive procedures. *JAMA Intern. Med.* 175:1163–1168.
Collins, M.D. and G.E. Mao. 1999. Teratology of retinoids. *Annu. Rev. Pharmacol. Toxicol.* 39:399–430.
Combs, G.F. 2012. *The Vitamins: Fundamental Aspects in Nutrition and Health.* Academic Press, New York, NY.
Corpe, C.P., P. Eck, J. Wang, H. Al-Hasani, and M. Levine. 2013. Intestinal dehydroascorbic acid (DHA) transport mediated by the facilitative sugar transporters, GLUT2 and GLUT8. *J. Biol. Chem.* 288:9092–9101.
Coxon, K.M., E. Chakauya, H.H. Ottenhof, H.M. Whitney, T.L. Blundell, C. Abell, and A.G. Smith. 2005. Pantothenate biosynthesis in higher plants. *Biochem. Soc. Trans.* 33:743–746.
Cronan, J.E. 2016. Assembly of lipoic acid on its cognate enzymes: An extraordinary and essential biosynthetic pathway. *Microbiol. Mol. Biol. Rev.* 80:429–450.
DeGaris, P.J. and I.J. Lean. 2008. Milk fever in dairy cows: A review of pathophysiology and control principles. *Vet. J.* 176:58–69.
Dekaney, C.M., G. Wu, Y.L. Yin, and L.A. Jaeger. 2008. Regulation of ornithine aminotransferase gene expression and activity by all-trans retinoic acid in Caco-2 intestinal epithelial cells. *J. Nutr. Biochem.* 19:674–681.
DeLuca, H.F. 2016. Vitamin D: Historical overview. *Vitam. Horm.* 100:1–20.
Deluca, H.F., J.M. Prahl, and L.A. Plum. 2011. 1,25-Dihydroxyvitamin D is not responsible for toxicity caused by vitamin D or 25-hydroxyvitamin D. *Arch. Biochem. Biophys.* 505:226–230.
DiPalma, J.R. and D.M. Ritchie. 1977. Vitamin toxicity. *Annu. Rev. Pharmacol. Toxicol.* 17:133–148.
Durán, J.M., M.J. Peral, M.L. Calonge, and A.A. Ilundáin. 2005. OCTN3: A $Na^+$-independent L-carnitine transporter in enterocytes basolateral membrane. *J. Cell Physiol.* 202:929–935.
Ducker, G.S. and J.D. Rabinowitz. 2017. One-carbon metabolism in health and disease. *Cell Metab.* 25:27–42.
Egaas, E. and G. Lambertsen. 1979. Naturally occurring vitamin D3 in fish products analysed by HPLC, using vitamin D2 as an international standard. *Int. J. Vitam. Nutr. Res.* 49:35–42.
Englard, S. and S. Seifter. 1986. The biochemical functions of ascorbic acid. *Annu. Rev. Nutr.* 6:365–406.
Ennis, E.A. and R.D. Blakely. 2016. Choline on the move: Perspectives on the molecular physiology and pharmacology of the presynaptic choline transporter. *Adv. Pharmacol.* 76:175–213.
Esmon, C.T., S. Vigano-D'Angelo, A. D'Angelo, and P.C. Comp. 1987. Anticoagulation proteins C and S. *Adv. Exp. Med. Biol.* 214:47–54.
Fang, Y.Z., S. Yang, and Wu, G. 2002. Free radicals, antioxidants, and nutrition. *Nutrition* 18:872–879.

Ferland, G. 2012. The discovery of vitamin K and its clinical applications. *Ann. Nutr. Metab.* 61:213–218.
Finkel, M.J. 1961. Vitamin K, and the vitamin K analogues. *Clin. Pharmacol. Ther.* 2:794–814.
Fleming, A. and A.J. Copp. 1998. Embryonic folate metabolism and mouse neural tube defects. *Science* 280:2107–2108.
Ford, J.E., K.J. Scott, B.F. Sansom, and P.J. Taylor. 1975. Some observations on the possible nutritional significance of vitamin B12 and folate-binding proteins in milk. Absorption of ($^{58}$Co)cyanocobalamin by suckling piglets. *Br. J. Nutr.* 34:469–492.
Fugate, C.J. and J.T. Jarrett. 2012. Biotin synthase: Insights into radical-mediated carbon-sulfur bond formation. *Biochim. Biophys. Acta* 1824:1213–1222.
García-Angulo, V.A. 2017. Overlapping riboflavin supply pathways in bacteria. *Crit. Rev. Microbiol.* 43:196–209.
Geiger, J.H. and X. Jin. 2006. The structure and mechanism of *myo*-inositol-1-phosphate synthase. *Subcell. Biochem.* 39:157–180.
Georgievskii, V.I. 1982. The physiological role of microelements. In: *Mineral Nutrition of Animals*. Edited by V.I. Georgievskii, B.N. Annenkov, and V.T. Samokhin. Butterworths, London, U.K.
Gill, D.L., T.K. Ghosh, and J.M. Mullaney. 1989. Calcium signaling mechanisms in endoplasmic reticulum activated by inositol-1,4,5 triphosphate and GTP. *Cell Calcium* 10:363–374.
Gille, D. and A. Schmid. 2015. Vitamin B12 in meat and dairy products. *Nutr. Rev.* 73:106–115.
Gopalan, C. and K.S. Jaya Rao. 1975. Pellagra and amino acids imbalance. *Vitam. Horm.* 33:505–28.
Gross, J. and P. Budowski. 1966. Conversion of carotenoids into vitamins $A_1$ and $A_2$ in two species of freshwater fish. *Biochem. J.* 101:747–754.
Gross, C.J., L.M. Henderson, and D.A. Savaiano. 1986. Uptake of L-carnitine, D-carnitine and acetyl-L-carnitine by isolated guinea-pig enterocytes. *Biochim. Biophys. Acta* 886:425–433.
Gruber, K., B. Puffer, and B. Kräutler. 2011. Vitamin B12-derivatives-enzyme cofactors and ligands of proteins and nucleic acids. *Chem. Soc. Rev.* 40:4346–463.
Hall, C.A. 1977. The carriers of native vitamin B12 in normal human serum. *Clin. Sci. Mol. Med.* 53:453–457.
Halsted, C.H. 2003. Absorption of water-soluble vitamins. *Curr. Opin. Gastroenterol.* 19:113–117.
Halsted, C.H. and V. Medici. 2011. Vitamin-dependent methionine metabolism and alcoholic liver disease. *Adv. Nutr.* 2:421–427.
Hayashi, H. 1995. Pyridoxal enzymes: Mechanistic diversity and uniformity. *J. Biochem.* 118:463–473.
Helmreich, E.J. 1992. How pyridoxal 5′-phosphate could function in glycogen phosphorylase catalysis. *Biofactors* 3:159–172.
Hippe, E. and M. Schwartz. 1971. Intrinsic factor activity of stomach preparations from various animal species. *Scand. J. Haematol.* 8:276–281.
Hirota, Y., N. Tsugawa, K. Nakagawa, Y. Suhara, K. Tanaka, Y. Uchino, A. Takeuchi et al. 2013. Menadione (vitamin K3) is a catabolic product of oral phylloquinone (vitamin K1) in the intestine and a circulating precursor of tissue menaquinone-4 (vitamin K2) in rats. *J. Biol. Chem.* 288:33071–33080.
Hopkins, F.G. 1912. Feeding experiments illustrating the importance of accessory factors in normal dietaries. *J. Physiol.* 44:425–460.
How, K.L., H.A. Hazewinkel, and J.A. Mol. 1994. Dietary vitamin D dependence of cat and dog due to inadequate cutaneous synthesis of vitamin D. *Gen. Comp. Endocrinol.* 96:12–18.
Imai, T., K. Tanaka, T. Yonemitsu, Y. Yakushiji, and K. Ohura. 2017. Elucidation of the intestinal absorption of para-aminobenzoic acid, a marker for dietary intake. *J. Pharm. Sci.* 106:2881–2888. doi: 10.1016/j.xphs.2017.04.070.
Irie, T., T. Sugimoto, N. Ueki, H. Senoo, and T. Seki. 2010. Retinoid storage in the egg of reptiles and birds. *Comp. Biochem. Physiol. B* 157:113–118.
Jones, G., S.A. Strugnell, and H.F. DeLuca. 1998. Current understanding of the molecular actions of vitamin D. *Physiol. Rev.* 78:1193–1231.
Jones, T.C. and R.D. Hunt. 1983. *Veterinary Pathology*. Lea & Febiger, Philadelphia, PA.
Kamanna, V.S., S.H. Ganji, and M.L. Kashyap. 2013. Recent advances in niacin and lipid metabolism. *Curr. Opin. Lipidol.* 24:239–245.
Kato, Y., M. Sugiura, T. Sugiura, T. Wakayama, Y. Kubo, D. Kobayashi, Y. Sai, I. Tamai, S. Iseki, and A. Tsuji. 2006. Organic cation/carnitine transporter OCTN2 (Slc22a5) is responsible for carnitine transport across apical membranes of small intestinal epithelial cells in mouse. *Mol. Pharmacol.* 70:829–837.
Killgore, I. 1989. Nutritional importance of pyrroloquinoline quinine. *Science* 245:850–852.
Kono, N. and H. Arai. 2015. Intracellular transport of fat-soluble vitamins A and E. *Traffic* 16:19–34.
Lucock M. 2000. Folic acid: Nutritional biochemistry, molecular biology, and role in disease processes. *Mol. Genet. Metab.* 71:121–138.

MacKay, D., J. Hathcock, and E. Guarneri. 2012. Niacin: Chemical forms, bioavailability, and health effects. *Nutr. Rev.* 70:357–366.

Maeda, Y., S. Kawata, Y. Inui, K. Fukuda, T. Igura, and Y. Matsuzawa. 1996. Biotin deficiency decreases ornithine transcarbamylase activity and mRNA in rat liver. *J. Nutr.* 126:61–66.

Mahan, D.C., S. Ching, and K. Dabrowski. 2004. Developmental aspects and factors influencing the synthesis and status of ascorbic acid in the pig. *Annu. Rev. Nutr.* 24:79–103.

Mai, K.S., G.T. Wu, and W. Zhu. 2001. Abalone, *Haliotis discus hannai Ino*, can synthesize *myo*-inositol *de novo* to meet physiological needs. *J. Nutr.* 131:2898–2903.

Manzetti, S., J. Zhang, and D. van der Spoel. 2014. Thiamin function, metabolism, uptake, and transport. *Biochemistry* 53:821–835.

March, B.E., V. Coates, and J. Biely. 1968. Reticulocytosis in response to dietary antioxidants. *Science* 164:1398–1399.

March, B.E., E. Wong, L. Seier, J. Sim, and J. Biely. 1973. Hypervitaminosis E in the chick. *J. Nutr.* 103:371–77.

Marchioli, R., G. Levantesi, A. Macchia, R.M. Marfisi, G.L. Nicolosi, L. Tavazzi, G. Tognoni, F. Valagussa, and GISSI-Prevenzione Investigators. 2006. Vitamin E increases the risk of developing heart failure after myocardial infarction: Results from the GISSI-Prevenzione trial. *J. Cardiovasc. Med.* 7:347–350.

Maurice, D.V., S.F. Lightsey, and J.E. Toler. 2004. Ascorbic acid biosynthesis in hens producing strong and weak eggshells. *Br. Poultry Sci.* 45:404–408.

McDonald, P., R.A. Edwards, J.F.D. Greenhalgh, J.F.D. Greenhalgh, C.A. Morgan, L.A. Sinclair. 2011. *Animal Nutrition*, 7th ed. Prentice Hall, New York.

McKay, E.J. and L.M. McLeay. 1981. Location and secretion of gastric intrinsic factor in the sheep. *Res. Vet. Sci.* 30:261–265.

McMahon, R.J. 2002. Biotin in metabolism and molecular biology. *Annu. Rev. Nutr.* 22:221–239.

Meadows, J.A. and M.J. Wargo. 2015. Carnitine in bacterial physiology and metabolism. *Microbiology* 161:1161–1174.

Meydani, M. and K.R. Martin. 2001. Intestinal absorption of fat-soluble vitamins. In: *Intestinal Lipid Metabolism.* Edited by C.M. Mansbach, P. Tso and A. Kuksis. Kluwer Academic, New York, pp. 367–381.

Miller, E.R.3rd, R. Pastor-Barriuso, D. Dalal, R.A. Riemersma, L.J. Appel, and E. Guallar. 2005. Meta-analysis: High-dosage vitamin E supplementation may increase all-cause mortality. *Ann. Intern. Med.* 142:37–46.

Moura, F.A., K.Q. de Andrade, J.C. dos Santos, and M.O. Goulart. 2015. Lipoic acid: Its antioxidant and anti-inflammatory role and clinical applications. *Curr. Top. Med. Chem.* 15:458–483.

Nabokina, S.M., K. Inoue, V.S. Subramanian, J.E. Valle, H. Yuasa, and H.M. Said. 2014. Molecular identification and functional characterization of the human colonic thiamine pyrophosphate transporter. *J. Biol. Chem.* 289:4405–4416.

Nabokina, S.M., M.L. Kashyap, and H.M. Said. 2005. Mechanism and regulation of human intestinal niacin uptake. *Am. J. Physiol. Cell Physiol.* 289:C97–C103.

Nakagawa, K., Y. Hirota, N. Sawada, N. Yuge, M. Watanabe, Y. Uchino, N. Okuda, Y. Shimomura, Y. Suhara, and T. Okano. 2010. Identification of UBIAD1 as a novel human menaquinone-4 biosynthetic enzyme. *Nature* 468:117–121.

National Research Council (NRC). 1998. *Nutrient Requirements of Swine*, National Academy Press, Washington, D.C.

Nau, H. 2001. Teratogenicity of isotretinoin revisited: Species variation and the role of all-*trans*-retinoic acid. *J. Am. Acad. Dermatol.* 45:S183–187.

Niehoff, I.D., L. Hüther, and P. Lebzien. 2009. Niacin for dairy cattle: A review. *Br. J. Nutr.* 101:5–19.

Nielsen, M.J., M.R. Rasmussen, C.B.F. Andersen, E. Nexø, and S.K. Moestrup. 2012. Vitamin B 12 transport from food to the body's cells—A sophisticated, multistep pathway. *Nat. Rev. Gastroenterol. Hepatol.* 9:345–354.

Niki, E. and M.G. Traber. 2012. A history of vitamin E. *Ann. Nutr. Metab.* 61:207–212.

Nilsson, A. and R.D. Duan. 2006. Absorption and lipoprotein transport of sphingomyelin. *J. Lipid Res.* 47:154–171.

O'Byrne, S.M., N. Wongsiriroj, J. Libien, S. Vogel, I.J. Goldberg, W. Baehr, K. Palczewski, and W.S. Blaner. 2005. Retinoid absorption and storage is impaired in mice lacking lecithin:retinol acyltransferase (LRAT). *J. Biol. Chem.* 280:35647–35657.

Okano, T., E. Kuroda, H. Nakao, S. Kodama, T. Matsuo, Y. Nakamichi, K. Nakajima, N. Hirao, and T. Kobayashi. 1986. Lack of evidence for existence of vitamin D and 25-hydroxyvitamin D sulfates in human breast and cow's milk. *J. Nutr. Sci. Vitaminol. (Tokyo)* 32:449–462.

Ouchi, A., M. Nakano, S. Nagaoka, and K. Mukai. 2009. Kinetic study of the antioxidant activity of pyrroloquinolinequinol (PQQH(2), a reduced form of pyrroloquinoline quinone) in micellar solution. *J. Agric. Food Chem.* 57:450–456.

Owens, C.A. Jr. 1971. Pharmacology and toxicology. In: *The Vitamins: Chemistry, Physiology, Pathology, Methods.* Edited by W.H. Sebrell and R.S. Harris. Academic Press, New York, NY, pp. 492–509.

Padayatty, S.J. and M. Levine. 2016. Vitamin C: The known and the unknown and Goldilocks. *Oral Dis.* 22:463–493.

Panche, A.N., A.D. Diwan, and S.R. Chandra. 2016. Flavonoids: An overview. *J. Nutr. Sci.* 5:e47.

Panter, R.A. and J.B. Mudd. 1969. Carnitine levels in some higher plants. *FEBS Lett.* 5:169–170.

Penniston, K.L. and S.A. Tanumihardjo. 2006. The acute and chronic toxic effects of vitamin A. *Am. J. Clin. Nutr.* 83:191–201.

Pesti, G.M., G.N. Rowland 3rd, and K.S. Ryu. 1991. Folate deficiency in chicks fed diets containing practical ingredients. *Poult. Sci.* 70:600–604.

Peterlik, M. 2012. Vitamin D insufficiency and chronic diseases: Hype and reality. *Food Funct.* 3:784–794.

Pinto, J.T. and A.J. Cooper. 2014. From cholesterogenesis to steroidogenesis: Role of riboflavin and flavoenzymes in the biosynthesis of vitamin D. *Adv. Nutr.* 5:144–163.

Politis, I. 2012. Reevaluation of vitamin E supplementation of dairy cows: Bioavailability, animal health and milk quality. *Animal* 6:1427–1434.

Pond, W.G., D.C. Church, and K.R. Pond. 1995. *Basic Animal Nutrition and Feeding*, 4th ed. John Wiley & Sons, New York.

Powers, H.J. 2003. Riboflavin (vitamin B-2) and health. *Am. J. Clin. Nutr.* 77:1352–1360.

Proszkowiec-Weglarz, M. and R. Angel. 2013. Calcium and phosphorus metabolism in broilers: Effect of homeostatic mechanism on calcium and phosphorus digestibility. *J. Appl. Poult. Res.* 22:609–627.

Puehringer, S., M. Metlitzky, and R. Schwarzenbacher. 2008. The pyrroloquinoline quinone biosynthesis pathway revisited: A structural approach. *BMC Biochem.* 9:8.

Quick, M. and L., Shi. 2015. The sodium/multivitamin transporter: A multipotent system with therapeutic implications. *Vitam. Horm.* 98:63–100.

Ragaller, V., P. Lebzien, K.H. Südekum, L. Hüther, and G. Flachowsky. 2011. Pantothenic acid in ruminant nutrition: A review. *J. Anim. Physiol. Anim. Nutr.* 95:6–16.

Rai, R.K., J. Luo, and T.H. Tulchinsky. 2017. Vitamin K supplementation to prevent hemorrhagic morbidity and mortality of newborns in India and China. *World J. Pediatr.* 13:15–19.

Rahman, M.M.A. and P. Hongsprabhas. 2016. Genistein as antioxidant and antibrowning agents in *in vivo* and *in vitro*: A review. *Biomed. Pharmacother.* 82:379–392.

Ranjan, R., A. Ranjan, G.S. Dhaliwal, and R.C. Patra. 2012. L-Ascorbic acid (vitamin C) supplementation to optimize health and reproduction in cattle. *Vet. Q.* 32:145–150.

Raux, E., H.L. Schubert, and M.J. Warren. 2000. Biosynthesis of cobalamin (vitamin B12): A bacterial conundrum. *Cell. Mol. Life Sci.* 57:1880–1893.

Rebhun, W.C., B.C. Tennant, S.G. Dill, and J.M. King. 1984. Vitamin K3-induced renal toxicosis in the horse. *J. Am. Vet. Med. Assoc.* 184:1237–1239.

Reboul, E. 2015. Intestinal absorption of vitamin D: From the meal to the enterocyte. *Food Funct.* 6:356–362.

Reboul, E., A. Berton, M. Moussa, C. Kreuzer, I. Crenon, and P. Borel. 2006. Pancreatic lipase and pancreatic lipase-related protein 2, but not pancreatic lipase-related protein 1, hydrolyze retinyl palmitate in physiological conditions. *Biochim. Biophys. Acta* 1761:4–10.

Reshkin, S.J., S. Vilella, G.A. Ahearn, and C. Storelli. 1989. Basolateral inositol transport by intestines of carnivorous and herbivorous teleosts. *Am. J. Physiol.* 256:G509–G516.

Roche. 1991. *Vitamin Nutrition for Swine.* Hoffmann-La Roche Inc. Nutley, NJ.

Sahr, T., S. Ravanel, and F. Rébeillé. 2005. Tetrahydrofolate biosynthesis and distribution in higher plants. *Biochem. Soc. Trans.* 33:758–762.

Said, H.M. 2011. Intestinal absorption of water-soluble vitamins in health and disease. *Biochem. J.* 437:357–372.

Said, H.M., H. Chatterjee, R.U. Haq, V.S. Subramanian, A. Ortiz, L.H. Matherly, F.M. Sirotnak, C. Halsted, and S.A. Rubin. 2000. Adaptive regulation of intestinal folate uptake: Effect of dietary folate deficiency. *Am. J. Physiol. Cell Physiol.* 279:C1889–C1895.

Samuel, K.G., H.J. Zhang, J. Wang, S.G. Wu, H.Y. Yue, L.L. Sun, and G.H. Qi. 2015. Effects of dietary pyrroloquinoline quinone disodium on growth performance, carcass yield and antioxidant status of broiler chicks. *Animal* 9:409–416.

Schmid, A. and B. Walther. 2013. Natural vitamin D content in animal products. *Adv. Nutr.* 4:453–462.

Schmitt, C.A. and V.M. Dirsch. 2009. Modulation of endothelial nitric oxide by plant-derived products. *Nitric Oxide* 21:77–91.

Semba, R.D. 2012. The discovery of the vitamins. *Int. J. Vitam. Nutr. Res.* 82:310–315.

Shane B. 2008. Folate and vitamin B12 metabolism: Overview and interaction with riboflavin, vitamin B6, and polymorphisms. *Food Nutr. Bull.* 29(2 Suppl.):S5–16.

Shearer, M.J., A. Bach, and M. Kohlmeier. 1996. Chemistry, nutritional sources, tissue distribution and metabolism of vitamin K with special reference to bone health. *J. Nutr.* 126(4 Suppl.):1181S–1186S.

Sherwood, T.A., R.L. Alphin, W.W. Saylor, and H.B. White 3rd. 1993. Folate metabolism and deposition in eggs by laying hens. *Arch. Biochem. Biophys.* 307:66–72.

Shibata, K., C.J. Gross, and L.M. Henderson. 1983. Hydrolysis and absorption of pantothenate and its coenzymes in the rat small intestine. *J. Nutr.* 113:2107–2115.

Shiraki, M., N. Tsugawa, and T. Okano. 2015. Recent advances in vitamin K-dependent Gla-containing proteins and vitamin K nutrition. *Osteoporosis Sarcopenia* 1:22–38.

Shukla, S., C.-P. Wu, K. Nandigama, and S.V. Ambudkar. 2007. The naphthoquinones, vitamin $K_3$ and its structural analogue plumbagin, are substrates of the multidrug resistance-linked ATP binding cassette drug transporter ABCG2. *Mol. Cancer Ther.* 6:3279–3286.

Smidt, C.R., C.J. Unkefer, D.R. Houck, and R.B. Rucker. 1991. Intestinal absorption and tissue distribution of ($^{14}$C)pyrroloquinoline quinone in mice. *Proc. Soc. Exp. Biol. Med.* 197:27–31.

Smith, C.M. and W.O. Song. 1996. Comparative nutrition of pantothenic acid. *J. Nutr. Biochem.* 7:312–321.

Smith, R.M. and H.R. Marston. 1970. Production, absorption, distribution and excretion of vitamin B12 in sheep. *Br. J. Nutr.* 24:857–877.

Soprano, D.R. and K.J. Soprano. 1995. Retinoids as teratogens. *Annu. Rev. Nutr.* 15:111–132.

Stadtman, T.C. 2002. Discoveries of vitamin $B_{12}$ and selenium enzymes. *Annu. Rev. Biochem.* 71:1–16.

Steinberg, F.M., M.E. Gershwin, and R.B. Rucker. 1994. Dietary Pyrroloquinoline quinone: Growth and immune response in BALB/c mice. *J Nutr.* 124:744–753.

Stephensen, C.B. 2001. Vitamin A, infection, and immune function. *Annu. Rev. Nutr.* 21:167–192.

Stites, T.E., A.E. Mitchell, and R.B. Rucker. 2000. Physiological importance of quinoenzymes and the *O*-quinone family of cofactors. *J. Nutr.* 130:719–727.

Suttle, N.F. 2010. *Mineral Nutrition of Livestock*, 4th ed. CABI, Wallingford, U.K.

Thakur, K., S.K. Tomar, A.K. Singh, S. Mandal, and S. Arora. 2016. Riboflavin and health: A review of recent human research. *Crit. Rev. Food Sci. Nutr.* 57:3650–3660. doi: 10.1080/10408398.2016.1145104.

Tong, L. 2013. Structure and function of biotin-dependent carboxylases. *Cell Mol. Life Sci.* 70:863–891.

Traber, M.G. 2007. Vitamin E regulatory mechanisms. *Annu. Rev. Nutr.* 27:347–362.

Trugo, N.M., J.E. Ford, and D.N. Salter. 1985. Vitamin B12 absorption in the neonatal piglet. 3. Influence of vitamin B12-binding protein from sows' milk on uptake of vitamin B12 by microvillus membrane vesicles prepared from small intestine of the piglet. *Br. J. Nutr.* 54:269–283.

Uchida, Y., K. Ito, S. Ohtsuki, Y. Kubo, T. Suzuki, and T. Terasaki. 2015. Major involvement of Na(+)-dependent multivitamin transporter (SLC5A6/SMVT) in uptake of biotin and pantothenic acid by human brain capillary endothelial cells. *J. Neurochem.* 134:97–112.

Ueland, P.M., A. Ulvik, L. Rios-Avila, Ø. Midttun, and J.F. Gregory. 2015. Direct and functional biomarkers of vitamin B6 status. *Annu. Rev. Nutr.* 35:33–70.

Ulatowski, L. and D. Manor. 2013. Vitamin E trafficking in neurologic health and disease. *Annu. Rev. Nutr.* 33:87–103.

Van Bennekum, A., M. Werder, S.T. Thuahnai, C.H. Han, P. Duong, D.L. Williams, P. Wettstein, G. Schulthess, M.C. Phillips, and H. Hauser. 2005. Class B scavenger receptor-mediated intestinal absorption of dietary β-carotene and cholesterol. *Biochemistry* 44:4517–4525.

Vadlapudi, A.D., R.K. Vadlapatla, and A.K. Mitra. 2012. Sodium dependent multivitamin transporter (SMVT): A potential target for drug delivery. *Curr. Drug Targets* 13:994–1003.

Vaz, F.M. and R.J.A. Wanders. 2002. Carnitine biosynthesis in mammals. *Biochem. J.* 361:417–429.

Vedder, L.C., J.M. Hall, K.R. Jabrouin, and L.M. Savage. 2015. Interactions between chronic ethanol consumption and thiamine deficiency on neural plasticity, spatial memory, and cognitive flexibility. *Alcohol Clin. Exp. Res.* 39:2143–2153.

Vogel, S., M.V. Gamble, and W.S. Blaner. 1999. Biosynthesis, absorption, metabolism and transport of retinoids. In: Retinoids. Edited by H. Nau and W.S. Blaner. Springer, New York, NY.

Waldrop, G.L., H.M. Holden, and M. St Maurice. 2012. The enzymes of biotin dependent $CO_2$ metabolism: What structures reveal about their reaction mechanisms. *Protein Sci.* 21:1597–1619.

Wang, J., H.J. Zhang, K.G. Samuel, C. Long, S.G. Wu, H.Y. Yue, L.L. Sun, and G.H. Qi. 2015. Effects of dietary pyrroloquinoline quinone disodium on growth, carcass characteristics, redox status, and mitochondria metabolism in broilers. *Poult. Sci.* 94:215–225.

Wang, J.J., Z.L. Wu, D.F. Li, N. Li, S.V. Dindot, M.C. Satterfield, F.W. Bazer, and G. Wu. 2012. Nutrition, epigenetics, and metabolic syndrome. *Antioxid. Redox Signal.* 17:282–301.

Weir, R.R., J.J. Strain, M. Johnston, C. Lowis, A.M. Fearon, S. Stewart, and L.K. Pourshahidi. 2017. Environmental and genetic factors influence the vitamin D content of cows' milk. *Proc. Nutr. Soc.* 76:76–82.

Wells, W.W. and D.P. Xu. 1994. Dehydroascorbate reduction. *J. Bioenerg. Biomembr.* 26:369–377.

Wells, W.W., D.P. Xu, Y.F. Yang, and P.A. Rocque. 1990. Mammalian thioltransferase (glutaredoxin) and protein disulfide isomerase have dehydroascorbate reductase activity. *J. Biol. Chem.* 265:15361–15364.

Wongsiriroj, N., R. Piantedosi, K. Palczewski, I.J. Goldberg, T.P. Johnston, E. Li, and W.S. Blaner. 2008. The molecular basis of retinoid absorption—A genetic dissection. *J. Biol. Chem.* 283:13510–13519.

Wrong, O.M., C.J. Edmonds, and V.S. Chadwick. 1981. *The Large Intestine: Its Role in Mammalian Nutrition and Homeostasis.* Wiley and Sons, New York.

Wu, G. 2013. *Amino Acids: Biochemistry and Nutrition*, CRC Press, Boca Raton, Florida.

Wu, G. and C.J. Meininger. 2002. Regulation of nitric oxide synthesis by dietary factors. *Annu. Rev. Nutr.* 22:61–86.

Wu, G., J. Fanzo, D.D. Miller, P. Pingali, M. Post, J.L. Steiner, and A.E. Thalacker-Mercer. 2014. Production and supply of high-quality food protein for human consumption: Sustainability, challenges and innovations. *Ann. N.Y. Acad. Sci.* 1321:1–19.

Wyatt, R.D., H.T. Tung, W.E. Donaldson, and P.B. Hamilton. 1973. A new description of riboflavin deficiency syndrome in chickens. *Poult. Sci.* 52:237–244.

Yao, K., Y.L. Yin, Z.M., Feng, Z.R., Tang, J. Fang, and G. Wu. 2011. Tryptophan metabolism in animals: Important roles in nutrition and health. *Front. Biosci.* S3:286–297.

Yeum, K.J. and R.M. Russell. 2002. Carotenoid bioavailability and bioconversion. *Annu. Rev. Nutr.* 22:483–504.

Yin, Z., Z. Huang, J. Cui, R. Fiehler, N. Lasky, D. Ginsburg, and G.J. Broze, Jr. 2000. Prothrombotic phenotype of protein Z deficiency. *Proc. Natl. Acad. Sci. USA* 97:6734–6738.

Zeisel, S.H. and K. da Costa. 2009. Choline: An essential nutrient for public health. *Nutr. Rev.* 67:615–623.

Zempleni, J., J.W. Suttie, J.F. Gregory III, and P.J. Stover. 2013. *Handbook of Vitamins*, 5th ed. CRC Press, Boca Raton, FL.

Zhao, R. and I.D. Goldman. 2013. Folate and thiamine transporters mediated by facilitative carriers (SLC19A1-3 and SLC46A1) and folate receptors. *Mol. Aspects Med.* 34:373–385.

Zhao, R., N. Diop-Bove, M. Visentin, and I. David Goldman. 2011. Mechanisms of membrane transport of folates into cells and across epithelia. *Annu. Rev. Nutr.* 31:177–201.

Zingg, J.M. 2015. Vitamin E: A role in signal transduction. *Annu. Rev. Nutr.* 35:135–173.

Zou, F., Y. Liu, L. Liu, K. Wu, W. Wei, Y. Zhu, and J. Wu. 2007. Retinoic acid activates human inducible nitric oxide synthase gene through binding of RARalpha/RXRalpha heterodimer to a novel retinoic acid response element in the promoter. *Biochem. Biophys. Res. Commun.* 355:494–500.

# 10 Nutrition and Metabolism of Minerals

The word "mineral" is derived from the English word "mine" or a substance in the earth's crust that can be obtained through "mining." They are the second to the eighth most abundant elements in the earth's crust, only after oxygen (% by weight): oxygen, 46.6; silica, 27.7; aluminum, 8.1; iron, 5.0; calcium, 3.6; sodium, 2.8; potassium, 2.6; magnesium, 2.1; and others, 1.5 (Lutgens and Tarbuck 2000). Minerals are inorganic elements that are present in both foods and animals. In contrast to carbohydrates, fatty acids, and amino acids (AAs), minerals are neither synthesized nor degraded by animals or microbes (Harris 2014). There are about 47 different minerals in organisms and feeds (Pond et al. 1995). Some minerals are present in the body at concentrations ≥400 mg/kg body weight (BW), and are called macrominerals: sodium (Na), potassium (K), chlorine (Cl), calcium (Ca), phosphorus (P), sulfur (S), and magnesium (Mg) (Table 10.1). Phosphorus usually exists as phosphates in cells and physiological fluids (Takeda et al. 2012). Animals contain small amounts of about 40 minerals at concentrations <100 mg/kg BW, which are termed microminerals or trace minerals (Mertz 1987). To date, the following 16 microminerals have been shown to have important physiological functions in animals: iron (Fe), copper (Cu), cobalt (Co), manganese (Mn), zinc (Zn), iodine (I), selenium (Se), molybdenum (Mo), chromium (Cr), fluorine (F), tin (Sn), vanadium (V), silicon (Si), nickel (Ni), boron (B), and bromine (Br) (McCall et al. 2014; McDonald et al. 2011; Mertz 1974). These microminerals and the seven macrominerals noted previously are classified as nutritionally essential for animals. Their deficiencies cause specific symptoms, such as reduced feed intake, growth restriction, impaired development, and even death (Suttle 2010). While some of the above minerals may become toxic to animals when fed at high levels, other minerals (e.g., cadmium [Cd], mercury [Hg], lead [Pb], beryllium [Be], arsenic [As], and aluminum [Al]) are toxic to animals at much lower levels and should be avoided at all times in their diets.

The chemical properties of minerals affect their nutritional and physiological functions (Harris 2014). They can gain or lose electrons. Some minerals are metals (e.g., Na and Fe), which become cations by loss of electrons and have good electrical and thermal conductivity. Many of the metals are transition metals (e.g., Fe, Cu, and Zn), which are in Groups 3 through 12 of the periodic table (Figure 10.1) and have a strong tendency to form coordination compounds (Rayner-Canham and Overton 2006). However, many minerals are nonmetals (e.g., Cl, I, and P), which lack the characteristics of a metal and become anions by gaining electrons. Most minerals form complexes with proteins for transport and biological functions, or interact with each other in the body. Metal-binding proteins are uniquely rich in cysteine, further underscoring the role of sulfur-containing AAs in mineral metabolism and function (Harris 2014). Thus, some minerals may affect the absorption and function of other minerals, and some can regulate gene expression in animal cells (Beckett et al. 2014; Cousins 1994). Furthermore, some minerals form coordination compounds with AAs, such that the complexes are absorbed into enterocytes and extraintestinal cells at high rates. These kinds of interactions, which can be beneficial or detrimental, are an important aspect of mineral nutrition in animals. An imbalance of minerals, distinct from a simple deficiency, is a cause of certain nutritional disorders in livestock, poultry, and fish (Georgievskii et al. 1982). Likewise, because minerals are not degraded, even those that are nutritionally essential can cause toxicity when their dietary intakes exceed requirements. Therefore, knowledge of the chemistry and metabolism of minerals is essential to understanding animal nutrition and feeding practices. The major objective of this chapter is to highlight the sources, absorption, transport, utilization, and functions of minerals in animals.

**TABLE 10.1**
**Content of Macrominerals in Newborn and Adult Animals (Amounts/kg of Fat-Free Body Weight)**

| Mineral | Man | Pig | Dog | Cat | Rabbit | Guinea Pig | Rat | Mouse | Cattle | Chicken |
|---|---|---|---|---|---|---|---|---|---|---|
| Body weight (kg) | 3.56 | 1.25 | 0.328 | 0.118 | 0.054 | 0.080 | 0.0059 | 0.0016 | 55 | 0.04 |
| Water (g) | 823 | 820 | 845 | 822 | 865 | 775 | 862 | 850 | 748 | 805 |
| Calcium (g) | 9.6 | 10.0 | 4.9 | 6.6 | 4.6 | 12.3 | 3.1 | 3.4 | 12 | 4.0 |
| Phosphorus (g) | 5.6 | 5.8 | 3.9 | 4.4 | 3.6 | 7.5 | 3.6 | 3.4 | 7 | 3.3 |
| Magnesium (g) | 0.56 | 0.32 | 0.17 | 0.26 | 0.23 | 0.46 | 0.25 | 0.34 | 0.30 | 0.3 |
| Sodium (mmol) | 82 | 93 | 81 | 92 | 78 | 71 | 84 | 72 | 80 | 83 |
| Potassium (mmol) | 53 | 50 | 58 | 60 | 53 | 69 | 65 | 70 | 49 | 56 |
| Chloride (mmol) | 55 | 52 | 60 | 66 | 56 | 60 | 67 | 61 | 52 | 60 |
| Body weight (kg) | 65 | 125 | 6.0 | 4.0 | 2.6 | 0.50 | 0.35 | 0.027 | 545 | 2.5 |
| Water (g) | 720 | 750 | 740 | 740 | 730 | 646 | 720 | 780 | 705 | 740 |
| Calcium (g) | 22.4 | 12.0 | 14.0 | 13.0 | 13.0 | 14.8 | 12.4 | 11.4 | 18.0 | 13.0 |
| Phosphorus (g) | 12.0 | 7.0 | 6.8 | 8.0 | 7.0 | 9.43 | 7.5 | 7.4 | 10.0 | 7.1 |
| Magnesium (g) | 0.47 | 0.45 | 0.40 | 0.45 | 0.50 | 0.94 | 0.40 | 0.43 | 0.41 | 0.50 |
| Sodium (mmol) | 80 | 65 | 69 | 65 | 58 | 77 | 59 | 63 | 69 | 51 |
| Potassium (mmol) | 69 | 74 | 65 | 77 | 72 | 107 | 81 | 80 | 49 | 69 |
| Chloride (mmol) | 50 | 41 | 43 | 41 | 32 | 48 | 40 | 46 | 31 | 44 |

*Source:* Cheek, D.B. and A.B. Holt. 1963. *Am. J. Physiol.* 205:913–918; Engle, W.A. and J.A. Lemons. 1986. *Pediatr. Res.* 20:1156–1160; Georgievskii, V.I. et al. 1982. *Mineral Nutrition of Animals*. Butterworths, London, U.K.; Kienzle, E. et al. 1998. *J. Nutr.* 128:2680S–2683S; Pond, W.G. et al. 1995. *Basic Animal Nutrition and Feeding*. 4th ed., John Wiley & Sons, New York.

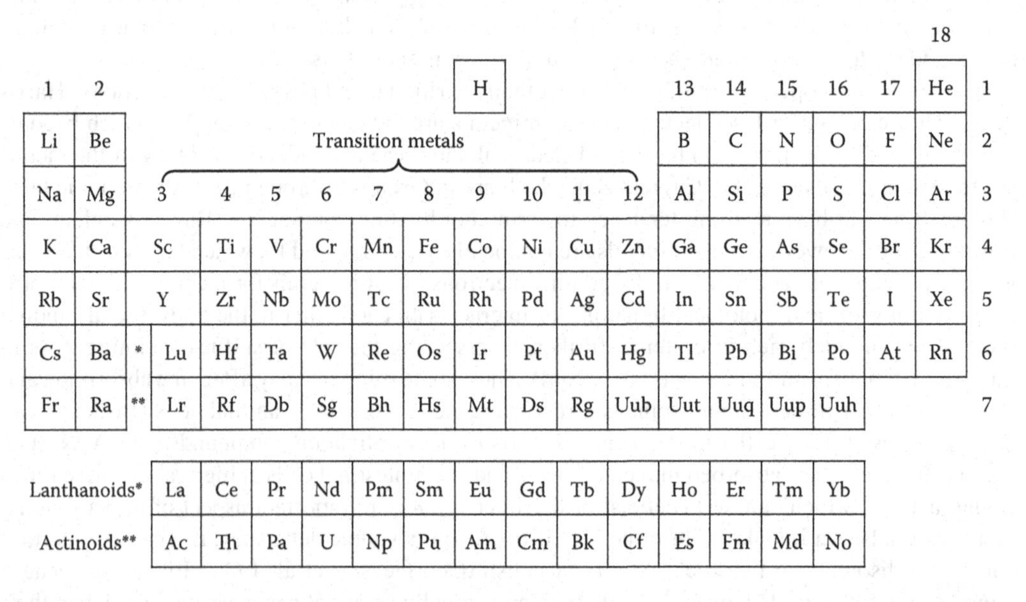


**FIGURE 10.1** The periodic table of elements. This table is an arrangement of the chemical elements by their atomic number (number of protons), electron configurations, and chemical properties. Elements with similar behavior are ordered in the same column, whereas elements within a row (period) are metals on the left, transition metals (columns 3 to 12) in the middle, and nonmetals on the right. (Adapted from Rayner-Canham, G. and T. Overton. 2006. *Descriptive Inorganic Chemistry.* W.H. Freeman and Company, New York, NY.)

# OVERALL VIEWS OF MINERALS

## Chemistry of Minerals

Minerals consist of elements, but not all elements are nutritionally essential. For example, hydrogen, which is the first element in the periodic table, is not considered a mineral in its elemental form. Like any nonhydrogen atom, an atom of a mineral is composed of a nucleus and the electrons surrounding the nucleus. The nucleus consists of protons that have positive charges and generally a similar number of neutrons that have no charge. An electron has one negative charge. More than 99.94% of an atom's mass is in the nucleus (Brown et al. 2003). The proton number is also known as the atomic number (e.g., 11 for sodium and 17 for chlorine). Atomic mass is the total mass of protons and neutrons in an atom, whereas atomic weight is the average mass of all of the naturally occurring isotopes of an element, with the unit being dalton (Da). If the number of protons and electrons is equal, an atom is electrically neutral and has no net electric charge. However, if an atom has more or fewer electrons than protons, it has one or more net negative or positive charges, respectively, and is called an ion. In other words, by gaining an electron, an atom becomes an anion, and by losing an electron, an atom becomes a cation. Two or more atoms form a compound (e.g., NaCl). After being dissolved in water, all binary ionic mineral compounds (e.g., NaCl) are ionized to yield their constituent ions (e.g., $Na^+$ and $Cl^-$). The stable valence states of nutritionally essential minerals are shown in Table 10.2.

Niels Bohr's prototypical model of atomic structure based on quantum theory explains the structure of an atom. In 1913, Bohr proposed that electrons of an atom occupy circular orbits (shells) with different energy levels around its nucleus. Each of these shells is identified with an integer (e.g., 1, 2, 3, 4, … , *n*), which is called a principal quantum number. The maximum number of electrons in a shell is $2 \times n^2$ (i.e., 2, 8, 18, 32, … for shell 1, 2, 3, 4, … , respectively), where *n* is the principal

**TABLE 10.2**
**Chemical Properties of Nutritionally Essential Minerals in Animals**

| Metals | | | | | Nonmetals | | | | |
|---|---|---|---|---|---|---|---|---|---|
| Name | Symbol | Valence State[a] | Atomic Number | Atomic Weight | Name | Symbol | Valence State[a] | Atomic Number | Atomic Weight |
| | | | | Macrominerals | | | | | |
| Calcium | Ca | +2 | 20 | 40.08 | Chlorine | Cl | −1 | 17 | 35.45 |
| Magnesium | Mg | +2 | 12 | 24.31 | Phosphorus | P | +3, +5, −3 | 15 | 30.97 |
| Potassium | K | +1 | 19 | 30.10 | Sulfur | S | +4, +6, −2 | 16 | 32.07 |
| Sodium | Na | +1 | 11 | 22.90 | | | | | |
| | | | | Microminerals | | | | | |
| Chromium | Cr | +2, +3, +6 | 24 | 52.00 | Boron | B | +3 | 5 | 10.81 |
| Cobalt | Co | +1, +2, +3 | 27 | 58.93 | Bromine | Br | −1 | 35 | 79.90 |
| Copper | Cu | +1, +2, +4 | 29 | 63.54 | Fluorine | F | −1 | 9 | 19.00 |
| Iron | Fe | +2, +3 | 26 | 55.85 | Iodine | I | −1 | 53 | 126.91 |
| Manganese | Mn | +2, +3 | 25 | 54.94 | Selenium | Se | +4, +6, −2 | 34 | 78.96 |
| Molybdenum | Mo | +4, +5, +6 | 42 | 95.94 | Silicon | Si | +2, +4 | 14 | 28.09 |
| Nickel | Ni | +1, +2 | 28 | 58.69 | Tin | Sn | +2, +4 | 50 | 118.71 |
| Vanadium | V | +2 to +5 | 23 | 50.94 | | | | | |
| Zinc | Zn | +2 | 30 | 65.39 | | | | | |

[a] Stable valence state.

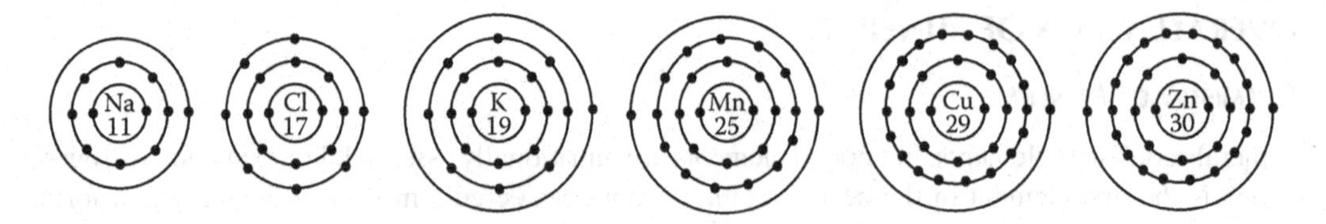


**FIGURE 10.2** The atomic structures of sodium, chlorine, potassium, manganese, copper, and zinc. Electrons of an atom occupy circular orbits (shells) with different energy levels around its nucleus. The maximum number of electrons in a shell is $2 \times n^2$ (i.e., 2, 8, 18, 32, … , for shell 1, 2, 3, 4, … , respectively), where $n$ is the principal quantum number (i.e., the number of shells). The higher a principal quantum number (or energy level), the farther the shell is from the nucleus. In all atoms, electrons that are in the outermost shell are called valence electrons, which are involved in chemical bonding.

quantum number (i.e., the number of shells). The higher a principal quantum number (or energy level), the farther the shell is from the nucleus. The atomic structures of sodium, chlorine, potassium, manganese, copper, and zinc are shown in Figure 10.2.

Within each shell, there are different spaces (called orbitals) with different shapes. The orbitals are denoted by a letter *s*, *p*, *d*, or *f*. The number of orbitals within a shell is equal to the shell number. For example, the first shell of an atom has 1 orbital (i.e., 1*s*); the second shell has 2 orbitals (i.e., 2*s* and 2*p*); the third shell has three orbitals (i.e., 3*s*, 3*p*, and 3*d*); and the fourth shell has four orbitals (i.e., 4*s*, 4*p*, 4*d*, and 4*f*). Orbitals *s*, *p*, *d*, and *f* have 1, 3, 5, and 7 suborbitals, respectively, with each suborbital holding up to two electrons (Rayner-Canham and Overton 2006). Thus, orbitals *s*, *p*, *d*, and *f* can have up to 2, 6, 10, and 14 electrons, respectively. The *s*-orbital primarily denotes elements in Groups 1 and 2 of the periodic Table, the *d*-orbital denotes Groups 3–12 elements (transition metals), the *p*-orbital denotes Group 13, 14, 15, 16, 17, and 18 elements, and the *f*-orbital denotes the lanthanides and actinides group. Electrons generally fill the lowest energy-level orbital first and then a higher energy-level orbital, constituting an electron filling pattern of 1*s*, 2*s*, 2*p*, 3*s*, 3*p*, 4*s*, 3*d*, 4*p*, 5*s*, 4*d*, 5*p*, 6*s*, 4*f*, 5*d*, 6*p*, 7*s*, and 5*f*. Note the different energy levels of *d*, *p*, and *f* orbitals: $3d > 4s$, $4d > 5s$, $4f > 6s$, and $5f > 7s > 6p$. There are, however, exceptions for chromium and copper, where the energy level of the 3*d* orbital is only slightly higher than that of the 4*s* orbital. An element is more stable when a *d* suborbital is either half-full (e.g., $4s^1$ and $3d^5$ for chromium) or completely full (e.g., $4s^1$ and $3d^{10}$ for copper), compared to a partially filled *d* suborbital. In all atoms, electrons that are in the outermost shell are called valence electrons, which are involved in chemical bonding.

Electron configuration, which is the distribution of electrons of an atom in orbitals, is shown in Table 10.3 for nutritionally essential macro- and microminerals. Na, which has a single electron in its outer 3*s* orbital, can lose that electron to form a cation ($Na^+$), whereas chlorine, which has seven valence electrons, can gain one electron to form an anion ($Cl^-$). These two ions have low-energy states, are chemically stable, and exist as an ionic salt (NaCl) used in animal diets. Likewise, K cation ($K^+$), Ca dication ($Ca^{2+}$), and P in the form of phosphate ($PO_4^{3-}$) are chemically stable. Of note, $Na^+$, $Cl^-$, $K^+$, $Ca^{2+}$, and $PO_4^{3-}$ are not redox-active. In contrast, many transition metals, which can occur in more than one oxidation state (e.g., $Fe^{2+}$ and $Fe^{3+}$), participate in redox reactions. As noted previously, all transition metals have incomplete 3*d* orbitals. Partially filling 3*d* orbitals allow a transition metal to accept or donate electrons and, therefore, these elements play an important role in cellular oxidation–reduction reactions (e.g., the mitochondrial electron transport system). Thus, the theory of atomic structure aids in the understanding of the electronic states and chemical properties of minerals as related to animal nutrition and metabolism.

## Overall View of Absorption of Dietary Minerals

The composition of minerals in common feedstuffs is summarized in Table 10.4. During feeding, a large amount of water is secreted into the lumen of the small intestine to facilitate food digestion;

**TABLE 10.3**
**Electron Configuration of Nutritionally Essential Minerals**

| Element (Atomic Number) | Electron Configuration | Abbreviated Form |
|---|---|---|
| Boron (5) | $1s^22s^22p^1$ | $[He]2s^22p^1$ |
| Fluorine (9) | $1s^22s^22p^5$ | $[He]2s^22p^5$ |
| Sodium (11) | $1s^22s^22p^63s^1$ | $[Ne]3s^1$ |
| Magnesium (12) | $1s^22s^22p^63s^2$ | $[Ne]3s^2$ |
| Silicon (14) | $1s^22s^22p^63s^23p^2$ | $[Ne]3s^23p^2$ |
| Phosphorus (15) | $1s^22s^22p^63s^23p^3$ | $[Ne]3s^23p^3$ |
| Sulfur (16) | $1s^22s^22p^63s^23p^4$ | $[Ne]3s^23p^4$ |
| Chlorine (17) | $1s^22s^22p^63s^23p^5$ | $[Ne]3s^23p^5$ |
| Potassium (19) | $1s^22s^22p^63s^23p^64s^1$ | $[Ar]4s^1$ |
| Calcium (20) | $1s^22s^22p^63s^23p^64s^2$ | $[Ar]4s^2$ |
| Vanadium (23) | $1s^22s^22p^63s^23p^64s^23d^3$ | $[Ar]4s^23d^3$ |
| Chromium (24) | $1s^22s^22p^63s^23p^64s^13d^5$ | $[Ar]4s^13d^5$ |
| Manganese (25) | $1s^22s^22p^63s^23p^64s^23d^5$ | $[Ar]4s^23d^5$ |
| Iron (26) | $1s^22s^22p^63s^23p^64s^23d^6$ | $[Ar]4s^23d^6$ |
| Cobalt (27) | $1s^22s^22p^63s^23p^64s^23d^7$ | $[Ar]4s^23d^7$ |
| Nickel (28) | $1s^22s^22p^63s^23p^64s^23d^8$ | $[Ar]4s^23d^8$ |
| Copper (29) | $1s^22s^22p^63s^23p^64s^13d^{10}$ | $[Ar]4s^13d^{10}$ |
| Zinc (30) | $1s^22s^22p^63s^23p^64s^23d^{10}$ | $[Ar]4s^23d^{10}$ |
| Selenium (34) | $1s^22s^22p^63s^23p^64s^23d^{10}4p^4$ | $[Ar]4s^23d^{10}4p^4$ |
| Bromine (35) | $1s^22s^22p^63s^23p^64s^23d^{10}4p^5$ | $[Ar]4s^23d^{10}4p^5$ |
| Tin (50) | $1s^22s^22p^63s^23p^64s^23d^{10}4p^65s^24d^{10}5p^2$ | $[Kr]5s^24d^{10}5p^2$ |
| Iodine (53) | $1s^22s^22p^63s^23p^64s^23d^{10}4p^65s^24d^{10}5p^5$ | $[Kr]5s^24d^{10}5p^5$ |

Electron configurations: Ar (argon), $1s^22s^22p^63s^23p^6$; He (helium), ($1s^2$); Kr (krypton), $1s^22s^22p^63s^23p^64s^23d^{10}4p^6$; Ne (neon), $1s^22s^22p^6$. These are all noble gases in Group 18 of the periodic table.

almost all of this water, along with dietary nutrients, is subsequently reabsorbed by the small intestine. Digestion of protein, lipids and carbohydrates in the stomach and small intestine releases minerals from their food matrix. Phytase plays an important role in the release of minerals from plant-source ingredients, because most minerals (particularly phosphorus) are bound to phytate and are entrapped within the complex fibers (Humer et al. 2015). Except for hydrogen fluoride (HF) and the truly chelated mineral complexes, the ions of free minerals are absorbed into enterocytes through specific or common transporters. The minerals that are truly chelated with organic compounds (e.g., heme and AAs) are absorbed intact as part of their carriers via endocytosis or specific transporters. Because it is easier to release minerals from animal- than plant-source ingredients, the bioavailabilities of various minerals (<1% for vanadium in food to nearly 100% for fluorine in water) in the former are generally higher than those in the latter (Georgievskii 1982; Pond et al. 1995). In nonruminants, when the bacteria in the lumen of the small intestine cannot produce sufficient phytase or fiber-digesting enzymes, exogenous sources of these enzymes through dietary supplementation can improve the bioavailability of dietary minerals (Chapter 13).

In ruminants, the ruminal epithelium can absorb certain minerals (e.g., Na and Mg); however, most minerals, except for Mg, are absorbed primarily in the small intestine (Leonhard-Marek et al. 2005). There are reports that most of the dietary Mg is absorbed by the reticulo-rumen in sheep (Tomas and Potter 1976) and steers (Greene et al. 1983). In nonruminants, most minerals, except for a few (e.g., cobalt and Ca), are absorbed primarily by the enterocytes of the jejunum through specific transporters (either facilitated or active transporters) or receptor-mediated endocytosis

**TABLE 10.4**
**Content of Minerals in Feedstuffs[a]**

| Feedstuff | Ca (%) | P (%) | Na (%) | Cl (%) | K (%) | Mg (%) | S (%) | Cu (ppm) | Fe (ppm) | Mn (ppm) | Se (ppm) | Zn (ppm) |
|---|---|---|---|---|---|---|---|---|---|---|---|---|
| Alfalfa, 17% CP | 1.53 | 0.26 | 0.09 | 0.47 | 2.3 | 0.23 | 0.29 | 10 | 333 | 32 | 0.34 | 24 |
| Barley grain | 0.06 | 0.35 | 0.04 | 0.12 | 0.45 | 0.14 | 0.15 | 7 | 78 | 18 | 0.19 | 25 |
| Blood meal[b] | 0.37 | 0.27 | 0.50 | 0.30 | 0.11 | 0.11 | 0.48 | 11 | 1922 | 6 | 0.58 | 38 |
| Blood meal[c] | 0.41 | 0.30 | 0.44 | 0.25 | 0.15 | 0.11 | 0.47 | 8 | 2919 | 6 | – | 30 |
| Canola meal | 0.63 | 1.01 | 0.07 | 0.11 | 1.22 | 0.51 | 0.85 | 6 | 142 | 49 | 1.10 | 69 |
| Casein, dried | 0.61 | 0.82 | 0.01 | 0.04 | 0.01 | 0.01 | 0.60 | 4 | 14 | 4 | 0.16 | 30 |
| Corn grain | 0.03 | 0.28 | 0.02 | 0.05 | 0.33 | 0.12 | 0.13 | 3 | 29 | 7 | 0.07 | 18 |
| CSM[d] | 0.19 | 1.06 | 0.04 | 0.05 | 1.40 | 0.50 | 0.31 | 18 | 184 | 20 | 0.80 | 70 |
| Feather meal | 0.33 | 0.50 | 0.34 | 0.26 | 0.19 | 0.20 | 1.39 | 10 | 76 | 10 | 0.69 | 111 |
| Fish meal, Menhaden | 5.21 | 3.04 | 0.40 | 0.55 | 0.70 | 0.16 | 0.45 | 11 | 440 | 37 | 2.10 | 147 |
| Flax meal | 0.39 | 0.83 | 0.13 | 0.06 | 1.26 | 0.54 | 0.39 | 22 | 270 | 41 | 0.63 | 66 |
| MBM[e] | 9.99 | 4.98 | 0.63 | 0.69 | 0.65 | 0.41 | 0.38 | 11 | 606 | 17 | 0.31 | 96 |
| Milk powder[f] | 1.31 | 1.00 | 0.48 | 1.00 | 1.60 | 0.12 | 0.32 | 5 | 8 | 2 | 0.12 | 42 |
| Oat grain | 0.07 | 0.31 | 0.08 | 0.10 | 0.42 | 0.16 | 0.21 | 6 | 85 | 43 | 0.30 | 38 |
| Peanut meal, sol. extr. | 0.22 | 0.65 | 0.07 | 0.04 | 1.25 | 0.31 | 0.30 | 15 | 260 | 40 | 0.21 | 41 |
| PBM[g] | 4.46 | 2.41 | 0.49 | 0.49 | 0.53 | 0.18 | 0.52 | 10 | 442 | 9 | 0.88 | 94 |
| Rice bran | 0.07 | 1.61 | 0.03 | 0.07 | 1.56 | 0.90 | 0.18 | 9 | 190 | 228 | 0.40 | 30 |
| Rice grain[h] | 0.04 | 0.18 | 0.04 | 0.07 | 0.13 | 0.11 | 0.06 | 21 | 18 | 12 | 0.27 | 17 |
| Safflower meal, sol. extr. | 0.34 | 0.75 | 0.05 | 0.08 | 0.76 | 0.35 | 0.13 | 10 | 495 | 18 | – | 41 |
| Sorghum grain | 0.03 | 0.29 | 0.01 | 0.09 | 0.35 | 0.15 | 0.08 | 5 | 45 | 15 | 0.20 | 15 |
| SBM[i] | 0.32 | 0.65 | 0.01 | 0.05 | 1.96 | 0.27 | 0.43 | 20 | 202 | 29 | 0.32 | 50 |
| Sunflower meal, sol. extr. | 0.36 | 0.86 | 0.02 | 0.10 | 1.07 | 0.68 | 0.30 | 26 | 254 | 41 | 0.50 | 66 |
| Wheat bran | 0.16 | 1.20 | 0.04 | 0.07 | 1.26 | 0.52 | 0.22 | 14 | 170 | 113 | 0.51 | 100 |
| Wheat grain[j] | 0.06 | 0.37 | 0.01 | 0.06 | 0.49 | 0.13 | 0.15 | 6 | 39 | 34 | 0.33 | 40 |
| Yeast (brewer's dried ) | 0.16 | 1.44 | 0.10 | 0.12 | 1.80 | 0.23 | 0.40 | 33 | 215 | 8 | 1.00 | 49 |

*Source:* National Research Council (NRC), *Nutrient Requirements of Swine*, National Academy Press, Washington, D.C., 1998

[a] Values are expressed on the as-fed basis.
[b] Conventional blood meal.
[c] Blood meal, spray or ring dried (93% dry matter).
[d] Cottonseed meal (solvent extract [sol. extr.], 41% CP).
[e] Meat and bone meal (93% dry matter).
[f] Bovine milk (skim, dried; 96% dry matter).
[g] Poultry by-product meal (93% dry matter). Calcium content is 3.0% (dry matter basis) in some PBM products.
[h] Polished, broken.
[i] Soybean meal (solvent extracted, 89% dry matter).
[j] Hard red, winter.

(Tables 10.5 and 10.6). This is called transcellular transport or absorption (Chapter 1). In a healthy gut with functional tight junctions between two enterocytes, passive diffusion of small molecules and ions through the tight junctions into the extracellular space, which is known as paracellular transport or absorption, is rather limited (Khanal and Nemere 2008). In fish, absorption of minerals also occurs through their gills. Upon entering the enterocyte, macrominerals exit as free ions, whereas microminerals are carried by vesicles or protein transporters across its cytosol (Suttle 2010). All minerals exit the enterocyte through its basolateral membrane via exocytosis or specific transporters into the lamina propria (Table 10.4), and ultimately enter the portal vein. These

**TABLE 10.5**
**Absorption of Macrominerals by the Enterocyte, Their Transport in Plasma, and Their Uptake by Tissues**

| Elements | Transporter in the Apical Membrane of Enterocyte | Transporter in the Cytosol of Enterocyte | Transporter in the Basolateral Membrane of Enterocyte | Transport in Plasma | Uptake by Extraintestinal Cells |
|---|---|---|---|---|---|
| Sodium | SGLT1, AMSC, NCT NHE2/3, AATs, NPT | No; free cation | $Na^+/K^+$-ATPase, NHE1 Na-K-2Cl CT (in) | Free cation | Sodium channels SGLT2 (kidney) |
| Potassium | K channels[a] | No; free cation | K channels K-Cl cotransporter Na-K-2Cl CT (in) $Na^+/K^+$-ATPase (in) | Free cation | K channels[a] K-Cl cotransporter |
| Chloride | Cl channels[b], NCT ($HCO_3^-/Cl^-$ exchange) | No; free anion | Cl channels (e.g., ClC-2) Na-K-2Cl CT (in) | Free anion | CACC (mainly) |
| Calcium | Ca transporter-1 | Calbindin | $Ca^{2+}$-ATPase | Free and PB | $Ca^{2+}$ channels |
| Phosphate | NaPi2b, PiT1, PiT2 | No; free anion as $PO_4^{2-}$ | $Na^+$-dependent transport | Free cation | NaPi2a, NaPi2c PiT1, PiT2 |
| Magnesium | TRPM6/7 | No; free cation | CNNM4 | Free cation | TRPM6/7 |
| Sulfur | AA transporters | No; as AAs | AA transporters | Free AAs | AA transporters |

AA(s), amino acid(s); AATs, sodium-dependent amino acid transporters; AMSC, amiloride-sensitive $Na^+$ channels; CACC, calcium-activated Cl channels; Cav, voltage-gated $Ca^{2+}$ channels; CNNM4, ancient conserved domain protein 4; NHE, $Na^+/H^+$ exchanger; NPT, sodium-phosphate cotransporter; NCT, electroneutral $Na^+$-$Cl^-$ absorption mediated by $Na^+/H^+$ (NHE2/3) and $Cl^-/HCO_3^-$; Na-K-2Cl CT (in), $Na^+$-$K^+$-$2Cl^-$ cotransporter; NaPi2b, sodium-phosphate cotransporter; PB, protein-bound; PiT1, phosphate transporter-1; PiT2, phosphate transporter-1; SLGT1, sodium-linked glucose transporter-1; TRPM6, transient receptor potential melastatin-related protein-6. The sign (in) indicates that minerals are transported from the lamina propria (ultimately the blood) into the intestinal epithelial cell.

[a] Potassium channels include $K^+/H^+$-ATPase, $Na^+$-$Cl^-$-$K^+$ transporter, and $K^+$ conductance channels.

[b] Ligand- or voltage-gated chloride channels. CFTR (cystic fibrosis transmembrane conductance regulator) is the major $Cl^-$ transporter in the apical membrane of the intestine.

nutrients are transported in the plasma as free or protein-bound ions, or in both forms, and are taken up by extraintestinal cells through exocytosis or specific transporters. In the blood plasma or the cells, most minerals (particularly microminerals) are present in a variety of complex forms, and only a few exist entirely as free elemental ions (i.e., $Na^+$, $K^+$, and $Cl^-$). Concentrations of macroelements in the serum of animals are shown in Table 10.7. Absorbed minerals, except for cobalt, copper, manganese, and mercury (which are excreted mainly via fecal excretion), are excreted from the body primarily through the urine (Georgievskii et al. 1982; Suttle 2010). Due to their low rates of intestinal absorption, many non-electrolyte minerals (e.g., Ca, Mg, P and Zn) in diets are generally excreted in greater amounts in feces than in urine.

## General Functions of Minerals

Minerals have many physiological and metabolic functions (Engle and Lemons 1986; Fang et al. 2002; Suttle 2010). These nutrients are (1) the major structural components of bones and teeth, with the content of minerals in the ash (%) of adult animals being as follows: Ca, 28.5; P, 16.6; K, 4.8; S, 3.6; Cl, 3.5; Na, 3.7; Mg, 1.1; and Fe, 0.15 (Georgievskii et al. 1982); (2) contributors to the

**TABLE 10.6**
**Absorption of Microminerals by the Enterocyte, Their Transport in Plasma, and Their Uptake by Tissues**

| Elements | Transporter in the Apical Membrane of Enterocyte | Transporter in the Cytosol of Enterocyte | Transporter in the Basolateral Membrane of Enterocyte | Transport in Plasma | Uptake by Extraintestinal Cells |
|---|---|---|---|---|---|
| Iron | DCT1 for $Fe^{2+}$ HCP1 for heme $Fe^{2+}$ Heme-R (for EDC) | Paraferritin complex | Ferroportin (only recognizing $Fe^{2+}$) | Transferrin (TF) | Transferrin receptor |
| Zinc | ZIP4, DCT-1, DMT-1 | CRIP | Zinc transporter-1 (ZnT1) ZnT2 | Albumin (60% Zn), MG (30% Zn), other factors (10% Zn) | Zip2/3 (liver) Zip4 (kidneys) Zips (other cells), $Ca_v$ |
| Copper | CTR1 (for $Cu^{1+}$) DCT1 (for $Cu^{2+}$) | ATOX1, ATP7a COX-17, CCS Glutathione, MTs | Vesicle discharge powered by ATP7a (a Cu-ATPase)c | Albumin (10% Cu), Ceruloplasmin (90% Cu) | CTR1 |
| Manganese | DCT1 | Vesicles, PMR1P ZIP8 | Vesicle discharge PMR1P | Primarily TF (~50%) | $Mn^{2+}$ transporter NRAMP1 in MΦ |
| Cobalt (free) | See $Fe^{2+}$ transport | Cytosolic protein | See $Fe^{2+}$ transport | Albumin | See $Fe^{2+}$ transport |
| Cobalt ($B_{12}$) | See Chapter 9 | | | | |
| Molybdenum | Active transporter | No; free cation | Unknown | $MoO_4^{2-}$, RBC | Active transporter |
| Selenium[a] | NaS1/2, Fa diffusion | Selenoprotein P | Exocytosis | Selenoprotein P | Seppl receptor |
| Selenium[b] | AA transporters | No; free AAs | AA transporters | (Seppl) | (endocytosis) |
| Chromium | Passive diffusion | Chromodulin | Vesicle discharge | TF, albumin | TF receptor (endocytosis) |
| Iodine | $Na^+/I^-$ symporter | No; free anion | Unknown | Albumin | $Na^+/I^-$ symporter |
| Fluorine | $F^-/H^+$ cotransporter anion exchange | $Ca^{2+}$, $Mg^{2+}$ | Fluc protein (FEX) | $Ca^{2+}$, $Mg^{2+}$ | $F^-$, $Ca^{2+}$, and $Mg^{2+}$ channels |
| Boron | NaBC1 | Unknown | Unknown | Unknown | NaBC1 |
| Bromine | $Cl^-$ and $I^-$ transporters | Unknown | Unknown | Unknown | $Na^+$-$K^+$-$2Cl^-$ |
| Nickel | DCT1 | No; free cation | Unknown | Albumin | Unknown |
| Silicon | NaPi2b; AQPs 3, 7, 9 | No; as $Si(OH)_4$ | Unknown | $Si(OH)_4$ | NaPi2b; AQPs 3, 7, 9 |
| Vanadium | Phosphate and other anion transporters | Ferritin (as vanadyl, $V^{4+}$) | Unknown, possibly non-heme iron pathways | Vanadyl-TF, -ferritin, HG | Unknown |

AA(s), amino acid(s); CRIP, cysteine-rich intracellular protein; CTR1, copper transporter-1; DCT1, divalent cation transporter-1; EDC, endocytosis; Fluc, fluoride carrier (also known as FEX, fluoride export protein); HCP1, heme carrier protein-1; HG, hemoglobin; heme-R, heme receptor; $\alpha_2$-MG, $\alpha_2$-macroglobulin; MΦ, macrophage and monocyte; MTs, metallothioneins; NaBC1, ($Na^+$-driven boron channel-1); NaS1/2, $Na^+$-sulfate cotransporters 1 and 2; PMR1P, manganese transporting ATPase; RBC, red blood cells.

[a] Inorganic forms of selenium, with selenate and selenite being transported by NaS1/2 and facilitated (Fa) diffusion, respectively.

[b] Organic forms of selenium (seleno-methionine and seleno-cysteine).

**TABLE 10.7**
**Concentrations of Macrominerals in the Serum of Animals (mM)**

| Mineral | Cattle | Chickens | Dogs | Goats | Mice | Pigs | Rabbits | Rats | Sheep |
|---|---|---|---|---|---|---|---|---|---|
| Sodium | 132–152 | 158 | 150 | 142–155 | 157–166 | 139 | 125–150 | 148–150 | 140–149 |
| Potassium | 3.9–5.8 | 5.7 | 4.7–4.9 | 3.5–6.7 | 7.8–8.0 | 5.2 | 3.5–7.0 | 6.1–7.0 | 6.0 |
| Chloride | 97–111 | 118 | 113 | 99–110 | 125–130 | 100 | 90–120 | 103–104 | 100–120 |
| Calcium | 2.4–3.1 | 3.0 | 2.7–2.8 | 2.2–2.9 | 2.2–2.6 | 3.0 | 1.4–3.0 | 3.0 | 2.5–3.0 |
| Phosphorus | 1.8–2.1 | 2.3 | 1.2–1.8 | 1.4–2.9 | 2.6–2.7 | 2.3 | 1.3–1.9 | 1.9–2.4 | 1.3–1.9 |
| Magnesium | 0.75–0.96 | 1.2–1.3 | 0.86 | 1.2–1.5 | 0.58–1.28 | 1.6–2.1 | 0.82–2.2 | 1.1–1.3 | 0.74–1.7 |

*Source:* Values for pigs are obtained from Rezaei, R. et al. 2013. *Amino Acids* 44:911–923. Values for other species are adapted from Fox, J.G. et al. 2002. *Laboratory Animal Medicine*. Academic Press, New York, NY; Georgievskii, V.I. et al. 1982. *Mineral Nutrition of Animals*. Butterworths, London, U.K.; Herzig, I. et al. 2009. *Czech. J. Anim. Sci.* 54:121–127; Morgan, V.E. and D.F. Chichester. 1935. *J. Biol. Chem.* 110:285–298.

mechanical stability of the body (e.g., Ca, P, Mg, F, and Si); (3) electrolytes in the body (e.g., Na, K, and Cl) essential for the electrical charges of cells, regulation of acid–base balance and osmotic pressure; (4) modulators of transport activity, permeability, and excitability of cell membranes (e.g., Na, K, Cl, and P); (5) facilitators of the digestion of foods in the gastrointestinal tract; (6) regulators of food intake (e.g., Cl, Na, P, and Zn); (7) cofactors or components of enzymes (e.g., Se, Ca, Mg, Mn, Zn, and Cu) and other molecules (e.g., iron in hemoglobin, cobalt in vitamin $B_{12}$, and iodine in thyroid hormones); and (8) participants in redox reactions (e.g., S, Cu, and Fe). Although Cr, V, Si, B, Br, Ni and Sn have biochemical roles in cell metabolism, these micro-minerals are widely present in feedstuffs and, therefore, are not of particular importance to the formulation of animal diets.

About 40% of all proteins crystallized to date have a metal bound either loosely or tightly (Waldron et al. 2009). Enzymes that use metal ions as cofactors are classified as metal-activated enzymes or metalloenzymes. Metal-activated enzymes exhibit a greater catalytic activity in the presence of a mono- or divalent metal ion, compared with its absence; examples include alkaline phosphatase ($Mg^{2+}$), ATPase ($Mg^{2+}$), choline kinase ($Mg^{2+}$), DNAse ($Mg^{2+}$), hexokinase ($Mg^{2+}$), inosine monophosphate dehydrogenase ($K^+$), leucine aminopeptidase ($Mn^{2+}$), phosphoglucomutase ($Mg^{2+}$), pyruvate kinase ($K^+$), RNAse ($Mg^{2+}$), thrombin ($Na^+$), and β-xylosidase ($Ca^{2+}$). Metalloenzymes are enzyme proteins containing metal ions that are directly bound to the proteins; examples include alcohol dehydrogenase ($Zn^{2+}$), aminopeptidase ($Zn^{2+}$), α-amylase ($Ca^{2+}$), arginase ($Mn^{2+}$), carbonic anhydrase ($Zn^{2+}$), catalase ($Fe^{2+}$), cytochrome *c* oxidase (Fe), DNA polymerase ($Zn^{2+}$), lysyl oxidase ($Cu^{2+}$), RNA polymerase ($Zn^{2+}$), protein phosphatase-1 ($Mn^{2+}$), pyruvate carboxylase ($Mn^{2+}$), superoxide dismutase ($Cu^{2+}$, $Zn^{2+}$), and tyrosinase ($Cu^{2+}$). About one-third of all enzymes known so far are metalloenzymes (Valdez et al. 2014). There are differences between metal-activated enzymes and metalloenzymes. Metals have only a weak association with metal-activated enzymes, but are tightly bound to metalloenzymes and retained by the enzymes on purification (Holm et al. 1996).

## MACROMINERALS

### SODIUM

Sodium was discovered by Humphry Davy in 1807. Its name is derived from the Latin "sodanum" meaning headache remedy, and its chemical symbol Na from the Latin "natrium." Sodium was used by ancient Egyptians and Chinese to preserve animal- and plant-source foods. $Na^+$ is the principal cation in extracellular fluid. In domestic animals, the concentrations of sodium are about 140 mM in the plasma, and about 14 mM in the intracellular fluid. It is the fourth most abundant mineral in the animal body (Table 10.6).

*Sources*

Much of the sodium is ingested in the form of NaCl (common salt). Most foods of vegetable origin have low Na content, while animal products are rich sources of this mineral (Pond et al. 1995). Thus, Na is usually added as 0.20%–0.35% NaCl to corn- and soybean meal-based diets for poultry and swine. For grazing animals, NaCl is generally supplemented to their diets in free-choice mineral salts.

*Absorption and Transport*

In the lumen of the small intestine, NaCl is ionized to give rise to $Na^+$ and $Cl^-$. In mammals (e.g., pigs and ruminants), birds, and fish, $Na^+$ enters the enterocyte from the intestinal lumen via $Na^+$-glucose cotransporter-1 (SGLT1); sodium channels (e.g., AMSC; amiloride-sensitive $Na^+$ channels [also known as epithelial sodium channels, ENaC]); sodium-dependent AA transporters; and the sodium-phosphate cotransporter (Carey et al. 1994; Song et al. 2016; Wright and Loo 2000). Furthermore, $Na^+$, along with $Cl^-$, is absorbed across the apical membrane of the enterocyte or colonocyte through two electroneutral exchangers: $Na^+/H^+$ (NHE2/3) and $Cl^-/HCO_3^-$ (Kato and Romero 2011). The absorption of $Na^+$ and $Cl^-$ via the transmembrane exchangers does not result in transepithelial currents, which contrasts with other modes of $Na^+$ and $Cl^-$ transport by the intestine (Gawenis et al. 2002). Sodium is present in the enterocyte as a free cation and is transported out of the cell by the basolateral $Na^+$-$K^+$-ATPase into the lamina propria (Manoharan et al. 2015). NHE-1, which is present in the basolateral membrane of the enterocyte, plays a role in transporting intracellular Na into the lamina propria in exchange for the entry of $H^+$ ions. Sodium is absorbed into the portal vein and carried in the plasma as a free cation for uptake by extraintestinal cells through sodium channels (Zakon 2012) or transporters (e.g., SGLT2 in kidneys). Intestinal absorption of sodium is coupled with water absorption and, therefore, plays an important role in preventing diarrhea (Field 2003).

*Functions*

The biochemical functions of sodium are summarized as follows:

*Regulation of Extracellular Osmolarity* In animals, plasma osmolarity is essentially the same as interstitial osmolarity or intracellular osmolarity. Because of its abundance, NaCl plays an important role in regulating extracellular osmotic pressure. Based on the concentrations of solutes in the plasma, its osmolarity is calculated to be 302 mOsmol/L. However, NaCl is not entirely ionized to $Na^+$ and $Cl^-$ in a physiological solution, and has an osmotic coefficient of 0.93. Accordingly, the measured value of plasma osmolarity is 282 mOsmol/L (Guyton and Hall 2000). Of note, Na contributes to about 46% of plasma osmolarity. When plasma osmolarity is low, water enters from the plasma into erythrocytes and other blood cells, and moves into the interstitial fluid and then into cells in tissues, causing the lysis of blood cells and edema. In contrast, when plasma osmolarity is high, water enters from the interstitial fluid and cells into the blood, resulting in cell shrinkage and hypertension. Thus, Na is important for maintaining cell volume and viability, as well as blood volume.

*Nutrient Transport Systems* The transport of glucose, AAs, and various ions (e.g., $I^-$, $Cl^-$, and phosphate) across cell membranes requires the cotransport of $Na^+$ ions. The transport proteins recognize and bind both $Na^+$ and other specific substrates. ATP is usually required for $Na^+$-dependent transport processes (e.g., glucose absorption by the small intestine [Figure 10.3]). The relatively high concentration of extracellular $Na^+$ is used to drive various nutrient transport systems. Thus, rehydration solutions usually contain NaCl and glucose, and possibly glutamine, glutamate, and glycine (Rhoads 1999; Wang et al. 2013).

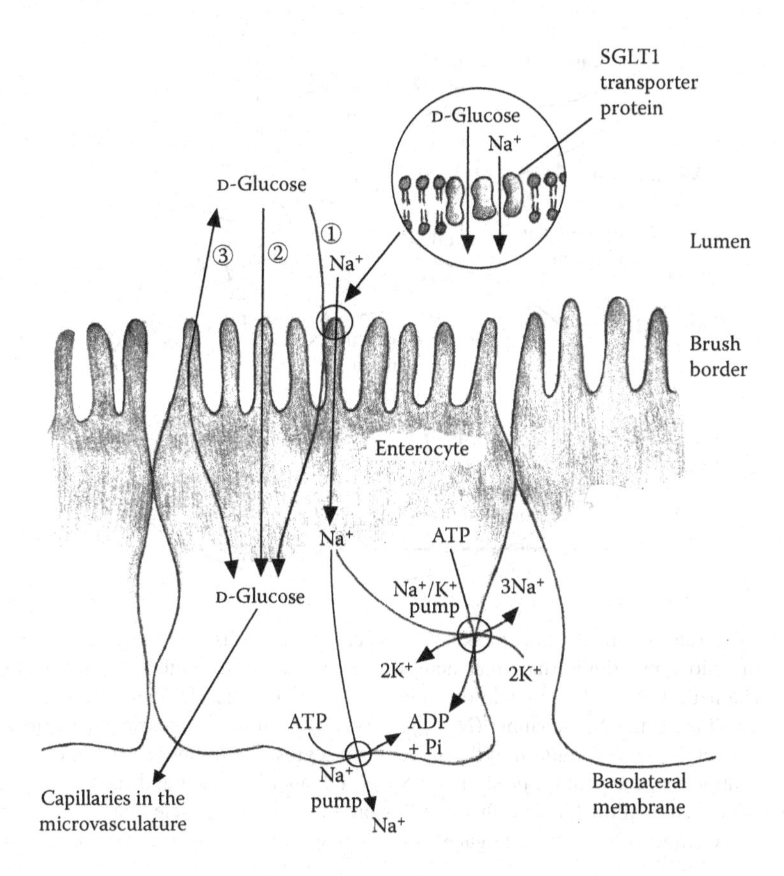


**FIGURE 10.3** Intestinal absorption of glucose through $Na^+$-dependent mechanisms. In the small intestine, Na-K-ATPase in the basolateral membrane is responsible for maintaining a low Na concentration in the enterocyte that is necessary to promote Na-coupled solute cotransport by sodium-glucose cotransporter (SGLT1).

*Activity of Sodium Pump* (Na-K-ATPase). This enzyme is a membrane-bound protein, and catalyzes the transport of $Na^+$ ions out of the cell in exchange for $K^+$ ions into the cell (Chapter 1). In the small intestine, Na-K-ATPase in the basolateral membrane is responsible for maintaining a low Na concentration in the enterocyte that is necessary to promote Na-coupled solute cotransport by SGLT1, $Na^+$-dependent AA transporters, and other $Na^+$-dependent transporters in the apical membrane, as noted previously. Importantly, the Na-K-ATPase is required for the functioning of nerves and muscle cells because the electrical impulses that occur in these cells depend on the relatively high concentrations of extracellular Na and intracellular concentrations of K (Pirkmajer and Chibalin 2016). Thus, an inhibition of Na-K-ATPase ouabain results in reduced ion transport by the small intestine and other tissues (e.g., the placenta).

*$Na^+/H^+$ Exchange* $Na^+/H^+$ exchange, along with $HCO_3^-$-based transport mechanisms, is a major mechanism for regulating intracellular pH in mammalian cells (Kato and Romero 2011). Thus, Na plays a role in regulating intracellular acid–base balance. As noted previously, in the small intestine, different isoforms of the NHE are localized in different membranes of the enterocyte to promote $Na^+$ absorption.

*Blood Pressure* Water retention in the body, particularly the blood, is associated with its Na concentration. Concentrations of $Na^+$ in the plasma affect (1) the entry of water into blood vessels by osmosis; (2) the renal reabsorption of $Na^+$ and water; (3) the integrity of red blood cells and vascular endothelial cells; and (4) blood flow and hemodynamics (O'Shaughnessy and Karet 2004).

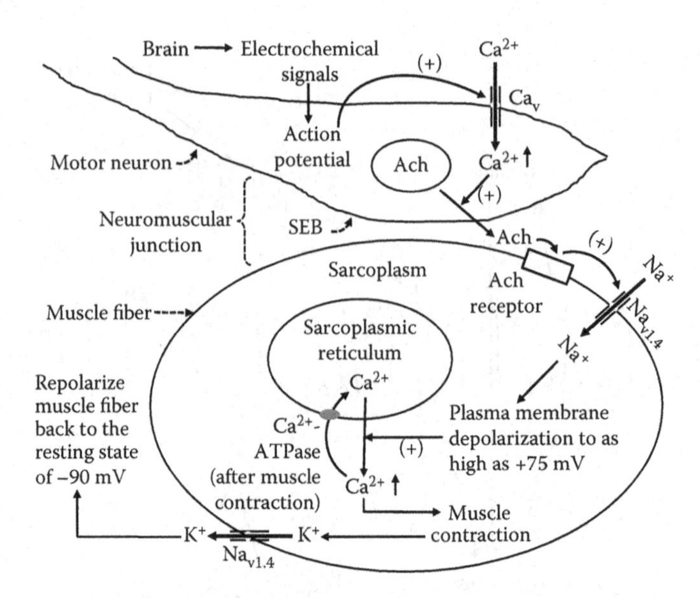


**FIGURE 10.4** The role of ion channels in skeletal muscle contractions. Electrochemical signals from the brain result in an action potential in the motor neuron, which causes $Ca^{2+}$ influx and the releases of acetylcholine (Ach). The neurotransmitter binds to the Ach receptor in the muscle fiber, resulting in the influx of $Na^+$ through the voltage-gated $Na^+$-channel ($Na^+_{v1.4}$), depolarization of the muscle plasma membrane, $Ca^{2+}$ efflux from the sarcoplasmic reticulum into the sarcoplasm (cytosol), and muscle contraction. Immediately after a muscle contraction, the sodium pore of the $Na^+_{v1.4}$ channel is closed and the potassium pore of the $Na^+_{v1.4}$ channel is opened to allow for $K^+$ efflux and repolarization of the muscle fiber to its resting state. $Ca_v$, voltage-gated $Ca^{2+}$-channel; $Na^+_{v1.4}$, voltage-gated $Na^+$-channel; SEB, synaptic end bulb; ↑, increase; and (+) activation.

*Action Potentials in Skeletal Muscle* Voltage-gated $Na^+$-channels provide the biochemical basis for electrical excitability in animals (Zakon 2012). $Na^+$ plays an important role in the contraction of skeletal muscle, so that mammals, birds, and fish can stand, walk, run, and do other physical work (Figure 10.4). Under normal physiological conditions, the neuromuscular junction in skeletal muscle is activated by signals from the central nervous system. This is followed by the influx of extracellular $Na^+$ ions into skeletal muscle fibers through a voltage-gated sodium channel ($Na_v1.4$). The entry of $Na^+$ into the muscle fibers depolarizes them, which increases their membrane potential from −90 mV at the resting state to as high as +75 mV. This triggers the efflux of calcium from the sarcoplasmic reticulum into the sarcoplasm (cytosol) to cause the contraction of skeletal muscle. To prevent the muscle from being perpetually contracted, the $Na_v1.4$ channel contains a fast inactivation gate to close the sodium pore very quickly after it opens, preventing the further entry of $Na^+$ ions into the cells. To balance intracellular cations, $K^+$ ion will exit the muscle fibers to repolarize them. This results in the pumping of $Ca^{2+}$ from the contractile apparatus to the sarcoplasmic reticulum, thereby relaxing the skeletal muscle. Thus, $Na^+$ acts in concert with $K^+$ and $Ca^{2+}$ to regulate muscle contraction.

*Regulation of Food Intake* As noted previously, Na is required for the intestinal absorption of dietary glucose, AAs, and some minerals, thereby affecting the rates of the passage of digesta through the gastrointestinal tract. This, in turn, has a profound effect on food and dry matter (DM) intake by animals (Chapter 12). In addition, Na taste receptors (epithelial sodium channels) are present in the apical membrane of the taste cells (which are not neurons) in the taste buds of the tongue (Chandrashekar et al. 2010). Interaction of $Na^+$ with a Na taste receptor allows $Na^+$ to move down a concentration gradient into the taste cell. This results in an increase in intracellular

Na concentration to depolarize the cell membrane, causing the opening of a voltage-gated $Ca^{2+}$ channel on the basolateral membrane of the taste cell for the influx of $Ca^{2+}$. An increase in intracellular $Ca^{2+}$ concentration causes the release of neurotransmitter molecules (in the form of synaptic vesicles), which are received by receptors on the nearby primary sensory neurons. A resulting electrical signal is transmitted along nerve cells to reach the brain's feeding center, which perceives and interprets the Na stimulus in the tongue. Low dietary intake of Na impairs the activation of sodium taste receptors, leading to reduced food intake. However, excess dietary intake of Na (e.g., supplementing 0.54% Na as 1.37% NaCl to a corn- and soybean meal-based diet [containing 0.25% NaCl] for postweaning pigs) reduces food intake by animals (Rezaei et al. 2013). In practice, high levels of NaCl in free-choice protein or energy supplements are used to restrict their consumption by grazing cattle.

#### *Deficiency Symptoms*

In animals, sodium deficiency (also known as hyponatremia) occurs in many parts of the world, particularly in tropical areas of Africa and the arid inland areas of Australia where pastures contain a low Na content (McDonald et al. 2011). A deficiency of Na results in a decrease in osmotic pressure, dehydration of the body, and hypotension. Symptoms of Na deficiency include reduced feed intake, low BW gain, reduced utilization of digested proteins and energy, nausea, headache, impaired egg production, eye lesions, and reproductive dysfunction (Lien and Shapiro 2007). Severe hyponatremia can cause confusion, seizures, coma, heart failure, and even death (Jones and Hunt 1983). Intravenous or oral administration of NaCl is effective in treating Na deficiency.

#### *Excess*

A major concern over sodium nutrition in animals is the role of high sodium intake in the development of hypertension due to increased water volume in blood vessels. High concentrations of $Na^+$ in the plasma (also known as hypernatremia) enhance both the passage of water into blood vessels and the circulating levels of angiotensinogen I (Kumar and Berl 1998). The latter undergoes limited hydrolysis in the vasculature of the lungs to become angiotensinogen II, which stimulates the release of aldosterone from the adrenal gland to augment renal reabsorption of $Na^+$ and water (Figure 10.5). Thus, high concentrations of $Na^+$ in the plasma result in increased urinary losses of Na. In addition, excessive intake of dietary Na reduces the feed intake and growth of animals. Mammals, birds, and fish with hypernatremia exhibit hypertonicity, which causes such severe clinical manifestations as neurological and cardiovascular disorders due to cell shrinking, and even death (Kumar and Berl 1998; Rondon-Berrios et al. 2017). Adequate drinking water should be provided to animals in cases of high Na intake.

### **POTASSIUM**

Potassium was first isolated from potash (the ashes of plants) by Humphry Davy in 1807. Thus, the word "potassium" is derived from *potash*. The chemical symbol of this element, K, is derived from the Latin "kalium" meaning alkali. Potassium is the most abundant cation in the intracellular fluid. The concentration of potassium is about 140 mM in the intracellular fluid, and is about 3.5–5.0 mM in the plasma.

#### *Sources*

Plants usually contain high levels of K (e.g., 25 g K/kg DM of grass). Thus, K deficiency in animals is rare. One exception is distillers' grains, with K supplementation being required in these cases. Of note, the soil of certain areas in the world (e.g., Brazil, Panama, and Uganda) contains low concentrations of $K^+$, and plants in these regions may be deficient in $K^+$ (Suttle 2010). In addition, dormant grasses are much lower in K and may not provide sufficient K to animals.

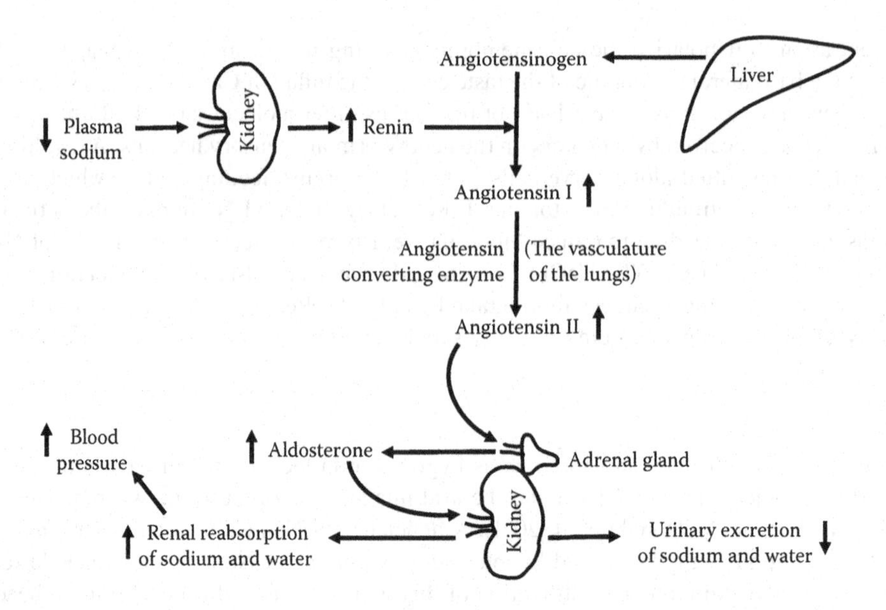


**FIGURE 10.5** Regulation of renal water excretion by concentrations of sodium in the plasma. When the concentration of sodium in the plasma is low, the release of renin by the kidneys is augmented to enhance the production of angiotensin II and aldosterone. The latter promotes renal reabsorption of sodium and water in an attempt to restore the concentration of sodium in the plasma to a normal value.

### *Absorption and Transport*

Potassium channels on the apical membranes of the enterocyte, which include $K^+/H^+$ ATPase, $Na^+$-$Cl^-$-$K^+$ transporter, and $K^+$ conductance channels, are responsible for $K^+$ absorption by the small intestine. They are widely expressed in both excitable and nonexcitable cells (Heitzmann and Richard. 2008). $K^+/H^+$ ATPase uses ATP to drive the inward flow of $K^+$ into the enterocyte in exchange for the outward flux of $H^+$ into the intestinal lumen. $Na^+$-$Cl^-$-$K^+$ transporter can bind all the three ions and use a sodium gradient to transport 1 $Na^+$, 1 $K^+$, and 2 $Cl^-$ ions into the cell. $K^+$ conductance channels use the electrochemical energy across the enterocyte membrane as the driving force to transport $K^+$; these channels are activated by $Ca^{2+}$ or gated by nucleotides, voltage, or specific ligands. Furthermore, K, along with Cl, is absorbed across the apical membrane of the enterocyte or colonocyte through two electroneutral exchangers: $K^+/H^+$ and $Cl^-/HCO_3^-$. Potassium is present in the enterocyte as a free cation and is transported out of the cell by the basolateral $K^+$ channels and the electroneutral K–Cl cotransporter into the lamina propria. $K^+$ exits the enterocyte together with $Cl^-$, with water following these osmolytes. Potassium is absorbed into the portal vein and carried in the plasma as a free cation for uptake by extraintestinal cells through $K^+$ channels and K–Cl cotransporters.

### *Functions*

The biochemical functions of potassium are summarized as follows:

*Regulation of Intracellular Osmolarity* Because of its abundance, K plays an important role in regulating intracellular osmotic pressure. Specifically, K contributes to about 50% of intracellular osmolarity.

*Activity of Sodium Pump and the Functions of the Nerves and Muscle Cells* Potassium is involved in the sodium pump activity and in the functioning of the nerves and muscle cells, as noted previously. Like $Na^+$, $K^+$ is also used in the conduction of impulses along nerves and muscle cells. This critical role of potassium is illustrated by hyperkalemic periodic paralysis (HYPP), which is a genetic disease associated with an increase in serum potassium concentration in humans and horses (Nollet and Deprez 2005).

The HYPP disease results from genetic mutations in transmembrane domains III and IV, which make up the fast inactivation gate of $Na_v1.4$ at the neuromuscular junction (Lehmann-Horn and Jurkat-Rott 1999). In patients with genetic mutations of $Na_v1.4$, the sodium channel is unable to inactivate. As a result, sodium conductance is sustained and the muscle remains permanently tense. This condition becomes worse in the presence of high concentrations of potassium in the plasma, because an elevated level of extracellular potassium reduces the exit of potassium from the muscle cells, further prolonging the sodium conductance and keeping the muscle in the continuous contraction state. Thus, HYPP is characterized by hyperexcitability or extreme weakness of skeletal muscle, leading to uncontrolled shaking followed by paralysis. This disease occurs in 2% of Quarter Horses with a single stallion ancestor named Impressive (Nollet and Deprez 2005). The HYPP syndromes can be alleviated by decreasing dietary intake of potassium and its concentrations in the plasma (Kollias-Baker 1999; Reynolds et al. 1998).

*Hormone Synthesis* Potassium stimulates the conversion of cholesterol into pregnenolone and the conversion of corticosterone into aldosterone (Chapter 6). As a result, potassium plays an important role in regulating sodium concentrations in the plasma, as noted previously.

*$H^+$-$K^+$-ATPase* In parietal cells of the stomach, the secretion of $H^+$ ions into the lumen in exchange for K uptake to generate HCl depends on $H^+$-$K^+$-ATPase. Thus, K is required to maintain a low gastric-luminal pH and facilitate protein digestion in animals (Chapter 7).

### *Deficiency Symptoms*

Potassium deficiency (plasma K concentration <3.5 mM), which is known as hypokalemia, results from inadequate dietary intake, gastrointestinal loss (e.g., through vomiting and diarrhea), urinary loss (e.g., diabetic ketoacidosis), hypomagnesemia, or hyperaldosteronism (Sweeney 1999). Renal $K^+$-channel efflux is inhibited by $Mg^{2+}$ (Huang and Kuo 2007); therefore, hypomagnesemia results in an increased excretion of $K^+$ by the kidneys, possibly leading to hypokalemia. In animals, syndromes of potassium deficiency include muscle weakness, spasms, tetany, paralysis, numbness (particularly in legs and hands), excessive loss of body water (due to an inability to concentrate urine), low blood pressure, frequent urination, and thirst. Finally, hypokalemia can also cause cardiac rhythm abnormalities, cardiac arrest, and even death in animals. Intravenous and oral administration of potassium, in addition to therapies aimed at correcting the associated endocrine and metabolic diseases, are necessary to treat K deficiency (Jones and Hunt 1983).

### *Excess*

A concentration of $K^+$ in the plasma greater than 5.5 mM is defined as hyperkalemia, which can result from excessive intake, excessive release from cells due to hemolysis and tissue injury, kidney failure (reduced $K^+$ excretion), hypoaldosteronism (which impairs $K^+$ excretion in the distal tubule and the collecting duct; common in dogs), and use of angiotensin-converting enzyme inhibitors (Kovesdy 2017). In animals, syndromes of hyperkalemia include reduced feed intake and impaired growth; fatigue and muscle weakness; hypomagnesemia (due to depolarization of the membrane potential of gastrointestinal cells [e.g., ruminal epithelial cells of the rumen] and the subsequent reduction in the absorption of dietary magnesium via the electrodiffusion mechanism [Schweigel et al. 1999]); and abnormal heart rhythm (arrhythmia), slow heart rate, and cardiac arrest; and even death. Toxicity of K is not likely if adequate drinking water is provided to animals (Greene et al. 1983).

## CHLORIDE

Chlorine (Cl) was discovered by Carl W. Schelle in 1774 through heating HCl with $MnO_2$. Chloride ($Cl^-$), which is the anion of Cl, is the principal anion in the extracellular fluid. In 1834, William Prout discovered that HCl is produced by the stomach. Chloride concentration is about 100–110 mM in the plasma, and about 4–5 mM in the intracellular fluid. Chloride is one of the halides (the others halides are fluoride, bromide, and iodide). The nonionized elemental forms of the halides are called halogens. (The term "halogen" comes from a Greek word meaning "salt-producing"). The movement of chloride ions across a membrane is often seen as a passive movement that serves to balance a charge difference caused by the movement of sodium or potassium. However, active transport mechanisms exist for the chloride anion.

*Sources*

With the exception of fish and meat meals, most foods have a low chloride content. In contrast, animal products are rich sources of this mineral. The major source of chloride for animal diets is NaCl, as noted previously.

*Absorption and Transport*

In the lumen of the small intestine, the chloride-containing salts (e.g., NaCl, KCl, $CaCl_2$, and $MgCl_2$) are ionized to give rise to $Cl^-$. In mammals (e.g., pigs and ruminants), birds, and fish, $Na^+$ enters the enterocyte from the intestinal lumen via (1) Cl channels (primarily cystic fibrosis transmembrane conductance regulator [CFTR]) and (2) electroneutral $Na^+$-$Cl^-$ absorption mediated by $Na^+/H^+$ (NHE2/3) and $Cl^-/HCO_3^-$ exchangers (Gawenis et al. 2002; Kato and Romero 2011). In the small intestine, the $Na^+/H^+$ exchanger takes up $Na^+$ and releases $H^+$, whereas the $Cl^-/HCO_3^-$ exchanger releases $HCO_3^-$ and takes up $Cl^-$. Thus, a major part of $Cl^-$ absorption is due to $Na^+$ absorption, and normally there is net water absorption together with $HCO_3^-$ secretion from the enterocyte into the lumen in exchange for the entry of luminal $Cl^-$ into the cell. This helps to neutralize the acidic digesta that moves from the stomach into the duodenum. Chloride is present in the enterocyte as a free anion and is transported out of the cell by the basolateral Cl channels (e.g., Cl channel-2; Pena-Munzenmayer et al. 2005). Chloride is absorbed into the portal vein and carried in the plasma as a free cation for uptake by extraintestinal cells through chloride channels, primarily calcium-activated Cl channels (Huang et al. 2012).

*Functions*

The biochemical functions of chloride are outlined as follows:

*Acid–base Balance* Chloride is associated with Na and K in the regulation of the acid–base balance in animals.

*Production of Gastric Hydrochloric Acid (HCl)* The parietal (oxyntic) cells of the stomach are the sources of gastric HCl. Gastric juice is a clear, yellow fluid of 0.2%–0.5% HCl, with a pH of about 1.0. HCl denatures proteins and peptides, which is important for their hydrolysis by proteases and peptidases. HCl also kills bacteria, which helps to prevent infection.

*Intestinal Secretion* In a postabsorptive state, the intestine secretes $Cl^-$ into the lumen to maintain osmolarity and acid–base balance in the lumen. The transporters involved in the secretion include (1) the basolateral $Na^+$-$K^+$-$2Cl^-$ cotransporter, which transports one $Na^+$, one $K^+$, and two $Cl^-$ ions from the lamina propria (ultimately the blood) into the intestinal epithelial cell, and (2) CFTR on the apical membrane of the intestinal epithelial cell. As noted previously, the $Na^+$ gradient, established by the basolateral $Na^+/K^+$-ATPase, provides the energy for the transport of ions into the cell. For a cotransporter, the presence of one substrate enhances the transport of the other. In the cases of infection or intake of a noxious compound into the intestine, fluid (water and $Cl^-$) secretion into the lumen is enhanced due to the cAMP-mediated activation of $Cl^-$ channel within intestinal epithelial cells.

*Maintaining a Hydrated State of the Mucus* The transport of $Cl^-$ ions across epithelial cells is associated with the movement of $Na^+$ and water, which helps to maintain a hydrated state of the mucus. This role is epitomized by the disease called "cystic fibrosis," one of the most common genetic disorders among Caucasians (Whites) (5% of population carries the defective gene). Swine models of cystic fibrosis have been developed for research purposes (Rogers et al. 2008). The disease results from a genetic mutation of the chloride transport channel in the apical membrane of airway epithelial cells such that the channel is not activated in a normal fashion by cAMP and protein kinase (Cutting 2015). The failure to transport $Cl^-$ ions from the lung epithelium into the air passage causes the failure of $Na^+$ and water to move passively into the airway. The impaired transport of water into the airway results in the development of a thick and dehydrating mucus in the lungs. This mucus impairs breathing and invites recurrent infections that eventually destroy the lungs.

#### *Deficiency Symptoms*

In all animals, a deficiency of chloride (also known as hypochloremia) reduces extracellular osmolarity and impairs acid–base balance (de Morais and Biondo 2006). Dietary Cl deficiency may result in an abnormal increase of the alkali reserve of the blood (alkalosis) caused by an excess of bicarbonate. This is because inadequate levels of $Cl^-$ in the body are partly compensated for by an increase in bicarbonate concentration. Animals with hypochloremia also exhibit increases in the urinary excretions of calcium and magnesium. Furthermore, reduced food intake, impaired protein digestion, growth restriction, muscle weakness, and dehydration occur in $Cl^-$-deficient animals (Jones and Hunt 1983). Intravenous and oral administration of NaCl are effective in treating Cl deficiency.

#### *Chloride Excess*

A concentration of $Cl^-$ in the plasma greater than 110 mM is defined as hyperchloremia, which can result from excessive intake of dietary salts (e.g., NaCl, KCl, and $NH_4Cl$), high concentrations of sodium in the plasma, and kidney failure. In animals, syndromes of hyperchloremia include nausea, vomiting, and diarrhea; reduced feed intake and impaired growth; sweating, dehydration, and high body temperature; fatigue and muscular weakness; high sodium concentrations in the plasma, hypertonicity, metabolic acidosis, and thirst; kidney disorders and failure; impaired blood flow; brain injury; and impaired oxygen transport by red blood cells (Cambier et al. 1998; Scarratt et al. 1985).

### Calcium

Calcium was discovered by Humphry Davy in 1808. In 1840, Jean Boussigault (a French chemist) and Justus von Liebig (a German chemist) recognized that bone consists of calcium and phosphorus. Calcium is a divalent cation and derives its name from the Latin "calx" meaning "lime." This metal is now known to be a major component of the skeleton (bone) and teeth as a salt with phosphate. A 70 kg animal contains about 1.3 kg of calcium, with about 99% present in the skeleton. Depending on animal species, concentrations of total calcium in plasma are 4.5–5.5 mM (approximately half of it binds to albumin), with calcium concentrations in serum being about 2.2–3.1 mM.

#### *Sources*

Milk, green leafy vegetables (especially legumes), and animal products (e.g., fish meal and meat and bone meal) containing bones are good sources of Ca. Cereals and roots are poor sources of Ca. Ground limestone, dicalcium phosphate, calcium carbonate, calcium citrate, calcium lactate, and calcium lactose are often used as Ca supplements for farm animals. Calcium oxalate is relatively insoluble and poorly absorbed by the intestine. Any calcium salt is more soluble in acid than at neutral pH.

#### *Absorption and Transport*

Calcium in the intestinal lumen is absorbed by the small intestine via calcium transporter-1 (CaT1, a calcium channel protein). The duodenum, jejunum, and ileum are responsible for the absorption of 5%, 15%, and 80% of calcium, respectively (Khanal and Nemere 2008). Upon entering the

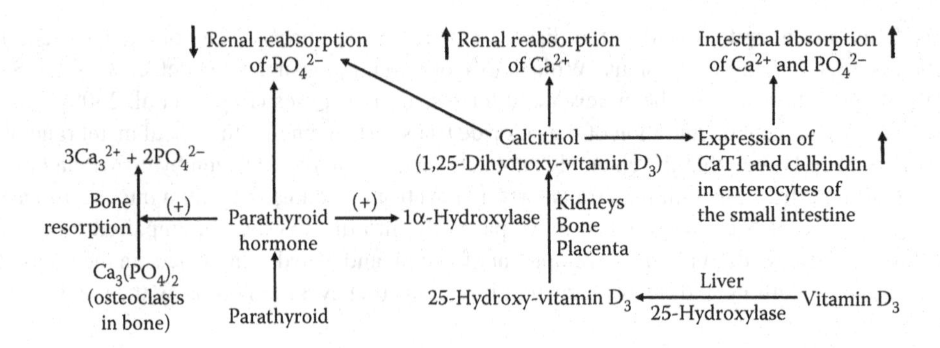


**FIGURE 10.6** Regulation of intestinal absorption of calcium and phosphate, as well as renal reabsorption in the kidneys by vitamin D (a sterol) and parathyroid hormone. Vitamin $D_3$ is converted into calcitriol, through interorgan metabolism involving mainly the liver and kidneys. Calcitriol and parathyroid hormone have anabolic effects on bone growth by enhancing intestinal absorption of calcium and phosphate, as well as renal reabsorption of calcium. ↑, increase; (+), activation; (−), inhibition.

enterocyte, $Ca^{2+}$ is transported to intracellular organelles by a cytosolic protein called calbindin. $Ca^{2+}$ exits the enterocyte across its basolateral membrane into the lamina propria via $Ca^{2+}$-ATPase. This basolateral membrane transporter is an antiporter, which transports $Ca^{2+}$ out of the enterocyte in exchange for the entry of $Mg^{2+}$ or $Na^+$ from the lamina propria (ultimately the blood). Thus, the hydrolysis of ATP drives intestinal $Ca^{2+}$ absorption. $Ca^{2+}$ enters the portal vein from the lamina propria, is transported in the plasma in both free and protein-bound forms, and is taken up by extraintestinal cells through specific $Ca^{2+}$ channels. Note that the relatively high content of fat or oxalic acid in animal diets results in the formation of calcium–fatty acid soaps or calcium oxalate, which reduces the intestinal absorption of $Ca^{2+}$.

Calcitriol (1,25-dihydroxy-vitamin $D_3$) and parathyroid hormone (PTH) play an important role in regulating $Ca^{2+}$ homeostasis in animals (Figure 10.6). Specifically, calcitriol, which is formed from vitamin $D_3$ or vitamin $D_2$, plays an important role in $Ca^{2+}$ homeostasis in animals. Specifically, physiological concentrations of calcitriol enhance intestinal $Ca^{2+}$ absorption by stimulating the expression of CaT1 and calbindin in enterocytes, the renal reabsorption of $Ca^{2+}$, and, in the case of low plasma $Ca^{2+}$ concentration, the mobilization of $Ca^{2+}$ from the bone matrix (Blaine et al. 2015). PTH, which is secreted by the parathyroid gland in response to low plasma $Ca^{2+}$ concentration, increases the concentration of $Ca^{2+}$ in the plasma through (1) upregulating the expression of 25-hydroxy-vitamin D hydroxylase (which converts 25-dihydroxy-vitamin D into 1,25-dihydroxy-vitamin D) and (2) activating osteoclasts to promote bone resorption (the mobilization of bone $Ca_3(PO_4)_2$ to $Ca^{2+}$ for entry into the plasma) (Blaine et al. 2015). PTH cell signaling involves the activation of protein kinases A and C (Swarthout et al. 2002).

The concentrations of magnesium and sodium in the plasma also regulate calcium homeostasis in the body (Agus 1999). Low dietary intake of $Mg^{2+}$ decreases its concentrations in the plasma and cells, as well as ATP production and PTH activity. This leads to reductions in: (1) energy-dependent intestinal absorption of Ca and renal reabsorption of Ca, and (2) concentrations of Ca in the plasma. Hypermagnesemia also results in hypocalcemia, and the underlying mechanisms include: (1) inhibiting the secretion of PTH from the parathyroid gland and (2) promoting the excretion of $Ca^{2+}$ by the kidneys due to low circulating levels of PTH. Similarly, hypernatremia (elevated $Na^+$ concentration in the plasma) reduces the concentration of $Ca^{2+}$ in the plasma (Alexander et al. 2013). In the lumen of the renal tubule, $Na^+$ competes with $Ca^{2+}$ for reabsorption into the blood. Thus, a high concentration of luminal $Na^+$ resulting from a high circulating level of $Na^+$ reduces the reabsorption of $Ca^{2+}$, leading to enhanced excretion of $Ca^{2+}$ by the kidneys. Thus, high-salt diets increase the risk for kidney stones and osteoporosis in animals.

**TABLE 10.8**
**Calcium-Activated Enzymes and Calcium-Binding Proteins**

| Enzyme or Protein | Function |
|---|---|
| Annexins | Cell adhesion |
| Blood-clotting proteins | Ca binds to γ-carboxyglutamic acid residues of proteins |
| Ca-ATPase | Release Ca from the sarcoplasmic reticulum in skeletal muscle |
| Ca-activated proteases (calpain) | Protein degradation in skeletal and cardiac muscles |
| Cadherins | Epithelial cell adhesion |
| Calbindin | Cytosolic calcium transport |
| Calcitonin | Regulator of blood calcium and phosphate concentrations |
| Calmodulin | Calmodulin-dependent protein kinases and in Ca-dependent cell signaling. Calmodulin-dependent enzymes (e.g., NO synthase) |
| Caspases | Protease activation (widely present in cells) |
| $Ca^{2+}$ transporter-1 | Membrane calcium transport |
| Cell adhesion molecules | Binds with other cells or with the extracellular matrix |
| Lipase | Triacylglycerols → Fatty acids + Monoacylglycerol (the lumen of the small intestine) |
| Nitric oxide (NO) synthase | Arginine + $O_2$ → NO + Citrulline |
| Pancreatic α-amylase | Hydrolysis of dietary starches |
| Pancreatic phospholipase $A_2$ | Hydrolysis of dietary phospholipids |
| Phospholipase $A_2$ | Release of fatty acid (e.g., arachidonic acid) from membrane-bound lipids |
| Phospholipase C | Hydrolysis of the inositol phosphate group of phosphatidyl-4,5-diphosphate |
| Protein kinase C | Phosphorylate enzymes in cell signaling |
| Phosphorylase kinase | Glycogen breakdown and synthesis |
| Thermolysin (*Bacillus* species)[a] | Microbial hydrolysis of peptide bonds containing hydrophobic amino acids |
| Troponin C (TpC) | Muscle contraction |
| Trypsin | Protein → Amino acids + Small peptides (the lumen of the small intestine) |
| Trypsinogen | Trypsinogen (inactive) → Trypsin (active protease) |

[a] This protease requires one zinc ion for enzymatic activity and four calcium ions for structural stability.

### *Functions*

The phosphates of $Ca^{2+}$ are the major minerals in bones, which protect internal organs and provide structural integrity to the body (Pond et al. 1995). The rigidity provided by the bones permits locomotion, and the support of loads against gravity. In addition, the formation of calcium carbonate from $Ca^{2+}$ and carbonate in the process of biomineralization is essential for eggshell production in laying birds. Furthermore, many enzymes and proteins require $Ca^{2+}$ for their biological activities (Table 10.8). For example, in some blood-clotting proteins, $Ca^{2+}$ is bound to residues of γ-carboxyglutamic acid, where this metal is required for their functions. Furthermore, as a cofactor of protein kinase C in different cell types, $Ca^{2+}$ participates in signal transduction pathways (serving as a second messenger) in response to extracellular signals (e.g., hormones and neurotransmitters). Finally, $Ca^{2+}$ is essential for skeletal muscle contractions, heartbeats, nerve transmission, and maximum milk production by lactating mammary glands. Thus, $Ca^{2+}$ plays a vital role in nutrition and physiology.

*Deficiency Symptoms*

In animals, the syndromes of Ca deficiency are similar to those of vitamin D deficiency, including abnormal skeletal growth and development, as well as rickets (Chapter 9). Additionally, milk fever (parturient paresis) may occur in lactating sows shortly after calving (Chapter 9). This metabolic disease is characterized by low serum Ca levels (causing hyper-excitability of the nervous system and weakened muscle contractions), muscular spasms, and, in severe cases, paralysis and unconsciousness. Intravenous administration of calcium gluconate or vitamin D along with dietary cation-anion balance helps to restore serum Ca concentrations and treat this disease. When Ca is supplemented to animal diets, it is important to consider their Ca/P ratios. For most non-ruminant farm animals, except laying hens, dietary ratios of bioavailable Ca to bioavailable P are usually in the range of 1:1 to 2:1 (e.g., 1.5:1 for growing mammals and fish). The proportion of Ca in the diet for laying hens (Ca:P ratio = 13:1) is much higher than that for 3- to 6-week-old growing broilers (Ca:P = 2.6:1), because of eggshell formation in the former (NRC 1994). Ruminants are not as sensitive to dietary Ca:P ratio as nonruminants. This is because some dietary Ca may be absorbed from the rumen and a large amount of plasma P is secreted back into the rumen, making the Ca/P ratio at the site of absorption in the small intestine much different than the dietary Ca/P ratio (Greene 2016). Excess P in diets reduces intestinal absorption of $Ca^{2+}$ and should be avoided for all animals.

*Excess*

As noted previously, the concentration of $Ca^{2+}$ in the plasma is regulated by dietary intake of calcium, bone resorption and remodeling, intestinal absorption, and renal tubule resorption. Hypercalcemia most commonly results from the overproduction of PTH by overactive parathyroid glands (hyperparathyroidism), but also from malignant diseases (e.g., cancer), as well as excessive use of calcium and vitamin D supplements. In animals, syndromes of hypercalcemia include (1) constipation, nausea, and vomiting; (2) reduced feed intake and impaired growth; (3) excessive deposition of calcium in blood vessels to form plaques that lead to the dysfunction of the heart and brain; and (4) muscle pain, abdominal pain, and kidney stones (Žofková 2016). Severe hypercalcemia can be life-threatening. Of interest, concentrations of $Ca^{2+}$ (as CaCl) in the ruminal fluid $\geq$450 μg/mL are toxic to ruminal microbes as assessed by the rate of cellulose digestion in all animals and dietary P at levels higher than dietary Ca should be avoided (Georgievskii et al. 1982).

## Phosphorus

Phosphorus was discovered from human urine by Hennig Brand in 1669. This mineral is derived from the Greek words "Phôs" (light) and "phorus" (bearer). Phosphorus is highly reactive and, therefore, is not found as a free element on the earth. In animals, phosphorus exists as phosphate, which consists of a central atom of phosphorus, four atoms of oxygen, and zero to three atoms of hydrogen. The concentration of inorganic phosphate (Pi) is 1.2–2.0 mM in the plasma. The total amount of intracellular phosphate (e.g., phosphate in ATP, ADP, AMP, GTP, UTP, creatine phosphate, phosphorylated protein, nucleic acids, and glucose-6-phosphate) is equivalent to 50–75 mM in animal cells. About 85% of the body's phosphate occurs in the bones, with about 14% in soft tissues and 1% in the extracellular fluid.

Phosphate resonates among several forms. A few forms of phosphate are shown below.

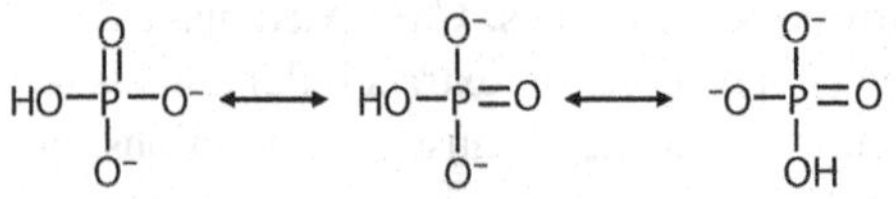

$$HO{-}P(=O)(O^-){-}O^- \longleftrightarrow HO{-}P(O^-)(O^-){=}O \longleftrightarrow {}^-O{-}P(O^-)(OH){=}O$$

Phosphate occurs in equilibrium with $H_3PO_4$, $H_2PO_4^-$, $HPO_4^{2-}$, and $PO_4^{3-}$, as shown below.

$$HO-P(=O)(OH)-OH \rightleftharpoons HO-P(=O)(OH)-O^- \rightleftharpoons HO-P(=O)(O^-)-O^- \rightleftharpoons {}^-O-P(=O)(O^-)-O^- \quad (\pm H^+ \text{ at each step})$$

The predominant form of phosphate at a neutral pH is $HPO_4^{2-}$. The fully protonated form, which is the predominant form in an environment of low pH, is phosphoric acid ($H_3PO_4$). In animals, phosphate reacts with calcium to form calcium phosphate in bones, and is also covalently bound to sugars, proteins, lipids, vitamins, and other organic molecules. Phosphate homeostasis is tightly controlled through the interorgan cooperation of the small intestine, kidneys, and bone.

### *Sources*

Animal products are good sources of P. Except for seeds which can have a substantial amount of P, plants and their products (e.g., hays and straws) generally have a low content of P. Insoluble Ca and Mg phytates in cereals and other plant products reduce P bioavailability to animals.

### *Absorption and Transport*

Phosphate in the intestinal lumen is absorbed by the small intestine via three $Na^+$-dependent phosphate transporters against an electrochemical gradient: sodium-phosphate cotransporter (NaPi2b), phosphate transporter-1 (PiT1), and phosphate transporter-2 (PiT2) (Candeal et al. 2017). NaPi2b, the major transporter of phosphate in the gut, transports phosphate across the apical membrane of the enterocyte with a stoichiometry of 3:1 $Na^+$:$HPO_4^{2-}$ at a relative low $K_M$ of ~10 μM (Sabbagh et al. 2011). The $Na^+$ concentration in the luminal fluid is greater than that in the cytosol of the enterocyte through the action of the $Na^+/K^+$-ATPase at the basolateral membrane, thereby providing a concentration gradient to drive $Na^+$-dependent phosphate absorption. PiT1 and PiT2 preferentially transport monobasic phosphate species with a 2:1 $Na^+$:$H_2PO_4^-$ stoichiometry (Khanal and Nemere 2008). Upon entering the enterocyte, phosphate is transported as a free anion to its basolateral membrane. At present, details of phosphate efflux across the basolateral membrane of the enterocyte into lamina propria are unknown. However, there is evidence for $Na^+$-dependent phosphate transport out of the intestinal basolateral membrane (Kikuchi and Ghishan 1987). Basolateral phosphate transport is bidirectional, depending on dietary intake of phosphate (Sabbagh et al. 2011). Phosphate is absorbed into the portal vein as a free anion and is taken up by extraintestinal cells through $Na^+$-dependent transporters, NaPi2a, NaPi2c, PiT1, and PiT2. Note that NaPi2a and NaPi2c in the apical membrane of the proximal tubule are responsible for the reabsorption of 80% of filtered phosphate (Sabbagh et al. 2011).

Phosphate homeostasis in animals is regulated by many factors, including intestinal absorption of dietary phosphate, renal reabsorption, and excretion of phosphate, as well as the exchange of phosphate between extracellular and bone storage pools (Marks et al. 2010). Physiological concentrations of calcitriol enhance intestinal phosphate absorption by stimulating the expression of NaPi2b in enterocytes, and, in the case of low plasma phosphate concentration, the mobilization of phosphate from the bone matrix (Figure 10.6). In addition, parathyroid hormone stimulates the release of phosphate from bones (Candeal et al. 2017). In response to hyperphosphatemia or hypocalcemia, the secretion of calcitriol and PTH is enhanced to decrease renal reabsorption of phosphate (Blaine et al. 2015). This physiological response helps to prevent an excessive elevation of plasma phosphate due to the bone resorption. In contrast, growth hormone, insulin, insulin-like growth factor 1, and thyroxine increase the renal reabsorption of phosphate. Thus, factors that favor muscle protein synthesis usually promote skeletal growth.

### *Functions*

Phosphorus has many biochemical functions in animals (Kornberg et al. 1999). A key role of phosphorus is the formation of calcium phosphate from $Ca^{2+}$ and phosphate in the process of biomineralization, which is critical in providing the skeleton of organisms and maintaining body structure. In addition, as a component of nucleotides (ATP, GTP, and UTP), phosphocreatine, nucleic acids (RNA and DNA), phospholipids, sphingosine 1-phosphate, and inositol-1,4,5-trisphosphate, phosphorus participates in (1) energy transfer, storage, and utilization; (2) covalent modifications of proteins and enzymes that are critical for the regulation of their biological activities; and (3) regulation of cellular signaling and physiological responses to hormonal and nutritional alterations. Furthermore, upon their entry into cells or production through metabolism, many low-molecular-weight substrates and metabolites are phosphorylated to prevent their leakage (e.g., phosphate groups of nucleotides, intermediates of glycolysis, pyridoxal phosphate, and 2,3-diphosphoglycerate), thereby maximizing the efficiency of product formation and modulating tissue oxygenation. Finally, phosphate is required as part of a coenzyme (e.g., pyridoxal phosphate) or an activator of an enzyme (phosphate-activated glutaminase and 1α-hydroxylase) to improve the efficiency of enzymatic reactions. Therefore, phosphorus occupies the central stage of cell metabolism.

#### *Deficiency Symptoms*

In animals, most syndromes of phosphorus deficiency (also known as hypophosphatemia) are similar to those of vitamin D deficiency. This nutritional problem commonly occurs in grazing livestock receiving no phosphate supplementation, especially in tropical and subtropical areas and North America, as a result of low P content in grass due to low P content available (e.g., present as tricalcium phosphate) to the local plants (Davidson 1945; McDonald et al. 2011). Feeding forages (e.g., alfalfa) that contain high Ca content but low P content can exacerbate P deficiency in ruminants. In addition, malnutrition, malabsorption, or disorders affecting renal phosphate reabsorption can result in hypophosphatemia. Animals with P deficiency exhibit whole-body phosphate depletion, as well as hemolysis, fatigue, reduced myocardial contractility, muscle weakness, respiratory failure, tremors, ataxia, anorexia, nausea, and vomiting (Allen-Durrance 2017). Prolonged P deficiency causes reduced feed intake; protein malnutrition due to reductions in the absorption, transport and synthesis of AAs, impaired growth and development of bones and the whole body (including skeletal muscle); bone resorption (demineralization); and skeletal defects (e.g., rickets in the young and osteomalacia in adults) (Harris 2014). Finally, male and female animals suffer from infertility when their diets are deficient in P (Greene et al. 1985; Morrow 1969).

#### *Excess*

Hyperphosphatemia is defined as an abnormally high phosphate concentration in the plasma. In animals, this metabolic disorder can result from excessive phosphate intake, inadequate calcium intake, decreased renal phosphate excretion (e.g., low levels of parathyroid hormone), or disorders (e.g., tissue injury and excessive bone resorption) that promote the exit of intracellular phosphate to extracellular space. Syndromes of hyperphosphatemia include reduced feed intake and impaired growth; poor digestibility of iron, calcium, magnesium, and zinc; impaired skeletal growth and development; anorexia, nausea, vomiting, and diarrhea; and low calcium concentrations in the plasma. Animals with phosphorus deficiency also exhibit abnormal neurological function and seizures; cardiovascular dysfunction; nonskeletal calcification of tissues (especially the kidneys); and acid–base imbalance (i.e., metabolic acidosis) and kidney stone (Ketteler et al. 2016; Spasovski 2015).

### Magnesium

Magnesium was first isolated by Humphry Davy in 1808. However, its discovery dates back to 1618, when a farmer in Epsom, England found that water from his well contained a bitter compound that could heal scratches and rashes. Interestingly, cows refused to drink this water and the unknown substance was later identified as $MgSO_4 \cdot 7H_2O$. Magnesium is a divalent cation, and is the sixth most abundant macromineral in living organisms (animal body: Ca>P>K>Na>S>Mg). Its concentration is about 0.8–2.2 mM in the plasma, and about 1–3 mM in the intracellular fluid. About 90% of the intracellular $Mg^{2+}$ is bound to ribosomes or polynucleotides (Wolf and Cittadini 2003).

### *Sources*

Magnesium is widely present in plant- and animal-source feedstuffs. Wheat bran, dried yeast, and most vegetable protein concentrates (e.g., cottonseed cake and linseed cake) are good sources of Mg. Clovers usually contain more Mg than grasses. Magnesium oxide is usually the form used for dietary supplementation to farm animals.

### *Absorption and Transport*

As noted previously, the reticulo-rumen is the major site for the absorption of dietary Mg in ruminants (Tomas and Potter 1976). In these species, there is no absorption of luminal $Mg^{2+}$ by their omasum or abomasum. In all animals, magnesium in the intestinal lumen is absorbed by the enterocyte via the apical transient receptor potential melastatin-related protein-6 (TRPM6), which is a cation channel protein (Voets et al. 2004). TRPM7 is required for the activity of TRPM6. Both TRPM6 and TRPM7 are unusual bifunctional proteins that consist of an ion channel and a cAMP-dependent protein kinase (Ryazanova et al. 2010). In the enterocyte, $Mg^{2+}$ is present as a free ion, as well as bound to proteins and nucleic acids. This mineral exits the enterocyte across its basolateral membrane into the lamina propria via CNNM4 (ancient conserved domain protein 4; Yamazaki et al. 2013), which is an electroneutral $Na^+/Mg^{2+}$ exchanger. This basolateral CNNM4 transports $Mg^{2+}$ out of the enterocyte in exchange for the entry of $Na^+$ without affecting transmembrane currents. $Mg^{2+}$ enters the portal vein from the lamina propria. This mineral is transported in the plasma in both free and protein (albumin)-bound forms, and is taken up by extraintestinal cells (including renal tubular epithelial cells) through $Mg^{2+}$ transporters, including TRPM6/7 (Ryazanova et al. 2010). Renal reabsorption of $Mg^{2+}$ is stimulated by PTH via the cAMP-dependent cell signaling, and is reduced in hypercalcemia due to the inhibition of PTH synthesis and release. Thus, $Mg^{2+}$ homeostasis is regulated by gastrointestinal absorption, utilization (e.g., milk production), and excretion via the kidneys. Although about 80% of plasma Mg is filtered at the glomerulus during a single pass, only 3% of it is excreted in the urine, and most of Mg in the renal tubule lumen is reabsorbed into the blood via the apical TRPM6/7 (Musso 2009).

### *Functions*

$Mg^{2+}$ interacts with ATP, DNA, and RNA to stabilize these polyphosphate compounds. This divalent ion is needed to alleviate electrostatic repulsion between phosphates, thereby stabilizing ATP structure, as well as base pairing and stacking in nucleic acids (Wolf and Cittadini 2003). In addition, $Mg^{2+}$ is bound to many proteins in cells, including membrane proteins. More than 300 enzymes require $Mg^{2+}$ as a cofactor for their catalytic activity, including those that synthesize and utilize ATP. Examples of these enzymes are given as follows:

1. Glycolysis pathway
   Glucose + ATP → G-6-P + ADP (Hexokinase)
   F-6-P + ATP → F-1,6-P + ADP (Phosphofructose kinase)
   1,3-Bis-P-glycerate + ADP ↔ 3-P-glycerate + ATP (Phosphoglycerate kinase)
   2-Phosphoglycerate ↔ Phosphoenolpyruvate (Enolase)
   Phosphoenolpyruvate ↔ Pyruvate (Pyruvate kinase)
2. Pyruvate dehydrogenase kinase: Active form → Inactive form
3. Pyruvate dehydrogenase phosphatase: Inactive form → Active form
4. Glycogen metabolism: G-1-P ↔ G-6-P (Phosphoglucomutase)
5. Gluconeogenesis: Propionate + ATP → Propionyl-CoA + AMP (Acyl-CoA synthase)
6. Pentose cycle
   G-6-P → 6-Phosphogluconolactone (Glucose-6-P dehydrogenase)

6-Phosphogluconolactone → 6-Phosphogluconate (Gluconolactone hydrolase)
Ribose 5-P → 5-Phosphoribosyl-1-pyrophosphate (PRPP) (PRPP synthetase)
Ribose 5-P + Xylulose 5-P ↔ Sedoheptulose 7-P + Glyceraldehyde 3-P (Transketolase, vitamin $B_6$)

7. Fatty acid degradation: Fatty acid + ATP → R-SCoA + AMP (Acyl-CoA synthase)
8. Urea cycle: Cit + Asp + ATP → Argininosuccinate (AS) + AMP (AS synthase)
9. Pathways of syntheses of purines and pyrimidines: Many enzymes require $Mg^{2+}$
10. DNA and RNA syntheses: Deoxyribonucleotides → DNA (DNA polymerase)
    DNA → RNA (RNA polymerase)
11. Protein synthesis: $Mg^{2+}$ is required for binding mRNA to ribosomes

$Mg^{2+}$ conducts electrical (nerve) impulses and alters the firing threshold of neurons in the central nervous system (CNS). The physiological concentrations of $Mg^{2+}$ block the binding of glutamate and aspartate to, and thus the activation of, N-methyl-D-aspartate (NMDA) receptors in neurons (Morris 1992). Glutamate and aspartate are the principal neurotransmitters for excitatory synaptic transmission in the CNS of vertebrates. A low concentration of $Mg^{2+}$ in the brain or cerebro spinal fluid (< 0.25 mM) causes the NMDA receptors to be activated by glutamate and aspartate, and reduces the threshold at which neurons repetitively fire nerve impulses (action potentials), resulting in nervous disorders and, consequently, tetany.

#### *Deficiency Symptoms*

Mg deficiency (also known as hypomagnesemia) reduces ATP production, endothelial nitric oxide synthesis, and antioxidative reactions, as well as feed intake, growth, immunity, and survival of animals. Mammals, birds, and fish with hypomagnesemia also exhibit neuromuscular irritability, tetany, seizures, depression, abnormal carbohydrate and AA metabolism, impaired blood flow in the microvasculature, and infertility (Al-Ghamdi et al. 1994; Kubena and Durlach 1990). Grass tetany frequently occurs in ruminants fed magnesium-inadequate forages or diets, particularly when ruminal $NH_4^+$ concentrations are elevated to reduce Mg absorption (Martens and Schweigel 2000). Hypomagnesemia can result in the activation of neurons, leading to sustained excitations and muscle cramps. Furthermore, Mg deficiency can induce hypocalcemia and hypokalemia by decreasing PTH activity, the resorption of bone, increasing the calcification of soft tissues, and augmenting the renal excretion of $Ca^{2+}$ and $K^+$. Excess of dietary potassium interferes with the absorption and metabolism of $Mg^{2+}$ in animals, therefore increasing risk for hypomagnesemia and tetany. Magnesium deficiency can be treated by oral administration of magnesium (as magnesium citrate, magnesium oxide, magnesium sulfate, or magnesium chloride). In clinics, intravenous Mg treatment is advocated to treat preeclampsia and acute myocardial infarction (Musso 2009).

#### *Excess*

Hypermagnesemia is defined as an abnormally high magnesium concentration in the plasma. This metabolic disorder is rare in farm animals, but can result from excessive magnesium intake, impaired renal excretion of magnesium, and excessive magnesium mobilization in animals. Syndromes of hypermagnesemia include nausea and vomiting; reduced DM digestibility, profuse diarrhea (because of the water flowing into the large intestine), and dehydration; reduced feed intake and impaired growth; muscle weakness and impaired breathing; and low blood pressure, low heart rate, and cardiac arrest (Topf and Murray 2003). Of note, concentrations of $Mg^{2+}$ (as $MgSO_4$) in the ruminal fluid $\geq$320 μg/mL are toxic to ruminal microbes as assessed by the rate of cellulose digestion (Georgievskii et al. 1982).

### SULFUR (S)

A natural form of sulfur known as *shiliuhuang* (a traditional Chinese medicine) was known in China since the sixth century BC. In 1777, Antoine Lavoisier reported that sulfur was an element, not a compound. The name of sulfur is derived from the Latin word *sulpur*, meaning "brimstone." Elemental sulfur is a bright and yellow crystal at room temperature. It has a chemical reactivity with all elements, except for gold, platinum, iridium, tellurium, and the noble gases. In nature, sulfur usually exists as sulfide and sulfate minerals.

#### *Sources*

Most of the sulfur in animals occurs in organic forms, for example, in sulfur-containing AAs (cysteine, cystine, methionine, homocysteine, and taurine), glutathione, and protein (Hoffer 2002). Disulfide compounds with S–S bonds confer the mechanical strength and insolubility of keratin, which occurs in outer skin, hair, and feathers (Chapter 4). Tissue and milk proteins have a ratio of N to S of ~13:1 to 15:1 (g/g). Wool, which is rich in cystine, contains ~4% sulfur. Sulfur is also present in two vitamins (biotin and thiamin), coenzyme A, and chondroitin sulfate (a structural component of cartilage, bone, tendons, and walls of blood vessels). In contrast to animal products, sulfur content is generally low in plants (Pond et al. 1995). However, plants grown on soils containing high sulfur content or fertilized with sulfur (e.g., ammonium sulfate) have an adequate or even relatively high amount of sulfur, and, in ruminants, may exacerbate a copper deficiency especially in the presence of molybdenum (Hardt et al. 1991). Most natural feedstuffs in some regions of the world (e.g., North America) contain sufficient sulfur to meet the requirements of grazing ruminants (Greene et al. 2016). The concentration of inorganic sulfur in water varies greatly among regions, ranging from <10 mg/L to 75 mg/L.

In the rumen of ruminants, the sources of sulfur for bacteria are either inorganic sulfate or organosulfur substances (e.g., sulfonates, sulfate esters, or sulfur-containing AAs). Sulfur content in the diets of most ruminants must be between 0.18% and 0.24% of DM to allow for sufficient synthesis of sulfur-containing compounds by ruminal bacteria (Suttle 2010). Sulfate is transported into the microorganisms through (1) ATP binding cassette (ABC)-type transporters and (2) major facilitator superfamily-type transporters (Kertesz et al. 2001). In contrast, ABC-type transporters are responsible for the uptake of all sulfonates and sulfate esters. The synthesis of these transporters is regulated by sulfur supplies. Because of the limited synthesis of sulfur-containing AAs from sulfur by nonruminants, inorganic sulfur in the diet has virtually no nutritional value for pigs, poultry, dogs, cats, rats, and fish.

#### *Absorption and Transport*

In animals, organic forms of sulfur are absorbed by the small intestine as cysteine, methionine, taurine, and glutathione, which are transported among different tissues (Chapter 7). In ruminants, inorganic forms of sulfur are used by ruminal microbes to synthesize cysteine and methionine, which are then used by the host (Chapter 7). However, the efficiency of sulfur utilization for microbial synthesis of AAs and proteins is affected by its sources (Suttle 2010). Absorbed sulfur enters the portal circulation. Large amounts of sulfur are stored as taurine in skeletal muscle, heart, and eyes, and as glutathione in tissues of digestive and reproductive systems (Wu 2013).

#### *Functions*

Traditionally, little attention has been paid to the nutrition of the sulfur element in nonruminants because these animals ingest sulfur mainly in the form of protein or supplemental methionine. In ruminants, sulfur (including supplemental inorganic compounds) is used for the microbial synthesis of cysteine and methionine, as noted previously (Felix et al. 2014). This mineral in the forms of sulfur-containing AAs is essential to the life of all organisms. Furthermore, physiological levels of $H_2S$, a metabolite of cysteine, and a gaseous signaling molecule in animal cells play an important role in regulating neurotransmission, blood flow, immune response, and nutrient metabolism in the body (Wu 2013).

#### *Deficiency Symptoms*

In animals, a deficiency of sulfur is generally associated with protein deficiency, as described in Chapter 7. In ruminants, dietary sulfur is a limiting factor for the microbial synthesis of cysteine and methionine (and therefore microbial protein synthesis) in ruminants when nonprotein nitrogen (e.g., urea) is supplemented to the diet (Suttle 2010). Replacement of some protein in ruminant rations with non-AA nitrogen (e.g., urea) may increase the risk of a sulfur deficiency, because the substituted protein contains methionine and cysteine. For efficient utilization of urea by lactating cows, a N/S ratio of 12:1 in the diet is adequate and a ratio of 10:1 is acceptable for all other kinds of ruminants (NRC 1976). In addition, sulfur supplementation must be considered for ruminant production in regions where the sulfur content in soil or plants is low.

#### *Excess*

Sulfate concentrations of <600 ppm (mg/L) in drinking water and a sulfur content of <0.4% of DM in diets are generally safe for animals, including swine, poultry and ruminants (Suttle 2010). Horses and rodents can tolerate 0.5% sulfur (DM basis) in their diets. Because total sulfur content is high (0.4–1.5% of DM) in dried distillers grains with solubles (DDGS) that is now often included in ruminant and nonruminant diets, producers have concern over sulfur toxicity. Excess sulfur in diets disturbs the acid–base balance in animals, reduces their feed intake and growth performance, and causes lesions of the gray matter in the brain (Drewnoski et al. 2014). Because inorganic sulfur is often supplemented to ruminants, producers have concern over the adverse effects of its excess. Georgievskii et al. (1982) reported that concentrations of sulfur (as $Na_2SO_4$) in the ruminal fluid ≥1 mg/mL are toxic to ruminal microbes as assessed by the rate of cellulose digestion. NRC (2005) suggested that the maximum tolerable limit for sulfur in beef cattle diets was 0.3% in diets containing greater than 85% concentrate, or 0.5% in diets containing greater than 40% forage. Pogge et al. (2014) reported that feeding a high-S diet (containing 0.68% S as sodium sulfate) to growing steers for 28 days reduced the absorption of Cu, Mn, and Zn by the small intestine but had no effect on the absorption or retention of Ca, K, Mg, and Na. Ruminants (e.g., cattle, sheep and goats) consuming elevated levels of sulfur may display "stargazing" as a symptom of polioencephalomalacia due to necrosis of the cerebrocortical region of the brain (Gould et al. 2002). In ruminants, toxicity of sulfur occurs because of the following reasons: (1) formation of hydrogen sulfite (a toxic agent) by the gastrointestinal flora to kill bacteria and induce excessive production of reactive oxygen species to cause oxidative damage; (2) production of sulfuric acid to reduce pH in the ruminal fluid and host tissues; and (3) reduced absorption of other minerals, such as copper, zinc and manganese by the small intestine because the ruminal reduction of sulfur produces intermediates that form water-insoluble complexes with the minerals, such as copper sulfide ($Cu_2S$), zinc sulfide (ZnS), and manganese sulfide (MnS) (Drewnoski et al. 2014). Thus, high sulfur content is a major factor limiting the inclusion of DDGS in animals (e.g., feedlot cattle) diets, and drinking water can also be a problematic source of sulfur especially in certain regions of the world (e.g., western ranges in the United States).

## MICROMINERALS

### Iron ($Fe^{2+}$ and $Fe^{3+}$)

There is a rich history of work on iron (Sheftel et al. 2012). Iron objects were found in Egypt around 3500 BC. However, René Antoine Ferchault de Réaumur was the first person to write about the various types of iron when he published his book in 1722. Iron is the most abundant trace mineral in animals (Table 10.9). Except for newborn pigs, which have a relatively low iron content at birth, neonates contain relatively high levels of iron, about 70 mg per kg BW. In mammals, birds, and fish, almost all iron (>90%) is present in protein-bound forms as iron, oxo–diiron (Fe–O–Fe), oxo–iron–zinc (Fe–O–Zn), iron–sulfur clusters (Fe–S), and heme (Ward and Kaplan 2012). Free iron concentrations are particularly low for two reasons: (1) $Fe^{3+}$ is barely water soluble and (2) $Fe^{2+}$ is toxic to cells.

#### *Sources*

Iron is widely distributed in foods, but its content varies greatly. Concentrates, green leafy materials, and roughage generally provide sufficient quantities of iron for farm animals (McDonald et al.

**TABLE 10.9**
**Content of Microminerals in the Bodies of Animals[a]**

| Microminerals | mg/kg Body Weight | Microminerals | mg/kg Body Weight |
|---|---|---|---|
| Iron | 30–80 | Cobalt | 0.02–0.10 |
| Zinc[a] | 8–45 | Nickel | 0.04–0.05 |
| Copper | 2–3.5 | Selenium | 0.02–0.025 |
| Molybdenum | 1–4 | Boron | <0.02 |
| Manganese | 0.48–0.56 | Bromine | <0.02 |
| Iodine | 0.2–0.5 | Vanadium | <0.02 |

*Source:* Georgievskii, V.I. et al. 1982. *Mineral Nutrition of Animals*. Butterworths, London, U.K.; Mertz, W. 1987. *Trace Elements in Human and Animal Nutrition*, Vol. 1, edited by Mertz, W., Academic Press, New York, NY.

[a] The content of zinc in the body varies markedly with animal species and physiological states (e.g., 8.5 mg/kg BW in newborn calves, 20 mg/kg BW in newborn piglets, and 45 mg/kg BW in laying hens [Georgievskii 1982; Herzig et al. 2009]).

2011). Leguminous plant species have more iron (200–400 ppm on a dry matter basis) than grasses (~40 ppm). Ferritin, which is a protein complexed with $Fe^{3+}$, is a major form of iron in food legumes such as soybeans (Theil 2004). Cereal grains are also good sources of iron (30–60 ppm). However, the bioavailability of iron in plant-source foods is low for mammals, birds, and fish (Haider et al. 2016). Animal products contain more bioavailable iron than plant products.

### *Absorption*

In the stomach, iron binds to a glycoprotein called gastroferrin, which is secreted by the oxyntic cells of the gastric mucosa; the iron-complexed gastroferrin flows into the duodenum along with food. In the lumen of the small intestine, $Fe^{3+}$ is reduced to $Fe^{2+}$ by vitamin C or duodenal cytochrome *b* (DCYTB, also called duodenal ferric reductase) on the apical membrane surface. DCYTB is a transmembrane oxidoreductase that utilizes intracellular vitamin C as an electron donor to reduce extracellular $Fe^{3+}$ to $Fe^{2+}$ (Asard et al. 2013). Subsequently, $Fe^{2+}$ is taken up into the enterocyte through the apical membrane divalent cation transporter-1 (DCT1; also known as divalent metal ion transporter-1 [DMT1] and natural resistance-associated macrophage protein-2 [NRAMP2]). DCT1 also transports $Zn^{2+}$, $Cu^{2+}$, and $Mn^{2+}$, but plays only a minor role in transporting $Ca^{2+}$ or $Mg^{2+}$. Upon entering the enterocyte, $Fe^{2+}$ binds to the paraferritin complex (a protein complex) and is then transferred to the basolateral membrane for exit into the lamina propria via ferroportin-1 (Figure 10.7). Because ferroportin only recognizes $Fe^{2+}$, $Fe^{3+}$ must be reduced to $Fe^{2+}$ in the paraferritin complex (Ward and Kaplan 2012). This protein complex does not store iron, but only mediates the passage of iron to the basolateral membrane of the enterocyte for export. Finally, $Fe^{3+}$ that is bound to mucins in the lumen of the small intestine enters the enterocyte through the mobilferrin-mediated ferric iron pathway. In this pathway, $\beta_3$-integrin facilitates the influx of $Fe^{3+}$ into the cell. Within the cytosol of the enterocyte, mobilferrin, which is localized in vesicles near the apical membrane in a complex linked to $\beta_3$-integrin and gastroferrin, shuttles $Fe^{3+}$ from $\beta_3$-integrin to gastroferrin. Eventually, $Fe^{3+}$ is transferred to the paraferritin complex.

Heme iron (heme-$Fe^{2+}$), which is bound to the heme's porphyrin ring, is absorbed as an intact complex from the small-intestinal lumen into the enterocyte via its apical membrane heme carrier protein-1 (HCP1). Note that the HCP1-mediated iron transport functions independently of the putative heme receptor and receptor-mediated heme endocytosis, which was proposed in the 1970s for heme uptake by the small intestine of both pigs and humans (Grasbeck et al. 1979). Once inside the enterocyte, heme is degraded by heme oxygenase to release $Fe^{2+}$ and biliverdin. $Fe^{2+}$ binds to the paraferritin complex.

Intracellular $Fe^{2+}$ exits the enterocyte across its basolateral membrane via ferroportin-1. Hephaestin, which is a transmembrane protein in the basolateral membrane of the enterocyte,

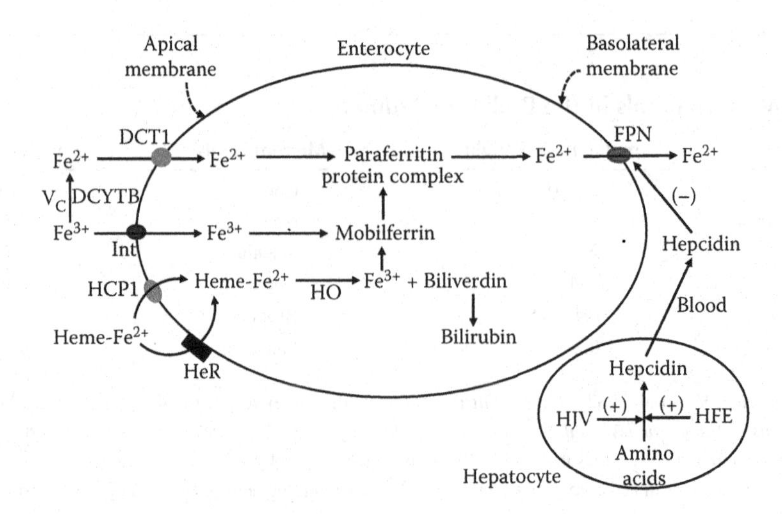


**FIGURE 10.7** Intestinal absorption of dietary iron. In the lumen of the small intestine, $Fe^{3+}$ is reduced to $Fe^{2+}$ by vitamin C ($V_c$) or duodenal cytochrome *b* (DCYTB) on the apical membrane surface. Inorganic $Fe^{2+}$ is absorbed by the enterocyte via divalent cation transporter-1 (DCT1), whereas $Fe^{3+}$ binds mucins and then enters the cell via $\beta_3$-integrin (Int). Heme-$Fe^{2+}$ is taken up by the enterocyte through heme carrier protein-1 (HCP1) or a heme receptor (HeR)-mediated endocytosis. Inside the enterocyte, heme-$Fe^{3+}$ is oxidized by heme oxygenase (HO). $Fe^{3+}$ is reduced to $Fe^{2+}$, which is transported by the paraferritin protein complex to the basolateral membrane and exits the cell via ferroportin (FPN). FPN is inhibited by hepcidin (a 25-AA polypeptide), which is synthesized from amino acids in hepatocytes. Hepatic synthesis of hepcidin is activated by human hemochromatosis protein (HFE) and hemojuvelin (HJV). Under inflammatory conditions, hepcidin production is elevated to reduce intestinal iron absorption and result in anemia. (+), activation; (−), inhibition.

facilitates the basolateral export of copper (Vulpe et al. 1999). The abundance of ferroportin in enterocytes is regulated by a 25-AA polypeptide called hepcidin, which is synthesized by hepatocytes (Ward and Kaplan 2012). The hepatic expression of hepcidin is upregulated by two proteins: HFE (human hemochromatosis protein) and HJV (hemojuvelin) (Barton et al. 2015). Hepcidin inhibits ferroportin activity by promoting the trafficking of ferroportin from the plasma membrane into the cytosol and then the degradation of ferroportin. Under inflammatory conditions, hepcidin concentration in the plasma is abnormally high, the intestinal absorption of iron is reduced, and iron is trapped within macrophages and the liver (Ganz 2003). This results in anemia due to a low concentration of iron in erythrocytes. In contrast, when hepcidin concentration in the plasma is abnormally low (e.g., in hemochromatosis, a hereditary disease associated with excessive build-up of iron in the plasma), the circulating levels of iron are high primarily because of an increase in ferroportin-mediated efflux of iron from cells (including enterocytes, hepatocytes, and immunocytes).

### *Transport in the Blood*

The absorbed iron enters the portal circulation. In the blood, $Fe^{2+}$ is oxidized to $Fe^{3+}$ by ferroxidase II, and $Fe^{3+}$ is transported by binding to transferrin (iron-binding protein [a glycoprotein] released by hepatocytes), which contains two sites for binding $Fe^{3+}$ ions but binds $Fe^{2+}$ weakly (Harris 2014). Of note, transferrin binds $Fe^{3+}$ tightly, but reversibly. Transferrin receptors on the plasma membrane of extraintestinal cells bind transferrin for its uptake into the cytoplasm via endocytosis. The entrapped transferrin merges with an endosome, where $Fe^{3+}$ is reduced to $Fe^{2+}$ by STEAP3 (six transmembrane epithelial antigen of the prostate protein-3; a metalloreductase [Sendamarai et al. 2008]). $Fe^{2+}$ exits the endosome, via DCT1, into the cytosol, where $Fe^{2+}$ binds two proteins (ferritin and hemosiderin) for storage. Hemosiderin is a water-insoluble protein complex, and is typically found in lysosomes. During pregnancy, uteroferrin (a progesterone-induced iron-binding protein) plays an important role in the storage and transport of iron in the conceptus (Bazer et al. 1991; Roberts et al. 1986).

**TABLE 10.10**
**Concentrations of Microminerals in the Serum of Animals (μg/100 mL)**

| Animal | Mn | Zn | Mo | Cu | Co | I | Fe |
|---|---|---|---|---|---|---|---|
| Dairy cows | 1.5–2.5 | 80–150 | 0.3–0.6 | 50–120 | 0.5–0.7 | 4–8 | 100 |
| Calves | 3–5 | 100–150 | 1.0 | 80–120 | 1.0 | 6.1–7.4 | 120–160 |
| Sheep | 4–5 | 100–120 | 3 | 60–100 | 0.5–1.0 | 4–8 | 100–150 |
| Pigs | 4–5 | 160 | 0.6–1.4 | 200 | 17–40 | 5–8 | 180 |
| Horses | 1.7–2.5 | 60–70 | 2–5 | 100–190 | 0.7–2.2 | 2–4 | 110–200 |
| Chickens | 10–24 | 150–210 | 10–34 | 20–30 | 0.5–0.8 | 5–10 | 102–516[a] |

*Source:* Georgievskii, V.I. et al. 1982. *Mineral Nutrition of Animals.* Butterworths, London, U.K; Huck, D.W. and A.J. Clawson. 1976. *J. Anim. Sci.* 43:1231–1246; Hunt, C.D. 1989. *Biol. Trace Elem. Res.* 22:201–220; Mondal, S., S. Haldar, P. Saha, T.K. Ghosh. 2010. *Biol. Trace Elem. Res.* 137:190–205; Ronis, M.J.J. et al. 2015. *Exp. Biol. Med.* 240:58–66; Smith, P. 1982. *Vet. Rec.* 111:149; Stanier, P. 1983. *Vet. Rec.* 113:518; Yörük, I. et al. 2007. *Biol. Trace Elem. Res.* 118:38-42.

[a] Concentrations of iron in the serum of chickens (μg/100 ml) are: growing chicks = 102; nonlaying hens = 158; laying hens = 516.

### *Content in the Body and Tissues*

The content of iron in animals (mg/kg BW) is as follows: cows, 60; horses, 66; sows, 50; 0- to 35-day-old pigs, 36–40; and chickens, 80 (Georgievskii et al. 1982). The content of iron in the blood plasma (mg/L) of animals is as follows: adult beef cattle, 1.4–1.5; calves, 1.2–1.6; chickens, 1.0 (nonlaying hens) to 5.2 (laying hens); mice, 0.9; pigs, 1.23; and sheep, 1.52–1.82. Its concentrations in serum are shown in Table 10.10. Of note, concentrations of micro-minerals (including iron) in serum or plasma are generally not good indicators of their nutritional status in animals, because micro-minerals are sequestered within cells and are released from the cells into the plasma under various physiological and pathological conditions. The content of iron in the tissues of mammals (mg/100 g fresh weight) is as follows: whole blood, 20–45; spleen, 20–40; liver, 10–20; kidneys, 4–6; heart, 4–8; skeletal muscle, 1.5–3; brain, 2–2.5; and bones, 3.5–4 (Georgievskii et al. 1982).

### *Functions*

Iron is essential for erythropoiesis (the formation of red blood cells), which occurs in fetal livers (mammals), erythroid cells (embryos of birds), red bone marrow (postnatal mammals and birds), and kidneys of fish (Bruns and Ingram 1973; Palis and Segel 1998; Roberts et al. 1986). Iron is a component of heme (Figure 10.8). Heme proteins include hemoglobin and myoglobin (which are used for $O_2$ binding, transport, and storage), metalloenzymes, and cytochromes. Furthermore, iron is required for the activities of some non-heme enzymes (Sheftel et al. 2012). Irons also participate in oxidoreduction reactions. In cytochromes, the oxidation and reduction of the iron atom are essential to their biological function. In contrast, oxidation of $Fe^{2+}$ to $Fe^{3+}$ in hemoglobin or myoglobin inhibits their biological activity.

*Hemoglobins* Concentrations of hemoglobins in the blood of healthy animals are 100–140 mg/L (Fox et al. 2002; Sheftel et al. 2012). These proteins contain 60% of the body's iron in horses, 68% in dogs and cattle, 73% in rats, and 80% in pigs (Georgievskii et al. 1982). Hemoglobins are tetrameric proteins (MW, 64,500): HbA (normal adult hemoglobin, $\alpha_2\beta_2$), HbF (fetal hemoglobin, $\alpha_2\gamma_2$), and HbS (sickle cell hemoglobin, $\alpha_2S_2$, on residue 6 of the β-chain, Val replaces Glu) (Thom et al. 2013). Hemoglobin, which contains 0.34% iron by weight, represents more than 95% of the proteins of the red blood cell (ARC 1981; Sheftel et al. 2012). Hemoglobins of vertebrate erythrocytes transport (1) $O_2$ from the respiratory organ to peripheral tissues; (2) $CO_2$ and protons from peripheral

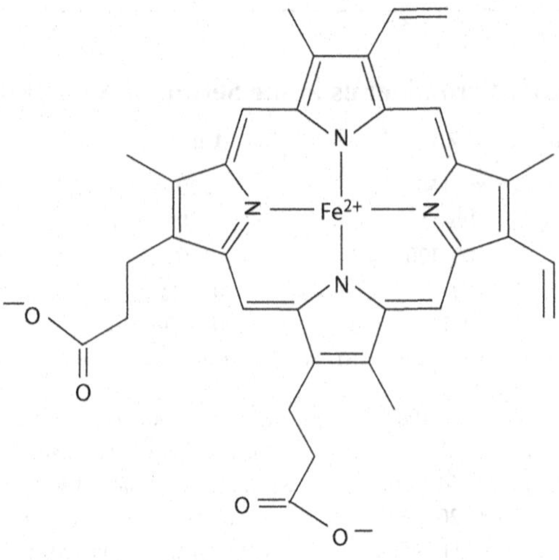

**FIGURE 10.8** The structure of heme. The pyrrole rings and methylene bridge carbons are coplanar, and the iron atom ($Fe^{2+}$) resides in almost the same plane. The fifth and sixth coordination positions of $Fe^{2+}$ are directed perpendicular to, and directly above and below, the plane of the heme ring. Thus, heme acts as a chelator of iron. Heme is synthesized in the liver from succinyl-CoA and glycine.

tissues to the lung for subsequent excretion; and (3) nitric oxide, which is synthesized from arginine in almost all cell types (Glanz 1996). 2,3-Bisphosphoglycerate, an intermediate in glycolysis, stabilizes the tetrameric structure of hemoglobin (Arnone 1972), indicating another important function of glycolysis in the functions of red blood cells.

*Myoglobin* Myoglobin is a single polypeptide chain (MW 16,900). It contains 10% of the body's iron in dogs and cattle, and 20% in rats and horses (Georgievskii et al. 1982). Myoglobin is a minor protein in muscle cells, and is used for the short-term storage of oxygen. In diving mammals such as dolphins and seals, the myoglobin content of skeletal muscle can reach 3%–8% of total protein.

*Cytochromes* Cytochromes are iron-containing heme proteins (Georgievskii et al. 1982). Several cytochromes occur in the respiratory chain, that is, cytochromes $b$, $c_1$, $c$, and $aa_3$ in animal cells. Cytochrome $aa_3$ is also known as cytochrome oxidase, which is the terminal component of the mitochondrial electron transport system. Cytochromes $b$, $c_1$, and $c$ are also classified as dehydrogenases, which are involved as carriers of electrons from flavoproteins to cytochrome $aa_3$ (cytochrome oxidase). Cytochromes P450 and $b_5$ are involved in the microsomal hydroxylation of many drugs, pesticides, carcinogens, and other xenobiotics via the cytochrome P450 monooxygenase systems. Cytochrome $b_5$ is involved in the microsomal $\Delta^9$ desaturation of long-chain fatty acids. In bacteria, nitric oxide reductase (heme-cytochrome $c$) converts NO into nitrous oxide ($N_2O$), and nitrite reductase (heme-cytochrome $c$) catalyzes the formation of $NH_3$ from $NO_2^-$ (Averill 1996).

$$2NO + 2e^- + 2H^+ \text{ (from 2 reduced cytochrome } c) \rightarrow N_2O + H_2O$$
$$+ \text{ 2 oxidized cytochrome } c \quad \text{(nitric oxide reductase containing cytochrome } c\text{-heme, bacteria)}$$

$$NO_2^- + 6e^- \text{ (from 6 reduced cytochrome } c) + 7H^+ \rightarrow NH_3 + \text{6 oxidized cytochrome } c$$
$$+ 2H_2O \quad \text{(nitrite reductase containing cytochrome } c\text{-heme)}$$

*Heme Enzymes* Heme enzymes depend on heme for their biological activities (Poulos 2014). They include peroxidase, catalase, prostaglandin endoperoxide synthase, guanylate cyclase, and myeloperoxidase in animals (Table 10.11). Bacteria contain these enzymes as well as nitrite

**TABLE 10.11**
**Heme and Non-Heme Iron Enzymes**

| Enzymes | Function |
|---|---|
| | **Heme Enzymes** |
| Catalase | $2H_2O_2 \rightarrow 2H_2O + O_2$ |
| Guanylate cyclase | GTP → cGMP + PPi |
| Indoleamine 2,3-dioxygenase (IDO) | Tryptophan catabolism (Tryptophan → *N*-formylkynurenine) |
| Myeloperoxidase | $H_2O_2 + Cl^- \rightarrow H_2O + HOCl$ (hypochlorous acid) |
| Nitrite reductase (heme, bacteria) | $NO_2^-$ (nitrite) + $2e^- + H^+ \rightarrow$ NO (nitric oxide) + $H_2O$ |
| Nitrite reductase (heme, bacteria) | $O_2 + 4e^- + 4H^+ \rightarrow 2H_2O$ |
| Peroxidase | $ROOR' + 2e^- + 2H^+ \rightarrow ROH + R'OH$ (e.g., $H_2O_2 + AH_2 \rightarrow 2H_2O + A$) |
| Prostaglandin endoperoxide synthase | Arachidonic acid + $2O_2 \rightarrow PGH_2$ |
| Tryptophan 2,3-dioxygenase (TDO) | Tryptophan catabolism (Tryptophan → *N*-formylkynurenine) |
| | **Non-Heme Iron Enzymes (Iron–Sulfur Proteins)** |
| Aconitase | Citrate → Isocitrate (Krebs cycle) |
| Adrenodoxin | Cholesterol → Steroid hormones |
| Coenzyme Q reductase | Mitochondrial respiratory chain |
| $\Delta^9$-Desaturase | Synthesis of polyunsaturated fatty acids |
| Dihydroxybiphenyl dioxygenase | Estradiol deoxygenation |
| Ferredoxin hydrogenase (bacteria) | $H_2$ + Oxidized ferredoxin ↔ $2H^+$ + Reduced ferredoxin |
| [Fe]-Hydrogenase (bacteria) | $H_2 \leftrightarrow 2H^+ + 2e^-$ |
| [Fe–Fe]-Hydrogenase (bacteria) | $H_2 \leftrightarrow 2H^+ + 2e^-$ |
| [Ni–Fe]-Hydrogenase (bacteria) | $H_2 \leftrightarrow 2H^+ + 2e^-$ |
| Hydrogenase (bacteria) | $2H_2 + NAD(P)^+$ + 2 Oxidized ferredoxin (Fd) ↔ $5H^+$ + NAD(P)H + 2 Reduced Fd |
| 3-Hydroxyanthranilate dioxygenase | Tryptophan catabolism (3-Hydroxyanthranilate → ACMS) |
| Lipoxygenases | Hydroperoxidation |
| NADH dehydrogenase | Mitochondrial respiratory chain |
| Phenylalanine hydroxylase | Hydroxylation of phenylalanine to tyrosine |
| Proline hydroxylase | Hydroxylation of proline residues in collagen |
| Ribonucleotide reductase | RNDP → Deoxy-RNDP (DNA synthesis) |
| Succinate dehydrogenase | Succinate + FAD ↔ Fumarate + $FADH_2$ (Krebs cycle) |
| Xanthine dehydrogenase | Xanthine → Uric acid (NAD-dependent, purine degradation) |

*Note:* ACMS, 2-amino-3-carboxymuconate semialdehyde; Deoxy-RNDP, deoxyribonucleotide diphosphate (dADP, dUDP, dGDP, and dCDP), which are converted to dATP, dTTP, dGTP, and dCTP for DNA synthesis; RNDP, ribonucleotide diphosphate (ADP, UDP, GDP, and CDP).

reductase. These enzymes have important physiological and immunological functions. For example, NO increases cGMP production by activating guanylate cyclase, whereas hypochlorous acid (HOCl, a strong oxidant) is used by phagocytic cells to kill pathogenic microorganisms. This may explain, in part, why severe iron deficiency is associated with increased incidence of infections.

*Heme-binding Protein* Hemopexin is a heme-binding protein synthesized by hepatocytes (Ascenzi and Fasano 2007). This protein can bind free heme in the hepatocytes and plasma. Therefore, hemopexin plays an important role in heme metabolism and transport.

*Non-heme Iron Enzymes and Proteins* Animals contain many non-heme iron enzymes (Table 10.10). The iron in these enzymes is generally tightly bound to the sulfur atoms of cysteine residues. Hence, these enzymes are called "iron–sulfur proteins," with the iron–sulfur center being 2Fe–2S, 4Fe–4S, or 3Fe–4S. These proteins are located in mitochondria, cytosol, and nucleus to exert their diverse functions (Stehling and Lill 2013).

*Iron Enzymes and Proteins Containing Neither Heme Nor the Iron–Sulfur Center* Prolyl hydroxylase (Fe), lysyl hydroxylase (Fe), and lipoxygenase (Fe) do not contain heme or the iron–sulfur center. However, these enzymes require $Fe^{2+}$ for their catalytic activities. Lipoxygenase oxidizes lipids into hydroperoxide, endoperoxide, and peroxyl free radicals. In animals, iron-binding proteins that do not contain heme or the iron–sulfur center include transferrin (iron-binding protein in blood), uteroferrin (iron-binding protein in the porcine conceptus), and lactoferrin (iron-binding protein in milk). In bacteria, nitrogenase (Fe and Mo) reduces $N_2$ to $NH_3$.

### *Fenton Reaction*

The Fenton reaction is named after Henry John Horstman Fenton, who discovered the formation of a reactive oxygen species from $H_2O_2$ and ferrous iron in 1894. This reaction, which results in the generation of the hydroxyl radical and oxidative stress, is activated under conditions of inflammation (increased intracellular iron concentrations) and tissue injury (increased extracellular iron concentrations) (Hanschmann et al. 2013).

$$Fe^{2+} + H_2O_2 \rightarrow Fe^{3+} + OH^- + OH\cdot$$

### *Interaction with Copper*

Both iron and copper have two oxidation states and are highly redox active. Thus, it is not surprising that iron–copper interactions exist in animal cells (Gulec and Collins 2014). The first nutritional evidence was provided in the 1920s by Conrad Elvehjem and colleagues that rats with anemia induced by dietary iron deficiency required dietary provision of both iron and copper to restore the concentration of hemoglobin in the blood (Hart et al. 1928). When dietary iron is deficient, copper uptake by enterocytes and hepatocytes is elevated, resulting in increased concentrations of copper in these cells (Gulec and Collins 2014). Copper accumulation in the liver can stimulate the synthesis and release of ferroxidase, which catalyzes the oxidation of $Fe^{2+}$ to $Fe^{3+}$ in the plasma, thereby impairing the export of iron from hepatocytes into the blood. When dietary copper is deficient, iron is accumulated in the liver (Williams et al. 1983), because the export of this mineral from hepatocytes into the blood is impaired due to the hepcidin-mediated internalization of ferroportin from the plasma membrane into the cytosol (Kono et al. 2010). Because the iron absorbed from the intestine is retained by the liver, plasma iron concentration is reduced in copper-deficient animals, thereby limiting iron supply to the bone marrow and causing anemia (Reeves and DeMars 2006).

### *Deficiency Symptoms*

In animals, iron deficiency results from inadequate intake and impaired absorption of dietary iron, impaired efflux of iron from the liver, reduced availability of iron-binding and transport proteins due to protein malnutrition, as well as antagonism of iron absorption and transport by other divalent metals (Sheftel et al. 2012). Gestating mammals are highly sensitive to iron deficiency because of their rapidly expanding body fluid volume and rapid fetal growth (Wu et al. 2012). Likewise, compared with adults, neonates are more vulnerable to iron deficiency due to their rapid tissue growth. Nursing animals consuming milk born from iron-deficient dams are at great risk for iron deficiency if not provided with an exogenous source of iron because milk is very low in iron. Low appetite, reduced growth, anemia, reduced blood flow, and impaired immune function are symptoms of iron deficiency. Because of the essential roles of iron in oxygen transport and storage, as well as energy metabolism, animals with iron deficiency exhibit extreme fatigue, weakness, shortness of breath, dizziness, pale skin, chest pain, fast heartbeat, cold feet, and unusual cravings for dirt (Haider et al. 2016; Theil 2004).

Among farm animals, piglets reared in confinement or entirely dependent on unsupplemented milk-based diets are particularly susceptible to anemia (Pond et al. 1995). Pigs are born with a very limited iron reserve and grow very rapidly during the neonatal period (Table 10.12), but sow's milk provides $<8$ mg of iron per day for a 2 kg piglet (compared with its requirement for 70 mg iron per day) (Georgievskii et al. 1982). Thus, newborn piglets must receive an intramuscular injection of 200 mg iron (in the form of an iron–dextran complex) within the first few days after birth. In contrast, anemia is not common in lambs and calves because they usually receive supplemental feeding. The amount of 25–30 mg soluble iron/kg dietary DM is sufficient for the appetite, growth, and development of preruminants (Bremner et al. 1976).

*Excess*

Iron toxicity is not a common problem in farm animals, but may result from a prolonged period of oral administration of iron (Pond et al. 1995). Dietary content of iron at 5 g/kg DM is toxic to 20 kg pigs, and intramuscular administration of a single dose of 0.6 g iron (as ferrous sulfate) per kg BW to 20 kg pigs causes death (Georgievskii et al. 1982). Chronic iron toxicity results in copper and phosphorus deficiencies; stomach pain and gastrointestinal dysfunction (because iron is corrosive to the lining of the gastrointestinal tract); nausea and vomiting; depression, reduced feed intake, and impaired growth; excess generation of reactive oxygen species, oxidative stress, and tissue (e.g., liver and brain) damage; and cardiomyopathy, hypotension, and seizures (Georgievskii et al. 1982; Gozzelino and Arosio 2016; Papanikolaou and Pantopoulos 2005). Animals with iron toxicity may die due to liver failure (Papanikolaou and Pantopoulos 2005).

## Zinc (Zn)

Pure metallic zinc was discovered in 1746 by the German chemist Andreas S. Marggraf. Its name is derived from the German word *Zinke* meaning "spiked" for the shape of zinc crystals. However, centuries earlier, zinc ores were used for making brass (a mixture of copper and zinc), which was found between 1400–1000 BC in Palestine. In the 1930s, Conrad Elvehjem and colleagues discovered that zinc was essential for rat growth (Todd et al. 1934). Two decades later, zinc deficiency due to the consumption of phytate-rich unleavened bread was found to be associated with a type of human dwarfism in Egypt (Prasad et al. 1963). To date, zinc is routinely included in the diets of mammals, birds, and fish.

**TABLE 10.12**
**Content of Iron in the Hemoglobin and Bodies of Young Pigs**

| Age (Days) | Body Weight (BW) (kg) | Hemoglobins in the Body | | Iron in Hemoglobin | | Iron in the Body | |
|---|---|---|---|---|---|---|---|
| | | Amount (g) | Content (mg/kg BW) | Amount (mg) | Content (mg/kg BW) | Amount (mg) | Content (mg/kg BW) |
| 0 | 1.3 | 12.3 | 9.46 | 41.8 | 32.2 | 52.3 | 40.2 |
| 7 | 2.7 | 28.8 | 10.7 | 97.9 | 36.3 | 122.4 | 45.3 |
| 14 | 4.2 | 38.4 | 9.14 | 130.6 | 31.1 | 163.3 | 38.9 |
| 21 | 6.0 | 52.1 | 8.68 | 177.1 | 29.5 | 221.4 | 36.9 |
| 28 | 7.8 | 66.1 | 8.47 | 224.7 | 28.8 | 280.9 | 36.0 |
| 35 | 9.8 | 80.9 | 8.26 | 275.1 | 28.1 | 343.9 | 35.1 |

*Source:* Adapted from Georgievskii, V.I. et al. 1982. *Mineral Nutrition of Animals.* Butterworths, London, U.K.

Zinc does not donate or accept electrons, and therefore zinc is not involved in oxidation–reduction reactions. However, $Zn^{2+}$ has strong attraction to electron pairs (Georgievskii et al. 1982). In the plasma and intracellular fluid, free zinc reacts rapidly with water to yield an insoluble zinc hydroxide:

$$Zn^{2+} + H_2O \rightarrow Zn(OH)_2\downarrow + 2H^+$$

Therefore, proteins are required to transport Zn in animals. In animals, the whole-body content of zinc ranks second among trace minerals behind iron (i.e., 2–2.5 g of zinc/70 kg BW), with most of zinc being present in skeletal muscle (47%), bone (29%), skin (6%), liver (5%), brain (1.5%), kidneys (0.7%), and heart (0.4%) (Harris 2014). Zinc is rich in the seminal fluid of males. In all cells, zinc exists primarily as a complex with proteins and nucleic acids.

*Sources*

Seafood (e.g., oysters, crab, lobster, and other shellfish), meat, eggs, dairy products, fish meal, yeast, seeds, nuts, and legumes (cooked dried beans and peas), as well as the bran and germ of cereal grains are good sources of zinc (Harris 2014). Most practical diets that contain a well-balanced mineral premix can supply sufficient zinc for farm animals. Forage-based diets for ruminants and horses are generally deficient in zinc, and, therefore, are usually supplemented with a free-choice mineral premix (Greene et al. 2000).

*Absorption and Transport*

In gastric fluid with an acidic environment, zinc can exist as a free ion. In the lumen of the small intestine with an alkaline solution, zinc binds to gastroferrin to increase its solubility. Zinc is absorbed into the enterocyte via the apical membrane transporters: ZIP4 (a member of the zinc family of transporters) and DCT-1 (Hojyo and Fukada 2016). Expression of ZIP4 is stimulated by dietary zinc intake. Upon entering the enterocyte, zinc binds primarily to a cytosolic protein called cysteine-rich intracellular protein and possibly a nonspecific binding protein (NSBP) for transport to the basolateral membrane. This mineral may also bind to cytosolic metallothionein for temporary storage in enterocytes. Zinc exits the enterocyte across its basolateral membrane into the lamina propria via Zn transporter-1, then enters the portal circulation. Intestinal absorption of zinc is reduced by various minerals (e.g., calcium and copper) and phytate.

Absorbed zinc enters the portal circulation. In the plasma, 60% and 30% of the zinc binds to albumin and $\alpha_2$-macroglobulin, respectively, and about 10% of the zinc binds to other serum factors (Harris 2014). Free Zn is present in serum at about 0.1 μM. Zinc in the blood is taken up by the liver via ZIP2/3, and exits this organ via ZnT-1 into the systemic circulation. Various other organs take up zinc via ZIPs (e.g., kidneys, ZIP4; pancreas, ZIP1; spleen and bone marrow, ZIP2/3) (Dempski 2012). There is evidence that voltage-gated $Ca^{2+}$ channels take part in the transport of $Zn^{2+}$ into animal cells (Bouron and Oberwinkler 2014). Once entering the cells, zinc is assimilated into various metalloproteins, including metallothionein. Metallothionein is a small protein (MW, 10,000), and about 1/3 of its AA residues are cysteine. Metallothionein may act as a reservoir for zinc, and as a detoxifying agent for toxic heavy metals, such as cadmium.

*Content in the Body and Tissues*

A newborn calf, newborn piglet, and newly hatched chick contain 500, 24–25, and 0.35–0.4 mg zinc, respectively (Georgievskii et al. 1982). The content of zinc in tissues (mg/100 g fresh weight) of adult mammals is as follows: liver, 4–8; kidneys, 1.3–1.8; spleen, 1.5–2.0; heart, 1.4–1.8; skeletal muscle, 0.8–1.2; brain, 0.8–1.3; bones, 6–12; and hide, 2–3. The content of zinc in tissues (mg/100 fresh weight) of 22 kg pigs is as follows: skeletal muscle, 2.2; bones, 5.0; liver, 7.7; whole blood, 0.38; heart, 1.7; hide, 1.2; stomach, 2.1; small intestine, 1.8; and colon, 1.8 (Georgievskii et al. 1982). The concentrations of zinc in the whole blood and plasma are 2.5–6.0 and 1–2 mg/L, respectively.

*Functions*

There are about 100 zinc enzymes associated with the mammalian genome (Harris 2014). Examples of the zinc-dependent enzymes and zinc-binding proteins are summarized in Table 10.13. To maintain a zinc finger structure (a structural configuration that contains zinc ions to stabilize a polypeptide

**TABLE 10.13**
**Zinc-Dependent Enzymes and Binding Proteins in Animals**

| Enzyme | Function |
|---|---|
| Alanyl-glycine dipeptidase | Hydrolysis of alanyl-glycine dipeptide |
| Alcohol dehydrogenase | Alcohol catabolism |
| Alkaline phosphatase | Hydrolyzes phosphate monoesters |
| Aminolevulinic acid dehydrogenase | Biosynthesis of heme |
| Aminopeptidase ($Zn^{2+}$, $Co^{2+}$, $Mo^{2+}$) | Hydrolysis of polypeptides |
| Angiotensin-converting enzyme | Regulation of Na balance and blood pressure |
| Carbonic anhydrase | $CO_2 + H_2O \rightarrow H_2CO_3 \leftrightarrow H^+ + HCO_3^-$ |
| Carboxypeptidase A | Digestion of dietary protein |
| Carboxypeptidase B | Digestion of dietary protein |
| Carnosidase ($Zn^{2+}$, $Mn^{2+}$) | Carnosine + $H_2O$ → L-Histidine + β-Alanine |
| Component 9 of complement | Immune system |
| Dehydroquinate synthase | Microbial synthesis of aromatic amino acids |
| DNAase | DNA degradation |
| DNA polymerase | DNA synthesis from deoxyribonucleotides |
| Enolase ($Zn^{2+}$, $Mg^{2+}$, $Mn^{2+}$) | 2-Phospho-D-glycerate ↔ Phosphoenolpyruvate + $H_2O$ |
| Fructose-1,6-bisphosphatase | Gluconeogenesis |
| Galactosyltransferase complex | Synthesis of lactose |
| Glutamate dehydrogenase | Glutamate + $NAD^+$ ↔ $NH_4^+$ + α-Ketoglutarate + NADH + $H^+$ |
| Glycyl-glycine dipeptidase | Hydrolysis of glycyl-glycine |
| Glycyl-leucine dipeptidase ($Zn^{2+}$, $Mn^{2+}$) | Hydrolysis of glycyl-leucine |
| Glyoxalase | Detoxification of aldehydes |
| Insulin in secretory vesicles | Used in stabilizing insulin |
| Lactate dehydrogenase | Pyruvate ↔ Lactate |
| Mannosidase | Hydrolysis of mannose |
| Metallothionein | Storage or detoxification of zinc |
| 5′-Nucleotidase | Cleavage of phosphate from nucleoside 5′-monophosphates |
| [a]Poly(ADP-ribose)polymerase | Repairs DNA damage |
| Protein kinase C | Cell signal transduction |
| Phospholipase C | $PIP_2$ → 1,2-Diacylglycerol + $IP_3$ |
| [a]Retinoic acid receptor | DNA binding and genetic regulation |
| RNAase | RNA degradation |
| RNA polymerase | RNA synthesis from ribonucleotides |
| [a]Steroid hormone receptor | DNA binding and genetic regulation |
| Superoxide dismutase (cytosol) | Removal $O_2^-$ |
| Thymulin | Hormone of the immune system |
| [a]Transcription factors | Regulation of synthesis of many mRNAs |
| Triosephosphate isomerase | Dihydroxyacetone-P ↔ D-Glyceraldehyde 3-P |
| Tripeptidase ($Zn^{2+}$ or $Co^{2+}$) | Hydrolysis of tripeptides |

$PIP_2$, phosphatidylinositol 4,5-bisphosphate; $IP_3$, inositol 1,4,5-trisphosphate.
[a] Indicates the presence of zinc finger structure.

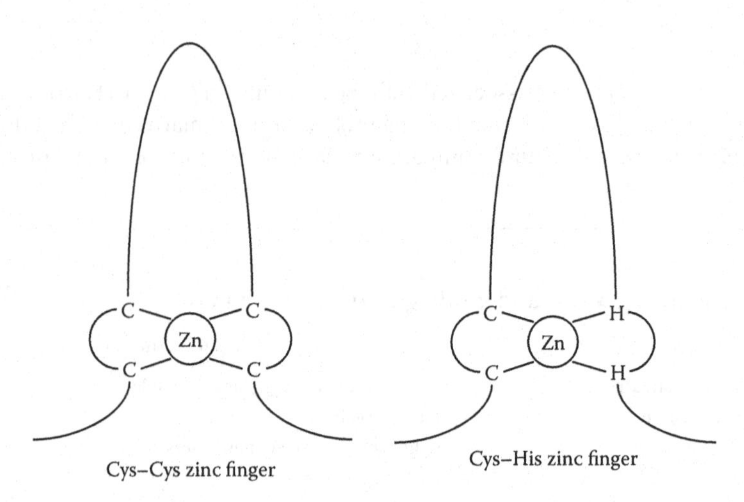


**FIGURE 10.9** The zinc finger structure in protein. This unique structure coordinates zinc ions with cysteine and histidine residues in proteins to stabilize them.

molecule) in proteins (Figure 10.9), zinc stabilizes the macromolecules (e.g., insulin and nucleic acids) and regulates gene expression in cells. Thus, zinc plays a significant role in genomic stability; the metabolism of protein (both protein synthesis and degradation), nucleic acids, carbohydrate, lipids, and energy; integrity and function of cells (including epithelial cells); transport of vitamins A and E in the blood; immune response; and reproduction (e.g., male and female fertility); and collagen and keratin formation, as well as healthy development and repair of hair, skin and nails. Furthermore, high dietary zinc (e.g., 2425–3000 ppm ZnO) can reduce the number of bacteria (e.g., Enterobacteriaceae, the *Escherichia* group, and *Lactobacillus* spp.) in the stomach, small intestine, and large intestine of weaned piglets (Starke et al. 2014). The inclusion of 0.3% ZnO (3000 ppm) in diets can prevent diarrhea, while enhancing the growth and feed efficiency of weanling pigs.

### *Deficiency Symptoms*

Zinc deficiency is widespread in farm animals if their diets are not supplemented with adequate zinc. Zinc is essential for many metabolic pathways (including protein synthesis and cell division), as noted previously. Thus, in animals, zinc deficiency results in reduced food intake, growth restriction, and poor food utilization; gastrointestinal ulcerative colitis, diarrhea, and anorexia; hypogonadism, low sperm counts, fetal abnormalities, and infertility; skin abnormalities, dermatitis, and impaired wound healing; impaired growth and development of the cells that mediate innate immunity and of T- and B-lymphocytes, leading to impaired immune function; impaired activation of the extracellular signal-regulated kinases (ERK1/2) in the brain, leading to neurological dysfunction; eye lesions and photophobia; and behavioral change (Harris 2014; Hojyo and Fukada 2016).

### *Excess*

Zinc toxicity rarely occurs in farm animals under practical feeding conditions, but may result from excessive zinc supplementation to diets (Pond et al. 1995). Excessive intake of zinc results in oxidative stress and apoptosis in animal cells (Formigari et al. 2007). Because the absorption of zinc, iron, copper and nickel by the apical membrane of the enterocyte shares the same transporter DCT1 (Table 10.6), excessive zinc results in impaired absorption of iron, copper and nickel by the small intestine. Many of the toxic effects of zinc result from copper and iron deficiencies. Syndromes of zinc toxicity include reduced feed intake and impaired growth; gastric irritation, abdominal pain, nausea, vomiting, and diarrhea; impaired absorption of dietary iron and copper, abnormal metabolism of iron and copper, and anemia; increased risk for infectious disease; cardiovascular and neurological dysfunction; and damage to reproductive tracts and impaired reproduction in both males and females (Cai et al. 2005; Georgievskii et al. 1982). Of note, Georgievskii et al. (1982) reported that concentrations of iron (as $FeSO_4 \cdot 7H_2O$) in the ruminal fluid ≥0.3 mg/mL are toxic to ruminal microbes as assessed by the rate of cellulose digestion.

## Copper (Cu)

Copper was discovered in the Middle East around 9000 BC. It is a reddish-orange, soft, malleable, and ductile metal. Copper is involved in oxidation–reduction reactions and occurs in the cuprous ($Cu^+$) and cupric ($Cu^{2+}$) states. Copper does not react with water, but it does slowly react with atmospheric oxygen to form a layer of brown-black copper oxide. O'Dell et al. (1961) found that dietary copper deficiency resulted in anemia, reduced growth, and aortic rupture in chicks. This seminal work extended the physiological role of copper beyond its action as an electron donor or acceptor in the mitochondrial electron transport system.

### *Sources*

Copper is present in most foods. Seeds, seed by-products, nuts, whole-grain cereals, legumes, soybean products, dark chocolate, and leafy green vegetables are good sources of copper. The copper content in plants is greatly affected by copper content in soil. Meats (including pork, poultry, and beef), liver, and eggs are rich in copper. In contrast, milk contains relatively low concentrations of copper.

### *Absorption*

In the lumen of the small intestine, $Cu^{2+}$ is reduced to $Cu^{1+}$; $Cu^{1+}$ and $Cu^{2+}$ are absorbed into the enterocyte through copper transporter-1 and DCT1, respectively. Inside the enterocyte, copper is transported by reduced glutathione to metallothionein for storage; and by three copper chaperones to its target sites: by Cox-17 to mitochondria, by copper chaperone for cytosolic superoxide dismutase (CCS) to the enzyme, and by ATOX-1 to ATP7a. The latter is a Cu-ATPase that is embedded in the surface of vesicles of the trans-Golgi network (TGN). The TGN vesicles move copper to the basolateral membrane of the enterocyte for discharge into the lamina propria, with the exit being powered by ATP hydrolysis. Copper is absorbed by the small intestine into the portal vein.

Many substances present in the diet affect the bioavailability of its copper. Specifically, copper from inorganic compounds is poorly absorbed in animals, with only ~5%–10% of ingested copper being absorbed and retained. Most of the fecal copper is unabsorbed dietary copper, but some of it is derived from bile acid. The bile is the major pathway for the secretion of endogenous copper. Dietary molybdenum also affects copper absorption and retention in animals in the presence of sulfur. Specifically, sulfite (formed from sulfate or organic sulfur compounds by microorganisms) reacts with molybdenum to form thiomolybdate, which then binds with copper to form an insoluble copper thiomolybdate (tetrathiomolybdate, $CuMo_2S_8$), thereby limiting the absorption of dietary copper (Pitt 1976). Tetrathiomolybdate may also affect copper metabolism in animals.

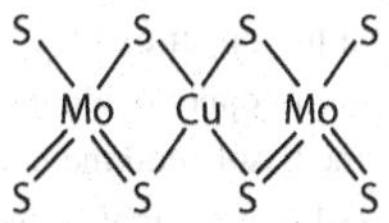

Tetrathiomolybdate

Baker (1999) reported that cupric oxide (CuO), which contains 80% Cu and, therefore, occupies less "space" in a trace-mineral premix, is not soluble in water and is unavailable for absorption by the small intestine. The bioavailability of Cu in CuO is not significantly different from zero. Good sources of utilizable forms of Cu in the diets for animals are $Cu_2O$ (88% Cu), CuCl (64.2% Cu), $CuCO_3 \cdot Cu(OH)_2$ (known as alkaline Cu carbonate; 57% Cu), $CuCl_2$ (47.3% Cu), cupric acetate (35.0% Cu), and $CuSO_4 \cdot 5H_2O$ (25.5% Cu) (Cromwell et al. 1998; Suttle 2010).

### *Transport in the Blood*

In the portal blood, 90% of copper is bound to plasma ceruloplasmin (binding primarily $Cu^{2+}$) for transport to tissues, and the remaining copper is bound to plasma albumin. Ceruloplasmin, which was discovered in the 1940s by Holmberg and Laurell (1948), is a single polypeptide chain (MW, 132,000) synthesized and released by the liver. This large size prevents the loss of this protein into the glomerular filtrate, and thus loss of the bound copper in the urine. Absorbed copper enters the portal circulation. In the blood, copper is taken up by the liver via CTR1 for distributing copper to extrahepatic tissues and excreting copper into the bile. The trafficking of copper in hepatocytes is essentially the same as that in enterocytes, except that (1) hepatocytes express ATP7b (a Cu-ATPase) rather than ATP7a; (2) the ATP7b releases copper into the bile and the blood; and (3) hepatocytes also release copper in its ceruloplasmin-bound form into the blood. Before being taken up into peripheral tissues, $Cu^{2+}$ in the plasma is reduced by vitamin C to $Cu^{+}$, which is then transported across the plasma membrane of animal cells via CTR1. Within animal cells, copper is stored in a metallothionein-bound form (Table 10.14).

### *Content in the Body and Tissues*

The content of copper in the tissues of farm animals (mg/kg fresh weight) is as follows: whole blood, 0.8–1.2; liver, 8–100; spleen, 1.2–12; kidneys, 2–4; heart, 3–4; skeletal muscle, 2–3; brain, 0.5–5.3; and bones, 3.7–40, depending on dietary intake of copper (Georgievskii et al. 1982). The concentrations of copper in the plasma (mg/L) are as follows: dogs, 0.67; pigs, 2.15; cattle, 0.91; and sheep, 1.15. Because of an increase in its mobilization from tissues, concentrations of copper in serum are elevated when animals are subjected to infectious diseases and other stressful conditions (Orr et al. 1990).

### *Functions*

As a cofactor of enzymes, copper participates in redox and hydroxylation reactions with important physiological functions. These roles of copper are highlighted in the following sections.

*Mitochondrial Electron Transport System* The oxidation state of copper can shift between $Cu^{+}$ and $Cu^{2+}$. Thus, copper acts as an electron donor or acceptor in cytochrome *c* and cytochrome

**TABLE 10.14**
**Copper Metalloenzymes and Binding Proteins**

| Enzyme or Protein | Function |
|---|---|
| Amine oxidase | Catabolism of amines, including histamine and polyamines |
| Ascorbate oxidase | Converts L-ascorbate and $O_2$ into dehydroascorbate and $H_2O$ |
| Cytochrome *c* oxidase | Mitochondrial respiratory chain |
| Cytochrome oxidase | Mitochondrial respiratory chain |
| Dopamine ß-hydroxylase | Conversion of dopamine into norepinephrine |
| Ceruloplasmin (a ferroxidase) | Multi-copper oxidase in plasma |
| Hephaestin (a ferroxidase) | Multi-copper oxidase that facilitates the export of Cu across the basolateral membrane of the enterocyte |
| Lysyl oxidase | Hydroxylation of lysine residues in collagen |
| Nitrite reductase (Cu, bacteria) | $NO_2^-$ (nitrite) + $2e^-$ + $2H^+$ → NO (nitric oxide) + $H_2O$ |
| PAM | Amidation of the glycine residue in neuropeptides |
| Superoxide dismutase (cytosol) | Requires $Cu^{2+}$ and $Zn^{2+}$. Removal of $O_2^-$ |
| Tyrosine oxidase | Melanin synthesis |
| Uricase (not in humans) | Uric acid → Allantoin |

PAM, peptidylglycine α-amidating monooxygenase.

oxidase of the mitochondrial electron transport system. These oxidation–reduction reactions are essential for ATP production in animals.

*Growth and Development of Connective Tissue* Copper is an essential cofactor of lysyl oxidase (Table 10.14). This enzyme catalyzes the cross-linking of collagen and elastin that is essential for the formation of mature extracellular proteins in connective tissue. Thus, through the action of lysyl oxidase, copper maintains the strength of connective tissue in various organs (e.g., the heart, skeletal muscle, and blood vessels) and supports bone formation.

*Antioxidative Reactions* Copper is a cofactor of a cytosolic antioxidant enzyme, copper-zinc superoxide dismutase (Cu,Zn-SOD) (Table 10.14). This enzyme catalyzes the conversion of the superoxide ($O_2^-$) free radical into molecular oxygen ($O_2$) and hydrogen peroxide ($H_2O_2$). The latter is degraded by catalase to form water. High levels of superoxide, which is produced by reactions involving oxygen metabolism, irreversibly oxidize macromolecules and cell membranes, resulting in cell and tissue damage. Therefore, copper, like zinc, is required for antioxidant defense in animal cells.

$$O_2^- + Cu^{2+} \rightarrow Cu^+ + O_2$$

$$O_2^- + Cu^+ + 2\,H^+ \rightarrow H_2O_2 + Cu^{2+}$$

$$\textit{Net reaction: } 2\,O_2^- + 2\,H^+ \rightarrow O_2 + H_2O_2$$

*Iron Metabolism* Ferroxidase oxidizes $Fe^{2+}$ to $Fe^{3+}$, which is carried by transferrin in the blood to tissues, such as liver and bone marrow. Four different proteins that possess ferroxidase activity require copper as their cofactor for their enzymatic activities in animals: the circulating ceruloplasmin, the membrane-bound ceruloplasmin (also called glycosylphosphatidylinositol-anchored ceruloplasmin), hephaestin (in the intestine, spleen, placenta, and kidneys), and zyklopen (in multiple tissues, including placenta and mammary gland). Copper deficiency results in iron overload in selected tissues, including the intestine, liver, brain, and retina. This is consistent with the notion that copper plays an important role in iron metabolism in animals.

*Other Enzymes* Some enzymes also depend on copper for their biological activities (Table 10.14). For example, as a cofactor of dopamine ß-hydroxylase, copper is required for the synthesis of norepinephrine (a neurotransmitter) from dopamine (Figure 10.10) and, therefore, for neurological function (Mertz 1987). Likewise, tyrosine oxidase depends on copper for enzymatic activity to catalyze melanin synthesis from tyrosine; thus, copper is necessary for pigment formation. In addition, ascorbate oxidase converts L-ascorbate and $O_2$ into dehydroascorbate and $H_2O$, thereby participating in vitamin C metabolism. Furthermore, copper is the cofactor of peptidyl-glycine α-amidating monooxygenase, which amidates the glycine residues in neuropeptides to render the peptides more hydrophilic and biologically active. These signaling peptides are crucial for neurological development and function.

$$\text{Peptide-C(O)NHCH}_2\text{CO}_2^- + O_2 + 2\,[H] \rightarrow \text{Peptide-C(O)NH}_2 + \text{CH(O)CO}_2^- + H_2O$$

*Antimicrobial Effects* Copper has an antimicrobial effect to inhibit the growth of molds, fungi, algae, and harmful microbes (Dollwet and Sorenson 1985). Indeed, copper had been used as an antibiotic long before the concept of microbes became understood in the nineteenth century. The underlying mechanisms may include structural alteration and dysfunction of proteins in bacteria and viruses; production of hydroxyl radical and radical–copper complexes to inactivate microorganisms; interference of microbial metabolism; antagonizing the actions of other essential elements, such as zinc and iron; and interaction with lipids to cause their peroxidation and opening holes in the cell membranes of bacteria. Of note, dietary supplementation with copper sulfate (200 ppm Cu from copper sulfate) prevents diarrhea and improves growth in postweaning piglets.

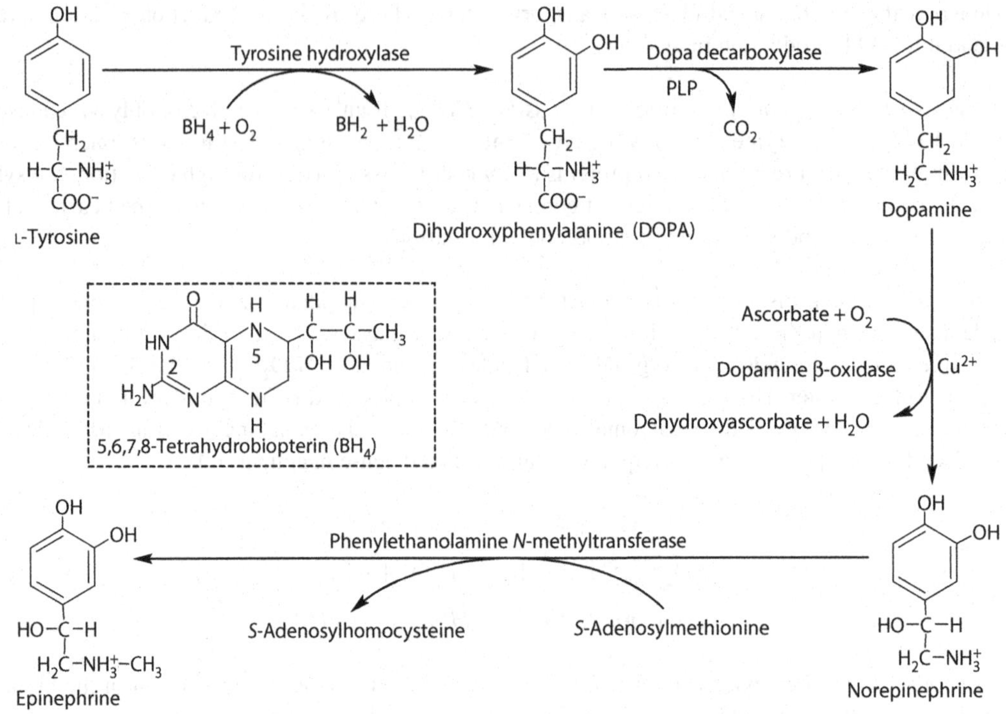

OH
CH2
H-C-NH3+
COO−
L-Tyrosine
Tyrosine hydroxylase
BH4 + O2
BH2 + H2O
OH
OH
CH2
H-C-NH3+
COO−
Dihydroxyphenylalanine (DOPA)
Dopa decarboxylase
PLP
CO2
OH
OH
CH2
H2C-NH3+
Dopamine
5,6,7,8-Tetrahydrobiopterin (BH4)
Ascorbate + O2
Dopamine β-oxidase
Cu2+
Dehydroxyascorbate + H2O
OH
OH
HO-C-H
H2C-NH3+
Norepinephrine
Phenylethanolamine N-methyltransferase
S-Adenosylhomocysteine
S-Adenosylmethionine
OH
OH
HO-C-H
H2C-NH3+-CH3
Epinephrine


**FIGURE 10.10** The synthesis of norepinephrine from dopamine via copper-dependent dopamine ß-hydroxylase in animals. Norepinephrine is both a hormone and a neurotransmitter. This pathway occurs in (1) the adrenal medulla, which releases norepinephrine into the blood as a hormone, and (2) noradrenergic neurons of the central and sympathetic nervous systems, which use norepinephrine as a neurotransmitter.

*Pigmentation* Copper is a reddish-brown color, which contributes to the pigment of feathers in certain birds. For example, turacin, a red porphyrin pigment in the feathers of the bird family Musophagidae, the turacos, contains 7% copper (Blumberg and Peisach 1965). The porphyrin (uroporphyrin III) is insoluble in water, but is soluble in an alkaline solution. In crustaceans such as shrimp, crabs, and lobsters, copper is an essential component of hemocyanin (a protein pigment), which is not bound to blood cells but is suspended in the hemolymph to carry oxygen to tissues (Conant et al. 1933). Oxygenated hemocyanin (oxyhemocyanin) has an intense blue color, while deoxygenated hemocyanin (deoxyhemocyanin) is colorless.

### *Deficiency Symptoms*

*Dietary Deficiency of Copper* Any animal is deficient in copper when its diet contains inadequate copper. Abnormal wool (easily broken) occurs in sheep raised on a diet deficient in copper, as occurs in Australia where the soil has a low copper content. This nutritional disease can be treated by increasing the dietary intake of copper. Copper deficiency in animals (particularly sheep) can also be triggered by high intake of dietary molybdenum (Dick 1952). Much evidence shows that copper deficiency is widespread in grazing ruminants, particularly in tropical regions, because of the low Cu content in diets and the relatively high content of antagonistic minerals (e.g., molybdenum, sulfur, and iron; Suttle 2010). Likewise, nonruminants that are fed corn- and soybean meal-based diets without copper supplementation and housed in confined pens are susceptible to copper deficiency. General metabolic disorders and diseases resulting from dietary copper deficiency include reduced feed intake and growth restriction; impaired iron utilization and anemia; oxidative stress; connective tissue degeneration, bone mineral loss, and cardiovascular dysfunction; thinning and weak hair, skin abnormalities, and pale skin pigment; impaired immunity; and demyelination of the central nervous system, destruction of the cerebral white matter, lack of coordination of the legs, seizures, as well as lesions of the brain stem and spinal cord motor tracts (Jones and Hunt 1983).

### *Genetic Diseases*

Severe defects in copper transport occur in two genetic diseases: Wilson's disease (which was first recognized by an English physician in 1906) and Menkes' disease (which was identified by John Menkes in 1960). Both diseases result from mutations in a gene encoding a copper-binding P-type ATPase, and are characterized by a low concentration of copper in the plasma.

### *Menke's Disease*

In normal subjects, a copper-binding P-type ATPase is expressed in all tissues, except the liver. This enzyme is responsible for directing the efflux of copper from cells. In Menke's disease, the efflux of copper from the basolateral membrane of the enterocyte into the portal vein is impaired (Figure 10.11). This results in (1) the accumulation of copper in the intestine and the kidney; (2) decreases in copper concentrations in the liver, serum, and brain, as well as ceruloplasmin concentration in serum; (3) a deficiency of copper-dependent enzymes; and (4) abnormal (easily broken) and steely hair (kinky hair) (Patel et al. 2017). Despite the accumulation of copper in the intestine and kidneys, the activities of many copper-dependent enzymes are decreased because of a defect in its incorporation into the apoenzymes. Menke's disease is X-linked and affects only male infants. Infants with this disease exhibit disorders in the nervous system (mental dysfunction), connective tissue, and vasculature, as well as hypotonia, seizures, and failure to thrive. No effective treatment is available for treating Menke's disease. However, treatment with daily copper injections may ameliorate syndromes of Menke's disease (Kaler et al. 2008).

### *Wilson's Disease*

The liver has a different type of copper-binding P-type ATPase (ATP7b), which is responsible for directing the efflux of copper out of hepatocytes into the blood. In Wilson's disease, this ATPase is defective in (1) the liver, which inhibits copper efflux from the liver into the bile or blood circulation (Figure 10.11), and (2) the kidneys, brain, placenta, red blood cells, and retina. This results in (1) the accumulation of copper in the liver, brain, kidney, red blood cells, retinal cells, and urine and (2) decreases in serum $Cu^{2+}$ and ceruloplasmin concentrations. The consequences are hepatic and neurological damages. Patients with Wilson's disease also have a green or golden pigmented ring around the corner of their eyes, due to the deposition of copper in the cells (Rodriguez-Castro et al. 2015). The treatment of Wilson's disease may include low dietary copper, along with lifelong administration of D-penicillamine, which chelates copper and depletes the body of the excess of this mineral (Rodriguez-Castro et al. 2015). Zinc salts are also supplemented to affected patients to

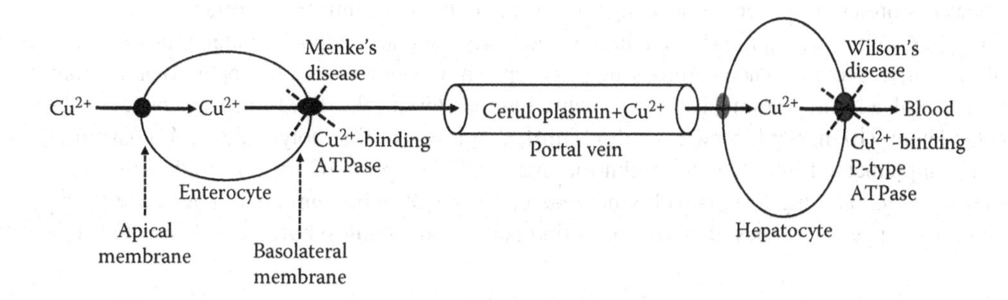


**FIGURE 10.11** Menkes' disease and Wilson's disease. In Menkes' disease, the efflux of copper from the basolateral membrane of the enterocyte into the portal vein is impaired because of a deficiency in Cu-binding ATPase. In Wilson's disease, the efflux of copper out of hepatocytes into the blood is impaired because of a deficiency in Cu-binding P-type ATPase (ATP7b).

attenuate the intestinal absorption of copper and induce expression of metallothionein to bind copper, thereby reducing the concentration of free copper in the blood.

*Excess*

Copper is a strong oxidizing agent. Thus, its excess results in stomach pains, nausea, and diarrhea, as well as tissue injury and disease in animals (Formigari et al. 2007). After entering the blood, copper partitions into red blood cells and plasma, with a 5- to 10-fold greater increase in its concentration in red blood cells than in plasma (Jones and Hunt 1983). Copper binds, and induces oxidative damage to, proteins (including hemoglobin in red blood cells that carry oxygen throughout the body), as well as proteins in plasma and other tissues (such as the liver, kidneys, and small intestine). Thus, high dietary intake of copper is toxic to animals.

(a) Species differences in sensitivity to nutritional copper toxicity.

There are two forms of copper toxicity: acute or chronic copper toxicity. Acute copper toxicity results from exceedingly high consumption of copper from diets (e.g., 20–100 mg/kg diet in sheep and young calves, and 200–800 mg/kg diet in adult cattle) (Jones and van der Merwe 2008). Chronic copper toxicity occurs when high amounts of copper at doses below the acutely toxic level are consumed over a period of time (e.g., copper levels in diets >25 ppm; a ratio of copper to molybdenum >10:1). Because copper can be stored in the liver for an extensive period (e.g., up to 18 months), the current and past feeds may be the sources of toxicity. Among domestic animals, sheep are most susceptible to chronic copper toxicity (Todd 1969). This is because ovine hepatocytes have a high affinity for copper and excrete copper into the bile at a low rate, leading to an accumulation of copper in the cells. Goats are not similar to sheep in their sensitivity to high copper diets, but are more similar to cattle. Goats and cattle can tolerate higher copper intake than sheep, but are more sensitive to high copper diets than swine and poultry.

Copper toxicity is relatively uncommon in nonruminant farm animals (swine and poultry). They can tolerate excess dietary copper better than ruminants. As stated previously, copper has an antimicrobial effect to inhibit the growth of bacteria, fungi (e.g., molds), algae and other harmful microbes, and its dietary supplementation is effective in enhancing the growth of nonruminants. Swine and poultry can be fed up to 250 and 400 mg Cu (as $CuSO_4$) per kg of diet, respectively, to improve their intestinal health and feed efficiency.

(b) Syndromes of nutritional copper toxicity and its treatment.

Animals with nutritional copper toxicity exhibit elevated copper concentration in serum (>2.0 ppm), anorexia, pallor, weakness, recumbence, red or brown urine, anemia, brown or dark blood, and pink serum. Untreated animals are often found dead, and their necropsy can show hepatocellular injury, bile duct occlusion, icterus (jaundice), and blue kidneys. Icterus (e.g., in the sclera of the eye) is caused by the disintegration of blood corpuscles (Jones and Hunt 1983). If copper concentrations in serum <2.0 ppm, a possibility of copper toxicity cannot be excluded because most copper is stored in the liver and a change in serum copper concentration is often transient.

Copper toxicity in animals can be treated. First, dietary copper content must be reduced substantially. Second, when animals (e.g., sheep) show syndromes of copper toxicity, they can receive oral administration of either D-penicillamine (50 mg/kg BW) once a day for 6 days or molybdenum (10 mg/kg BW twice daily). Third, safe levels of thiomolybdates and/or sulfur can be either supplemented into diets to inhibit the intestinal absorption of copper or administered intravenously (e.g., 0.83 mg Mo [as trithiomolybdate] per kg BW) into animals to decrease the uptake of plasma copper by tissues, thereby preventing copper poisoning syndromes (Wang et al. 1992).

## MANGANESE (Mn)

Manganese was proposed as a new element by Carl Scheele in 1774. However, Johan Gahn is generally recognized for its discovery. This mineral derives its name from the Greek "magnesia," a region in southeastern Greece. Both manganese and magnesium are divalent metals, but they differ in chemical and biochemical properties. The early work of Kemmerer et al. (1931) led to the discovery that dietary Mn is required for ovulation in female mice. Subsequent studies also found that Mn is essential for the growth, lactation, and fertility of both ruminants (Hidiroglou 1979) and swine (Grummer et al. 1950). These investigations highlight an important role for minerals in animal production.

#### *Sources*

Manganese is present naturally in ores as oxides, hydroxides, carbonates, and silicates. Animal products, as well as plant foods (e.g., nuts, green leafy vegetables, and most whole grains), are good sources of manganese. However, corn contains a very low content of this mineral. The concentrations of Mn in water and forages vary with locations.

#### *Absorption and Transport*

Less than 10% of ingested manganese (e.g., 3%–5% in poultry) is absorbed by the small intestine of animals. In the small intestine, $Mn^{2+}$ is absorbed into enterocytes primarily by DCT1 (Bai et al. 2012). ZIP8 may also play a role in the transport of $Mn^{2+}$ across the apical membrane of the cells. Within the enterocytes, $Mn^{2+}$ is transported into its target sites by a Golgi transporter PMR1P (manganese transporting ATPase) and vesicles. Both PMR1P and vesicle discharge mediate the exit of $Mn^{2+}$ across the basolateral membrane of the enterocyte into the lamina propria. Dietary intake of divalent metals, such as $Ca^{2+}$, $Cu^{2+}$, $Mg^{2+}$, and $Zn^{2+}$, negatively inhibits $Mn^{2+}$ absorption by the small intestine. Absorbed manganese enters the portal circulation. During transport in the blood, $Mn^{2+}$ is carried to peripheral tissues by transferrin (~50%) as well as albumin (~5%), α2-macroglobulin, heavy γ-globulins, lipoproteins, citrate, and carbonate (Davidsson et al. 1989; Scheuhammer and Cherian 1985). Extraintestinal tissues take up $Mn^{2+}$ by specific transporters. NRAMP1 is the major transporter of $Mn^{2+}$ in macrophages and monocytes.

#### *Content in the Body and Tissues*

Newborn calves, newborn piglets, and newly hatched chicks contain 65–70 mg, 0.65–0.7 mg, and 10–20 μg Mn, respectively (Georgievskii et al. 1982). Concentrations of Mn in the whole blood and plasma of cattle are 50–100 and 5–6 μg/L, respectively. The content of Mn in tissues of animals (μg/100 g fresh weight) is as follows: liver, 200–300; kidneys, 120–150; bones, 300–370; pancreas, 140–160; spleen, 20–25; heart, 25–30; brain, 34–40; and skeletal muscle, 15–25. The distribution of Mn in the body (%) is as follows: skeleton, 55–57; liver, 17–18; skeletal muscle, 10–11; hide, 5–6; and other organs, 10–13 (Georgievskii et al. 1982).

#### *Functions*

$Mn^{2+}$ is required for a number of enzymes involved in AA and glucose metabolism, ammonia detoxification, antioxidative reactions, bone development, and wound healing (Table 10.15). For example, $Mn^{2+}$ is an essential cofactor for arginase, which hydrolyzes arginine into ornithine (a precursor of polyamines and proline) plus urea (Brook et al. 1994). In addition, glycosyltransferase catalyzes the synthesis of proteoglycans that are needed for the formation of cartilage and bone. Furthermore, the catalytic center of prolidase, which catalyzes the hydrolysis of proline- or hydroxyproline-containing dipeptides, contains $Mn^{2+}$ (Besio et al. 2013).

#### *Deficiency Syndromes*

In animals, manganese deficiency results in low appetite and growth restriction; abnormal metabolism of AAs, glucose, and lipids (e.g., hyperammonemia, impaired gluconeogenesis, and reduced plasma HDL levels); skeletal and bone defects (i.e., bone malformation in calves and piglets); oxidative stress and reduced insulin sensitivity; scaly skin and dermatitis; degeneration of reproductive tracts and reduced reproductive function in both males and females; and impaired immunity (Georgievskii et al. 1982; Harris 2014). Young birds also exhibit perosis. These abnormalities can be treated by dietary supplementation with manganese.

**TABLE 10.15**
**Manganese-Dependent Enzymes in Animals**

| Enzyme or Protein | Function |
|---|---|
| Arginase | Arginine + $H_2O$ → Ornithine + Urea |
| Acetyl-CoA carboxylase | Enz-biotin + $HCO_3^-$ + ATP → Enz-biotin–$COO^-$ + ADP + Pi |
| Glutamine synthetase | Glutamate + $NH_4^+$ → Glutamine |
| Glycosyltransferase | Synthesis of proteoglycans |
| Manganese superoxide dismutase | $2O_2^-$ + $2H^+$ → $H_2O_2$ + $O_2$ (mitochondria) |
| PEPCK | Oxaloacetate + GTP → Phosphoenolpyruvate + GDP + $CO_2$ |
| Prolidase | Hydrolysis of proline- or hydroxyproline-containing dipeptides |
| Propionyl-CoA carboxylase | Enz-biotin + $HCO_3^-$ + ATP → Enz-biotin–$COO^-$ + ADP + Pi |
| Pyruvate carboxylase | Pyruvate + $HCO_3^-$ + ATP → Oxaloacetate + ADP + Pi |

PEPCK, phosphoenolpyruvate carboxykinase.

### *Excess*

High concentrations of manganese in tissues, particularly the brain, result in neurological disorders in animals. Symptoms of manganese toxicity include reduced feed intake and growth restriction; headaches, violent psychotic behavior, and Parkinson-like symptoms; and muscle rigidity, leg cramps, and irritation (Santamaria and Sulsky 2010). Excessive manganese (e.g., 250–500 mg/kg diet for sheep and 2.6–3 g/kg diet for calves; or 0.32 mg/mL in ruminal fluid) adversely alters the microbial population, concentrations of total short-chain fatty acids, and the ratio of propionate to total short-chain fatty acids in the rumen, while reducing growth and the concentration of hemoglobin in blood (Georgievskii et al. 1982). Risk for neurotoxicity of manganese is increased in animals receiving total parenteral nutrition.

## Cobalt

Georg Brandt is credited with discovering cobalt in 1735. Its name is derived from the German word *Kobalt*, meaning "goblin," a superstitious term used for the ore of cobalt. However, centuries earlier, cobalt was used in Egyptian sculptures and Persian jewelry. The discovery that cobalt is present in the corrin ring of vitamin $B_{12}$ pointed to an important role for this mineral in animal nutrition.

### *Sources*

Seafoods (e.g., clams, oysters, scallops, and shrimp), meats (beef, pork, and poultry), liver, milk, yeast, and leafy vegetables are good sources of cobalt. The cobalt content of plants varies with their species and the cobalt content of the soil. The inorganic forms of cobalt include cobalt arsenide, cobalt arsenosulfide, cobalt oxide, cobalt sulfide, cobalt chloride, and cobalt sulfate (WHO 2006). The organic form of cobalt in plants and animals is primarily vitamin $B_{12}$. Ruminants obtain cobalt from both forages and soil. However, the content of cobalt in plants depends on their species (more cobalt in legumes than in cereals), soil type, and vegetative stages.

### *Absorption and Transport*

Inorganic $Co^{3+}$ and $Fe^{2+}$ have identical electronic configurations, and share a common intestinal absorptive pathway (Naylor and Harrison. 1995). Iron, which is usually more prevalent than cobalt in foods, out-competes cobalt for intestinal absorption. The absorption of cobalt as vitamin $B_{12}$ occurs via complex pathways involving specific binding proteins, as described in Chapter 9. Absorbed cobalt enters the portal circulation. In the blood, non-vitamin $B_{12}$ and vitamin $B_{12}$ are carried, respectively, through albumin and specific binding proteins into tissues, which take them up through iron and vitamin $B_{12}$ transporters, respectively. Assimilation of dietary cobalt by nonruminants is usually low (e.g., birds 3%–7%; pigs 5%–10%; and horses 15%–20%) (Georgievskii et al. 1982).

In the rumen, bacteria take up cobalt through cobalt transporters 1 and 2 (Kobayashi and Shimizu. 1999), as well as an ATP binding cassette (ABC)-type cobalt transport system (Cheng et al. 2011). COT2, also known as GRR1, is responsible for glucose-dependent divalent cation transport. Bacteria use cobalt to synthesize vitamin $B_{12}$.

### *Content in the Body and Tissues*

The content of cobalt in the body of animals (μg/kg BW) is as follows: adult cows, 83; newborn pigs, 110; and newly hatched chicks, 60 (Georgievskii et al. 1982). The content of cobalt in the tissues (μg/kg fresh weight) of farm animals is as follows: liver, 30–100; kidneys, 20–30; bones, 20–30; heart, 12–35; spleen, 20–40; skeletal muscle, 3–7; and pancreas, 10–30. For example, the content of cobalt in tissues (μg/kg DM) of sheep fed a cobalt-adequate regular diet is as follows: liver, 150; spleen, 90; kidneys, 250; heart, 60; and pancreas, 110 (Georgievskii et al. 1982).

### *Functions*

Methyl cobalamin and 5′-deoxyadenosyl cobalamin are required by methionine synthetase and methylmalonyl-CoA mutase as cofactors, respectively (Chapter 9). Methionine synthetase plays an important role in reducing the concentrations of homocysteine (an oxidant) in the liver and plasma, whereas methylmalonyl-CoA mutase is essential for the synthesis of glucose from propionate. The latter is crucial to maintain glucose homeostasis in ruminants. In eukaryotes and prokaryotes, cobalt is a cofactor of methionine aminopeptidase, which removes N-terminal methionine from polypeptides to render them biologically active (Arfin et al. 1995). In yeast, methionine aminopeptidase uses either cobalt or zinc as a cofactor.

### *Deficiency Syndromes*

Various parts of the world have a low content of cobalt in the soil, and its forage vegetation is deficient in cobalt (<0.88 mg/kg DM; Georgievskii et al. 1982). Animals grazing in these regions have a low content of cobalt in the body (30–60 μg/kg BW). Syndromes of cobalt deficiency in animals are similar to those of vitamin $B_{12}$ deficiency (Chapter 9). Cobalt deficiency can be treated by dietary supplementation with cobalt and vitamin $B_{12}$ in ruminants and nonruminants, respectively.

### *Excess*

Toxic threshold levels of dietary cobalt intake differ among animals (mg/kg BW per day): 0.5 for calves, 1.0 for cows, 2–3 for sheep, and 3.0–3.5 for chicks (Georgievskii et al. 1982). Growing-finishing pigs can tolerate up to 200 ppm cobalt in corn-soybean meal diets containing 82 to 178 ppm iron (Huck and Clawson 1976). Cobalt excess results in reduced feed intake, growth restriction, dermatitis, cardiomyopathy, and goiter (Harris 2014). The latter occurs because cobalt reduces the uptake of iodine and, therefore, thyroid hormone synthesis by the thyroid gland.

## MOLYBDENUM

Molybdenum was discovered by Carl Welhelm Scheele in 1778. Molybdenum can occur as $Mo^{4+}$, $Mo^{5+}$, and $Mo^{6+}$. The most common form of molybdenum is molybdate ($MoO_4^-$). Tungsten, which is similar to molybdenum in chemical structure, competes with molybdenum for binding to molybdopterin (a pterin that is eventually complexed with molybdenum).

### *Sources*

Seafoods, meats, milk and dairy products, egg yolk, legumes (e.g., beans and peas), leafy vegetables, and whole grains are good sources of molybdenum.

### *Absorption and Transport*

Molybdenum is absorbed by the stomach and small intestine through an active, carrier-mediated process, which is inhibited by sulfate (Mason and Cardin 1977). This may explain why high dietary sulfate content reduces the absorption and retention of dietary molybdenum in ruminants and why these animals are more susceptible to molybdenum toxicity when dietary sulfate is reduced to sulfide in the rumen (Suttle 2010). Molybdenum exits the enterocyte across its basolateral membrane via unknown transporters, which may include multidrug resistance-associated proteins 3 and 4 (MRPs 3 and 4) for transporting GSH conjugates. Absorbed molybdenum enters the portal circulation and is transported in the blood either as the free hexavalent molybdate anion ($MoO_4^{2-}$) in the plasma or attached to proteins in red blood cells. Molybdenum is taken up by tissues through yet unknown transporters, which may include a $Na^+$-dependent active transporter.

### *Content in the Body and Tissues*

The blood of animals contains 10–20 μg Mo/L, with 70% of Mo being in erythrocytes and 30% in the plasma (Georgievskii et al. 1982). Thus, concentrations of Mo in the plasma are 3–6 μg/L. The content of Mo in tissues (mg/kg fresh weight) of animals fed Mo-adequate diets is as follows: bones, 15–40; liver, 2–13; kidneys, 2–3.4; spleen, 0.4–1.2; skeletal muscle, 0.4–1.2; heart, 0.5–0.8; brain, 0.1–0.15; and hide, 2.5–5.0 (Georgievskii et al. 1982). The distribution of Mo in the body of animals (%) is as follows: bones, 60–65; hide, 10–11; wool (sheep), 5–6; skeletal muscle, 5–6; liver, 2–3; and other tissues, 9–18 (Georgievskii et al. 1982).

### *Functions*

Three molybdenum-dependent enzymes require iron as iron–sulfur centers or heme for intraelectron transfer, and one molybdenum-dependent enzyme uses $NAD^+$ as the electron acceptor. These enzymes in animal cells, which are indicated in the following reactions, play an important role in purine catabolism and uric acid synthesis, aldehyde detoxification, and the metabolism of sulfur-containing AAs. As noted previously, molybdenum can be used to treat copper toxicity in animals.

$$\text{Hypoxanthine} + O_2 + H_2O \rightarrow \text{Xanthine} + H_2O_2 \quad \text{(Xanthine oxidase, Mo, Fe/S)}$$

$$\text{R-CHO} + O_2 + H_2O \rightarrow \text{R-COO}^- + H_2O_2 + H^+ \quad \text{(Aldehyde oxidase, Mo)}$$

$$SO_3^{2-} \text{ (sulfite)} + H_2O \rightarrow SO_4^{2-} \text{ (sulfate)} + 2H^+ + 2e^- \quad \text{(Sulfite oxidase, Mo, heme-Fe)}$$

$$\text{Xanthine} + NAD^+ + H_2O \rightarrow \text{Uric acid} + NADH + H^+ \quad \text{(Xanthine dehydrogenase, Mo, NAD}^+\text{)}$$

$$NO_3^- + NADPH + H^+ \rightarrow NO_2^- + NADP^+ + H_2O \quad \text{(Nitrate reductase, Mo; bacteria)}$$

$$N_2 + 8e^- + 8H + \rightarrow H_2 + 2NH_3 \quad \text{(Nitrogenase, Fe and Mo [or vanadium]; bacteria])}$$

Molybdenum plays an important role in the utilization of nitrate and nitrogen gas by bacteria through the following two molybdenum-dependent reactions. Nitrate reductase, which is a transmembrane respiratory enzyme in bacteria, fungi, and yeast, contains FAD and heme-iron. Nitrogenase contains a non-heme Fe–sulfur center.

$$\text{Nitrate reductase: } NO_3^- \text{ (nitrate)} + NADH + H^+ \rightarrow NO_2^- \text{ (nitrite)} + NAD^+ + H_2O$$
$$\text{Nitrogenase: } N_2 + 8H^+ + 8e^- + 16\text{Mg-ATP} \rightarrow 2NH_3 + H_2 + 16\text{Mg-ADP} + 16\text{Pi}$$

### *Deficiency Syndromes*

Molybdenum deficiency is rare in farm animals under practical production conditions. Animals with experimentally induced molybdenum deficiency exhibit elevated concentrations of xanthine and sulfite in the plasma, as well as an abnormal heart rhythm and neurological dysfunction (Harris 2014).

### *Excess*

High levels of molybdenum, which can result in molybdenum toxicity (known as molybdenosis), interfere with the absorption and utilization of dietary copper, leading to anemia, diarrhea, fatigue, and exhaustion in animals. There are reports that 200 ppm molybdenum in diets or 5 mg molybdenum/kg BW is safe for steers (Kessler et al. 2012).

## SELENIUM

Selenium was discovered by Jöns Jacob Berzelius in 1817 as a nonmetal element that was present with sulfur-containing compounds. Its name is derived from the Greek word *selene*, meaning "moon." Because the chemical property of selenium is similar to that of sulfur (e.g., nearly identical atomic radius), selenium can partly replace sulfur in methionine and cysteine, as well as sulfide ores. Thus, the inorganic form of selenium is present in metal sulfide ores, whereas the organic form of cysteine occurs in certain AAs. Selenium was initially thought to be a toxic metal until Schwarz and Foltz (1957) discovered that a dietary deficiency of selenium-induced liver necrosis in rats.

Selenium is the only dietary mineral that is regulated by the U.S. Food and Drug Administration (FDA) because of its historical recognition as a toxic substance. In 1929, the USDA identified selenium as a toxic substance in animal feeds. However, based on the results of subsequent studies, the FDA approved the addition of selenium as a nutritional supplement to swine and certain poultry diets in 1974 and to ruminant diets in 1979 (Ullrey 1980). The inability to supplement selenium-deficient diets prior to FDA approval had cost the U.S. animal industry hundreds of millions of dollars.

### *Sources*

Selenium content in concentrate feeds varies greatly with plant species (e.g., 0.1 mg to 4 g Se per kg DM), soils (generally <1–100 mg Se per kg soil), and seasons (Georgievskii et al. 1982). Some regions of the world are deficient, but some are rich, in this mineral. The concentration of Se in groundwater ranges from <3 to 340 μg/L (Bajaj et al. 2011; Naftz and Rice 1989). The dominant forms of selenium in feeds and forages are seleno-methionine, and seleno-cysteine. Seafoods, meats, liver, milk, nuts, and green leafy vegetables are good sources of this mineral. Organic forms of selenium are better utilized by animals, as compared with inorganic forms (Bodnar et al. 2016). This mineral exists as selenious ($H_2SeO_3$) and selenic ($H_2SeO_4$) acids, and their salts are called selenites and selenates, respectively. Selenium can also occur as $H_2Se$ (hydrogen selenide) and $(CH_3)_3Se^+$ (trimethylselenonium ion).

### *Absorption and Transport*

The inorganic form of selenium, selenate, is absorbed rapidly by the small intestine via the apical $Na^+$-sulfate cotransporters 1 and 2, whereas another form of selenium, selenite, is absorbed into the enterocyte via facilitated diffusion (Burk and Hill 2015). Selenite absorption varies from 50% to 90%, and selenate absorption is nearly complete. Inside enterocytes, inorganic selenium is incorporated into selenoprotein P (Seppl). The latter is exported across the basolateral membrane of the cells into the lamina propria via exocytosis. The absorbed inorganic selenium enters the portal circulation as Seppl, which is subsequently taken up by the liver via Seppl receptor (apolipoprotein E receptor-2)-mediated endocytosis. In hepatocytes, Seppl is degraded through proteolysis to release selenium, which is used for the synthesis of selenoproteins, including liver-type Seppl. The latter is exported from the liver into the blood via receptor-mediated exocytosis. In the systemic circulation, Seppl is the major transport form of the diet-derived inorganic selenium. Seppl in the blood is taken up by extrahepatic tissues via Seppl receptor-mediated endocytosis. Intracellular catabolism of Seppl releases selenium, which then participate in biochemical reactions.

Dietary seleno-methionine and seleno-cysteine (the organic forms of selenium in which the S atom is replaced by Se) are absorbed by the enterocyte via methionine and cysteine transporters, respectively (Chapter 7). These two AAs exit the enterocyte across its basolateral membrane into the lamina propria via methionine and cysteine transporters, respectively. The absorbed organic selenium enters the portal circulation as seleno-methionine and seleno-cysteine, which are subsequently taken up by the liver via methionine and cysteine transporters, respectively. In hepatocytes, these two AAs are degraded to release selenium, which is used for the synthesis of selenoproteins, including liver-type Seppl. The metabolic fate of Seppl is the same as described previously.

### *Content in the Body and Tissues*

Georgievskii et al. (1982) reported the content of Se in the bodies and tissues of animals. The concentration of Se in the whole blood is 50–180 μg/L, with about 70% of Se being present in erythrocytes and 30% in plasma. The concentrations of Se in tissues (μg/100 g fresh weight) of sheep fed a diet containing 0.3 ppm Se are as follows: kidneys, 78; liver, 19; pancreas, 14; spleen, 12; heart, 9.7; skeletal muscle, 8.9; lungs, 8.4; brain, 6.9; hooves, 2.7; and hair, 21. The concentrations of Se in tissues (μg/100 g fresh weight) of sheep fed a diet containing 2–4 ppm Se are as follows: kidneys, 87; liver, 60; pancreas, 39; spleen, 30; heart, 30; skeletal muscle, 23; lungs, 23; brain, 26; hooves, 72; and hair, 49. The increases in Se concentrations in response to its dietary intake are not uniform throughout the tissues. The content of Se in farm animals is 20–25 μg/kg BW and varies with dietary Se content. The distribution of Se in the body (%) is as follows: skeletal muscle and heart, 50–52; bones, 10; liver, 8; hide, hair, and horny tissues, 14–15; and other tissues, 15–18.

### *Functions*

Selenium is a cofactor of glutathione peroxidase (4 Se atoms/protein) (Figure 10.12) and many other selenoproteins with redox signaling functions (Table 10.16). For example, thioredoxin converts oxidized peroxiredoxin and oxidized protein into reduced peroxiredoxin and reduced protein, respectively, whereas glutaredoxin reduces $H_2O_2$, lipid hydroperoxide, and oxidized protein (Figure 10.13). Thus, this mineral plays an important role in antioxidative reactions (Hanschmann et al. 2013). In addition, selenium can regulate the expression of genes related to antioxidative defense in animal cells (Burk and Hill 2015).

### *Deficiency Syndromes*

Selenium deficiency results in oxidative stress and tissue damage in animals. In animals, syndromes include: (1) enhanced hemolysis; (2) white muscle disease (gross skeletal muscle degeneration and loss of pigmentation); (3) Keshan disease (named after a region in Northeast China), which is characterized by poor blood circulation, cardiomyopathy, and myocardium necrosis; (4) Kashin–Beck disease (a degenerative osteoarthritis with skeletal deformations and dwarfism); (5) impairment of cell-mediated and humoral immune responses; (6) male infertility; and (7) increased risk for cancer development (Hanschmann et al. 2013; Harris 2014; Wrobel et al. 2016). Selenium deficiency can be treated by dietary supplementation with selenium.

### *Excess*

Although selenium is essential for health, high doses of selenium induce oxidative stress and, therefore, are highly toxic to mammals, birds, fish and shrimp. Selenium toxicity (selenosis) in animals

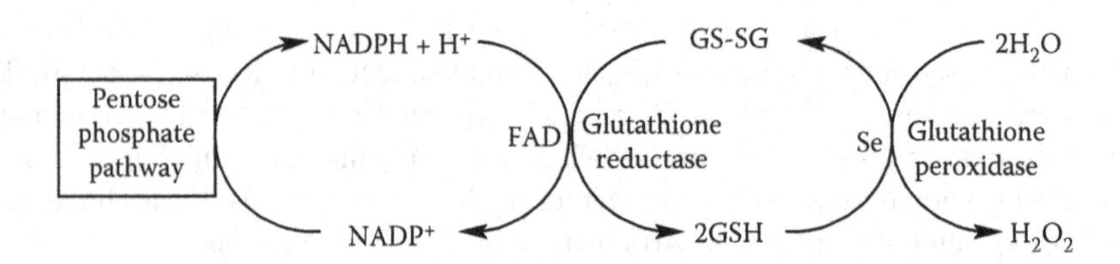


**FIGURE 10.12** Role of glutathione in antioxidative reactions in cells. Selenium (Se) is a cofactor of glutathione peroxidase (4 Se atoms/protein). Thus, a deficiency of Se results in oxidative stress in animals.

**TABLE 10.16**
**Seleno-Enzymes and Proteins in Animals**

| Enzyme or Protein | Function |
|---|---|
| **Enzymes** | |
| Classical GSH peroxidase (GPX1) | $2GSH + H_2O_2 \rightarrow GS\text{–}SG + 2H_2O$ |
| Gastrointestinal GSH peroxidase (GPX2) | $2GSH + H_2O_2 \rightarrow GS\text{–}SG + 2H_2O$ |
| Plasma GSH peroxidase (GPX3) | $2GSH + H_2O_2 \rightarrow GS\text{–}SG + 2H_2O$ |
| Phospholipid-hydroperoxide (PLH) GSH peroxidase (GPX4) | $2GSH + PLH \rightarrow GS\text{–}SG + Lipid + 2H_2O$ |
| Iodothyronine 5′-deiodinase-1 (liver, kidney) | Thyroxine ($T_4$) → 3,5,3′-Triiodothyronine ($T_3$) |
| Iodothyronine 5′-deiodinase-2 (thyroid gland, muscle, heart) | Thyroxine ($T_4$) → 3,5,3′-Triiodothyronine ($T_3$) |
| Iodothyronine 5′-deiodinase-3 (brain, fetal tissues, placenta) | Thyroxine ($T_4$) → 3,5,3′-Triiodothyronine ($T_3$) |
| Thioredoxin reductase (containing $FAD^+$) | $OTR + NADPH + H^+ \rightarrow RTR + NADP^+$ |
| Methionine sulfoxide (MSO) reductase | MSO (Protein) + $NADPH + H^+ \rightarrow$ Methionine (Protein) + $NADP^+ + H_2O$ |
| **Proteins** | |
| Selenoprotein P (plasma) | A secreted, antioxidative glycoprotein |
| Selenoprotein W (initially identified in sheep muscle and heart) | An antioxidative protein |

GSH, reduced glutathione; GS-SG, oxidized glutathione; OTR, oxidized thioredoxin; RTR, reduced thioredoxin.

can occur after acute or chronic ingestion of excess selenium (Georgievskii et al. 1982). Symptoms include nausea and vomiting; reduced food intake and growth restriction; nail discoloration, brittleness, and loss; hair loss; fatigue; irritability; neurological dysfunction; garlic-like breath odor (due to the volatile metabolite dimethylselenide); and cirrhosis of the liver, pulmonary edema, or even death (Wrobel et al. 2016). In animals, plasma selenium concentrations 10 to 15 times greater than normal values can be fatal (Horsetalk 2009). Because selenium poisoning does not have an antidote, recognizing the symptoms is crucial for the effective management of affected subjects. Based on clinical studies, chelation or emesis is not recommended for treatment of selenium toxicity. However, once the cause has been identified, it is essential to prevent a further exposure.

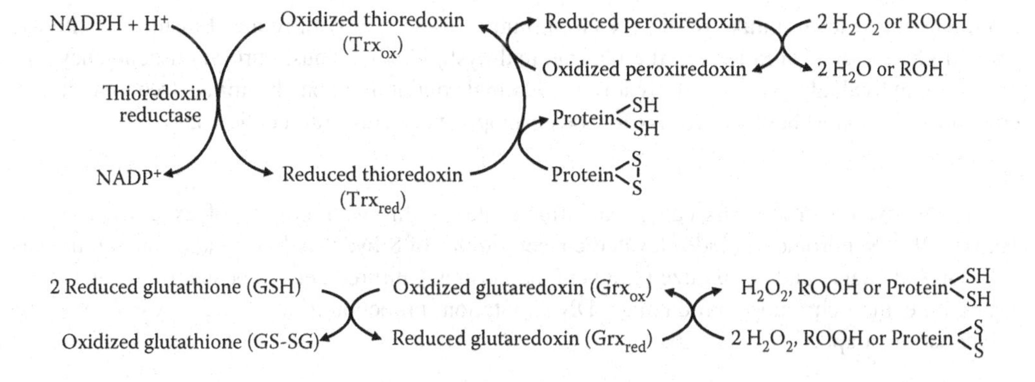


**FIGURE 10.13** Roles of thioredoxin, peroxiredoxin, and glutaredoxin in antioxidative reactions in animals. LOH, lipid; LOOH, lipid hydroperoxide. Reduced thioredoxin catalyzes the conversion of oxidized peroxiredoxin and oxidized protein into reduced peroxiredoxin and reduced protein, respectively. Reduced glutaredoxin catalyzes the conversion of $H_2O_2$, lipid hydroperoxide, and oxidized protein into $H_2O$, lipid hydroperoxide, and reduced protein, respectively.

## Chromium

Chromium was discovered by Louis-Nicolas Vaquelin in 1897. Its name is derived from the Greek word "chrōma," meaning color. Many chromium compounds are intensely colored, with chromium being in different oxidation states. Chromium metal and Cr(III) ions are not considered toxic, but hexavalent chromium (Cr(VI), $Cr_2O_7^{2-}$), such as a chromate or dichromate, is a powerful oxidant and highly soluble in water. Almost all chromium is obtained from the single commercially viable ore chromite, chromium oxide ($FeCr_2O_4$). A biological role of chromium was unknown until Schwarz and Mertz (1959) discovered that a dietary deficiency of this mineral impaired glucose utilization in rats.

### *Sources*

Seafoods, meats, liver, egg yolk, yeast, nuts, legumes, potatoes, and green leafy vegetables are good sources of chromium(III).

### *Absorption and Transport*

In the stomach's acidic environment, the hexavalent form of chromium is reduced to $Cr^{3+}$. In the small intestine, the trivalent chromium is absorbed into the enterocytes via passive diffusion (Dowling et al. 1989). In the enterocytes, chromium is bound to chromodulin, which is a low-molecular-weight oligopeptide (Gly–Cys–Asp–Glu) synthesized by nearly all tissues, particularly the liver (Vincent 2000). One molecule of chromodulin binds four equivalents of chromic ions. Discharge of chromium-containing vesicles may be responsible for the export of chromium out of the enterocyte. Only 0.4%–2.8% of ingested chromium is absorbed by animals (Harris 2014). Absorbed chromium enters the portal circulation. In the blood, chromium is carried by transferrin and albumin for transport to tissues, which take up chromium via transferrin receptor-mediated endocytosis. Chromium is bound to chromodulin for storage in the cells.

### *Functions*

In skeletal muscle, heart, adipocytes, and hepatocytes, chromium tightly binds to chromodulin, forming the chromium–chromodulin complex. The latter binds the insulin receptor, thereby maintaining and amplifying the tyrosine kinase activity of the insulin receptor (Vincent 2000). Thus, chromium plays an important role in regulating the metabolism of glucose and lipids in animals, including the stimulation of glucose uptake and utilization by skeletal muscle, as well as fatty acid and cholesterol synthesis in the liver.

### *Deficiency Syndromes*

In animals, insufficient intake of dietary chromium is associated with reduced insulin sensitivity, elevated glucose concentrations in the plasma, and dyslipidemia. Thus, chromium deficiency can predispose individuals to metabolic syndrome. Animals maintained on chromium-free total parenteral nutrition support have a high risk for the development of chromium deficiency.

### *Excess*

Chromium toxicity in animals can occur after acute or chronic ingestion of excess chromium (Harris 2014). Syndromes include elevated concentrations of 8-hydroxydeoxyguanosine (an indicator of DNA damage) and peroxidized lipids in the plasma. Cultured cells exposed to toxic levels of chromium exhibit chromosomal damage, DNA mutation, mitochondrial damage, oxidative stress, and induction of apoptosis.

## Iodine

Iodine was discovered by the French chemist Barnard Courtois in 1811. Its name is derived from the Greek word "ιωδης," meaning "violet-colored." Iodine exists as a gas ($I_2$) or as salts (e.g., KI and NaI), and has many oxidation states, including iodide ($I^-$), iodate ($IO_3^-$), and the various periodate anions (e.g., metaperiodate [$IO_4^-$] and orthoperiodate [$IO_6^{5-}$]). In animals, about 70%–80% of iodine is present in the thyroid gland, with the remainder being mostly in skeletal muscle. As early as 1850, Jean Boussingault found that dietary iodine was effective in preventing and treating goiter.

### *Sources*

Iodine is present in plants at trace amounts. It occurs mainly as inorganic iodide. For example, plants grown in iodine-deficient soils have as low as 10 μg/kg DM, while plants grown in iodine-rich soils contain 1 mg/kg DM. The richest sources of iodine are seafoods, mushrooms, and sunflower seeds. Eggs, freshwater fish, meats, liver, peanuts, and bone meal are good sources of this mineral. Grains, vegetables, and nuts contain a low iodine content. In areas where goiter is endemic and the consumption of seafoods is limited, diets are usually supplemented with iodine in the form of iodized salt to humans. The hydrogen iodide derivative of ethylenediamine (ethylenediamine dihydriodide [EDDI]) is the main supplement to livestock and poultry diets. EDDI can be added to diets to prevent foot rot in cattle (Berg et al. 1984).

### *Absorption and Transport*

Dietary iodine is converted into the iodide ion before it is absorbed by the stomach (a minor site of $I^-$ absorption) and the small intestine (the major site of $I^-$ absorption) via the sodium/iodide ($Na^+$/$I^-$) symporter (NIS, also known as sodium/iodide cotransporter, a glycoprotein) into the enterocyte (Nicola et al. 2009). Note that NIS is not present in the basolateral membrane of the enterocyte. The $Na^+$ gradient drives the entry of extracellular $I^-$ into the cell, with a $2Na^+/1I^-$ stoichiometry (Eskandari et al. 1997). $I^-$ exits the enterocyte across its basolateral membrane into the lamina propria and enters the portal circulation. To date, a vesicle or basolateral membrane transporter of $I^-$ has not been identified. In the blood, $I^-$ is bound to albumin and is taken up by tissues, such as the liver and thyroid gland, through NIS (Nicola et al. 2015). About 85% of absorbed $I^-$ is utilized by the thyroid gland.

NIS expression and activity are subject to nutritional regulation (Nicola et al. 2015). For example, high dietary intake of iodine or intracellular $I^-$ concentrations in enterocytes reduce NIS-mediated uptake of $I^-$ through several posttranscriptional mechanisms: (1) reduced expression of the NIS gene; (2) increased degradation of the NIS protein; and (3) reduced mRNA levels for NIS due to a reduction in its stability. To date, there are no experimental data regarding hormonal regulation of NIS expression in the small intestine. However, there is a suggestion that thyroid hormones enhance intestinal NIS expression to maximize dietary $I^-$ absorption (Nicola et al. 2015).

### *Content in the Body and Tissues*

The content of iodine in mammals is 35–200 μg/kg BW and varies with dietary iodine content. A 100 kg pig and a 500 kg cow contain 4.5 and 17 mg iodine, respectively (Georgievskii et al. 1982). In animals fed $I^-$-adequate diets, the distribution of $I^-$ in the body (%) is as follows: thyroid gland, 70–80; skeletal muscle, 10–12; hide, 3–4; bones, 3; and other organs, 5–10. The content of $I^-$ in tissues (μg/100 g fresh weight) of calves is as follows: thyroid gland, 24–38; whole blood, 6.3–7.8; serum, 6.1–7.4; hair, 1.7–3.2; hide, 2.7–4.0; liver, 8.0–8.1; kidneys, 7.0–7.2; and lungs, 5.0–5.2 (Georgievskii et al. 1982).

### *Functions*

Iodine plays an important role in the synthesis of thyroid hormones (Leung and Braverman 2014). This metabolic pathway begins with a protein called thyroglobulin. Its tyrosine residues are iodized by $I^+$, which is formed from $I^-$ by $H_2O_2$-dependent thyroperoxidase. Thyroxine- and triiodothyronine-containing thyroglobulin enters the lysosome for proteolysis to release thyroxine and triiodothyronine. In the plasma, 99% of these two hormones are bound to the thyroid-binding proteins. The thyroid hormones regulate the metabolism of protein, lipids, and glucose, as well as basal metabolism, and are essential to the proper development and differentiation of all animal cells that are required for the maturation of tissues (particularly the brain, heart, skeletal muscle, small intestine, kidneys, and lungs) (Nicola et al. 2015).

### *Deficiency Syndromes*

In animals, insufficient dietary $I^-$ reduces the synthesis of thyroxine and triiodothyronine, leading to hypothyroidism. The deficiency of thyroid hormones impairs negative feedback control of pituitary gland activity, resulting in increased production of thyroid-stimulating hormone. The latter causes the thyroid to enlarge with the onset of the disease called goiter, as an attempt for the thyroid gland to trap more iodide and to compensate for the iodine deficiency (Dumont et al. 1992). In addition, animals with iodine deficiency exhibit dry and scaly skin, stunted growth, excess fat deposition, retarded psychomotor development, impaired reproduction, and neurological dysfunction (Zimmermann 2009). These adverse effects occur at all stages of the life cycle and, when occurring *in utero*, can have transgenerational impacts. Of note, the metabolic disorders resulting from dietary iodine deficiency can be prevented and treated through dietary supplementation with iodine.

### *Excess*

Like dietary deficiency of iodine, chronic overconsumption of iodine also results in hypothyroidism and goiter (Leung and Braverman 2014). Such a finding, known as the Wolff–Chaikoff effect, was initially reported by Jan Wolff and Israel Lyon Chaikoff (1948). The underlying mechanisms include (1) the production of several substances (e.g., intrathyroidal iodolactones, iodoaldehydes, and iodolipids) that inhibit thyroid peroxidase activity; (2) reduced activity of intrathyroidal deiodinase; and (3) reduced abundance of NIS in the apical membrane of enterocytes and the basolateral membrane of thyroid follicular cells due to reduced gene expression (Nicola et al. 2015).

Iodine excess is uncommon in livestock, poultry, and fish nutrition. However, this nutritional problem can occur with high supplemental doses of iodine. Excessive intake of dietary iodine (e.g., iodine content [from KI] of $\geq$600 mg/kg diet in chicks) causes the thyroid gland to become overactive and produce excess thyroid hormones (hyperthyroidism). Affected animals lose BW (particularly muscle, bone, and adipose tissue), and suffer from neurological dysfunction, growth depression, and reduced feed efficiency (Jones and Hunt 1983; Leung and Braverman 2014). In chicks, the toxic effect of supplemental iodine (1000–1500 mg/kg diet) could be fully reversed by dietary addition of 50 or 100 mg/kg bromine provided as NaBr (Baker et al. 2003). This is because bromide, like thiocyanate, is an inhibitor of $I^-$ transport and utilization by the small intestine and thyroid gland (Abraham 2005).

## Fluorine

Fluorine was discovered by Henri Moissan in 1886. Its name is derived from the Latin word "fluere" meaning "to flow." Fluorite (calcium fluoride, $CaF_2$), the primary mineral source of fluorine, was first described in 1529, when the mineral product was added to metal ores to lower their melting points. As the most electronegative element, it is extremely reactive toward $H^+$ at a low pH, and toward $Ca^{2+}$ and $Mg^{2+}$ at neutral pH. In terms of charge and size, the fluoride ion resembles the hydroxide ion. In cells, fluoride reacts with $Ca^{2+}$ to form calcium fluoride, which combines with phosphate to form fluorapatite ($FCa_5(PO_4)_3$). The latter is present in the bones and teeth (Nielsen 2009). In animals, about 99% of fluoride is found in bones, with the rest in soft connective tissue and other cell types.

### *Sources*

Fluoride is widely present in plant- and animal-source feedstuffs, as well as ground–surface water. Naturally occurring fluoride concentrations in surface waters are generally low (<0.5 ppm), depending on the locations. At neutral pH, hydrogen fluoride is usually fully ionized to $F^-$ and $H^+$.

### *Absorption and Transport*

In the gastric lumen with a low pH, $F^-$ reacts with $H^+$ to form HF, which is taken up by the stomach via nonionic carrier-mediated diffusion (Barbier et al. 2010). In the small intestine, $F^-$ is transported into the enterocyte across its apical membrane by a transmembrane carrier (likely an $F^-/H^+$ cotransporter) and possibly by an anion exchanger. In the enterocyte, $F^-$ binds to $Ca^{2+}$ and $Mg^{2+}$ to form calcium and magnesium ionospheres, respectively. $F^-$ exits the cell across its basolateral membrane via the export Fluc protein, a fluoride carrier (also known as FEX, fluoride export protein), which is a single-barreled transmembrane channel in animals (Berbasova et al. 2017). Absorbed $F^-$ enters the portal circulation. In the blood, $F^-$ binds to $Ca^{2+}$ and $Mg^{2+}$ for transport into tissues, which take up (1) free $F^-$ via an $F^-$ channel and (2) the $Ca^{2+}$- or $Mg^{2+}$-complexed $F^-$ via $Ca^{2+}$ and $Mg^{2+}$ channels, respectively.

Absorption of fluorine by the gastrointestinal tract is very rapid. About 40% and 45% of ingested fluoride are absorbed by the stomach and the small intestine, respectively (Barbier et al. 2010). High dietary content of $Ca^{2+}$ and $Mg^{2+}$, which form insoluble salts with $F^-$, can reduce the absorption of $F^+$ by the small intestine.

### *Functions*

Fluoride is an integral component of calcified tissues. This mineral enhances $Na^+$-dependent phosphate transport by osteoblasts (Selz et al. 1991) and tyrosine kinase activity in these cells (Burgener et al. 1995) to promote their proliferation and bone formation. Adequate intake of $F^-$ is essential for the hardening, normal structure, and strength of bones and teeth.

### *Deficiency Syndromes*

Because diets and drinking water with added iodine monofluoride usually contain fluoride, its deficiency is rare in animals under practical feeding conditions. However, farm sources of water may not provide adequate fluoride. In cases of fluoride deficiency induced under experimental conditions (e.g., <12 ppm fluoride in diets for dairy cows), deficiency syndromes include tooth decay and dental caries, as well as possibly osteoporosis (Nielsen 2009). The latter is characterized by a decrease in bone mass and an increase in bone fragility.

### *Excess*

Fluoride and fluoroacetate inhibit enolase (an enzyme in glycolysis) and aconitase (an enzyme of the Krebs cycle), respectively (Whitford 1996). Chronic exposure to high levels of $F^-$ (e.g., >93 ppm fluoride in diets for dairy cows) affects (1) the formation of enamel (the outer covering of the tooth), leading to dental fluorosis that is characterized by mottled, discolored, and porous enamel, and (2) osteoblast growth and structure, causing osteoporosis in bones (Jones and Hunt 1983). There are reports of endemic fluorosis in both teeth and bones in lactating cows, beef cattle, sheep, and dogs due to their chronic exposure to fluoride in the neighborhood of fluorine industries (Krishnamachari 1987). Excess $F^-$ also results in enhanced production of reactive oxygen species, reduced intracellular concentrations of glutathione, and release of cytochrome *c* from mitochondria (Barbier et al. 2010). The toxicity of $F^-$ can be treated by (1) oral administration of dilute calcium hydroxide or calcium chloride to prevent intestinal $F^-$ absorption and (2) intramuscular injection of calcium gluconate to increase calcium concentrations in the plasma, which in turn block $F^-$ uptake by bones and other tissues.

## **Boron**

Boron was discovered by Humphry Davy, Joseph-Louis Gay-Lussac, and L.J. Thénard in 1808. Its name is derived from the Arabic word "buraq" and the Persian word "burah," meaning borax. Boron is not a metal. The chemical properties of boron resemble those of silicon (Cotton and Wilkinson, 1988). In nature, boron exists predominantly as boric acid ($H_3BO_3$) and the salts of polyboric acids (e.g., sodium tetraborate decahydrate, $Na_2B_4O_7 \cdot 10H_2O$, also called borax).

### *Sources*

Boron is widely present in natural water as undissociated boric acid with some borate ions, and concentrations of boron in groundwater range widely from <0.3 to >100 mg/L, depending on the regions of the world (WHO 2003). The richest sources of boron are fruits, vegetables, pulses, legumes, and nuts. Meats, fish, dairy products, and most grains (e.g., corn and rice) are poor sources of this mineral. Boron occurs primarily as boron oxides (e.g., $B_2O_3$) and borate anions complexed with $Ca^{2+}$ and pectin in plants, and as calcium salts in the bones of animals.

### *Absorption and Transport*

Dietary boron is absorbed by the small intestine via NaBC1 ($Na^+$-driven boron channel-1), with a $2Na^+/1B(OH)_4^-$ stoichiometry (Liao et al. 2011; Park et al. 2004). This mineral exits the enterocyte across its basolateral membrane via unknown transporters. About 85% of ingested boron is absorbed into the portal circulation. Little is known about boron transport in the blood. Extraintestinal tissues, for example, kidneys (Liao et al. 2011) and bones, take up boron from the plasma via NaBC1, which is a ubiquitous electrogenic $Na^+$-coupled borate transporter (Park et al. 2004).

### *Functions*

Boron stimulates the synthesis of 17β-estradiol, testosterone, 25-hydroxy-vitamin $D_3$, calcitonin, and osteocalcin, thereby playing an important role in reproduction, calcium and magnesium metabolism, bone structure and mineralization, and muscle strength (Harris 2014; Nielsen 2008). In addition, boron plays an essential role in osteoblast growth and in maintaining the normal structure and function of bones and joints (Newnham 1994). Furthermore, there is evidence that boron is essential for the growth of bones and other connective tissues and that it stimulates intestinal magnesium absorption, reduces the production of inflammatory molecules, improves neurological function, and enhances wound healing in animals (Pizzorno 2015).

### *Deficiency Syndromes*

Boron is widely present in plant- and animal-source feedstuffs, as well as drinking water, and, therefore, its deficiency is rare in livestock, poultry, and fish under practical feeding conditions. However, boron deficiency in animals can be induced under experimental conditions. Dietary boron deficiency results in growth restriction, a loss of bone mass (osteoporosis), decreased electrical conductivity in the brain, impaired reproductive function, and oxidative stress in animals (Pizzorno 2015). For example, in chicks with a marginal intake of vitamin D, dietary deprivation of boron exacerbated gross bone abnormalities, impaired the initiation of cartilage calcification, and decreased chondrocyte density in the zone of the growth plate (Nielsen 2008). In addition, compared with a diet containing 0.31–1.85 mg boron/kg, boron deprivation or a low boron content in diets (0.045–0.062 mg/kg) resulted in testicular atrophy, low sperm counts, and sperm abnormality in male frogs, as well as ovarian atrophy and impaired oocyte maturation in female frogs (Fort et al. 2002). Furthermore, impaired embryogenesis and high rates of embryonic mortality occurred in zebrafish fed a boron-depleted brine shrimp diet and maintained for six months in water containing only 1.1 μg boron/L, compared to those maintained in water containing about 490 μg boron/L (Rowe and Eckhert 1999). At present, the biochemical mechanisms responsible for the beneficial effects of boron on improving bone growth and reproductive performance in animals are unknown.

### *Excess*

High concentrations of boron bind to $NAD^+$ and *S*-adenosylmethionine, and also inhibit oxidoreductases, xanthine oxidase, glyceraldehyde-3-phosphate dehydrogenase, and aldehyde dehydrogenase (Hunt 2012). Thus, excess boron in diets and the environment is toxic to animals, as shown for rats (dietary intake of 17.5 mg boron/kg BW per day) (Kabu and Akosman 2013). Syndromes include low appetite, nausea, and weight loss; testicular cell damage and atrophy; infertility in males and females; oxidative stress and damages to tissues (e.g., the brain, liver and kidneys); impaired growth of bones; and decreases in hemoglobin levels and splenic hematopoiesis.

## Bromine

Bromine was discovered by Carl Jacob Löwig in 1825. Its name is derived from the Ancient Greek "stench," based on its disagreeable smell. Its chemical properties are intermediate between those of chlorine and iodine, being less reactive than chlorine and more reactive than iodine. Bromine is a strong oxidizing agent, reacting with many elements in order to complete its outer shell. Because elemental bromine is very reactive, it usually occurs as compounds (e.g., hydrogen bromide [HB] and sodium bromide [NaB]) in nature.

### *Sources*

Seaweed is a rich source of bromine. Marine organisms are the main source of organobromine compounds, which are synthesized by a unique algal enzyme, vanadium-dependent bromoperoxidase (Carter-Franklin and Butler 2004). Plants also contain this mineral. Bromide is present in groundwater at various concentrations (from <0.05 to 11 mg/L), depending on the regions of the world (Brindha and Elango 2013). Of note, the Dead Sea, in which plants and animals cannot survive, contains 0.5% bromide ions (Kesner 1999).

### *Absorption and Transport*

Dietary bromine is absorbed as bromide by the small intestine. Specific intestinal transporters for bromide have not been identified. However, there is indirect evidence that bromide shares the chloride and iodide transporters for absorption from the intestinal lumen into the enterocytes (Abraham 2005; Mahajan et al. 1996). Bromide exits the enterocyte across its basolateral membrane via unknown transporters. Absorbed bromide enters the portal circulation, but little is known about bromide transport in the blood. Extraintestinal tissues take up bromide possibly via chloride channels (e.g., $Na^+$-$K^+$-$2Cl^-$ cotransporters) and iodide transporters.

### *Functions*

In eosinophils, peroxidase (a haloperoxidase) preferentially uses bromide over chloride as the cofactor to produce hypobromite (hypobromous acid), which kills multicellular parasites and some bacteria. In addition, animal studies indicate that bromine is essential for the cross-linking (maturation) of type IV collagen, which is predominantly a basal lamina component in arterioles, venules, and capillaries (McCall et al. 2014).

### *Deficiency Syndromes*

Because bromine is present in feeds and drinking water, its deficiency is rare in mammals, birds, and fish under practical feeding conditions. Under experimental conditions, in animals, dietary deficiency of bromine impairs immunity, as well as the growth and function of the connective tissue. For example, compared to goats fed a 20 mg Br/kg diet, goats fed a 0.8 mg Br/kg diet exhibited growth depression, reduced fertility, increased abortions, and reduced life expectancy, as well as structural abnormalities of the thyroid gland, heart, lungs, pancreas, and ovaries (Ceko et al. 2016).

### *Excess*

Because bromine shares the same transporter with iodine for intestinal absorption and transport by extraintestinal tissues, bromine competes with iodine for metabolic pathways. Thus, excess bromine interferes with the uptake and utilization of iodine by the thyroid gland for the synthesis of thyroid hormones. DNA damage in cells, neurological dysfunction, skin defects, and renal failure also occur in animals with chronic exposure to excess bromine (Abraham 2005). As noted previously, bromine is used as an antidote of iodine poisoning.

## Nickel

Nickel was discovered by Axel Fredrik Cronstedt in 1751. However, its use for making bronzes and nickel–copper alloys dates back as far as 3500 BCE. The name of this mineral is derived from the German word "kupfernickel," meaning Devil's copper or St Nicholas's (Old Nick's) copper. The most common oxidation state of nickel is +2, and is chemically active. $Ni^{2+}$ forms compounds with many anions, including sulfide, sulfate, carbonate ($CO_3^{2-}$), hydroxide, carboxylates, and halides.

### *Sources*

Nickel is widely spread in plants (Nielsen 1987). Nuts (including peanuts) and leguminous seeds are good sources of nickel. Most plant-source feedstuffs contain this mineral. Common forages contain 0.5–3.5 mg nickel per kg DM. In contrast, animal products are poor sources of nickel.

### *Absorption and Transport*

Dietary nickel is absorbed by the small intestine via DCT1. In rats with a mutation in the DCT1 protein, there is no intestinal transport of nickel via the apical membrane of the enterocyte (Knöpfel et al. 2005). Nickel exits the enterocyte across its basolateral membrane via yet unidentified transporter(s). Less than 10% of ingested nickel is absorbed into the portal circulation, and the remainder is excreted in the feces (Nielsen 1987). In the blood, this mineral is transported by albumin to tissues, which take up nickel via yet unknown transporters.

### *Functions*

A role of this mineral in microbial metabolism is well known. For example, by serving as a cofactor of nine bacterial enzymes: urease, superoxide dismutase, glyoxalase I, acireductone dioxygenase, [NiFe]-hydrogenase, carbon monoxide dehydrogenase, acetyl-CoA A synthase/decarbonylase, methyl-coenzyme M reductase, and lactate racemase (Boer et al. 2014), nickel affects the metabolism of AAs, carbohydrates, and lipids in intestinal bacteria. Thus, nickel plays an important role in the utilization of nonprotein nitrogen and urea recycling in ruminants. Nickel is selected by these diverse enzymes because of its plasticity in coordination and redox chemistry (Ragsdale 2009). In animal cells, nickel activates heme oxygenase to produce carbon monoxide, a gaseous signaling molecule (Sunderman et al. 1983). Results from some animal studies have shown that nickel acts in synergy with vitamin $B_{12}$ to stimulate DNA synthesis and hematopoiesis in bone marrows (Nielsen 1991). Furthermore, a dietary deficiency of nickel impairs the growth of several animal species, including chicks, cows, goats, pigs, rats, and sheep (Nielsen 1991).

### *Deficiency Syndromes*

Because of its relatively high content in plant feedstuffs and its presence in animal-source products and drinking water, nickel is normally not deficient in livestock, poultry, or fish under practical feeding conditions. When nickel deficiency is experimentally induced in six animal species (cattle, chicks, goats, pigs, rats, and sheep), they exhibit growth restriction, impaired hematopoiesis, reduced hematocrit, oxidative stress, or structural abnormalities of tissues (Nielsen 1987). The deficiency syndromes can be fully alleviated by dietary supplementation with nickel.

### *Excess*

Toxic levels of nickel inhibit dioxygenases, including histone demethylases. Excess dietary intake of nickel (e.g., $\geq$250 mg/kg diet for chicks, dogs, ducks, mice, monkeys, rabbits, pigs, and rats) results in toxic effects (Nielsen 1987). Syndromes include depressed food intake partly due to low palatability, growth restriction, diarrhea, dark-colored feces, coarse and shaggy hair, vomiting, anemia, and tissue (e.g., liver, lung, and skin) lesions. Of note, cattle (including lactating cows and dairy calves) are less sensitive to nickel toxicity, as dietary supplementation with $\leq$250 mg Ni/kg does not affect feed consumption, milk production (cows), or growth (calves) (O'Dell et al. 1970a, b). In animals, high dietary nickel reduces the intestinal absorption of iron, copper, zinc, and magnesium, and consequently exacerbates their dietary deficiencies. High dietary intake of vitamins or protein may alleviate nickel toxicity in animals, including rats and chicks (Nielsen 1987).

## SILICON

Silicon was discovered by Jöns Jakob Berzelius in 1823. Its name is derived from the Latin word "silicis," meaning "flint." It is the second most abundant element in the earth's crust, only after oxygen, as noted previously. This mineral has great chemical affinity for oxygen and forms long or circular chains with oxygen atoms or the "–OH" group. In addition, silicon has a strong anion character to bind $Ca^{2+}$, $Fe^{2+}$, $Mg^{2+}$, and $Mn^{2+}$, as well as aluminum. In animals, this mineral forms complexes with collagen for biomineralization in bones. Although silicon is present in all tissues, it is most prevalent in bones and other connective tissues, including skin and arteries.

### *Sources*

Silicon is widely present in plant- and animal-source feedstuffs. Silica content in plants is generally higher than that in animals. For example, whole grasses and cereals contain 30–60 g silica per kg DM. However, fruits and bone-free animal products contribute little silica to diets. In nature, silica exists as silicon dioxide ($SiO_2$, also known as silica) and silicates (silicic acid esters). Silicon dioxide is poorly soluble in water. In neutral water, silicates are broken down to orthosilicic acid ($Si(OH)_4$), which is the major silicon species absorbed by the small intestine. A synthetic compound consisting of silicon is silicone, which is a polymer with a silicon–oxygen–silicon (Si–O–Si) backbone and is not absorbed by the intestine due to its poor solubility in water.

### *Absorption and Transport*

In animals, dietary silica as $Si(OH)_4$ is absorbed by the small intestine via (1) NaPi2b, a known sodium-phosphate cotransporter (Ratcliffe et al. 2017) and (2) aquaporins (AQPs) 3, 7, and 9 (Garneau et al. 2015). $Si(OH)_4$ exits the enterocyte across its basolateral membrane into the lamina propria. A specific basolateral $Si(OH)_4$ transporter has not been identified, but it may be a $Na^+$-dependent transporter for the phosphate export. Absorbed silica enters the portal circulation. In the blood, $Si(OH)_4$ is not bound to proteins and is taken up by extraintestinal tissues possibly via (1) tissue-specific AQPs 3, 7, 9, and 10 (Garneau et al. 2015) and possibly NaPi2a and NaPi2c, as reported for phosphate ions. In the extracellular matrix of many tissues, including the aorta, trachea, tendon, bone, and skin, $Si(OH)_4$ is largely bound to glycosaminoglycans (Price et al. 2013).

Dietary forms of silicon affect its absorption by the small intestine. About 50%–60% of the soluble $Si(OH)_4$ in drinking water and ingested green beans is absorbed by the small intestine (Sripanyakorn et al. 2009). In contrast, only 2% of silicon in ingested bananas, where the mineral forms large complex polymers, is taken up by the gut (Price et al. 2013). Silica nanoparticles can be absorbed through the intestine, but particle diameter and surface properties are major determinants of the rates of their absorption.

### *Functions*

Silicon enhances the activities of (1) prolyl hydroxylase for posttranslational hydroxylation of proline residues in collagen and, therefore, the maturation of this protein; (2) alkaline phosphatase to dephosphorylate compounds under alkaline conditions; and (3) acid phosphatase to dephosphorylate compounds under acidic conditions (Price et al. 2013). This mineral also stimulates the synthesis of type-1 collagen and elastin, osteoblast differentiation, and the incorporation of $Ca^{2+}$ and phosphate into bones. Furthermore, silicon binds to glycosaminoglycans and plays an important role in the formation of cross-linkages between collagen and proteoglycans (Sripanyakorn et al. 2009). Collectively, silicon is essential for the formation and rigidity of bones, as well as the maintenance of the normal structure of connective tissues.

### *Deficiency Syndromes*

Because silica is widely present in feeds and drinking water, its deficiency is rare in mammals, birds, and fish under practical feeding conditions. Under experimental conditions, dietary silicon deficiency has the following adverse effects: (1) reducing the content of collagen, glycosaminoglycan, articular cartilage, hexosamines, and hydroxyproline in bones and (2) impairing bone calcification and formation, connective tissue development, cardiovascular function, and wound healing (Schwarz 1978). A lack of silicon in purified diets reduced the average daily weight gain of 1- to 21-day-old chicks by 50% (Carlisle 1972) and caused bone abnormalities (Carlisle 1980). Similar results were reported for young rats (Schwarz and Milne 1972). The growth depression and impaired bone biomineralization of silicon-deficient chicks and rats can be prevented by dietary supplementation with silicon (e.g., 100 ppm silicon as $Na_2SiO_3 \cdot 9H_2O$; Carlisle 1972, 1980; Schwarz and Milne 1972).

### *Excess*

In animals, inhalation of $SiO_2$ leads to irritation, fibrogenic reaction, and phagocytosis of silica particles by alveolar macrophages in lungs (Jones and Hunt 1983). The engulfed silica fuses with the lysosomes, resulting in the damage of the lysosomal membrane and the subsequent release of lysosomal enzymes to kill the phagocytes. Free $SiO_2$ released from the lysed cells is engulfed again to initiate another vicious cycle to eventually damage the lungs. This disease is called silicosis. Oral intake of silica from naturally occurring foods generally does not pose a risk of adverse effects (Harris 2014; Sripanyakorn et al. 2009). However, chronic intake of excess $SiO_2$ or other silica compounds (e.g., magnesium trisilicate) can result in its deposits in the renal tubules to develop a disease called calculi.

## VANADIUM

Vanadium (V) was discovered in Mexico by Andrés Manuel del Rio in 1801. It was named for Vanadis, the Scandinavian goddess of beauty due to the multiple valance states (–3 to +5) of this mineral. The elemental metal is rarely found in nature, and vanadium exists as complexes with oxygen, nitrogen, and other elements (Crans et al. 2004). $V^{2+}$ compounds are reducing agents, and $V^{5+}$ compounds are oxidizing agents. $V^{+4}$ compounds exist as vanadyl derivatives that contain the $VO^{2+}$ center. Vanadium with the valance states of +4 and +5 is more relevant to biology (Tsiani and Fantus 1997). Vanadates ($VO_4^{2-}$) are similar to molybdates ($MoO_4^{2-}$) and phosphates ($PO_4^{3-}$) in chemical structure.

### *Sources*

Vanadium is present in plant- and animal-source feedstuffs, as well as drinking water. The average vanadium concentration in freshwater, groundwater, and potable water is 0.5 μg/L, with the highest concentrations being up to 130 μg/L in volcanic areas (Rehder 2015). Some mineral water springs contain high concentrations of vanadium ions (e.g., 54 μg/L in springs near Mount Fuji [Rehder 2008]). The average vanadium content in foods (where vanadium is mainly present in the form of the vanadyl species) is 5–30 μg/kg DM (Rehder 2015). Rich food sources of this mineral are shellfish, whole grains, and black pepper. Meats, dairy products, legumes, and fruits contain a low content of vanadium. In animal diets, vanadium occurs mainly as $VO^{2+}$ (vanadylate, $V^{4+}$) and $HVO_4^{2-}$ (vanadate, $V^{5+}$). The air and the stainless-steel equipment used for feed processing may also be sources of vanadium.

### *Absorption and Transport*

Absorption of dietary vanadium by the small intestine is mediated by transmembrane carriers (Nielsen 1995). In the stomach, $V^{5+}$ is reduced by vitamin C to $V^{4+}$, which is less toxic than the former. $V^{4+}$ enters the duodenum. In the small intestine, $V^{4+}$ and $V^{5+}$ are absorbed by phosphate and other anion transporters, as well as possibly non-heme iron absorption pathways. The rate of $V^{5+}$ transport by enterocytes is 3 to 5 times greater than that of $V^{4+}$ (Nielsen 1987). Thus, the amount of dietary vanadium that is absorbed by animals depends on gastric conditions and the time of the transit of food through the stomach. Upon entering the enterocyte, vanadium binds to ferritin. Vanadium exits the enterocyte across its basolateral membrane via yet unidentified transporter(s), which may include non-heme iron export pathways. Absorbed vanadium enters the portal circulation. In the blood, this mineral is transported mainly as $V^{4+}$–transferrin and $V^{4+}$–ferritin complexes in the plasma and as the $V^{4+}$–hemoglobin complex within erythrocytes. Vanadium exits the capillaries of the microvasculature into the interstitial fluid, where $V^{4+}$ is the predominant form of vanadium. Extraintestinal tissues take up $V^{4+}$ and $V^{5+}$ via yet unknown transporters, which may include phosphate transporters and other anion transporters (e.g., $Cl^-/HCO_3^-$ exchangers and divalent anion–sodium cotransporter). Within animal cells, $V^{5+}$ is reduced by vitamin C, glutathione, and NADH to $V^{4+}$, which is the primary form of vanadium. Ferritin may be the major intracellular binding protein for $V^{4+}$ and $V^{5+}$.

Less than 5% of ingested vanadium is absorbed by the intestine of fed animals, and the remainder is excreted in the feces. For example, only 0.34% of ingested vanadium as ammonium metavanadate was absorbed by the intestine of fed sheep (Hansard et al. 1982), and 2.6% of ingested vanadium as $V_2O_5$ (vanadium pentoxide) was absorbed by fed rats (Conklin et al. 1982). In contrast, in fasted rats, 30% of orally administered vanadium as $Na_3VO_4$ was absorbed by the small intestine, with the remainder being recovered in the feces (Wiegmann et al. 1982). Thus, the rate of the intestinal absorption of vanadium varies greatly with animal species, nutritional state, and dietary composition. Under fed conditions, only a small amount of dietary vanadium is available to animals.

### *Functions*

The role of vanadium as an essential cofactor of bromoperoxidase in marine algae has stimulated great interest in its biological function (Butler 1998). In this reaction, $R\text{-}H + Br^- + H_2O_2 \rightarrow R\text{-}Br + H_2O + OH^-$, the brominated hydrocarbon product is essential for algal growth and survival. To date, a vanadium-dependent enzyme has not been identified in animal cells. Pharmacological but safe doses of vanadium (0.1 mg $V_2O_5$/mL in drinking water for 14 days) reduce intestinal transport of glucose in both normal and diabetic rats (Madsen et al. 1993), which likely results from an inhibition of $Na^+/K^+$-ATPase activity in the basolateral membrane of enterocytes (Hajjar et al. 1987). Furthermore, vanadium enhances insulin action in animal cells through stimulating the phosphorylation of the insulin receptor, thereby augmenting glucose utilization by skeletal muscle, heart, and adipose tissue (Crans et al. 2004).

### *Deficiency Syndromes*

Because vanadium is widely present in feeds and drinking water, its deficiency is rare in animals under practical feeding conditions. Under experimental conditions, dietary vanadium deficiency reduces growth and reproductive performance, as reported for rats fed a vanadium-free purified diet (Schwarz and Milne 1971). Addition of vanadium to the diet enhanced chicken growth by over 40%. Vanadium deficiency in chickens also leads to a reduction in feather growth, as well as bone abnormalities in the tibia (Mertz 1974). Furthermore, Anke et al. (1990) found that goats fed a vanadium-deficient diet (10 μg vanadium/kg) had a higher abortion rate and produced less milk during the first 56 days of lactation, compared with goats fed a diet containing 2 mg vanadium/kg. In addition, kids from vanadium-deprived goats exhibited a high rate of mortality, skeletal deformations in the forelegs, and swollen tarsal joints of the forefeet (Anke et al. 1990).

### *Excess*

Toxic levels of dietary vanadium (mg/kg diet) differ among animals: rats, 25; growing chicks, 30; laying hens, 20; and sheep, 400 (Nielsen 1987). High concentrations of vanadium inhibit the activities of alkaline, acid, and protein phosphatases, as well as protein phosphorylases, diphosphoesterase, ribonuclease, and $Na^+/K^+$-ATPase, with Ki values being 0.4–2.5 μM (Crans et al. 2004). Thus, excess vanadium interferes with cell signal transduction and metabolism. There are reports that 200 ppm ammonium metavanadate in drinking water impairs male fertility and enhances embryonic death in rats (Morgan and El-Tawil 2003). In addition, excess vanadium in diets results in (1) gastrointestinal discomfort, reduced food intake, diarrhea, and growth restriction; (2) green coloring of the tongue; (3) oxidative stress; and (4) renal failure, respiratory dysfunction, and cardiovascular defects (Assem and Levy 2009). Vanadium toxicity can be alleviated by dietary EDTA, chromium, protein, ferrous iron, and NaCl (Nielsen 1987).

## Tin (Sn)

The discoverer and discovery date of tin are unknown. However, the peoples of Egypt, Mesopotamia, and the Indus valley started to use this mineral for manufacturing alloys (e.g., bronze) around 3000 BC. The name of tin is derived from the Latin word "stannum." Tin has two main oxidation states, $Sn^{2+}$ and $Sn^{4+}$. Tin is widely used to plate steel cans for food-processing equipment (e.g., cooking utensils) and food containers. Cassiterite ($SnO_2$, $Sn^{4+}$), the naturally occurring tin oxide form of tin that is soluble in acids but insoluble in water, is the most important raw material for chemical research and the commercial production of tin. The salts of tin (e.g., $SnCl_2$ and $SnF_4$) are soluble in water.

### *Sources*

Tin is present at a very low concentration in plant- and animal-source feedstuffs, as well as drinking water. Dissolved in water, tin generally occurs as $SnO(OH)_3^-$. Concentrations of tin in the water of rivers are usually 6–10 ng/L, with much higher concentrations of up to 300 ng/L in some regions, such as the Rhine (WHO 2004). In most unprocessed foods, the content of tin (mainly as $Sn^{4+}$) is generally <1 mg/kg DM, but higher content is present in canned foods as a result of dissolution of the tin coating or tin plate. Stannous fluoride (tin fluoride, $SnF_4$) is used as a vehicle for fluoride to improve oral health.

### *Absorption and Transport*

Little is known about the cellular and molecular characteristics of intestinal tin absorption in animals. Dietary tin (+2 and +4) is absorbed by the small intestine via a passive transporter. Only a small amount of dietary tin (3%–40% depending on content) is absorbed into the portal circulation, and the remainder is excreted in the feces (Salant and Rieger 1914). Through the blood circulation, tin is transported to tissues, which take up tin via yet unknown transporters. In animals, tin occurs mainly in bones and the skin (also feather in birds), and, to a much lesser extent, other tissues (e.g., liver, kidneys, lungs, spleen, and lymph nodes) (Johnson and Greger 1985; Salant et al. 1914). During intestinal absorption, transport in the blood, and storage in tissues, tin does not undergo change in its oxidation state.

### *Deficiency Syndromes*

Because tin is present in feeds, its deficiency is rare in mammals, birds, and fish under practical feeding conditions. However, tin deficiency in animals can be induced under experimental conditions. Schwarz et al. (1970) reported that rats fed a tin-free purified diet exhibited poor growth and loss of hair. Addition of Sn compounds (e.g., stannic sulfate and potassium stannate) supplying 1–2 mg Sn/kg diet increased growth rates of the rats by 50%–60%, compared with tin-deficient rats, because the experimental diet did not contain adequate riboflavin. Compared to rats fed a diet containing 2 mg tin/kg, rats fed a diet containing 17 μg tin/kg exhibited poor growth and decreased food efficiency (Yokoi et al. 1990). Dietary supplementation with tin fully restored the normal rates of food intake and growth in the animals.

### *Excess*

Excess tin causes metabolic and physiological abnormalities in animals. For example, the activity of δ-aminolevulinic acid dehydratase in the erythrocytes of rats was reduced by 45% in response to high tin intake (Johnson and Greger 1985). In addition, compared with the control, dietary supplementation with 720 mg tin/kg diet to growing chickens decreased BW gain, feed intake, and feed efficiency, as well as the content of hemoglobin, red blood cells, and hematocrit in the blood (Sun et al. 2014). Furthermore, oral administration of excess stannous chloride (30 mg tin/kg every 12 h) for 3 days reduced intestinal calcium absorption (Yamaguchi et al. 1979). Finally, activities of antioxidative enzymes (e.g., GSH peroxidase and superoxide dismutase) in tissues are reduced by high dietary intake of tin (Sun et al. 2014).

## Toxic Metals

Aluminum, arsenic, cadmium, lead, and mercury have no biological or nutritional function, but are highly toxic to animals. They are potential environmental pollutants in the air, ground and drinking water, and soil, and can readily enter the body through the mouth, lungs, skin, and eyes via feeding, inhalation, and contact. These minerals are usually present at a trace amount in animal feeds (Table 10.17). Maximum tolerable levels of dietary minerals are summarized in Table 10.18. However, accidental exposure of animals to high doses of aluminum, arsenic, cadmium, lead, and mercury is extremely harmful and can be fatal (Vázquez et al. 2015).

## Aluminum (Al)

Aluminum is the third most abundant element in the earth's crust, as noted previously. It was discovered by Humphry Davy in 1808. Aluminum metal is chemically reactive with over 100 different minerals, and has a strong affinity for oxygen to form oxides. Its most common oxidation state is +3, but this mineral also exists as $Al^{1+}$ and $Al^{2+}$. At a neutral pH, aluminum forms $Al(OH)_3$, which is barely soluble in water.

### *Sources*

Aluminum is present in the air, water, and many plant-source foods (CDC 2017). Concentrations of aluminum in drinking water range from <0.001 to 1.029 mg/L, depending on the region, whereas those in groundwater at a neutral pH generally fall below 0.1 mg/L. Forages contain 0.3–3.3 g aluminum/kg DM, and these levels of mercury do not pose a risk to grazing ruminants (Niles 2017). The content of aluminum in cereal grains is generally <5 ppm. This mineral does not accumulate in the products and tissues of healthy animals to any significant extent.

### *Absorption and Transport*

In the small intestine, $Al^{+}$ is oxidized to $Al^{2+}$ by membrane-bound oxidase. $Al^{2+}$ is absorbed by the enterocyte via the apical membrane DCT1. Within the enterocyte, aluminum is transported by ferritin to the basolateral membrane. This mineral exits the enterocyte across its basolateral membrane into lamina propria via unknown transporters, which may include MRPs 3 and 4 for transporting GSH conjugates. Absorbed aluminum enters portal circulation. The rate of intestinal absorption of dietary aluminum is generally low (0.5% of ingested Al in food matrix; 0.3% of Al in drinking water), except when aluminum is complexed with organic ligands (e.g., citrate, tartarate, and glutamate) (Cunat et al. 2000; Krewski et al. 2007). In the blood, aluminum is bound to proteins, such as albumin and transferrin. Through receptor-mediated endocytosis, the aluminum–transferrin complex crosses (1) the blood–brain barrier into brain cells and (2) the plasma membrane of osteoblasts into the bones. The aluminum not absorbed by the intestine is excreted in the feces. In the blood circulation, >95% of aluminum is excreted via the urine.

**TABLE 10.17**
**Total Content of Toxic Metals in Animal Feeds (mg/kg Dry Matter)**

| Feed | Cadmium | Lead | Arsenic | Mercury |
|---|---|---|---|---|
| | | **Ingredient** | | |
| Barley grain | 0.11 | 0.97 | – | 0.006 |
| Citrus pulp meal | 0.19 | 0.76 | – | – |
| Fish meal | 0.40 | 0.52 | 4.7 | 0.10 |
| Corn grain | 0.06 | 0.56 | 0.26 | – |
| Rapeseed, extracted | 0.15 | 0.60 | – | – |
| Soybean meal | 0.07 | 0.93 | – | 0.022 |
| Sugar beet pulp | 0.14 | 1.47 | – | – |
| Sunflower meal | 0.41 | – | – | 0.003 |
| Sunflower seeds | – | 0.37 | – | – |
| Mineral premix, unspecified | 0.58 | 3.38 | 6.8 | 0.02 |
| Meat and bone meal | – | 0.81 | – | – |
| Wheat | 0.19 | 0.26 | – | 0.003 |
| | | **Forages** | | |
| Grass/herbage (fresh) | 0.62 | 4.93 | – | 0.02 |
| Hay | 0.73 | 3.89 | 0.05 | 0.005 (alfalfa) |
| Grass silage | 0.09 | 2.02 | 0.12 | – |
| Corn silage | 0.28 | 2.19 | 0.05 | – |
| | | **Complete Feeds** | | |
| Ruminants, unspecified | 0.11 | 0.34 | 0.27 | 0.012 |
| Poultry, unspecified | 0.16 | 1.16 | 1.83 | 0.039 |
| Poultry, layers | 0.16 | 0.87 | 0.20 | – |
| Poultry, broilers | 0.19 | 0.52 | 0.34 | – |
| Pigs, unspecified | 0.09 | 1.03 | 0.62 | 0.032 |
| Pigs, <17 weeks | 0.16 | 0.77 | 0.72 | – |
| Pigs, >16 weeks | 0.07 | 0.38 | 0.31 | – |
| Pigs, sows | 0.09 | 0.70 | 0.85 | – |

*Source:* López-Alonso, M. 2012. *Animal Feed Contamination*, Edited by J. Fink-Gremmels. Woodhead Publishing, U.K., pp. 183–204.

#### *Toxicity*

Aluminum inhibits $Ca^{2+}$-, iron-, and $Mg^{2+}$-dependent enzymes, and interact with cell membrane proteins and lipids, thereby impairing cell signaling pathways, interfering with cell metabolism, inhibiting nucleic acid and protein synthesis, enhancing the production of reactive oxygen species, and impairing neurotransmission (Jaishankar et al. 2014). The latter causes oxidative stress and damages tissues. A dietary level of >500 ppm aluminum (DM basis) is toxic to animals (Jones and Hunt 1983). The greatest complications of aluminum toxicity occur in the brain (Niles 2017). In fish, high levels of aluminum also inhibit gill enzymes that are essential for the uptake of ions from the surrounding water (Rosseland et al. 1990). In all animals, excess aluminum results in digestive disorders, low appetite, growth restriction, and low feed efficiency. Of practical importance in nutrition, elevated intakes of aluminum reduce phosphorus absorption and bioavailability, as well as feed intake, growth and development in animals (Crowe et al. 1990).

**TABLE 10.18**
**Maximum Tolerable Levels of Dietary Minerals for Farm Animals (on As-Fed Basis)**

| Microminerals | Cattle | Sheep | Swine | Poultry | Rabbits | Horses |
|---|---|---|---|---|---|---|
| Aluminum (ppm) | 1000 | 1000 | 200 | 200 | 200 | 200 |
| Arsenic (ppm) | | | | | | |
| Inorganic | 50 | 50 | 50 | 50 | 50 | 50 |
| Organic | 100 | 100 | 100 | 100 | 100 | 100 |
| Boron (ppm) | 150 | 150 | 150 | 150 | 150 | 150 |
| Bromine (ppm) | 200 | 200 | 200 | 2500 | 200 | 200 |
| Cadmium (ppm) | 0.5 | 0.5 | 0.5 | 0.5 | 0.5 | 0.5 |
| Calcium (%) | 2 | 2 | 1<br>1.2 (Other) | 4 (Laying hen) | 2 | 2 |
| Chromium (ppm) | | | | | | |
| Chloride form | 1000 | 1000 | 1000 | 1000 | 1000 | 1000 |
| Oxide form | 3000 | 3000 | 3000 | 3000 | 3000 | 3000 |
| Cobalt (ppm) | 10 | 10 | 10 | 10 | 10 | 10 |
| Copper (ppm) | 100 | 25 | 250 | 300 | 800 | 200 |
| Fluorine (ppm) | 40 (Young)<br>100 (Finishing)<br>50 (Adult) | 60 (Breeding)<br>150 (Finishing) | 150 | 150 (Turkey)<br>200 (Chickens) | 40 | 40 |
| Iodine (ppm) | 50 | 50 | 400 | 300 | 5 | – |
| Iron (ppm) | 1000 | 500 | 3000 | 1000 | 500 | 500 |
| Lead (ppm) | 30 | 30 | 30 | 30 | 30 | 30 |
| Magnesium (%) | 0.5 | 0.5 | 0.3 | 0.3 | 0.3 | 0.3 |
| Manganese (ppm) | 1000 | 1000 | 400 | 2000 | 400 | 400 |
| Mercury (ppm) | 2 | 2 | 2 | 2 | 2 | 2 |
| Molybdenum (ppm) | 10 | 10 | 20 | 100 | 5 | 500 |
| Nickel (ppm) | 50 | 50 | 100 | 300 | 50 | 50 |
| Phosphorus (%) | 1 | 0.6 | 1.5 | 0.8 (Laying hen)<br>1 (Other) | 1 | 1 |
| Potassium (%) | 3 | 3 | 2 | 2 | 3 | 3 |
| Selenium (ppm) | 2 | 2 | 2 | 2 | 2 | 2 |
| Silicon (%) | 0.2 | 0.2 | – | – | – | – |
| Sodium chloride (%) | 4 (Lactating)<br>9 (Nonlactating) | 9 | 8 | 2 | 3 | 3 |
| Sulfur (%) | 0.4 | 0.4 | – | – | – | – |
| Vanadium (ppm) | 50 | 50 | 10 | 10 | 10 | 10 |
| Zinc (ppm) | 500 | 300 | 1000 | 1000 | 500 | 500 |

*Source:* Georgievskii, V.I. et al. 1982. *Mineral Nutrition of Animals*. Butterworths, London, U.K.; Mertz, W. 1987. *Trace Elements in Human and Animal Nutrition*, Vol. 1, Academic Press, New York, NY; NRC. 2005. *Mineral Tolerance of Animals*. 2nd ed. National Academies Press, Washington, DC; Pond, W.G. et al. 1995. *Basic Animal Nutrition and Feeding*. 4th ed., John Wiley & Sons, New York.

## Arsenic (As)

Arsenic was discovered by Albertus Magnus in 1250 through extracting a gold-like pigment from an arsenic ore ($As_2S_3$). In 1649, Johann Schröder published methods for preparing arsenic from arsenic oxides. The name of arsenic is derived from the Latin "arsenicum" or Greek "arsenikon," meaning a strong or muscular character. The most common oxidation states for arsenic are −3 in the arsenides, which are alloy-like intermetallic compounds, +3 in the arsenites, and +5 in the arsenates and most organoarsenic compounds. Arsenic can occur as $As_4O_6$ (a gas) or as $AsO_3$ (a crystal) that gives rise to arsenic acid ($H_3AsO_4$ or $AsO(OH)_3$) in water. Arsenic acid is similar to phosphoric acid in chemical structure, such that arsenate and phosphate salts behave very similarly in biochemical reactions. In foods and animal tissues, arsenic usually occurs in combination with sulfur and metals.

### *Sources*

Arsenic is present in the air, water, and many plant-source foods (López-Alonso 2012; Welch et al. 2000). Concentrations of arsenic in drinking water range from <5 to 150 μg/L, depending on the region, whereas those in groundwater range from <1 to 10 μg/L. Forages contain 0.25 to 3.5 mg arsenic/kg DM, and these levels of arsenic do not pose a risk to grazing ruminants (López-Alonso 2012). The content of arsenic in cereal grains ranges from 3 to 285 μg/kg, depending on the plant species and region (Zhao et al. 2010). In cereal grains, arsenic exists as 30% inorganic As (mainly arsenite) and 70% dimethylarsinic acid (Moore et al. 2010). This mineral does not accumulate in the products and tissues of healthy animals to any significant extent.

### *Absorption and Transport*

In the stomach and small intestine, dietary $As^{5+}$ is reduced to $As^{3+}$ by vitamin C. $As^{3+}$ and $As^{5+}$ are absorbed by the apical phosphate transporters into the enterocyte, where any $As^{5+}$ is further reduced to $As^{3+}$ by intracellular vitamin C and GSH. In the enterocyte, $As^{3+}$ may bind to metallothionein and GSH. This mineral exits the enterocyte across its basolateral membrane via unknown transporters, which may include MRPs 3 and 4 for transporting GSH conjugates. Absorbed $As^{3+}$ enters the portal circulation, where any $As^{5+}$ is further reduced to $As^{3+}$. In the portal blood, $As^{3+}$ binds to albumin and is subsequently taken up by the liver (hepatocytes), where $As^{3+}$ is converted into arsenobetaine and dimethylarsenic by *S*-adenosylmethionine-dependent methyltransferase. The liver releases arsenobetaine and dimethylarsenic into the blood, where dimethylarsenic binds to haptoglobin and the hemoglobin α-chain (released from erythrocytes) to form a ternary dimethylarsinous–hemoglobin–haptoglobin complex (Naranmandura and Suzuki 2008). This complex and arsenobetaine (which does not bind to any protein) are transported via the blood circulation to the kidneys, which then excrete arsenobetaine and dimethylarsenic via the urine.

Very little arsenic is stored in the tissues of healthy animals. For example, two days after the administration of arsenic into rats, only 0.3% of the administered arsenic is retained in the body (Harris 2014). Because of their roles in arsenic metabolism and transport, methionine and GSH play an important role in the detoxification of inorganic arsenic to nontoxic or weakly toxic organoarsenics in animals (Figure 10.11).

### *Toxicity*

Arsenic toxicity is one of the most common cases of heavy metal poisoning in cattle and other domestic animals, which results from dipping powder, herbicides, hide preservatives, insecticides, and timber preservatives (Moxham and Coup 1968). On farms, arsenic poisoning is associated with trash dumps, old sheds where arsenicals may have been stored (and forgotten), and old containers of arsenicals discarded inappropriately. Inorganic arsenic is a very toxic metal because it binds with the sulfhydryl groups of about 200 enzymes, thereby inactivating them (Ratnaike 2003). These enzymes are involved in a wide array of reactions, including energy metabolism, protein synthesis, DNA synthesis and repair, immunity, antioxidative response, and neurotransmission. In addition, as an anion structurally analogous to phosphate anion, inorganic arsenic is an inhibitor of $Na^+$-dependent phosphate transport (NaPi-2b-mediated transport) in the small intestine (Villa-Bellosta and Sorribas 2010), and possibly of phosphate-activated glutaminase. A dietary level of >5 ppm As (DM basis) is toxic to animals (Jones and Hunt 1983). Acute arsenic poisoning is associated initially with nausea, vomiting, abdominal pain, severe diarrhea, and a burning sensation in the mouth.

Chronic exposure to arsenic results in multiorgan failure (including headaches, muscle weakness, chronic pain, and peripheral neuropathy), skin lesions, as well as skin, lung, and bladder cancers (Jaishankar et al. 2014).

## CADMIUM (Cd)

Cadmium was discovered by Friedrich Strohmeyer in 1817. Its name is derived from the Latin word "cadmia" meaning calamine (zinc carbonate, $ZnCO_3$), or from the Greek word *kadmeia* with the same meaning. Cadmium occurs in the oxidation state +2 in most of its compounds. This mineral is chemically similar to zinc and forms complexes with zinc and lead in sulfide ores. Cadmium and its compounds are highly water soluble compared to other metals. Cadmium sulfide and selenide are commonly used as pigments in plastics.

### *Sources*

Cadmium is present in the air, water, and many plant-source foods (WHO 2011a). Concentrations of cadmium in unpolluted natural water are generally <1 μg/L, whereas those in drinking water range from <0.2 to 26 μg/L, depending on the region. Of note, in contaminated water, concentrations of cadmium are generally >1 μg/L, such as the maximum value 100 μg/L recorded in the Rio Rimao, Peru. Forages contain 2–12 mg cadmium/kg DM, and these levels of mercury do not pose a risk to grazing ruminants (López-Alonso 2012). The content of cadmium is usually <10 μg/kg DM in fruits and vegetables, and about 25 μg/kg wet weight in cereals. Cadmium is accumulated in tissues of animals, being 10–100 and 100–1000 μg/kg wet weight in the liver and kidneys, respectively.

### *Absorption and Transport*

Dietary cadmium ($Cd^{2+}$) is absorbed by the small intestine into the lamina propria via the apical transporter CDT1 (Ryu et al. 2004). In the enterocyte, $Cd^{2+}$ is carried by metallothionein to the basolateral membrane. This mineral exits the enterocyte across its basolateral membrane via an exporter called metal transporter protein 1 (MTP1) (Ryu et al. 2004). Absorbed $Cd^{2+}$ enters the portal circulation, where it is transported bound to transferrin and albumin. In the blood, $Cd^{2+}$ is taken up by extraintestinal tissues via iron transporters and receptors. Inside the cells, this mineral binds to metallothionein for storage. The Cd not absorbed by the intestine is excreted in the feces. However, this metal can accumulate in the liver and kidney, where it has multiple cytotoxic effects. In the blood circulation, most Cd is excreted via the urine.

The rate of intestinal absorption of dietary cadmium is generally low (usually 0.5%–3% of ingested Cd in animals and 5%–7% in humans) (Asagba 2013), and is negatively affected by dietary iron content. Dietary deficiency of iron leads to an elevation of intestinal absorption of dietary Cd.

### *Toxicity*

Cadmium is a metabolic antagonist to zinc, copper, and calcium in animals, therefore inhibiting enzymes involved in energy metabolism, protein synthesis, DNA synthesis and repair, immune response, antioxidative reactions, and neurotransmission (Jaishankar et al. 2014; Vázquez et al. 2015). A dietary level of 50 ppm Cd (DM basis), which is provided as $CaCl_2$, Cd succinate, or Cd propionate, can result in intoxication to animals, whereas a dietary level of 640 ppm (DM basis) causes rapid deterioration in their health status (Jones and Hunt 1983). Syndromes of acute Cd poisoning include stomach irritation, vomiting, and diarrhea. Inhaling higher levels of Cd can result in severe damage to the lungs and in respiratory dysfunction. Chronic exposure to excess Cd causes (1) necrotizing enteritis and intestinal atrophy; (2) damage to endothelial cells of the microvasculature, leading to hemorrhagic necrosis in some organs (e.g., testes and skin); (3) disturbances in calcium metabolism, osteoporosis (skeletal damage), and fragile bones; (4) formation of renal stones, and renal dysfunction; and (5) damages to the liver and lungs (Jaishankar et al. 2014; Jones and Hunt 1983; Vázquez et al. 2015).

## Lead (Pb)

It is unknown when humans first discovered lead, but this mineral has been mined for over 6000 years. Lead has two main oxidation states (+4 and +2), and does not react with oxygen. In the earth, lead rarely occurs as an element and instead is present in ores (e.g., lead sulfide [PbS]). Compounds of lead ($PbF_2$, $PbCl_2$, and $PbSO_4$, which are poorly soluble in water) are usually found in the +2 oxidation state.

### *Sources*

Lead is present in the air, water, and many plant-source foods (WHO 2011b). Concentrations of lead in drinking water range from 1 to 100 μg/L, whereas mean values in groundwater range from 1 to 70 μg/L, depending on the region. Forages contain 0.3–16 mg lead/kg DM, depending on the region, and these levels of lead do not pose a risk to grazing ruminants (Khan et al. 2012). The content of lead in vegetables ranges from <0.2 to 2 mg/kg DM (McBride et al. 2014), and the content of lead in cereal grains is generally <60 μg/kg DM (Zhang et al. 1998).

### *Absorption and Transport*

In the stomach and small intestine, dietary $Pb^{4+}$ is reduced to $Pb^{2+}$ by vitamin C. $Pb^{2+}$ is absorbed by the small intestine into the lamina propria via the apical transporter CDT1 (Bressler et al. 2004). In the enterocyte, $Pb^{2+}$ binds to metallothionein and possibly GSH for transport to the basolateral membrane. This mineral exits the enterocyte across its basolateral membrane via unknown transporters, which may include MRPs 3 and 4 for transporting GSH conjugates. Absorbed lead enters the portal circulation. In the blood, lead binds to hemoglobin in red blood cells for transport to extraintestinal tissues. This mineral can accumulate in tissues due to its low rate of clearance from the body. The half-life of lead in the blood and soft tissues is about 40 days for adults, and this increases to about 20 years in the bones (Jaishankar et al. 2014).

The rate of intestinal absorption of dietary lead is generally low (usually 1%–2% of ingested Pb), and is negatively affected by dietary intakes of iron, calcium, and phosphorus (Bressler et al. 2004). Dietary deficiency of iron, calcium, and phosphorus facilitates intestinal absorption of dietary Pb and, therefore, exacerbates the toxicity of dietary Pb.

### *Toxicity*

Lead binds to the sulfhydryl groups of many enzymes and displaces calcium, iron, zinc, magnesium, and sodium as a cofactor for many enzymes (Vázquez et al. 2015). In addition, lead inhibits key enzymes involved in heme synthesis from glycine and succinate. Thus, excess lead inactivates a wide array of enzymes involved in energy metabolism, protein synthesis, DNA synthesis and repair, immunity, antioxidative response, and neurotransmission, while enhancing the production of reactive oxygen species and damaging lipids, proteins, and nucleic acids in cell membranes and organelles (Jaishankar et al. 2014). Dietary intake of 6 mg Pb/kg BW per day is toxic to postweaning mammals, and dietary intake of 2.7 mg Pb/kg BW can be fatal to neonates (Jones and Hunt 1983). Acute lead poisoning results in low appetite, headache, hypertension, abdominal pain, nausea, vomiting, renal dysfunction, and fatigue, as well as weakness in the fingers, wrists, or ankles (Assi et al. 2016). Chronic exposure of lead can cause anemia, hypertension, infertility, birth defects, muscular weakness, brain damage and neurological dysfunction, renal failure, bone loss and abnormalities, and cancers (Assi et al. 2016; Jones and Hunt 1983).

## Mercury (Hg)

It is unknown when humans first discovered mercury, but the use of this mineral by Egyptians dates back to about 1500 BC. Mercury resists a loss of an electron from its outer orbital to form a cation, and behaves similarly to noble gases. However, mercury reacts with atmospheric hydrogen sulfide, whereas ionic mercury and organomercury have a high affinity for reduced sulfhydryl groups,

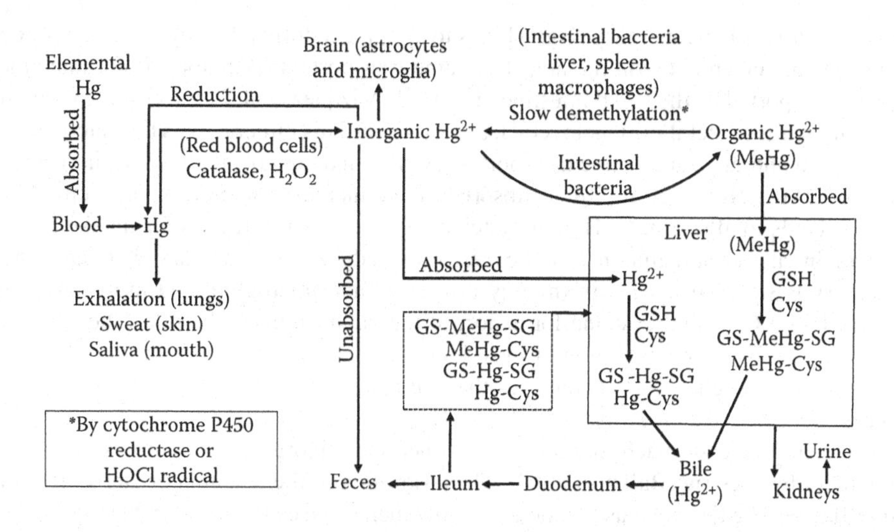


**FIGURE 10.14** Metabolism of elemental, inorganic, and organic mercury in animals via different pathways. Intestinal bacteria, erythrocytes, liver, and kidneys play an important role in the detoxification of mercury through the formation of glutathione and cysteine derivatives. These end products are released from the liver to the bile and then to the small intestine for excretion in the feces. Because of the enterohepatic circulation, most of mercury's glutathione and cysteine derivatives are absorbed from the ileum into the liver, thereby prolonging the life of mercury in animals. Excess mercury is stored in the brain and can cause neurological toxicity. * Methylmercury is demethylated by organomercury lyase to form inorganic mercury, which is poorly absorbed by the intestine.

including those of cysteine and GSH (Ballatori 2002). In nature, mercury occurs in +1 (e.g., HgCl) and +2 (e.g., $HgCl_2$ and HgS) oxidation states, with $Hg^{2+}$ being the major species of mercury. Note that $HgCl_2$ is readily soluble in water, HgCl has a low solubility in water, and HgS (mercury sulfide) is barely soluble in water. The mercury element (Hg) is a liquid at room temperature (e.g., 20–25°C). Different forms of mercury have very different metabolic fates in animals (Figure 10.14).

### *Sources*

Mercury is present in the air, water, and many plant-source foods mainly in three forms: metallic element, inorganic salts (mostly $Hg^{2+}$), and organic compounds ($Hg^{2+}$) (Clarkson 2002). They possess different toxicity and bioavailability to animals. Microorganisms can convert inorganic mercury into methyl mercury. Organomercury compounds, which include methylmercury (MeHg; $CH_3HgX$), are soluble in water and occur in the +2 oxidation state. Concentrations of mercury in drinking water range from 5 to 100 ng/L (with a mean value of 25 ng/L), whereas those in ground and surface water are generally <0.5 μg/L and can reach >2 μg/L, depending on the region (WHO 2005). Forages generally contain <0.1 mg mercury/kg DM, depending on the region, and this low level of mercury does not pose a risk to grazing ruminants (EFSA 2008). The content of mercury in vegetables ranges from 5 to 75 μg/kg DM, and the content of mercury in cereal grains ranges from 4 to 30 μg/kg DM (Tkachuk and Kuzina 1972). Fish meal may contain <0.5 ppm Hg (EFSA 2008).

### *Absorption and Transport*

*Elemental Mercury (a liquid)* The epithelial cells of the gastrointestinal tract are barriers to elemental mercury in diets due to the absence of its transporter. The tight junctions of the gut are virtually impermeable to elementary mercury. Studies with rats indicate that <0.01% of the ingested elemental mercury is absorbed from the gastrointestinal tract (Clarkson 2002). In erythrocytes, elemental mercury is oxidized by catalase and $H_2O_2$ to form inorganic $Hg^{2+}$. The element is excreted from animals via exhalation, sweat, and saliva, respectively, through the lungs, sweat, and feces.

*Inorganic Mercury* Ionic mercury ($Hg^{2+}$) binds to cysteine to form a Hg–cysteine complex, which is taken up by the enterocyte via the apical cysteine transporters (Ballatori 2002). Ionic mercury can also be transported by the small intestine via DCT1 (Vázquez et al. 2015). Inside the enterocyte, ionic mercury binds to metallothionein, GSH, and cysteine. This mineral exits the enterocyte across its basolateral membrane via cysteine transporters, MRPs, and possibly the organic anion transporters (Ballatori 2002; Nigam et al. 2015). Absorbed ionic mercury enters the portal circulation. In the blood, it binds to albumin, GSH, and cysteine and is carried to tissues for uptake by cysteine transporters. In rats, a small amount of ionic mercury is reduced to elementary Hg (Clarkson 2002). Ionic mercury is stored in the brain (mainly astrocytes and microglia), and most ionic mercury is conjugated with GSH and cysteine for export to the duodenum via the bile. The enterohepatic circulation allows for the reabsorption of most inorganic mercury by the ileum into the liver. The GS–$Hg^{2+}$–SG and cysteine–$Hg^{2+}$ complexes that are not absorbed by the ileum are then excreted in the feces.

In the lumen of the stomach and small intestine, some inorganic mercury is converted into methylmercury by bacteria (Ballatori 2002). The absorption of the resultant organomercury by the small intestine will be the same as the dietary methylmercury (see the sections below).

The rate of the absorption of dietary inorganic mercury depends on its solubility and ease of dissociation in the gastrointestinal tract. About 7%–20% of ingested inorganic mercury is absorbed by the small intestine of animals (Clarkson 2002; Jaishankar et al. 2014; Suttle 2010). Dietary intake of divalent minerals negatively affects the intestinal absorption of inorganic mercury. Adequate dietary intake of AAs facilitates the excretion of inorganic mercury from the body. The half-life of inorganic mercury in animals ranges from 2 to 3 months.

*Organic Mercury* Monomethyl mercury is the predominant form of organic mercury in plant and fish products. In the lumen of the small intestine, a small amount of organic mercury is demethylated by luminal bacteria to inorganic mercury (Clarkson 2002), which is absorbed by the small intestine, as described previously. Organic mercury ($Hg^{2+}$) binds to cysteine to form a $CH_3$–Hg–cysteine complex, which is structurally similar to methionine. The $CH_3$–Hg–cysteine complex is taken up by the enterocyte via the apical methionine transporters (Ballatori 2002). Inside the enterocyte, the organic mercury binds mainly to metallothionein and, to a lesser extent, to GSH and cysteine. This mineral exits the enterocyte across its basolateral membrane via methionine transporters and MRPs (Vázquez et al. 2015). Absorbed organic mercury enters the portal circulation. In the blood, it binds to albumin, GSH, and cysteine and is transported to tissues, where the $CH_3$–Hg–cysteine complex is taken up by methionine transporters. In certain extraintestinal tissues and cells, such as the liver, spleen, and macrophages, methylmercury undergoes slow demethylation to form inorganic mercury (NAS 2000), which is excreted from the body, as described previously. In the liver, some organic mercury is conjugated with GSH and cysteine in the liver for excretion to the bile for export to the duodenum. Similar to inorganic mercury, the enterohepatic circulation allows for the reabsorption of most organic mercury by the ileum into the liver. The GS–$MeHg^{2+}$–SG and cysteine–$MeHg^{2+}$ complexes that are not absorbed by the ileum are then excreted in the feces. About 90% of dietary MeHg absorbed by the small intestine is excreted from animals in the form of inorganic mercury (NAS 2000).

About 90%–95% of ingested organic mercury is absorbed by the small intestine of animals (Jaishankar et al. 2014; NAS 2000; Suttle 2010). Through competitive interaction with the transmembrane methionine transporters, dietary methionine and large neutral AAs negatively affect the intestinal absorption of organic mercury. In addition, adequate dietary intake of AAs facilitates the excretion of organic mercury from the body. The half-life of organic mercury in animals ranges from 2 to 3 months.

Dimethylmercury and diethylmercury, which are used for laboratory research, are volatile and lipid-soluble liquids. They are extremely poisonous and dangerous to animals. Dimethylmercury and diethylmercury readily diffuse into the enterocytes and, thereafter, enter the systemic circulation.

These two compounds are transported in the blood as lipoprotein complexes. In the liver, spleen, and macrophages, dimethylmercury and diethylmercury are converted into monomethyl mercury, which is subsequently excreted from the body, as described previously.

*Toxicity*

Mercury has a high capacity for binding to the sulfhydryl groups of proteins, thereby inhibiting their enzymatic and other biological activities (Vázquez et al. 2015). In addition, mercury causes oxidative stress, DNA damage, microtubule destruction, mitochondrial defects, and lipid peroxidation (Jaishankar et al. 2014). Thus, mercury in any form is poisonous by severely affecting the neurological, digestive, and renal organ systems. A dietary level of >2 ppm Hg (DM basis) is toxic to animals (Jones and Hunt 1983). Syndromes of mercury intoxication include diarrhea, headache, abdominal pain, nausea, vomiting, muscle twitching and atrophy, tremors, weakness, impaired neurological function, loss of coordination, kidney malfunction, respiratory failure, vision impairment, and even death. Treatment of mercury toxicity includes (1) the use of selenium, which binds Hg and improves antioxidative capacity, as an antidote (Bjørklund 2015) and (2) chelation drugs (including edetate calcium disodium and penicillamine) to reduce mercury absorption and facilitate its excretion in the feces.

## SUMMARY

Minerals are inorganic substances that are important for (1) skeletal growth, development, and function (e.g., Ca, P, and F); (2) cellular metabolism by serving as cofactors of a plethora of enzymes (e.g., $Na^+$-$K^+$-ATPase, $Ca^{2+}$-dependent protein kinase, and arginase [Mn]); and (3) physiological functions by regulating gene expression and biological activities of proteins (e.g., Zn in the zinc Figure structure, Cu and Fe in the mitochondrial respiratory chain, and boron in the cross-linking of collagens). Based on their quantitative needs, nutritionally essential minerals are classified as macrominerals (Na, Cl, K, Ca, P, Mg, and S) or microminerals (Fe, Cu, Co, Mn, Zn, I, Se, Mo, Cr, F, Sn, V, Si, Ni, B, and Br). Toxic minerals that have no physiological or nutritional function include Al, As, Cd, Pb, and Hg. All minerals are stable in feeds and animal tissues. Transition metals have multiple oxidation states and, therefore, participate in intracellular oxidation–reduction reactions. Because of their similar electron configurations, many minerals have similar chemical properties. Although requirements of animals for these nutrients are quantitatively low, all of them must be supplied in diets for mammals, birds, fish, and other animals. Compared with mature animals, dietary requirements of animals for all nutritionally essential minerals are much higher for growing, gestating, and lactating animals.

Minerals are absorbed primarily by the small intestine and transported in the blood through different mechanisms (Figure 10.15). Specifically, minerals are absorbed into the intestinal epithelial cell (primarily the jejunum of the small intestine for most minerals) through its apical membrane via specific transporters (e.g., ZIP4 for Zn, Na channels for $Na^+$, Cl channels for $Cl^-$, CTR1 for $Cu^{2+}$, and Ca transporter for $Ca^{2+}$), as well as transporters with a broad specificity for a group of ions (e.g., DCT1 for divalent metals; phosphate transporters for phosphate, vanadium, and As; and NaPi2b for silicon and phosphate). For trafficking in enterocytes, all macrominerals but $Ca^{2+}$ occur as free ions, whereas most microminerals bind cytosolic proteins (e.g., ferritin and metallothionein), GSH, or cysteine. Minerals exit the intestinal epithelial cell across its basolateral membrane into the lamina propria via specific transmembrane transporters (e.g., $Na^+$-$K^+$-ATPase for $Na^+$, ZnT1 for $Zn^{2+}$, and ferroportin for $Fe^{2+}$), vesicle discharge, receptor-mediated exocytosis, or MRPs 3 and 4 that transport GSH conjugates. Absorbed minerals enter the portal circulation. In the blood, all macrominerals but $Ca^{2+}$ occur as free ions, whereas most microminerals bind cytosolic proteins (e.g., ferritin and metallothionein), GSH, or cysteine. Tissues take up minerals from the blood via specific transporters, transporters with a broad specificity for a group of ions, or receptor-mediated endocytosis.

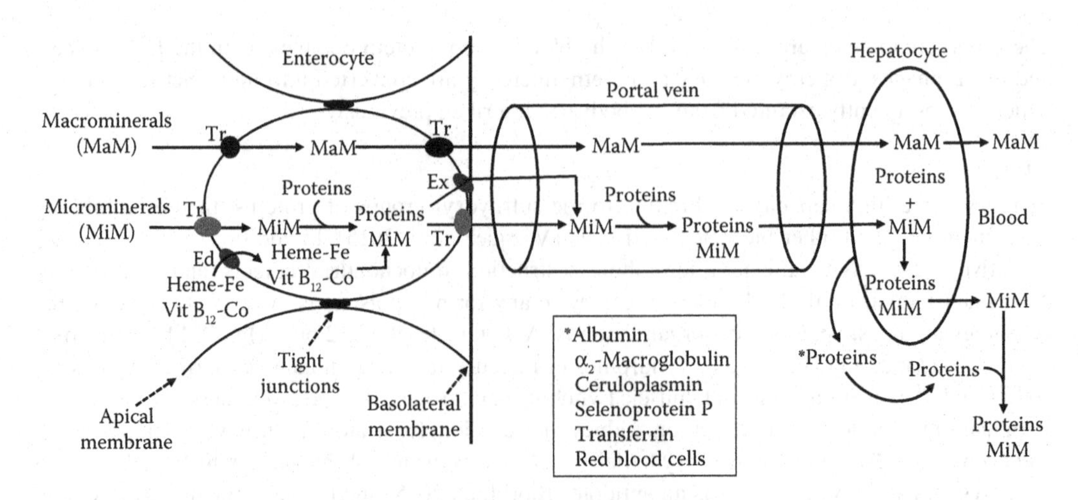


**FIGURE 10.15** Intestinal absorption of dietary minerals and their transport in blood. In the lumen of the small intestine, dietary macrominerals (MaM) and microminerals (MiM) are absorbed by enterocytes through various apical membrane transporters (Tr). Heme-iron and vitamin $B_{12}$-complexed cobalt enter the cells via endocytosis (Ed). Inside the enterocyte, MaM exist as free ions, whereas MiM bind to specific proteins for transport to the basolateral membrane. MaM and MiM exit the enterocytes through the basolateral membrane, whereas exocytosis (Ex) may mediate the export of some MiM. Absorbed minerals enter the portal vein and are subsequently taken up by hepatocytes. The liver releases the minerals into the blood, where MaM are transported as free ions, and MiM bind to albumin and specific proteins (synthesized by hepatocytes) for transport to tissues. * The types of proteins are indicated in the insert box.

It is important to choose suitable biological samples to assess the mineral status of an animal. For example, concentrations of Ca, inorganic P, and Mg in serum or plasma are good indicators of their dietary intakes by an animal, but their hepatic concentrations are not. In contrast, concentrations of Zn, Cu, and Mn in serum or plasma do not necessarily reflect their deficiency or excess in an animal, but their hepatic concentrations are useful indicators of their nutritional status. Furthermore, whole blood Se is valuable to assess the Se status of an animal, but concentrations of Se in serum or plasma are not. Finally, while elevated intakes of some minerals (e.g., Na, Cl, K, and S) are associated with increases in their urinary excretion, fecal excretion of other minerals (e.g., Mg, Ca, P, and Zn) is generally more than their urinary output because of relatively low rates of intestinal absorption.

Except for selenium, nutritionally essential minerals are utilized in the form in which they are absorbed from the intestine. As electrolytes, the minerals are essential for (1) the maintenance of extracellular and intracellular osmolarity, water balance, and blood pressure and flow and (2) the conduction of electrical impulses that control the physiological activities of the heart, skeletal muscle, and brain. Furthermore, metals play structural roles in proteins, participate in oxidation–reduction reactions, transport and store $O_2$, and function in the active sites of enzymes involved in nutrient and energy metabolism. Dietary requirements of animals for these nutrients are affected by physiological states, environment, and disease. The common syndromes of their dietary deficiencies include poor appetite, growth restriction, and low feed efficiency; nausea and vomiting; compromised immune response; reduced fertility; the impairment of bone growth and development; oxidative stress; and, in severe cases, death. Of note, these problems also occur in response to excess intakes of minerals. In feeding practices, caution must be taken to (1) recognize mineral-mineral and mineral-organic constituent interactions that are important in animal nutrition (e.g., Mg-K, Ca-P, Mg-Ca, Zn-Cu, Zn-Fe, Cu-Mo-S, Cu-Fe, Zn-Cu-Fe, and Fe-vitamin C); and (2) minimize the entry of toxic metals without physiological or nutritional function into animals via feedstuffs, drinking water, and other environmental sources (e.g., volcanic eruptions, mining, and smelting).

## REFERENCES

Abraham, G.E. 2005. The historical background of the iodine project. *The Original Internist.* 12:57–66.

Agricultural Research Council (ARC). 1981. *The Nutrient Requirements of Pigs.* Commonwealth Agricultural Bereaux, Slough, England.

Agus, Z. 1999. Hypomagnesemia. *J. Am. Soc. Nephrol.* 10:1616–1622.

Alexander, R.T. H. Dimke, and E. Cordat. 2013. Proximal tubular NHEs: Sodium, protons and calcium? *Am. J. Physiol.* 305:F229–236.

Al-Ghamdi, S.M., E.C. Cameron, and R.A. Sutton. 1994. Magnesium deficiency: Pathophysiologic and clinical overview. *Am. J. Kidney Dis.* 24:737–752.

Allen-Durrance, A.E. 2017. A quick reference on phosphorus. *Vet. Clin. North Am. Small Anim. Pract.* 47:257–262.

Anke, M., B. Groppel, W. Arnhold, M. Langer, and U. Krause. 1990. The influence of the ultratrace element deficiency (Mo, Ni, As, Cd, V) on growth, reproduction, and life expectance. In: *Trace Elements in Clinical Medicine*, Edited by H. Tomita. Springer-Verlag, Tokyo, Japan, pp. 361–376.

Arfin, S.M., R.L. Kendall, L. Hall, L.H. Weaver, A.E. Stewart, B.W. Matthews, and R.A. Bradshaw. 1995. Eukaryotic methionyl aminopeptidases: Two classes of cobalt-dependent enzymes. *Proc. Natl. Acad. Sci. USA* 92:7714–7718.

Arnone, A. 1972. X-ray diffraction study of binding of 2,3-diphosphoglycerate to human deoxyhaemoglobin. *Nature* 237:146–149.

Asagba, S.O. 2013. Cadmium absorption. In: *Encyclopedia of Metalloproteins*, Edited by R.H. Kretsinger, V.N. Uversky, and E.A. Permyakov, Springer, New York, NY, pp. 332–337.

Asard, H., R. Barbaro, P. Trost, and A. Berczi. 2013. Cytochromes $b_{561}$: Ascorbate-mediated trans-membrane electron transport. *Antioxid. Redox. Signal.* 19:1026–1035.

Ascenzi, P. and M. Fasano. 2007. Heme-hemopexin: A "chronosteric" heme-protein. *IUBMB Life* 59:700–708.

Assem, F.L. and S. Levy. 2009. A review of current toxicological concerns on vanadium pentoxide and other vanadium compounds: Gaps in knowledge and directions for future research. *J. Toxicol. Environ. Health B. Crit. Rev.* 12:289–306.

Assi, M.A., M.N.M. Hezmee, A.W. Haron, M.Y.M. Sabri, and M.A. Rajion. 2016. The detrimental effects of lead on human and animal health. *Vet. World* 9:660–671.

Averill, B.A. 1996. Dissimilatory nitrite and nitric oxide reductases. *Chem. Rev.* 96:2951–2964.

Bai, S.P., L. Lu, R.L. Wang, L. Xi, L.Y. Zhang, and X.G. Luo. 2012. Manganese source affects manganese transport and gene expression of divalent metal transporter 1 in the small intestine of broilers. *Br. J. Nutr.* 108:267–276.

Bajaj, M., E. Eiche, T. Neumann, J. Winter, and C. Gallert. 2011. Hazardous concentrations of selenium in soil and groundwater in North-West India. *J. Hazard Mater.* 189:640–646.

Baker, D.H. 1999. Cupric oxide should not be used as a copper supplement for either animals or humans. *J. Nutr.* 129:2278–2279.

Baker, D.H., T.M. Parr, and N.R. Augspurger. 2003. Oral iodine toxicity in chicks can be reversed by supplemental bromine. *J. Nutr.* 133:2309–2312.

Ballatori, N. 2002. Transport of toxic metals by molecular mimicry. *Environ. Health Perspect.* 110(Suppl. 5):689–694.

Barbier, O., L. Arreola-Mendoza, and L. María Del Razo. 2010. Molecular mechanisms of fluoride toxicity. *Chem.-Biol. Interact.* 188:319–333.

Barton, J.C., C.Q. Edwards, and R.T. Acton. 2015. HFE gene: Structure, function, mutations, and associated iron abnormalities. *Gene* 574:179–192.

Bazer, F.W., D. Worthington-White, M.F. Fliss, and S. Gross. 1991. Uteroferrin: A progesterone-induced hematopoietic growth factor of uterine origin. *Exp. Hematol.* 19:910–915.

Beckett, E.L., Z. Yates, M. Veysey, K. Duesing, and M. Lucock. 2014. The role of vitamins and minerals in modulating the expression of microRNA. *Nutr. Res. Rev.* 27:94–106.

Berbasova, T., S. Nallur, T. Sells, K.D. Smith, P.B. Gordon, S.L. Tausta, and S.A. Strobel. 2017. Fluoride export (FEX) proteins from fungi, plants and animals are "single barreled" channels containing one functional and one vestigial ion pore. *PLoS One* 12(5):e0177096.

Berg, J.N., J.P. Maas, J.A. Paterson, G.F. Krause, and L.E. Davis. 1984. Efficacy of ethylenediamine dihydriodide as an agent to prevent experimentally induced bovine foot rot. *Am. J. Vet. Res.* 45:1073–1078.

Besio, R., M.C. Baratto, R. Gioia, E. Monzani, S. Nicolis, L. Cucca, A. Profumo et al. 2013. A Mn(II)-Mn(II) center in human prolidase. *Biochim. Biophys. Acta* 1834:197–204.

Bjørklund, G. 2015. Selenium as an antidote in the treatment of mercury intoxication. *Biometals* 28:605–614.

Blaine, J., M. Chonchol, and M. Levi. 2015. Renal control of calcium, phosphate, and magnesium homeostasis. *Clin. J. Am. Soc. Nephrol.* 10:1257–1272.

Blumberg, W.E. and J. Peisach. 1965. An electron spin resonance study of copper uroporphyrin III and other touraco feather components. *J. Biol. Chem.* 240:870–876.

Bodnar, M., M. Szczyglowska, P. Konieczka, and J. Namiesnik. 2016. Methods of selenium supplementation: Bioavailability and determination of selenium compounds. *Crit. Rev. Food Sci. Nutr.* 56:36–55.

Boer, J.L., S.B. Mulrooney, and R.P. Hausinger. 2014. Nickel-dependent metalloenzymes. *Arch. Biochem. Biophys.* 544:142–152.

Bouron, A. and J. Oberwinkler. 2014. Contribution of calcium-conducting channels to the transport of zinc ions. *Pflugers Arch.* 466:381–387.

Bremner, I., J.M. Brockway, and H.T. Donnelly. 1976. Anaemia and veal calf production. *Vet. Rec.* 99:203–205.

Bressler, J.P., L. Olivi, J.H. Cheong, Y. Kim, and D. Bannona. 2004. Divalent metal transporter 1 in lead and cadmium transport. *Ann. N.Y. Acad. Sci.* 1012:142–152.

Brindha, K. and L. Elango. 2013. Causes for variation in bromide concentration in groundwater of a granitic aquifer. *Int. J. Res. Chem. Environ.* 3:163–171.

Brook, A.A., S.A. Chapman, E.A. Ulman, and G. Wu. 1994. Dietary manganese deficiency decreases rat hepatic arginase activity. *J. Nutr.* 124:340–344.

Brown, T.L., H.E. LeMay Jr, B.E. Bursten, and J.R. Burdge. 2003. *Chemistry* Prentice Hall, Upper Saddle River, NJ.

Bruns, G.A.P. and V.M. Ingram. 1973. Erythropoiesis in the developing chick embryo. *Dev. Biol.* 30:455–459.

Burgener, D., J.-P. Bonjour, and J. Caverzasio. 1995. Fluoride increases tyrosine kinase activity in osteoblast-like cells: Regulatory role for the stimulation of cell proliferation and Pi transport across the plasma membrane. *J. Bone Mineral Res.* 10:164–171.

Burk, R.F. and K.E. Hill. 2015. Regulation of selenium metabolism and transport. *Annu. Rev. Nutr.* 35:109–134.

Butler, A. 1998. Vanadium haloperoxidases. *Curr. Opin. Chem. Biol.* 2:279–285.

Cai, L., X.K. Li, Y. Song, and M.G. Cherian. 2005. Essentiality, toxicology and chelation therapy of zinc and copper. *Curr. Med. Chem.* 12:2753–2763.

Cambier, C., B. Detry, D. Beerens, S. Florquin, M. Ansay, A. Frans, T. Clerbaux, and P. Gustin. 1998. Effects of hyperchloremia on blood oxygen binding in healthy calves. *J. Appl. Physiol.* 85:1267–1272.

Candeal, E., Y.A. Caldas, N. Guillén, M. Levi, and V. Sorribas. 2017. Intestinal phosphate absorption is mediated by multiple transport systems in rats. *Am. J. Physiol. Gastrointest. Liver Physiol.* 312:G355–G366.

Carey, H.V., U.L. Hayden, S.S. Spicer, B.A. Schulte, and D.J. Benos. 1994. Localization of amiloride-sensitive $Na^+$ channels in intestinal epithelia. *Am. J. Physiol.* 266:G504–510.

Carlisle, E.M. 1972. Silicon: An essential element for the chick. *Science* 178:619–621.

Carlisle, E.M. 1980. Biochemical and morphological changes associated with long bone abnormalities in silicon deficiency. *J. Nutr.* 110:1046–1056.

Carter-Franklin, J.N. and A. Butler. 2004. Vanadium bromoperoxidase-catalyzed biosynthesis of halogenated marine natural products. *J. Am. Chem. Soc.* 126:15060–15066.

CDC (Center for Disease Control). 2017. Aluminum. https://www.atsdr.cdc.gov/toxprofiles/tp22-c6.pdf

Ceko, M.J., S. O'Leary, H.H. Harris, K. Hummitzsch, and R.J. Rodgers. 2016. Trace elements in ovaries: Measurement and physiology. *Biol. Reprod.* 94:86.

Chandrashekar, J., C. Kuhn, Y. Oka, D.A. Yarmolinsky, E. Hummler, N.J.P. Ryba, and C.S. Zuker. 2010. The cells and peripheral representation of sodium taste in mice. *Nature* 464:297–301.

Cheek, D.B. and A.B. Holt. 1963. Growth and body composition of the mouse. *Am. J. Physiol.* 205:913–918.

Cheng, J., B. Poduska, R.A. Morton, and T.M. Finan. 2011. An ABC-type cobalt transport system is essential for growth of *Sinorhizobium meliloti* at trace metal concentrations. *J. Bacteriol.* 193:4405–4416.

Clarkson, T.W. 2002. The three modern faces of mercury. *Environ. Health Perspect.* 110 (Suppl. 1):11–23.

Conant, J.B., B.F. Chow, and E.B. Schoenbach. 1933. The oxidation of hemocyanin. *J. Biol. Chem.* 101:463–473.

Conklin, A.W., Skinner, C.S., Felten, T.L., and Sanders, C.L. 1982. Clearance and distribution of intratracheally instilled vanadium compounds in the rat. *Toxicol. Lett.* 11:199–203.

Cotton, P.A. and L. Wilkinson. 1988. *Advanced Inorganic Chemistry*, 5th ed. John Wiley & Sons, New York, NY, pp. 162–165.

Cousins, R.J. 1994. Metal elements and gene expression. *Annu. Rev. Nutr.* 14:449–469.

Crans, D.C., J.J. Smee, E. Gaidamauskas, and L. Yang. 2004. The chemistry and biochemistry of vanadium and the biological activities exerted by vanadium compounds. *Chem. Rev.* 104:849–902.

Crowe, N.A., M.W. Neathery, W.J. Miller, L.A. Muse, C.T. Crowe, J.L. Varnadoe, and D.M. Blackmon. 1990. Influence of high dietary aluminum on performance and phosphorus bioavailability in dairy calves. *J. Dairy Sci.* 73:808–818.

Cromwell, G.L., M.D. Lindemann, H.J. Monegue, D.D. Hall, and D.E. Orr, Jr. 1998. Tribasic copper chloride and copper sulfate as copper sources for weanling pigs. *J. Anim. Sci.* 76:118–123.

Cunat, L., M.-C. Lanhers, M. Joyeux, and D. Burnel. 2000. Bioavailability and intestinal absorption of aluminum in rats. *Biol. Trace Elem. Res.* 76:31–55.

Cutting, G.R. 2015. Cystic fibrosis genetics: From molecular understanding to clinical application. *Nat. Rev. Genet.* 16:45–56.

Davidson, W.B. 1945. Nutritional deficiency diseases, their sources and effects. *Can. J. Comp. Med.* 9:155–162.

Davidsson, L., B. Lönnerdal, B. Sandström, C. Kunz, and C.L. Keen. 1989. Identification of transferrin as the major plasma carrier protein for manganese introduced orally or intravenously or after *in vitro* addition in the rat. *J. Nutr.* 119:1461–1464.

de Morais, H.A. and A.W. Biondo. 2006. Disorders of chloride: Hyperchloremia and hypochloremia. In: *Fluid, Electrolyte, and Acid–Base Disorders*, 3rd ed, Edited by S.P. DiBartola. Elsevier, New York, NY, pp. 80–91.

Dempski, R.E. 2012. The cation selectivity of the ZIP transporters. *Curr. Top. Membr.* 69:221–245.

Dick, A.T. 1952. The effect of diet and of molybdenum on copper metabolism in sheep. *Aust. Vet. J.* 28:30–33.

Dollwet, H.H.A. and J.R.J. Sorenson. 1985. Historic uses of copper compounds in medicine. *Trace Elem. Med.* 2:80–87.

Dowling, H.J., E.G. Offenbacher, and F.X. Pi-Sunyer. 1989. Absorption of inorganic, trivalent chromium from the vascularly perfused rat small intestine. *J. Nutr.* 119:1138–1145.

Drewnoski, M.E., D.J. Pogge, and S.L. Hansen. 2014. High-sulfur in beef cattle diets: A review. *J. Anim. Sci.* 92:3763–3780.

Dumont, J.E., F. Lamy, P. Roger, and C. Maenhaut. 1992. Physiological and pathological regulation of thyroid cell proliferation and differentiation by thyrotropin and other factors. *Physiol. Rev.* 72:667–697.

EFSA. 2008. Mercury as undesirable substance in animal feed: Scientific opinion of the panel on contaminants in the food chain. *EFSA J.* 654:1–76.

Engle, W.A. and J.A. Lemons. 1986. Composition of the fetal and maternal guinea pig throughout gestation. *Pediatr. Res.* 20:1156–1160.

Eskandari, S., D.D. Loo, G. Dai, O. Levy, E.M. Wright, and N. Carrasco. 1997. Thyroid $Na^+/I^-$ symporter. Mechanism, stoichiometry, and specificity. *J. Biol. Chem.* 272:27230–27238.

Fang, Y.Z., S. Yang, and G. Wu. 2002. Free radicals, antioxidants, and nutrition. *Nutrition* 18:872–879.

Felix, T.L., C.J. Long, S.A. Metzger, and K.M. Daniels. 2014. Adaptation to various sources of dietary sulfur by ruminants. *J. Anim. Sci.* 92:2503–2510.

Field, M. 2003. Intestinal ion transport and the pathophysiology of diarrhea. *J. Clin. Invest.* 111:931–943.

Formigari, A., P. Irato, and A. Santon. 2007. Zinc, antioxidant systems and metallothionein in metal mediated-apoptosis: Biochemical and cytochemical aspects. *Comp. Biochem. Physiol. C.* 146:443–459.

Fort, D.J., R.L. Rogers, D.W. McLaughlin, C.M. Sellers, and C.L. Schlekat. 2002. Impact of boron deficiency on *Xenopus laevis*. A summary of biological effects and potential biochemical roles. *Biol. Trace Elem. Res.* 90:117–142.

Fox, J.G., L.C. Anderson, F.M. Loew, and F.W. Quimby. 2002. *Laboratory Animal Medicine*. Academic Press, New York, NY.

Ganz, T. 2003. Hepcidin, a key regulator of iron metabolism and mediator of anemia of inflammation. *Blood* 102:783–788.

Garneau, A.P., G.A. Carpentier, A.A. Marcoux, R. Frenette-Cotton, C.F. Simard, W. Rémus-Borel, L. Caron et al. 2015. Aquaporins mediate silicon transport in humans. *PLoS One* 10(8):e0136149.

Gawenis, L.R., X. Stien, G.E. Shull, P.J. Schultheis, A.L. Woo, N.M. Walker, and L.L. Clarke. 2002. Intestinal NaCl transport in NHE2 and NHE3 knockout mice. *Am. J. Physiol.* 282:G776–G784.

Georgievskii, V.I., B.N. Annenkov, and V.T. Samokhin. 1982. *Mineral Nutrition of Animals*. Butterworths, London.

Glanz, J. 1996. Hemoglobin reveals new role as blood pressure regulator. *Science* 271:1670.

Gould, D.H., D.A. Dargatz, F.B. Garry, D.W. Hamar, and P.F. Ross. 2002. Potentially hazardous sulfur conditions on beef cattle ranches in the United States. *J. Am. Vet. Med. Assoc.* 221:673–677.

Gozzelino, R. and P. Arosio. 2016. Iron homeostasis in health and disease. *Int. J. Mol. Sci.* 17(130):1–14.

Grasbeck, R., I. Kouvonen, M. Lundberg, and R. Tenhunen. 1979. An intestinal receptor for heme. *Scand. J. Haematol.* 23:5–9.

Greene, L.W. 2016. Assessing the mineral supplementation needs in pasture-based beef operations in the Southeastern United States. *J. Anim. Sci.* 94:5395–5400.

Greene, L.W., P.G. Harms, G.T. Schelling, F.M. Byers, W.C. Ellis, and D.J. Kirk. 1985. Growth and estrous activity of rats fed adequate and deficient levels of phosphorus. *J. Nutr.* 115:753.

Greene, L.W. 2000. Designing mineral supplementation of forage programs for beef cattle. *J. Anim. Sci.* 77 (E-Suppl):1–9.

Greene, L.W., J.P. Fontenot, and K.E. Webb Jr. 1983. Site of magnesium and other macromineral absorption in steers fed high levels of potassium. *J. Anim. Sci.* 57:503–510.

Grummer, R.H., O.G. Bentley, P.H. Phillips, and G. Bohstedt. 1950. The role of manganese in growth, reproduction, and lactation of swine. *J. Anim. Sci.* 9:170–175.

Gulec, S. and J.F. Collins. 2014. Molecular mediators governing iron–copper interactions. *Annu. Rev. Nutr.* 34:95–116.

Guyton, A.C. and J.E. Hall. 2000. *Textbook of Medical Physiology.* W.B. Saunders Company, Philadelphia, PA.

Haider, L.M., L. Schwingshackl, G. Hoffmann, and C. Ekmekcioglu. 2016. The effect of vegetarian diets on iron status in adults: A systematic review and meta-analysis. *Crit. Rev. Food Sci. Nutr.* [Epub ahead of print].

Hajjar, J.J., J.C. Fucci, W.A. Rowe, and T.K. Tomicic. 1987. Effect of vanadate on amino acid transport in rat jejunum. *Proc. Soc. Exp. Biol. Med.* 184:403–409.

Hansard, S.L., II, C.B. Ammerman, and P.R. Henry. 1982. Vanadium metabolism in sheep. *J. Anim. Sci.* 55:350–356.

Hanschmann, E.-M., J.R. Godoy, C. Berndt, C. Hudemann, and C.H. Lillig. 2013. Thioredoxins, glutaredoxins, and peroxiredoxins—Molecular mechanisms and health significance: From cofactors to antioxidants to redox signaling. *Antioxid. Redox. Signal.* 19:1539–1605.

Hardt, P.F., W.R. Ocumpaugh, and L.W. Greene. 1991. Forage mineral concentration, animal performance, and mineral status of heifers grazing cereal pastures fertilized with sulfur. *J. Anim. Sci.* 69:2310–2320.

Harris, E.D. 2014. *Minerals in Foods.* DEStech Publications, Inc. Lancaster, PA.

Hart, E.B., H. Steenbock, J. Waddell, and C.A. Elvehjem. 1928. Iron in nutrition. VII. Copper as a supplement to iron for hemoglobin building in the rat. *J. Biol. Chem.* 277:797–812.

Heitzmann, D. and W. Richard. 2008. Physiology and pathophysiology of potassium channels in gastrointestinal epithelia. *Physiol. Rev.* 88:1119–1182.

Herzig, I., M. Navrátilová, J. Totušek, P. Suchý, V. Večerek, J. Blahová, and Z. Zralý. 2009. The effect of humic acid on zinc accumulation in chicken broiler tissues. *Czech. J. Anim. Sci.* 54:121–127.

Hidiroglou, M. 1979. Trace element deficiencies and fertility in ruminants: A review. *J. Dairy Sci.* 62:1195–1206.

Hoffer, L.J. 2002. Methods for measuring sulfur amino acid metabolism. *Curr. Opin. Clin. Nutr. Metab. Care* 5:511–517.

Hojyo, S. and T. Fukada. 2016. Zinc transporters and signaling in physiology and pathogenesis. *Arch. Biochem. Biophys.* 611:43–50.

Holm, R.H., P. Kennepohl, and E.I. Solomon. 1996. Structural and functional aspects of metal sites in biology. *Chem. Rev.* 96:2239–2314.

Holmberg, C.G and C.B. Laurell. 1948. Investigations in serum copper. II. Isolation of the copper containing protein, and a description of some of its properties. *Acta Chem. Scand.* 2:550–556.

Horsetalk. 2009. Polo pony selenium levels up to 20 times higher than normal. http://www.horsetalk.co.nz. Accessed on May 28, 2017.

Huang, C.L. and E. Kuo. 2007. Mechanism of hypokalemia in magnesium deficiency. *J. Am. Soc. Nephrol.* 18:2649–2652.

Huang, F., X.M. Wong, and L.Y. Jan. 2012. Calcium-activated chloride channels. *Pharmacol. Rev.* 64:1–15.

Huck, D.W. and A.J. Clawson. 1976. Excess dietary cobalt in pigs. *J. Anim. Sci.* 43:1231–1246.

Humer, E., C. Schwarz, and K. Schedle. 2015. Phytate in pig and poultry nutrition. *J. Anim. Physiol. Anim. Nutr.* 99:605–625.

Hunt, C.D. 1989. Dietary boron modified the effects of magnesium and molybdenum on mineral metabolism in the cholecalciferol-deficient chick. *Biol. Trace Elem. Res.* 22:201–220.

Hunt, C.D. 2012. Dietary boron: Progress in establishing essential roles in human physiology. *J. Trace Elem. Med. Biol.* 26:157–160.

Jaishankar, M., T. Tseten, N. Anbalagan, B.B. Mathew, and K.N. Beeregowda. 2014. Toxicity, mechanism and health effects of some heavy metals. *Interdiscip. Toxicol.* 7:60–72.

Jones, T.C. and R.D. Hunt. 1983. *Veterinary Pathology.* Lea & Febiger, Philadelphia, PA.

Jones, M. and D. van der Merwe. 2008. Copper toxicity in sheep is on the rise in Kansas and Nebraska. Comparative Toxicology, Kansas State Veterinary Diagnostic Laboratory, Kansas.

Johnson, M.A. and J.L. Greger. 1985. Tin, copper, iron and calcium metabolism of rats fed various dietary levels of inorganic tin and zinc. *J. Nutr.* 115:615–624.

Kabu, M. and M.S. Akosman. 2013. Biological effects of boron. *Rev. Environ. Contam. Toxicol.* 225:57–75.

Kaler, S.G., C.S. Holmes, D.S. Goldstein, J. Tang, S.C. Godwin, A. Donsante, C.J. Liew, S. Sato, and N. Patronas. 2008. Neonatal diagnosis and treatment of Menkes disease. *N. Engl. J. Med.* 358:605–614.

Kato, A. and M.F. Romero. 2011. Regulation of electroneutral NaCl absorption by the small intestine. *Annu. Rev. Physiol.* 73:261–281.

Kemmerer, A.R., C.A. Elvehjem, and E.B. Hart. 1931. Studies on the relation of manganese to the nutrition of the mouse. *J. Biol. Chem.* 92:623–630.

Kertesz, M.A. 2001. Bacterial transporters for sulfate and organosulfur compounds. *Res. Microbiol.* 152:279–290.

Kesner, M. 1999. *Bromine and Bromine Compounds from the Dead Sea.* Weizmann Institute of Science, Jerusalem, Israel.

Kessler, K.L., K.C. Olson, C.L. Wright, K.J. Austin, P.S. Johnson, and K.M. Cammack. 2012. Effects of supplemental molybdenum on animal performance, liver copper concentrations, ruminal hydrogen sulfide concentrations, and the appearance of sulfur and molybdenum toxicity in steers receiving fiber-based diets. *J. Anim. Sci.* 90:5005–5012.

Ketteler, M., O. Liangos, and P.H. Biggar. 2016. Treating hyperphosphatemia—Current and advancing drugs. *Expert Opin. Pharmacother.* 17:1873–1879.

Khan, Z.I., M. Ashraf, K. Ahmad, A. Bayat, M.K. Mukhtar, S.A.H. Naqvi, R. Nawaz, M.J. Zaib, and M. Shaheen. 2012. Lead toxicity evaluation in rams grazing on pasture during autumn and winter: A case study. *Pol. J. Environ. Study* 21:1257–1260.

Khanal, R.C. and I. Nemere. 2008. Regulation of intestinal calcium transport. *Annu. Rev. Nutr.* 28:1791–1796.

Kienzle, E., J. Zentek, and H. Meyer. 1998. Body composition of puppies and young dogs. *J. Nutr.* 128:2680S–2683S.

Kikuchi, K. and F.K. Ghishan. 1987. Phosphate transport by basolateral plasma membranes of human small intestine. *Gastroenterology* 93:106–113.

Knöpfel, M., L. Zhao, and M.D. Garrick. 2005. Transport of divalent transition-metal ions is lost in small-intestinal tissue of *b/b* Belgrade rats. *Biochemistry* 44:3454–3465.

Kobayashi, M. and S. Shimizu. 1999. Cobalt proteins. *Eur. J. Biochem.* 261:1–9.

Kollias-Baker, C. 1999. Therapeutics of musculoskeletal disease in the horse. *Vet. Clin. North Am. Equine Pract.* 15:589–602.

Kono, S. K. Yoshida, N. Tomosugi, T. Terada, Y. Hamaya, S. Kanaoka, and H. Miyajima. 2010. Biological effects of mutant ceruloplasmin on hepcidin-mediated internalization of ferroportin. *Biochim. Biophys. Acta* 1802:968–975.

Kornberg, A., N.N. Rao, and D. Ault-Riché. 1999. Inorganic polyphosphate: A molecule of many functions. *Annu. Rev. Biochem.* 68:89–125.

Kovesdy, C.P. 2017. Updates in hyperkalemia: Outcomes and therapeutic strategies. *Rev. Endocr. Metab. Disord.* 18:41–47.

Krewski, D., R.A. Yokel, E. Nieboer, D. Borchelt, J. Cohen, J. Harry, S. Kacew, J. Lindsay, A.M. Mahfouz, and V. Rondeau. 2007. Human health risk assessment for aluminium, aluminium oxide, and aluminium hydroxide. *J. Toxicol. Environ. Health B Crit. Rev.* 10(Suppl. 1):1–269.

Krishnamachari, K.A.V.R. 1987. Fluorine. In: *Trace Elements in Human and Animal Nutrition*, Vol. 1, Edited by W. Mertz, Academic Press, New York, NY, pp. 365–415.

Kubena, K.S. and J. Durlach. 1990. Historical review of the effects of marginal intake of magnesium in chronic experimental magnesium deficiency. *Magnes. Res.* 3:219–226.

Kumar, S. and T. Berl. 1998. Sodium. *Lancet* 352:220–228.

Lehmann-Horn, F. and K. Jurkat-Rott. 1999. Voltage-gated ion channels and hereditary disease. *Physiol. Rev.* 79:1317–1372.

Leonhard-Marek, S., F. Stumpff, I. Brinkmann, G. Breves, and H. Martens. 2005. Basolateral $Mg^{2+}/Na^+$ exchange regulates apical nonselective cation channel in sheep rumen epithelium via cytosolic $Mg^{2+}$. *Am. J. Physiol.* 288:G630–G645.

Leung, A.M. and L.E. Braverman. 2014. Consequences of excess iodine. *Nat. Rev. Endocrinol.* 10:136–142.

Liao, S.F., J.S. Monegue, M.D. Lindemann, G.L. Cromwell, and J.C. Matthews. 2011. Dietary supplementation of boron differentially alters expression of borate transporter (NaBCl) mRNA by jejunum and kidney of growing pigs. *Biol. Trace Elem. Res.* 143:901–912.

Lien, Y.H. and J.I. Shapiro. 2007. Hyponatremia: Clinical diagnosis and management. *Am. J. Med.* 120:653–658.

López-Alonso, M. 2012. Animal feed contamination by toxic metals. In: *Animal Feed Contamination*, Edited by J. Fink-Gremmels. Woodhead Publishing, U.K., pp. 183–204.

Lutgens, F.K. and E.J. Tarbuck. 2000. *Essentials of Geology*, 7th ed. Prentice Hall, Upper Saddle River, NJ.

Madsen, K.L, V.M. Porter, and R.N. Fedorak. 1993. Oral vanadate reduces $Na^+$-dependent glucose transport in rat small intestine. *Diabetes* 42:1126–1132.

Mahajan, R.J., M.L. Baldwin, J.M. Harig, K. Ramaswamy, and P.K. Dudeja. 1996. Chloride transport in human proximal colonic apical membrane vesicles. *Biochim. Biophys. Acta* 1280:12–18.

Manoharan, P., S. Gayam, S. Arthur, B. Palaniappan, S. Singh, G.M. Dick, and U. Sundaram. 2015. Chronic and selective inhibition of basolateral membrane Na-K-ATPase uniquely regulates brush border membrane Na absorption in intestinal epithelial cells. *Am. J. Physiol. Cell Physiol.* 308:C650–656.

Marks, J., E.S. Debnam, and R.J. Unwin. 2010. Phosphate homeostasis and the renal-gastrointestinal axis. *Am. J. Physiol. Renal Physiol.* 299:F285–F296.

Martens, H. and M. Schweigel. 2000. Pathophysiology of grass tetany and other hypomagnesemias. Implications for clinical management. *Vet. Clin. North Am. Food Anim. Pract.* 16:339–368.

Mason, J. and C.J. Cardin. 1977. The competition of molybdate and sulphate ions for a transport system in the ovine small intestine. *Res. Vet. Sci.* 22:313–315.

McBride, M.B., H.A. Shayler, H.M. Spliethoff, R.G. Mitchell, L.G. Marquez-Bravo, G.S. Ferenz, J.M. Russell-Anelli, L. Casey, and S. Bachman. 2014. Concentrations of lead, cadmium and barium in urban garden-grown vegetables: The impact of soil variables. *Environ. Pollut.* 194:254–261.

McCall, A.S., C.F. Cummings, G. Bhave, R. Vanacore, A. Page-McCaw, and B.G. Hudson, 2014. Bromine is an essential trace element for assembly of collagen IV scaffolds in tissue development and architecture. *Cell* 157:1380–1392.

McDonald, P., R.A. Edwards, J.F.D. Greenhalgh, C.A. Morgan, and L.A. Sinclair. 2011. *Animal Nutrition*, 7th ed. Prentice Hall, New York, NY.

Mertz, W. 1974. The newer essential trace elements, chromium, tin, vanadium, nickel and silicon. *Proc. Nutr. Soc.* 33:307–313.

Mertz, W. 1987. *Trace Elements in Human and Animal Nutrition*, Vol. 1, Academic Press, New York, NY.

Mondal, S., S. Haldar, P. Saha, T.K. Ghosh. 2010. Metabolism and tissue distribution of trace elements in broiler chickens fed diets containing deficient and plethoric levels of copper, manganese, and zinc. *Biol. Trace Elem. Res.* 137:190–205.

Moore, K.L, M. Schröder, E. Lombi, F.-J. Zhao, S.P. McGrath, M.J. Hawkesford, P.R. Shewry, and C.R.M. Grovenor. 2010. NanoSIMS analysis of arsenic and selenium in cereal grain. *New Phytologist* 185:434–445.

Morgan, A.M. and O.S. El-Tawil. 2003. Effects of ammonium metavanadate on fertility and reproductive performance of adult male and female rats. *Pharmacol. Res.* 47:75–85.

Morgan, V.E. and D.F. Chichester. 1935. Properties of the blood of the domestic fowl. *J. Biol. Chem.* 110:285–298.

Morris, M.E. 1992. Brain and CSF magnesium concentrations during magnesiumdeficit in animals and humans: Neurological symptoms. *Magnes. Res.* 5:303–313.

Morrow, D.A. 1969. Phosphorus deficiency and infertility in dairy heifers. *J. Am. Vet. Med. Assoc.* 154:761–768.

Moxham, J.W. and M.R. Coup. 1968. Arsenic poisoning of cattle and other domestic animals. *New Zealand Vet. J.* 16:161–165.

Musso, C.G. 2009. Magnesium metabolism in health and disease. *Int. Urol. Nephrol.* 41:357–362.

Naftz, D.L. and J.A. Rice. 1989. Geochemical processes controlling selenium in ground water after mining, Powder River Basin, Wyombg, U.S.A. *Appl. Geochem.* 4:4565–4575.

Naranmandura, H. and K.T. Suzuki. 2008. Identification of the major arsenic-binding protein in rat plasma as the ternary dimethylarsinous-hemoglobin-haptoglobin complex. *Chem. Res. Toxicol.* 21:678–685.

National Academy of Sciences (NAS). 2000. *Toxicological Effects of Methylmercury.* National Academies Press, Washington, D.C.

National Research Council (NRC). 1976. *Nutrient Requirements of Beef Cattle.* National Academies Press, Washington, DC.

National Research Council (NRC). 1994. *Nutrient Requirements of Poultry.* National Academies Press, Washington, D.C.

Naylor, G.P.L. and J.D. Harrison. 1995. Gastrointestinal iron and cobalt absorption and iron status in young rats and guinea pigs. *Hum. Exp. Toxicol.* 14:959–954.

Newnham, R.E. 1994. Essentiality of boron for healthy bones and joints. *Environ. Health Perspect.* 102 (Suppl. 7):83–85.

Nicola, J.P., C. Basquin, C. Portulano, A. Reyna-Neyra, M. Paroder, and N. Carrasco. 2009. The $Na+/I^-$ symporter mediates active iodide uptake in the intestine. *Am. J. Physiol. Cell Physiol.* 296:C654–662.

Nicola, J.P., N. Carrasco, and A.M. Masini-Repiso. 2015. Dietary I(–) absorption: Expression and regulation of the Na(+)/I(–) symporter in the intestine. *Vitam. Horm.* 98:1–31.

Nielsen, F.H. 1987. Nickel. In: *Trace Elements in Human and Animal Nutrition*, Vol. 1, Edited by W. Mertz, Academic Press, New York, NY, pp. 245–273.

Nielsen, F.H. 1991. Nutritional requirements for boron, silicon, vanadium, nickel, and arsenic: Current knowledge and speculation. *FASEB J.* 5:2661–2667.

Nielsen, F.H. 1995. Vanadium absorption. In: *Handbook of Metal-Ligand Interactions in Biological Fluids. Bioinorganic Medicine*. Vol. 1, Edited by G. Berthon, Marcell Dekker, Inc., New York, NY, pp. 425–427.

Nielsen, F.H. 2008. Is boron nutritionally relevant? *Nutr. Rev.* 66:183–191.

Nielsen, F.H. 2009. Micronutrients in parenteral nutrition: Boron, silicon, and fluoride. *Gastroenterology* 137(5 Suppl.):S55–S60.

Nigam, S.K., K.T. Bush, G. Martovetsky, S.Y. Ahn, H.C. Liu, E. Richard, V. Bhatnagar, and W. Wu. 2015. The organic anion transporter (OAT) family: A systems biology perspective. *Physiol. Rev.* 95:83–123.

Niles, G.A. 2017. Toxicoses of the ruminant nervous system. *Vet. Clin. North Am. Food Anim. Pract.* 33:111–138.

NRC. 2005. *Mineral Tolerance of Animals.* 2nd ed. National Academies Press, Washington, D.C.

Nollet, H. and P. Deprez. 2005. Hereditary skeletal muscle diseases in the horse. A review. *Vet. Q.* 27:65–75.

O'Dell, B.L., B.C. Hardwick, G. Reynolds, and J.E. Savage. 1961. Connective tissue defect in the chick resulting from copper deficiency. *Proc. Soc. Exp. Biol. Med.* 108:402–405.

O'Dell, G.D., W.J. Miller, W.A. King, J.C. Ellers, and H. Jurecek. 1970a. Effect of nickel supplementation on production and composition of milk. *J. Dairy Sci.* 53:1545–1548.

O'Dell, G.D., W.J. Miller, W.A. King, S.L. Moore, and D.M. Blackmon. 1970b. Nickel toxicity in the young bovine. *J. Nutr.* 100:1447–1453.

Orr, C.L., D.P. Hutcheson, R.B. Grainger, J.M. Cummins, and R.E. Mock. 1990. Serum copper, zinc, calcium and phosphorus concentrations of calves stressed by bovine respiratory disease and infectious bovine rhinotracheitis. *J. Anim. Sci.* 68:2893–2900.

O'Shaughnessy, K.M. and F.E. Karet. 2004. Salt handling and hypertension. *J. Clin. Invest.* 113:1075–1081.

Palis, J. and G.B. Segel. 1998. Developmental biology of erythropoiesis. *Blood Rev.* 12:106–114.

Papanikolaou, G. and K. Pantopoulos. 2005. Iron metabolism and toxicity. *Toxicol. Appl. Pharmacol.* 202:199–211.

Park, M., Q. Li, N. Shcheynikov, W. Zeng, and S. Muallem. 2004. NaBC1 is a ubiquitous electrogenic $Na^+$-coupled borate transporter essential for cellular boron homeostasis and cell growth and proliferation. *Mol. Cell.* 16:331–341.

Patel, P., A.V. Prabhu, and T.G. Benedek. 2017. The history of John Hans Menkes and kinky hair syndrome. *JAMA Dermatol.* 153(1):54.

Pena-Munzenmayer, G., M. Catalan, I. Cornejo, C.D. Figueroa, J.E. Melvin, M.I. Niemeyer, L.P. Cid, and F.V. Sepulveda. 2005. Basolateral localization of native ClC-2 chloride channels in absorptive intestinal epithelial cells and basolateral sorting encoded by a CBS-2 domain di-leucine motif. *J. Cell Sci.* 118:4243–4252.

Pirkmajer, S. and A.V. Chibalin. 2016. Na,K-ATPase regulation in skeletal muscle. *Am. J. Physiol. Endocrinol. Metab.* 311:E1–E31.

Pitt, M.A. 1976. Molybdenum toxicity: Interactions between copper, molybdenum and sulphate. *Agents and Actions* 6:758–769.

Pizzorno, L. 2015. Nothing boring about boron. *Integr. Med (Encinitas).* 14:35–48.

Pogge, D.J., M.E. Drewnoski, and S.L. Hansen. 2014. High dietary sulfur decreases the retention of copper, manganese, and zinc in steers. *J. Anim. Sci.* 92:2182–2191.

Pond, W.G., D.C. Church, and K.R. Pond. 1995. *Basic Animal Nutrition and Feeding.* 4th ed., John Wiley & Sons, New York, NY.

Poulos, T.L. 2014. Heme enzyme structure and function. *Chem. Rev.* 114:3919–3962.

Prasad, A.S., A. Schulert, A. Miale, Z. Farid, and H.H. Sandstead. 1963. Zinc and iron deficiencies in male subjects with dwarfism and hypogonadism but without ancylostomiasis, schistosomiasis or severe anemia. *Am. J. Clin. Nutr.* 12:437–444.

Price, C.T., K.J. Koval, and J.R. Langford. 2013. Silicon: A review of its potential role in the prevention and treatment of postmenopausal osteoporosis. *Int. J. Endocrinol.* 2013:Article ID 316783.

Ragsdale, S.W. 2009. Nickel-based enzyme systems. *J. Biol. Chem.* 284:18571–18575.

Ratcliffe, S., R. Jugdaohsingh, J. Vivancos, A. Marron, R. Deshmukh, J.F. Ma, N. Mitani-Ueno et al. 2017. Identification of a mammalian silicon transporter. *Am. J. Physiol. Cell Physiol.* 312:C550–C561.

Ratnaike, R.N. 2003. Acute and chronic arsenic toxicity. *Postgrad. Med. J.* 79:391–396.

Rayner-Canham, G. and T. Overton. 2006. *Descriptive Inorganic Chemistry.* W.H. Freeman and Company, New York, NY.

Reeves, P.G. and L.C. DeMars. 2006. Signs of iron deficiency in copper-deficient rats are not affected by iron supplements administered by diet or by injection. *J. Nutr. Biochem.* 17:635–642.

Rehder, D. 2008. *Bioinorganic Vanadium Chemistry.* John Wiley & Sons, New York, NY.

Rehder, D. 2015. The role of vanadium in biology. *Metallomics* 7:730–742.

Reynolds, J.A., G.D. Potter, L.W. Greene, G. Wu, G.K. Carter, M.T. Martin, T.V. Peterson, M. Murray-Gerzik, G. Moss, and R.S. Erkert. 1998. Genetic-diet interactions in the hyperkalemic periodic paralysis syndrome in quarter horses fed varying amounts of potassium. IV. Pre-cecal and post-ileal absorption of potassium and sodium. *J. Equine Vet. Sci.* 18:827–831.

Rezaei, R., D.A. Knabe, C.D. Tekwe, S. Dahanayaka, M.D. Ficken, S.E. Fielder, S.J. Eide, S.L. Lovering, and G. Wu. 2013. Dietary supplementation with monosodium glutamate is safe and improves growth performance in postweaning pigs. *Amino Acids* 44:911–923.

Rhoads, M. 1999. Glutamine signaling in intestinal cells. *J. Parenter. Enteral. Nutr.* 23(Suppl. 5):S38–40.

Roberts, R.M., T.J. Raub, and F.W. Bazer. 1986. Role of uteroferrin in transplacental iron transport in the pig. *Fed. Proc.* 45:2513–2518.

Rodriguez-Castro, K.I., F.J. Hevia-Urrutia, and G.C. Sturniolo. 2015. Wilson's disease: A review of what we have learned. *World J. Hepatol.* 7:2859–2870.

Rogers, C.S., D.A. Stoltz, D.K. Meyerholz, L.S. Ostedgaard, T. Rokhlina, P.J. Taft, M.P. Rogan et al. 2008. Disruption of the CFTR gene produces a model of cystic fibrosis in newborn pigs. *Science* 321:1837–1841.

Rondon-Berrios, H., C. Argyropoulos, T.S. Ing, D.S. Raj, D. Malhotra, E.I. Agaba, M. Rohrscheib et al. 2017. Hypertonicity: Clinical entities, manifestations and treatment. *World J. Nephrol.* 6:1–13.

Ronis, M.J.J., I.R. Miousse, A.Z. Mason, N. Sharma, M.L. Blackburn, and T.M. Badger. 2015. Trace element status and zinc homeostasis differ in breast and formula-fed piglets. *Exp. Biol. Med.* 240:58–66.

Rosseland, B.O., T.D. Eldhuset, and M. Staurnes. 1990. Environmental effects of aluminium. *Environ. Geochem. Health* 12:17–27.

Rowe, R.I. and C.D. Eckhert. 1999. Boron is required for zebrafish embryogenesis. *J. Exp. Biol.* 202:1649–1654.

Ryazanova, L.V., L.J. Rondon, S. Zierler, Z. Hu, J. Galli, T.P. Yamaguchi, A. Mazur, A. Fleig, and A.G. Ryazanov. 2010. TRPM7 is essential for $Mg^{2+}$ homeostasis in mammals. *Nat. Commun.* 1:109.

Ryu, D.-Y., S.-J. Lee, D.W. Park, B.-S. Choi, C.D. Klaassen, and J.-D. Park. 2004. Dietary iron regulates intestinal cadmium absorption through iron transporters in rats. *Toxicol. Lett.* 152:19–25.

Sabbagh, Y., H. Giral, Y. Caldas, M. Levi, and S.C. Schiavi. 2011. Intestinal phosphate transport. *Adv. Chronic Kidney Dis.* 18:85–90.

Salant, W., J.B. Rieger, and E.L.P. Treuthardt. 1914. Absorption and fate of tin in the body. *J. Biol. Chem.* 17:265–273.

Santamaria, A.B. and S.I. Sulsky. 2010. Risk assessment of an essential element: Manganese. *J. Toxicol. Environ. Health A* 73:128–155.

Scarratt, W.K., T.J. Collins, and D.P. Sponenberg. 1985. Water deprivation-sodium chloride intoxication in a group of feeder lambs. *J. Am. Vet. Med. Assoc.* 186:977–978.

Scheuhammer, A.M. and M.G. Cherian. 1985. Binding of manganese in human and rat plasma. *Biochim. Biophys. Acta* 840:163–169.

Schryver, H.F., H.F. Hintz, P.H. Craig, D.E. Hogue, and J.E. Lowe. 1972. Site of phosphorus absorption from the intestine of the horse. *J. Nutr.* 102:143–147.

Schwarz, K. 1978. Significance and function of silicon in warm-blooded animals: Review and outlook. In: *Biochemistry of Silicon and Related Problems*, Edited by G. Bendz and I. Lindquist, Plenum Press, New York, NY, pp. 207–230.

Schwarz, K. and C.M. Foltz. 1957. Selenium as an integral part of factor 3 against dietary necrotic liver degeneration. *J. Am. Chem. Soc.* 79:3292–3293.

Schwarz, K. and W. Mertz. 1959. Chromium (III) and glucose tolerance factor. *Arch. Biochem. Biophys.* 85:292–295.

Schwarz, K., D.B. Milne, and E. Vinyard. 1970. Growth effects of tin compounds in rats maintained in a trace element-controlled environment. *Biochem. Biophys. Res. Commun.* 40:22–29.

Schwarz, K. and D.B. Milne. 1971. Growth effects of vanadium in the rat. *Science* 174:426–428.
Schwarz, K. and D.B. Milne. 1972. Growth-promoting effects of silicon in rats. *Nature* 239:333–334.
Schweigel, M., I. Lang, and H. Martens. 1999. $Mg^{2+}$ transport in sheep rumen epithelium: evidence for an electrodiffusive uptake mechanism. *Am. J. Physiol.* 277: G976–G982.
Selz, T., J. Caverzasio, and J.P. Bonjour. 1991. Fluoride selectively stimulates Na-dependent phosphate transport in osteoblast-like cells. *Am. J. Physiol.* 260:E833–E838.
Sendamarai, A.K., R.S. Ohgami, M.D. Fleming, and C.M. Lawrence. 2008. Structure of the membrane proximal oxidoreductase domain of human Steap3, the dominant ferrireductase of the erythroid transferrin cycle. *Proc. Natl. Acad. Sci. USA* 105:7410–7415.
Sheftel, A.D., A.B. Mason, and P. Ponka. 2012. The long history of iron in the universe and in health and disease. *Biochim. Biophys. Acta* 1820:161–187.
Sheng, H.P., R.A. Huggins, C. Garza, H.J. Evans, A.D. LeBlanc, B.L. Nichols, and P.C. Johnson. 1981. Total body sodium, calcium, and chloride measured chemically and by neutron activation in guinea pigs. *Am. J. Physiol.* 241:R419–422.
Smith, P. 1982. Cobalt concentrations in equine serum. *Vet. Rec.* 111:149.
Song, P., A. Onishi, H. Koepsell, and V. Vallon. 2016. Sodium glucose cotransporter SGLT1 as a therapeutic target in diabetes mellitus. *Expert Opin. Ther. Targets* 20:1109–1125.
Spasovski, G. 2015. Advances in pharmacotherapy for hyperphosphatemia in renal disease. *Expert Opin. Pharmacother.* 16:2589–2599.
Sripanyakorn, S., R. Jugdaohsingh, W. Dissayabutr, S.H.C. Anderson, R.P.H. Thompson, and J.J. Powell. 2009. The comparative absorption of silicon from different foods and food supplements. *Br. J. Nutr.* 102:825–834.
Stanier, P. 1983. Molybdenum concentrations in equine serum. *Vet. Rec.* 113:518.
Starke, I.C., R. Pieper, K. Neumann, J. Zentek, and W. Vahjen. 2014. The impact of high dietary zinc oxide on the development of the intestinal microbiota in weaned piglets. *FEMS Microbiol. Ecol.* 87:416–427.
Stehling, O. and R. Lill. 2013. The role of mitochondria in cellular iron–sulfur protein biogenesis: Mechanisms, connected processes, and diseases. *Cold. Spring. Harb. Perspect. Biol.* 5:a011312.
Sun, L.-H., N.-Y. Zhang, Q.-H. Zhai, X. Gao, C. Li, Q. Zheng, C.S. Krumm, and D. Qi. 2014. Effects of dietary tin on growth performance, hematology, serum biochemistry, antioxidant status, and tin retention in broilers. *Biol. Trace Elem. Res.* 162:302–308.
Sunderman, F.W. Jr, L.M. Bibeau, and M.C. Reid. 1983. Synergistic induction of microsomal heme oxygenase activity in rat liver and kidney by diethyldithiocarbamate and nickel chloride. *Toxicol. Appl. Pharmacol.* 71:436–444.
Suttle, N.F. 2010. *Mineral Nutrition of Livestock*, 4th ed. CABI, Wallingford, U.K.
Swarthout, J.T., R.C. D'Alonzo, N. Selvamurugan, and N.C. Partridge. 2002. Parathyroid hormone-dependent signaling pathways regulating genes in bone cells. *Gene* 282:1–17.
Sweeney, R.W. 1999. Treatment of potassium balance disorders. *Vet. Clin. North Am. Food Anim. Pract.* 15:609–617.
Takeda, E., H. Yamamoto, H. Yamanaka-Okumura, and Y. Taketani. 2012. Dietary phosphorus in bone health and quality of life. *Nutr. Rev.* 70:311–321.
Theil, E.C. 2004. Iron, ferritin, and nutrition. *Annu. Rev. Nutr.* 24:327–343.
Thom, C.S., C.F. Dickson, D.A. Gell, and M.J. Weiss. 2013. Hemoglobin variants: Biochemical properties and clinical correlates. *Cold Spring Harb. Perspect. Med.* 3(3):a011858.
Tkachuk, R. and F.D. Kuzina. 1972. Mercury levels in wheat and other cereals, oilseed and biological samples. *J. Sci. Food. Agric.* 23:1183–1195.
Todd, J.R. 1969. Chronic copper toxicity of ruminants. *Proc. Nutr. Soc.* 28:189–198.
Todd, W.R., C.A. Elvehjem, and E.B. Hart. 1934. Zinc in the nutrition of the rat. *Am. J. Physiol.* 107:146–156.
Tomas, F.M. and B.J. Potter. 1976. The site of magnesium absorption from the ruminant stomach. *Br. J. Nutr.* 36:37–45.
Topf, J.M. and P.T. Murray. 2003. Hypomagnesemia and hypermagnesemia. *Rev. Endocr. Metab. Disord.* 4(2):195–206.
Tsiani, E. and I.G. Fantus. 1997. Vanadium compounds. Biological actions and potential as pharmacological agents. *Trends. Endocrinol. Metab.* 8:51–58.
Ullrey, D.E. 1980. Regulation of essential nutrient additions to animal diets (selenium—a model case). *J. Anim. Sci.* 51:645–651.
Valdez, C.E., Q.A. Smith, M.R. Nechay, and A.N. Alexandrova. 2014. Mysteries of metals in metalloenzymes. *Acc. Chem. Res.* 47:3110–3117.
Vázquez, M., M. Calatayud, C. Jadán Piedra, G.M. Chiocchetti, D, Vélez, and V. Devesa. 2015. Toxic trace elements at gastrointestinal level. *Food Chem. Toxicol.* 86:163–175.

Villa-Bellosta, R. and V. Sorribas. 2010. Arsenate transport by sodium/phosphate cotransporter type IIb. *Toxicol. Appl. Pharmacol.* 247:36–40.

Vincent, J.B. 2000. The biochemistry of chromium. *J. Nutr.* 130:715–718.

Voets, T., B. Nilius, S. Hoefs, A.W. van der Kemp, G. Droogmans, R.J. Bindels, and J.G. Hoenderop. 2004. TRPM6 forms the $Mg^{2+}$ influx channel involved in intestinal and renal $Mg^{2+}$ absorption. *J. Biol. Chem.* 279:19–25.

Vulpe, C.D., Y.M. Kuo, T.L. Murphy, L. Cowley, C. Askwith, N. Libina, J. Gitschier, and G.J. Anderson. 1999. Hephaestin, a ceruloplasmin homologue implicated in intestinal iron transport, is defective in the sla mouse. *Nat. Genet.* 21:195–199.

Waldron, K.J., J.C. Rutherford, D., Ford, and N.J. Robinson. 2009. Metalloproteins and metal sensing. *Nature* 460:823–830.

Wang, W.W., Z.L. Wu, Z.L. Dai, Y. Yang, J.J. Wang, and G. Wu. 2013. Glycine metabolism in animals and humans: Implications for nutrition and health. *Amino Acids* 45:463–477.

Wang, Z.Y., Y.L. Yang, W.F. Wu, H.D. Wang, D.H. Shi, and J. Mason. 1992. Treatment of copper poisoning in goats by the injection of trithiomolybdate. *Small Rumin. Res.* 8:31–40.

Ward, D.M. and J. Kaplan. 2012. Ferroportin-mediated iron transport: Expression and regulation. *Biochim. Biophys. Acta* 1823:1426–1433.

Welch, A.H., D.B. Westjohn, D.R. Helsel, and R.B. Wanty. 2000. Arsenic in ground water of the United States: Occurrence and geochemistry. *Groundwater* 38:589–604.

Whitford, GM. 1996. The metabolism and toxicity of fluoride. *Monogr. Oral Sci.* 16 (Rev. 2):1–153.

WHO (World Health Organization). 2003. *Boron in Drinking Water.* Geneva, Switzerland.

WHO (World Health Organization). 2004. *Inorganic Tin in Drinking Water.* Geneva, Switzerland.

WHO (World Health Organization). 2005. *Mercury in Drinking Water.* Geneva, Switzerland.

WHO (World Health Organization). 2006. *Cobalt and Inorganic Cobalt Compounds.* Geneva, Switzerland.

WHO (World Health Organization). 2011a. *Cadmium in Drinking Water.* Geneva, Switzerland.

WHO (World Health Organization). 2011b. *Lead in Drinking Water.* Geneva, Switzerland.

Wiegmann, T.B., H.D. Day, and R.V. Patak. 1982. Intestinal absorption and secretion of radioactive vanadium ($^{48}VO_3^-$) in rats and effect of $Al(OH)_3$. *J. Toxicol. Environ. Health* 10:233–245.

Williams, D.M., F.S. Kennedy, and B.G. Green. 1983. Hepatic iron accumulation in copper-deficient rats. *Br. J. Nutr.* 50:653–660.

Wolf, F.I. and A. Cittadini. 2003. Chemistry and biochemistry of magnesium. *Mol. Aspects. Med.* 24:3–9.

Wolff, J. and I.L. Chaikoff. 1948. Plasma inorganic iodide as a homeostatic regulator of thyroid function. *J. Biol. Chem.* 174:555–564.

Wright, E.M. and D.D. Loo. 2000. Coupling between $Na^+$, sugar, and water transport across the intestine. *Ann. N.Y. Acad. Sci.* 915:54–66.

Wrobel, J.K., R. Power, and M. Toborek. 2016. Biological activity of selenium: Revisited. *IUBMB Life* 68:97–105.

Wu, G. 2013. *Amino Acids: Biochemistry and Nutrition*, CRC Press, Boca Raton, FL.

Wu, G., B. Imhoff-Kunsch, and A.W. Girard. 2012. Biological mechanisms for nutritional regulation of maternal health and fetal development. *Paediatr. Perinatal. Epidemiol.* 26(Suppl. 1):4–26.

Yamaguchi, M., Y. Kubo, and T. Yamamoto. 1979. Inhibitory effect of tin on intestinal calcium absorption in rats. *Toxicol. Appl. Pharmacol.* 47:441–444.

Yamazaki, D., Y. Funato, J. Miura, S. Sato, S. Toyosawa, K. Furutani, Y. Kurachi et al. 2013. Basolateral $Mg^{2+}$ extrusion via CNNM4 mediates transcellular $Mg^{2+}$ transport across epithelia: A mouse model. *PLoS Genet.* 9(12):e1003983.

Yokoi, K., M. Kimura, and Y. Itokawa. 1990. Effect of dietary tin deficiency on growth and mineral status in rats. *Biol. Trace Elem. Res.* 24:223–231.

Yörük, I., Y. Deger, H. Mert, N. Mert, and V. Ataseven. 2007. Serum concentration of copper, zinc, iron, and cobalt and the copper/zinc ratio in horses with equine herpesvirus-1. *Biol. Trace Elem. Res.* 118:38–42.

Zakon, H.H. 2012. Adaptive evolution of voltage-gated sodium channels: The first 800 million years. *Proc. Natl. Acad. Sci. USA* 109(Suppl. 1):10619–25.

Zhang, Z.W., T. Watanabe, S. Shimbo, K. Higashikawa, and M. Ikeda. 1998. Lead and cadmium contents in cereals and pulses in north-eastern China. *Sci. Total Environ.* 220:137–145.

Zhao, F.J., J.L. Stroud, T. Eagling, S.J. Dunham, S.P. McGrath, and P.R. Shewry. 2010. Accumulation, distribution, and speciation of arsenic in wheat grain. *Environ. Sci. Technol.* 44:5464–5468.

Zimmermann, M.B. 2009. Iodine deficiency. *Endocr. Rev.* 30:376–408.

Žofková, I. 2016. Hypercalcemia. Pathophysiological aspects. *Physiol. Res.* 65:1–10.

# 11 Nutritional Requirements for Maintenance and Production

Mammals (e.g., cattle, pigs, rats, and sheep) and birds (e.g., chickens, ducks, and geese) are warm-blooded animals, and maintain a constant internal temperature through changes in internal heat production in response to a cold or warm environment (Collier and Gebremedhin 2015). Most mammals and birds have body temperatures of around 37°C and 40°C, respectively. In contrast, cold-blooded animals (e.g., fish, shrimp, amphibians, reptiles, insects, and worms) do not maintain a constant body temperature, with their body temperature changing with their environment (van de Pol et al. 2017). Thus, per kg body weight (BW), metabolic rates differ markedly between warm- and cold-blooded animals (Blaxter 1989). However, all animals have basal requirements for energy and nutrients to sustain their physiological needs for survival and physical activities. In livestock, poultry, and fish production, nutritional requirements of animals generally refer to their requirements for nutrients in diets.

Dietary energy is contained in the three major classes of macronutrients: carbohydrates, lipids, and protein/amino acids (AAs) (Chapter 8). The requirement for energy or nutrients that keeps the animal at zero energy or nutrient balance is defined as the maintenance requirement for energy or nutrients. Different animal species, individuals of the same species, and the same animals at different physiological states have different maintenance requirements for energy, AAs, glucose, fatty acids, vitamins, minerals, and water (Pond et al. 1995). When nutrient intake exceeds maintenance requirement, animals grow, or produce (Campbell 1988). Thus, the total requirement for energy or nutrients is the sum of the requirements for maintenance plus production (including growth, lactation, gestation, and work), which is of practical importance in animal nutrition (NRC 2001, 2011, 2012). The same nutrients are needed for both maintenance and production. However, the amounts of energy or nutrients required for maintenance generally differ from those for production. Likewise, the efficiencies of energy or nutrient utilization for maintenance are different from those for production (McDonald et al. 2011). In practice, the requirements of animals for energy and nutrients can be determined through a combination of several techniques, including calorimetry, feeding trials, comparative slaughter experiments, and isotope studies.

For healthy, physically active adult animals (e.g., mature dogs, cats, horses, and boars) that do not gain tissue protein or produce a product (e.g., eggs, milk, conceptus, or wool), requirements for energy and nutrients should be above their maintenance requirements. This is because muscular activity requires energy and is also associated with enhanced metabolism of nutrients in a tissue-specific manner (Newsholme and Leech 2009). Protein and fats are deposited in growing animals only when: (1) the dietary intake of energy and AAs exceeds the maintenance requirements for energy and AAs; and (2) the requirements for all other nutrients are met. However, in gestating dams, their fetuses can grow despite inadequate maternal intake of energy, dry matter (DM) or macronutrients, because the mothers mobilize nutrients from their tissues to provide an endogenous source of nutrients (Wu et al. 2006). Similarly, lactating cows produce a large amount of milk even though they exhibit a negative energy balance in the first month after calving (Maltz et al. 2013). This illustrates dynamic changes, or plasticity, in nutrient metabolism and requirements of animals in their life cycles. Inadequate intake of nutrients reduces the growth and productivity of the animal, whereas excesses in their intake have environmental consequences such as contributions to nitrogen and phosphorus pollution, as well as global warming (Wu et al. 2014c).

Either undernutrition or overnutrition causes poor animal health, results in metabolic disorders, and increases risks for infectious diseases. Optimizing animal nutrition is essential to maximizing the production of high-quality animal products for human consumption, economic returns in animal agriculture, and the longevity of animals. The major objective of this chapter is to highlight the principles of nutritional requirements of animals for maintenance and production.

## NUTRITIONAL REQUIREMENTS FOR MAINTENANCE

### Energy Requirements for Maintenance

The basal metabolic rate (BMR) of an animal is used to estimate its maintenance requirement for energy (Baldwin 1995). The BMR is the energy expended in the fasting animal, which is also known as fasting catabolism (Chapter 8). When expressed as net energy (NE), the BMR represents the maintenance requirement for energy. However, when expressed as metabolizable energy (ME) for fed animals, the maintenance requirement includes the BMR plus the heat increment of the diet (see Chapter 8). Energy requirements for the basal metabolism are explained by (1) intracellular protein turnover (protein synthesis and degradation); (2) maintenance of cellular ionic gradients, especially the Na and K gradients; (3) substrate cycles (e.g., substrate cycles in glucose and fat intermediary metabolism); (4) biosynthetic processes (e.g., gluconeogenesis, protein synthesis, ureagenesis); (5) active transport of organic nutrients (e.g., AA transport by cells, glucose reabsorption by renal epithelial cells, and urea excretion by the kidneys); and (6) contraction of skeletal, cardiac, and smooth muscles (Baldwin and Bywater 1984; Kelly et al. 1991; Milligan and Summers 1986). These variables are summarized in Table 11.1.

The BMR is determined using direct or indirect calorimetry. Any factors that influence fasting metabolism should be eliminated (Blaxter 1989). In addition, previous feeding levels, which can affect gene expression and substrate concentrations in tissues, influence plateau heat production and BMR in fasted animals (de Lange et al. 2006). Therefore, it is important that the test animal be in the postabsorptive, resting, and healthy state, fed balanced diets before the testing, and housed in its thermoneutral zone. Specifically, the gastrointestinal tract of the animal must first be free of feed residues. The excretion of feed residues from the gastrointestinal tract can be monitored by observing the disappearance of a marker (e.g., dye) in feed particles, and it takes a longer time in ruminants than in nonruminants (Chapter 1). For example, in cows, about 80% of the feed particles ingested through the mouth are excreted within 80 h, and the excretion rate is reduced thereafter; therefore, the BMR in ruminants is often measured 10 days after the last meal (Chapter 1). Second, the metabolic rate of an animal is a function of its physiological state in which the body temperature should be constant. However, under disease conditions (e.g., fever and infections) or exposure to toxins, substrate oxidation is altered, contributing to changes in basal energy requirements. Third, the

**TABLE 11.1**
**Energy Requirements for Basal Metabolism in Animals**

| Physiological Activity | Maximum Contribution (%) |
|---|---|
| Intracellular protein turnover | 25 |
| Maintenance of cellular ionic gradients | 25 |
| Substrate cycles in metabolism | 15 |
| Biosynthetic processes in metabolism | 15 |
| Active transport of organic nutrients | 10 |
| Contraction of skeletal, cardiac, and smooth muscles | 10 |

*Source:* Baldwin, R.L. 1995. *Modeling Ruminant Digestion and Metabolism*. Chapman & Hall, New York, NY; Kelly, J.M. et al. 1991. *J. Dairy Sci.* 74:678–694; Milligan, L.P. and M. Summers. 1986. *Proc. Nutr. Soc.* 45:185–193.

**TABLE 11.2**
**Typical Thermoneutral Zones (TNZ) of Animals**

| Species | TNZ (°C) | Species | TNZ (°C) |
|---|---|---|---|
| Rat | 26–28 | Sheep | 20–25 |
| Dog (with long hair) | 13–16 | Cow | 15–20 |
| Fowl | 15–26 | Goat | 15–20 |
| Turkey poults | 20–28 | Swine | 20–26 |
| Calves | 15–20 | Man | 26–28 |

*Source:* Bondi, A.A. 1987. *Animal Nutrition*. John Wiley & Sons, New York, NY.

test animal must be placed within its thermoneutral (comfort) zone (Table 11.2), within which heat production by the resting animal is minimal and is sufficient to offset heat loss. The thermoneutral zone may be reduced when humidity is high (Mount 1978). At a high temperature, high humidity prevents cooling by reducing the evaporation of sweat. Technically, the relative humidity inside an animal calorimeter should not exceed 50% (e.g., 37%–45% for sheep) (Pinares and Waghorn 2012). Therefore, care should be taken to account for these variables when measuring the BMR of animals.

## Additional Factors Affecting the BMR

### Metabolic Size of Animals

In mammals and birds, an important element in determining the BMR is to assure that the animal maintains a constant body temperature, as noted previously. In fish, the BMR is also important to sustain life. Heat loss to the environment is proportional to (a) the difference between body temperature and ambient temperature; and (b) body surface area. Since the body temperatures of all farm mammals are nearly the same, their body surface area is the major factor that determines their heat loss (Blaxter 1989). This notion also applies to birds and fish, whose body temperatures are usually higher and lower, respectively, than those of mammals. The surface area of the animal, which is often difficult to measure, is generally proportional to the 2/3 power of the BW (White and Seymour 2002). However, much evidence from the studies of mammalian species ranging from the 20 g mouse to the 4 ton elephant indicates that heat loss is proportional to the 3/4 power of the BW (Brody 1945). Thus, the 3/4 power of the BW ($W^{0.75}$) is generally referred to as the metabolic BW or metabolic size (Chapter 8). Some authors also have used $W^{0.73}$ to express the BMR in certain species. Of interest, variations of BMR per metabolic body size among animal species are much lower than values expressed per kg BW (Table 11.3).

### Age and Sex of Animals

The age of an animal is another major factor affecting its BMR. The BMR usually decreases with postnatal age (Turner and Taylor 1983), which corresponds to a decrease in circulating concentrations of thyroid hormones (Segal et al. 1982). For example, the BMRs (MJ/kg $W^{0.73}$) of cattle at different ages are: 0.586 (1 month, mo); 0.565 (3 mo); 0.523 (6 mo); 0.419 (18 mo); 0.398 (24 mo); 0.377 (36 mo); and 0.356 (48 mo) (Bondi 1987). The BMR also decreases with a reduction in lean body mass. An increase in skeletal muscle mass and activity has the effect of enhancing the BMR, but an increase in white adipose tissue has the opposite effect (Blaxter 1989). Of interest, the metabolic rate of the fetus is relatively low, compared with that of newborns. For example, the rate of heat production per kg tissue in fetal lambs is about the same as that of mature ewes at rest (Bondi 1987). However, within 24 h after birth, the BMR of the newborn lamb is 2 times greater than that of the fetus because of needs for heat production to maintain the body temperature in the extrauterine life.

**TABLE 11.3**
**BMRs of Adult Animals**

| Species | Body Weight (BW) (kg) | Basal Metabolic Rate (MJ/Day) | | |
|---|---|---|---|---|
| | | Per Animal | Per kg BW | Per kg BW$^{0.75}$ |
| Cow | 500 | 34.1 | 0.0682 | 0.323 |
| Pig | 70 | 7.5 | 0.107 | 0.310 |
| Man | 70 | 7.1 | 0.101 | 0.293 |
| Sheep | 50 | 4.3 | 0.0860 | 0.229 |
| Fowl | 2 | 0.60 | 0.300 | 0.357 |
| Rat | 0.3 | 0.12 | 0.400 | 0.53 |

*Source:* Bondi, A.A. 1987. *Animal Nutrition.* John Wiley & Sons, New York, NY.

Oxidation of fatty acids by brown adipose tissue contributes to the non-shivering thermogenesis in neonatal lambs and many other animals such as cattle, rats, and humans (Satterfield and Wu 2011). Some species (e.g., pigs and chicks) lack brown adipose tissue before or after birth.

Hormonal profiles in plasma differ between males and females during the growing-finishing periods and adult life. For example, the concentrations of thyroid hormones in plasma are greater in males than in females (Segal et al. 1982). Thus, the BMR of males is generally higher than that of nonpregnant females of similar age and size. Similarly, intact males (e.g., boars) have a greater BMR and gain less body fat than castrated males (e.g., barrows) (Knudson et al. 1985). Furthermore, factors (e.g., ambient temperatures, disease, and dietary intakes of tyrosine, phenylalanine, and iodine) that affect the synthesis and degradation of thyroid hormones can also greatly influence the BMR (Kim 2008).

### Normal Living Conditions of Animals

The BMR is measured in fasting animals (Blaxter 1989). It is difficult to translate the values of the BMR into practical recommendations for maintenance requirements of normal living animals, because of (a) the heat increment of feeding; (b) the muscular activity of the free-moving animal; and (c) changes in the habitual environment that deviate from the thermoneutral zones for the animals (Bondi 1987). Thus, it is preferable to determine the net energy (NE) requirement for maintenance using fed animals with an energy balance of zero. Alternatively, the rate of fasting heat production may be multiplied by a factor of greater than 1 (i.e., 1.15 for housed animals, and 1.25–1.5 for outdoor grazing animals) to obtain the true BMR of animals under feeding conditions (Osuji 1974). The factors of 1.15 to 1.25–1.5 are recommended because (1) the acts of eating, chewing, gut motility, standing, and walking, and other physical activities in the housed animals produce some heat, which amounts to ~15% of the heat produced by fasting metabolism; and (2) grazing animals, which spend more energy on walking longer distances to forage foods than their housed counterparts, generate a large amount of heat, which amounts to ~25%–50% of the heat produced by fasting metabolism (Osuji 1974).

## Protein and AA Requirements for Maintenance

AAs are building blocks of proteins and regulators of protein kinases, including the mechanistic target of rapamycin (MTOR; the master activator of protein synthesis) (Chapter 7). Animals degrade protein and AAs continuously, and therefore there must be a maintenance requirement for AAs to replace their daily losses (Campbell 1988). In addition, the mammalian small intestine requires glutamate, glutamine, and aspartate as major metabolic fuels for maintenance and growth (Wu 1998), and the fish small intestine requires both glutamate and glutamine to fulfill metabolic needs for ATP and nucleotide synthesis (Jia et al. 2017). Although avian enterocytes have a limited ability to degrade glutamine due to low glutaminase activity (Wu et al. 1995), those cells may extensively oxidize glutamate and aspartate for ATP production. The maintenance requirement for protein is the sum of the amounts of nitrogen excreted in the urine, feces, and lungs and skin when the animal is at nitrogen equilibrium (Reeds and Garlick 2003). In practice, the maintenance requirement for AAs can be determined by feeding the test animal two or more levels of dietary protein or AAs and then extrapolating the BW to zero AA intake (ARC 1981). Note that the energy requirement for maintenance must be met in these studies to minimize the use of body protein as an energy source to reduce urinary nitrogen excretion. Under ideal conditions, urinary nitrogen excretion (so-called endogenous nitrogen, meaning that its immediate precursors are derived from tissues rather than feed) should be minimal. The minimum excretion of urinary nitrogen is proportional to metabolic body size (McDonald et al. 2011). Since different AAs are utilized through different metabolic pathways and at different rates, and since many AAs are synthesized de novo from common substrates in animals, it is technically challenging to determine the true maintenance requirements for AAs.

Fecal nitrogen excretion derived from the gastrointestinal epithelium and bacteria, as well as other endogenous sources, is called metabolic nitrogen (Chapter 7). In nonruminants, amounts of the metabolic nitrogen are estimated by feeding a nitrogen-free diet to the animals and measuring fecal nitrogen excretion. However, estimates obtained with AA-free diets may be lower than the true maintenance protein requirements of animals receiving normal amounts of dietary AAs, due to lower rates of whole-body protein turnover and AA catabolism in animals fed AA-free diets. Furthermore, feeding a nitrogen-free diet inhibits fermentation in the rumen of ruminants (Chapter 5), and therefore this method is not applicable to ruminants. Rather, the regression technique, in which fecal N (g/100 g fecal DM; Y axis) is plotted as a function of feed N (g/100 g fecal DM; X axis) and extrapolated to zero N intake, is often used to estimate the amount of metabolic nitrogen in ruminants (Hironaka et al. 1970).

Ruminants produce more metabolic nitrogen than nonruminants. For example, the amount of fecal nitrogen excreted per day is about 1–2 g/kg DM in nonruminants and about 4–6 g/kg DM intake in mature ruminants (e.g., 280 g metabolizable protein/day in a 600 kg cow). This reflects a much larger gastrointestinal tract and a much greater number of bacteria in the digestive tract of ruminants than nonruminants. Depending on species and age, the maintenance requirements of various animals for true protein are 1–6 g/$BW^{0.75}$ kg per day, and are affected by their living environment (ARC, 1981; NRC 1995, 2001). This is equivalent to 1.8–11 g true dietary protein/$BW^{0.75}$ kg per day, given that their true digestibility is 85% and the efficiency of utilization of truly digestible protein for maintenance is 65% (i.e., 1 or 6 $\div$ 85% $\div$ 65% $=$ 1.8 or 11). Corresponding to changes in the rates of whole-body protein turnover and AA oxidation, the maintenance requirements of dietary protein or AAs are decreased with age but increased with cold or heat stress and disease.

## Fatty Acid Requirements for Maintenance

Like other organic nutrients, fatty acids in an animal undergo turnover constantly and are lost from the body via oxidation to $CO_2$ and $H_2O$ (Chapter 6). Thus, fatty acids, particularly ω3 and ω6 polyunsaturated fatty acids (PUFAs), must be provided to animals ultimately from the diet to maintain membrane fluidity, basal metabolism, and survival of the cells. Since long-chain fatty acids are stored for a prolonged period of time (at least days) in white adipose tissue, liver, and other tissues, maintenance requirements for these nutrients cannot be readily determined in a short-term experiment (Bondi 1987). A long-term study is required to achieve this goal, and at the same time, both the energy and nitrogen balances of the animal must be maintained. The minimum requirements for PUFAs by animals can be determined through feeding different dietary levels of the PUFAs and then observing growth performance, as well as the appearance of skin and hair. A deficiency of PUFAs often results in dermatitis, bleeding gums, skin necrosis, and hair loss. The ARC (1981) reported the minimal (maintenance) requirements of 30–90 kg pigs for linoleic acid (0.31 g/kg BW per day) or arachidonic acid (0.21 g/kg BW per day).

### Vitamin Requirements for Maintenance

Vitamins are excreted in the urine and feces. Thus, it is customary to determine the maintenance requirement for water- and lipid-soluble vitamins by measuring their excretion (including metabolites) in urine and feces under conditions of dietary depletion (Combs 1998), analogous to those used for estimating the maintenance requirements for AAs (Chapter 7). Since the digestion and absorption of lipid-soluble vitamins requires fats, dietary provision of lipids is a prerequisite for assessing the bioavailability of those vitamins. The ARC (1981) summarized the minimum (maintenance) requirements for vitamins by pigs. For example, the minimum requirements for retinol by 5–40 kg pigs, 40–90 kg pigs, and breeding sows (or gilts) are 22, 16, and 14 μg/kg BW per day, respectively. In addition, the minimum requirements of thiamin, riboflavin, pantothenic acid, pyridoxine, and vitamin $B_{12}$ by 90 kg pigs are 17, 28, 110, 28, and 0.10 μg/kg BW per day, respectively. Ruminants consuming plant-based diets with sufficient carbohydrates, proteins, and cobalt have no maintenance requirements for dietary vitamins because of their synthesis by ruminal bacteria (NRC 2011). It is noteworthy that a deficiency of most water-soluble vitamins can occur rapidly in animals, with such syndromes as skin lesions, neurological disorders, anemia, and fatigue (Chapter 9). Like the deficiencies of PUFAs, it takes a prolonged period of time for animals to exhibit the syndromes due to deficiencies of lipid-soluble vitamins, such as blurry vision, failure of blood clotting after a cut, injury, anemia, and abnormal bone development (Combs 1998).

### Mineral Requirements for Maintenance

In animals, minerals are essential for extracellular and intracellular osmolarity, as well as the growth and development of bones and teeth (Chapter 10). These nutrients are excreted primarily in the urine and, to a much lesser extent, in the feces (Chapter 10). Since minerals are not degraded in animals, their maintenance requirements by the animal can be determined by measuring their obligatory losses in urine plus feces under conditions of dietary depletion (Harris 2014). Alternatively, radioactive or stable isotopes can be used to determine the excretion of endogenous minerals. Let us use calcium as an example. The excretion of endogenous calcium by an adult non-lactating cow weighing 500 kg is 8.1 g/day (Bondi 1987). Assuming that the true absorption rate of dietary calcium in cattle is 45%, the maintenance requirement for dietary calcium would be 36 mg/kg BW per day [i.e., (8.1 g/day ÷ 0.45)/500 kg]. The mineral requirement for maintenance is generally proportional to metabolic body size. For example, the maintenance requirement for calcium by the non-lactating cow is about 0.325 mg/kJ of fasting heat production. The ARC (1981) summarized the obligatory losses of minerals from growing pigs as follows (μg/kg BW per day): calcium, 32; phosphorus, 20; magnesium, 400; sodium, 1140; and potassium, 130. These values indicate the maintenance requirements for the minerals.

### Water Requirements for Maintenance

Water ($H_2O$) is the most abundant nutrient in animals. This polar molecule contains one oxygen and two hydrogen atoms (Figure 11.1). The oxygen atom is connected to each hydrogen atom by a covalent bond, with the oxygen atom carrying a partial negative charge and each of the hydrogen atoms having a partial positive charge. Water exists in a liquid (between 0°C and 100°C at the standard pressure of 1 atm), solid (ice, <0°C), or vaporous (>100°C) state. At physiological temperatures, water is a chemically stable liquid in animals. Owing to its polarity, each water molecule can potentially form four intermolecular hydrogen bonds with surrounding water molecules.

Water content in the fat-free body is 72%–75% in various animal species (Table 11.4). Most of the water in the body is present inside the cells (intracellular water), but a significant proportion of water is outside the cells (extracellular water). Intracellular water, interstitial water, and blood-plasma water account for 50%, 15%, and 5% of the BW, respectively (Maynard et al. 1979). Dietary water is absorbed primarily by the small intestine and the large intestine. It was assumed for years that water passes through biological membranes only by simple diffusion through lipid bilayers until the

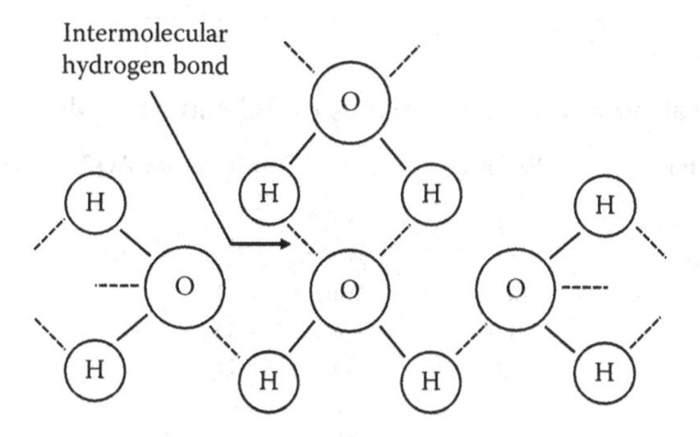


**FIGURE 11.1** The structure of the water molecule. Water ($H_2O$) is a small bent molecule consisting of one oxygen and two hydrogen atoms. The oxygen atom is connected to each hydrogen atom by a covalent bond. Each water molecule can potentially form four intermolecular hydrogen bonds with surrounding water molecules.

## TABLE 11.4
## The Composition of Water, Crude Protein, and Ash in the Fat-Free Body of Different Animal Species[a]

| Species | Body Weight (kg) | Water (%) | Crude Protein (%) | Ash (%) |
|---|---|---|---|---|
| Cat | 4 | 74.4 | 21.0 | 4.6 |
| Cattle | 500 | 71.4 | 22.1 | 6.0 |
| Hen | 2.5 | 71.9 | 22.0 | 3.9 |
| Horse | 650 | 73.0 | 20.5 | 5.8 |
| Man | 65 | 72.8 | 19.4 | 7.8 |
| Pig | 125 | 75.6 | 19.6 | 4.7 |
| Rat | 0.35 | 73.7 | 22.1 | 4.2 |
| Rabbit | 2.6 | 72.8 | 23.2 | 4.0 |
| Sheep | 80 | 71.1 | 21.9 | 4.2 |

*Source:* Blaxter, K.L. 1989. *Energy Metabolism in Animals and Man*. Cambridge University Press, New York, NY.

[a] Crude protein (%) = N% × 6.25.

discovery of water channel proteins known as aquaporins (AQPs) (Agre and Kozono 2003). Since water passes through cell membranes relatively slowly by simple diffusion, the rapid and specific water flow across biological membranes is primarily mediated by AQPs, the water-transporting protein channels. AQPs are a family of small (28–30 kD) integral membrane proteins that primarily transport water, but some APQs also transport glycerol, urea, and other solutes across the plasma membrane of cells (Zhu et al. 2015). The movement of water via AQPs is driven by osmotic gradients. To date, 13 AQP isoforms (AQPs 0–12) have been identified in mammals. On the basis of their structural and functional properties, AQPs are divided into three subgroups: classical aquaporins (AQPs 0, 1, 2, 4, 5, 6, and 8), aquaglyceroporins (AQPs 3, 7, 9, and 10), and superaquaporins (AQPs 11 and 12) (Table 11.5). AQPs are widely distributed in reproductive (both male and female), respiratory, digestive, excretory, circulatory, muscular, and other systems of animals (Zhu et al. 2015).

Water is lost from the animal body periodically through urine and feces, and constantly through evaporation from the skin and the respired air via the lungs (McDonald et al. 2011). The loss of water through the skin and lungs is known as insensible perspiration. Water losses are positively related to body size and are affected by nutritional, physiological, and environmental factors. For example, water loss from the feces increases as the proportion of undigested dietary material increases

**TABLE 11.5**
**Classification and Characteristics of AQP in Animals**

| Classification | Isoform | Substrates for AQP Transport |
|---|---|---|
| Aquaporin | AQP0 | Water |
| | AQP1 | Water, $CO_2$, NO, and $NH_3$ |
| | AQP2 | Water |
| | AQP4 | Water, $CO_2$, $O_2$, and NO |
| | AQP5 | Water and $CO_2$ |
| | AQP6 | Water, anions, urea, and glycerol |
| | AQP8 | Water, urea, and $NH_3$ |
| Aquaglyceroporin | AQP3 | Water, urea, glycerol, and $NH_3$ |
| | AQP7 | Water, urea, glycerol, and $NH_3$ |
| | AQP9 | Water, urea, glycerol, other solutes, and $NH_3$ |
| | AQP10 | Water, urea, and glycerol |
| Superaquaporin | AQP11 | Uncertain |
| | AQP12 | Uncertain |

*Source:* Zhu, C. et al. 2015. *Front. Biosci.* 20:838–871.

(Bondi 1987). In addition, as the concentrations of glucose, ketone bodies, and urea in plasma increase, water loss via urination increases. Furthermore, water loss through evaporation and respiration increases as the ambient temperature increases. For example, Maynard et al. (1979) reported that the average *Bos taurus* cow weighing 450 kg and consuming 10 kg dry feed per day drank 28, 41, and 66 L of water when the ambient temperature was 4°C, 21°C, and 32°C, respectively. Average requirements of animals for water in a temperate climate are summarized in Table 11.6.

Water is essential to life (Maynard et al. 1979). This nutrient dissolves many salts and hydrophilic organic molecules (e.g., sugars, AAs, nucleic acids, and enzymes), and is the solvent in all

**TABLE 11.6**
**Average Daily Requirements of Animals for Water at a Temperate Climate**

| | Daily Water Requirements | |
|---|---|---|
| Species | L | L/kg Body Weight |
| Beef cow (lactating, 500 kg) | 60 | 0.12 |
| Beef cattle (450 kg) | 40 | 0.09 |
| Dairy cow (lactating, 500 kg) | 90 | 0.18 |
| Dairy cow (maintenance, 500 kg) | 60 | 0.12 |
| Horse (medium work, 450 kg) | 40 | 0.09 |
| Horse (lactating, 450 kg) | 50 | 0.11 |
| Poultry, hen (2 kg) | 0.5 | 0.25 |
| Rat (0.3 kg) | 0.075 | 0.25 |
| Swine (growing, 30 kg) | 6 | 0.20 |
| Swine (growing, 60–100 kg) | 8 | 0.10 |
| Swine (lactating sow, 150 kg) | 18 | 0.12 |
| Sheep (lactating ewe, 50 kg) | 6 | 0.12 |
| Sheep (fattening lamb, 50 kg) | 4 | 0.08 |

*Source:* Maynard, L.A. et al. 1979. *Animal Nutrition*. McGraw-Hill, New York, NY.

biochemical reactions. When acids (e.g., HCl, glutamic acid, aspartic acid) dissolve in water, they yield their corresponding anions. An adequate volume of water in the body is necessary to maintain the intracellular and extracellular concentrations of all nutrients (including AAs, glucose, fatty acids, and electrolytes) within physiological ranges. Thus, water is required to maintain osmo-equilibrium in all animals. In addition, as a component of synovial fluid, water plays an important role in lubricating the joints to facilitate muscle locomotion. Also, as the major constituent of cerebrospinal fluid, water helps to provide a cushion for protecting the nervous system. Furthermore, water absorbs heat produced from chemical reactions to minimize increases in body temperature. Therefore, animals must consume sufficient water for health and production. This is particularly important for: (1) lactating dams; (2) young mammals within the first week after weaning; (3) all animals living at high ambient temperatures; and (4) all sick animals with fever and an elevated body temperature. Thus, severe dehydration in animals results in their death.

### Use of Energy and Its Substrates for Maintenance

Different nutrients are utilized in animals through different pathways (Chapters 5–10). For example, the rumen ferments carbohydrates to produce short-chain fatty acids (SCFAs) (Chapter 6). As discussed in Chapter 8, the energetic efficiency of ATP production from the oxidation of protein in mammals (which synthesize urea from ammonia) is higher than that in birds (which synthesize uric acid from ammonia). In both mammals and birds, but not fish, the energetic efficiency of ATP production from the oxidation of fats or glucose is higher than that for proteins or AAs (Chapter 8). Thus, protein is generally not used as the major metabolic fuel in the whole body of mammals and birds. However, this is not the case with fish, as certain AAs (e.g., Glu, Gln, and Asp) may be important energy substrates for their metabolically active tissues, such as the small intestine, liver, and kidneys (Jia et al. 2017).

Even at maintenance requirements, animals synthesize proteins and fats. However, both proteins and fats undergo continuous degradation (Chapters 6 and 7). In growing or producing animals, the maintenance requirement is coupled to the production requirement. Therefore, the total requirement is generally used to formulate diets for farm animals (NRC 2001, 2011, 2012). Since the energetic efficiencies of synthetic processes vary with precursors and products (Chapter 8), energy substrates have different efficiencies with which they are used for maintenance and production. For example, in pigs, the efficiencies of AAs and fatty acids for maintenance are 78% and 95% of those for glucose, respectively, whereas the efficiencies of AAs and glucose for fat deposition are 61% and 83% of those for fatty acids (ARC 1981). In growing beef cattle, the efficiencies of ME used for both maintenance and BW gain increase with increasing ME in the diet within a physiological range (2.0–3.2 Mcal/kg diet) (Blaxter 1989). This is because dietary intake of energy (primarily in the forms of water-soluble and insoluble polysaccharides) by ruminants above the maintenance level can enhance microbial protein yields and SCFA production in the rumen (de Faria and Huber 1983; Hackmann and Firkins 2015). This results in (1) reduced production of gases (e.g., $CH_4$) by the gastrointestinal tract; (2) increased hepatic gluconeogenesis from propionate; (3) increased lipogenesis from acetate and butyrate in white adipose tissue; (4) increased ATP production from acetate and butyrate in diverse tissues; and (5) increased availability of AAs for protein synthesis in skeletal muscle and other tissues, leading to reduced excretion of nitrogenous wastes in the urine and feces. When a quantity of dietary energy is not used by animals for maintenance and production, an energetic inefficiency in feed utilization occurs (van Milgen et al. 2001). This concept helps us to better understand nutritional requirements of animals for production.

## NUTRITIONAL REQUIREMENTS FOR PRODUCTION

Diets for productive animals must meet the requirements for energy and specific nutrients (AAs, fatty acids, carbohydrates, minerals, vitamins, and water) for: (1) the formation of milk (mammals), eggs (poultry), and wool (e.g., sheep); (2) the growth of tissues, such as skeletal muscle; and

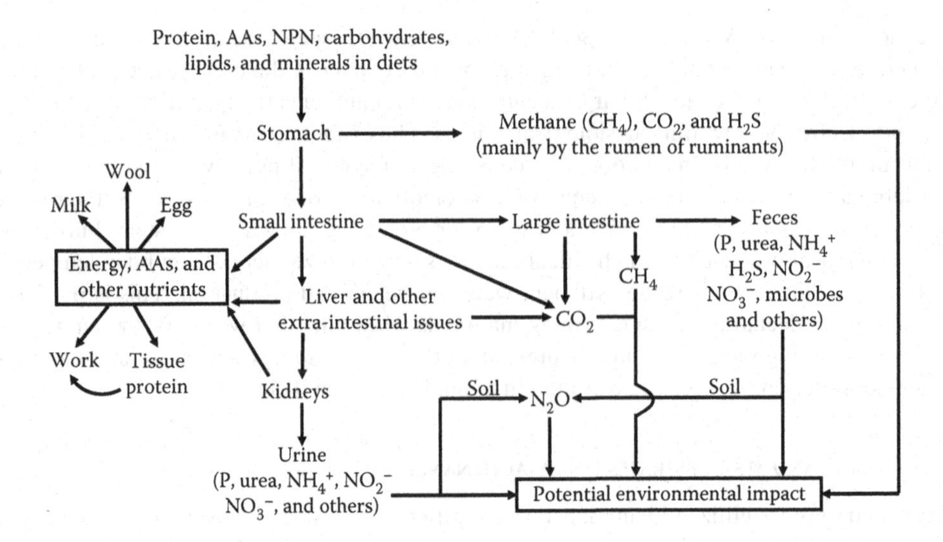


**FIGURE 11.2** Metabolism of nutrients to methane ($CH_4$), carbon dioxide, urea, ammonia, hydrogen sulfide ($H_2S$), nitrous oxide ($N_2O$), and other products in animals. Dietary nutrients are terminally digested and absorbed in the small intestine. The kidneys and liver contribute AAs and glucose for utilization. The metabolism of protein, carbohydrates, and lipids in the gastrointestinal tract (particularly the rumen of ruminants) generates methane and $CO_2$, whereas the metabolism of protein also produces ammonia and $H_2S$. Nitrogenous substances in urine and feces are fermented by bacteria in the soil to form $N_2O$. Optimizing the formulation of diets is an attractive means to mitigate the potential impact of animal production on greenhouse gas emissions and the environment. AAs, amino acids; NPN, nonprotein and non-AA nitrogen.

(3) work (horses and cattle) (Figure 11.2). Since AAs cannot be synthesized solely from fatty acids and carbohydrates, animals must consume protein or AAs from diets (Wu et al. 2014a,b,c). Protein deficiency results in low appetite, poor growth (fetuses and young animals), depressed reproductive performance, reduced milk production, and impaired egg laying. Providing adequate protein or AAs in ruminant (e.g., beef cattle and cow) and nonruminant (e.g., pig and poultry) diets is essential for optimal animal health and productivity (the ability of an animal to grow, reproduce, and produce useful outputs [e.g., milk, eggs, wool, and muscular work]), as well as farm profitability.

Nutritional requirements of animals for production are often determined from factorial analysis of their products (e.g., tissue protein accretion, milk, wool, and eggs), and must be considered along with their nutritional requirements for maintenance. The efficiency of utilization of dietary energy and nutrients for production depends on animal species, tissue, and nutritional adequacy. While all nutrients are essential for animal production, the dietary ratios of protein:energy, arginine:lysine, calcium:phosphorus, and ω3 PUFAs:ω6 PUFAs are of particular interest to producers when practical ration are formulated. Enhancing the efficiency of nutrient utilization can help sustain the global animal industry, while mitigating its adverse impact on the environment.

### Suboptimal Efficiencies of Animal Protein Production in Current Agricultural Systems

A major goal of animal nutrition is to fully realize the genetic potential of livestock, poultry, and fish for reproduction, growth (including accretion of protein in skeletal muscle), and resistance to disease, while preventing the excessive accumulation of white adipose tissue (Wu et al. 2014c). In mammals, birds, and fish, mitochondria play an important role in ATP production, and mitochondrial function greatly influences energetic efficiency and therefore feed efficiency (Bottje and Carstens 2009). Biological efficiency of animal production, which refers to the effectiveness in use of feed to produce tissues (e.g., skeletal muscle), milk, or eggs in agricultural operations, is a

**TABLE 11.7**
**Suboptimal Efficiencies of Production of Animal Protein in Current Agricultural Systems[a,b]**

| Animal | Weeks of Production | Efficiency for Protein Gain (%) (Based on Edible Protein)[b] | Efficiency for Protein Gain (%) (Based on Whole-Body Protein)[c] |
|---|---|---|---|
| Broiler chickens | 6 | 33.3 | 39.9 |
| Laying hens (eggs) | 55 | 31.3 | 34.0 |
| Pigs | 25 | 23.3 | 29.6 |
| Cows (milk) | 44 | 19.7 | 19.7 |
| Feedlot beef cattle | 54 | 12.1 | 18.9 |
| Grazing beef cattle | 76 | 6.7 | 10.5 |

[a] Adapted from Wu, G. et al. 2014a. *Ann. N.Y. Acad. Sci.* 1328:18–28.

[b] Animals were fed their conventional diets. Calculated as edible protein in product (e.g., tissue, eggs, or milk)/protein intake from diet × 100%. Protein is expressed as crude protein. Crude protein content (g/100 g fresh weight) in cow's milk, beef meat, pig meat, poultry meat, and eggs is 3.62, 19.7, 20.5, 19.1, and 12.7, respectively. The ratio of live BW to edible meat (kg/kg) is 515:288 for grazing beef cattle, 540:302 for feedlot ("cereal") beef cattle, 109:78.1 for pigs, and 2.54:2.0 for poultry. A laying hen produces 17.7 kg edible eggs (295 eggs × 60 g/egg) in 55 weeks. In edible meat and eggs, the weight of bone and shell is deducted from the total weight of carcass and egg, respectively.

[c] Calculated as whole-body protein in animal/protein intake from diet × 100%. These data are physiologically meaningful. Protein is expressed as crude protein. The CP content in the nonedible part of beef, pork, or poultry is 14%.

major determinant of economic efficiency to minimize costs for livestock, poultry, and fish production (Campbell 1988). Natural resources for growing feedstuffs and pasture plants are becoming increasingly limited. Owing to physiological and biochemical constraints, the digestion of feeds and the conversion of dietary proteins to tissue proteins in animals remain suboptimal (Table 11.7). Irreversible catabolism of AAs generates carbon dioxide, ammonia, hydrogen sulfide, methane, urea, and uric acid, further reducing the efficiencies of animal growth, lactation, and reproduction (Chapter 7). Although bacteria in the rumen have a high capacity for converting nonprotein nitrogen into AAs, this process generates a large amount of ammonia, and its use for the synthesis of AAs and protein occurs at suboptimal rates. Thus, the efficiency of utilizing dietary protein to produce whole-body protein is less than 40% for nonruminants and less than 25% for ruminants (Wu et al. 2014a). In addition to species differences, the efficiency of protein synthesis from dietary AAs in skeletal muscle and other tissues decreases with increasing age. For example, approximately 70%, 55%, 50%, and 45% of dietary protein is converted into tissue protein in 14-day-old sow-reared pigs, 30-day-old pigs (weaned at 21 days of age to a corn- and soybean meal-based diet), 110-day-old pigs, and 180-day-old pigs, respectively (Wu et al. 2014a). Similarly, approximately 52%, 48%, 45%, and 41% of dietary protein is converted into tissue protein in 1-, 2-, 4-, and 6-week-old broiler chickens fed corn- and soybean meal-based diets, respectively. Furthermore, the sensitivity of skeletal muscle to insulin decreases as the age of the animal increases (Chapter 7). Thus, we are facing enormous challenges to sustain the production of high-quality protein by farm animals, as feedstuff resources are becoming increasingly limited. Optimizing dietary formulations is an attractive means to mitigate the potential impact of animal production on greenhouse gas emissions and the environment.

## Nutritional Requirements for Reproduction of Females

Improving the efficiency of reproduction is of great economic importance in animal production (Wu et al. 2006). In both males and females, fertility depends on genetic traits and environmental factors. Adequate nutrition is essential for the normal reproductive functions of all animals, including sperm production, ovulation (controlled by gonadotropin-releasing hormone [GnRH] and

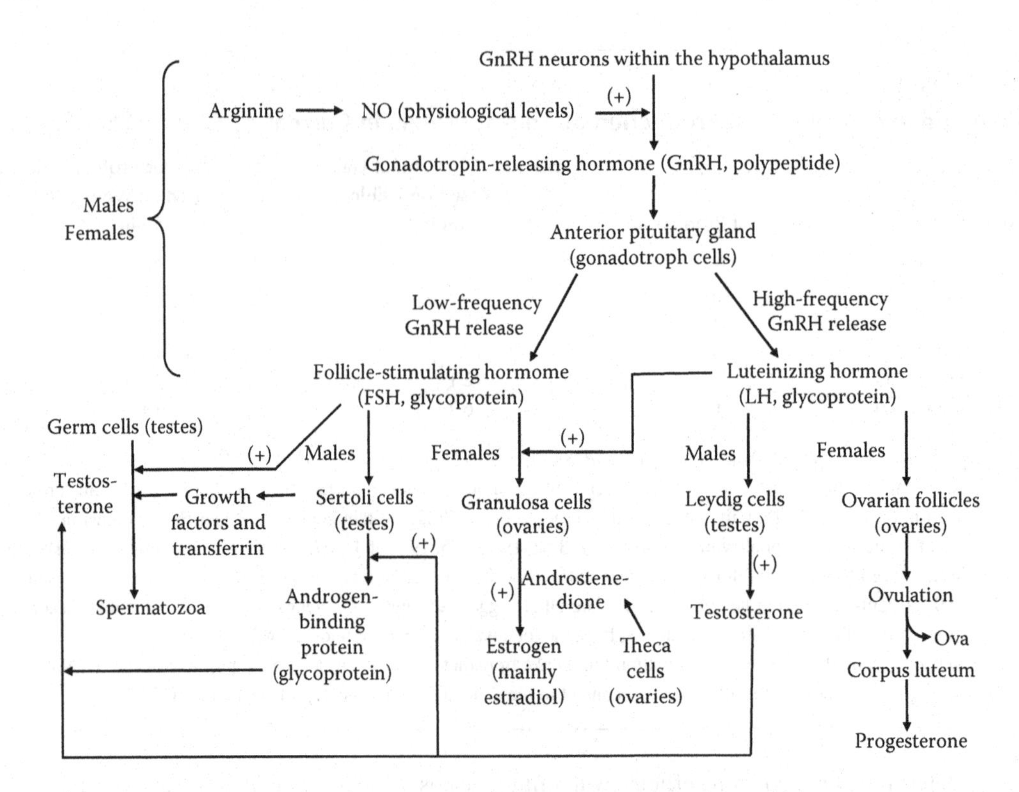


**FIGURE 11.3** The hypothalamic–pituitary–gonadal axis and hormones for animal reproduction. The frequency of release (pulses) of gonadotropin-releasing hormone (GnRH) from the hypothalamus is critical to stimulate the production of follicle-stimulating hormone (FSH) and LH by the anterior pituitary gland. In males, GnRH is secreted in pulses at a low constant frequency. In females, the frequency of GnRH pulse varies from low during most of the estrous cycle to high to induce a surge in LH required for ovulation of ova from ovarian follicles and the formation of corpora lutea that produce progesterone. Both FSH and LH act synergistically to enhance: (1) the release of estrogen and progesterone from the ovaries of females; and (2) the generation of testosterone and spermatogenesis in the testes of males. Each ovarian follicle contains an oocyte (ovum) with surrounding granulosa cells and theca cells in the ovaries, whereas spermatogonia, Sertoli cells, and Leydig cells are present in the testes. Estrogen, progesterone, and testosterone have negative feedback effects on GnRH release. These reproductive hormones are synthesized from cholesterol, a metabolite of fatty acids. Physiological levels of nitric oxide (NO, a metabolite of arginine) and adequate white adipose tissue for leptin production, for example, play important roles in regulating reproduction in both males and females by stimulating the cGMP-dependent NO signaling pathway.

luteinizing hormone [LH]) (Figure 11.3), conception, and parturition (Evans and Anderson 2017). Conversely, undernutrition delays the maturation of the reproductive system and impairs its function after puberty. Physiological levels of nitric oxide (NO, a metabolite of arginine) play an important role in reproduction by stimulating the release of GnRH from the hypothalamus (Dhandapani and Brann 2000). In addition, through cell signaling and nutrient utilization, metabolic hormones, such as leptin, insulin, and ghrelin, are key mediators of fertility in males and females. Furthermore, progesterone released by the ovaries and placenta is an essential hormone for establishing and maintaining pregnancy in mammals (Bazer et al. 2008). For example, in pigs and sheep, progesterone, along with other factors including estrogen, acts on the endometrial luminal and glandular epithelia to regulate the synthesis and secretion of certain components of histotroph (Figure 11.4). The latter is a mixture of molecules that includes proteins (e.g., secreted phosphoprotein 1 [osteopontin]), growth factors, hormones, cytokines, AAs, and other molecules that support the growth and development of the conceptus (embryo/fetus and associated placental membranes) (Johnson et al. 2014b).

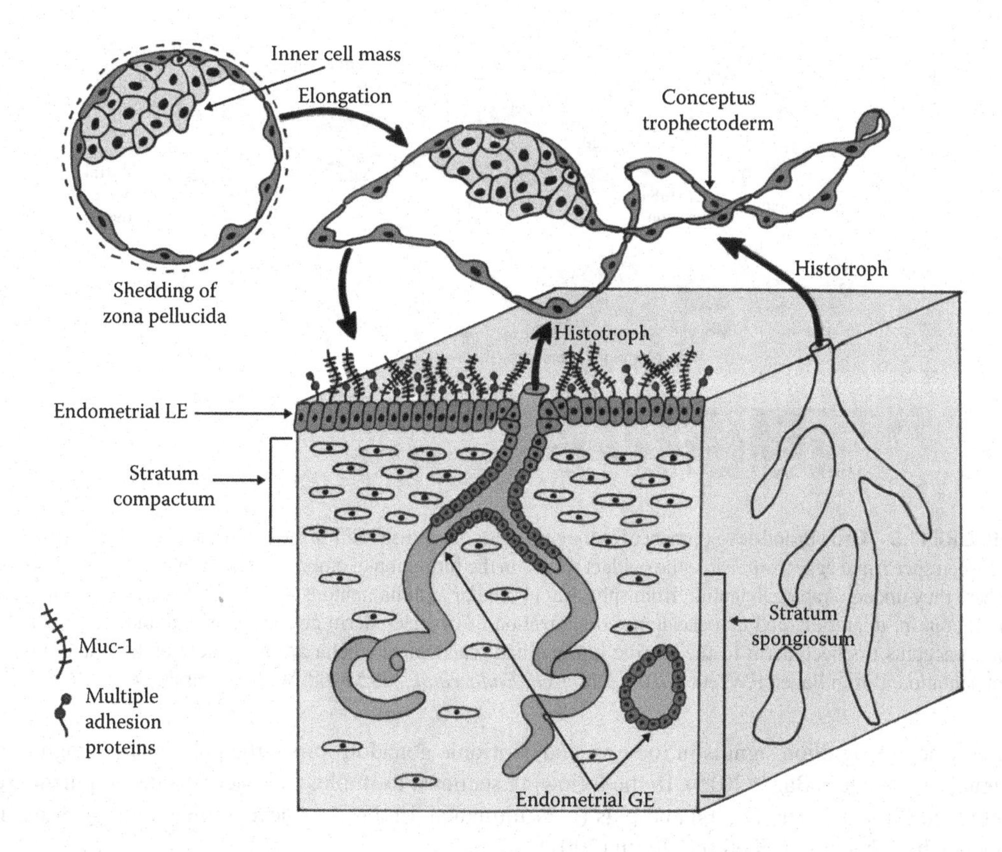


**FIGURE 11.4** Uterine secretions for embryonic survival, growth, and development in mammals. During pregnancy, progesterone, estrogen, and other factors stimulate the endometrial luminal and glandular epithelia to secrete proteins, hormones, cytokines, nutrients, and other substances, which are collectively called histotroph. These molecules support the growth and development of the conceptus (embryo/fetus and associated placental membranes). (From Bazer, F.W. et al. 2014. *Mol. Cell. Endocrinol.* 398:53–68. With permission.)

## Early Developmental Events of Conceptuses

### *Stages of Embryonic Development*

Development of conceptuses in different mammalian species differs in: (1) the duration of the preimplantation period; and (2) the type of implantation (noninvasive vs. invasive) and placentation (epitheliochorial in pigs, synepitheliochorial in ruminants, endotheliochorial in rodents, and hemochorial in primates) (Bazer et al. 2014). However, the early stages of embryonic development and phases of blastocyst implantation are similar among mammalian species (Figure 11.5). For early development of the zygote (a fertilized ovum), successive cleavage events occur at Stage 1, resulting in the formation of a 32- to 64-cell morula. At Stage 2 of development, the morula forms a blastocyst characterized by two distinct cell populations: (1) the inner cell mass, which develops into the embryo, and (2) the trophectoderm, which gives rise to the chorion of the placenta. Within the uterine lumen, the events of blastocyst development prior to implantation are divided into five phases: (1) shedding of the zona pellucida; (2) pre-contact and blastocyst orientation; (3) apposition of the trophectoderm and uterine luminal epithelium; (4) adhesion of trophectoderm to the uterine luminal epithelium; and (5) invasion of the blastocyst into the uterine endometrium, which is unique to species (e.g., rodents and primates) that have invasive implantation (Bazer et al. 2008). Interferon tau is the pregnancy recognition signal produced and secreted by trophectoderm cells of ruminant conceptuses (Days 12–13 in sheep and 16–17 in cattle). In contrast, estrogens are the pregnancy recognition signals in pigs (Days 11–12 of gestation), while prolactin and placental lactogen are

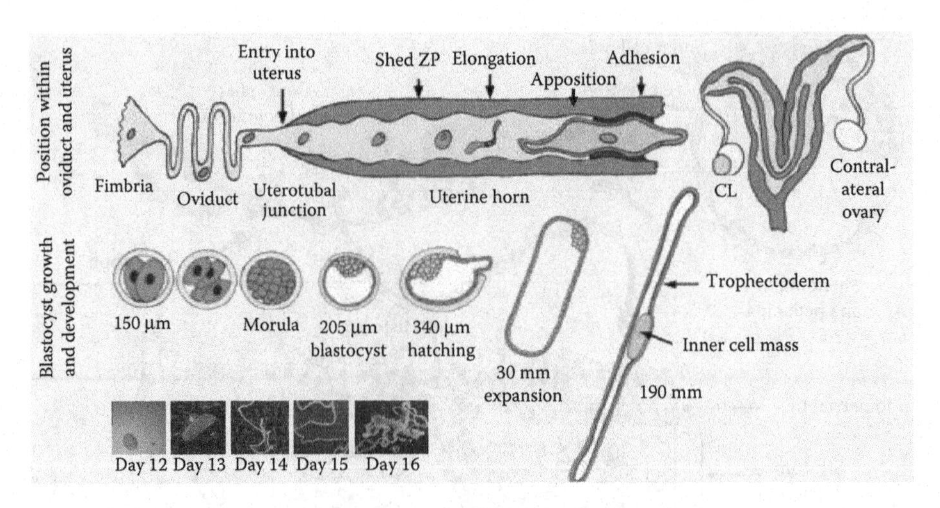


**FIGURE 11.5** Growth and development of ovine embryos/conceptuses within the oviduct and uterus. Fertilization between sperm and eggs (ova) inside the oviduct results in the formation of embryos. The embryos enter the uterus, where they undergo rapid elongation from spherical to tubular and filamentous forms as conceptuses that require proliferation, migration, and cytoskeleton reorganization of trophectoderm cells. Apposition and attachment of the conceptus trophectoderm to the uterine luminal and glandular epithelia are intricately orchestrated during implantation. (From Bazer, F.W. et al. 2014. *Mol. Cell. Endocrinol.* 398:53–68. With permission.)

pregnancy recognition signals in rodents, and chorionic gonadotropin is the pregnancy recognition signal in primates (Bazer 2015). In the following sections, examples of conceptus development are provided for sheep (ruminants) and pigs (nonruminants). Embryonic development and hatching in poultry have been described by Moran (2007).

In sheep, embryos enter the uterus on Day 3 after breeding, develop to spherical blastocysts, and then transform to large spherical (Day 10, 0.4 mm), tubular, and filamentous forms between Days 12 (1 × 33 mm), 14 (1 × 68 mm), and 15 (1 × 150–190 mm) of pregnancy (Bazer et al. 2012a,b). Meanwhile, extra-embryonic membranes extend into the contralateral uterine horn between Days 16 and 20 of pregnancy. Elongation of ovine conceptuses is a prerequisite for central implantation involving apposition and adhesion between the trophectoderm of the conceptus and uterine luminal and superficial glandular epithelia. Later, there is loss of the luminal epithelium, which allows intimate contact between the trophectoderm and the uterine basal lamina proximal to uterine stromal cells between Days 18 and 50–60 of gestation. These events in development of the ovine conceptus are illustrated in Figure 11.5.

In swine, following fertilization, zygotes develop and cleave into 2- and 4-cell stage embryos in the oviduct (Bazer et al. 2010). After entering the uterus around Day 3 of gestation, embryos continue to cleave, develop to blastocysts by Days 7–8 of gestation, and then hatch from the zona pellucida. Thereafter, blastocysts migrate within the uterine lumen to achieve equal spacing among themselves and then undergo dramatic changes in morphology from an expanded spherical shape to tubular and filamentous forms between Days 10 and 15 of pregnancy. The diameter of spherical blastocysts is only 5–10 mm by Day 10 of gestation. However, when reaching a spherical diameter of 10 mm on about Day 11 of gestation, it takes only 3 or 4 h for blastocysts to elongate to tubular and then filamentous conceptuses that are 150–200 mm in length; and by Day 15, they approach approximately 1000 mm in length (Geisert and Yelich 1997). This dramatic morphological change occurs initially through cellular remodeling rather than cellular hyperplasia, but the final phase of elongation between Days 12 and 15 involves both cellular hyperplasia and cellular remodeling (Geisert et al. 1982). Porcine conceptuses initiate attachment of trophectoderm to uterine luminal epithelia on Day 13 of pregnancy, and implantation is accomplished by about Day18 of gestation in advance of placentation and formation of a true epitheliochorial placenta. The chorioallantoic

**TABLE 11.8**
**Stages of the Fetal and Postnatal Development of Porcine Skeletal Muscle**

| Stage | Days of Gestation | Major Events |
|---|---|---|
| 1 | From conception to 25 d of gestation | Embryonic myogenesis from a common mesenchymal precursor |
| 2 | From 25 to 50 d of gestation | Formation of primary muscle fibers (rapid fusion of primary myoblasts) |
| 3 | From 50 to 90 d of gestation | Formation of secondary muscle fibers (formed on the surface of primary fibers) |
| 4 | From 90 to 95 d of gestation | Establishment of muscle fiber numbers |
| 5 | d 114 of gestation | Total numbers of muscle fibers are fixed at birth |
| 6 | After birth | Growth of skeletal muscle by increasing the size of its fibers (hypertrophy)[a]; and maturation of skeletal muscle |

*Source:* Ji, Y. et al. 2017. *J. Anim. Sci. Biotechnol.* 8:42.

[a] Hypertrophy is defined as an increase in the size of the skeletal muscle cell (also known as muscle fiber), whereas hyperplasia refers to an increase in the number of cells.

placenta is evident by Day 20 of gestation and grows rapidly thereafter. Of note, the uterine-placental bilayer develops progressively complex folds to augment the surface area of contact between the chorionic membrane and luminal epithelial cells. The placental and uterine microvasculature lies immediately beneath these epithelia, and therefore the development of placental folds is important for efficient transport of nutrients from the mother to the developing conceptus. Before Day 35 of gestation, porcine conceptuses are uniformly distributed within each uterine horn. After this time in gestation, uterine capacity becomes a limiting factor for fetal growth even though the fetuses are distributed relatively uniformly (Ford et al. 2002). In fetal pigs, primary muscle fibers form from the rapid fusion of primary myoblasts on Days 25–50 of gestation, whereas secondary muscle fibers form on the surface of primary fibers on Days 50 to 90 of gestation (Table 11.8).

### *Embryonic Origins of Fetal Tissues*

The embryo differentiates to form three germ layers: endoderm (the innermost layer), mesoderm (the middle layer), and ectoderm (the outer layer) (Senger 1997). The endoderm is the origin of the digestive tract, liver, lungs, pancreas, thyroid gland, and other glands. The mesoderm is the origin of the circulatory system, skeletal muscle, bones, reproductive tracts, kidneys, and urinary ducts (Pownall et al. 2002). The lineage of skeletal muscle development is shown in Figure 11.6. The ectoderm is the origin of the central nervous system, sense organs, mammary glands, sweat glands, skin, hair, and hooves. Before placentation, the embryo receives nutrients from uterine secretions and oxygen from its surrounding environment. The timelines of conceptus development differ among mammals, such as swine and sheep (Bazer et al. 2010). However, maternal undernutrition or overnutrition during early gestation negatively affects conceptus development in all species (Hoffman et al. 2016; Wu et al. 2006).

### *Functions of the Placenta*

As noted previously, the placenta starts to develop during early gestation in mammals (e.g., as early as Day 18 of gestation in pigs) and then placental blood vessels are clearly visible (e.g., Day 25 of gestation in pigs). In all species, a functional placenta transports nutrients, respiratory gases, and products of their metabolism between the maternal and fetal circulations, which is crucial for fetal survival, growth, and development (Wang et al. 2012). Rates of utero-placental blood flow depend on placental vascular growth (a result of angiogenesis and vasodilation of blood vessels) and placental vascularization, which are greatly enhanced by physiological concentrations of NO and polyamines (Reynolds et al. 2006). To support increased uterine and placental blood flows, placental angiogenesis increases markedly from the first to the second and third trimesters of gestation

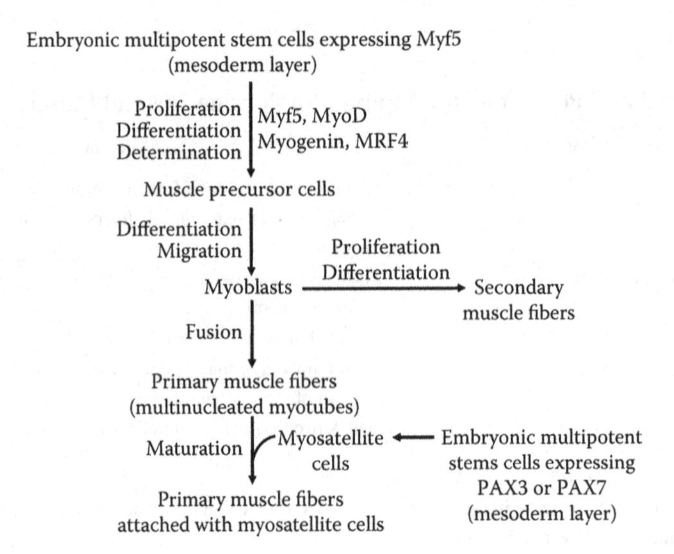


**FIGURE 11.6** Embryonic lineage for development of skeletal muscle in animals. MRF4, muscle regulatory factor 4; PAX3, paired box protein 3; PAX7, paired box protein 7.

(e.g., term = 114 days in pigs and 147 days in sheep) and continues to increase during the last days of gestation. Uptake of nutrients by the uterus or the fetus is determined by both the rate of blood flow and concentrations of nutrients in the arterial and venous blood. Thus, uptakes of both macro- and micro-nutrients by the uterus are greater in pregnant women than in nonpregnant women (Reynolds et al. 2006). Conversely, impaired placental blood flow contributes to IUGR (intrauterine growth restriction) in mammalian pregnancies (Wu et al. 2004).

## Effects of Nutrients and Related Factors on Reproductive Performance of Females

1. *Overall Undernutrition or Overnutrition.* Undernutrition not only affects the onset of puberty and sexual development but also impairs ovulation and fertilization. Maternal undernutrition, particularly protein deficiency, reduces the weight of the dam more than that of her offspring, because maternal tissues are mobilized to provide nutrients to the fetus, which has a high priority for nutrients (Ashworth 1991; Pond et al. 1991). The protection of the fetus may not occur when the mother is deficient in nutrients, particularly arginine, folic acid, vitamin A, and iron (Wu et al. 2012). The early gestation period is critical for placental growth, differentiation, angiogenesis, vascularization, and fetal organogenesis, whereas most of the fetal growth occurs in the last trimester of pregnancy (Reynolds et al. 2006). Before birth, the fetus is nurtured in the sterile, protected, moist, and warm environment of the uterus, and receives nutrients via the umbilical vein (parenteral nutrition) and also by swallowing amniotic fluid (enteral nutrition).

   Either undernutrition or overnutrition increases the incidence of early embryonic mortality (Ji et al. 2017). In animal production, it is desirable for females to conceive soon after parturition to maximize economic returns. As a result, breeding and conception must occur in ruminants when cows are lactating or within the first week after the termination of lactation in nonruminants. For example, cows are often bred shortly after the peak of lactation, and pigs are bred within 5 days following a 21 day period of lactation. The challenge is that milk production often induces a temporary negative energy and protein balance in most females, which is not conducive to successful reproduction (Wu et al. 2006). Indeed, in dairy breeds of cattle, sheep, and goats, high milk output interferes with reproduction, because of negative energy and protein balances in the dams. For this reason, in dairy cattle, the conception rates of heifers are usually much higher than those for lactating cows, although fertility rates are low for both beef and dairy cows under stress conditions (e.g., heat stress and malnutrition) (Santos et al. 2016; Thatcher et al. 2010).

Nutrition affects the early resumption of the ovarian cycle during the postpartum period after females give birth, as well as the success of conception (Chen et al. 2012). For example, adequate body condition and positive energy balance are important for the onset of estrus, fertilization of the oocyte, and high conception rates in animals. Note that suckling delays the resumption of the ovarian cycle in both ruminants and nonruminants through its effect on the central nervous system to disrupt the pattern of pulsatile release of GnRH from the hypothalamus and hence LH from the pituitary (McNeilly et al. 1994). However, overfeeding dams in late lactation or during the dry period may result in the so-called metabolic syndrome (e.g., dyslipidemia) associated with impaired reproductive function. In litter-bearing species, such as pigs and prolific ewes, the level of nutrition greatly affects the ovulation rate and therefore fertility and fecundity. Feeding sows and ewes with a poor body condition a high-level energy diet for a few weeks before mating can enhance ovulation rates and the number of fertilized embryos. However, this practice, which is known as "flushing," increases oxidative stress in the conceptus and the rate of embryonic mortality, and is no longer recommended to producers.

2. *Maternal Protein and Arginine Intake.* Low intake of protein delays puberty in females (Muñoz-Calvo and Argente 2016). A deficiency in dietary protein reduces the fertility of females after puberty. In addition, a deficiency in dietary protein decreases food intake and is therefore associated with deficiencies in intake of other nutrients. Producers must pay attention to adverse effects of a high-level intake of protein by gestating dams because high levels of ammonia are particularly toxic to embryos and cause large metabolic burdens on maternal organs (e.g., liver and kidneys). For example, in gestating gilts, increasing the dietary content of crude protein from 12% to 16% progressively reduces the number of live-born piglets per litter (Ji et al. 2017). In addition, an excess of dietary protein, which is supplemented in the form of soybean meal, is associated with reduced conception rates and increased embryonic losses in dairy cows (Butler 1998; Laven and Drew 1999). The underlying mechanisms may include: (1) increased production of ammonia, which induces oxidative stress (Haussinger and Görg 2010), depletion of α-ketoglutarate (an intermediate of the Krebs cycle for ATP production) via glutamate dehydrogenase, and elevated pH in cells (Wu 2013); (2) increased generation of $H_2S$ and homocysteine to cause further oxidative stress; (3) reduced secretion of histotroph from the uterus; (4) impairment of blood flow (including utero-placental blood flow) and nutrient transport due to decreased NO availability; and (5) low production of progesterone from ovaries (Butler 1998). Dietary supplementation with arginine (e.g., 0.4%–0.8% in swine diets) after Day 14 of gestation can improve embryonic and fetal survival through enhancing placental angiogenesis and growth, utero-placental blood flow, folding at the uterine–placental interface and its structural development, MTOR cell signaling in the conceptus, and removal of excess ammonia (Wu et al. 2013, 2017).
3. *Deficiencies of Minerals and Vitamins.* Diets that are deficient in minerals and vitamins, particularly phosphorus, calcium, manganese, copper, zinc, cobalt, vitamin A, and vitamin E, impair fertility in females (Clagett-Dame and Knutson 2011). Dietary supplementation with a deficient mineral or vitamin can improve reproductive performance. A deficiency of phosphorus, which is common in ruminants grazing on forages or herbage grown in phosphorus-deficient soil, delays puberty, inhibits estrus, and reduces the numbers and weights of calves or lambs. This effect of phosphorus deficiency is often associated with low food intake and inadequate provision of other nutrients. In both ruminants and nonruminants, retention of the placenta following parturition, which delays the next conception by causing uterine infection, may also result from nutritional deficiencies in selenium, copper, vitamin A, and vitamin E.

4. *Diseases, Toxins, Stress, and Excess Minerals.* Diseases (e.g., infections by bacteria, viruses, or parasites), toxins, air pollution, stress (physical or psychological), and goitrogens (causing enlargement of the thyroid), as well as high levels of plant estrogens (e.g., isoflavones) and nitrates, can reduce conception rates in both ruminants and nonruminants (Bazer et al. 2014; Jefferson and Williams 2011). These negative factors impair the metabolic activities and functions of the uterus, placenta, and ovaries. Of note, soybean meal, the most common protein supplement for all farm animals, contains genistein (an isoflavone) and weak goitrogens (possibly 1-methyl-2-mercaptoimidazole and potassium thiocyanate) that inhibit thyroid peroxidase (an enzyme required for the synthesis of thyroid hormones). Thus, genistein may contribute to infertility when high levels of dietary soybean meal are fed to females of reproductive age. The goitrogens in soybeans can be partially inactivated by heat. Just like the adverse effects of their deficiencies, excessive intakes of sodium, phosphorus, calcium, and fluorine can also reduce conception rates in animals.

## Intrauterine Growth Restriction

1. *Definition and Occurrence of IUGR.* Intrauterine growth restriction (IUGR) is defined as impaired growth and development of the mammalian embryo/fetus or its organs during pregnancy (Wu et al. 2006). In practice, IUGR is identified as fetal or birth weight less than two standard deviations of the mean BW for gestational age. For example, for crossbred sows (Yorkshire × Landrace dams and Duroc × Hampshire boars), the mean birth weight is 1.4 kg, and a piglet with a birth weight of less than 1.1 kg is considered to have IUGR (Ji et al. 2017). Multiple genetic and environmental factors contribute to IUGR. Although the fetal genome plays an important role in growth potential *in utero*, convincing evidence shows that the intrauterine environment is a major determinant of fetal growth (Wu et al. 2006). For example, results of embryo transfer studies clearly indicate that the recipient mother, rather than the donor mother, strongly influences fetal growth (Brooks et al. 1995). Among intrauterine environmental factors, under- or over-nutrition plays the most critical role in influencing placental and fetal growth. Among livestock species, pigs exhibit the highest rates of embryonic mortality, IUGR, and neonatal deaths. These problems are further exacerbated by: (1) restricting the feed intake of gestating swine (e.g., by 50%–60% compared with ad libitum intake) to prevent excess maternal fat accretion; and (2) a variety of factors encountered in the different phases of swine production, including extreme ranges in environmental temperatures, feed hygiene and safety, suboptimal nutrition, and disease (Ji et al. 2017).
2. *Consequences of IUGR.* IUGR has permanent negative impacts on organ structure, neonatal adjustments, preweaning survival, postnatal growth, feed efficiency, lifetime health, skeletal muscle composition, physical strengths, excessive accumulation of white adipose tissue, meat quality, reproductive performance, and the onset of adult diseases (Oksbjerg et al. 2013; Wu et al. 2006). Altered organ mass and structure, such as reduced numbers of pancreatic islets, reduced numbers of kidney glomeruli, or reduced numbers of secondary (but not primary) muscle fibers, are consequences of IUGR and equally important to functional consequences (Foxcroft et al. 2006). How IUGR negatively affects embryonic and fetal development is unknown, but this problem likely involves an impairment of protein synthesis in skeletal muscle. Although IUGR may be a natural mechanism to protect the dam in case of maternal undernutrition, it has adverse effects on the survival and growth performance of the progeny and the efficiency of animal production. Effective solutions must be developed to prevent and treat IUGR in mammals.

## Determination of Nutrient Requirements by Gestating Dams

Nutrient requirements during pregnancy can be estimated by combining the maternal and fetal requirements for maintenance and growth (i.e., the factorial method). Estimation of dietary needs for energy and nutrients during gestation can be based on: (1) the rates of accretion of placental, fetal, and uterine tissues; and (2) the efficiency of utilization of energy and nutrients for gains in the growth of those tissues. The additional needs for the growth of maternal tissues must be met for females that are bred before reaching a mature size.

## Nutritional Requirements for Reproduction of Males

### Overall Undernutrition or Overnutrition

After a prolonged period of overall undernutrition (e.g., global reduction in food or energy intake), semen quality in males (including bulls, rams, and boars) is reduced. For example, the concentrations of fructose (the source of energy for sperm motility) and citrate are reduced in the seminal fluid of undernourished males. Undernutrition impairs development of the testes and the synthesis of testosterone in males. At the other spectrum of nutrition, overnutrition induces oxidative stress and decreases semen quality, thereby contributing to male infertility.

### Protein and Arginine Intake

Physiological levels of NO stimulate GnRH release from the hypothalamus and therefore testosterone production and spermatogenesis in the testes (Figure 11.2). Similar to the problems seen in females, low intake of protein and energy also delays puberty in males (Dance et al. 2015). In addition, a deficiency in dietary protein reduces food intake, leading to deficiencies in other nutrients that are necessary for spermatogenesis (Ghorbankhani et al. 2015). The maintenance requirement of males for energy and protein is greater than that for females, because males have a greater proportion of lean tissue than females due to testosterone-induced muscular hypertrophy (Herbst and Bhasin 2004). Furthermore, as reported for mammals including boars (Louis et al. 1994), low protein intakes reduce libido and semen volume. Of note, although the average ejaculate of an adult male (e.g., bull and boar), including spermatozoa and accessory secretions, contains only a relatively small amount of DM, the seminal fluid contains relatively high levels of polyamines and arginine (Wu et al. 2013). For example, concentrations of polyamines in porcine seminal fluid are 90 μM in comparison with those in plasma 3–5 μM, and dietary supplementation with 1% Arg-HCl to sexually active boars for 30 days enhanced concentrations of polyamines in seminal fluid by 63% compared with the control group (Wu et al. 2009). Concentrations of polyamines and arginine may be reduced in the seminal fluid of malnourished males. In humans, low levels of polyamines and arginine in the semen are known to be associated with infertility. For example, feeding an arginine-deficient diet to adult men for 9 days decreased sperm counts and the percentage of motile sperm by 90% (Holt and Albanese 1944). Remarkably, oral administration of L-arginine (e.g., 0.5 g/day for 6–8 weeks) to infertile men increased the number and motility of sperm, resulting in successful pregnancies for their female partners (Tanimura 1967). Furthermore, dietary supplementation with L-arginine or L-citrulline (e.g., 5 g/day over 6 weeks) to impotent men with impaired endogenous synthesis of nitric oxide can enhance sexual function (Cormio et al. 2011; Kobori et al. 2015).

### Deficiencies of Minerals and Vitamins

A deficiency of vitamin A causes degeneration of the germinal epithelium of the testes, thereby reducing or eliminating spermatogenesis (Clagett-Dame and Knutson 2011). As in females, a severe and prolonged deficiency of vitamin A results in the complete failure of reproduction in males (Chapter 9). The testicular tissue and spermatozoa contain high levels of zinc, and thus the zinc requirement for testicular growth and normal sperm production is higher than that for animal growth. Inadequate intake of zinc impairs Leydig cell function and reduces sperm counts in males (Abbasi et al. 1980). In addition, deficiencies in phosphorus, selenium, and copper (Chapter 10), as well as in vitamin C, folate, and vitamin E (Chapter 9), also contribute to infertility in males.

### Diseases, Toxins, Stress, and Excess Minerals

Diseases, toxins, air pollution, stress (physical or psychological), and goitrogens reduce reproductive performance in males, as in females (Meldrum et al. 2016). All of these factors impair the metabolic activities and functions of testes and other parts of the reproductive tract. In addition, excessive intakes of iron and copper are highly toxic in males and females (Chapter 10). Large amounts of those two minerals damage the structure of male gonads and spermatozoa, cause defective spermatogenesis, reduce *libido*, and induce oxidative injury in multiple cell types, thereby impairing fertility (Tvrda et al. 2015).

## Fetal and Neonatal Programming

Alterations in maternal and fetal nutrition and endocrine status during gestation result in developmental adaptations that may permanently change structure, physiology, and metabolism of offspring, therefore predisposing the individuals to metabolic defects and reduced food efficiency for lean tissue growth, as well as cardiovascular, metabolic, and endocrine diseases in adult life (Wu et al. 2004). These adverse effects may be carried over to the next generation or beyond. This phenomenon of transgenerational impacts is known as fetal programming, which is mediated by stable and heritable alterations in gene expression through covalent modifications of DNA and histones without changes in DNA sequences (namely, epigenetics). The mechanisms responsible for the epigenetic regulation of protein expression and functions include: chromatin remodeling; DNA methylation (occurring at the 5′-position of cytosine residues within CpG dinucleotides); and histone modifications (acetylation, methylation, phosphorylation, and ubiquitination) (Ji et al. 2016). Like maternal malnutrition, undernutrition during the neonatal period also reduces growth performance and feed efficiency (e.g., by 5%–10% in postweaning pigs), increasing the days necessary to reach market BW (Ji et al. 2017). Supplementing functional AAs (e.g., arginine and glutamine) and vitamins (e.g., folate) plays a key role in activating the mammalian target of rapamycin signaling and regulating the provision of methyl donors for DNA and protein methylation. For example, dietary supplementation with arginine reduces the incidence of IUGR and the within-litter variations in birth weights of piglets (Wu et al. 2013). Therefore, these nutrients are beneficial for the dietary treatment of metabolic disorders in offspring with IUGR or neonatal malnutrition. The mechanism-based strategies hold great promise for the improvement of the efficiency of animal production.

## Nutritional Requirements for Postnatal Growth of Animals

Rapid growth of skeletal muscle, mainly protein accretion, is economically important for livestock, poultry, and fish industries worldwide (Wu et al. 2014c). As noted in Chapter 7, the balance between the rates of protein synthesis and degradation is the determinant of tissue growth. Therefore, over the past 50 years, extensive research has focused on the regulation of intracellular protein turnover in skeletal muscle (Hernandez-García et al. 2016; Reeds and Mersmann 1991). The maximal growth rate of animal tissues depends on both genetic and environmental factors. An animal can fully express its genetic potential only when its requirements for energy and all nutrients (e.g., AAs, fatty acids, carbohydrates, minerals, and vitamins) are met, as noted previously.

### Components of Animal Growth

The general sigmoid curve of animal growth, expressed as increases in absolute body or tissue weight with age, is shown in Figure 11.7. This curve consists of four phases: lag, log or exponential, maturity, and stationary. In farm animals, the head and extremities develop early, and the hindquarters and loin region develop very late during the growing-finishing period (Wagner et al. 1999). The patterns of accretion of protein and fat in animals vary with species and developmental stages (Gerrard and Grant 2002). However, as age advances, weight gain generally consists of an increasing percentage of fat and a decreasing percentage of water (ARC 1981; NRC 2001, 2011, 2012). In contrast, the percentage of protein in the body generally increases gradually after birth until

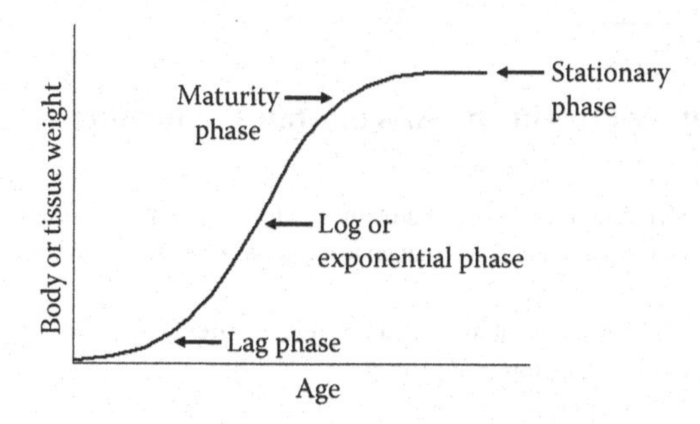


**FIGURE 11.7** The general curve describing animal growth over time (age). This sigmoid curve consists of lag, log, or exponential, maturity, and stationary phases.

animals reach sexual maturity (Susenbeth and Keitel 1988). In fully mature animals, excess energy is stored almost entirely as fats, and only a relatively small amount of proteins may be deposited as a cellular component of white adipocytes, muscle fibers, hair, and keratinized cells of skin.

An increase in BW is the most common measure of growth due to its simplicity. However, the growth of any animal is characterized by increases in the weight of its muscles, white adipose tissue, bones, and internal organs that are associated with the enhanced accretion of protein, minerals, water, and fats (van Es 1976). Since the deposition of 1 g protein in the body is associated with the retention of 3 g water (Wu et al. 2014a), a net synthesis of 1 g protein in tissues (primarily skeletal muscle, which is 40%–45% of the BW) results in a weight gain of 4 g. Rapid muscle protein accretion leads to fast animal growth. For example, young animals have a higher rate of net protein synthesis and therefore a higher rate of growth than older ones (Davis et al. 1998). However, the opposite may not always hold true. This is because weight gain may not necessarily result from lean tissue growth and rather may simply be caused primarily by fat accumulation in the body.

As a hydrophobic molecule, triacylglycerol (TAG, fat) is deposited in the animal body free of water. Although fat may be deposited in various tissues, it is stored mainly in the subcutaneous white adipose tissue, abdominal cavity, and connective tissue (Smith and Smith 1995). A certain amount of fat among muscle fibers within skeletal muscle (called marbling fat) confers a good taste to meats eaten by consumers. As more fat is accumulated in animals than protein, water content in the body decreases. Thus, in ruminants and pigs, water content is generally 75%–80% at birth but decreases to 45%–50% at their market weights (ARC 1981, NRC 2001). The expansion of fats during the finishing period results primarily from an increase in the size of white adipocytes. Results from growth studies involving cattle and pigs indicate that the deposition of 1.4 g fat in the animal body is associated with the replacement of 0.4 g water and that the actual gain in the whole body is only 1 g (Pond et al. 1995; van Es 1976). Thus, weight gain increases to a lesser extent when fat is accreted in the body, compared to the accretion of the same amount of protein.

Despite concern over adverse effects of overweight or obesity on health, animals require fats for normal physiological function (Chapter 6). For example, although obesity increases the risk for infertility in both males and females (Norman 2010), an adequate amount of body fat is necessary for reproduction, such as the pulsatile GnRH release (Sam and Dhillo 2010). This can be explained by the facts that: (1) leptin secretion from white adipose tissue is necessary for attainment of puberty (Cardoso et al. 2014); and (2) testosterone, estradiol, progesterone, and all other steroid hormones are synthesized from cholesterol, which is a lipid synthesized from fatty acids (Kiess et al. 2000).

## Absolute versus Relative Rate of Animal Growth

The absolute growth rate refers to the amount of weight gain per unit of time (e.g., g/day). The relative growth rate of animals is commonly expressed in terms of changes in BW within a given period of time (e.g., %/day). The absolute rates of whole body growth in animals increase, but the relative rates

## TABLE 11.9
## Important Roles of Dietary Protein and AAs in Animal Nutrition

1. Metabolic and hormone profiles
   a. Maintaining optimal concentrations of AAs and proteins (including albumin) in plasma
   b. Maintaining endocrine balance, as well as optimal concentrations of insulin, growth hormone, IGF-I, and thyroid hormones in plasma
   c. Maintaining optimal anti-oxidative reactions; reducing oxidative stress
   d. Maintaining optimal synthesis of neurotransmitters
   e. Reducing excess deposition of white adipose tissue
   f. Maintaining optimal whole-body energy expenditure
2. Nutrient absorption and transport
   a. Promoting intestinal absorption of nutrients, including vitamins, minerals, AAs, glucose, and fatty acids
   b. Promoting the transport of vitamins, minerals, and long-chain fatty acids in blood and among various tissues
   c. Helping to store vitamins and minerals in cells
3. Protein synthesis and growth
   a. Promoting protein synthesis and increasing proteolysis in skeletal muscle and whole body
   b. Preventing growth stunting of the young; improving development (including cognitive development) of the young
   c. Preventing intrauterine growth restriction and its lifelong negative consequences on postnatal growth, metabolism, and health (e.g., increasing risk for obesity, infection, and cardiovascular abnormalities)
   d. Increasing skeletal muscle mass; maintaining physical strengths
   e. Enhancing feed efficiency
4. Organ structure
   a. Preventing cardiac structural abnormalities
   b. Preventing the loss of calcium and bones, and dental abnormalities
   c. Preventing hair breakage and loss; maintaining optimal production of pigment; maintaining normal hair structure and appearance
   d. Preventing pale skin, dry or flaking skin, and skin atrophy
   e. Maintaining optimal immune responses; reducing risk for, and mortality of, infectious diseases
5. Health and reproduction
   a. Improving cardiovascular function; preventing hypertension or hypotension; reducing risks for headache and fainting
   b. Preventing excess fluid retention in tissues; preventing peripheral and periorbital edema (particularly swelling in the abdomen, leg, hands, and feet)
   c. Preventing emotional disorders (e.g., moodiness, severe depression, and anxiety), irritability, and insomnia
   d. Preventing a loss of libido; improving fertility (including spermatogenesis in males and conception in females); reducing embryonic loss; enhancing pregnancy outcomes

of their whole body growth decrease, as they approach sexual maturity. However, the absolute or relative rates of fat and protein depositions in the body may not necessarily follow the pattern of growth for the whole body (Table 11.9). A combination of feed efficiency, animal price, and meat yield determines the market weight of farm animals (Thornton 2010). Thus, animals are sold to the market at a heavier BW than usual, when their numbers are lower due to disease outbreak or other causes, so that more meat can be produced per animal at the expense of a reduced efficiency of nutrient utilization.

### Regulation of Animal Growth by Anabolic Agents

As noted in Chapter 7, many hormones play an important role in animal growth primarily by regulating skeletal muscle protein synthesis and catabolism. A net increase in tissue protein synthesis (i.e., the rate of protein synthesis is greater than the rate of protein degradation) results in weight gain. Insulin, growth hormone, and insulin-like growth factor-I are anabolic hormones (Etherton and Bauman 1998). Interestingly, tissue sensitivity to hormones decreases with advancing age in animals and humans. Thus, the frequency of feeding can affect the pulse of these hormones and other anabolic nutrients in plasma (Boutry et al. 2013; El-Kadi, et al. 2012). This concept can have important

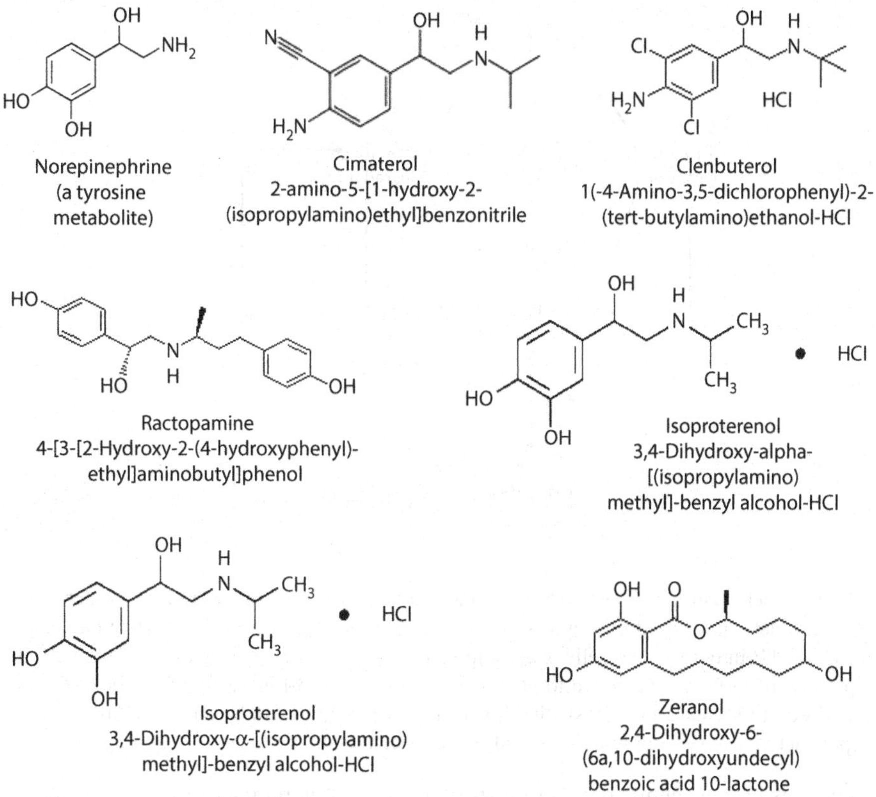

Norepinephrine
(a tyrosine
metabolite)

Cimaterol
2-amino-5-[1-hydroxy-2-
(isopropylamino)ethyl]benzonitrile

Clenbuterol
1(-4-Amino-3,5-dichlorophenyl)-2-
(tert-butylamino)ethanol-HCl

Ractopamine
4-[3-[2-Hydroxy-2-(4-hydroxyphenyl)-
ethyl]aminobutyl]phenol

Isoproterenol
3,4-Dihydroxy-alpha-
[(isopropylamino)
methyl]-benzyl alcohol-HCl

Isoproterenol
3,4-Dihydroxy-α-[(isopropylamino)
methyl]-benzyl alcohol-HCl

Zeranol
2,4-Dihydroxy-6-
(6a,10-dihydroxyundecyl)
benzoic acid 10-lactone

**FIGURE 11.8** The chemical structures of β-agonists used in animal production. These are analogues of norepinephrine (a metabolite of tyrosine), but are not steroids.

implications for improving the efficiency of feed utilization and reducing the costs of animal production. The higher the rate of gain in BW, the shorter the time required for the animal to reach a slaughter weight or full productive performance, and the smaller the proportion of feed used for maintenance (Ji et al. 2017). Insulin resistance often occurs in aging animals and in gestating dams during the last trimester of gestation, which leads to their mobilization of fats and a reduction in protein synthesis.

Growth-promoting agents can improve the efficiency of meat production and produce leaner meat. These agents are of two major types in ruminants and nonruminants: (1) hormone-like substances [e.g., β-agonists (Figure 11.8)]; and (2) antibiotic-like substances (Reeds and Mersmann 1991). They also reduce white adipose tissue in the body and enhance the growth of the animals through different mechanisms (Gerrard and Grant 2002).

### *β-Agonists*

Ractopamine (known as Paylean for swine and Optaflexx for cattle) is a feed additive that promotes lean tissue growth in swine and cattle (Bohrer et al. 2013; Lean et al. 2014). This agent acts as a trace amine-associated receptor 1 (TAAR1) agonist and also as a β-adrenoreceptor agonist that stimulates both $\beta_1$ and $\beta_2$ adrenergic receptors to enhance lipolysis in skeletal muscle (Johnson et al. 2014a). Ractopamine has been banned as a feed additive in many countries, including the European Union, China, and Russia because of concern over adverse effects of its residue in meat on human health. However, ractopamine has been approved for use in some countries, such as the United States, Japan, and Canada to improve meat production by livestock fed an adequate protein diet. Other growth promoters available for cattle and sheep include zeranol and trienbolone (Figure 11.5); they may be administered as feed additives, oil-based injections, or subcutaneous implants to the animals.

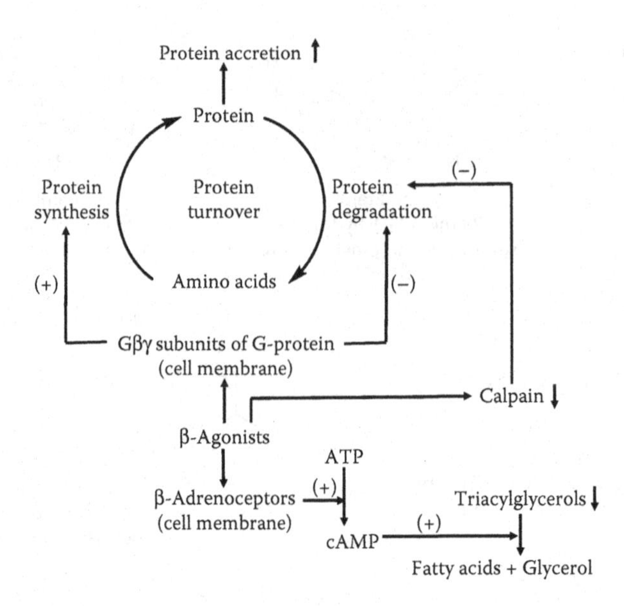


**FIGURE 11.9** Mechanisms for β-agonists to enhance lean tissue growth and reduce fat deposition in animals. β-Agonists act on: (1) β-adrenoceptors on the cell membrane to activate adenylate (adenylyl) cyclase, which converts ATP into cAMP in cells (e.g., adipocytes); and (2) the Gβγ subunits of the cell membrane-bound G-protein, resulting in the activation of the phosphoinositol 3-kinase (PI3K)–protein kinase B (Akt) signaling pathway to increase protein synthesis and inhibit protein degradation. In addition, the β-agonists reduce calpain activity in skeletal muscle via unknown mechanisms.

All β-agonists have a chemical structure similar to that of norepinephrine, which is a metabolite of tyrosine and a catecholamine (Reeds and Mersmann 1991). The modes of actions of these agents involve β-adrenoceptors and the Gβγ subunits of G-protein, both of which are localized on the cell membrane. β-Agonists bind to the membrane-bound β-adrenoceptors, thereby activating the adenylate cyclase to produce cAMP from ATP and then promote cAMP-dependent lipolysis in cells (e.g., white adipocytes) via protein kinase A signaling (Figure 11.9). In addition, β-agonists promote protein synthesis and reduce protein degradation in skeletal muscle via stimulation of the Gβγ subunits of the cell membrane-bound G-protein, which leads to activation of the phosphoinositol 3-kinase (PI3K)-protein kinase B (Akt) signaling pathway (Koopman et al. 2010). The growth signal is integrated via the MTOR, which is a master regulator of protein synthesis and an inhibitor of autophagy (a pathway of lysosomal proteolysis) (Chapter 7). β-Agonists (including catecholamines) inhibit calpain (calcium-dependent proteases) in skeletal muscle through β2-adrenoceptors and cAMP signaling (Navegantes et al. 2001). Owing to their anabolic effects on enhancing net protein accretion, β-agonists could provide an effective treatment for ameliorating skeletal muscle wasting in a catabolic state and promoting muscle hypertrophy in healthy animals.

#### *Specific Growth-Promoting Agents for Ruminants*

In ruminant nutrition, antibiotic-like substances have been used as growth-promoting agents, through acting on the ruminal and/or intestinal microflora to modify the quantity and quality of the fermentation products (Cameron and McAllister 2016). Furthermore, monensin, an antibiotic produced by certain bacteria, has gained wide acceptance as a feed additive for ruminants because it improves feed utilization efficiency by altering rumen fermentation in favor of propionate production (Chapter 13).

### Compensatory Growth

Compensatory growth (the ability of an animal to recover growth after periods of underfeeding) is an interesting area of investigation in animal biology. Animals that have been subjected to a period of undernutrition and thus to restricted growth exhibit compensatory growth during a subsequent period of re-alimentation (Hornick et al. 2000). Expressed as a percent increase in body or tissue weight, such animals grow faster than other animals of similar age when an adequate feed supply becomes available. This biological phenomenon has been observed in mammals, birds, fish, and reptiles (Boersma and Wit 1997). Over time, the body weights of animals with prior nutritional restriction may become similar to those of animals that did not experience such stress (Gerrard and Grant 2002). However, high rates of compensatory growth often result in excessive fat deposition in white adipose tissue and therefore negatively affect animal health (Gerrard and Grant 2002). The major reasons for the compensatory growth may result from increases in feed intake upon re-alimentation, the absorptive capacity of the gastrointestinal tract, the hepatic production of insulin-like growth factor-I, and feed efficiency, in association with concomitant decreases in intestinal microbial activity and the rates of whole-body catabolism of AAs (Boersma and Wit 1997; Heyer and Lebret 2007; Won and Borski 2013; Zhu et al. 2017). Whether IUGR offspring can fully catch up with those with a normal birth weight in terms of weight gains will depend on the severity of fetal growth restriction, as well as weight gains (particularly protein accretion) during the suckling period and the first weeks postweaning (Ji et al. 2017). The earlier in life nutritional deficiencies occur and the longer the period of food deprivation, the less the compensatory growth will be. Since the metabolic status (particularly hepatic or gastrointestinal function) of IUGR offspring differs from that of offspring with a normal birth weight, different dietary formulations must be developed for each phenotype of animals.

### Critical Role of Dietary AA Intake in Animal Growth

AAs are the building blocks of protein. As indicated previously, changes in the abundance of skeletal muscle account for most animal growth. Since protein is the most abundant component of DM in muscle, and since AAs are the constituents of protein, dietary AA intake plays a critical role in influencing the growth, feed efficiency, and health of all animals (Table 11.9). Thus, an active area of research in nutrition is dietary protein and AA requirements for growing animals (Escobar et al. 2006; Humphrey et al. 2008; Liao et al. 2018), particularly ruminants which exhibit a low feed efficiency (Brake et al. 2014; Wilkinson 2011). Dietary protein or AA intake is of great importance for animal producers on the basis of both biological and economic considerations. The efficiency of utilization of dietary energy, fat, and carbohydrates depends on the quantity and quality of dietary protein (Campbell 1988; Reeds and Mersmann 1991). Beef cattle are known for their low rate of conversion of dietary protein into body protein, and the efficiency of grazing cattle is only 1/2 that of high-producing dairy cows (Table 11.10). Depending on the species, the efficiency of dietary protein used for tissue protein deposition is about 70%–75% in milk-fed neonates and 40%–45% in animals approaching a market weight and consuming corn- and soybean meal-based diets (Wu 2013; Wu et al. 2014a). Thus, sufficient knowledge of protein metabolism and requirements of growing animals (especially ruminants) will increase the efficiency of feed utilization and prevent the waste of energy and AAs.

As discussed in Chapter 7, classic feeding trials involving several levels of dietary protein or AAs are required to determine total protein requirements for animal growth. The measured endpoints are usually nitrogen retention and weight gain. When energy is insufficient, nitrogen balance may become negative even if sufficient protein is fed (McDonald et al. 2011). This necessitates adequate provision of dietary lipids, carbohydrates, vitamins, and minerals, as well as drinking water, when studies of nitrogen balance or growth trials are conducted. On the other hand, an excess of dietary protein or AA intake is wasteful, and feeding a surplus of protein or AAs may not increase the protein content of the tissue accounting for live-weight gain and may result in negative impacts on animal health and the environment (Wu et al. 2014b).

Recommendations of dietary NEAA requirements for animals should depend on expected rates of growth, optimal reproduction, optimal health and, in the case of livestock, poultry and fish, production performance and feed efficiency (Wu et al. 2014b). Recent advances in the analysis of all proteinogenic AAs in food and animal-tissue proteins have made it possible to determine dietary

**TABLE 11.10**
**Daily Gains of the Whole Body, Fat and Protein and Feed:Gain Ratios in Barrows and Gilts between 18 and 125 kg BW**

| Variable | Changes between 18 and 125 kg BW |
|---|---|
| Daily weight gain | Increases progressively between 18 and 82 kg BW for barrows and gilts |
| | Decreases gradually between 82 and 125 BW for barrows and gilts |
| | Barrows > gilts between 18 and 125 BW |
| Daily protein gain | Increases progressively between 18 and 73 kg BW for barrows and gilts |
| | Decreases gradually between 73 and 125 BW for barrows and gilts |
| | Barrows > gilts before 90 kg BW; barrows = gilts between 90 and 125 BW |
| Daily fat gain | Increases progressively between 18 and 90 kg BW for barrows and gilts |
| | Little change between 90 and 125 BW for barrows and gilts |
| | Barrows > gilts between 18 and 125 BW |
| Feed:Gain (g/g) | Increases progressively between 18 and 125 kg BW for barrows and gilts |
| | Barrows = gilts between 18 and 50 kg BW; Barrows > gilts between 50 and 15 kg BW |

*Source:* Adapted from Wagner, J.R. et al. 1999. *J. Anim Sci.* 77:1442–1466.

intakes of these AAs by animals. On the basis of published studies, Wu (2014) proposed Texas A&M University's optimal ratios of AAs (formerly known as ideal AA patterns) in typical corn- and soybean meal-based diets for pigs (Table 11.11) and chickens (Table 11.12) at various phases of growth and production. These recommended values are based on the true ileal digestibilities for dietary AA and can be readily converted to percentages of total AA in the diet (g/100 g diet).

## Nutritional Requirements for Milk Production

Newborn mammals depend on milk for survival and growth; therefore, lactation is critical for their survival, growth, and development. The composition of nutrients in the milk of mammals varies among species (Table 11.13) or breeds within a species, stage of lactation, and different milking intervals. Colostrum is the first secretion from the mammary gland immediately and within a few days after parturition. Colostrum is characterized by high concentrations of immunoglobulins necessary for conferring passive immunity due to the underdeveloped immune system of the newborn (Table 11.14). Besides immunoglobulins and oligosaccharides, colostrum and mature milk also contain non-nutrient substances (e.g., osteopontin, insulin-like growth factor I [IGF-I], and other bioactive factors). Of note, nitrogen-containing substances (primarily β-casein, α-lactalbumin, other proteins, and free AAs) are highly abundant organic nutrients in the milk of farm animals (Table 11.15), but the content of fat and lactose in milk is also high on a DM basis. Adequate production of milk is essential to a high efficiency of livestock production. However, in livestock species (e.g., sows and cows), milk production is often a limiting factor for maximum preweaning growth of offspring (Dunshea et al. 2005; Rezaei et al. 2016). To meet maximum milk production, lactating dams need to increase their feed intake per kg BW by 50%–80%, compared with their non-lactating counterparts, depending on lactation stage (Bell 1995; Kim et al. 2013). Therefore, an important goal of animal nutrition research is to understand lactation biology.

### Mammary Gland

The lactating mammary gland is metabolically active and requires considerably more nutrients than the whole body on a per kg basis, although this organ represents only 5%–7% of the BW (Akers 2002). The lactating gland is a highly organized organ with a compound, tubulo–alveolar structure. Proteins, as well as some AAs, fats and lactose, are synthesized and secreted by mammary

**TABLE 11.11**
**Texas A&M University's Optimal Ratios of True Digestible Amino Acids for Swine Diets[a]**

| Amino Acid | Growing Pigs (kg)[b] | | | | Gestating Pigs[c] | | Lactating Sows[b] |
|---|---|---|---|---|---|---|---|
| | 5–10 | 10–20 | 20–50 | 50–110 | d 0–90 | d 90–114 | |
| | % of Diet (As-Fed Basis) | | | | | | |
| Alanine | 1.14 | 0.97 | 0.80 | 0.64 | 0.69 | 0.69 | 0.83 |
| Arginine | 1.19 | 1.01 | 0.83 | 0.66 | 1.03 | 1.03 | 1.37 |
| Asparagine | 0.80 | 0.68 | 0.56 | 0.45 | 0.50 | 0.50 | 0.66 |
| Aspartate | 1.14 | 0.97 | 0.80 | 0.64 | 0.61 | 0.61 | 0.94 |
| Cysteine | 0.32 | 0.28 | 0.24 | 0.20 | 0.19 | 0.19 | 0.26 |
| Glutamate | 2.00 | 1.70 | 1.39 | 1.12 | 0.89 | 0.89 | 1.81 |
| Glutamine | 1.80 | 1.53 | 1.25 | 1.00 | 1.00 | 1.60 | 1.38 |
| Glycine | 1.27 | 1.08 | 0.89 | 0.71 | 0.48 | 0.48 | 0.75 |
| Histidine | 0.46 | 0.39 | 0.32 | 0.26 | 0.29 | 0.29 | 0.39 |
| Isoleucine | 0.78 | 0.66 | 0.54 | 0.43 | 0.45 | 0.45 | 0.66 |
| Leucine | 1.57 | 1.33 | 1.09 | 0.87 | 1.03 | 1.03 | 1.41 |
| Lysine | 1.19 | 1.01 | 0.83 | 0.66 | 0.51 | 0.51 | 0.80 |
| Methionine | 0.32 | 0.28 | 0.24 | 0.20 | 0.16 | 0.16 | 0.25 |
| Phenylalanine | 0.86 | 0.73 | 0.60 | 0.48 | 0.54 | 0.54 | 0.77 |
| Proline | 1.36 | 1.16 | 0.95 | 0.76 | 0.89 | 0.89 | 1.24 |
| Serine | 0.70 | 0.60 | 0.49 | 0.39 | 0.45 | 0.45 | 0.74 |
| Threonine | 0.74 | 0.65 | 0.55 | 0.46 | 0.41 | 0.41 | 0.56 |
| Tryptophan | 0.22 | 0.19 | 0.17 | 0.14 | 0.11 | 0.11 | 0.18 |
| Tyrosine | 0.67 | 0.57 | 0.46 | 0.37 | 0.40 | 0.40 | 0.62 |
| Valine | 0.85 | 0.72 | 0.59 | 0.47 | 0.55 | 0.55 | 0.72 |

*Source:* Wu, G. 2014. *J. Anim. Sci. Biotechnol.* 5:34.

[a] Except for glycine, all AAs are L-isomers. Values are based on true ileal digestible AAs. Crystalline AAs (e.g., feed-grade arginine, glutamate, glutamine, and glycine), whose true ileal digestibility is 100%, can be added to a diet to obtain their optimal ratios. The molecular weights of intact AAs were used for all the calculations. The content of DM in all the diets is 90%. The content of metabolizable energy in the diets of growing pigs, gestating pigs, and lactating pigs is 3330, 3122, and 3310 Kcal/kg diet, respectively.

[b] Fed ad libitum (90% DM).

[c] Fed 2 kg/day on Days 0–90, and 2.3 kg/day on Days 90–114 (90% DM).

epithelial cells (MECs) in response to hormones (e.g., prolactin, insulin, and glucocorticoids). The alveoli are connected to a duct system through which the secreted milk flows into the teat canal, where it can be removed by suckling or milking (Figure 11.10). The stroma of a lactating gland is composed of connective tissue surrounding the epithelial structure. The cellular components of the connective tissue consist of fibroblasts, blood vessels, and leukocytes, while noncellular components include collagen and other connective tissue proteins (Inman et al. 2015). In addition, an extensive white adipose tissue exists as part of the stroma of the developing gland. This fat pad (an extraparenchymal tissue) is enlarged during the early phases of fetal and postnatal development, but decreased progressively in mass during the periods of puberty, pregnancy, and lactation.

Structural development of the mammary gland occurs in utero during fetal growth, and the prepubertal and post-pubertal periods, pregnancy, and lactation (Figure 11.11). This process is known as mammogenesis. The mammary gland develops rapidly during sexual maturation under the influence of hormones such as estrogen, progesterone, adrenal corticoids, prolactin, growth hormone, and thyroxine (Musumeci et al. 2015). Most of mammogenesis occurs during gestation under the

**TABLE 11.12**
**Texas A&M University's Optimal Ratios of True Digestible Amino Acids in Diets for Chickens[a]**

| Amino Acid | Age of Chickens | | |
|---|---|---|---|
| | 0 to 21 Days[b] | 21 to 42 Days[c] | 42 to 56 Days[d] |
| | | % of Lysine in Diet | |
| Alanine | 102 | 102 | 102 |
| Arginine | 105 | 108 | 108 |
| Asparagine | 56 | 56 | 56 |
| Aspartate | 66 | 66 | 66 |
| Cysteine | 32 | 33 | 33 |
| Glutamate | 178 | 178 | 178 |
| Glutamine | 128 | 128 | 128 |
| Glycine | 176 | 176 | 176 |
| Histidine | 35 | 35 | 35 |
| Isoleucine | 67 | 69 | 69 |
| Leucine | 109 | 109 | 109 |
| Lysine | 100 | 100 | 100 |
| Methionine | 40 | 42 | 42 |
| Phenylalanine | 60 | 60 | 60 |
| Proline | 184 | 184 | 184 |
| Serine | 69 | 69 | 69 |
| Threonine | 67 | 70 | 70 |
| Tryptophan | 16 | 17 | 17 |
| Tyrosine | 45 | 45 | 45 |
| Valine | 77 | 80 | 80 |

*Source:* Wu, G. 2014. *J. Anim. Sci. Biotechnol.* 5:34.
[a] Except for glycine, all AAs are L-isomers. Values are based on true ileal digestible AAs.
[b] Patterns of AA composition in the ideal protein are the same for male and female chickens. The amounts of digestible lysine in diet (as-fed basis; 90% DM) are 1.12% and 1.02% for male and female chickens, respectively.
[c] Patterns of AA composition in the ideal protein are the same for male and female chickens. The amounts of digestible lysine in diets (as-fed basis; 90% DM) are 0.89% and 0.84% for male and female chickens, respectively.
[d] Patterns of AA composition in the ideal protein are the same for male and female chickens. The amounts of digestible lysine in diets (as-fed basis; 90% DM) are 0.76% and 0.73% for male and female chickens, respectively.

control of various hormones (particularly estrogen, growth hormone, insulin-like growth factor-I, progesterone, placental lactogen, and prolactin) in a species- and stage-dependent manner. Thus, progesterone and prolactin promote lobuloalveolar development to form alveolar buds. Following parturition, the cessation of progesterone secretion is necessary for the initiation of milk production, because progesterone inhibits the secretion of hormones from the anterior lobe of the pituitary gland (Girmus and Wise 1992). Thus, at the onset of lactation, mature alveoli capable of producing and secreting milk are formed. Milk secretion is maintained by suckling and/or milking, which stimulates the secretion of prolactin and other hormones active in the mechanism of milk secretion. Suckling of the nipple by the neonate also causes the oxytocin-induced contraction of the myoepithelial cells around the alveoli to eject the milk through the ducts into the nipple. Upon weaning,

**TABLE 11.13**
**Composition of Mature Milk of Domesticated and Wild Mammals[a]**

| Species | Fat | Casein | Whey Protein | Total Protein | NPN Subs | Lactose | Total Carb | Ca | Ash | DM[b] |
|---|---|---|---|---|---|---|---|---|---|---|
| Antelope[c] | 72 | 48 | 14 | 62 | 18 | 42 | 47 | 2.6 | 13 | 212 |
| Baboon | 46 | 4.7 | 7.3 | 12 | 3.0 | 60 | 77 | 0.44 | 3.0 | 141 |
| Bat | 133 | x | x | 80 | 5.0 | 34 | 40 | x | 6.8 | 265 |
| Bear (black) | 220 | 88 | 57 | 145 | 7.5 | 3.0 | 27 | 3.6 | 19 | 419 |
| Bear (grizzly) | 185 | 68 | 67 | 135 | 7.0 | 4.0 | 32 | 3.4 | 13 | 372 |
| Bear (polar) | 331 | 71 | 38 | 109 | 5.6 | 4.0 | 30 | 3.0 | 12 | 488 |
| Beaver | 182 | 85 | 23 | 108 | 6.3 | 17 | 22 | 2.4 | 20 | 338 |
| Bison | 35 | 37 | 8.0 | 45 | 3.0 | 51 | 57 | 1.2 | 9.6 | 150 |
| Buffalo | 77 | 38 | 7.0 | 45 | 5.2 | 40 | 47 | 1.9 | 8.0 | 192 |
| Blue whale | 423 | 73 | 36 | 109 | 6.6 | 10 | 13 | 3.4 | 16 | 568 |
| Camel | 45 | 29 | 10 | 39 | 5.6 | 49 | 56 | 1.4 | 7.0 | 153 |
| Cat (domestic) | 108 | 31 | 60 | 91 | 10 | 42 | 49 | 1.8 | 6.2 | 264 |
| Chimpanzee | 37 | 4.8 | 7.2 | 12 | 2.0 | 70 | 82 | 0.36 | 11 | 144 |
| Cow (domestic)[d] | 37 | 28 | 6.0 | 34 | 2.2 | 49 | 56 | 1.2 | 7.1 | 136 |
| Coyote | 107 | x | x | 99 | x | 30 | 32 | x | 9.0 | 247 |
| Deer | 197 | 94 | 10 | 104 | 14 | 26 | 30 | 2.6 | 14 | 359 |
| Dog (domestic) | 95 | 51 | 23 | 74 | 23 | 33 | 38 | 2.0 | 12 | 242 |
| Dolphin | 330 | 39 | 29 | 68 | 3.0 | 10 | 11 | 1.5 | 7.5 | 420 |
| Donkey (Ass) | 14 | 11 | 9.0 | 20 | 3.2 | 61 | 68 | 0.91 | 4.5 | 110 |
| Elephant | 116 | 19 | 30 | 49 | 4.1 | 51 | 60 | 0.80 | 7.6 | 237 |
| Ferret | 80 | 32 | 28 | 58 | 6.7 | 38 | 44 | x | 8.0 | 197 |
| Fin whale | 286 | 82 | 38 | 120 | 6.2 | 2.0 | 26 | 3.0 | 16 | 454 |
| Fox | 63 | x | x | 63 | 4.0 | 47 | 50 | 3.4 | 10 | 190 |
| Giant panda | 104 | 50 | 21 | 71 | 10 | 12 | 15 | 1.3 | 9.4 | 209 |
| Giraffe | 125 | 48 | 8.0 | 56 | 2.2 | 34 | 40 | 1.5 | 8.7 | 232 |
| Goat (domestic) | 45 | 29 | 5.0 | 34 | 5.8 | 43 | 47 | 1.4 | 7.9 | 139 |
| Goat (mountain) | 57 | 24 | 7.0 | 31 | 5.3 | 28 | 32 | 1.3 | 12 | 136 |
| Gorilla | 19 | 13 | 9.0 | 22 | 1.9 | 62 | 73 | 3.2 | 6.0 | 122 |
| Guinea pig | 39 | 66 | 15 | 81 | 12 | 30 | 36 | 1.6 | 8.2 | 176 |
| Hamster | 126 | 58 | 32 | 90 | 11 | 32 | 38 | 2.1 | 14 | 279 |
| Horse (domestic) | 19 | 14 | 8.3 | 22 | 3.6 | 62 | 69 | 0.95 | 5.1 | 119 |
| Human[e] | 42 | 4.4 | 6.6 | 11 | 2.8 | 70 | 80 | 0.32 | 2.2 | 138 |
| Kangaroo | 21 | 23 | 23 | 46 | 4 | <0.01 | 47 | 1.6 | 12 | 130 |
| Lion | 189 | 57 | 36 | 93 | 6.6 | 27 | 34 | 0.82 | 14 | 337 |
| Llama | 42 | 62 | 11 | 73 | 9.6 | 60 | 66 | 1.7 | 7.5 | 198 |
| Mink | 80 | x | x | 74 | 12 | 69 | 76 | 1.3 | 10 | 252 |
| Moose | 105 | x | x | 135 | 18 | 33 | 38 | 3.6 | 16 | 312 |
| Mouse (Lab) | 121 | 70 | 20 | 90 | 11 | 30 | 36 | 2.5 | 15 | 273 |
| Mule[f] | 18 | x | x | 20 | 3.0 | 55 | 62 | 0.76 | 4.8 | 108 |
| Musk ox | 110 | 35 | 18 | 53 | 7.0 | 27 | 33 | 3.0 | 18 | 221 |
| Opossum | 61 | 48 | 44 | 92 | 4.6 | 16 | 20 | 4.2 | 16 | 194 |
| Peccary | 36 | 40 | 15 | 55 | 5.7 | 66 | 71 | 1.2 | 6.4 | 174 |
| Pig (domestic) | 80 | 28 | 20 | 48 | 5.4 | 52 | 58 | 3.1 | 9.2 | 201 |
| Pronghorn | 130 | x | x | 69 | 7.2 | 40 | 43 | 2.5 | 13 | 262 |
| Rabbit | 183 | 104 | 32 | 136 | 11 | 18 | 21 | 6.3 | 20 | 371 |
| Rat (Lab) | 126 | 64 | 20 | 84 | 6.3 | 30 | 38 | 3.2 | 15 | 269 |

*(Continued)*

**TABLE 11.13 (*Continued*)**
**Composition of Mature Milk of Domesticated and Wild Mammals[a]**

| Species | Fat | Casein | Whey Protein | Total Protein | NPN Subs | Lactose | Total Carb | Ca | Ash | DM[b] |
|---|---|---|---|---|---|---|---|---|---|---|
| Reindeer | 203 | 86 | 15 | 101 | 14 | 28 | 35 | 3.1 | 14 | 367 |
| Rhesus monkey | 40 | 11 | 5.0 | 16 | 1.6 | 70 | 82 | 0.40 | 26 | 166 |
| Rhinoceros | 4.0 | 11 | 3.0 | 14 | 2.3 | 66 | 72 | 0.56 | 3.7 | 96 |
| Sea lion | 349 | x | x | 136 | 4.1 | 0.0 | 6.0 | 0.76 | 6.4 | 502 |
| Seal (fur) | 251 | 46 | 43 | 89 | 6.9 | 1.0 | 24 | 0.70 | 5.0 | 376 |
| Seal (gray) | 532 | 50 | 52 | 102 | 10 | 1.0 | 26 | 2.0 | 7.0 | 677 |
| Seal (harp) | 502 | 38 | 21 | 59 | 2.4 | 8.9 | 23 | 1.2 | 3.9 | 590 |
| Seal (hooded) | 404 | x | x | 67 | 5.0 | 0.0 | 10 | 1.2 | 8.6 | 496 |
| Sheep (domestic) | 74 | 46 | 10 | 56 | 2.7 | 48 | 55 | 1.9 | 9.2 | 195 |
| Sperm whale[g] | 153 | 32 | 50 | 82 | 6.3 | 20 | 22 | 1.5 | 8.0 | 270 |
| Squirrel (gray) | 121 | 50 | 24 | 74 | 16 | 30 | 34 | 3.6 | 12 | 257 |
| Tree shrew | 170 | x | x | 85 | 19 | 15 | 20 | x | 8.0 | 302 |
| Water buffalo | 74 | 32 | 6.0 | 38 | 5.8 | 48 | 55 | 1.9 | 7.8 | 181 |
| Water shrew | 200 | x | x | 100 | x | 1.0 | 30 | x | 20 | 350 |
| White whale | 220 | 82 | 38 | 120 | 3.7 | 2.0 | 18 | 3.6 | 16 | 378 |
| Wolf | 96 | x | x | 92 | 4.8 | 32 | 35 | 4.0 | 25 | 253 |
| Yak | 68 | 36 | 7.0 | 43 | 2.5 | 50 | 54 | 1.3 | 8.0 | 176 |
| Zebra | 21 | 12 | 11 | 23 | 2.6 | 74 | 82 | 0.8 | 3.5 | 132 |

*Source:* Rezaei, R. et al. 2016. *J. Anim. Sci. Biotechnol.* 7:20.

[a] Values are g/kg whole milk. Nonprotein nitrogen = total nitrogen − protein nitrogen. Nitrogen content in milk protein is 15.67%. The amount of nonprotein nitrogenous substances (g/kg whole milk) is calculated as the amount of nonprotein nitrogen (g/kg whole milk) × 6.25. Caseins include $\alpha_{S1}$-casein, $\alpha_{S2}$-casein, β-casein, γ-casein, and *k*-casein. Whey proteins include α-lactoalbumin, β-lactoglobulin, serum albumin, immunoglobulins, lactoferrins, lysozymes, AA oxidases, xanthine oxidase, and other enzymes.

[b] Including fat, protein, NPN, lactose plus other carbohydrates, and minerals (total ash). When data on total carbohydrates have not been reported, ratios of lactose to other carbohydrates in milk are estimated to be 15:1 (g/g).

[c] Gemsbok antelope.

[d] Concentrations of urea, creatinine, and amino sugars are 317, 127, and 392 mg/L whole milk, respectively.

[e] Concentrations of urea, creatinine, and amino sugars are 274, 209, and 1111 mg/L whole milk, respectively.

[f] *Mule* is a domesticated hybrid animal produced by crossing a female horse with a male *donkey*.

[g] Pygmy sperm whale.

AA = amino acids; Ca = calcium; Carb = carbohydrates; DM = dry matter; NPN subs = nonprotein nitrogenous substances (including free AAs, small peptides, urea, ammonia, uric acid, creatine, creatinine, and other low-molecular weight nitrogenous substances). The symbol "x" denotes the lack of data in the literature.

lactation stops, and the mammary gland undergoes involution through apoptosis and autophagy to its non-lactating state (Rezaei et al. 2016).

## Milk Synthesis by MECs

The milk is produced in MECs arranged in alveoli (or acini) and is drained through a system of arborizing ducts toward the body surface. The natural length of lactation differs among mammals. For example, cows lactate for about 40 weeks with the peak of lactation at 6–8 weeks after calving, ewes lactate for about 12–20 weeks with the peak of lactation at 2–3 weeks after lambing, and sows lactate for about 6–8 weeks, with the peak of lactation at 3–4 weeks after farrowing (Akers 2002; Bell 1995; Manjarin et al. 2014). In all mammals, the synthetic capacity of the mammary gland depends largely on the number and efficiency of functional MECs, and milk synthesis is regulated

**TABLE 11.14**
**Composition of Immunoglobulins (Ig) in Colostrum and Mature Milk**

| Species | Type of Milk | Ig A (g/L) | Ig G (g/L) | Ig M (g/L) |
|---|---|---|---|---|
| Cow | Colostrum | 3.9 | 50.5 | 4.2 |
| | Mature milk | 0.20 | 0.80 | 0.05 |
| Goat | Colostrum | 0.9–2.4 | 50–60 | 1.6–5.2 |
| | Mature milk | 0.03–0.08 | 0.1–0.4 | 0.01–0.04 |
| Sheep | Colostrum | 2.0 | 61 | 4.1 |
| | Mature milk | 0.06 | 0.3 | 0.03 |
| Sow | Colostrum | 10–26 | 62–94 | 3–10 |
| | Mature milk | 3.4–5.6 | 1.0–1.9 | 1.2–1.4 |
| Human | Colostrum | 17.4 | 0.43 | 1.6 |
| | Mature milk | 1.0 | 0.04 | 0.1 |

*Source:* Rezaei, R. et al. 2016. *J. Anim. Sci. Biotechnol.* 7:20.

at both transcriptional and post-transcriptional levels (Osorio et al. 2016). As part of the systemic circulation, a pair of major arteries provides the blood to the mammary gland. Uptake of nutrients from a large volume of blood is required for milk production. For example, in lactating cows, the production of 1 L milk requires the passage of approximately 500 L blood through the mammary gland (Braun and Forster 2012). During lactation, blood flow through the mammary gland is very rapid, and blood nutrients are actively taken up by the mammary gland.

Different methods have been developed to study the biosynthesis of milk constituents in the mammary gland. Determination of the arteriovenous (A-V) differences in a substance entering and leaving the mammary gland is the simplest method (Trottier et al. 1997). On the basis of the A-V differences in a substance, the rate of its extraction can be calculated as (A-V)/A × 100%. If the rate of blood flow (mL/min) is known, it is multiplied by the rate of extraction to obtain the absolute rate of uptake of molecules by the mammary gland. The mammary glands of lactating goats take

**TABLE 11.15**
**Composition of Proteins in Mature Milk of Mammals**

| Protein | Cow (g/L Milk) | Pig (g/L Milk) | Sheep (g/L Milk) | Goat (g/L Milk) | Horse (g/L Milk) | Human (g/L Milk) |
|---|---|---|---|---|---|---|
| Caseins | 28 | 28 | 46 | 29 | 13.6 | 4.4 |
| α-S1 | 10.6 | 20 | 16.6 | 4.3 | 2.4 | 0.52 |
| α-S2 | 3.4 | 2.4 | 6.4 | 5.8 | 0.2 | 0.0 |
| β | 10.1 | 2.3 | 18.3 | 11.2 | 10.7 | 2.8 |
| κ | 3.9 | 3.3 | 4.5 | 7.7 | 0.24 | 1.0 |
| Whey proteins | 6.0 | 20 | 10 | 5.0 | 8.3 | 6.6 |
| α-Lactalbumin | 1.2 | 3.0 | 2.4 | 0.85 | 2.4 | 2.8 |
| β-Lactoglobulin | 3.2 | 9.5 | 6.4 | 2.3 | 2.6 | 0.0 |
| Lactoferrin | 0.02–0.2 | 0.1–0.25 | 0.1 | 0.02–0.2 | 0.58 | 3–4 |
| Transferrin | 0.02–0.2 | 0.02–0.2 | 0.1 | 0.02–0.2 | 0.1 | 0.02–0.03 |
| Immunoglobulins | 1.1 | 6.6 | 0.4 | 0.4 | 1.6 | 1.2 |
| Serum albumin | 0.4 | 0.5 | 0.5 | 0.6 | 0.4 | 0.5 |

*Source:* Rezaei, R. et al. 2016. *J. Anim. Sci. Biotechnol.* 7:20.

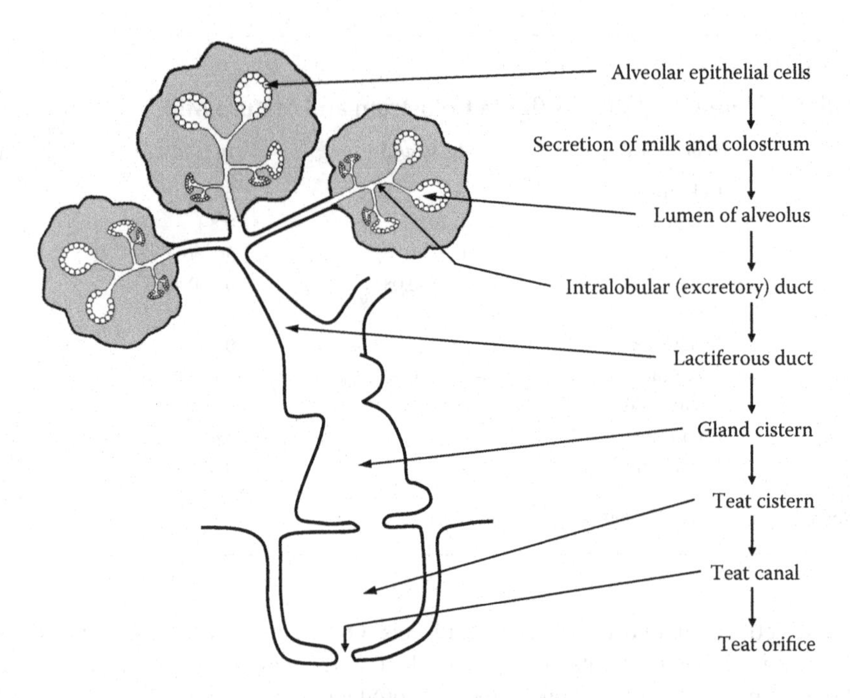


**FIGURE 11.10** The basic structure of the mammary gland. MECs are responsible for the synthesis and release of milk by lactating mammals. The alveoli are connected to a duct system through which the secreted milk flows into the teat canal, from which it can be removed by suckling or milking. (Rezaei, R. et al. 2016. *J. Anim. Sci. Biotechnol.* 7:20.)

up, from the arterial blood, a large amount of acetate, glucose, lactate, AAs, β-hydroxybutyrate and TAG, but only a small quantity of glycerol, long-chain fatty acids, and phospholipids (Table 11.16).

1. *Proteins and AAs in milk. True protein in milk.* Approximately 80%–95% of the nitrogen in milk is present in true protein (casein, lactalbumin, and lactoglobulin) and free AAs, with the remaining nitrogen primarily as urea, ammonia, creatine, and creatinine (Rezaei et al. 2016). Albumin, κ-casein, and immunoglobulins (acting as antibodies) in the colostrum and milk are derived from their direct passage from the maternal blood to the lumen of the alveoli. Protein concentrations are greater in colostrum than in mature milk. In colostrum, concentrations of albumin and globulins are greater than those of casein (Tables 11.13 and 11.14). In milk, about 25% of DM and a similar proportion of energy are in the protein fraction (Table 11.16). A high-producing cow produces 1–1.5 kg protein per day, and a rapidly growing calf or steer deposits about 250 g protein per day (Tucker 2000). Thus, milk production requires a large amount of dietary protein.
   *Processing of milk protein in the MECs.* Proteins that are synthesized at the rough endoplasmic reticulum (RER) are either secreted proteins (e.g., casein, β-lactoglobulin, and α-lactalbumin), membrane-bound proteins (e.g., extracellular matrix proteins involved in cell–cell contacts and membrane-bound enzymes), or intracellular proteins (e.g., enzymes, structural proteins [e.g., keratin], and fatty acid-binding proteins) (Ollivier-Bousquet 2002). Within MECs, the newly synthesized proteins are transferred from the RER to the Golgi apparatus where they are processed for transport out of the cells. Casein is secreted as a micelle, which is formed in the Golgi from casein, calcium, and phosphorus. Casein, which exists in several forms, represents the bulk of the protein in the mature milk of all nonhuman species: 82%–86% in ruminants, 52%–80% in nonruminants, and 40% in

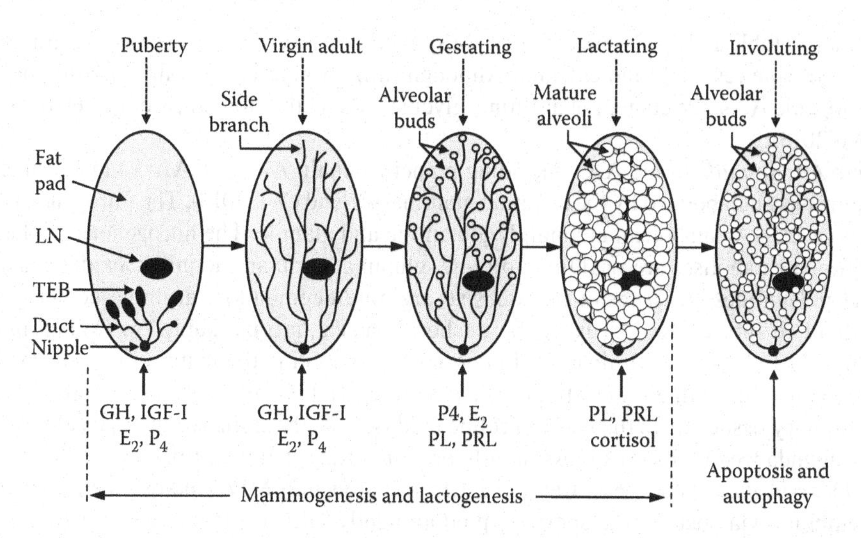


**FIGURE 11.11** Development of the mammary gland in mammals. Mammogenesis begins during fetal development. After birth, mammary ducts elongate through cell proliferation. At the onset of puberty, high concentrations of growth hormone and insulin-like growth factor in plasma stimulate mammary duct proliferation to form terminal end buds (TEBs) at the tips of the ducts. Under the influence of estrogen, TEBs actively proliferate to form ductal branches, which fill the mammary fat pad. After this stage, the TEBs regress. During pregnancy, progesterone and prolactin promote lobuloalveolar development to form alveolar buds. At the onset of lactation, mature alveoli capable of producing and secreting milk are formed. Suckling of the nipple by the neonate results in contractions of the myoepithelial cells around the alveoli, causing the milk to be ejected through the ducts into the nipple. Upon weaning, lactation stops and the mammary gland undergoes involution through apoptosis and autophagy to its nonlactating state. E2 = estrogen; GH = growth hormone; IGF-I = insulin-like growth factor-I; LN = lymph node; P4 = progesterone; PL = placental lactogen; PRL = prolactin. (Courtesy of Rezaei, R. et al. 2016. *J. Anim. Sci. Biotechnol.* 7:20.)

**TABLE 11.16**
**Concentrations of Milk Precursors in the Mammary Arteries and the Rates of Extraction of Nutrients by the Mammary Glands of Lactating Goats**

| Substance | Arterial Concentration (mg/L) | Extraction Rate (%) |
|---|---|---|
| | **Blood** | |
| Acetate | 89 | 63 |
| Glucose | 445 | 33 |
| Lactate | 67 | 30 |
| Oxygen (volume as liter) | 119 | 45 |
| | **Plasma** | |
| AAs | 2.7–68.5 | 15–72 |
| Glycerol | 3.4 | 7 |
| β-Hydroxybutyrate | 58 | 57 |
| Long-chain free fatty acids | 87 | 3 |
| Phospholipids | 1600 | 4 |
| Sterols | 1040 | 0 |
| Triglycerides | 219 | 40 |

*Source:* Mepham, T.B. and J.L. Linzell. 1966. *Biochem. J.* 101:76–83.

humans (Table 11.15). Casein contains phosphorylated AA residues (e.g., serine, threonine, and tyrosine residues) and calcium. Although milk protein is generally rich in most proteinogenic AAs, the content of arginine, glycine, and methionine in casein is relatively low (Wu 2013).

*Free AAs in milk.* Some AAs, including branched-chain AAs (BCAAs) and arginine, are extensively catabolized by the lactating mammary gland (Wu 2013). The nitrogenous products of BCAA catabolism are mainly glutamine and alanine. The nitrogenous products of arginine catabolism are ornithine, proline, glutamate, glutamine, nitric oxide, citrulline, and polyamines. As a result of extensive arginine degradation, arginine content in the milk of all species studied, except for the horse and cat, is remarkably low (Manjarin et al. 2014). Milk-borne polyamines are important for promoting the maturation and growth of the neonatal intestine. Interestingly, there is little catabolism of proline and glutamine in mammary tissue due to the lack of proline oxidase and glutaminase, and this helps explain the abundance of those two AAs in milk proteins (Rezaei et al. 2016).

2. *Lactose in milk.* Glucose is transported from blood into MECs across their basolateral membrane via specific transporters (predominantly GLUT1) (Zhao and Keating 2007). Approximately 60% or more of the glucose extracted by the lactating mammary gland is used for lactose synthesis, with the remaining portion of the glucose being used for fat synthesis, oxidation, and perhaps alanine synthesis. Studies with $^{14}$C-glucose have shown that blood glucose is the major precursor for both moieties (i.e., glucose and galactose) of the lactose molecule (Baxter et al. 1956). Glycerol, a hydrolytic product of triglycerides, is a precursor of glucose synthesis in the liver of the lactating dam and thus plays a role in galactose and lactose production by MECs. In these cells, both glucose and galactose enter the Golgi to form lactose via a series of enzyme-catalyzed reactions (Chapter 5). The formation of lactose in the Golgi results in the movement of water from the extracellular space (and thus the blood) into the cytoplasm and then into the Golgi, where lactose ultimately becomes a component of milk. Lactose contributes to most of the osmotic pressure in milk (Table 11.12) and therefore is of nutritional and physiological importance for suckling neonates.
3. *Lipids in milk.* In the milk of most mammals (including cows and swine), except for a few (including horses), 98% of the lipids are TAG (Palmquist 2006). The lipids of the equine milk contain 80% TAG (Stoneham et al. 2017). Sterols, including cholesterol (the major milk sterol), represent less than 0.5% of the total milk lipid fraction, and the concentrations of phospholipids are low in milk (Jensen 2002). However, phospholipids are essential components of the milk fat globule. Fats are not water soluble, do not contribute to the osmotic pressure of milk, and are present in milk as an emulsion. Concentrations of fats and fatty acids in the milk of different species vary greatly. For example, the milk of ruminants has relatively high concentrations of butyrate, other SCFAs, odd-numbered fatty acids, and branched-chain fatty acids (Park and Haenlein 2006). A unique component of the milk of ruminants is conjugated linoleic acid, which has many important roles in nutrition (Chapter 6). $C_{18:1}$, $C_{16:0}$, and $C_{18:0}$ are the most abundant fatty acids in bovine milk, as are $C_{18:1}$ and $C_{16:0}$ in sow's milk (Palmquist 2006). The fatty acids in milk have two major sources: blood triglycerides as lipoproteins and/or de novo synthesis.

*Fatty acids from lipoproteins in the MECs.* During the passage of triglycerides from blood to the mammary tissue, fatty acids and glycerol are released by lipoprotein lipase bound to the endothelial surface of the capillary wall (Chapter 6). Following their passage through the capillary wall into the MECs, fatty acids and glycerol are taken up by these cells. The circulating low-density lipoproteins (LDLs) also enter the mammary tissue via the process of endocytosis mediated by the membrane-bound LDL receptor (Osorio et al. 2016). Approximately 50% of the fatty acids in milk are derived from blood lipoproteins (Palmquist 2006).

*De novo synthesis of fatty acids in the MECs.* In the MECs of lactating animals, fatty acids are synthesized from glucose, acetate, butyrate, acetoacetate, and β-hydroxybutyrate in a species-dependent manner (Chapter 6). De novo synthesis by MECs contributes about 50% of the fatty acids in milk (Palmquist 2006). Glucose metabolism through the pentose cycle generates the NADPH required for fatty acid synthesis. The ketone bodies are important precursors for the synthesis of fatty acids in the milk of ruminants, rodents, and humans, but not in that of pigs. This is because ketogenesis is limited in swine (including lactating sows) due to a deficiency of 3-hydroxy-3-methyl-glutaryl-CoA synthase in the liver (Chapter 5). In the mammary tissue of lactating sows, fatty acids (up to $C_{18}$) in sow's milk can be synthesized from blood glucose and acetate (Linzell and Mepham 1969). In contrast, there is little conversion of glucose into fatty acids in the mammary gland of ruminants (Chapter 6).

*Synthesis of phospholipids and cholesterol by the MECs.* The phospholipids in milk are synthesized from diacylglycerol and phosphatidic acid by the MECs (Chapter 6). Phospholipids are transported among organelles of the MECs via spontaneous membrane diffusion, cytosolic phospholipid transfer proteins, vesicles, and membrane contact sites (Vance 2015). The cholesterol in milk lipids originates predominantly from blood and, to a lesser extent, de novo synthesis in the MECs (Ontsouka and Albrecht 2014).

*Synthesis of fats by the MECs.* Fatty acids, glycerol, and monoacylglycerides are taken up by the MECs for the synthesis of triglycerides in the smooth endoplasmic reticulum (Chapter 6), leading to the formation of small lipid droplets. Numerous small lipid droplets fuse to yield larger droplets, which move toward the apical membrane. The large lipid droplets exit the MEC across its apical membrane into the lumen of alveoli and the duct system of the mammary gland. Except for the horse, fat is the major energy substrate for the suckling neonates of mammals (Table 11.17). The concentration of lipids in the milk of horses is only about 50% of that in the cow's milk.

4. *Minerals in milk.* Minerals in blood pass into the mammary gland to become components of milk (Shennan and Peaker 2000). For farm mammals, colostrum may contain about twice the amount of most minerals as mature milk, and the concentration of iron in colostrum may exceed that in milk by 10- to 17-fold. However, concentrations of potassium are lower in colostrum than in milk (Park and Haenlein 2006). Concentrations of calcium and phosphorus are much higher in milk than in blood (13 times higher for calcium and 10 times for phosphorus). Milk differs from plasma in mineral concentrations and is more like those in intracellular fluid. Dietary intake of most trace minerals greatly influences their concentrations in milk (Suttle 2010). However, the concentrations of copper, iron, and zinc in milk may not be altered significantly in response to dietary supplements.
5. *Milk's organic substances not synthesized in MECs.* A number of organic substances in maternal plasma are transported across the MEC into the duct system essentially unchanged. These substances include vitamins and immunoglobulins, which are the same as those found in the blood or mucosal secretions (Hurley and Theil 2011). Vitamins in the blood enter the MEC through its basolateral membrane via specific transporters or receptor-mediated endocytosis (Chapter 9). Immunoglobulins bind to specific receptors on the basolateral surface of the MEC, enter the cell, and are then exported into the lumen of the alveolus through the apical side of the cell via endocytic vesicles (or transport vesicles) (Hurley and Theil 2011). In this process, the membrane of the transport vesicles fuses with the inner surface of the apical membrane of the MEC and releases immunoglobulins into the lumen of the alveolus. As the transport vesicles traverse the cell, they do not seem to interact with the Golgi, secretory vesicles, or lipid droplets. Serum albumin may also be transported across MEC via this clathrin-mediated mechanism (Monks and Neville 2004). Since there is no serum albumin receptor, serum albumin molecules are probably internalized into the MEC along with immunoglobulins in the transport vesicles.

**TABLE 11.17**
**Percentage of Total Calories Represented by Fat, Protein, and Carbohydrates in the Milks of Some Mammals**

| Species | Fat (kcal/ kg Milk) | Protein + AAs (kcal/kg Milk) | Carb (kcal/ kg Milk) | Total Energy (kcal/kg Milk) | % Calories as Fat | % Calories as Protein + AAs | % Calories as Carb |
|---|---|---|---|---|---|---|---|
| Cat | 1014 | 518 | 192 | 1725 | 58.8 | 30.1 | 11.1 |
| Cow | 347 | 189 | 220 | 756 | 46.0 | 25.0 | 29.0 |
| Deer | 1850 | 599 | 118 | 2567 | 72.1 | 23.4 | 4.6 |
| Dog | 892 | 464 | 149 | 1505 | 59.3 | 30.8 | 9.9 |
| Dolphin | 3099 | 378 | 43 | 3520 | 88.0 | 10.7 | 1.2 |
| Donkey | 131 | 119 | 267 | 517 | 25.4 | 23.0 | 51.6 |
| Elephant | 1089 | 275 | 235 | 1600 | 68.1 | 17.2 | 14.7 |
| Goat | 423 | 200 | 184 | 807 | 52.4 | 24.8 | 22.8 |
| Guinea pig | 366 | 470 | 141 | 977 | 37.5 | 48.1 | 14.4 |
| Hamster | 1183 | 518 | 149 | 1851 | 63.9 | 28.0 | 8.0 |
| Horse | 178 | 130 | 270 | 578 | 30.8 | 22.4 | 46.8 |
| Human | 394 | 65 | 314 | 773 | 51.0 | 8.4 | 40.6 |
| Kangaroo | 197 | 259 | 184 | 641 | 30.8 | 40.5 | 28.8 |
| Mouse | 1136 | 518 | 141 | 1796 | 63.3 | 28.9 | 7.9 |
| Pig | 751 | 275 | 227 | 1254 | 59.9 | 22.0 | 18.1 |
| Rabbit | 1718 | 767 | 82 | 2567 | 66.9 | 29.9 | 3.2 |
| Rat | 1183 | 470 | 149 | 1802 | 65.7 | 26.1 | 8.3 |
| Reindeer | 1906 | 583 | 137 | 2627 | 72.6 | 22.2 | 5.2 |
| Rhesus monkey | 376 | 92 | 321 | 789 | 47.6 | 11.6 | 40.7 |
| Sea lion | 3277 | 745 | 24 | 4046 | 81.0 | 18.4 | 0.6 |
| Sheep | 695 | 313 | 216 | 1224 | 56.8 | 25.6 | 17.6 |
| Squirrel (gray) | 1136 | 443 | 133 | 1712 | 66.4 | 25.9 | 7.8 |
| Wolf | 901 | 238 | 212 | 1351 | 66.7 | 17.6 | 15.7 |
| Yak | 639 | 238 | 212 | 1088 | 58.7 | 21.8 | 19.5 |

The energy values of fat, protein + AAs, and total carbohydrates were calculated on the basis of their combustion energy of 9.39, 5.40, and 3.92 kcal/g, respectively.
Carb, carbohydrates.

## Release of Milk Proteins, Lactose, and Fats from MECs to the Lumen of the Alveoli

In the MECs, the Golgi apparatus participates in the processing of milk proteins as glycosylated proteins, the synthesis of lactose and fats, and osmotic gradients for transport of water, and therefore plays an important role in the synthesis of milk components (Rezaei et al. 2016). Milk proteins and lactose are transported to the apical area of the MECs via secretory vesicles, which make their way to the apical membrane via a mechanism involving microtubules made of polymerized tubulin (Shennan and Peaker 2000). Tubulin is one of several cytoskeletal proteins which form the cellular scaffolding that provides structure to the cell. Keratin is another cytoskeletal protein. The apical membrane of MECs and the membrane of the secretory vesicle fuse, resulting in an opening through which the vesicle contents are discharged into the lumen of the alveoli.

Since fats and long-chain fatty acids are insoluble in water, the lipid droplets in milk are covered by a thin membrane consisting of protein and phospholipids to form milk fat globules on the endoplasmic reticulum membrane (Palmquist 2006). Approximately 13% of protein binds to lipids in milk (Wu and Knabe 1994). These lipid droplets are released from the endoplasmic reticulum into the cytosol and transported to the apical membrane of the MEC for secretion into the lumen of the alveoli via exocytosis.

### Efficiency of Energy Utilization for Milk Production

Energy (primarily ATP) is required for milk synthesis. In the MECs, about 90% of the ATP is generated via the mitochondrial electron transport system (Rezaei et al. 2016). When there are no changes in body reserves of the lactating animals, the gross efficiency of milk production is the ratio of the energy in milk (output) to the energy in the feed consumed (input) during a given period. The net efficiency of milk production is the ratio of energy in milk to the energy in feed excluding maintenance requirements. Energy requirements for lactation are calculated factorially by summing those for maintenance, milk production, and changes in BW. In essence, milk yield and its energy content [e.g., bovine and sow's milk (Table 11.16)] determine energy requirements for lactation. In milk, fat content varies the most, protein content varies less, and minerals and lactose vary the least (Table 11.13).

There is a negative energy balance in lactating cows, goats, ewes, and sows during early lactation (Baldwin and Bywater 1984). In cows, the efficiency of utilization of energy during early lactation is as follows: feed ME to milk = 0.644; body fats to milk = 0.824; feed ME to body fats = 0.747; and feed ME to body fats during the dry period = 0.587 (Bondi 1987). Thus, fat deposition during lactation is 27% more efficient than that in the dry period. The efficiency in the conversion of feed into milk in high-producing cows is increased by 10% through intramuscular administration of recombinant bovine growth hormone to high-producing dairy cows (Etherton and Bauman 1998). A possible alternative solution is dietary supplementation with rumen-protected arginine, as this technique is highly effective in enhancing milk production by sows (Mateo et al. 2008). Besides DM intake, water consumption by lactating mothers greatly affects the volume of milk produced daily. Overall, the efficiency of milk production decreases with advanced lactation, because of the decreasing metabolic activity in the MECs (Gorewit 1988).

## Nutritional Requirements for Production of Muscular Work

In underdeveloped nations, cattle are still used to plough the soil (Pearson et al. 2003). In developed countries, increasing numbers of horses are used for racing and other recreational purposes. In many regions of the world, horses, donkeys, mules (male donkeys × female horses), yaks, and camels are used for transport. Physical performance is the major output of the working cattle, horses, and riding animals in agriculture and transport (Pearson et al. 2003). As noted in Chapter 1, cattle are ruminants, whereas horses are monogastric herbivores with a relatively small stomach and a voluminous cecum and colon. The large intestine of horses has digestive functions similar to those of ruminants (Chapter 1). However, horses do not ruminate, and the gases produced by fermentation in the cecum and colon escape from the gastrointestinal tract through the rectum (Chapter 1). Owing to the posterior compartments of fiber digestion in horses, ingested intact fiber enters the large intestine. Consequently, the rate of passage of digesta from the stomach to the distal end of the small intestine is greater in horses than in cattle (McDonald et al. 2011). Although the microflora and its biochemical activity in the cecum and colon of horses are similar to those in ruminants, fiber digestion in horses is not as efficient as in ruminants (Bondi 1987). Diets containing <15% fiber are well digested by horses, which utilize dietary fiber more efficiently than rabbits (Chapter 6). Donkeys, mules (offspring of male donkeys × female horses), yaks, and camels are all herbivores, which consume plants (e.g., grass and vegetables) as their diets.

### Energy Conversion in Skeletal Muscle

Skeletal muscle is chemodynamic, as it converts chemical energy directly into mechanical (dynamic) energy (Lieber and Bodine-Fowler 1993). Thus, muscle differs from the steam engine and the internal combustion engine, because these engines convert chemical energy first into thermal energy (heat) and the latter into dynamic energy. Skeletal muscle consists of fibers made of myofibrils. There are two major important proteins in the myofibrils: actin and myosin. During contraction, bundles of actin and myosin filaments slide into each other to generate force. The energy required for contractions of skeletal muscle is supplied directly by the enzymatic hydrolysis of ATP to ADP plus phosphate in the presence of calcium and magnesium (Newsholme and Leech 2009). Interestingly, myosin, in association with actin, has an ATPase activity.

$$\text{ATP} \rightarrow \text{ADP} + \text{Pi} + \text{Mechanical Energy} + \text{Heat}$$

Under normal feeding conditions, fatty acids and glucose are the major sources of energy for skeletal muscle in mammals and birds (Jobgen et al. 2006). Whether this is also true for fish and shrimp is unknown. Glycogen, ketone bodies, and free AAs (e.g., glutamine and BCAAs) are also sources of energy for the muscle. In the contracting muscle, the amount of glycogen is gradually reduced. Under predominantly anaerobic conditions, ATP is produced in skeletal muscle through glycolysis, an inefficient pathway for ATP production (Chapter 5).

Although contractions of skeletal muscle specifically require ATP and its concentration in the muscle is greater than that in the liver, creatine phosphate is the major high-energy phosphate stored in the muscle and brain. Indeed, the concentration of phosphocreatine (also known as creatine phosphate) in skeletal muscle (19 mmol/kg or 25 mM) is much greater than that of ATP (4.5 mmol/kg or 6 mM). Creatine is synthesized from arginine, glycine, and methionine through an interorgan cooperation (mainly the liver, kidney, and muscle) (Wu 2013). Thus, adequate protein nutrition is crucial for maintaining muscular work.

$$\text{ATP} + \text{Creatine} \leftrightarrow \text{ADP} + \text{Phosphocreatine (Creatine kinase)}$$

When ATP is used by skeletal muscle for contraction, this reaction proceeds from the right to the left (Newsholme and Leech 2009). With the depletion of ATP, fatigue sets in and, after prolonged muscular activity, the accumulation of lactic acid results in muscle cramps (Allen et al. 2008). At rest, the energy in ATP is transferred to creatine and is then stored in phosphocreatine; namely the reaction proceeds from the left to the right.

### High Requirements for Dietary Energy, Protein, and Minerals for Muscular Work

1. *Muscular work-induced increases in nutrient metabolism.* A working animal expends more energy than a resting one and therefore requires higher intakes of dietary energy substrates (fats, glucose, and AAs) (Jobgen et al. 2006). In addition, rates of muscle protein turnover are enhanced in response to muscular work, with outcomes depending on its intensity and dietary intake of energy and protein (Allen et al. 2008). Thus, additional dietary AAs for protein synthesis to offset the loss of body protein must be supplied in diets. There are suggestions that dietary intake of protein and energy by subjects be increased by 30% and 60%, respectively, for moderate and intense exercise (Wu 2016). Furthermore, the rates of production of oxidants are greater in the working animal, compared with the resting one. Thus, requirements for dietary antioxidant nutrients (e.g., vitamins E, A, and C) must also be augmented accordingly for the working animal, compared with the resting one (Allen et al. 2008). Note that vitamin E is particularly important for the maintenance of the structural integrity of skeletal muscle.
   Intensive work is associated with sweating, and thus the loss of large amounts of water, sodium, and chloride as well as small amounts of potassium, magnesium, calcium, and phosphorus (Keen 1993). This requires supplementation of water, sodium chloride, and other minerals in a continuous and balanced manner. Dehydration is the major danger under conditions of hard work or intensive heat. For example, a horse with intense exercise may need up to 60 L of water and 100 g of sodium chloride per day to avoid dehydration (Zeyner et al. 2017). A consequence of severe dehydration is collapse and death.

**TABLE 11.18**
**Efficiency in the Use of Metabolic Fuels for Muscular Power Production in Horses**

1. A 500 kg horse worked 8 h per day to pull a 67 kg plough at the speed of 4 km/h (32 km/day).
2. Total requirement for metabolizable energy (ME) = 135,208 kJ/day.
3. Maintenance requirement for ME = 47,301 kJ/day.
4. ME requirement for walking = 19,968 kJ/day (624 kJ/km × 32 km/day = 19,968 kJ/day)[a].
5. ME requirement for muscular power production = 67,939 kJ/day (135,208 − 47,301 − 19,968 kJ/day = 67,939 kJ/day).
6. Energy value of the useful work done (ploughing) = 21,026 kJ/day [67 kg × 32 km/day = 2,144 (kg·km)/day = 21,026 kJ/day][b]
7. Efficiency of ME for the useful work done (ploughing) = 31% (21,026 kJ/day ÷ 67,939 kJ/day × 100% = 31%)
8. Efficiency of ME beyond maintenance for the useful work done (ploughing) = 24% [21,026 kJ/day/(19,968 + 67,939 kJ/day)×100% = 24%]

*Source:* Adapted from Bondi. A.A. 1987. *Animal Nutrition*. John Wiley & Sons, New York, NY.

[a] ME requirement for walking by a 500 kg horse is 624 kJ/km. Thus, 32 km/day × 624 kJ/km = 19,968 kJ/day.

[b] Calculated on the basis of 1 kg·km = 9.807 kJ. Thus, 2,144 (kg·km)/day × 9.807 kJ/(kg·km) = 21,026 kJ/day.

2. *Energetic efficiency of muscular work.* The upper limit of the efficiency of the conversion of dietary energy into work is set by the maximum efficiency of the conversion of fats, glucose, and AAs into ATP (e.g., 55% for fatty acids and glucose; 37% for glutamine; 46% for BCAAs) (Wu 2013). In fish and shrimp that lack the urea cycle and directly excrete ammonia into the surrounding water, fat, glucose, and proteins have similar energetic efficiencies (Chapter 8). The working animal must also walk, and fish must swim regularly, and these activities require energy expenditure. Unlike an engine, the working animal or swimming fish must spend energy on maintenance regardless of working, walking, other physical activities, or resting. Thus, dietary nutrients are required by exercising animals for both maintenance and muscular power production.

   In mammals and birds, the efficiency of the conversion of dietary fat or glucose into work is greater than that for protein or AAs, as noted previously. For a 500 kg horse that works 8 h per day to pull a 67 kg plough at the speed of 4000 m/h, the efficiency in the use of ME for ploughing (the useful work done, muscular power production) is 31%, and the efficiency in the use of ME beyond maintenance for the useful work done is 24% (Table 11.18). The latter value is similar to the efficiency of converting dietary protein into milk protein in lactating cows (Table 11.9).
3. *Benefits of moderate muscular activity in enhancing animal growth and feed efficiency.* Moderate muscular work (e.g., walking or swimming) increases the rates of whole-body oxidation of fatty acids and glucose to minimize fat accretion in the body, while enhancing tissue insulin sensitivity and activating the MTOR signaling pathway to promote protein synthesis and deposition in skeletal muscle (Jobgen et al. 2006). As noted previously, a fat reduction in tissues is not associated with a loss of water, but protein accretion is accompanied by water retention in a ratio of 1–3 (g/g) in the body. Thus, in response to moderate exercise, animals with adequate intakes of energy and nutrients (including AAs) exhibit a greater growth rate and a higher feed efficiency, compared with animals with minimal physical activity. For example, Murray et al. (1974) reported that female pigs (12–60 kg) with a 6 × 10 min treadmill-exercise regimen three afternoons a week (Monday, Wednesday, and Friday) for 9 weeks exhibited a 15% increase for both weight gain and feed efficiency (weight gain/feed intake) during weeks 7 to 9 of the experiment, compared to the control group. Furthermore, regular swimming enhances growth rates and feed efficiencies in several fish species, including rainbow trout, Masu salmons, striped bass, and zebra fish

(Davison and Herbert 2013). These findings indicate an important role for moderate muscular activity in improving the efficiency of feed utilization for lean tissue growth in animals.

## Nutritional Requirements for Production of Wool and Feathers

### Wool Production in Sheep and Goats

The term wool is usually restricted to describing the fibrous protein derived from the specialized skin cells (follicles) in animals. Sheep (e.g., Merino sheep) and goats (e.g., Cashmere and Angora goats) produce wool for making high-quality clothes. The wool consists of wool fiber (almost entirely protein and wool α-keratins produced by the epidermal cells), wool wax (mainly esters of cholesterol and other alcohols produced by the sebaceous glands), and water (Reis and Gillespie 1985). Keratin contains a high content of cysteine, which is synthesized from methionine in the liver (Chapter 7). Of note, the content of the sulfur-containing AAs in keratin is about 15% (14% cysteine plus 0.4% methionine), which is 12- and 10-times that in soybean meal and microbial proteins, respectively (Bradbury 1973). Thus, wool production requires a large amount of both cysteine and methionine. To produce a fleece containing 3 kg protein in 1 year, the sheep would need to deposit 8.2 g protein/day in the wool.

In sheep and goats, wool growth depends on the quality and quantity of dietary protein digested, as well as the profile of AAs absorbed in the small intestine. The efficiency of truly digestible protein for wool/hair growth (including water retention) is about 60%, and the protein deposited in wool accounts for ~20% of the total protein synthesis in the skin (Liu et al. 1998). A 50 kg Merino ewe must absorb ~135 g protein/day to achieve her maximum rate of wool growth (Qi and Lupton 1994). If such a ewe is provided with a diet containing the metabolizable energy of 12 MJ/day (i.e., twice its maintenance requirement), 101 g of microbial protein would be synthesized per day to yield only 69 g of AAs absorbed by the small intestine (i.e., $101 \times 0.8 \times 0.85 = 69$ g). To achieve maximum growth of wool, the diet of the sheep must be supplemented with a good source of undegraded protein and an additive rich in the sulfur-containing AAs. Thus, wool growth in sheep responds well to dietary intakes of protein, energy, minerals and vitamins, and the response is affected by the genotype and reproductive status of the animal (Reis and Sahlu 1994). Similar findings have been reported for Cashmere and Angora goats (Galbraith 2000).

## Nutritional Requirements for Production of Eggs in Poultry

Egg production is of great economic importance in the poultry industry. Egg production provides a unique opportunity to augment the supply of some nutrients (e.g., ω-3 PUFAs, taurine, and arginine) for human consumption. The egg with completed shell contains all nutrients necessary to produce a viable embryo, and is the sole reproductive product of birds.

### Composition of the Egg

The egg consists of three basic parts: yolk, egg white, and shell (membranes) (Table 11.19). The white portion is the major part of the egg. Calcium carbonate, protein, and lipids are the main DM components of the egg's shell, white, and yolk, respectively (Gilbert 1971a). The egg white contains about 40 different proteins, such as ovalbumin (54%); ovotransferrin (12%–13%, an antimicrobial agent); ovomucoid (11%, an inhibitor of trypsin); globulins (8%); lysozymes (3.4%–3.5%, which split β-(1,4)-D-glucosaminides and lyse bacteria); ovomucin (1.5%–2.9%, antiviral hemagglutination); flavoprotein (0.8%, which binds riboflavin); ovomacroglobulin (0.5%); ovoglycoprotein (0.5%–1%); ovoinhibitor (0.1%–1.5%, an inhibitor of trypsin, chymotrypsin, and other proteases); avidin (0.05%, which binds biotin); and papain inhibitor (0.1%, an inhibitor of papain and other proteases) (Gilbert 1971b). Egg white contains only a trace amount of lipids (0.02%), which includes triglycerides, diglycerides, free fatty acids, cholesterol ester, cholesterol, phosphatidylcholine, lysophosphatidylcholine, phosphatidylethanolamine, and sphingomyelin (Sato et al. 1973).

**TABLE 11.19**
**Chemical Composition of Eggs from Hens[a]**

| Substance | Shell (%) | White (%) | Yolk (%) | Egg without Shell (%) | Egg with Shell (%) |
|---|---|---|---|---|---|
| Water | 1.5 | 88.5 | 49.0 | 73.6 | 67.1 |
| Protein | 4.2 | 10.5 | 16.7 | 12.8 | 11.8 |
| Lipid | Trace | Trace | 31.6 | 11.8 | 9.8 |
| Other OM | Trace | 0.50 | 1.1 | 1.0 | 0.64 |
| Minerals[b] | 94.3 | 0.50 | 1.6 | 0.80 | 10.6 |

*Source:* Gilbert, A.B. 1971a. In: *Physiology and Biochemistry of the Domestic Fowl*, edited by D.J. Bell and B.M. Freeman. Academic Press, London, pp.1153–1162.

[a] A 58 g egg consists of shell, 6.1 g (10.5%); yolk, 18 g (31.0%); and white 33.9 g (58.5%).

[b] Mainly as calcium carbonate.

OM, organic matters (including carbohydrate).

In egg yolk, the ratio of protein to lipids is 1:2, with the lipids being present as lipoproteins (e.g., LDLs, which contain 90% lipids, as well as high-density lipoproteins) (McIndoe 1971). Egg yolk proteins consist of lipovitellin a (58%); lipovitellin b (11%); livetin a (4%); livetin b (5%); livetin g (2%); phosvitin (7%; a principal phosphoprotein that can bind iron and calcium); and apo low-density lipoprotein (12%) (McIndoe 1971). Egg yolk lipids include neutral lipids (65%), phospholipids (30%), cholesterol (5%), and carotenoids (8–20 mg/g yolk) (Anton 2013; Blesso 2015). The phospholipids comprise phosphatidylcholine (83%), phosphatidylethanolamine (14%), sphingomyelin (0.8%), and phosphatidylinositol (0.15%) (Anton 2013; Blesso 2015).

## Formation of the Egg

Eggs are produced in the female reproductive tract through the interorgan metabolism of nutrients (Figure 11.12). The formation of one egg by a laying hen requires ~24 h (Cunningham et al. 1984). Specifically, proteins and lipids in yolk are synthesized in the liver of a laying hen under the influence of estrogen, and then transported to her ovary. The rates of hepatic protein synthesis and lipogenesis in mature laying hens may be 5- to 10-times those in the liver of immature females, and the concentrations of free fatty acids in plasma increase approximately 10-fold immediately prior to the laying of an egg. The composition of fatty acids in the liver and plasma is substantially altered in laying hens with respect to the composition of fatty acids in the yolk, with the proportions of palmitic and oleic acids being increased, while those of stearic and linoleic acids are decreased (Anton 2013; Gilbert 1971a).

The yolk proteins and lipids from the liver are deposited in the ovary, along with water, AAs, carbohydrates, vitamins, and minerals that are all ultimately derived from maternal blood (Anton 2013). As in mammals, under the influence of high concentrations of LH, a mature follicle of the ovary ovulates to release a yolk into the oviduct. Ovulation of the mature follicle requires not only LH, but also progesterone (Cunningham et al. 1984). In chickens, 4–6 h prior to the LH surge, the circulating concentrations of progesterone (released from the largest and most mature ovarian follicle) are the greatest during a laying cycle. This peak in plasma concentrations of progesterone is necessary for the subsequent surge of LH to induce ovulation.

The next stage of egg formation involves the synthesis of egg white proteins from blood-derived AAs in the oviduct tissues, which is stimulated and maintained by steroid hormones (e.g., estrogen and progesterone) (Palmiter 1972). The egg white (also called albumen) is then formed from the oviduct-derived proteins, a trace amount of liver-derived lipids, as well as water, minerals, and vitamins, that are all ultimately derived from maternal blood. The egg white is added to the surface of the yolk to form a complex. The coated yolk then enters the shell gland (or uterus).

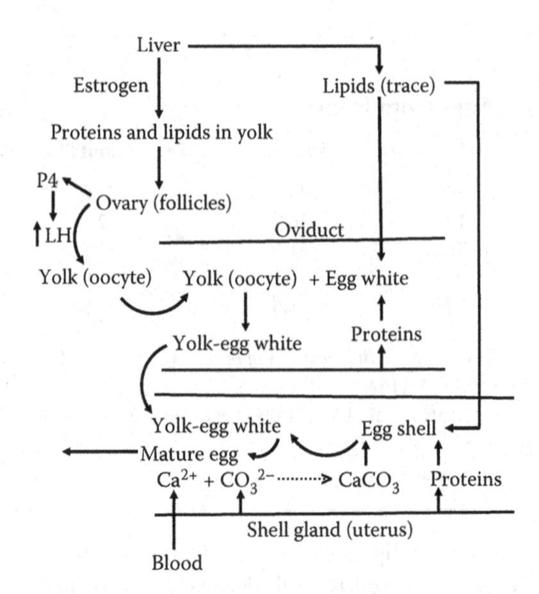


**FIGURE 11.12** Formation of eggs by laying poultry. Under the influence of estrogen, the liver of a laying hen synthesizes and releases proteins and lipids (components of the yolk), which are transported to the follicles of the ovary for deposition and formation of yolk. Through the action of luteinizing hormone (LH), which peaks in response to a progesterone surge, the mature follicle releases the yolk into the oviduct, in which both estrogen and progesterone stimulate and maintain the synthesis of egg white proteins. In the oviduct, the egg white is formed from the egg white proteins, a trace amount of liver-derived lipids, as well as water, vitamins, and minerals. After the yolk is coated with the egg white, this complex enters the shell gland (or uterus), where the eggshell is generated from the deposition of calcium carbonate (main component) and other minerals. In domestic chickens, the formation of one egg requires about 24 h.

In the shell gland, the eggshell is formed from the deposition of calcium carbonate (the main component) and other minerals, and this process requires about 17–20 h in hens (Burley and Vadehra 1989). Vitamin D and parathyroid hormone stimulate the intestinal absorption of calcium and its transport by the shell gland for eggshell formation. The protein in the eggshell is synthesized and secreted by the shell gland. Since the shell gland in the uterus does not store significant amounts of calcium, the shell gland derives calcium (2–2.5 g calcium per egg) and other minerals from the blood. The deposition of calcium carbonate ($CaCO_3$; containing 40% calcium) in the developing eggshell is maintained through continuous secretion of bicarbonate from the shell gland to produce a mature egg (Burley and Vadehra 1989). Note that carbon dioxide exists in the blood as dissolved gas ($CO_2$), carbonic acid ($H_2CO_3$), and bicarbonate ($HCO_3^-$). Eggshell color results from pigment deposition and therefore is affected by the diets of hens.

$$CO_2 + H_2O \rightarrow H_2CO_3 \text{ (carbonic anhydrase)}$$

$$H_2CO_3 \rightarrow H^+ + HCO_{3-}$$

$$HCO_{3-} \rightarrow H^+ + CO_3^{2-}$$

$$Ca^{2+} + CO_3^{2-} \rightarrow CaCO_3$$

### High Requirements for Dietary Energy, Protein, and Calcium for Egg Production

Requirements of energy, protein, and calcium by laying hens are particularly high (Burley and Vadehra 1989). Syntheses of egg yolk protein and lipids by the liver and of egg white proteins by the oviduct require a large amount of ATP. In addition, vitamins (particularly vitamin D) and other minerals must be supplied in adequate amounts to ensure high production of eggs and high rates of hatchability and survival. The following calculations are examples of minimum requirements for dietary energy, protein, and calcium by a 2 kg laying hen.

1. *Dietary energy requirement.* A 58 g egg contains 91.8 cal of gross energy (Pond et al. 1995). On the basis of the production of a 58 g egg per day and the digestibility of dietary energy (90%), at least 102 cal of energy in the diet are used for egg production by a 2.0 kg hen. The dietary energy requirement for maintenance is 79.4 (=71.5/0.90) cal/kg BW per day (159 cal/day for a 2 kg hen) in a laying hen that does not gain BW (Table 11.3). Thus, the requirement of dietary energy is at least 261 cal/day (102 + 159; production + maintenance) for the 2 kg laying hen. If the laying hen produces 250 eggs per year, at least 65.25 Kcal of dietary energy (equivalent to 6.94 kg fat) are used for this purpose.
2. *Dietary protein requirement.* On the basis of the production of a 58 g egg per day and the digestibility of dietary protein (85%), at least 8.1 g of protein in the diet are used for egg production by a 2.0 kg hen (Pond et al. 1995). The dietary protein requirement for maintenance is 1.95 (=1.66/0.85) g/kg BW per day (3.9 g/day for a 2 kg hen) in a laying hen that does not gain BW (Pond et al. 1995). Thus, the requirement of dietary protein is at least 12 g/day (8.1 + 3.9; production + maintenance) for the 2 kg laying hen. If the laying hen produces 250 eggs per year, at least 3.0 kg of dietary protein are used for this purpose.
3. *Dietary calcium requirement.* The eggshell consists of about 95% calcium carbonate and 5% organic material (Burley and Vadehra 1989). On the basis of the production of a 58 g egg per day and the digestibility of dietary calcium (50%), at least 4.64 g of calcium in the diet are used for egg production by a 2.0 kg hen. The dietary calcium requirement for maintenance is estimated to be 0.02 g/kg BW per day (0.04 g/day for a 2 kg hen) in a laying hen that does not gain BW (Pond et al. 1995). Thus, the requirement of dietary calcium is at least 4.68 g/day (4.64 + 0.04; production + maintenance) for the 2 kg laying hen. If a laying hen produces 250 eggs per year, at least 1.17 kg of calcium in the diet are used for this purpose.

### Feather Growth and Color of Birds

In birds, feathers are formed in the follicles of the epidermis which produce β-keratin proteins and wax, and have distinctive colors (Haake et al. 1984). These complex integumentary structures cover ~75% of the bird's skin and aid in flight, thermal insulation, and waterproofing. The wax consists of short-, medium-, and long-chain fatty acids (Chapter 3). The colors of feathers are produced by pigments, which are tyrosine metabolites (melanins [brown and beige pheomelanins, as well as black and grey eumelanins]), plant substances known as carotenoids (red, yellow, or orange), or copper-containing porphyrins (Bennett and Thery 2007). Tetrahydrobiopterin, oxygen, copper, iron, and zinc are cofactors for the synthesis of melanins from tyrosine (Wu 2013). In animals, vitamin C stabilizes tetrahydrobiopterin and promotes the intestinal absorption of iron, and therefore is required for feather growth. The pigments refract, reflect, or scatter selected wavelengths of light to produce various colors.

Feathers comprise 85%–90% protein, 1.5% lipids, 8%–10% water, and 1%–2.5% minerals (Murphy et al. 1990). The most abundant AAs in the β-keratin proteins of feathers are glycine, proline, serine, cystine, and BCAAs, as reported for the rachis (central shafts) and barbs (serial paired branches) of penguin feathers (Table 11.20). Similar results were reported for feathers of fowl (Akahane et al. 1977). It is noteworthy that the three most abundant AAs are those AAs which can be synthesized *de novo*, but it is unknown whether their *de novo* synthesis is sufficient for feather development in birds. Since cysteine, tyrosine, and BCAAs are not synthesized de novo in animals, avian diets must contain not only high levels of small neutral AAs, but also aromatic,

**TABLE 11.20**
**Composition of AAs in Feathers of Birds**

| AA | Rachis of Three Species of Penguins | | | Barbs of Three Species of Penguins | | | Whole Feather of Fowl |
|---|---|---|---|---|---|---|---|
| | *P. adeliae* | *P. antarctica* | *P. papua* | *P. adeliae* | *P. antarctica* | *P. papua* | |
| | μmol/g Dry Mass | | | μmol/g Dry Mass | | | % of AA Residues |
| Ala | 722 | 634 | 641 | 499 | 503 | 506 | 5.6 |
| Arg | 328 | 321 | 326 | 337 | 335 | 339 | 4.7 |
| Asp[a] | 464 | 496 | 525 | 628 | 630 | 615 | 6.3 |
| Cys[b] | 717 | 707 | 776 | 782 | 878 | 786 | 4.2 |
| Glu[c] | 498 | 557 | 570 | 685 | 709 | 684 | 8.6 |
| Gly | 1477 | 1386 | 1405 | 1155 | 1096 | 1109 | 11.5 |
| His | 81 | 73 | 72 | 78 | 33 | 30 | 0.3 |
| Ile | 374 | 389 | 405 | 424 | 436 | 431 | 4.3 |
| Leu | 986 | 923 | 924 | 727 | 729 | 741 | 7.4 |
| Lys | 44 | 45 | 40 | 78 | 80 | 75 | 1.2 |
| Met | 73 | 68 | 73 | 103 | 112 | 101 | 0.3 |
| Phe | 216 | 203 | 235 | 203 | 178 | 199 | 3.6 |
| Pro | 1035 | 986 | 1002 | 1044 | 1074 | 1046 | 11.7 |
| Ser | 933 | 785 | 792 | 703 | 716 | 727 | 15.7 |
| Thr | 392 | 409 | 436 | 437 | 452 | 452 | 5.3 |
| Tyr | 222 | 254 | 230 | 243 | 257 | 215 | 1.6 |
| Val | 724 | 737 | 737 | 839 | 860 | 845 | 7.7 |

*Sources:* Adapted, for the three species of penguins, from Murphy, M.E. et al. 1990. *The Condor* 92:913–921; and, for the whole feather of fowl, from Akahane, K. et al. 1977. *J. Biochem.* 81:11–18.

[a] Aspartate plus asparagine.
[b] Cystine.
[c] Glutamate plus glutamine.

sulfur-containing, and large neutral AAs to ensure the optimal growth of feathers. There is evidence that dietary intake of protein affects the development of feather colors in birds (Meadows et al. 2012).

## SUMMARY

The daily requirements of gestating, lactating, growing, egg-producing, or working animals for energy or nutrients consist of maintenance and production requirements. The energy requirement for maintenance is the amount of energy needed to keep the animal in energy equilibrium. Likewise, the nutrient requirement for maintenance refers to the amount of a specific nutrient needed to keep a zero balance of the nutrient in the animal. Animals grow or produce only after their maintenance requirements are met. The requirements of animals for dietary energy and nutrients vary with their genetic backgrounds and physiological states (e.g., gestation, lactation, and growth), as well as the environments in which they are living. The maintenance and production requirements (total requirements) are usually determined through experiments (e.g., calorimetry, feeding trials, or isotope approaches), as illustrated for swine at different stages of production (Table 11.21). However, the recommended values should be used only as references because dynamic changes in nutrient metabolism occur in animals under various conditions that are different from the settings of scientific experiments. In all cases, the physiology and metabolism of animals (e.g., milk production

**TABLE 11.21**
**Total Requirements (Maintenance Plus Production) of Swine for Nutrients at Different Stages of Production**

| Item | Growing Pigs at Different BW Range (kg) | | | | | | | G Sows (P1)[a] | | G Sows (P4+)[b] | | La Sows[c] | |
|---|---|---|---|---|---|---|---|---|---|---|---|---|---|
| | 5–7 | 7–11 | 11–25 | 25–50 | 50–75 | 75–100 | 100–135 | <d90 | >d90 | <d90 | >d90 | P1 | P2+ |
| **Dietary Energy Content, kcal/kg Diet (As-Fed Basis, 90% DM)** | | | | | | | | | | | | | |
| NE | 2448 | 2448 | 2412 | 2475 | 2475 | 2475 | 2475 | 2518 | 2518 | 2518 | 2518 | 2518 | 2518 |
| DE | 3542 | 3542 | 3490 | 3402 | 3402 | 3402 | 3402 | 3388 | 3388 | 3388 | 3388 | 3388 | 3388 |
| ME | 3400 | 3400 | 3350 | 3300 | 3300 | 3300 | 3300 | 3300 | 3300 | 3300 | 3300 | 3300 | 3300 |
| **Feed Intake (FI, As-Fed Basis), BW Gain, and Body Protein (BP) Deposition, g/Day** | | | | | | | | | | | | | |
| FI + wastage | 280 | 493 | 953 | 1582 | 2229 | 2636 | 2933 | 2130 | 2530 | 2200 | 2600 | 5.95 | 6.61 |
| BW gain | 210 | 335 | 585 | 758 | 900 | 917 | 867 | 578 | 543 | 410 | 340 | 71 | 176 |
| BP deposition | – | – | – | 128 | 147 | 141 | 122 | – | – | – | – | – | – |
| **Dietary Content of Total AA and Total Crude Protein (CP), % (As-Fed Basis)** | | | | | | | | | | | | | |
| Arginine | 0.75 | 0.68 | 0.62 | 0.50 | 0.44 | 0.38 | 0.32 | 0.31 | 0.40 | 0.20 | 0.27 | 0.48 | 0.47 |
| Histidine | 0.58 | 0.53 | 0.48 | 0.39 | 0.34 | 0.30 | 0.25 | 0.21 | 0.25 | 0.13 | 0.17 | 0.35 | 0.34 |
| Isoleucine | 0.88 | 0.79 | 0.73 | 0.59 | 0.52 | 0.45 | 0.39 | 0.34 | 0.41 | 0.22 | 0.28 | 0.49 | 0.47 |
| Leucine | 1.75 | 1.54 | 1.41 | 1.13 | 0.98 | 0.85 | 0.71 | 0.52 | 0.71 | 0.34 | 0.50 | 0.96 | 0.92 |
| Lysine | 1.70 | 1.53 | 1.40 | 1.12 | 0.97 | 0.84 | 0.71 | 0.58 | 0.76 | 0.37 | 0.52 | 0.86 | 0.83 |
| Methionine | 0.49 | 0.44 | 0.40 | 0.32 | 0.28 | 0.25 | 0.21 | 0.17 | 0.22 | 0.11 | 0.14 | 0.23 | 0.23 |
| Met + Cys | 0.96 | 0.87 | 0.79 | 0.65 | 0.57 | 0.50 | 0.43 | 0.39 | 0.51 | 0.27 | 0.38 | 0.47 | 0.46 |
| Phenylalanine | 1.01 | 0.91 | 0.83 | 0.68 | 0.59 | 0.51 | 0.43 | 0.32 | 0.42 | 0.21 | 0.30 | 0.47 | 0.46 |
| Phe + Tyr | 1.60 | 1.44 | 1.32 | 1.08 | 0.94 | 0.82 | 0.70 | 0.58 | 0.75 | 0.39 | 0.53 | 0.98 | 0.94 |
| Threonine | 1.05 | 0.95 | 0.87 | 0.72 | 0.64 | 0.56 | 0.49 | 0.44 | 0.55 | 0.32 | 0.42 | 0.58 | 0.56 |
| Tryptophan | 0.28 | 0.25 | 0.23 | 0.19 | 0.17 | 0.15 | 0.13 | 0.10 | 0.14 | 0.07 | 0.11 | 0.16 | 0.15 |
| Valine | 1.10 | 1.00 | 0.91 | 0.75 | 0.65 | 0.57 | 0.49 | 0.42 | 0.55 | 0.29 | 0.40 | 0.75 | 0.72 |
| CP (N × 6.25) | 22.7 | 20.6 | 18.9 | 15.7 | 13.8 | 12.1 | 10.4 | 9.6 | 12.8 | 6.8 | 9.6 | 20.5 | 17.9 |
| **Dietary Content of Total Minerals, % or Amount/kg Diet (As-Fed Basis)** | | | | | | | | | | | | | |
| Calcium, % | 0.85 | 0.80 | 0.70 | 0.66 | 0.59 | 0.52 | 0.46 | 0.58 | 0.79 | 0.41 | 0.64 | 0.59 | 0.57 |
| Phosphorus, % | 0.70 | 0.65 | 0.60 | 0.56 | 0.52 | 0.47 | 0.43 | 0.47 | 0.58 | 0.36 | 0.49 | 0.53 | 0.52 |
| Sodium, % | 0.40 | 0.35 | 0.28 | 0.10 | 0.10 | 0.10 | 0.10 | 0.15 | – | – | – | 0.20 | – |

*(Continued)*

**TABLE 11.21 (*Continued*)**

**Total Requirements (Maintenance Plus Production) of Swine for Nutrients at Different Stages of Production**

| Item | Growing Pigs at Different BW Range (kg) | | | | | | | G Sows (P1)[a] | | G Sows (P4+)[b] | | La Sows[c] | |
|---|---|---|---|---|---|---|---|---|---|---|---|---|---|
| | 5–7 | 7–11 | 11–25 | 25–50 | 50–75 | 75–100 | 100–135 | <d90 | >d90 | <d90 | >d90 | P1 | P2+ |
| Chloride, % | 0.50 | 0.45 | 0.32 | 0.08 | 0.08 | 0.08 | 0.08 | 0.12 | – | – | – | 0.16 | – |
| Magnesium, % | 0.04 | 0.04 | 0.04 | 0.04 | 0.04 | 0.04 | 0.04 | 0.06 | – | – | – | 0.06 | – |
| Potassium, % | 0.30 | 0.28 | 0.26 | 0.23 | 0.19 | 0.17 | 0.17 | 0.20 | – | – | – | 0.20 | – |
| Copper, mg/kg | 6.00 | 6.00 | 5.00 | 4.00 | 3.50 | 3.00 | 3.00 | 10 | – | – | – | 20 | – |
| Iodine, mg/kg | 0.14 | 0.14 | 0.14 | 0.14 | 0.14 | 0.14 | 0.14 | 0.14 | – | – | – | 0.14 | – |
| Iron, mg/kg | 100 | 100 | 100 | 60 | 50 | 40 | 40 | 80 | – | – | – | 80 | – |
| Mn, mg/kg | 4.00 | 4.00 | 3.00 | 2.00 | 2.00 | 2.00 | 2.00 | 25 | – | – | – | 25 | – |
| Se, mg/kg | 0.30 | 0.30 | 0.25 | 0.20 | 0.15 | 0.15 | 0.15 | 0.15 | – | – | – | 0.15 | – |
| Zinc, mg/kg | 100 | 100 | 80 | 60 | 50 | 50 | 50 | 100 | – | – | – | 100 | – |
| **Dietary Content of Vitamins, IU or Amount/kg Diet (As-Fed Basis)** | | | | | | | | | | | | | |
| Vitamin A, IU | 2200 | 2200 | 1750 | 1300 | 1300 | 1300 | 1300 | 4000 | – | – | – | 2000 | – |
| Vitamin D, IU | 220 | 220 | 200 | 150 | 150 | 150 | 150 | 800 | – | – | – | 800 | – |
| Vitamin E, IU | 16 | 16 | 11 | 11 | 11 | 11 | 11 | 44 | – | – | – | 44 | – |
| Menadione, mg | 0.50 | 0.50 | 0.50 | 0.50 | 0.50 | 0.50 | 0.50 | 0.50 | – | – | – | 0.50 | – |
| Biotin, mg | 0.08 | 0.05 | 0.05 | 0.05 | 0.05 | 0.05 | 0.05 | 0.20 | – | – | – | 0.20 | – |
| Choline, mg | 600 | 500 | 400 | 300 | 300 | 300 | 300 | 1250 | – | – | – | 1000 | – |
| Folacin, mg | 0.30 | 0.30 | 0.30 | 0.30 | 0.30 | 0.30 | 0.30 | 1.3 | – | – | – | 1.3 | – |
| Niacin, mg | 30 | 30 | 30 | 30 | 30 | 30 | 30 | 10 | – | – | – | 10 | – |
| PA, mg | 12 | 10 | 9.0 | 8.0 | 7.0 | 7.0 | 7.0 | 12 | – | – | – | 12 | – |
| Riboflavin, mg | 4.0 | 3.5 | 3.0 | 2.5 | 2.0 | 2.0 | 2.0 | 3.75 | – | – | – | 3.75 | – |
| Thiamin, mg | 1.5 | 1.0 | 1.0 | 1.0 | 1.0 | 1.0 | 1.0 | 1.0 | – | – | – | 1.00 | – |
| Vitamin $B_6$, mg | 7.0 | 7.0 | 3.0 | 1.0 | 1.0 | 1.0 | 1.0 | 1.0 | – | – | – | 1.00 | – |
| Vitamin $B_{12}$, µg | 20 | 17.5 | 15 | 10 | 5.0 | 5.0 | 5.0 | 15 | – | – | – | 15 | – |

*Source:* National Research Council (NRC). 2012. *Nutrient Requirements of Swine*. National Academies Press, Washington, DC.

[a] Anticipated litter size of 12.5 and anticipated mean birth weight of 1.40 kg. For minerals other than calcium and phosphorus, as well as vitamins, values for >d90 gestating sows may be 100–125% of those for <d90 gestating sows. Dietary NE content is 2518 kcal/kg diet (ME = 3300 kcal/kg diet), and feed intake + wastage is 2.21 kg/day.

[b] Anticipated litter size of 13.5 and anticipated mean birth weight of 1.40 kg.

[c] Mean daily weight gain of nursing pigs = 190 g/day during a 21 day lactation period. For minerals other than calcium and phosphorus, as well as vitamins, values for P2+ lactating sows may be 100–125% of those for P1 lactating sows. Dietary NE content is 2518 kcal/kg diet (ME = 3300 kcal/kg diet), and feed intake + wastage is 6.28 kg/day.

G, gestating; La, lactating; P, parity; PA, pantothenic acid.

in mammals, work of cattle and horses, and feather formation and color in birds) must be borne in mind when assessing their energy and nutrient requirements during their life cycle.

Since a new life starts from a fertilized egg, optimizing maternal nutrition not only improves pregnancy outcomes, but may also be beneficial for the health, growth, and development of several generations of offspring. Also, maximal milk production by dams will ensure the successful nurturing and survival of their newborns, so that they will efficiently gain tissue protein during the growing-finishing period. Likewise, sustaining egg production by hens and promoting muscle growth are critical for the competitiveness of the poultry industry. Achieving these goals critically depends on adequate nutritional support to the animals, and can be facilitated by metabolic regulators (e.g., functional AAs, β-agonists, and anabolic hormones). In the life cycle, compensatory growth of animals commonly occurs, which refers to their accelerated growth following a fetal or postnatal period of slowed growth and development, particularly as a result of nutrient deprivation. Fetal (embryonic) or neonatal programming plays a key role in regulating postnatal growth and survival of mammals, birds, and possibly fish, as well as their feed efficiencies for lean tissue growth. Finally, the usefulness of any recommendations for dietary energy and nutrient requirements must be evaluated on a large scale under practical production conditions. Collectively, the science-based formulation of nutrient-balanced and adequate diets will not only improve the growth and productivity of animals, but will also mitigate the impact of livestock, poultry, and fish industries on the quality of the environment worldwide.

## REFERENCES


Abbasi, A.A., A.S. Prasad, P. Rabbani, and E. Du Mouchelle. 1980. Experimental zinc deficiency in man. Effect on testicular function. *J. Lab. Clin. Med.* 96:544–550.

Agre, P. and D. Kozono. 2003. Aquaporin water channels: molecular mechanisms for human diseases. *FEBS Lett.* 555:72–78.

Akahane, K., S. Murozono, K. Murayama. 1977. Soluble proteins from fowl feather keratin I. Fractionation and properties. *J. Biochem.* 81:11–18.

Akers, R.M. 2002. *Lactation and the Mammary Gland.* Iowa State University Press, Ames, Iowa.

Allen, D.G., G.D. Lamb, and H. Westerblad. 2008. Skeletal muscle fatigue: Cellular mechanisms. *Physiol. Rev.* 88:287–332.

Anton, M. 2013. Egg yolk: Structures, functionalities and processes. *J. Sci. Food Agric.* 93:2871–2880.

ARC (Agricultural Research Council). 1981. *The Nutrient Requirements of Pigs.* Commonwealth Agricultural Bereaux, Slough, England.

Ashworth, C.J. 1991. Effect of pre-mating nutritional status and post-mating progesterone supplementation on embryo survival and conceptus growth in gilts. *Anim. Reprod. Sci.* 26:311–321.

Baldwin, R.L. 1995. *Modeling Ruminant Digestion and Metabolism.* Chapman & Hall, New York, NY.

Baldwin, R.L. and A.C. Bywater. 1984. Nutritional energetics of animals. *Annu. Rev. Nutr.* 4:101–114.

Baxter, C.F., A.L. Black, and M. Kleiber. 1956. The blood precursors of lactose as studied with $^{14}$C-labeled metabolites in intact dairy cows. *Biochim. Biophys. Acta* 21:277–285.

Bazer, F.W., R.C. Burghardt, G.A. Johnson, T.E. Spencer, and G. Wu. 2008. Interferons and progesterone for establishment and maintenance of pregnancy: Interactions among novel cell signaling pathways. *Reprod. Biol.* 8:179–211.

Bazer, F.W. 2015. History of maternal recognition of pregnancy. *Adv. Anat. Embryol. Cell Biol.* 216:5–25.

Bazer, F.W., G.W. Song, J.Y. Kim, K.A. Dunlap, M.C. Satterfield, G.A. Johnson, R.C. Burghardt, and G. Wu. 2012a. Uterine biology in sheep and pigs. *J. Anim. Sci. Biotechnol.* 3:23.

Bazer, F.W., G.H. Song, J.Y. Kim, D.W. Erikson, G.A. Johnson, R.C. Burghardt, H. Gao, M.C. Satterfield, T.E. Spencer, and G. Wu. 2012b. Mechanistic mammalian target of rapamycin (MTOR) cell signaling: Effects of select nutrients and secreted phosphoprotein 1 on development of mammalian conceptuses. *Mol. Cell. Endocrinol.* 354:22–33.

Bazer, F.W., G. Wu, G.A. Johnson, and X.Q. Wang. 2014. Environmental factors affecting pregnancy: Endocrine disrupters, nutrients and metabolic pathways. *Mol. Cell. Endocrinol.* 398:53–68.

Bazer, F.W., G. Wu, T.E. Spencer, G.A. Johnson, R.C. Burghardt, and K. Bayless. 2010. Novel pathways for implantation and establishment and maintenance of pregnancy in mammals. *Mol. Hum. Reprod.* 16:135–152.

Bell, A.W. 1995. Regulation of organic nutrient metabolism during transition from late pregnancy to early lactation. *J. Anim. Sci.* 73:2804–2819.

Bennett, A.T.D. and M. Thery. 2007. Avian color vision and coloration: Multidisciplinary evolutionary biology. *Am. Nat.* 169:S1–S6.

Blaxter, K.L. 1989. *Energy Metabolism in Animals and Man.* Cambridge University Press, New York, NY.

Blesso, C.N. 2015. Egg phospholipids and cardiovascular health. *Nutrients* 7:2731–2747.

Boersma, B. and J.M. Wit. 1997. Catch-up growth. *Endocr. Rev.* 18:646–661.

Bohrer, B.M., J.M. Kyle, D.D. Boler, P.J. Rincker, M.J. Ritter, and S.N. Carr. 2013. Meta-analysis of the effects of ractopamine hydrochloride on carcass cutability and primal yields of finishing pigs. *J. Anim. Sci.* 91:1015–1023.

Bondi, A.A. 1987. *Animal Nutrition.* John Wiley & Sons, New York, NY.

Bottje, W.G. and G.E. Carstens. 2009. Association of mitochondrial function and feed efficiency in poultry and livestock species. *J. Anim. Sci.* 87(14 Suppl.):E48–E63.

Boutry, C., S.W. El-Kadi, A. Suryawan, S.M. Wheatley, R.A. Orellana, S.R. Kimball, H.V. Nguyen, and T.A. Davis. 2013. Leucine pulses enhance skeletal muscle protein synthesis during continuous feeding in neonatal pigs. *Am. J. Physiol. Endocrinol. Metab.* 305:E620–631.

Bradbury, J.H. 1973. The structure and chemistry of keratin fibers. *Adv. Protein Chem.* 27:111–211.

Brake, D.W., E.C. Titgemeyer, and D.E. Anderson. 2014. Duodenal supply of glutamate and casein both improve intestinal starch digestion in cattle but by apparently different mechanisms. *J. Anim. Sci.* 92:4057–4067.

Braun, U. and E. Forster. 2012. B-mode and colour Doppler sonographic examination of the milk vein and musculophrenic vein in dry cows and cows with a milk yield of 10 and 20 kg. *Acta Vet. Scand.* 54:15.

Brody, S. 1945. *Bioenergetics and Growth.* Reinhold Publishing, New York, NY.

Brooks, A.A., M.R. Johnson, P.J. Steer, M.E. Pawson, and H.I. Abdalla. 1995. Birth weight: Nature or nurture? *Early Human Dev.* 42: 29–35.

Burley, R.W. and D.V. Vadehra. 1989. *The Avian Egg: Chemistry and Biology.* John Wiley & Sons, New York, NY.

Butler, W.R. 1998. Review: effect of protein nutrition on ovarian and uterine physiology in dairy cattle. *J. Dairy Sci.* 81:2533–2539.

Cameron, A. and T.A. McAllister. 2016. Antimicrobial usage and resistance in beef production. *J. Anim. Sci. Biotechnol.* 7:68.

Campbell, R.G. 1988. Nutritional constraints to lean tissue accretion in farm animals. *Nutr. Res. Rev.* 1:233–253.

Cardoso, R.C., B.R. Alves, L.D. Prezotto, J.F. Thorson, L.O. Tedeschi, D.H. Keisler, M. Amstalden, and G.L. Williams. 2014. Reciprocal changes in leptin and NPY during nutritional acceleration of puberty in heifers. *J. Endocrinol.* 223:289–298.

Chen, T.Y., P. Stott, R.Z. Athorn, E.G. Bouwman, and P. Langendijk. 2012. Undernutrition during early follicle development has irreversible effects on ovulation rate and embryos. *Reprod. Fertil. Dev.* 24:886–892.

Clagett-Dame, M. and D. Knutson. 2011. Vitamin A in reproduction and development. *Nutrients* 3:385–428.

Collier, R.J. and K.G. Gebremedhin. 2015. Thermal biology of domestic animals. *Annu. Rev. Anim. Biosci.* 3:513–532.

Combs, G.F. 1998. *The Vitamins.* Academic Press, New York, NY.

Cormio, L., M. De Siati, F. Lorusso, O. Selvaggio, L. Mirabella, F. Sanguedolce, and G. Carrieri. 2011. Oral L-citrulline supplementation improves erection hardness in men with mild erectile dysfunction. *Urology* 77:119–122.

Cunningham, F.J., S.C. Wilson, P.G. Knight, and R.T. Gladwell. 1984. Chicken ovulation cycle. *J. Exp. Zool.* 232:485–494.

Dance, A., J. Thundathil, R. Wilde, P. Blondin, and J. Kastelic. 2015. Enhanced early-life nutrition promotes hormone production and reproductive development in Holstein bulls. *J. Dairy Sci.* 98:987–998.

Davis, T.A., D.G. Burrin, M.L. Fiorotto, P.J. Reeds, and F. Jahoor. 1998. Roles of insulin and amino acids in the regulation of protein synthesis in the neonate. *J. Nutr.* 128: 347S–350S.

Davison, W. and N.A. Herbert. 2013. Swimming-enhanced growth. In: *Swimming Physiology of Fish.* Edited by A.P. Palstra and J.V. Planas, Berlin: Springer, pp. 177–202.

de Faria, V.P. and J.T. Huber. 1983. Effect of dietary protein and energy levels on rumen fermentation in Holstein steers. *J. Anim. Sci.* 58:452–259.

de Lange, K., J. van Milgen, J. Noblet, S. Dubois, and S. Birkett. 2006. Previous feeding level influences plateau heat production following a 24 h fast in growing pigs. *Br. J. Nutr.* 95:1082–1087.

Dhandapani, K.M. and D.W. Brann. 2000. The role of glutamate and nitric oxide in the reproductive neuroendocrine system. *Biochem. Cell Biol.* 78:165–179.

Dunshea, F.R., D.E. Bauman, E.A. Nugent, D.J. Kerton, R.H. King, and I. McCauley. 2005. Hyperinsulinaemia, supplemental protein and branched-chain amino acids when combined can increase milk protein yield in lactating sows. *Br. J. Nutr.* 93:325–332.

El-Kadi, S.W., A. Suryawan, M.C. Gazzaneo, N. Srivastava, R.A. Orellana, H.V. Nguyen, G.E. Lobley, and T.A. Davis. 2012. Anabolic signaling and protein deposition are enhanced by intermittent compared with continuous feeding in skeletal muscle of neonates. *Am. J. Physiol. Endocrinol. Metab.* 302:E674–686.

Escobar, J., J.W. Frank, A. Suryawan, H.V. Nguyen, S.R. Kimball, L.S. Jefferson, and T.A. Davis. 2006. Regulation of cardiac and skeletal muscle protein synthesis by individual branched-chain amino acids in neonatal pigs. *Am. J. Physiol. Endocrinol. Metab.* 290:E612–621.

Etherton, T.D. and D.E. Bauman. 1998. Biology of somatotropin in growth and lactation of domestic animals. *Physiol. Rev.* 78:745–761.

Evans, M.C. and G.M. Anderson. 2017. Neuroendocrine integration of nutritional signals on reproduction. *J. Mol. Endocrinol.* 58:R107–R128.

Ford, S.P., K.A. Vonnahme, and M.E. Wilson. 2002. Uterine capacity in the pig reflects a combination of uterine environment and conceptus genotype effects. *J. Anim. Sci.* 80:E66–E73.

Foxcroft, G.R., W.T. Dixon, S. Novak, C.T. Putman, S.C. Town, and M.D.A. Vinsky. 2006. The biological basis for prenatal programming of postnatal performance in pigs. *J. Anim. Sci.* 84(E. Suppl.):E105–112.

Galbraith, H. 2000. Protein and sulphur amino acid nutrition of hair fibre-producing Angora and Cashmere goats. *Livest. Prod. Sci.* 64:81–93.

Geisert, R.D., J.W. Brookbank, R.M. Roberts, Bazer, F.W. 1982. Establishment of pregnancy in the pig: II. Cellular remodeling of the porcine blastocyst during elongation on day 12 of pregnancy. *Biol. Reprod.* 27:941–955.

Geisert, R.D. and J.V. Yelich. 1997. Regulation of conceptus development and attachment in pigs. *J. Reprod. Fertil. Suppl.* 52:133–149.

Gerrard, D.E. and A.L. Grant. 2002. *Principles of Animal Growth and Development.* Kendall Hunt, Dubuque, IA.

Ghorbankhani, F., M. Souri, M.M. Moeini, and R. Mirmahmoudi. 2015. Effect of nutritional state on semen characteristics, testicular size and serum testosterone concentration in Sanjabi ram lambs during the natural breeding season. *Anim. Reprod. Sci.* 153:22–28.

Gilbert, A.B. 1971a. The female reproductive effort. In: *Physiology and Biochemistry of the Domestic Fowl.* Edited by D.J. Bell and B.M. Freeman. Academic Press, London, pp. 1153–1162.

Gilbert, A.B. 1971b. Egg albumen as its formation. In: *Physiology and Biochemistry of the Domestic Fowl.* Edited by D.J. Bell and B.M. Freeman. Academic Press, London, pp. 1291–1329.

Girmus, R.L. and M.E. Wise. 1992. Progesterone directly inhibits pituitary luteinizing hormone secretion in an estradiol-dependent manner. *Biol. Reprod.* 46:710–714.

Gorewit, R.C. 1988. Lactation biology and methods of increasing efficiency. In: *Designing Foods: Animal Product Options in the Marketplace.* National Academies Press, Washington, DC, pp. 208–223.

Haake, A.R., G. Konig, and R.H. Sawyer. 1984. Avian feather development: Relationships between morphogenesis and keratinization. *Dev. Biol.* 106:406–413.

Hackmann, T.J. and J.L. Firkins. 2015. Maximizing efficiency of rumen microbial protein production. *Front. Microbiol.* 6:465.

Harris, E.D. 2014. *Minerals in Foods.* DEStech Publications, Inc., Lancaster, PA.

Haussinger, D. and B. Görg. 2010. Interaction of oxidative stress, astrocyte swelling and cerebral ammonia toxicity. *Curr. Opin. Clin. Nutr. Metab. Care* 13:87–92.

Herbst, K.L. and S. Bhasin. 2004. Testosterone action on skeletal muscle. *Curr. Opin. Clin. Nutr. Metab. Care* 7:271–277.

Hernandez-García, A.D., D.A. Columbus, R. Manjarín, H.V. Nguyen, A. Suryawan, R.A. Orellana, and T.A. Davis. 2016. Leucine supplementation stimulates protein synthesis and reduces degradation signal activation in muscle of newborn pigs during acute endotoxemia. *Am. J. Physiol. Endocrinol. Metab.* 311:E791–E801.

Heyer, A. and B. Lebret. 2007. Compensatory growth response in pigs: Effects on growth performance, composition of weight gain at carcass and muscle levels, and meat quality. *J. Anim. Sci.* 85:769–778.

Hironaka, R., C.B. Bailey, and G.C. Kozub. 1970. Metabolic fecal nitrogen in ruminants estimated from dry matter excretion. *Can. J. Anim. Sci.* 50:55–60.

Hoffman, M.L., K.N. Peck, M.E. Forella, A.R. Fox, K.E. Govoni, and S.A. Zinn. 2016. The effects of poor maternal nutrition during gestation on postnatal growth and development of lambs. *J. Anim. Sci.* 94:789–799.

Holt, L.E. Jr. and A.A. Albanese. 1944. Observations on amino acid deficiencies in man. *Trans. Assoc. Am. Physicians* 58:143–156.

Humphrey, B.D., S. Kirsch, and D. Morris. 2008. Molecular cloning and characterization of the chicken cationic amino acid transporter-2 gene. *Comp. Biochem. Physiol.* B 150:301–311.

Hornick, J.L., C. Van Eenaeme, O. Gérard, I. Dufrasne, and L. Istasse. 2000. Mechanisms of reduced and compensatory growth. *Domest. Anim. Endocrinol.* 19:121–132.

Hurley, W.L. and P.K. Theil. 2011. Perspectives on immunoglobulins in colostrum and milk. *Nutrients* 3:442–474.

Inman, J.L., C. Robertson, J.D. Mott, and M.J. Bissell. 2015. Mammary gland development: Cell fate specification, stem cells and the microenvironment. *Development* 142:1028–1042.

Jefferson, W.N. and C.J. Williams. 2011. Circulating levels of genistein in the neonate, apart from dose and route, predict future adverse female reproductive outcomes. *Reprod. Toxicol.* 31:272–279.

Jensen, R.G. 2002. The composition of bovine milk lipids: January 1995 to December 2000. *J. Dairy Sci.* 85:295–350.

Ji, Y., Z.L. Wu, Z.L. Dai, K.J. Sun, J.J. Wang, and G. Wu. 2016. Nutritional epigenetics with a focus on amino acids: Implications for the development and treatment of metabolic syndrome. *J. Nutr. Biochem.* 27:1–8.

Ji, Y., Z.L. Wu, Z.L. Dai, X.L. Wang, J. Li, B.G. Wang, and G. Wu. 2017. Fetal and neonatal programming of postnatal growth and feed efficiency in swine. *J. Anim. Sci. Biotechnol.* 8:42.

Jia, S.C., X.Y. Li, S.X. Zheng, and G. Wu. 2017. Amino acids are major energy substrates for tissues of hybrid striped bass and zebrafish. *Amino Acids.* doi: 10.1007/s00726-017-2481-7.

Jobgen, W.S., S.K. Fried, W.J. Fu, C.J. Meininger, and G. Wu. 2006. Regulatory role for the arginine-nitric oxide pathway in metabolism of energy substrates. *J. Nutr. Biochem.* 17:571–588.

Johnson, B.J., S.B. Smith, and K.Y. Chung. 2014a. Historical overview of the effect of $\beta$-adrenergic agonists on beef cattle production. *Asian-Australas. J. Anim. Sci.* 27:757–766.

Johnson, G.A., R.C. Burghardt, and F.W. Bazer. 2014b. Osteopontin: A leading candidate adhesion molecule for implantation in pigs and sheep. *J. Anim. Sci. Biotechnol.* 5:56.

Keen, C.L. 1993. The effect of exercise and heat on mineral metabolism and requirements. In: *Nutritional Needs in Hot Environments: Applications for Military Personnel in Field Operations.* Edited by B.M. Marriott. National Academy of Sciences, Washington, DC, pp. 117–135.

Kelly, J.M., M. Summers, H.S. Park, L.P. Milligan, and B.W. McBride. 1991. Cellular energy metabolism and regulation. *J. Dairy Sci.* 74:678–694.

Kiess, W., G. Müller, A. Galler, A. Reich, J. Deutscher, J. Klammt, and J. Kratzsch. 2000. Body fat mass, leptin and puberty. *J. Pediatr. Endocrinol. Metab.* 13 (Suppl. 1):717–22.

Kim, B. 2008. Thyroid hormone as a determinant of energy expenditure and the basal metabolic rate. *Thyroid* 18:141–144.

Kim, S.W., A.C. Weaver, Y.B. Shen, and Y. Zhao. 2013. Improving efficiency of sow productivity: Nutrition and health. *J. Anim. Sci. Biotechnol.* 4(1):26.

Knudson, B.K., M.G. Hogberg, R.A. Merkel, R.E. Allen, and W.T. Magee. 1985. Developmental comparisons of boars and barrows: II. Body composition and bone development. *J. Anim. Sci.* 61:797–801.

Kobori, Y., K. Suzuki, T. Iwahata, T. Shin, Y. Sadaoka, R. Sato, K. Nishio et al. 2015. Improvement of seminal quality and sexual function of men with oligoasthenoteratozoospermia syndrome following supplementation with L-arginine and Pycnogenol®. *Arch. Ital. Urol. Androl.* 87:190–193.

Koopman, R., S.M. Gehrig, B. Léger, J. Trieu, S. Walrand, K.T. Murphy, and G.S. Lynch. 2010. Cellular mechanisms underlying temporal changes in skeletal muscle protein synthesis and breakdown during chronic $\beta$-adrenoceptor stimulation in mice. *J. Physiol.* 588: 4811–4823.

Laven, R.A. and S.B. Drew. 1999. Dietary protein and the reproductive performance of cows. *Vet. Rec.* 145:687–695.

Lean, I.J., J.M. Thompson, and F.R. Dunshea. 2014. A meta-analysis of zilpaterol and ractopamine effects on feedlot performance, carcass traits and shear strength of meat in cattle. *PLoS One* 9(12): e115904.

Liao, S.F., N. Regmi, and G. Wu. 2018. Homeostatic regulation of plasma amino acid concentrations. *Front. Biosci.* 23:640–655.

Lieber, R.L. and S.C. Bodine-Fowler. 1993. Skeletal muscle mechanics: Implications for rehabilitation. *Physical Ther.* 73:844–856.

Linzell, J.L. and T.B. Mepham. 1969. Mammary metabolism in lactating sows: Arteriovenous differences of milk precursors and the mammary metabolism of [$^{14}$C]glucose and [$^{14}$C]acetate. *Br. J. Nutr.* 23:319–332.

Liu, S.M., G. Mata, H. O'Donoghue, and D.G. Masters. 1998. The influence of live weight, live-weight change and diet on protein synthesis in the skin and skeletal muscle in young Merino sheep. *Br. J. Nutr.* 79:267–274.

Louis, G.F., A.J. Lewis, W.C. Weldon, P.S. Miller, R.J. Kittok, and W.W. Stroup. 1994. The effect of protein intake on boar libido, semen characteristics, and plasma hormone concentrations. *J. Anim. Sci.* 72:2038–2050.

Maltz, E., L.F. Barbosa, P. Bueno, L. Scagion, K. Kaniyamattam, L.F. Greco, A. De Vries, and J.E. Santos. 2013. Effect of feeding according to energy balance on performance, nutrient excretion, and feeding behavior of early lactation dairy cows. *J. Dairy Sci.* 96:5249–5266.

Manjarin, R., B.J. Bequette, G. Wu, and N.L. Trottier. 2014. Linking our understanding of mammary gland metabolism to amino acid nutrition. *Amino Acids* 46:2447–2462.

Mateo, R.D., G. Wu, H.K. Moon, J.A. Carroll, and S.W. Kim. 2008. Effects of dietary arginine supplementation during gestation and lactation on the performance of lactating primiparous sows and nursing piglets. *J. Anim. Sci.* 86:827–835.

Maynard, L.A., J.K. Loosli, H.F. Hintz, and R.G. Warner. 1979. *Animal Nutrition*. McGraw-Hill, New York, NY.

McDonald, P., R.A. Edwards, J.F.D. Greenhalgh, J.F.D. Greenhalgh, C.A. Morgan, and L.A. Sinclair. 2011. *Animal Nutrition*, 7th ed. Prentice Hall, New York.

McIndoe, W.M. 1971. Yolk synthesis. In: *Physiology and Biochemistry of the Domestic Fowl*. Edited by D.J. Bell and B.M. Freeman. Academic Press, London, pp. 1209–1223.

McNeilly, A.S., C.C. Tay, and A. Glasier. 1994. Physiological mechanisms underlying lactational amenorrhea. *Ann. N.Y. Acad. Sci.* 709:145–155.

Meadows, M.G., T.E. Roudybush, and K.J. McGraw. 2012. Dietary protein level affects iridescent coloration in Anna's hummingbirds, *Calypte anna*. *J. Exp. Biol.* 215:2742–2750.

Meldrum, D.R., R.F. Casper, A. Diez-Juan, C. Simon, A.D. Domar, and R. Frydman. 2016. Aging and the environment affect gamete and embryo potential: Can we intervene? *Fertil. Steril.* 105:548–559.

Mepham, T.B. and J.L. Linzell. 1966. A quantitative assessment of the contribution of individual plasma amino acids to the synthesis of milk proteins by the goat mammary gland. *Biochem. J.* 101:76–83.

Milligan, L.P. and M. Summers. 1986. The biological basis of maintenance and its relevance to assessing responses to nutrients. *Proc. Nutr. Soc.* 45:185–193.

Monks, J. and M.C. Neville. 2004. Albumin transcytosis across the epithelium of the lactating mouse mammary gland. *J. Physiol.* 560:267–280.

Moran, E.T., Jr. 2007. Nutrition of the developing embryo and hatchling. *Poult. Sci.* 86:1043–1049.

Mount, E.L. 1978. Heat transfer between animals and environment. *Proc. Nutr. Soc.* 37:21–28.

Muñoz-Calvo, M.T. and J. Argente. 2016. Nutritional and pubertal disorders. *Endocr. Dev.* 29:153–173.

Murphy, M.E., J.R. King, T.G. Taruscio. 1990. Amino acid composition of feather barbs and rachises in three species of pygoscelid penguins: Nutritional implications. *The Condor* 92:913–921.

Murray, D.M., J.P. Bowland, R.T. Berg, and B.A. Young. 1974. Effects of enforced exercise on growing pigs: Feed intake, rate of gain, feed conversion, dissected carcass composition, and muscle weight distribution. *Can. J. Anim. Sci.* 54:91–96.

Musumeci, G., P. Castrogiovanni, M.A. Szychlinska, F.C. Aiello, G.M. Vecchio, L. Salvatorelli, G. Magro, and R. Imbesi. 2015. Mammary gland: From embryogenesis to adult life. *Acta Histoche.* 117:379–385.

National Research Council (NRC). 1995. *Nutrient Requirements of Laboratory Animals*. National Academy Press, Washington, DC.

National Research Council (NRC). 2001. *Nutrient Requirements of Dairy Cattle*. National Academy Press, Washington, DC.

National Research Council (NRC). 2011. *Nutrient Requirements of Fish and Shrimp*. National Academy Press, Washington, DC.

National Research Council (NRC). 2012. *Nutrient Requirements of Swine*. National Academies Press, Washington, DC.

Navegantes, L.C., N.M. Resano, R.H. Migliorini, and I.C. Kettelhut. 2001. Catecholamines inhibit $Ca^{2+}$-dependent proteolysis in rat skeletal muscle through $\beta_2$-adrenoceptors and cAMP. *Am. J. Physiol. Endocrinol. Metab.* 281:E449–454.

Newsholme, E.A. and T.R. Leech. 2009. *Functional Biochemistry in Health and Disease*. John Wiley & Sons, West Sussex, UK.

Norman, J.E. 2010. The adverse effects of obesity on reproduction. *Reproduction* 140:343–345.

Oksbjerg, N., P.M. Nissen, M. Therkildsen, H.S. Møller, L.B. Larsen, M. Andersen, J.F. Young. 2013. Meat science and muscle biology symposium: In utero nutrition related to fetal development, postnatal performance, and meat quality of pork. *J. Anim. Sci.* 91:1443–53.

Ollivier-Bousquet, M. 2002. Milk lipid and protein traffic in mammary epithelial cells: Joint and independent pathways. *Reprod. Nutr. Dev.* 42:149–162.

Ontsouka, E.C. and C. Albrecht. 2014. Cholesterol transport and regulation in the mammary gland. *J. Mammary Gland Biol. Neoplasia.* 19:43–58.

Osorio, J.S., J. Lohakare, and M. Bionaz. 2016. Biosynthesis of milk fat, protein, and lactose: Roles of transcriptional and posttranscriptional regulation. *Physiol. Genomics* 48:231–256.

Osuji, P.O. 1974. The physiology of eating and the energy expenditure of the ruminant at pasture. *J. Range Management.* 27:436–443.

Palmiter, R.D. 1972. Regulation of protein synthesis in chick oviduct. *J. Biol. Chem.* 247:6450–6461.

Palmquist, D.L. 2006. Milk fat: Origin of fatty acids and influence of nutritional factors. In: *Advanced Dairy Chemistry, Vol. 2: Lipids*, 3rd ed. Edited by P.F. Fox and P.L.H. McSweeney. Springer, New York.

Park, Y.W. and G.F.W. Haenlein. 2006. *Handbook of Milk of Non-bovine Mammals.* Blackwell Publishing, Oxford, UK.

Pearson, R.A., P. Lhoste, M. Saastamoinen, and W. Martin-Rosset. 2003. Working animals in agriculture and transport. *EAAP Tech. Ser.* 6:1–210.

Pinares, C. and G. Waghorn. 2012. *Technical Manual on Respiration Chamber Designs.* Ministry of Agriculture and Forestry of New Zealand. Wellington, New Zealand.

Pond, W.G., R.R. Maurer, and J. Klindt. 1991. Fetal organ response to maternal protein deprivation during pregnancy in swine. *J. Nutr.* 121:504–509.

Pond, W.G., D.C. Church, and K.R. Pond. 1995. *Basic Animal Nutrition and Feeding.* 4th ed., John Wiley & Sons, New York.

Pownall, M.E., M.K. Gustafsson, and C.P. Emerson, Jr. 2002. Myogenic regulatory factors and the specification of muscle progenitors in vertebrate embryos. *Annu. Rev. Cell Dev. Biol.* 18:747–783.

Qi, K. and C.J. Lupton. 1994. A review of the effect of sulfur nutrition in wool production and quality. *Sheep Goat Res. J.* 10:133–140.

Reeds, P.J. and P.J. Garlick. 2003. Protein and amino acid requirements and the composition of complementary foods. *J. Nutr.* 133:2953S–2961S.

Reeds, P.J. and H.J. Mersmann. 1991. Protein and energy requirements of animals treated with β-adrenergic agonists: A discussion. *J. Anim. Sci.* 69:1532–1550.

Reis, P.J. and J.M. Gillespie. 1985. Effects of phenylalanine and analogues of methionine and phenylalanine on the composition of wool and mouse hair. *Aust. J. Biol. Sci.* 38:151–63.

Reis, P.J. and T. Sahlu. 1994. The nutritional control of the growth and properties of mohair and wool fibers: A comparative review. *J. Anim. Sci.* 72:1899–1907.

Reynolds, L.P., J.S. Caton, D.A. Redmer, A.T. Grazul-Bilska, K.A. Vonnahme, P.B. Borowicz, J.S. Luther, J.M. Wallace, G. Wu, and T.E. Spencer. 2006. Evidence for altered placental blood flow and vascularity in compromised pregnancies. *J. Physiol. (London)* 572:51–58.

Rezaei, R., Z.L. Wu, Y.Q. Hou, F.W. Bazer, and G. Wu. 2016. Amino acids and mammary gland development: Nutritional implications for neonatal growth. *J. Anim. Sci. Biotechnol.* 7:20.

Sam, A.H. and W.S. Dhillo. 2010. Endocrine links between fat and reproduction. *Obstetr. Gynaecol.* 12:231236.

Santos, J.E., R.S. Bisinotto, and E.S. Ribeiro. 2016. Mechanisms underlying reduced fertility in anovular dairy cows. *Theriogenology* 86:254–262.

Sato, Y., K. Watanabe, and T. Takahashi. 1973. Lipids in egg white. *Poult. Sci.* 52:1564–1570.

Satterfield, M.C. and G. Wu. 2011. Growth and development of brown adipose tissue: Significance and nutritional regulation. *Front. Biosci.* 16:1589–1608.

Segal, J., B.R. Troen, S.H. Ingbar. 1982. Influence of age and sex on the concentrations of thyroid hormone in serum in the rat. *J. Endocrinol.* 93:177–181.

Senger, P.L. 1997. *Pathways to Pregnancy and Parturition.* Current Conceptions, Inc., Pullman, WA.

Shennan, D. and M. Peaker. 2000. Transport of milk constituents by the mammary gland. *Physiol. Rev.* 80:925–951.

Smith, S.B. and D.R. Smith. 1995. *The Biology of Fat in Meat Animals. Current Advances.* American Society of Animal Science, Champaign, Illinois, USA.

Stoneham, S.J., P. Morresey, and J. Ousey. 2017. Nutritional management and practical feeding of the orphan foal. *Equine Vet. Edu.* 29:165–173.

Susenbeth, A. and K. Keitel. 1988. Partition of whole body protein in different body fractions and some constants in body composition in pigs. *Livest. Prod. Sci.* 20:37–52.

Suttle, N.F. 2010. *Mineral Nutrition of Livestock*, 4th ed. CABI, Wallingford, U.K.

Tanimura, J. 1967. Studies on arginine in human semen. Part II. The effects of medication with L-arginine-HCl on male infertility. *Bull. Osaka Med. School* 13:84–89.

Thatcher, W.W., J.E. Santos, F.T. Silvestre, I.H. Kim, and C.R. Staples. 2010. Perspective on physiological/endocrine and nutritional factors influencing fertility in post-partum dairy cows. *Reprod. Domest. Anim.* 45 (Suppl. 3):2–14.

Thornton, P.K. 2010. Livestock production: Recent trends, future prospects. *Philos. Trans. R. Soc. Lond. B Biol. Sci.* 365:2853–2867.

Trottier, N.L., C.F. Shipley, and R.A. Easter. 1997. Plasma amino acid uptake by the mammary gland of the lactating sow. *J. Anim. Sci.* 75:1266–1278.

Tucker, H.A. 2000. Hormones, mammary growth, and lactation: A 41-year perspective. *J. Dairy Sci.* 83:874–884.

Turner, H.G. and C.S. Taylor. 1983. Dynamic factors in models of energy utilization with particular reference to maintenance requirement of cattle. *World Rev. Nutr. Diet.* 42:135–190.

Tvrda, E., R. Peer, S.C. Sikka, and A. Agarwal. 2015. Iron and copper in male reproduction: A double-edged sword. *J. Assist. Reprod. Genet.* 32:3–16.

van de Pol, I., G. Flik, and M. Gorissen. 2017. Comparative physiology of energy metabolism: Fishing for endocrine signals in the early vertebrate pool. *Front. Endocrinol (Lausanne).* 8:36.

van Es, A.J.H. 1976. Meat production from ruminants. *Meat Animals* 7:391–401.

van Milgen, J., J. Noblet, and S. Dubois. 2001. Energetic efficiency of starch, protein and lipid utilization in growing pigs. *J. Nutr.* 131:1309–1318.

Vance, J.E. 2015. Phospholipid synthesis and transport in mammalian cells. *Traffic* 16:1–18.

Wagner, J.R., A.P. Schinckel, W. Chen, J.C. Forrest, and B.L. Coe. 1999. Analysis of body composition changes of swine during growth and development. *J. Anim Sci.* 77:1442–1466.

Wang, J.J., Z.L. Wu, D.F. Li, N. Li, S.V. Dindot, M.C. Satterfield, F.W. Bazer, and G. Wu. 2012. Nutrition, epigenetics, and metabolic syndrome. *Antioxid. Redox. Signal.* 17:282–301.

White, C.R. and R.S. Seymour. 2002. Mammalian basal metabolic rate is proportional to body mass$^{2/3}$. *Proc. Natl. Acad. Sci. USA.* 100:4046–4049.

Wilkinson, J.M. 2011. Re-defining efficiency of feed use by livestock. *Animal* 5:1014–1022.

Won, E.T. and R.J. Borski. 2013. Endocrine regulation of compensatory growth in fish. *Front. Endocrinol (Lausanne)* 4:74.

Wu, G. 1998. Intestinal mucosal amino acid catabolism. *J. Nutr.* 128:1249–1252.

Wu, G. 2013. *Amino Acids: Biochemistry and Nutrition*, CRC Press, Boca Raton, Florida.

Wu, G. 2014. Dietary requirements of synthesizable amino acids by animals: A paradigm shift in protein nutrition. *J. Anim. Sci. Biotechnol.* 5:34.

Wu, G. 2016. Dietary protein intake and human health. *Food Funct.* 7:1251–1265.

Wu, G. and D.A. Knabe. 1994. Free and protein-bound amino acids in sow's colostrum and milk. *J. Nutr.* 124:415–424.

Wu, G., F.W. Bazer, and H.R. Cross. 2014a. Land-based production of animal protein: Impacts, efficiency, and sustainability. *Ann. N.Y. Acad. Sci.* 1328:18–28.

Wu, G., F.W. Bazer, T.A. Cudd, C.J. Meininger, and T.E. Spencer. 2004. Maternal nutrition and fetal development. *J. Nutr.* 134:2169–2172.

Wu, G., F.W. Bazer, Z.L. Dai, D.F. Li, J.J. Wang, and Z.L. Wu. 2014b. Amino acid nutrition in animals: Protein synthesis and beyond. *Annu. Rev. Anim. Biosci.* 2:387–417.

Wu, G., F.W. Bazer, T.A. Davis, S.W. Kim, P. Li, J.M. Rhoads, M.C. Satterfield, S.B. Smith, T.E. Spencer, and Y.L. Yin. 2009. Arginine metabolism and nutrition in growth, health and disease. *Amino Acids* 37:153–168.

Wu, G., F.W. Bazer, G.A., Johnson, C. Herring, H. Seo, Z.L. Dai, J.J. Wang, Z.L. Wu, and X.L. Wang. 2017. Functional amino acids in the development of the pig placenta. *Mol. Reprod. Dev.* 84:870–882.

Wu, G., F.W. Bazer, J.M. Wallace, and T.E. Spencer. 2006. Intrauterine growth retardation: Implications for the animal sciences. *J. Anim. Sci.* 84:2316–2337.

Wu, G., J. Fanzo, D.D. Miller, P. Pingali, M. Post, J.L. Steiner, and A.E. Thalacker-Mercer. 2014c. Production [Name]nd supply of high-quality food protein for human consumption: Sustainability, challenges and innovations. *Ann. N.Y. Acad. Sci.* 1321:1–19.

Wu, G., N.E. Flynn, W. Yan, and D.G. Barstow, Jr. 1995. Glutamine metabolism in chick enterocytes: Absence of pyrroline-5-carboxylate synthase and citrulline synthesis. *Biochem. J.* 306:717–721.

Wu, G., B. Imhoff-Kunsch, and A.W. Girard. 2012. Biological mechanisms for nutritional regulation of maternal health and fetal development. *Paediatr. Perinatal Epidemiol.* 26 (Suppl. 1): 4–26.

Wu, G., Z.L. Wu, Z.L. Dai, Y. Yang, W.W. Wang, C. Liu, B. Wang, J.J. Wang and Y.L. Yin. 2013. Dietary requirements of "nutritionally nonessential amino acids" by animals and humans. *Amino Acids* 44:1107–1113.

Zeyner, A., K. Romanowski, A. Vernunft, P. Harris, A.-M. Müller, C. Wolf, and E. Kienzle. 2017. Effects of different oral doses of sodium chloride on the basal acid–base and mineral status of exercising horses fed low amounts of hay. *PLoS One* 12(1):e0168325.

Zhao, F.Q. and A.F. Keating. 2007. Expression and regulation of glucose transporters in the bovine mammary gland. *J. Dairy Sci.* 90(E. Suppl.):E76–E86.

Zhu, C., Z.Y Jiang, F.W. Bazer, G.A. Johnson, R.C. Burghardt, and G. Wu. 2015. Aquaporins in the female reproductive system of mammals. *Front. Biosci.* 20:838–871.

Zhu, Y., Q. Niu, C. Shi, J. Wang, and W. Zhu. 2017. The role of microbiota in compensatory growth of protein-restricted rats. *Microb. Biotechnol.* 10:480–491.

# 12 Regulation of Food Intake by Animals

Food provides an animal with nutrients and energy. Food intake is essential to the maintenance, growth, development, and reproduction of all animals. Their voluntary food consumption is influenced by (1) dietary characteristics; (including nutrient composition and palatability) and availability; (2) energy supply; (3) blood metabolites (e.g., amino acids [AAs], glucose, and short-chain fatty acids [SCFAs]); (4) digestive tract capacity and gut-fill (food digestibility); (5) feedback signals from the gastrointestinal tract, liver, and brain in response to dietary intakes of nutrients and concentrations of hormones in the blood circulation (Figure 12.1); (6) physiological status (e.g., gestation, lactation and growth) and pathological conditions (e.g., fever, infection and cancer); and (7) ambient temperatures (Forbes 2007). These animal, food, and environmental factors are summarized in Table 12.1. In addition, animals learn about the metabolic consequences of consuming foods with certain physical or sensory properties, including appearance, flavor, and texture, and choose preferentially or avoid foods that they have previously experienced (Catanese et al. 2016; Wadhera and Capaldi-Phillips 2014). Recent studies have identified receptors for food flavors in the tongue (Niot and Besnard 2017) and the gastrointestinal tract (Breer et al. 2012), which provide a biochemical basis for food selection by animals. Thus, animals can reject, adapt to, or maintain food intake according to their nutritional and physiological needs.

Enteral nutrients are provided to animals through food intake via the mouth or direct infusion to the gastrointestinal tract. In modern intensive or extensive farming systems, livestock, poultry, and fish have free access to foods under most production conditions. Overall, the amount of feed (or dry matter [DM]) intake by an animal is a function of its body weight (BW) or the size and frequency of meals (Baile and Forbes 1974). In growing animals, food intake is generally proportional to their weight gains. Thus, food intake is closely related to two important issues in nutrition: the productivity of farm animals and obesity development. Therefore, animal producers strive to increase the voluntary food intake of farm animals at some phases of production, such as lactation, weaning, and postweaning growth, or when they are sick, while minimizing fat accretion in the body (Sartin et al. 2011). In contrast, owners of companion animals are increasingly concerned about the food consumption of their dogs, cats, and other pets to reduce obesity. Also, in all dams, maternal obesity before breeding impairs embryonic survival, whereas maternal obesity during pregnancy increases the risk for fetal mortality and perinatal complications (Wu et al. 2006). Thus, the regulation of feed intake by multiple factors at several levels is critical for health and productivity of mammals, birds, and fish (Table 12.1). The main objective of this chapter is to highlight the mechanisms responsible for the control of food intake by animals.

## REGULATION OF FOOD INTAKE BY NONRUMINANTS

### CONTROL CENTERS IN THE CENTRAL NERVOUS SYSTEM

#### Hypothalamus, Neurotransmitters, and Neuropeptides

The brain collects information from the special sensors and receptors in the gastrointestinal tract and other organs (Marx 2003). It was originally proposed that there were centers (the feeding center and satiety center) in the hypothalamus, which is located beneath the cerebrum of the brain (Auffray 1969). The feeding center (also known as the lateral hypothalamic area [LHA]) causes the animal to eat unless inhibited by the satiety center (also known as the ventromedial hypothalamus [VMH]) which receives signals from the body as a result of food consumption (Figure 12.2). Thus, lesions in the LHA result in underfeeding, whereas lesions in the VMH or the paraventricular nucleus (PVN) cause overfeeding

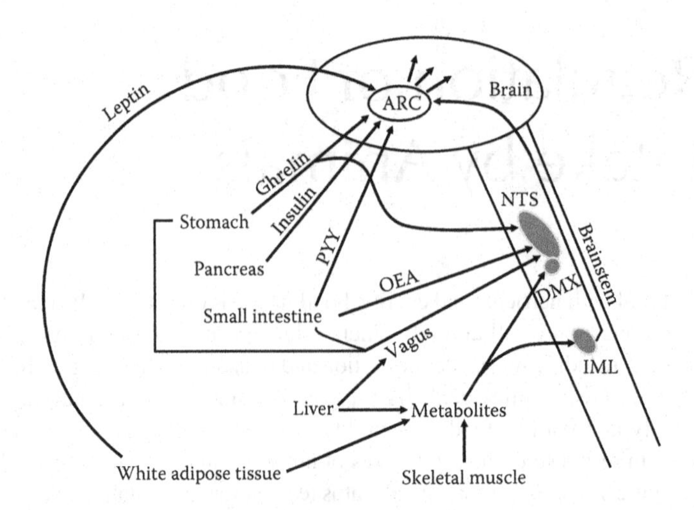


**FIGURE 12.1** Regulation of voluntary food intake by animals at the gastrointestinal tract, liver, and brain levels. DMX, dorsal motor nucleus of the vagus nerve; IML, intermediolateral cell column; NTS, nucleus tractus solitaries; OEA, oleoylethanolamide; PYY, peptide YY.

(Abdalla 2017). However, the LHA and VMH are not the only parts of the brain that control food intake. The paraventricular nuclei of the hypothalamus, just ventral to the ventromedial nuclei, are particularly sensitive to the effects of neurotransmitters, including noradrenaline, neuropeptide Y (NPY), and α-melanocyte-stimulating hormone (α-MSH, a melanocortin) (Kirouac 2015). Neurons within the central and peripheral nervous systems communicate with each other through these neurotransmitters. Most of them are metabolites of AAs that either inhibit or stimulate appetite (Table 12.2).

It is now widely recognized that the arcuate nucleus (ARC), which is located in the hypothalamus, contains two major types of neurons with opposing actions: agouti-related peptide (AgRP)/NPY

**TABLE 12.1**
**Factors Affecting Food Intake of Animals**

| Factors | Examples |
|---|---|
| Diets | Amount and type of AA; energy content; composition of carbohydrates, lipids, vitamins, and minerals; anti-nutritional factors and toxic substances; ingredients of diets; methods of food processing; physical characteristics of diets (e.g., temperature, particle size, color, smell, and taste); the form of diet (liquid, pellet, or powder); and water quality |
| Genes | Species (e.g., cattle, fish, horse, humans, pigs, poultry, and sheep), breeds (leghorn vs. broiler chickens; Meishan vs. offspring of Landrace × Yorkshire gilts and Duroc × Hampshire boars), and sex (males and females; boars vs. sows) |
| Physiological and metabolic factors in plasma | Age, pregnancy, and lactation; light, circadian clock, and melatonin; release of hormones and satiety signals from the gut and brain; concentrations of AAs, glucose, fatty acids, and their metabolites (e.g., ammonia, lactate and ketone bodies in plasma and brain; and motility of the gastrointestinal tract) |
| Pathology | Infection, trauma, neoplasia, diabetes, obesity, cardiovascular disease, fetal growth restriction, nausea, and vomiting |
| Environment | Ambient temperature (e.g., heat stress[a], cold, local heating); ambient humidity; air pollution (e.g., $PM_{2.5}$, ammonium sulfate, ammonia, $H_2S$, CO, and $CO_2$); and sanitation |
| Management and behavior | Frequency of meals, weaning, individual and group hygiene, noise, handling and treatment of animals, physical activity, dietary habits, and social behavior |

[a] This is a particularly severe problem for animals without sweat glands, such as dogs, sheep, and swine.

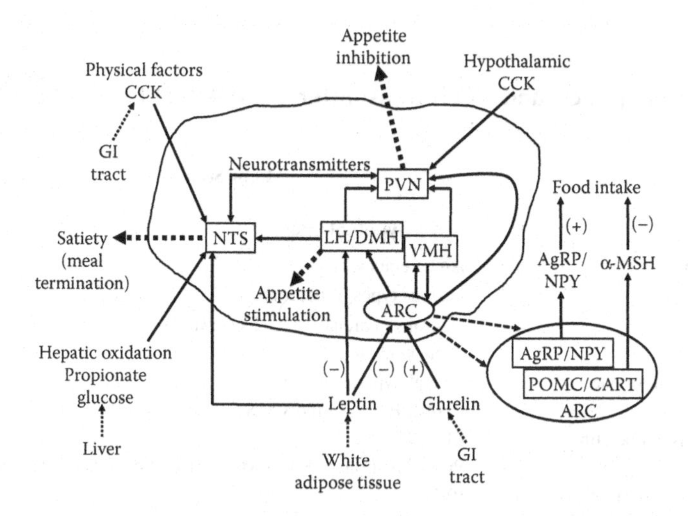


**FIGURE 12.2** The centers of food intake control in the brain. The arcuate is located in the hypothalamus and contains two major types of neurons with opposing actions: agouti-related peptide/neuropeptide Y neurons (stimulating appetite); and pro-opiomelanocortin/cocaine–amphetamine regulated transcript neurons (inhibiting appetite). Ghrelin stimulates, but leptin inhibits, food intake by animals. AgRP, agouti-related peptide; ARC, Arcuate; CART, cocaine-amphetamine regulated transcript; CCK, Cholecystokinin; DMH, Dorsomedial hypothalamus; LH, Lateral hypothalamus (also known as lateral hypothalamic area [LHA]); α-MSH, α-melanocyte-stimulating hormone; NPY, neuropeptide Y; POMC, pro-opiomelanocortin; PVN, paraventricular nucleus; NTS, nucleus tractus solitarius; VMN, ventromedial nucleus. (Adapted from Sartin, J.L. et al. 2011. *J. Anim. Sci.* 89:1991–2003. (+), stimulation; (−) inhibition.)

neurons; and pro-opiomelanocortin (POMC)/cocaine–amphetamine regulated transcript (CART) neurons (Sutton et al. 2016). Activation of the AgRP/NPY neurons stimulates appetite. In contrast, activation of the POMC/CART neurons reduces appetite by causing the release of α-melanocyte-stimulating hormone (α-MSH, an anorexigenic neuropeptide) from the presynaptic terminals of the POMC neurons. By binding to the melanocortin-3 and -4 receptors (MC3R, MC4R) on the second-order neurons, α-MSH reduces food intake and enhances energy expenditure (Figure 12.3). Thus, the POMC neurons connect with second-order neurons in other brain centers, which transmit the signals through the nucleus of the tractus solitarius (NTS) to the body. Many peptide-regulating hormones work through the ARC, but some may also have direct effects on the NTS and other brain centers. The roles of these neuropeptides as satiety signals are summarized in Table 12.2.

## Leptin and Insulin

Leptin (from Greek *leptos*, meaning "thin") is synthesized and secreted by white adipose tissue, whereas insulin is synthesized and secreted by β-cells of the pancreas (Thon et al. 2016). Leptin (the "satiety hormone") and insulin act on the receptors in the ARC of the hypothalamus to stimulate the production of POMC/CART, while inhibiting the release of AgRP/NPY, thereby suppressing food intake by animals (Figure 12.2). For example, administration of leptin into the ventral tegmental area (VTA; 15–500 ng/side) or ARC (15–150 ng/side) of female rats decreased food intake for 72 h, inducing weight loss during the first 48 h (VTA) or 24 h (ARC) after the infusions (Bruijnzeel, et al. 2011). There is evidence that leptin increases the frequency of action potentials in the anorexigenic POMC neurons through membrane depolarization and reduced inhibition by local orexigenic NPY/GABA neurons (Cowley et al. 2001). The administration of insulin (0.005–5 mU/side) into the VTA or ARC decreased food intake for 24 h, but did not affect body weights. Neither insulin nor leptin in the ARC affected brain reward thresholds. Thus, when fat stores and plasma concentrations of leptin and insulin are elevated, the feed intake of animals is reduced. However, when fat stores and plasma levels of leptin and insulin are reduced, AgRP/NPY neurons are activated and POMC/CART

**TABLE 12.2**
**Hormones, Neuropeptides, and Neurotransmitters That Affect Food Intake (FI) by Animals**

| Substance | Major Source | Effect on FI |
|---|---|---|
| | **Hypothalamus** | |
| Agouti-related protein | Arcuate nucleus | Increase |
| γ-Aminobutyrate | Various types of neurons | Increase |
| Dopamine | Neurons in arcuate nucleus (reward) | Increase |
| Neuropeptide Y | Arcuate nucleus | Increase |
| Melanin-concentrating hormone | Lateral hypothalamic area (LHA) and other regions in brain | Increase |
| Opioids[a] | LHA, PE, PVN, and VMN | Increase |
| Orexin (also known as hypocretin) | LHA, DMN | Increase |
| CART | POMC neurons, PVN, VMN, LHA, and median eminence | Decrease |
| Corticotrophin-releasing hormone (CRH) | PVN | Decrease |
| Melanocortin | VMN | Decrease |
| α-Melanocyte-stimulating hormone | POMC neurons | Decrease |
| Neurotransmitters | VMN | Decrease |
| Neurotransmitters | Dorsomedial nucleus (DMN) | Decrease |
| Norepinephrine | PVN and VMH | Decrease |
| Pro-opiomelanocortin (POMC) | POMC neurons | Decrease |
| Serotonin | PVN, LHA, and VMN | Decrease |
| Urocortin | PVN | Decrease |
| | **Brainstem** | |
| Neurotransmitters | Nucleus tractus solitarius (NTS)[b] | Decrease |
| Neurotransmitters | Intermediolateral cell column (IML) | Decrease |
| | **The Digestive System** | |
| Ghrelin | Epithelial cells of stomach and small intestine | Increase |
| Cholecystokinin (CCK) | Small intestine | Decrease |
| Gastrin | Enteroendocrine cells | Increase |
| Glucagon-like peptide-1 (GLP-1) | Small intestine | Decrease |
| Insulin | Pancreatic β-cells | Decrease |
| Peptide YY (36-AA peptide) | Enteroendocrine cells of the intestine | Decrease |
| Oleoylethanolamide (OEA, FA derivative) | Enterocytes | Decrease |
| Serotonin | Enteroendocrine cells of the intestine | ?? |
| Nitric oxide | Enteroendocrine cells of the intestine | Increase |
| | **White Adipose Tissue** | |
| Leptin | White adipocytes | Decrease |

CART = cocaine and amphetamine-related transcript; CRH = corticotrophin-releasing hormone; DMH, dorsomedial hypothalamus; NTS = nucleus tractus solitaries; PE = periventricular nucleus; PVN = paraventricular nucleus; VMN = ventromedial nucleus.

[a] Examples are endorphins and enkephalins in the hypothalamus.

[b] The communication from tissues in the digestive system to the NTS is transmitted along afferent fibers of the vagus nerve or sympathetic nerves.

neurons are inhibited, leading to increased food intake and weight gain (Figure 12.3). In obese sheep, plasma leptin concentrations are markedly increased, suggesting leptin resistance (Daniel et al. 2002). This results from the reduced transport of leptin into the brain as opposed to intrahypothalamic leptin insensitivity (Adam and Findlay 2009). Under conditions of overnutrition, obesity, and type 2 diabetes mellitus, insulin signaling in the central nervous system is impaired, leading to

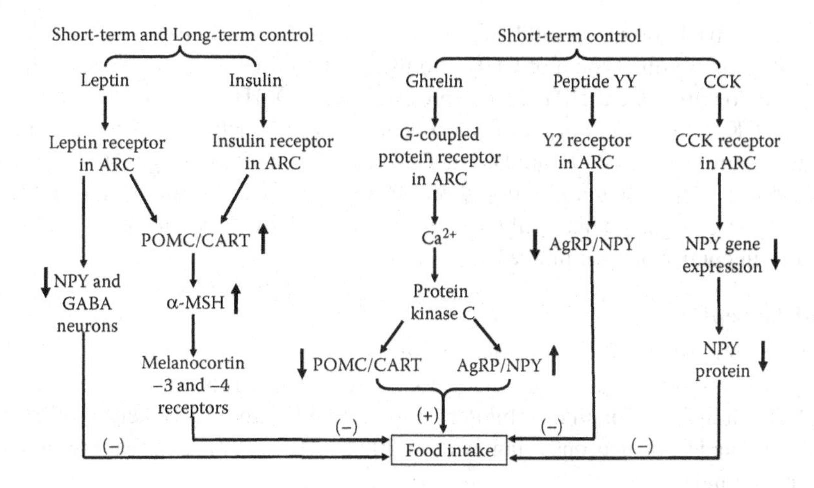


**FIGURE 12.3** Regulation of food intake by leptin, insulin, and gastrointestinal peptides in animals. AgRP, agouti-related peptide; ARC, Arcuate; CART, cocaine-amphetamine regulated transcript; CCK, Cholecystokinin; $\alpha$-MSH, $\alpha$-melanocyte-stimulating hormone; NPY, neuropeptide Y; POMC pro-opiomelanocortin; ↑, increase; ↓, decrease; (+), stimulation; (–), inhibition.

insulin resistance and augmenting disease progression (Vogt and Brüning 2013). Therefore, as acute and long-term satiety signals, both leptin and insulin play an important role in the control of energy homeostasis of the whole body.

## Ghrelin

Ghrelin is a peptide hormone (28 AAs) produced by the enteroendocrine X/A cells in the stomach and the small intestine (Steinert et al. 2017). In the central nervous system, ghrelin acts on a G-coupled protein receptor to increase the intracellular calcium concentration and protein kinase C activity through the inositol 1,4,5-triphosphate/phospholipase C and diacylglycerol signaling pathway. At the ARC, ghrelin activates the AgRP/NPY neurons and inactivates the POMC/CART neurons, thereby stimulating appetite (Kojima and Kangawa 2005). Thus, ghrelin is the "hunger hormone" that opposes the actions of leptin, and plays an important role in the short-term regulation of food intake (Chen et al. 2007; Steinert et al. 2017).

## Peptide YY

Peptide YY (peptide tyrosine tyrosine [PYY] with 36 AA residues) is synthesized and secreted primarily by the enteroendocrine L cells in the small intestine and the colon in response to food intake (Steinert et al. 2017). When the concentration of PYY is elevated in plasma, the binding of this peptide to the Y2 receptor in the ARC is increased to inhibit the AgRP/NPY neurons. A decrease in the production of AgRP/NPY leads to inhibition of food intake. Thus, in experimental animals, either administration of PYY into the systemic circulation or microinjection of PYY into the paraventricular hypothalamic nucleus or the hippocampus caused a decrease in food intake (Alhadeff et al. 2015). Fats, fatty acids, and many other luminal nutrients, as well as the chyme in the proximal small intestine induce PYY release by the small intestine. Thus, a large amount of food in the small intestine results in low appetite. Much evidence shows that PYY plays an important role in the short-term regulation of food intake (Steinert et al. 2017).

## Cholecystokinin

This peptide hormone is produced by the enteroendocrine I cells of the duodenum in response to food intake, and is also found in the brain (Steinert et al. 2017). Most of the cholecystokinin (CCK) receptors are present in the dorsomedial hypothalamic nucleus (DMH). Administration of CCK into the lateral ventricle of sheep inhibits feed intake (Baile and Della-Ferra 1984). Mechanistic studies indicate that administration of CCK into the DMH of rats resulted in Fos activation in the entire brain and downregulated NPY gene expression in the DMH (Chen et al. 2008). Peripherally administered CCK, which acts only for a short term, primarily activates neurons in the NST, but also stimulates neurons in the PVN and DMH. Thus, CCK is an afferent signal that acts on the NTS to reduce meal size. When the gut motility is low, the release of CCK from the intestine is increased as a peripheral satiety signal. This results in low appetite and low food intake. Thus, CCK contributes to short-term control of food intake by animals.

#### Glucagon-Like Peptide-1

Glucagon-like peptide-1 (GLP-1) is released from enteroendocrine L cells in the small intestine, particularly in the distal ileum and proximal colon, in response to food intake (Kaviani and Cooper 2017). It induces satiation through its inhibitory effects on NPY and AgRP neurons and stimulatory effects on POMC and CAR neurons (Stanley et al. 2004). GLP-1 is an acute satiety signal to inhibit food intake by animals.

### Control of Food Intake by Nutrients and Metabolites

#### Dietary Energy Content

Dietary energy content is a major nutritional factor that affects food intake by animals (Table 12.3). Since energy is not matter, it does not influence the food intake of animals by itself. Rather, the nutrients (e.g., fats, carbohydrates, and protein) that contain energy, as well as their metabolites, affect the neurological network that controls food intake. Nutrient metabolism requires AAs, vitamins, and minerals, as well as cellular signal transductions. Thus, the relationship between dietary energy content and food intake is complex. In both pigs and poultry, when dietary intakes of AAs, vitamins, and minerals are sufficient, food intake generally decreases as the dietary intake of metabolizable energy increases within a usual range, but increases as the dietary intake of metabolizable energy decreases within a usual range (Forbes 2007). Such a feeding behavior results in either the complete compensation of, or a moderate increase in, dietary energy intake. For example, in growing pigs, dietary DM intake is progressively reduced as the dietary content of digestible energy increases from 12.5 to 15.4 MJ/kg (Henry 1985). In laying hens, food intake progressively decreased from 127 to 107 g/day as the dietary content of metabolizable energy increased from 10.5 to 13.4 MJ/kg diet, but dietary intake of total metabolizable energy increased from 1.34 to 1.42 MJ/day (de Groot 1972).

#### Dietary Content of Sweet Sugars

A small amount of sweet sugars (e.g., glucose and sucrose) in diets confers a sweet taste, thus promoting food intake by animals. Sweet receptors, which are classified as the taste receptor, type 1 (T1R, G-protein-coupled receptor), are present in the apical membrane of taste cells in the taste bud of the tongue (Nelson et al. 2001). Interaction of sweet ligands with the T1R activates its coupled G-protein. The activated $G_s$ $\alpha$-subunit binds to and activates adenylate cyclase to produce cAMP. The latter activates protein kinase A to phosphorylate a voltage-gated $K^+$ channel, resulting in its closure, the depolarization of the taste cell, and the opening of $Ca^{2+}$ channels on the basolateral membrane of the cell. An increase in intracellular $Ca^{2+}$ concentration causes the release of neurotransmitter molecules (in the form of synaptic vesicles), which are received by receptors on the nearby primary sensory neurons. A resulting electrical signal is transmitted along nerve cells to reach the brain's feeding center that perceives and interprets the free-sugar stimulus in the tongue, thereby enhancing consumption of food by mammals, birds, and fish.

#### Glucose Concentrations in the Plasma

In contrast to dietary sweet sugars, Mayer (1953) reported that high circulating levels of glucose reduced appetite in monogastric animals. This author proposed a glucostatic theory in the control of

**TABLE 12.3**
**Nutrients That Affect Food Intake by Ruminants and Nonruminants**

| Nutrients | Feed Intake | Animals |
|---|---|---|
| Dietary content of protein and amino acids | | |
| Low | Reduced | Ruminants and nonruminants |
| Medium | Increased | Ruminants and nonruminants |
| High | Reduced | Ruminants and nonruminants |
| Dietary imbalance of amino acids | Reduced | Ruminants and nonruminants |
| Dietary content of energy | | |
| Low | Reduced | Ruminants and nonruminants |
| Medium | Increased | Ruminants and nonruminants |
| High | Reduced | Ruminants and nonruminants |
| Dietary content of total fatty acids | | |
| Low | Reduced | Nonruminants |
| Medium | Increased | Nonruminants |
| High | Reduced | Ruminants and nonruminants |
| Low dietary content of PUFAs | Reduced | Ruminants and nonruminants |
| Glucose concentration in GIT | | |
| High | Reduced | Nonruminants |
| Low | Increased | Nonruminants |
| High SCFAs in the rumen and blood | Reduced | Ruminants |
| High SCFAs and other weak OAs in diet | Reduced | Nonruminants (weanling) |
| GIT-fill | | |
| Low | Increased | Ruminants and nonruminants |
| High | Reduced | Ruminants and nonruminants |
| High concentrations of KB in blood | Reduced | Ruminants and nonruminants |
| Dehydration status in the body | Reduced | Ruminants and nonruminants |
| Dietary minerals (e.g., Na, Ca, P, Fe, and Zn) | | |
| Low | Reduced | Ruminants and nonruminants |
| High | Reduced | Ruminants and nonruminants |
| Dietary vitamins (e.g., B-complex vitamins) | | |
| Low | Reduced | Nonruminants |
| High | Reduced | Nonruminants |

GIT, gastrointestinal tract; KB, ketone bodies; OAs, organic acids; PUFAs, polyunsaturated fatty acids; SCFAs, short-chain fatty acids.

food intake;specifically, an increase or decrease in glucose concentration in the plasma can serve as a stimulus for satiety or hunger, respectively. Much evidence shows that it is the glucose concentration within the gastrointestinal tract or in the hepatic portal vein, but not in the systemic circulation, that regulates food intake by animals (Forbes 2007). For example, short-term infusion of a large amount of glucose into the gastrointestinal tract of growing pigs to increase its concentration in plasma also reduced food intake (Gregory et al. 1987). In contrast, neither hepatic portal nor jugular infusions of glucose affected short-term food intake by pigs (Houpt et al. 1979). Thus, glucose acts on sensors on the mucosae of the stomach or the small intestine to signal appetite inhibition. In poultry, infusion of glucose into the portal vein but not into peripheral veins suppressed food intake (Shurlock and Forbes 1981a, 1984). Similarly, duodenal infusion of glucose also inhibited food intake in chickens (Shurlock and Forbes 1981a). These results suggest that either glucose sensing by the small intestine or glucose uptake by the liver plays a role in controlling food intake. In dogs, infusion of glucose into the hepatic portal vein inhibits food intake, but the infusion of the

**TABLE 12.4**
**Effects of Dietary Protein Content on Food Intake by Male Sprague–Dawley Rats[a]**

| Day of Feeding | Body Weight (g) | | | Food Intake (g/100 g BW) | | |
|---|---|---|---|---|---|---|
| | 30% Casein | 20% Casein | 5% Casein | 30% Casein | 20% Casein | 5% Casein |
| d 0 | 98.2 ± 3.1 | 98.1 ± 3.2 | 98.3 ± 3.0 | – | – | – |
| d 2 | 124 ± 3.3[b] | 122 ± 3.2[b] | 104 ± 3.1[c] | 9.55 ± 0.39[d] | 10.9 ± 0.43[c] | 14.3 ± 0.53[b] |
| d 4 | 152 ± 3.7[b] | 148 ± 3.5[b] | 120 ± 3.3[c] | 9.16 ± 0.37[d] | 10.6 ± 0.42[c] | 13.9 ± 0.52[b] |
| d 6 | 175 ± 4.0[b] | 171 ± 3.8[b] | 129 ± 3.3[c] | 8.86 ± 0.35[d] | 10.2 ± 0.42[c] | 13.5 ± 0.49[b] |
| d 8 | 196 ± 4.2[b] | 190 ± 4.2[b] | 136 ± 3.4[c] | 8.57 ± 0.34[d] | 9.91 ± 0.45[c] | 13.1 ± 0.47[b] |
| d 10 | 216 ± 4.8[b] | 209 ± 4.5[b] | 146 ± 3.4[c] | 8.30 ± 0.32[d] | 9.72 ± 0.41[c] | 12.7 ± 0.48[b] |
| d 12 | 238 ± 4.9[b] | 230 ± 4.6[b] | 157 ± 3.6[c] | 7.79 ± 0.31[d] | 9.28 ± 0.38[c] | 12.3 ± 0.48[b] |
| d 14 | 256 ± 5.1[b] | 248 ± 4.9[b] | 167 ± 3.5[c] | 7.65 ± 0.32[d] | 8.97 ± 0.36[c] | 11.8 ± 0.44[b] |

[a] The semi-purified diet was prepared as described by Wu et al. (1999). Male Sprague–Dawley rats had free access to their respective diets. Body weight (BW) and food intake were measured every 2 days.

d 0 = 30 days of age. Values are means ± SEM, $n = 10$.

[b–d] Within a row, means not sharing the same letters differ ($P < 0.05$).

same amount of glucose into the general circulation through the jugular vein had no effect (Russek 1970). This finding further indicates a role of the liver in the control of food intake. Hepatic glucose oxidation may be required for this sugar to regulate food consumption of animals. An increase in glucose levels in the portal vein may change the rate of impulses generated in the afferent fibers of the autonomic nerves terminating in the liver (Forbes 2000; Shurlock and Forbes 1981b). When glucose and insulin concentrations in plasma are low, which occurs during fasting, the appetite of animals is stimulated.

### Protein and AAs

Some AAs themselves are neurotransmitters (Chapter 7). Amino acid levels in the brain and plasma affect the concentrations of the neurotransmitters and thus are expected to regulate food intake. For example, a low or high content of dietary protein (e.g., 5% or 30%) reduces food intake by young rats, when compared to a 20%-protein diet (Table 12.4). Inadequate levels of protein and methionine in diets also reduce feed intake by lactating cows (Table 12.5). Much evidence shows that animals

**TABLE 12.5**
**Effects of Dietary Protein and Methionine Levels on Feed Intake and Milk Production by Lactating Cows**

| Variable | Crude Protein Level in Diet | | Rumen-Protected Methionine in Diet | | Pooled SEM |
|---|---|---|---|---|---|
| | 15.8% | 17.1% | 0 g/Day | 9 g/Day | |
| DM intake | 24.4 | 25.5* | 24.6 | 25.3* | 0.37 |
| Milk yield | 40.0 | 41.7* | 40.0 | 41.4† | 0.72 |

*Source:* Broderick et al. *J. Dairy Sci.* 92:2719–28.

Values are kg/day. Holstein cows were fed corn silage-based experimental diets for 4 weeks.

* $P < 0.05$ and

† $P = 0.10$ versus the corresponding control.

**TABLE 12.6**
**Effects of Dietary Arginine Content on Food Intake by Male Sprague–Dawley Rats[a]**

| Day of Feeding | Body Weight (g) | | | Food Intake (g/100 g BW) | | |
|---|---|---|---|---|---|---|
| | 1% Arg | 0.3% Arg | 0% Arg | 1% Arg | 0.3% Arg | 0% Arg |
| d 0 | 96.1 ± 3.4 | 96.0 ± 3.5 | 96.2 ± 3.4 | – | – | – |
| d 2 | 114 ± 4.7[b] | 102 ± 4.0[c] | 99.0 ± 3.3[d] | 10.6 ± 0.32[d] | 11.8 ± 0.34[c] | 13.9 ± 0.35[b] |
| d 4 | 139 ± 5.0[b] | 111 ± 4.4[c] | 105 ± 3.4[c] | 10.1 ± 0.30[d] | 11.2 ± 0.32[c] | 13.3 ± 0.34[b] |
| d 6 | 160 ± 5.2[b] | 122 ± 4.7[c] | 112 ± 3.6[d] | 9.77 ± 0.31[d] | 10.8 ± 0.33[c] | 12.8 ± 0.37[b] |
| d 8 | 179 ± 5.5[b] | 135 ± 5.0[c] | 120 ± 3.7[d] | 9.46 ± 0.33[d] | 10.5 ± 0.35[c] | 12.2 ± 0.36[b] |
| d 10 | 199 ± 5.6[b] | 149 ± 5.2[c] | 128 ± 3.8[d] | 9.15 ± 0.31[d] | 10.1 ± 0.34[c] | 11.8 ± 0.35[b] |
| d 12 | 217 ± 5.8[b] | 161 ± 5.4[c] | 134 ± 4.0[d] | 8.87 ± 0.29[d] | 9.82 ± 0.32[c] | 11.4 ± 0.33[b] |
| d 14 | 232 ± 6.3[b] | 171 ± 5.5[c] | 140 ± 3.9[d] | 8.55 ± 0.28[d] | 9.48 ± 0.31[c] | 11.2 ± 0.33[b] |

[a] The semi-purified diet was prepared as described by Wu et al. (1999). Male Sprague–Dawley rats had free access to their respective diets. Body weight (BW) and food intake were measured every 2 days.
d 0 = 30 days of age. Values are means ± SEM.
[b–d] Within a row, means not sharing the same superscript letters differ ($P < 0.05$).

are very sensitive to dietary AA provision (Wu et al. 2014). For example, young rats fed an arginine-deficient diet consume less food per kg BW than the rats fed an arginine-adequate diet (Table 12.6). When arginine is deficient from the diet, the ratio of arginine: lysine may be imbalanced for young animals and systemic NO synthesis is impaired.

Poultry, pigs, and rats rejected a purified diet lacking one AA or a group of non-synthesizable AAs between 15 and 30 min after starting consumption of the diet (Edmonds and Baker 1987a, b; Edmonds et al. 1987; Harper et al. 1970). These animals continued to eat until satiation when the EAA-free diet was replenished with the missing EAA. Food intake of rats and pigs increased in response to a mild deficiency of dietary lysine, methionine, and threonine, but decreased in response to a mild deficiency of tryptophan. In contrast, excess AA in diets also reduced food intake by animals. For example, young rats ate 25%–60% less food if their diets contained 2% tryptophan; 3% histidine, methionine, phenylalanine, threonine, or lysine; or 4% leucine, isoleucine, or valine (Gietzen et al. 2007; Harper et al. 1970). Young pigs (8 kg BW) consumed 40%, 20%, and 30% less feed if their diets contain 4% DL-methionine, threonine, or tryptophan, respectively, but 4% leucine in the diet did not appear to affect their feed intake (Table 12.7). Interestingly, when young pigs were

**TABLE 12.7**
**Effects of Amino Acids on Feed Intake by Young Pigs (8 kg) Fed a Corn- and Soybean Meal-Based Diet (20% CP)**

| Amino Acid | Supplemental Dose of Amino Acid (%) | | | |
|---|---|---|---|---|
| | 0 | 1 | 2 | 4 |
| | % of feed intake in the control group (no supplementation) | | | |
| DL-Methionine | 100 | 95 | 83 | 61 |
| L-Leucine | 100 | 98 | 99 | 99 |
| L-Threonine | 100 | 95 | 80 | 80 |
| L-Tryptophan | 100 | 96 | 93 | 70 |

*Source:* Edmonds, M.S. and D.H. Baker. 1987. *J. Anim. Sci.* 64:1664–71.

**TABLE 12.8**
**Self-Selection of Corn- and Soybean Meal-Based Diets (20% CP) by Young Pigs (8 kg)**

| Amino Acid Supplementation to Diet | Feed Intake (g/Day) | |
|---|---|---|
| | Days 0–3 | Days 4–9 |
| Control | 358 | 484 |
| 4% L-Lysine | 30 | 224 |
| 4% L-Threonine | 15 | 220 |
| 4% L-Arginine | 27 | 130 |
| 4% DL-Methionine | 8 | 18 |
| 4% L-Tryptophan | 2.7 | 2.4 |

*Source:* Edmonds, M.S. et al. 1987. *J. Anim. Sci.* 65:179–185.

fed corn- and soybean meal-based diets containing supplemental 4% lysine, threonine, arginine, DL-methionine, or tryptophan, feed intake was reduced by 90%–95% within the first 3 days (Table 12.8). Within 4–9 days, the pigs fed the supplemental 4% lysine or threonine diets consumed 38% of feed for the control group, the pigs fed the supplemental 4% arginine diet consumed 20% of feed for the control group, and the pigs fed the supplemental 4% DL-methionine or tryptophan diet ate little feed (Table 12.8). Likewise, young chicks consumed 32% less feed if their diets contained 4% histidine, lysine, threonine, or tryptophan; 44% less feed if their diets contained 4% phenylalanine; or 50% less feed if their diets contained 4% methionine (Table 12.9). Finally, an imbalance among branched-chain AAs (e.g., leucine: isoleucine: valine > 8: 1: 1) or basic AAs (e.g., arginine: lysine: histidine > 2.5:1:0.4) greatly affected feed intake by all animals studied (including rats, pigs, and chicks) (Harper et al. 1970; Smith and Austic 1978). Thus, dietary protein or AA content influences the response of animals to an excess or deficiency of AAs, and different animal species have a different sensitivity to an excess or deficiency of AAs.

Most studies on food intake regulation have focused on AAs that are not synthesized *de novo* in animal cells (Gietzen et al. 2007). However, little is known about a role for synthesizable AAs in the control of feed consumption by animals. Wu et al. (1996) reported that adding 0.5% or 1% glutamine to a corn- and soybean meal-based diet for 2 weeks did not affect feed intake by postweaning pigs. Likewise, adding 0.5%–2% monosodium glutamate to the corn- and soybean meal-based diet (containing 21% crude protein [CP]) for 2 weeks did not affect feed intake by postweaning pigs

**TABLE 12.9**
**Effects of Amino Acid Supplementation on Feed Intake by Young Male Chicks (8-Day Old) Fed a Corn- and Soybean Meal-Based Diet (23% CP)**

| Amino Acid Supplementation | Feed Intake (g/Day) | Amino Acid | Feed Intake (g/Day) Supplementation |
|---|---|---|---|
| Control | 175 | Control | 175 |
| 4% L-Leucine | 175 | 4% L-Lysine | 121 |
| 4% L-Arginine | 165 | 4% L-Histidine | 119 |
| 4% L-Valine | 165 | 4% L-Tryptophan | 118 |
| 4% L-Isoleucine | 155 | 4% L-Phenylalanine | 105 |
| 4% L-Threonine | 125 | 4% L-Methionine | 77 |

*Source:* Edmonds, M.S. and D.H. Baker. 1987. *J. Anim. Sci.* 65:699–705.

**TABLE 12.10**
**Effects of Dietary Supplementation with Glutamine or Glutamic Acid on Feed Intake by Weanling Pigs[a]**

| Amino Acid | Dietary Supplementation (%) | | | | Pooled SEM |
|---|---|---|---|---|---|
| | 0.0 | 0.5 | 1.0 | 2.0 | |
| L-Glutamine | 348[b] | 353[b] | 342[b] | 287[c] | 19 |
| L-Glutamic acid | 352 | 356 | 361 | 358 | 22 |

[a] Values, expressed as g/day, are means with pooled SEM, $n = 12$. Pigs were weaned at 21 days of age (with an average body weight of 5.5 kg) to a corn- and soybean meal-based diet containing 21% CP (Wu et al. 1996) supplemented with 0.0 to 2% L-glutamine or L-glutamic acid.
Feed intake was measured during the second-week postweaning.
[b,c] $P < 0.05$.

(Rezaei et al. 2013). However, supplementing 2% glutamine (Table 12.10) or 4% monosodium glutamate (Rezaei et al. 2013) to a corn- and soybean meal-based diet reduced feed intake by postweaning pigs via different mechanisms. Excess glutamine increased the concentration of ammonia in the plasma, whereas excess monosodium glutamate supplementation increased the dietary intake of sodium (Rezaei et al. 2013). For comparison, supplementing 2% glutamic acid to the same corn- and soybean meal-based diet did not affect food intake by pigs (Table 12.10). Thus, like synthesizable AAs, different non-synthesizable AAs have different effects on feed intake by animals.

Mammals and birds respond similarly to dietary arginine:lysine imbalance. However, the species of fish must be borne in mind in discussing effects of dietary arginine:lysine ratios on feed intake. For example, there is an antagonism between arginine and lysine in certain fish (e.g., Cobia) in that either a high or low ratio of arginine:lysine in the diet (e.g., 1.25/1.00 or 0.56/1.00 vs. 0.91/1.00) reduced their feed intake and growth (Van Nguyen et al. 2014). In contrast, some fish (e.g., Midas *Amphilophus citrinellus*) are not sensitive to a wide range of arginine:lysine ratios in diets (e.g., 0.27/1.00, 0.82/1.00, or 1.63/1.00) (Dabrowski et al. 2007). Thus, supplementing up to 4% Arg to a casein–gelatin-based diet containing 28% CP for 6 weeks had no adverse effects on juvenile channel catfish (Buentello and Gatlin 2001).

### Fatty Acids and Ketone Bodies

High levels of fatty acids in the gastrointestinal tract stimulate the release of intestinal peptide hormones CCK, PYY, GLP-1, gastric insulinotropic polypeptide, and gastric inhibitory peptide but suppress the release of ghrelin (Kaviani and Cooper 2017), and therefore are expected to inhibit feed intake. Similarly, elevated concentrations of fatty acids in plasma enhance the circulating levels of glucose and insulin, which further contribute to reductions in meal size and frequency. Usually, high-fat diets reduce gastric and intestinal emptying, increase the concentrations of free-fatty acids in both the gastrointestinal tract and plasma, and promote the development of the fatty liver, thereby reducing food intake by animals. Such adverse effects of high-fat feeding occur despite no increase in dietary energy content. For example, in 4- to 16-week-old male rats fed ad libitum, food intake decreased from 36.3 to 29.6 g/kg BW per day, as the fat content increased from 4.3% to 23.6% at the same dietary energy content of 4746 kcal/kg diet (Jobgen et al. 2009). In this case, the total dietary energy intake of the rats in the low- and high-fat groups was the same (145 kcal/kg BW per day) (Jobgen et al. 2009).

High intake of dietary fats can result in increased production of acetoacetate and β-hydroxybutyrate (Chapter 6). In the fed state, elevated levels of these ketone bodies may also serve as a satiety signal to suppress food intake (Robinson and Williamson 1980). Intraperitoneal administration of β-hydroxybutyrate to 2-day-old chicks deprived of food for 3 h (0, 0.5, 1.0, or 1.5 g/kg BW) or intracerebroventricular administration of β-hydroxybutyrate (0, 0.25, 0.50, or 1.00 mg in 10 μL) under the same feeding conditions decreased subsequent food intake in a dose-dependent manner (Sashihara et al. 2001). Thus, in poultry, ketone bodies act as an inhibitory signal for food intake in both the central and peripheral nervous systems. In contrast, long-term intracerebroventricular infusion of β-hydroxybutyric acid to female rats for 28 days (fed either a high-fat/low-carbohydrate or a low-fat/high-carbohydrate diet [isocaloric]) reduced body weight but not food intake (Sun et al. 1997). It is possible that peripheral oxidation of ketone bodies may be necessary for them to inhibit the centers of food intake control in the brain. Alternatively, there may be species differences in the response to exogenous ketone bodies.

### Nitric Oxide

Nitric oxide (NO) is synthesized from arginine in nearly all cell types, including enterocytes and nitrergic neurons of the intestine (Chapter 7). By activating guanylate cyclase to produce cGMP, NO relaxes the smooth muscle of the gastrointestinal tract and stimulates the motility of the gut, thereby increasing food intake (Groneberg et al. 2016). Inhibition of NO synthesis impairs gastric accommodation and enhances meal-induced satiety (Tack et al. 2002). It is possible that NO plays a role in adaptive relaxation through a reflex response of the non-adrenergic, non-cholinergic nerves to an increase in intragastric pressure. Physiological levels of NO stimulate the food intake by many studied species, including chickens (Choi et al. 1994), mice (Czech et al. 2003), and rats (De Luca et al. 1995). These findings explain, in part, why dietary arginine deficiency reduces food intake by animals, including rats (Table 12.6).

### Serotonin

Serotonin (a metabolite of tryptophan) is a neurotransmitter that mediates signal transduction between two neurons in the central (e.g., the PVN or VMH neurons for the food intake control) and gastrointestinal nervous systems (Abdalla 2017). Within the synapse, the first nerve cell releases serotonin into the space between the two neurons, and the second nerve cell has receptors which recognize serotonin and elicit a series of physiological responses (e.g., happiness when serotonin levels are high) (Chapter 1). Inhibition of reuptake of serotonin from the intercellular space prolongs its action. Intracerebroventricular or intraperitoneal administration of serotonin into animals, such as rats (Miryala et al. 2011) and fish (Pérez-Maceira et al. 2016), suppresses food intake by inhibiting the POMC/CART neurons in the ARC.

In animals, approximately 90% of serotonin is present in the gastrointestinal tract, and this neurotransmitter directly regulates intestinal contraction and appetite. When the intestinal concentration of serotonin is low, animals crave food. Conversely, a high concentration of serotonin, which can be brought about by activation of gastrointestinal serotonergic neurons, inhibits food intake by animals. Thus, drugs that stimulate serotonergic activity (e.g., fenfluramine, fluoxetine, and 3,4-methylenedioximetanfetamine) or block its uptake (e.g., Sibutramine and opioid antagonists) reduce meal size without affecting the initiation of feeding or meal frequency (Voigt and Fink 2015). Similarly, supplementing 4% tryptophan to the diets of young pigs and chicks substantially decreases their food intake (Edmonds and Baker 1987a,b).

### Norepinephrine

Norepinephrine (a metabolite of tyrosine) is another neurotransmitter that regulates food intake by animals. The release of norepinephrine by the noradrenergic neurons (PVN or VMH) in the brain is stimulated by β-endorphin produced from the ARC neurons. Vagal inputs from peripheral tissues (e.g., the stomach and small intestine) can modulate norepinephrine release by neurons in the central nervous system, thereby integrating central and peripheral signals to control food intake (Voigt and Fink 2015). In general, norepinephrine inhibits food intake. Similar to serotonin, inhibition of norepinephrine reuptake by drugs (e.g., Sibutramine and GW320659) induces satiety and confers an antidepression effect (Kintscher 2012). These findings explain, in part, why dietary supplementation with 4% phenylalanine (a precursor of tyrosine) reduces food intake by animals, including pigs and chicks (Edmonds and Baker 1987a,b).

### Other Chemical Factors

A dietary deficiency or excess of vitamins (e.g., B complex vitamins) and minerals (e.g., Na, Ca, P, Fe, and Zn) reduces food intake by nonruminants (Chapters 9 and 10). In addition, the color and physical form of food (e.g., hardness and particle size) can affect food intake (Forbes 2007). This is particularly important for weanling mammals such as pigs, calves, and lambs. These neonates can consume a large amount of liquid milk but only a small amount of solid food. For example, weanling piglets may eat $< 10\%$ of their preweaning DM intake during the first 3 days postweaning (Wu et al. 1996). Thus, highly palatable, digestible, and sweet foods (e.g., whey powder, blood meal, and sucrose), preferably in a liquid form, should be provided to weanling pigs. Animals learn about the characteristics of their diets to develop conditioned preferences and aversions to meet their physiological needs in their life cycles. Finally, animals with sepsis, fever, inflammation, cancer cachexia, and many other diseases exhibit low feed intake, because endotoxins and inflammatory cytokines (e.g., interleukin-1$\alpha$, interleukin-1$\beta$, interleukin-6, tumor necrosis factor-$\alpha$, and interferon-$\gamma$) inhibit the AgRP/NPY neurons and stimulate the POMC/CART neurons to promote the release of the anorexic neurotransmitter $\alpha$-MSH in the hypothalamus (Burfeind et al. 2016).

Weak organic acids (e.g., lactic acid, formic acid, acetic acid, propionic acid, butyric acid, citric acid, fumaric acid, and benzoic acid) are often supplemented to the diets of weanling mammals (e.g., swine) to enhance their feed intake during the first 2 weeks postweaning (Pluske 2013; Suiryanrayna and Ramana 2015). These acids can be both bacteriostatic and bactericidal, depending on the levels of their inclusion in the diet. Additionally, 0.8% lactic acid has also been added to drinking water for weanling piglets to improve their growth performance and feed efficiency, while reducing the number of *E. coli* in the duodenum and jejunum (Cole et al. 1968). Early weaned piglets (3–4 weeks of age) generally exhibit a limited digestive and absorptive capacity due to: (1) insufficient production of gastric acid (HCl), as well as pancreatic and intestinal digestive enzymes; and (2) reductions in the small-intestinal villus area and the expression of intestinal transport proteins. Lowering dietary pH through the use of weak organic acids can alleviate the weaning-associated problems in young pigs.

## REGULATION OF FOOD INTAKE BY RUMINANTS

Neurotransmitters, neuropeptides, and nutrients that regulate food intake by nonruminants influence feed intake by ruminants in the same way. For example, feeding a diet containing rumen-protected fats between late lactation and calving, as well as after parturition, reduced feed and energy intakes by cows (Kuhla et al. 2016). Additionally, food intake by ruminants is constrained by (1) physical limits of the rumen and other compartments of the gastrointestinal tract; (2) physical and chemical characteristics of dietary ingredients (e.g., particle size, particle fragility, silage fermentation products, the content and ruminal hydrolysis rates of fiber and other carbohydrates, the content and type of fats, and the content and ruminal degradation rates of protein); and (3) metabolic transformations in the production and utilization of SCFAs (Allen 2000; Forbes 2000). Like non-ruminants, the productivity of ruminants is limited by food intake and particularly dietary intakes of protein and energy.

### Physical Limits of the Rumen

The bulk of food also affects the animal's appetite, particularly for ruminants, which typically depend on forages as a major source of nutrients (Ellis et al. 2000). Although the rumen has a very large capacity, the slow rates of digestion and passage of forage feeds mean that each particle of feed remains in the rumen for a very long time (typically 20–50 h) and that rumen capacity can be limiting to food intake. The more fibrous the forage is, the slower its digestion. There are stretch (tension) receptors in the smooth muscle layer of the rumen wall, as well as mechanoreceptors in the epithelium of the rumen. Of note, tension receptors and epithelial mechanoreceptors are also present in the reticulum, abomasum, the small intestine, and the large intestine of ruminants (Forbes 2007). Thus, rumen fill, acting through stretch receptors on the rumen wall, is a major factor regulating the intake of feed (including forages) by ruminants. In addition, entry of feed into the rumen and the increased amount of ruminal content can activate the ruminal epithelial mechanoreceptors. After feeding, physical distension and feed particles stimulate the tension receptors and mechanoreceptors in the rumen wall, respectively, to generate chemical signals through the vagus nerve. These signals are received and interpreted by satiety centers in the brain to terminate a meal (Abdalla 2017). Any factors which decrease the residence time of the particle in the rumen, including reduced particle size of the food, increased activity of the rumen microflora, and replacement of some of the forage with rapidly digested concentrate supplements, will increase voluntary food intake. In contrast, increased forage particle length, increased content of NDF in the diet, and reduced digestibility of dietary DM (including NDF), will reduce feed intake by ruminants (Khan et al. 2014).

## Control of Food Intake by Nutrients and Metabolites

### Dietary Energy Content

Regarding feed intake, ruminants exhibit two-phase responses to dietary energy content (Baumgardt and Peterson 1971; Forbes 2007). Specifically, the feed intake of ruminants increases as dietary energy content increases within a physiological range, whereas their feed intake decreases as dietary energy content increases above the upper physiological level. For example, feed intake and dietary energy intake of growing sheep progressively increased when the dietary content of digestible energy was raised from 6 to 12.5 MJ/kg DM, but gradually decreased when the dietary content of digestible energy was further raised from 12.5 to 14 MJ/kg DM (Baumgardt 1970). Similarly, feed intake and dietary energy intake of growing cattle increased with increasing dietary content of digestible energy from 8 to 13 MJ/kg DM, but their feed intake and dietary energy intake gradually decreased with further increasing dietary content of digestible energy from 13 to 15 MJ/kg DM (Baumgardt 1970).

### Dietary Nitrogen Content

Food intake of ruminants is reduced when they are fed diets containing either very low or very high content of nitrogen (Barker et al. 1988; Forbes 1996). Major function of dietary nitrogen (mostly protein and AAs) is to fulfill the growth of ruminal microbes, which digest dietary carbohydrates to provide energy for both ruminal bacteria and the host. Moore and Kunkle (1995) reported that the dietary DM intake of growing cattle increases progressively from 0% to 2.5% of BW as dietary CP content increases from 0% to 8% (DM basis). Food intake and growth of ruminants (e.g., sheep and cattle) fed protein-deficient diets are increased by infusions of protein into the duodenum (Egan 1977). Thus, adequate food intake is necessary for optimal ruminant production. For example, growing beef cattle (135 kg BW) gain 0.23 kg BW when fed a 10% CP diet (DM basis) but 1.36 kg BW when fed a 22% CP diet. However, excess protein intake, which increases ammonia concentration in the rumen and plasma, reduces food intake by ruminants (Provenza 1996).

### Glucose

In contrast to nonruminants, the concentration of glucose in plasma does not appear to play a role in regulating food intake by ruminants. For example, intraruminal, intravenous, or intracerebroventricular infusion of glucose did not influence food intake by cattle (Forbes 2007). An increase in plasma glucose concentration within a physiological range did not affect food intake by sheep or goats (Weston 1996). These results may be explained by a normally low circulating level of glucose in ruminants (2.3–3 mM), coupled with a low rate of glucose oxidation in the liver and other peripheral tissues.

### Short-Chain Fatty Acids

SCFAs inhibit chemical receptors in the rumen wall and play an important role in regulating feed intake by ruminants (Forbes 2007). When fed cereal grains that are highly digestible in the rumen, lactating cows consume 13% less feed (~3 kg DM/day) (Allen 2000). Similarly, feeding more rapidly fermented starch to the cows increased the proportion of propionate in the SCFAs and the contribution of SCFAs as a fuel, but reduced meal size by 17%, inter-meal intervals by 10%, and overall food intake by 8% (Oba and Allen 2003). Much evidence shows that SCFAs have hypophagic effects on ruminants, and propionate is more potent in reducing feed intake than acetate or butyrate when infused into the portal vein of sheep or the mesenteric veins of steers (Allen et al. 2005). For example, compared with the control, infusion of sodium acetate and sodium propionate (1–15 mol/3 h) into the rumen of cows and sheep reduces food intake in a dose-dependent manner (Grovum 1995). Some of these effects may be brought about by changes in osmotic pressure within the rumen. However, infusion of 1 mol of sodium acetate to the rumen depresses food intake more than the infusion of 1 mol sodium chloride to the rumen (Forbes 2007). Interestingly, denervation of the liver prevents the effect of SCFAs on food intake in ruminants.

Extensive oxidation of propionate in the liver to produce ATP has been proposed as the major mechanism responsible for the hypophagic action of this SCFA. This further supports the view that feeding behavior is regulated, in part, by the hepatic oxidation of metabolic fuels (Allen and Bradford 2012). Of note, the hypophagic response to propionate is amplified by dietary intake of fats and long-chain fatty acids (particularly unsaturated long-chain fatty acids), hyperlipidemia during the periparturient period, as well as gut-derived hormones, such as CCK and glucagon-like peptide 1 (Ingvartsen and Andersen 2000; Litherland et al. 2005).

## DIET SELECTION IN NONRUMINANTS AND RUMINANTS

Animals prefer highly digestible foods that are sources of energy and nutrients, and dislike poorly digestible foods that are bulky and low in energy or protein (Baile and Forbes 1974). Thus, digestibility or gut-fill and food intake are positively correlated (Baile and Forbes 1974). In practice, a marginal deficiency of a nutrient (particularly AAs) leads to an increase in food intake, but a severe deficiency or excess of an essential nutrient (particularly AAs, vitamins, and minerals) markedly reduces food intake. For example, animals choose diets containing a lower amount of protein as they get older to match the declining requirements for protein (Gietzen et al. 2007). Since most nutrients are toxic when present at very high levels in the diet, an excess of a nutrient may reduce food intake, growth performance, milk, and egg production. This is important for grazing animals and for animals offered different kinds of diets. In all animals, the quantity of their feed consumption and the content of nutrients in the self-selected diets reflect their nutritional requirements for maintenance, growth, and health. This involves the coordination of the gastrointestinal tract, the peripheral organs, and the central nervous system (San Gabriel and Uneyama 2013; Stanley et al. 2004). Diet selection is necessary for animals to survive during their evolution.

### Nonruminants

Rats, pigs, and chickens have the ability to select a diet that contains adequate protein or AA levels that are appropriate to their requirements (Baidoo et al. 1986; Baldwin 1985; Summers and Leeson 1979). For example, when rats had free access to diets containing 5%, 25%, 50%, 100%, or 200% of their lysine requirement, they foraged all the diets and selected the diet that contained 100% of their lysine requirement (Gietzen et al. 2007; Harper et al. 1970). When offered isocaloric 0.7%- and 1.0%-lysine diets, young pigs (7.5 kg) preferred a better balanced diet (1.0%-lysine) over a lysine-deficient (0.7% lysine) one (Ettle and Roth 2009). Similarly, pigs and chicks are able to distinguish among diets differing in the content of methionine, threonine, or tryptophan and prefer a better balanced diet over an AA-deficient one (Forbes 2007). When 4- to -9-week-old broilers were given a choice between two foods, both of which contained higher protein content (28% or 32%) than that required for optimal growth, the animals preferred the lower protein (28%) diet and avoided the higher protein (32%) diet (Shariatmadari and Forbes 1993). Of note, when the broilers were offered a choice of two diets: 6.5% versus 11.5%, 6.5% versus 22.5%, 11.5% versus 22.5%, or 22.5% versus 28% protein, they could differentiate successfully between two diets to meet their growth requirements for protein (Shariatmadari and Forbes 1993). Furthermore, poultry have an appetite for diets containing adequate levels of lysine, methionine, vitamin B1, vitamin B6, vitamin C, calcium, and zinc (Rose and Kyriazakis 1991). These findings demonstrate the "nutritional wisdom" of animals to choose between foods with adequate or low protein levels. The innate ability of animals to select food for optimal growth and health is orchestrated by changes in the concentrations of neurotransmitters in the central and peripheral nervous systems.

### RUMINANTS

Grazing ruminants must select forages wisely for growth and survival. They can discriminate among foods based on their color, taste, odor, texture, and shape; select nutritious foods from a diverse array of plant species to meet their nutritional requirements; and avoid foods with low nutrient content and toxins (Milne 1991; Provenza 1996). On the basis of feedbacks from positive and negative consequences of foraging, as well as neurally mediated interactions among the sense, digestive, and central nervous systems, ruminants develop their habits of successful grazing. Like nonruminants, ruminants also have the "nutritional wisdom" to choose between foods with adequate, low, or high protein levels. For example, lambs acquire aversions to foods that are not balanced in AA composition (Egan and Rogers 1978). Furthermore, Kyriazakis and Oldham (1993) reported that growing sheep fed diets containing the same energy content (11 MJ ME/kg feed) but different CP contents (7.8%, 10.9%, 14.1%, 17.2%, and 23.5%; fresh feed basis) gained 273, 326, 412, 418, and 396 g/day, respectively. Specifically, when the sheep were given a choice between a 7.8%- or 10.9%-CP feed and a 23.5%-CP feed, they consumed different proportions of the 23.5%-CP diet (33.9% vs. 18.7% of total feed intake) such that the CP content in the mixed feeds was 13.1% and 13.3%, respectively. When the sheep were given a choice between a 14.1%- or 17.2%-CP feed and a 23.5%-CP feed, they consumed different proportions of the 23.5%-CP diet (17.6% vs. 9% of total feed intake), such that the CP content in the mixed feeds was 15.8% and 17.8%, respectively. Clearly, when the animals were offered diets containing CP contents above the CP requirement, they preferred a diet with a lower CP content. Thus, sheep are able to select a diet that meets their CP requirement and avoid excessive protein intake. In addition to optimizing nutritional balance, ruminants also choose food with sufficient fiber content to stabilize rumen fermentation (e.g., pH, SCFAs, and nonprotein nitrogen).

## ECONOMIC BENEFITS OF FEED EFFICIENCY IMPROVEMENT

Feed efficiency may be expressed as product output/feed input. As noted previously, feed intake is the basis of livestock, poultry, and fish production. After food is ingested by animals, it is converted into protein and fats in tissues or other products (e.g., milk, wool, and eggs). By definition, optimal feed intake positively contributes to maximum feed efficiency. In general, feed cost contributes to ~70% of the total cost of animal production (e.g., 66% in calf feeding and 77% in yearling feeding; Spangler 2013), and feed efficiency is a major determinant of farm profits. For example, in the U.S. cattle production, a 10% improvement in feed efficiency results in a reduction of feed costs by U.S. $1.2 billion and a 43% increase in profits, whereas a 10% improvement in body-weight gain results in an 18% increase in profits (Spangler 2013). Furthermore, Taylor (2016) reported that, in the beef industry, a 1% improvement in feed efficiency has the same economic impact as a 3% increase in the rate of body-weight gain. Similar relationships either between feed efficiency and profits or between body-weight gain and profits also hold true for swine and poultry production (Williams 2012).

While actual feed intake by pigs, poultry, or dairy cows housed in pens can be easily measured, actual feed intake by grazing ruminants is difficult to quantify. Koch et al. (1963) recognized that rates of feed intake are related to the BW and weight gain of animals. These authors suggested that feed intake could be partitioned into two components: (1) the feed intake expected for the given level of production and (2) a residual portion. The residual portion of feed intake, namely residual feed intake (RFI), could be used to identify animals that deviate from their expected level of feed intake. The lower the RFI value, the more efficient the animal is for converting feed into animal tissues or products. Thus, RFI, which is a measure of feed efficiency, is defined as the difference between an animal's actual feed intake (FI) and its expected FI ($FI_{exp}$) based on its size and growth over a specified period.

Expected FI can be predicted from production data by using feeding standards formulae or by regression using actual feed test data (e.g., $FI_{exp} = b_0 + b_1ADG + B_2W^{0.75}$), where ADG is average daily body-weight gain, and $W^{0.75}$ is the metabolic weight of an animal. In cattle divergently selected for RFI, heat production, body composition, and physical activity explained 73% of the variation in RFI: namely, protein turnover plus tissue metabolism plus stress (37%); digestibility (10%); heat increment and fermentation (9%); physical activity (9%); body composition (5%); and feeding patterns (2%) (Herd and Arthur 2009). The mechanisms responsible for 27% of the variation in RFI are still not known, and may involve AA synthesis, gluconeogenesis, and ion transport. Since the heritability of RFI is higher than that of FI, the RFI is a useful variable for breeding and selection of domestic animals, including cattle (Herd and Arthur 2009) and pigs (Patience et al. 2015).

## SUMMARY

Eating through the mouth is the ordinary way for animals to obtain energy and nutrients. Food intake is essential to the growth, development, and survival of mammals, birds, fish, and shrimp. A limited amount of ration is provided to some livestock species during a certain phase of production (e.g., gestating sows, gestating ewes, and breeding stocks) in modern farming systems, so that they will not become obese or overweight. However, most ruminants and nonruminants have free access to their foods under practical housing, grazing, or feeding conditions. Knowledge about physiological and nutritional control of food intake by animals is critical for animal productivity and welfare, as well as feed efficiency. The latter can be measured as RFI in ruminants. Research over the past 50 years has shown that the feed intake of animals is regulated by complex interactions among nutrients (in both the gastrointestinal tract and plasma), gastrointestinal sensing and fill, hormones, neuropeptides, and neurotransmitters (Figure 12.4). Either a high dietary content of fats, protein, and energy or a low dietary content of vitamins (e.g., B-complex vitamins) and minerals (e.g., Na, Ca, P, and Zn) reduces food intake by animals. The relationship between dietary energy content and food intake is complex, because nutrient metabolism depends on AAs, vitamins, and minerals, as well as cellular regulatory machinery. In general, feed intake is reduced when dietary energy or nutrient content is low, increased when dietary energy or nutrient content is intermediate, and decreased when dietary energy or nutrient content is high.

Leptin (released from white adipose tissue) and insulin (released from the pancreatic β-cells) inhibit food intake by activating the POMC/CART neurons and suppressing the AgRP/NPY neurons. These two hormones play an important role in both the acute and long-term energy balance of animals. Three important gastrointestinal peptides that regulate food intake are ghrelin, PYY, and CCK. These molecules act through different mechanisms. Specifically, PYY and CCK (released from the endocrine cells in the gastrointestinal tract) suppress AgRP/NPY neurons and reduce expression of the NPY gene, respectively, thereby inhibiting food intake. In contrast, ghrelin (another gastrointestinal peptide) stimulates food intake of animals by suppressing the POMC/CART neurons and activating the AgRP/NPY neurons through the $Ca^{2+}$-protein kinase C signaling pathway. As the major "hunger hormone," ghrelin opposes the actions of leptin, which is the major "satiety hormone." Besides the neuropeptides and hormones that are synthesized from AAs, neurotransmitters are either AAs (e.g., aspartate, glutamate, and glycine) or their metabolites (e.g., NO, serotonin, GABA, and norepinephrine). Thus, dietary intake of protein or AAs profoundly influences the neurological network and thereby food intake by animals. This provides the biochemical basis for

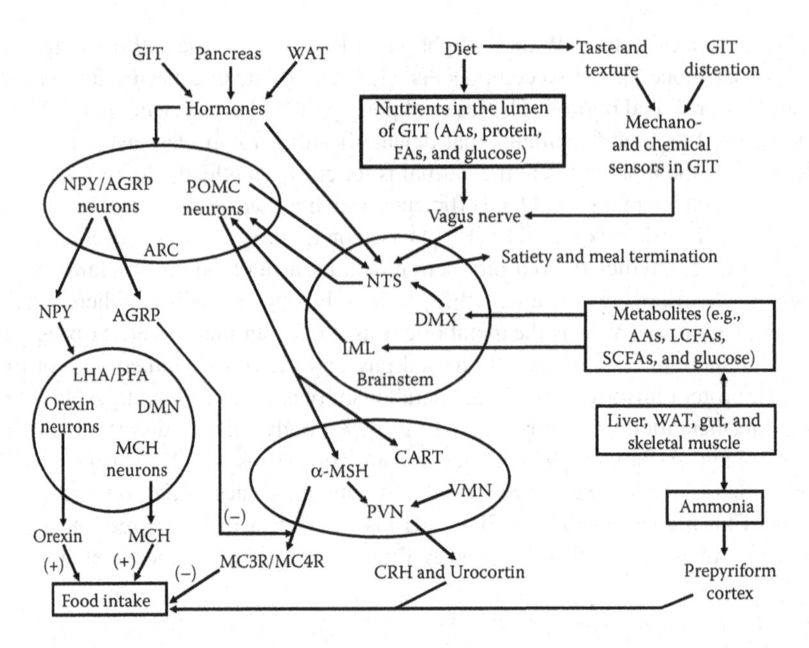


**FIGURE 12.4** A summary of mechanisms whereby food intake of animals is regulated by a complex interactive network among nutrients (in both the gastrointestinal tract and plasma), gastrointestinal sensing and filling, hormones, neuropeptides, and neurotransmitters. AAs, amino acids; AgRP, agouti-related peptide; ARC, Arcuate; CART, cocaine-amphetamine regulated transcript; CRH, corticotrophin-releasing hormone; DMN, dorsal medial nucleus of the hypothalamus; DMX, dorsal motor nucleus of the vagus nerve; FAs, fatty acids; GIT, gastrointestinal tract; IML, intermediolateral cell column; LCFAs, long-chain fatty acids; LHA, lateral hypothalamic area; MC, melanocortin; MC3R, melanocortin-3 receptor; MC4R, melanocortin-4 receptor; MCH, melanin-concentrating hormone; α-MSH, α-melanocyte-stimulating hormone; NPY, neuropeptide Y; PFA, perifornical area; POMC pro-opiomelanocortin; PVN, paraventricular nucleus; NTS, nucleus tractus solitarius; SCFAs, short-chain fatty acids; VMN, ventromedial nucleus; WAT, white adipose tissue; (+), stimulation; (–), inhibition.

self-selection or "foraging" of foods as an innate ability of both ruminants and nonruminants to meet their nutritional and physiological needs. Collectively, food intake is regulated by dietary, genetic, physiological, pathological, and environmental factors, as well as management and behavior.

## REFERENCES

Abdalla, M.M. 2017. Central and peripheral control of food intake. *Endocr. Regul.* 51:52–70.

Adam, C.L. and P.A. Findlay. 2010. Decreased blood-brain leptin transfer in an ovine model of obesity and weight loss: Resolving the cause of leptin resistance. *Int. J. Obes.* 34:980–988.

Alhadeff, A.L., D. Golub, M.R. Hayes, and H.J. Grill. 2015. Peptide YY signaling in the lateral parabrachial nucleus increases food intake through the Y1 receptor. *Am. J. Physiol. Endocrinol. Metab.* 309: E759–E766.

Allen, M.S. 2000. Effects of diet on short-term regulation of feed intake by lactating dairy cattle. *J. Dairy Sci.* 83:1598–1624.

Allen, M.S. and B.J. Bradford. 2012. Control of food intake by metabolism of fuels: A comparison across species. *Proc. Nutr. Soc.* 71:401–409.

Allen, M.S., B.J. Bradford, and K.J. Harvatine. 2005. The cow as a model to study food intake regulation. *Annu. Rev. Nutr.* 25:523–547.

Auffray, P. 1969. Effect of ventromedial hypothalamic lesions on food intake in the pig. *Annales de Biologie Animale, Biochimie et Biophysique* 9:513–526.

Baidoo, S.K., M.K., McIntosh, and F.X. Aherne. 1986. Selection preference of starter pigs fed canola meal and soyabean meal supplemented diets. *Can. J. Anim. Sci.* 66:1039–1049.

Baile, C.A. and J.M. Forbes. 1974. Control of feed intake and regulation of energy balance in ruminants. *Physiol. Rev.* 54:160–214.

Baile, C.A. and M.A. Della-Fera. 1984. Peptidergic control of food intake in food-producing animals. *Fed. Proc.* 43:2898–2902.

Baldwin, B.A. 1985. Neural and hormonal mechanisms regulating food intake. *Proc. Nutr. Soc.* 44:303–311.

Barker, D.J., P.J. May, and W.M. Jones. 1988. Controlling the intake of grain supplements by cattle, using ureasuperphosphate. *Proc. Aust. Sot. Anim. Prod.* 17:146–149.

Baumgardt, B.R. 1970. Control of feed intake in the regulation of energy balance. In: *Physiology of Digestion and Metabolism in the Ruminant.* Edited by A.T. Phillipson. Oriel Press Ltd., Newcastle, pp. 235–253.

Baumgardt, B.R. and Peterson, A.D. 1971. Regulation of food intake in ruminants. 1. Caloric density of diets for young growing lambs. *J. Dairy Sci.* 54:1191–1194.

Breer, H., J. Eberle, C. Frick, D. Haid, and P. Widmayer. 2012. Gastrointestinal chemosensation: Chemosensory cells in the alimentary tract. *Histochem. Cell Biol.* 138:13–24.

Bruijnzeel, A.W., L.W. Corrie, J.A. Rogers, and H. Yamada. 2011. Effects of insulin and leptin in the ventral tegmental area and arcuate hypothalamic nucleus on food intake and brain reward function in female rats. *Behav. Brain. Res.* 219:254–264.

Buentello, J. A. and D. M. Gatlin 3rd. 2001. Effects of elevated dietary arginine on resistance of channel catfish to exposure to *Edwardsiella ictaluri. J. Aquatic Animal Health* 13:194–201.

Burfeind, K.G., K.A. Michaelis, and D.L. Marks. 2016. The central role of hypothalamic inflammation in the acute illness response and cachexia. *Semin. Cell Dev. Biol.* 54:42–52.

Catanese, F., P. Fernández, J.J. Villalba, and R.A. Distel. 2016. The physiological consequences of ingesting a toxic plant (*Diplotaxis tenuifolia*) influence subsequent foraging decisions by sheep (*Ovis aries*). *Physiol. Behav.* 167:238–247.

Chen, L.L., Q.Y. Jiang, X.T. Zhu, G. Shu, Y.F. Bin, X.Q. Wang, P. Gao, and Y.L. Zhang. 2007. Ghrelin ligand-receptor mRNA expression in hypothalamus, proventriculus and liver of chicken (Gallus gallus domesticus): Studies on ontogeny and feeding condition. *Comp. Biochem. Physiol.* A 147:893–902.

Chen, J., K.A. Scott, Z. Zhao, T.H. Moran, and S. Bi. 2008. Characterization of the feeding inhibition and neural activation produced by dorsomedial hypothalamic cholecystokinin administration. *Neurosci.* 152:178–188.

Choi, Y.H., M. Furuse, J. Okumura, and D.M. Denbow. 1994. Nitric oxide controls feeding behavior in the chicken. *Brain Res.* 654:163–166.

Cole, D.J.A., R.M. Beal, and J.R. Luscombe. 1968. The effect on performance and bacterial flora of lactic acid, propionic acid, calcium propionate and calcium acrylate in the drinking water of the weaned pigs. *Vet. Rec.* 83:459–464.

Cowley, M.A., J.L. Smart, M. Rubinstein, M.G. Cerdán, S. Diano, T.L. Horvath, R.D. Cone, and M.J. Low. 2001. Leptin activates anorexigenic POMC neurons through a neural network in the arcuate nucleus. *Nature* 411:480–484.

Czech, D.A., M.R. Kazel, and J. Harris. 2003. A nitric oxide synthase inhibitor, *N*(G)-nitro-l-arginine methyl ester, attenuates lipoprivic feeding in mice. *Physiol. Behav.* 80:75–79.

Dabrowski, K., M. Arslan, B.F. Terjesen, and Y.F. Zhang. 2007. The effect of dietary indispensable amino acid imbalances on feed intake: Is there a sensing of deficiency and neural signaling present in fish? *Aquaculture* 268:136–142.

Daniel, J.A., T.H. Elsasser, C.D. Morrison, D.H. Keisler, B.K. Whitlock, B. Steele, D. Pugh, and J.L. Sartin. 2003. Leptin, tumor necrosis factor-alpha (TNF), and CD14 in ovine adipose tissue and changes in circulating TNF in lean and fat sheep. *J. Anim. Sci.* 81:2590–2599.

de Groot, G. 1972. A marginal income and cost analysis of the effect of nutrient density on the performance of White Leghorn hens in battery cages. *Br. Poult. Sci.* 13:503–520.

De Luca, B., M. Monda, and A. Sullo. 1995. Changes in eating behavior and thermogenic activity following inhibition of nitric oxide formation. *Am. J. Physiol.* 268:R1533–R1538.

Egan, A.R. 1977. Nutritional status and intake regulation in sheen VIII. Relationships between the voluntary intake of herbage by sheep and the protein/energy ratio in the digestion products. *Aust. J. Agr. Res.* 28:907–915.

Egan, A.R. and Q.R. Rogers. 1978. Amino acid imbalance in ruminant lambs. *Aust. J. Agr. Res.* 29:1263–1279.

Edmonds, M.S. and D.H. Baker. 1987a. Amino acid excesses for young pigs: Effects of excess methionine, tryptophan, threonine or leucine. *J. Anim. Sci.* 64:1664–1671.

Edmonds, M.S. and D.H. Baker. 1987b. Comparative effects of individual amino acid excesses when added to a corn-soybean meal diet: Effects on growth and dietary choice in the chick. *J. Anim. Sci.* 65:699–705.

Edmonds, M.S., Gonyou HW, and Baker DH. 1987. Effect of excess levels of methionine, tryptophan, arginine, lysine or threonine on growth and dietary choice in the pig. *J. Anim. Sci.* 65:179–185.
Ellis, W.C., Poppi, D. and Matis, J.H. 2000. Feed intake in ruminants: Kinetic aspects. In: *Farm Animal Metabolism and Nutrition*. Edited by J.P.F. D'Mello. CAPI Publishing, Oxon, UK, pp. 335–363.
Ettle, T. and F.X. Roth. 2009. Dietary selection for lysine by piglets at differing feeding regimen. *Livest. Sci.* 122:259–263.
Forbes, J.M. 1996. Integration of regulatory signals controlling forage intake in ruminants. *J. Anim. Sci.* 74:3029–3035.
Forbes, J.M. 2000. Physiological and metabolic aspects of feed intake control. In: *Farm Animal Metabolism and Nutrition*. Edited by J.P.F. D'Mello. CAPI Publishing, Oxon, UK, pp. 319–333.
Forbes, J.M. 2007. *Voluntary Food Intake and Diet Selection in Farm Animals.* CABI International, Wallingford, UK.
Gietzen, D.W., S. Hao, and T.G. Anthony. 2007. Mechanisms of food intake repression in indispensable amino acid deficiency. *Annu Rev Nutr.* 2007;27:63–78.
Gregory, P.C., M. McFadyen, and D.V. Rayner. 1987. The Influence of gastrointestinal infusions of glucose on regulation of food intake in pigs. *Q. J. Exp. Physiol.* 72:525–535.
Groneberg, D., B. Voussen, and A. Friebe. 2016. Integrative control of gastrointestinal motility by nitric oxide. *Curr. Med. Chem.* 23:2715–2735.
Grovum, W. L. 1995. Mechanisms explaining the effects of short chain fatty acids on feed intake in ruminants-osmotic pressure, insulin and glucagons. In: *Ruminant Physiology: Digestion, Metabolism, Growth and Reproduction*. Edited by W.V. Engelhardt, S. Leonhard-Marek, G. Breves and D. Giesecke. Ferdinand Enke Verlag, Stuttgart, pp. 137–197.
Harper, A.E., N.J. Benevenga, and R.M. Wohlhueter. 1970. Effects of ingestion of disproportionate amounts of amino acids. *Physiol. Rev.* 50:428–558.
Henry, Y. 1985. Dietary factors involved in feed intake regulation in growing pigs: A review. *Lives. Prod. Sci.* 12:339–354.
Herd, R.M. and P.F. Arthur. 2009. Physiological basis for residual feed intake. *J. Anim. Sci.* 87(E. Suppl.):E64–E71.
Houpt, T.R., S.M. Anika, and K.A. Houpt. 1979. Preabsorptive intestinal satiety controls of food intake in pigs. *Am. J. Physiol.* 236:R328–R337.
Ingvartsen, K.L. and J.B. Andersen. 2000. Integration of metabolism and intake regulation: A review focusing on periparturient animals. *J. Dairy Sci.* 83:1573–1597.
Jobgen, W.J., C.J. Meininger, S.C. Jobgen, P. Li, M.-J. Lee, S.B. Smith, T.E. Spencer, S.K. Fried, and G. Wu. 2009. Dietary L-arginine supplementation reduces white-fat gain and enhances skeletal muscle and brown fat masses in diet-induced obese rats. *J. Nutr.* 139:230–237.
Kaviani, S. and J.A. Cooper. 2017. Appetite responses to high-fat meals or diets of varying fatty acid composition: A comprehensive review. *Eur. J. Clin. Nutr.* doi: 10.1038/ejcn.2016.250.
Khan, M.A., A. Bach, L. Castells, D.M. Weary, and M.A. von Keyserlingk. 2014. Effects of particle size and moisture levels in mixed rations on the feeding behavior of dairy heifers. *Animal* 8:1722–1727.
Kintscher, U. 2012. Reuptake inhibitors of dopamine, noradrenaline, and serotonin. *Handb. Exp. Pharmacol.* 209:339–347.
Kirouac, G.J. 2015. Placing the paraventricular nucleus of the thalamus within the brain circuits that control behavior. *Neurosci. Biobehav. Rev.* 56:315–329.
Koch, R.M., L.A. Swiger, D. Chambers, and K.E. Gregory. 1963. Efficiency of feed use in beef cattle. *J. Anim. Sci.* 22:486–494.
Kojima, M. and K. Kangawa. 2005. Ghrelin: Structure and function. *Physiol. Rev.* 85:495–522.
Kuhla, B., C.C. Metges, and H.M. Hammon. 2016. Endogenous and dietary lipids influencing feed intake and energy metabolism of periparturient dairy cows. *Dom. Anim. Endocrinol.* 56:S2–S10.
Kyriazakis, I. and J.D. Oldham. 1993. Diet selection in sheep: The ability of growing lambs to select a diet that meets their crude protein (nitrogen×6.25) requirements. *Br. J. Nutr.* 69:617–629.
Litherland, N.B., S. Thire, A.D. Beaulieu, C.K. Reynolds, J.A. Benson, and J.K. Drackley. 2005. Dry matter intake is decreased more by abomasal infusion of unsaturated free fatty acids than by unsaturated triglycerides. *J. Dairy Sci.* 88:632–643.
Marx, J. 2003. Cellular warriors at the battle of the bulge. *Science* 299:846–849.
Mayer, J. 1953. Glucostatic regulation of food intake. *N. Engl. J. Med.* 249:13–16.
Milne, J.A. 1991. Diet selection by grazing animals. *Proc. Nutr. Soc.* 50:77–85.
Miryala, C.S.J., N. Maswood, and L. Uphouse. 2011. Fluoxetine prevents 8-OH-DPAT-induced hyperphagia in Fischer inbred rats. *Pharmacol. Biochem. Behav.* 98:311–315.

Moore, J.E. and W.E. Kunkle. 1995. Improving forage supplementation programs for beef cattle. *Proc. Florida Ruminant Nutr. Symposium*, University of Florida, Gainesville, FL, pp. 65–74.

Nelson, G., M.A. Hoon, J. Chandrashekar, Y. Zhang, N.J. Ryba, and C.S. Zuker. 2001. Mammalian sweet taste receptors. *Cell* 106:381–390.

Niot, I. and P. Besnard. 2017. Appetite control by the tongue-gut axis and evaluation of the role of CD36/SR-B2. *Biochimie* 136:27–32.

Oba, M. and M.S. Allen. 2003. Effects of corn grain conservation method on feeding behavior and productivity of lactating dairy cows at two dietary starch concentrations. *J. Dairy Sci.* 86:174–183.

Patience, J.F., M.C. Rossoni-Serão, and N.A. Gutiérrez. 2015. A review of feed efficiency in swine: Biology and application. *J. Anim. Sci. Biotechnol.* 6:33.

Pérez-Maceira, J.J., C. Otero-Rodiño, M.J. Mancebo, J.L. Soengas, and M. Aldegunde. 2016. Food intake inhibition in rainbow trout induced by activation of serotonin 5-HT2C receptors is associated with increases in POMC, CART and CRF mRNA abundance in hypothalamus. *J. Comp. Physiol. B* 186:313–321.

Pluske, J.R. 2013. Feed- and feed additives-related aspects of gut health and development in weanling pigs. *J. Anim. Sci. Biotechnol.* 4:1.

Provenza, F.D. 1996. Acquired aversions as the basis for varied diets of ruminants foraging on rangelands. *J. Anim. Sci.* 74:2010–2020.

Rezaei, R., D.A. Knabe, C.D. Tekwe, S. Dahanayaka, M.D. Ficken, S.E. Fielder, S.J. Eide, S.L. Lovering, and G. Wu. 2013. Dietary supplementation with monosodium glutamate is safe and improves growth performance in postweaning pigs. *Amino Acids* 44:911–923.

Robinson, A.M. and D.H. Williamson. 1980. Physiological roles of ketone bodies as substrates and signals in mammalian tissues. *Physiol. Rev.* 60:143–187.

Rose, S.P. and I. Kyriazakis. 1991. Diet selection of pigs and poultry. *Proc. Nutr. Soc.* 50:87–98.

Russek, M. 1970. Demonstration of the influence of an hepatic glucose-sensitive mechanism on food intake. *Physiol. Behavior* 5:1207–1209.

San Gabriel, A. and Uneyama, H. 2013. Amino acid sensing in the gastrointestinal tract. *Amino Acids* 45:451–461.

Sartin, J.L., B.K. Whitlock, and J.A. Daniel. 2011. Triennial growth symposium: Neural regulation of feed intake: Modification by hormones, fasting, and disease. *J. Anim. Sci.* 89:1991–2003.

Sashihara, K., M. Miyamoto, A. Ohgushi, D.M. Denbow, and M. Furuse. 2001. Influence of ketone body and the inhibition of fatty acid oxidation on the food intake of the chick. *Br. Poult. Sci.* 42:405–408.

Shariatmadari, F. and J.M. Forbes. 1993. Growth and food intake responses to diets of different protein contents and a choice between diets containing two levels of protein in broiler and layer strains of chicken. *Br. Poultry Sci.* 34:959–970.

Shurlock, T.G.H. and J.M. Forbes. 1981a. Factors affecting food intake in the domestic chicken: The effect of infusions of nutritive and non-nutritive substances into the crop and duodenum. *Br. Poultry Sci.* 22:323–331.

Shurlock, T.G.H. and J.M. Forbes. 1981b. Evidence for hepatic glucostatic regulation of food intake in the domestic chicken and its interaction with gastrointestinal control. *Br. Poultry Sci.* 22:333–346.

Shurlock, T.G.H. and J.M. Forbes. 1984. Effects on voluntary intake of infusions of glucose and amino acids into the hepatic portal vein of chickens. *Br. Poultry Sci.* 25:303–308.

Smith, T.K. and R.E. Austic. 1978. The branched-chain amino acid antagonism in chicks. *J. Nutr.* 108:1180–1191.

Spangler, M. 2013. Genetic improvement of feed efficiency: Tools and tactics. http://www.iowabeefcenter.org/proceedings/FeedEfficiencySelection.pdf. Accessed on April 10, 2017.

Stanley, S., K. Wynne, and S. Bloom. 2004. Gastrointestinal satiety signals III. Glucagon-like peptide 1, oxyntomodulin, peptide YY, and pancreatic polypeptide. *Am. J. Physiol. Gastrointest. Liver Physiol.* 286:G693–G697.

Steinert, R.E., C. Feinle-Bisset, L. Asarian, M. Horowitz, C. Beglinger, and N. Geary. 2017. Ghrelin, CCK, GLP-1, and PYY(3–36): Secretory controls and physiological roles in eating and glycemia in health, obesity, and after RYGB. *Physiol. Rev.* 97:411–463.

Summers, J.D. and S. Leeson. 1979. Diet presentation and feeding. In: *Food Intake Regulation in Poultry.* Edited by K.N. Boormanand B.M. Freeman. Longman, Edinburgh, pp. 445–469.

Sun, M., R.J. Martin, and G.L. Edwards. 1997. ICV beta-hydroxybutyrate: Effects on food intake, body composition, and body weight in rats. *Physiol. Behav.* 61:433–436.

Suiryanrayna, M.V.A.N. and J.V. Ramana. 2015. A review of the effects of dietary organic acids fed to swine. *J. Anim. Sci. Biotechnol.* 6:45.

Sutton, A.K., M.G. Myers, and D.P. Olson. 2016. The role of PVH circuits in peptin action and energy balance. *Annu. Rev. Physiol.* 78:207–221.

Tack, J., I. Demedts, A. Meulemans, J. Schuurkes, and J. Janssens. 2002. Role of nitric oxide in the gastric accommodation reflex and in meal induced satiety in humans. *Gut* 51:219–224.

Taylor, J. 2016. National program for genetic improvement of feed efficiency in beef cattle. *Beef Improvement Federation Annual Meeting and Symposium*. Manhattan, Kansas.

Thon, M., T. Hosoi, and K. Ozawa. 2016. Possible integrative actions of leptin and insulin signaling in the hypothalamus targeting energy homeostasis. *Front. Endocrinol* (*Lausanne*). 7:138.

Van Nguyen, M., I. Ronnestad, L. Buttle, H.V. Lai, and M. Espe. 2014. Imbalanced lysine to arginine ratios reduced performance in juvenile cobia (*Rachycentron canadum*) fed high plant protein diets. *Aquaculture Nutrition* 20:25–35.

Vogt, M.C. and J.C. Brüning. 2013. CNS insulin signaling in the control of energy homeostasis and glucose metabolism—From embryo to old age. *Trends Endocrinol. Metab.* 24:76–84.

Voigt, J.P. and H. Fink. 2015. Serotonin controlling feeding and satiety. *Behav. Brain. Res.* 277:14–31.

Wadhera, D. and E.D. Capaldi-Phillips. 2014. A review of visual cues associated with food on food acceptance and consumption. *Eat. Behav.* 15:132–143.

Weston, R.H. 1996. Some aspects of constraint to forage consumption by ruminants. *Aust. J. Agric. Res.* 47:175–197.

Williams, N. 2012. Feed efficiency potential for pigs and poultry. https://www.slideshare.net/trufflemedia/dr-noel-williams-feed-efficiency-potential-for-pigs-and-poultry. Accessed on April 10, 2017.

Wu, G., F.W. Bazer, Z.L. Dai, D.F. Li, J.J. Wang, and Z.L. Wu. 2014. Amino acid nutrition in animals: Protein synthesis and beyond. *Annu. Rev. Anim. Biosci.* 2:387–417.

Wu, G., N.E. Flynn, S.P. Flynn, C.A. Jolly, and P.K. Davis. 1999. Dietary protein or arginine deficiency impairs constitutive and inducible nitric oxide synthesis by young rats. *J. Nutr.* 129:1347–1354.

Wu, G., S.A. Meier, and D.A. Knabe. 1996. Dietary glutamine supplementation prevents jejunal atrophy in weaned pigs. *J. Nutr.* 126:2578–2584.

Wu G, F.W. Bazer, J.M. Wallace, and T.E. Spencer. 2006. Intrauterine growth retardation: Implications for the animal sciences. *J. Anim. Sci.* 84:2316–2337.

# 13 Feed Additives

Improving the efficiency of utilization of dietary nutrients is essential to enhance the efficiency of animal production (Wu et al. 2014) and farm profits (Spangler 2013). Digestion and metabolism of nutrients are two major targets for increasing nutrient utilization by ruminants, nonruminants, fish, and shrimp. Digestive enzymes are synthesized and secreted by the gastrointestinal tract, intestinal microbes, liver, and pancreas to digest feedstuffs (Chapter 1). However, the amounts of proteases, carbohydrases, and lipases in the stomach and the small intestine may be inefficient for optimal digestion of protein, fats, fibers, minerals, and vitamins in animals under certain production conditions (e.g., heat and cold stresses, disease, and weaning). Likewise, nutrients that are ordinarily present in feed may not be sufficient for maximal growth or feed efficiency of animals, and therefore are supplemented to diets to enhance productivity (Tan and Yin 2017). Furthermore, exogenous substances are often needed as anti-mold or anti-oxidative ingredients in rations under production conditions. Thus, dietary supplementation with digestive enzymes, functional ingredients, growth-promoting agents, or anti-mycotoxin absorbents can allow for more economic utilization of raw materials by livestock, poultry, and fish, while reducing the output of undigested nutrients (protein, carbohydrates, calcium, and phosphorus) and microbial fermentation products (e.g., ammonia, urea, and indoles) in manure (Bedford and Schulze 1998; Phillips et al. 1995; Weaver and Kim 2014).

By definition, any substance that is intentionally added to feed is a feed additive. Over the past five decades, feed additives (exogenous enzymes and nonenzymes, including amino acids [AAs], fatty acids, sugars, vitamins, minerals, probiotics, prebiotics, and antibiotics) have received increasing attention from both nutritionists and producers (Cowieson and Roos 2016; Hou et al. 2017; Jiang and Xiong 2016). Since most enzymes act on specific substrates, their use should be limited to certain diets (Beauchemin et al. 2001; Bedford 2000). How animals respond to a feed additive will depend on many factors, including (a) its source, form, and bioactivity; (b) the age, physiological conditions, digestive structure, and health status (e.g., bacterial, viral, or parasite infection); (c) dietary ingredients, their interactions and nutritional compositions, and amounts of anti-nutritional factors; and (d) the environment in which animals are housed and fed. Thus, the efficacy of feed additives varies with animal species, farms, feed composition, and methods of manufacture, and economic value must be verified under practical production conditions. The main objective of this chapter is to highlight the use of feed additives in animal production and the underlying mechanisms of actions, and to outline those conditions where their inclusion in diets is most likely to result in beneficial effects.

## ENZYME ADDITIVES

### Overview

Barley, rye, triticale, and wheat are common ingredients of poultry and swine diets in many regions of the world (Bedford 2000; Pettersson and Aman 1989). However, these cereals contain large amounts of soluble non-starch polysaccharides (NSPs), which form viscous gels in the presence of water (Chapter 2). Major adverse effects of NSPs result from their ability to increase digesta viscosity in the gastrointestinal tract, impair the digestion and absorption of nutrients, and interact with the gut microflora to alter the morphology and function of the digestive system (Chapter 5). Thus, the majority of commercial enzyme products that are used for poultry feeding are added to barley, oats, peas, rye, or wheat-based diets (Bedford and Schulze 1998), but some studies have been conducted to evaluate the enzyme preparations for swine diets (Kerr and Shurson 2013). The

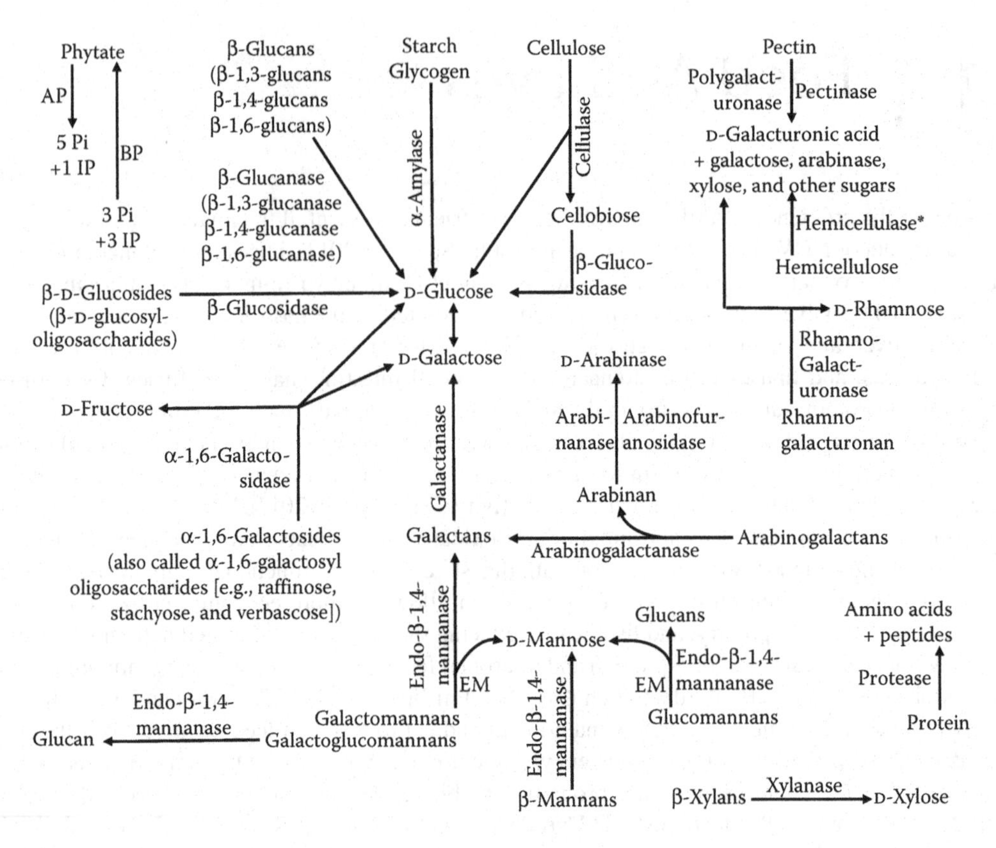


**FIGURE 13.1** Use of carbohydrases and proteases to hydrolyze polysaccharides and protein in diets, respectively. All these enzymes have been used as feed additives to nonruminant diets, whereas cellulase and hemicellulase are generally used for ruminant diets. Complete hydrolysis products are shown. However, in the digestive tract of nonruminants fed the feed carbohydrases, plant-source polysaccharides are partially hydrolyzed. *A complex mixture of enzymes is required to fully degrade hemicelluloses. AP, acidic phytase; BP, alkaline phytase; EM, exo-mannanase; IP, inositol phosphate; Pi, inorganic phosphate.

feed enzymes used in nonruminant diets include: (1) β-glucanases, pentosanases, or phytases; (2) a mixture of all these enzymes; (3) a mixture of proteases; and (4) a mixture of carbohydrases and proteases (Figure 13.1). In contrast, carbohydrases for ruminant diets generally fall into the classification of cellulases and hemicellulases (Kung 2001). Although hundreds of enzyme products are marketed for livestock and poultry to date, they are manufactured primarily from four bacterial species (*Bacillus subtilis*, *Lactobacillus acidophilus*, *L. plantarum*, and *Streptococcus faecium*, spp.) and three fungal species (*Aspergillus oryzae*, *Trichoderma reesei*, and *Saccharomyces cerevisiae*) (Meale et al. 2014). In nonruminants, a reduction in the viscosity of the small-intestinal contents is primarily responsible for the beneficial effect of supplementation with carbohydrases on nutrient digestion and absorption. In contrast, supplemental enzymes work mainly by facilitating the utilization of dietary fiber in ruminants (Beauchemin et al. 1997; Iwaasa et al. 1997). Thus, use of enzyme additives depends on animal species and their developmental stages.

## Special Thermozymes for Feeds

Like any proteins, feed enzymes can be inactivated by heating, acidification, alkaline treatment, and by interaction with certain metals. In recent years, some thermostable enzymes (called hyperthermophilic enzymes or thermozymes) have been produced by hyperthermophiles (bacteria and archaea with optimal growth temperatures of >80°C) or by *E. coli* through the DNA-recombinant techniques (Vieille and Zeikus 2001). To date, thermozymes for feeds include xylanase, phytase, endoglucanase, and cellobiohydrolase (Fakruddin 2017). Their biochemical properties have important implications for the feed industry. Specifically, in the manufacture of animal feeds, pelleting is often used to convert mash feeds into compressed pellets to confer several advantages, including convenient handling and transport, reduction of dust and waste, higher digestibility of carbohydrates, and reduction or elimination of dietary pathogens (Amerah et al. 2011). This process first involves a short conditioning period of exposure to high temperatures (e.g., 70–100°C for seconds to several minutes, depending on the type and formulation of the feed) and steam, followed by extrusion through a pelleting die that temporarily raises the temperature of the feed because of friction. Since thermozymes are stable under pelleting conditions, it is now feasible to incorporate these enzymes into feed pellets.

## Enzyme Additives for Nonruminants

### β-Glucanases

β-Glucanases, which are also called β-D-glucan glucanohydrolases, are synthesized from AAs by microbes. The stomach and the small intestine of poultry and swine do not produce animal-source enzymes to break down β-D-glucans, which are polymers of β-(1-3)-, β-(1-4)-, or β-(1-6)-linked glucose residues, to form β-D-glucose (Campbell and Bedford 1992). As indicated in Chapter 2, β-glucans are present in higher plants (e.g., barley, oats, and wheat) as components of special cell walls, and are rich in barley and oats. β-Glucan has a similar bond structure to highly indigestible cellulose. However, β-glucan does not have the same chemical properties (insolubility, hydrophobicity, and extensive lignification) as cellulose. When fed to poultry and swine, the viscous grains (e.g., barley and wheat) induce a condition of increased intestinal viscosity, thereby impairing nutrient digestion and absorption in the small intestine (Burnett 1966). The physical structure of the endosperm cell wall of these grains may also impede the access of digestive enzymes to the plant material. If β-glucans escape digestion and enter the large intestine (including the long ceca in poultry), most of them appear in the fecal excreta in the form of gels that cause undesirable "sticky droppings."

*Poultry.* The use of enzymes for poultry diets dates back to the 1920s when Clicker and Follwell (1925) supplemented crude enzymes, called "protozymes," from *Aspergillus oryzae* into the diet of poultry to improve their growth performance and feed efficiency. Studies in the 1940s and 1950s demonstrated that adding a crude "amylase" preparation (which contained β-glucanase activity) to barley-based diets for chicks resulted in a significant improvement in the body-weight gain and feed conversion ratio (Fry et al. 1957; Hastings 1946). These beneficial effects of β-glucanase on nutrient utilization and weight gains in young poultry fed barley-based diets have also been reported by other investigators (Edney et al. 1989; Grootwassink et al. 1989). Similarly, the addition of a combination of xylanase and β-glucanase to corn- and soybean meal-based diets deficient in ME, crude protein (CP), Ca, and P resulted in a significant increase in growth performance and utilization of dry matter (DM), energy, P, and N in broiler chickens (Lu et al. 2013).

Interestingly, there are reports that supplementation with a β-glucanase/pentosanase enzyme complex to barley-, oat-, or rye-based diets for laying hens does not consistently improve egg production (e.g., the number, weight, and specific gravity of eggs) (Brenes et al. 1993). It is possible that in older birds, β-glucanase released from microorganisms in the stomach and small intestine can digest β-glucans to some extent. In support of this view, mature cellulolytic microflora are established in the digestive tract of older poultry. In addition to the production criteria, reducing the adhesiveness of the fecal excreta from barley-fed birds is also a criterion for assessing the usefulness of dietary β-glucanase supplementation. A decrease in the adhesiveness of the fecal excreta is important for overall cleanliness in group-raised broilers and for sanitation in egg production.

*Swine.* Adding β-glucanase to a barley-based diet can enhance body-weight (BW) gain of 31- to 41-day-old postweaning pigs without affecting feed efficiency (Bedford et al. 1992). Importantly, the enzyme supplementation may reduce diarrhea in weanling piglets. In contrast, dietary supplementation with β-glucanase does not result in a significant beneficial effect on growth performance or feed efficiency in 2-month-old or older pigs (19–100 kg BW) (Graham et al. 1988; Thacker et al. 1988). Similarly, supplementation with β-glucanase to a corn- and soybean meal-based diet did not affect DM, energy, or CP digestibility in 6 kg pigs (Li et al. 1996), and supplementation with β-mannanase to corn–soybean meal diets had no effect on nutrient digestibility or growth performance of weanling and growing-finishing pigs (Pettey et al. 2002). These findings may be explained by: (1) denaturation of β-glucanase by the strong acid HCl in the stomach (with pH ~2); (2) relatively low contents of β-glucans in corn- and soybean meal-based diets; (3) the presence of β-glucanase in some feed ingredients; and (4) sufficient hydrolysis of β-glucans of such diets by microbial enzymes present in the stomach, small intestine, and large intestine of pigs, and possibly by diet-derived β-glucanase. Thus, the most likely application of β-glucanase to the swine industry may be its addition to barley-based diets for weanling pigs in which the intestinal microbiome is not well developed.

### Pentosanases (Arabinase and Xylanase)

Pentosans $[(C_5H_8O_4)_n]$ are homopolysaccharides consisting of β-(1-4)-linked pentose residues. Arabinans and xylans are two examples, and are hydrolyzed by arabinase and xylanase (pentosanases), respectively. Arabinase and xylanases are synthesized by a variety of fungi, bacteria, yeast, marine algae, protozoans, snails, crustaceans, insects, and plant seeds, but are not produced by mammalian or avian cells (Gírio et al. 2010; Kulkarni et al. 1999). Pentosans are rich in rye, wheat, and triticale (a hybrid of wheat and rye), and can also induce viscosity in the intestine of poultry and swine. When poultry and swine are fed diets which are based on these cereals that contain considerable amounts of arabinoxylans, their weight gains and feed efficiency may be improved in response to dietary supplementation with pentosanases.

*Poultry.* Dietary supplementation with pentosanase (arabinoxylanase) improved the feed efficiency and growth performance of broiler chickens fed rye-based diets (Grootwassink et al. 1989). Similarly, adding pentosanases to rye- or wheat-based diets improved energy and protein digestibility, as well as the weight gain and feed conversion ratio in young broiler chicks (Table 13.1).

**TABLE 13.1**
**Effects of Dietary Supplementation of Pentosanase Preparations on Growth Performance of Young Broiler Chicks**

| | | Enzyme Levels (g/kg) | | | | | | |
|---|---|---|---|---|---|---|---|---|
| | Days | 0 | 0.11 | 0.22 | 0.44 | 0.88 | SE | *P*-Value |
| Body weight (g) | 15 | 282 | 347 | 350 | 364 | 373 | 5.22 | <0.01 |
| | 27 | 810 | 893 | 914 | 941 | 951 | 9.50 | <0.01 |
| Weight gain (g) | 15–27 | 524 | 545 | 564 | 576 | 577 | 7.74 | <0.01 |
| Feed intake (g) | 1–15 | 413 | 470 | 464 | 477 | 482 | 7.71 | <0.01 |
| | 1–27 | 1410 | 1532 | 1519 | 1533 | 1531 | 19.0 | <0.01 |
| | 15–27 | 997 | 1062 | 1055 | 1056 | 1049 | 13.7 | <0.01 |
| Feed conversion[a] | 1–15 | 1.46 | 1.36 | 1.33 | 1.31 | 1.29 | 0.02 | <0.01 |
| | 1–27 | 1.74 | 1.72 | 1.66 | 1.63 | 1.61 | 0.02 | <0.01 |
| | 15–27 | 1.89 | 1.94 | 1.87 | 1.83 | 1.82 | 0.03 | <0.01 |

*Source:* Pettersson, D. and P. Aman. 1989. *Br. J. Nutr.* 62:139–149. Chicks were fed a rye- or wheat-based diet between days 15 and 27 of age.

[a] g feed/g body weight.

**TABLE 13.2**
**Effects of Dietary Supplementation with Different Sources of Xylanase on Small-Intestinal luminal Viscosity and Carbohydrate Concentrations, and Growth Performance of Broiler Chickens[a]**

| Enzyme Supplementation | Viscosity (mPa·s) | | Jejunal Luminal Carbohydrate[b] | | Body Weight Gain[c] (g/wk per Bird) | Feed Conversion Ratio (Feed: Gain, g/g) |
|---|---|---|---|---|---|---|
| | Jejunum | Ileum | Free Sugars | Soluble NSPs | | |
| Control (none) | 9.4[e] | 28.3[e] | 1381[f] | 445[e] | 345[e] | 2.16[d] |
| Xylanase A | 5.2[f] | 8.3[f] | 1700[d] | 689[d] | 392[d] | 1.97[e] |
| Xylanase B | 18.4[d] | 84.1[d] | 1782[d] | 696[d] | 395[d] | 2.01[e] |
| Xylanase C | 3.4[f] | 7.2[f] | 1635[e] | 426[e] | 383[d] | 2.04[d,e] |

*Source:* Choct, M. 2006. *World's Poult. Sci. J.* 62:5–16.

[a] Xylanase A was isolated from *Thermomyces lanuginosus*, Xylanase B from *Humicola insolens*, and Xylanase C from *Aspergillus aculeatus*.

[b] mg/g marker.

[c] Broiler chickens were fed a wheat-based diet containing the normal content of metabolizable energy (13.7–14.5 MJ/kg dry matter).

[d–f] Within a column, means not sharing the same superscript letters differ ($P < 0.05$).

NSPs, non-starch polysaccharides; mPa·s, millipascal second; wk, week.

Furthermore, feeding high levels of rye to laying hens reduced egg production, but their productive performance was improved in response to dietary supplementation with pentosanase. Compared with β-glucanase, pentosanases appear to be less effective in reducing the adhesiveness of the fecal excreta in birds, probably because (1) the pentosan fragments remaining after the action of pentosanase are relatively large and therefore contribute to the residual viscosity; and (2) there is continued pentosan solubilization throughout the lower gut. It may also be because pentosanases lack the β-glucanase activity that is required to degrade β-glucans. If the β-glucans are not degraded, they can contribute to sticky feces. Choct (2006) reported that various microbial sources of supplemental feed xylanase improved the body-weight gains of broiler chickens, despite having different effects on small-intestinal viscosity (Table 13.2). Interestingly, the anti-nutritive effects of rye appear to be reduced in older poultry when compared to young birds. This is likely because of the presence of a larger amount of microbial pentosanases and xylanase in the lumen of the crop, small and large intestines of older birds.

*Swine.* Pigs fed a rye-based diet gain less weight compared with those fed barley (Table 13.3). However, dietary supplementation with pentosanases to young pigs fed rye-based diets does not consistently improve growth performance (Bedford et al. 1992). Similarly, Thacker et al. (2002) have shown that dietary supplementation with pentosanases failed to improve growth performance of pigs (21.5–100.7 kg BW) or their carcass traits. This is likely a reflection of the ability of the fully established microbiome in older pigs to produce the enzymes required to degrade pentosans.

### *Phytase*

As noted in Chapter 10, phytate is a phosphate-conjugated inositol and the major storage form of phosphate in plants. Phytate phosphorus content in soybeans and rapeseed is about 6 times that in corn, wheat, and barley, whereas phytate phosphorus content in soybean meal is about 40% higher than that in corn (Woyengo and Nyachoti 2013). Phytate is often present as a protein–phytate complex in plants (Figure 13.2), rendering protein less susceptible to proteases in the small intestine and increasing the endogenous losses of nutrients (including AAs and minerals). Furthermore, phytate has a capacity to chelate positively charged cations, especially calcium, iron, zinc, magnesium,

**TABLE 13.3**
**Effects of Dietary Pentosanase or β-Glucanase Supplementation on the Growth Performance of Weanling Pigs**

| Treatment | Weight Gain (kg) | Feed Intake (kg) | Feed Efficiency (Gain: Feed Ratio) | Starch Digestibility (%) | Small-Intestine Lumen pH |
|---|---|---|---|---|---|
| | **High Rye-Based Diet (Experiment 1; Mean Initial Body Weight = 10.7 kg)** | | | | |
| Control | 4.24 | 6.94 | 0.608 | 81.9 | 6.04–6.10 |
| Pentosanase | 4.24 | 6.64 | 0.637 | 84.1 | 6.28–6.57 |
| | **Hulless Barley-Based Diet (Experiment 2; Mean Initial Body Weight = 12.1 kg)** | | | | |
| Control | 5.24 | 9.05 | 0.572 | 73.8 | 5.86–6.19 |
| β-Glucanase | 6.14* | 9.57 | 0.646 | 71.5 | 5.76–6.19 |

*Source:* Bedford, M.R. et al. 1992. *Can. J. Anim. Sci.* 72:97–105. Values are means, $n = 6$. *$P < 0.05$ versus the corresponding control group. Yorkshire × Landrace pigs were weaned at an average 26 days of age and housed in pairs in pens. Littermate pairs were randomly assigned to one of the two experimental treatments, providing 6 pens and 12 pigs per treatment. Following a 5 day period of acclimation, pigs had free access to their diets for 10 days.

potassium, and manganese (Figure 13.1). When phytate binds to digestive enzymes in the lumen of the gastrointestinal tract, these enzymes are less effective in hydrolyzing lipids, carbohydrates, proteins, minerals, and vitamins (Humer et al. 2015). By reducing the availability of dietary phosphorus and other nutrients, phytate has considerable anti-nutritive effects for animals and increases their requirements for dietary nutrients (Dersjant-Li et al. 2015).

Phytate itself is not a good source of phosphorus for nonruminants because of inadequate phytase activity in the gastrointestinal tract. In animals, the sources of phytase for phytate digestion may be endogenous mucosae, gut microflora, plant ingredients, and exogenous phytase preparations (Humer et al. 2015). Although phytase is present in the small intestine of broilers, laying hens, and swine, the enzyme activity may be insufficient to release phosphate from phytate under normal nutritional and physiological conditions. Phosphorus deficiency may occur when inorganic sources of phosphorus are not added to nonruminant diets. Owing to the uncertainty of the bioavailability of plant phosphorus, dietary formulations often rely on added inorganic phosphates to meet most of the animal's needs. Therefore, most diets for nonruminants contain ~50% more phosphorus than the animal's daily requirements. Any excess phosphorus is excreted in feces and urine, which, if not managed properly, can cause environmental pollution. The need to reduce phosphorus and N excretion levels led to a market opportunity for the introduction of exogenous phytases.

There are two types of phytases: acidic phytases (optimum pH, 3.0–5.5) and alkaline phytases (optimum pH, 7.0–8.0). Acidic phytases from bacteria, fungi, or plants hydrolyze phytase to generate five inorganic phosphate and one inositol-phosphate molecule or even myo-inositol. Alkaline phytases hydrolyze phytate into inositol-triphosphates and three inorganic phosphate molecules. Like any enzyme, phytase activity is affected by pH (acidic pH in gastric and neutral in small intestine), inhibitors (e.g., Ca, Fe, and Zn), and temperature. Through increasing phytate hydrolysis, supplementing phytase to diets for poultry and swine can enhance the bioavailability of dietary phosphorus by 20%–30%. As a result, the amount of added inorganic phosphorus can be reduced accordingly without adverse effects on the growth performance of the animals (Dersjant-Li et al. 2015; Humer et al. 2015). In nonruminants, the digestibility of AA is also positively correlated with the degree of phytate degradation (Amerah et al. 2014). In certain cases, the presence of natural phytase in some feed ingredients (e.g., wheat) may reduce the benefits of dietary phytase supplementation (Dersjant-Li et al. 2015).

Dietary calcium content affects phytase activity in the small intestine. The greater the calcium content of the diet, the lower the phytase activity. This is because calcium not only precipitates

Phytate–Mineral complex (neutral pH)

Phytate–Starch complex (neutral pH)

Phytate–Protein complex (neutral pH)

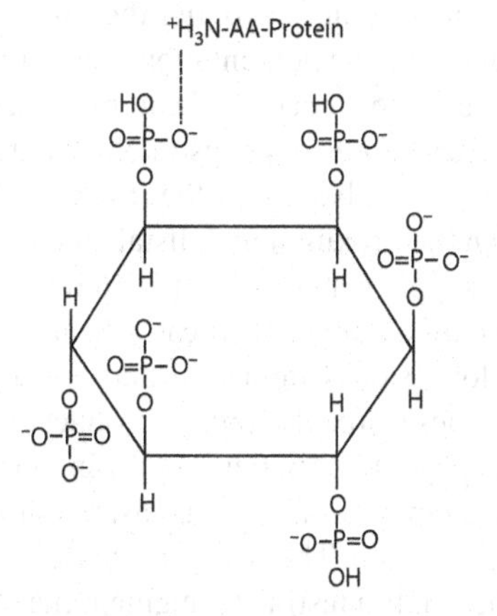


Phytate–Protein complex (acidic pH)

**FIGURE 13.2** Interaction of phytate with protein and minerals in feedstuffs at a neutral pH. Note that the interaction of phytase with protein at an acidic pH differs from that at a neutral pH. (Adapted from Humer, E. et al. 2015. *J. Anim. Physiol. Anim. Nutr.* 99:605–625.)

phytate but also inhibits phytase activity, thereby reducing the susceptibility of phytate to enzymatic hydrolysis. Use of chelators such as citric acid, which remove calcium from soluble phytate complexes, can be effective in increasing phytase activity in the small intestine. The ratio of calcium to phosphorus in diets is also important, as an exceedingly high Ca:P ratio may reduce the nutritional benefits of phytase supplementation. However, in broiler chickens, the beneficial effects of dietary phytase supplementation in improving the digestion of dietary P, dry matter, and protein are achieved at different dietary ratios of Ca to available P (1.43, 2.14, 2.86, and 3.57) (Amerah et al. 2014). Even though phytase is added to poultry and swine diets, they must still provide sufficient Ca and P to ensure proper skeletal (bone) growth and development.

## Other Enzymes

*β-Mannanase.* Corn- and soybean meal-based diet, which are widely used in the United States, China, and many other countries to feed nonruminants, contain a high amount of mannose-linked NSPs [e.g., 1.2% galactomannans (Kim et al. 2003)]. Thus, microbial β-mannanase (also called β-mannosidase), which hydrolyzes these polysaccharides, may be added to such diets for poultry and swine to improve their productivity. Jackson et al. (2004) conducted an experiment to determine the effects of graded levels of β-mannanase (0, 50, 80, and 110 MU/ton) on the growth of 0- to 21-day-old male broilers fed antibiotic-free diets that were based on corn and soybean meal. Dietary inclusion of the enzyme at 80 or 110 MU/ton improved BW gain by 3.9%–4.8% and feed efficiency by 3.5%–3.8% over the control group, but the inclusion of 50 MU/ton had no significant benefit. Similarly, supplementation with β-mannanase (400 IU/kg diet) to a corn- and soybean meal-based diet enhanced the daily weight gain of 2- to 22-day-old broiler chickens by 3.5% (Kong et al. 2011). Likewise, Lv et al. (2013) found that adding β-mannanase to a corn- and soybean meal-based diet (200, 400, or 600 U/kg diet) for growing pigs with an initial BW of 23.6 kg for 28 days increased: (1) the digestibility of dietary CP, fiber, Ca, and P; and (2) BW gain and feed efficiency in a dose-dependent manner. Collectively, these findings indicate that the small-intestinal bacteria of poultry or young swine do not produce sufficient β-mannanase and that an exogenous source of this enzyme is necessary to fully digest corn- and soybean meal-based diets.

*Enzyme mixtures.* While none of the commercial individual enzymes are likely pure preparations, the activities of associated enzymes may be much lower than those of the principal enzymes. Plant-source feed ingredients contain a variety of complex polysaccharides (e.g., α-1,6-galactosides in soybean meal) that are usually linked to proteins. Thus, a mix of enzymes may be more effective than a single enzyme in improving the digestibility of dietary nutrients. For example, Kim et al. (2003) reported that supplementation with a mixture of α-1,6-galactosidase, β-1,4 mannanase, and β-1,4 mannosidase to a corn–soybean meal-based diet enhanced DM and AA digestibility, as well as feed efficiency in nursery pigs (a 35 day trial, 6.3–19.1 kg BW; and a 21 day trial, 8.0–15.2 kg BW). These authors also found that the use of the enzyme mixture decreased the concentrations of stachyose in the proximal and distal small intestine and of raffinose in the distal small intestine. Furthermore, supplementation with different multienzyme preparations to corn and soybean meal-based diets (small amounts of wheat, wheat screenings, barley, mill-run, canola meal, and peas) fed to 7 kg pigs for 28 days improved nutrient digestibility and growth performance (Omogbenigun et al. 2004). These mixed enzyme products contained xylanase, β-glucanase, amylase, protease, invertase, and phytase activities, but differed in the type of plant cell wall-degrading activities (e.g., cellulase, galactanase, and mannanase; cellulase and pectinase; or cellulase, galactanase, mannanase, and pectinase). The use of protease is notable for enhancing the hydrolysis of plant-source proteins in the small intestine to augment the efficiency of their utilization for lean-tissue growth in nonruminants (Cowieson and Roos 2016). Thus, adding a mixture of β-glucanase and proteases to a corn–soybean meal diet can increase the digestibility of DM, energy, CP, and phosphorus in growing pigs (Ji et al. 2008). Likewise, 4 week dietary supplementation with a mixture of β-mannanase, α-amylase, and protease to growing barrows (mean initial body weights of 55.6–56.9 kg) augmented their daily BW gain by 3.3% and 2.6%, respectively, when fed a corn- and soybean meal-based or a complex diet (Jo et al. 2012). Collectively, these results indicate that the use of complex carbohydrases along with proteases can optimize the response of monogastric animals to feed enzymes.

## Enzyme Additives for Ruminants

Cellulase hydrolyzes cellulose to D-glucose. However, a complex mixture of enzymes is required to fully degrade hemicelluloses. Hemicellulases (e.g., L-arabinanases, D-galactanases, D-mannanases, and D-xylanases) hydrolyze the hemicellulose polymer backbone. Before or in conjunction with depolymerization of the hemicellulose backbone, many different debranching enzymes release its side chains, depending on the specific type of hemicellulose being hydrolysed. The debranching enzymes include arabinofuranosidase, feruloyl and coumaric esterases, acetylxylan esterase, α-glucuronidase, and xylosidases. A variety of enzymes plays an important role in the hydrolysis of ester, ether and glycosidic linkages between hemicellulose and lignin to release lignin. For example, glucuronoyl esterases hydrolyze the ester bond between the D-glucuronic acid or 4-O-methyl-D-glucuronic acid of glucuronoxylan and the hydroxyl groups of lignin (Biely 2016). Efficient hydrolysis of hemicelluloses by digestive enzymes in the gastrointestinal tract is essential for the utilization of dietary fiber by animals.

Over the past 60 years, many studies have been conducted to determine the effects of dietary supplementation with fiber-degrading enzymes on growth and lactation performance of ruminants. The early enzyme preparations were poorly defined, and animal responses were variable (Burroughs et al. 1960; Perry et al. 1960; Rust et al. 1965). For example, when cattle were fed diets consisting of ground ear corn, oat silage, corn silage, or alfalfa hay mixed with an enzyme cocktail containing amylolytic, proteolytic, and cellulolytic activities (Agrozyme®), they gained 6.8%–24.0% more body weight and exhibited a 6.0%–21.2% improvement in feed efficiency, compared with the cattle fed untreated control diets (Burroughs et al. 1960). In contrast, Perry et al. (1960) reported that supplementation with Agrozyme® reduced the daily weight gain of beef cattle by 20.4% when the enzyme product was fed with a corn silage diet. Clearly, interactions occur between dietary ingredients and enzyme preparations to affect their efficacy.

The opportunity to improve growth and lactation performance of ruminants through dietary supplementation with feed enzymes lies in complementing the rumen that already has an active microbiome to produce carbohydrases, proteases, peptidases and lipasess. The development of molecular biology techniques, reductions in fermentation costs, and the availability of better-defined enzyme preparations (e.g., cellulases and xylanases) have prompted a re-examination of the potential use of exogenous enzymes in ruminant production (Meale et al. 2014). Some published studies have provided sufficient evidence for the responses of beef and dairy cattle to exogenous enzymes with consistent and predictable increases in weight gains. Some examples are shown in Tables 13.4 and 13.5. These findings argue against the previous view that the endogenous activity of ruminal microbes to break down plant cell walls could not be augmented by supplementary exogenous enzymes. The beneficial effects of the enzyme preparations result mainly from improvements in ruminal fiber digestion and ultimately an increase in the availability of digestible DM to the host. However, there are reports of various effects of dietary supplementation with exogenous fibrolytic enzymes on lactation and growth performance in ruminants (e.g., dairy cows, beef cattle, goats, sheep, or buffalo) (Sujani and Seresinhe 2015). Clearly, much research is required to define the conditions under which consistent positive responses in ruminant production to enzyme preparations can be realized. With

**TABLE 13.4**
**Effects of Adding Commercial Feed Enzymes on Growth Performance of Feedlot Finishing Cattle**

| | Control | Enzyme Level | | Change |
|---|---|---|---|---|
| | | 1× | 2× | |
| Study 1 (no ionophore, no implant)[a] | | | | |
| Initial weight (kg) | 407 | 414 | – | – |
| Dry matter intake (kg/day) | 9.99 | 9.53 | – | −5% |
| Live-weight gain (kg/day) | 1.43 | 1.52 | – | +6% |
| Dry matter intake/live-weight gain | 7.11 | 6.33 | – | −11% |
| Study 2 (with ionophore and implant)[b] | | | | |
| Initial weight (kg) | 477 | 477 | 477 | – |
| Dry matter intake (kg/day) | 11.1 | 11.5 | 11.5 | +4% |
| Live-weight gain (kg/day) | 1.70 | 1.87 | 2.01 | +10% to 18% |
| Dry matter intake/live-weight gain | 6.50 | 6.18 | 5.70 | −5% to 12% |

[a] Beauchemin, K.A. et al. 1997. *Can. J. Anim. Sci.* 77: 645–653.

[b] Iwaasa, A.D. et al. 1997. *Proceedings of the Joint Rowett Research Institute and INRA Rumen Microbiology Symposium*. Aberdeen, Scotland.

Feedlot cattle were fed high-concentrate diets consisting of barley grain, supplement, and barley silage.

**TABLE 13.5**
**Effects of Supplementing Feed Enzymes to Diets for Cows in Early Lactation**

| | Rode et al. (1999) | | Yang et al. (2000) | | |
|---|---|---|---|---|---|
| | Control | Enzyme | Control | Enzyme in Conc. | Enzyme in TMR |
| Dry matter intake (kg/day) | 18.7 | 19.0 | 19.4 | 19.8 | 20.4 |
| Milk production (kg/day) | 35.9 | 39.5 | 35.3 | 37.4 | 35.2 |
| Milk composition (g/kg) | | | | | |
| Fat | 38.7 | 33.7 | 33.4 | 31.9 | 31.4 |
| Protein | 32.4 | 30.3 | 31.8 | 31.3 | 31.3 |
| Lactose | 47.3 | 46.2 | 46.5 | 46.5 | 45.6 |
| Live-weight change (kg/day) | −0.63 | −0.60 | 0.15 | 0.04 | 0.14 |
| Dry matter digestibility (%) | 61.7 | 69.1 | 63.9 | 66.6 | 65.7 |
| NDF digestibility (%) | 42.5 | 51.0 | 42.6 | 44.4 | 45.9 |

*Source:* Rode, L.M. et al. 1999. *J. Dairy Sci.* 82:2121–2126. Yang, W.Z. et al. 2000. *J. Dairy Sci.* 83:2512-2520.
Conc., concentrates; NDF, neutral detergent fiber; TMR, total mixed ration.

the gain of new knowledge, fibrolytic enzymes hold great potential to enhance feed utilization and productivity (e.g., growth and lactation performance) in ruminants.

## NONENZYME ADDITIVES

### NONRUMINANTS

There is a long history of the use of nonenzyme additives in poultry and swine diets. The additives include antibiotics, probiotics, prebiotics, mycotoxin absorbents, and crystalline AAs (Cromwell 2000; McDonald et al. 2011; Wang et al. 2012, 2016; Yue et al. 2017). Animal producers have successfully improved weight gain and feed efficiency of nonruminants through the use of antibiotics and chemotherapeutics. Over the past 50 years, 17 antimicrobial agents (12 antibiotics and 5 chemotherapeutics) have been used as feed additives (Table 13.6). Nearly all antibiotics used for feeding nonruminants contain nitrogen and some of them are aminoglycosides (Figure 13.3). The presence of N atoms in antibiotics alters the electronic configuration of the compounds and confers or enhances their antimicrobial activity (Patrick 1995). For example, in penicillin, the N atom of the β-lactam structure makes its carbonyl carbon highly electrophilic, thereby facilitating the binding of the antibiotic to transpeptidases (enzymes that catalyze the final step in cell-wall biosynthesis, i.e., the cross-linking of peptidoglycans) on the plasma membrane of bacteria (Sauvage et al. 2008).

**TABLE 13.6**
**Antimicrobial Organic Agents Used for Swine Diets**

| Antibiotics | Antibiotics | Chemotherapeutics |
|---|---|---|
| Apramycin | Neomycin | Arsanilic acid |
| Bacitracin methylene disalicylate | Oxytetracycline | Carbadox (synthetic) |
| Bacitracin zinc | Penicillin | Roxarsone |
| Bambermycins | Tiamulin | Sulfamethazine |
| Chlortetracycline | Tylosin | Sulfathiazole |
| Lincomycin | Virginiamycin | |

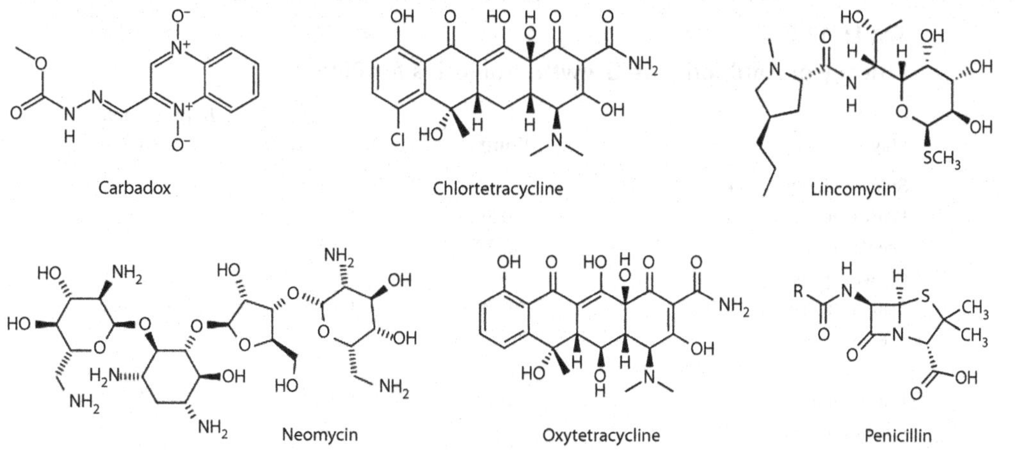

Carbadox Chlortetracycline Lincomycin

Neomycin Oxytetracycline Penicillin

**FIGURE 13.3** Antibiotics for feeding nonruminants. Nearly all antibiotics used for feeding nonruminants contain nitrogen and some of them are aminoglycosides.

This results in an inhibition of the transpeptidases and the killing of susceptible bacteria. Without a cell wall, a bacterium cannot maintain its homeostasis and dies quickly. N-Containing antibiotics generally have higher biological activity than non-N compounds (Bérdy 2012).

## Antibiotics

*Enhancers of feed efficiency.* Antimicrobial agents were first used as additives in diets for chickens (Moore et al. 1946) and pigs (Brauder et al. 1953) in the 1940s and 1950s, respectively. Antimicrobial agents, used as feed additives at low concentrations (subtherapeutic), inhibit the growth of intestinal microorganisms, improve the growth rate and efficiency of feed utilization, and reduce mortality and morbidity. Antimicrobial agents are also used at intermediate levels to prevent disease and at high (therapeutic) levels to treat diseases in animals (Cromwell 2002). This class of compounds includes antibiotics (which are naturally produced by yeasts, molds, and other microorganisms) and chemotherapeutics (which are chemically synthesized). Most antibiotics are synthesized from AAs. In addition to organic substances, high concentrations of zinc and copper have antimicrobial activities, and have been included in the diets of weanling pigs to prevent their intestinal dysfunction (e.g., diarrhea). The efficacy of antibiotics in improving growth performance and feed efficiency of pigs is well documented in the literature. An example is shown in Table 13.7. The results are usually more pronounced on commercial farms than at Research Experiment Stations in the United States, probably because of a cleaner environment in the latter. Antimicrobial agents play an important role in the efficient production of pork, beef, poultry meat, and other animal products worldwide.

*Modes of action on stimulating animal growth.* The mechanisms responsible for the beneficial action of antibiotics on enhancing animal growth and feed efficiency are not well understood, and may include: (1) inhibition of the growth of intestinal bacterial (including pathogenic microbes); (2) reduction in the thickness of the intestinal mucosa to enhance nutrient absorption and to decrease mucosal AA catabolism; (3) reduction of microbial use and catabolism of nutrients, particularly dietary AAs; (4) reduction of growth-depressing microbial metabolites; and (5) inhibition of subclinical infections (Gaskins et al. 2002; Visek 1978; Wu 1998). Since microorganisms in the small intestine are now known to play an important role in the catabolism of dietary AAs, decreasing the numbers and activity of small-intestinal microbes with the use of antibiotics will reduce AA degradation in the intestinal lumen, thereby increasing the bioavailability of dietary AAs for protein synthesis and other synthetic pathways.

*Concern over antibiotic-resistant bacteria.* As early as the 1950s, concern was expressed that continued use of antibiotics to promote growth of poultry and other food animals might result in antibiotic resistance of pathogenic bacteria in humans (Starr and Reynolds 1951). The concern

**TABLE 13.7**
**Efficacy of Antibiotics as Growth Promoters for Pigs[a]**

| Stage | Control | Antibiotic | Improvement (%) |
|---|---|---|---|
| Starting phase (7–25 kg) | | | |
| Daily gain (kg) | 0.39 | 0.45 | 16.4 |
| Feed/gain ratio | 2.28 | 2.13 | 6.9 |
| Growing phase (17–49 kg) | | | |
| Daily gain (kg) | 0.59 | 0.66 | 10.6 |
| Feed/gain ratio | 2.91 | 2.78 | 4.5 |
| Growing-finishing phase (24–89 kg) | | | |
| Daily gain (kg) | 0.69 | 0.72 | 4.2 |
| Feed/gain ratio | 3.30 | 3.23 | 2.2 |

*Source:* Cromwell, G.L. 2000. In: *Swine Nutrition.* Edited by A.J. Lewis and L.L. Southern. CRC Press, New York. pp. 401–426.

[a] Data collected from 453, 298, and 443 experiments involving 13,632, 5,783, and 13,140 pigs, for the starting, growing, and growing-finishing phases, respectively.

gained momentum in the late 1960s and subsequently developed into advocacy for governments to ban the use of antibiotics as feed additives. Antibiotic use in animals can have direct and indirect effects on human health due to (1) the presence of antibiotic residues in animal products (e.g., meat and milk) consumed by humans; (2) human contact with antibiotic-resistant bacteria from food animals; and (3) the spread of antibiotic-resistant bacteria to various components of the ecosystem (e.g., water and soil). The use of antibiotics as feed additives for growth promotion has been banned in member states of the European Union and is now being phased out in many countries. Thus, alternatives to feed antibiotics must be actively developed (Thacker 2013).

*Alternatives to feed antibiotics.* Improvements of intestinal health and immunity should serve as the guiding principles for the development of alternatives to feed antibiotics. The most widely researched alternatives include probiotics, prebiotics, acidifiers (e.g., formate, propionic acid, butyric acid, fumaric acid, citric acid, and benzoic acid), lipids (e.g., lauric acid, 1-monoglyceride, and tributyrate), plant extracts, minerals [e.g., 250 ppm copper sulfate ($CuSo_4$) and 2500 ppm zinc oxide (ZnO)], antimicrobial peptides, clay minerals, egg yolk antibodies (e.g., IgY), essential oils (aromatic oily liquids obtained from plant material), eucalyptus oil-medium chain fatty acids [e.g., octanoic acid ($C_{8:0}$) and caproic acid ($C_{6:0}$)], rare earth elements (e.g., lanthanum–yeast mixture), recombinant enzymes (e.g., feed enzymes as noted previously), spray-dried porcine plasma, yeast culture, bacteriophages, lysozymes, bovine colostrum, lactoferrin, conjugated fatty acids, chito-oligosaccarides, seaweed extracts, and certain AAs (Thacker 2013). Clay minerals, which consist of silicon, aluminum, and oxygen as in the natural extracted clays (bentonites, zeolite, and kaolin), can bind to toxic materials (e.g., aflatoxins, plant metabolites, heavy metals, and endotoxins) in the gastrointestinal tract of animals, thereby reducing their biological availability, absorption, and toxicity. Essential oils usually have a characteristic odor or flavor, and are mixtures of plant phenolic compounds (e.g., thymol, carvacrol, and eugenol), terpenes (e.g., citric and pineapple extracts), alkaloids (capsaicin), lectins, aldehydes (e.g., cinnamaldehyde), polypeptides, or polyacetylenes. Finally, like some peptides synthesized by the intestinal mucosa, certain protein hydrolysates from animal sources contain antimicrobial peptides (Chapter 4), which exert their actions by damaging the cell membrane of bacteria, interfering with the functions of their intracellular proteins, inducing the aggregation of cytoplasmic proteins, and affecting the metabolism of bacteria (Hou et al. 2017).

### Direct-Fed Microbials (Probiotics)

Animals are sterile in the womb. Recent well-controlled studies do not support the hypothesis that microbiomes exist within the healthy fetal milieu (Perez-Muñoz et al. 2017). Neonates acquire some of the members of intestinal microbiomes during passage through the birth canal. After birth, with the consumption of milk and other kinds of foods, the digestive tracts are naturally colonized by a variety of microorganisms from the environment. Under healthy conditions, "beneficial" microorganisms colonize the intestine (and the rumen in ruminants) in a symbiotic relationship with the host. Gut microbes compete with potential pathogenic microbes, and are essential for the normal development and well-being of the host. For example, poultry and pigs raised in a sterile environment are more susceptible to bacterial infections, probably due to under-development of the immune system and no competition of normal microbes against pathogenic organisms.

Direct-fed microorganisms, commonly referred to as "probiotics," are live, naturally occurring microorganisms that are beneficial to the animals through direct feeding. Probiotics can be defined as dietary supplements containing beneficial live bacteria or yeast that confer a health benefit to the gut flora and the host. *Lactobacillus* and *Bifidobacterium* are the most widely used probiotic bacteria for maintaining the intestinal microbial ecosystem and mucosal integrity. Lactobacilli are the predominant lactic acid bacteria found in the pig intestine and constitute a major proportion of the entire intestinal microbiota. As such, they are of particular importance for the maintenance of gut health. Probiotics serve as sources of digestive enzymes and improve the balance of the intestinal microflora. To date, direct-fed microbials approved for swine and other livestock are listed in Table 13.8 and should be used according to the approved doses. In poultry and pigs, the response to probiotics is considerably less consistent compared with the response to antibiotics.

The mechanisms proposed for the action of direct-fed microbials are summarized as follows: (1) production of antibacterial compounds (e.g., organic acids, bacteriocins, and antibiotics); (2) competition with undesirable organisms for colonization space and/or nutrients (competitive exclusion); (3) production of nutrients (e.g., AAs and vitamins) or other growth factors that stimulate other microorganisms in the digestive tract; (4) production and/or stimulation of enzymes; (5) metabolism and/or detoxification of undesirable compounds; (6) stimulation of immune response in host animals; (7) production of nutrients (e.g., AAs and vitamins) or other growth factors that stimulate the host

**TABLE 13.8**
**Direct-Fed Microbials Used for the Diets of Swine and Other Livestock Species**

| | | |
|---|---|---|
| *Aspergillus niger* | *B. infantis* | *L. enterii* |
| *A. oryzae* | *B. longum* | *Leuconostoc mesenteroides* |
| *Bacillus coagulans* | *B. thermophilum* | *Pediococcus acidilacticii* |
| *B. lentus* | *Lactobacillus acidophilus* | *P. cerevisiae* |
| *B. licheniformis* | *L. brevis* | *P. pentosaceus* |
| *B. pumilus* | *L. bulgaricus* | *Propionibacterium freudenreichii* |
| *B. subtilis* | *L. casei* | *P. shermanii* |
| *Bacteroides amphophilus* | *L. cellobiosus* | *Saccharomyces cerevisiae* |
| *B. capillosus* | *L. curvatus* | *Enterococcus cremoris* |
| *B. ruminocola* | *L. delbruekii* | *E. diacetylactis* |
| *B. suis* | *L. fermentum* | *E. faecium* |
| *Bifidobacterium adolescentis* | *L. helveticus* | *E. intermedius* |
| *B. animalis* | *L. lactis* | *E. lactis* |
| *B. bifidum* | *L. plantarum* | *E. thermophilus* |

*Source:* Cromwell, G.L. 2000. In: *Swine Nutrition*. Edited by A.J. Lewis and L.L. Southern. CRC Press, New York, pp. 401–426.

animal; and (8) increased digestibility of dietary protein and the absorption of AAs into the portal circulation (Bergen and Wu 2009). This knowledge is fundamental to the development of new strategies to prevent enteric disorders. For example, when pigs are weaned at an early age (e.g., $\leq$21 days), they are at increased risk for enteric disease, diarrhea, and malnutrition likely due to disruption in the establishment of a stable intestinal microbiota, thereby allowing pathogenic bacteria to flourish and cause disease. Dietary supplementation with 1% glutamine or 2% glutamate improves the gut immune function and mucosal integrity, thereby reducing the incidence of diarrhea, enhancing nutrient digestion and absorption, and promoting weight gains.

### Prebiotics

Prebiotics can be defined as food ingredients that are not digested by animal-source enzymes but can beneficially affect the host by selectively stimulating the growth and/or activity of one or a limited number of the bacterial species in the small and large intestines. Oligosaccharides (mainly fructooligosaccharides and mannanoligosaccharide) are commonly used as prebiotics for livestock species, poultry, and humans (Halas and Nochta 2012). Dietary supplementation with mannanoligosaccharide reduced the incidence of diarrhea in weanling piglets and enhanced their growth performance (Castillo et al. 2008). Similarly, adding chitosan oligosaccharides to the diets of young chicks and weanling pigs inhibited the growth of oral and intestinal pathogenic bacteria, improved immune status, and increased the density of small-intestinal microvilli (Deng et al. 2007; Wang et al. 2003). Furthermore, dietary lactose has previously been shown to act as a prebiotic, promoting the growth of beneficial commensal bacteria, such as *Bifidobacteria* and *Lactobacillus*, and improving gut health and growth performance in weaning piglets (Daly et al. 2014; Pierce et al. 2006). The mechanisms responsible for the beneficial effects of prebiotics include: (1) improvements in the digestion of nutrients (protein, DM, and minerals), the absorption of AAs and minerals by the small intestine, N economy in the intestine, and feed efficiency; (2) modulation of the metabolism of urea, ammonia, and AAs in the lumen of the large intestine; and (3) changes in the intestinal microflora to selectively promote the growth and activity of beneficial bacteria (e.g. *bifidobacteria*) and therefore the postnatal development of the intestinal and whole-body immune systems (Bergen and Wu 2009).

### Agents to Remove or Absorb Mycotoxins in Feeds

Mycotoxins are secondary metabolites produced by organisms of the fungal kingdom, such as Aspergillus, Penicillium, and Fusarium. Mycotoxin-producing molds are distributed widely throughout the world and actively grow in different environmental conditions. Contamination with mycotoxins can arise on a farm throughout the harvest, drying, and storage processes, and the risk increases under conditions of high temperature and moisture (CAST 2003). The major classes of toxic mycotoxins in foods are aflatoxins, deoxynivalenol, zearalenone, trichothecenes, fumonisins, ochratoxin A, and ergot alkaloids. Aflatoxins are a family of toxins produced by certain fungi (*Aspergillus flavus* and *Aspergillus parasiticus*) present in agricultural crops such as corn, peanuts, cottonseed, and tree nuts. There are four common aflatoxins: $B_1$, $B_2$, $G_1$, and $G_2$ (Figure 13.4), which can bind to protein and DNA to cause aflatoxicosis (general poisoning to animals). Acute severe intoxication causes direct damage to the intestine and liver and subsequent illness or death, whereas chronic sub symptomatic exposure results in inhibition of protein synthesis, chronic disease, and poor growth performance. Among livestock species, swine are most sensitive to aflatoxins. These substances are usually present at varying concentrations in feed ingredients used for swine, poultry and ruminant rations (Wu et al. 2016). The mean oral lethal dose ($LD_{50}$) for swine is 0.62 mg/kg, which is significantly lower than that for other livestock species (Pier 1992).

Methods for protecting animals from those toxic effects include grain testing, use of mold inhibitors, fermentation, microbial inactivation, physical separation, thermal inactivation, irradiation, ammoniation, ozonation, dilution, and use of adsorbents (Rezaei et al. 2013). Adsorbents have been used as one of the best and most practical methods, because they are relatively inexpensive, generally recognized as safe (GRAS), and can be easily added to animal feeds. Adsorbents added to aflatoxin-contaminated

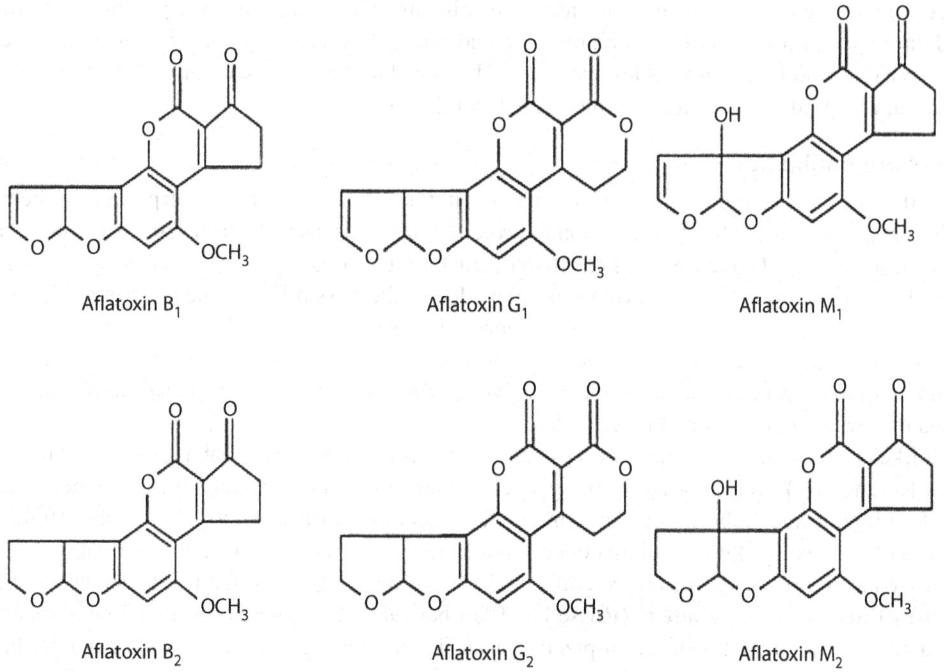

**FIGURE 13.4** Aflatoxin structures. There are four common aflatoxins, including $B_1$, $B_2$, $G_1$, and $G_2$, in animal feeds. These toxins are divided based on their fluorescence under UV light and the presence or absence of a double bond at the 8, 9 carbons. Aflatoxins $B_1$ and $G_1$ have a double bond at the 8, 9 carbons, while aflatoxins $B_2$ and $G_2$ do not. This double bond leads to formation of an epoxide, which is a more toxic form of aflatoxins $B_1$ and $G_1$. The B aflatoxins are named for their blue fluorescence, and the G aflatoxins for their green-blue fluorescence under UV irradiation on thin-layer chromatography plates. Of the four aflatoxins, aflatoxin $B_1$ is the most potent natural carcinogen and the most prevalent one.

feeds can bind to aflatoxin during the digestive process and cause the toxin to be excreted safely from the animal body (Phillips et al. 1995). Possible adsorbent materials that have been studied so far include silicate minerals, activated carbons, complex indigestible carbohydrates (e.g., cellulose, polysaccharides in the cell walls of yeast and bacteria such as glucomannans, peptidoglycans, and others), and synthetic polymers (e.g., cholestyramine, polyvinylpyrrolidone, and derivatives).

Silicate minerals are the most widely studied mycotoxin-sequestering agents. There are two important subclasses of these minerals: phyllosilicates and tectosilicates. Mineral clays of the phyllosilicate subclass include the montmorillonite/smectite group, the kaolinite group, and the illite (or clay-mica) group. Tectosilicates consist of the highly studied zeolites. Montmorillonites, the major component of bentonite, can be categorized as calcium, magnesium, potassium, or sodium bentonites. These products have been widely used as mycotoxin-sequestering agents due to their ion exchange effects (Abbès et al., 2008; Shi et al., 2007; Thieu et al., 2008). Zeolites are silicates that consist of interlocking tetrahedrals of $SiO_4$ and $AlO_4$. Large pores in zeolites have sufficient space for attracting and holding positive cations. Of the aluminosilicates, hydrated sodium calcium aluminosilicate is the most studied adsorbent which is characterized as "aflatoxin selective clay," and therefore is not considered as an effective adsorbent of other mycotoxins (Phillips et al. 1995).

## Ruminants

Owing to their unique gastrointestinal systems, ruminants digest diets differently than nonruminants do. Thus, the types of antibiotic-like substances (mainly ionophores) and direct-fed microbials for ruminants are different from those for nonruminants. These ruminant-specific products aim at modulating the production of short-chain fatty acids and microbial protein in the rumen to enhance the provision of both metabolizable energy and a balanced mix of AAs to enhance ruminant growth, lactation, and production (Cameron and McAllister 2016).

### Ionophore Antibiotics

In ruminants, an inhibition of all microorganisms in the rumen is often counterproductive because of their essential roles in the fermentation of protein, fatty acids, as well as structural and non-structural carbohydrates (Cameron and McAllister 2016). Likewise, there is also concern about the use of antibiotics as feed additives in ruminant diets due to the possibility of the evolution of resistant strains of disease-causing organisms. Ionophores (lipophilic compounds), which were originally used to control intestinal parasites in poultry (Bergen and Bates 1984), are now commonly added to ruminant diets. Examples for this group of polyether molecules are monensin, salinomycin, lasalocid, laidlomycin, and narasin (Figure 13.5).

Unlike animal cells, the membranes of bacteria are relatively impermeable to ions and use ionic (both $K^+$ and $Na^+$) gradients as a driving force for nutrient uptake. Specifically, ruminal bacteria maintain high intracellular potassium concentration and low intracellular sodium concentration in the face of high extracellular sodium concentration and low potassium concentration. Since ruminal pH is frequently acidic but the intracellular pH of ruminal bacteria is neutral, these cells have an inwardly directed proton gradient (Russell and Strobel 1989). Ionophores stimulate the transport of ions across cell membranes of Gram-positive bacteria, dissipating ion (e.g., $H^+$ and $Na^+$) gradients, and uncoupling energy expenditure from cell growth, thereby depleting intracellular ATP and killing these bacteria (Callaway et al. 2003). These antimicrobials specifically target Gram-positive ruminal bacterial populations and alter the microbial ecology of the intestinal microbial consortium to increase production efficiency. Gram-positive bacteria have the porous peptidoglycan layer that allows small molecules to reach the cytoplasmic membrane where an ionophore rapidly dissolves into the cell membrane (Newbold et al. 1993). Conversely, Gram-negative bacteria (e.g., *Escherichia coli*) are insensitive to ionophores.

Monensin is produced by *Streptomyces cinnamonensis*, whereas salinomycin is synthesized by *Streptomyces albus*. These two ionophore antibiotics (Figure 13.4) improve the feed efficiency of ruminants by modifying rumen fermentation to enhance the production of propionate and reduce the production of acetate and butyrate. In addition, monensin and salinomycin reduce methanogenesis

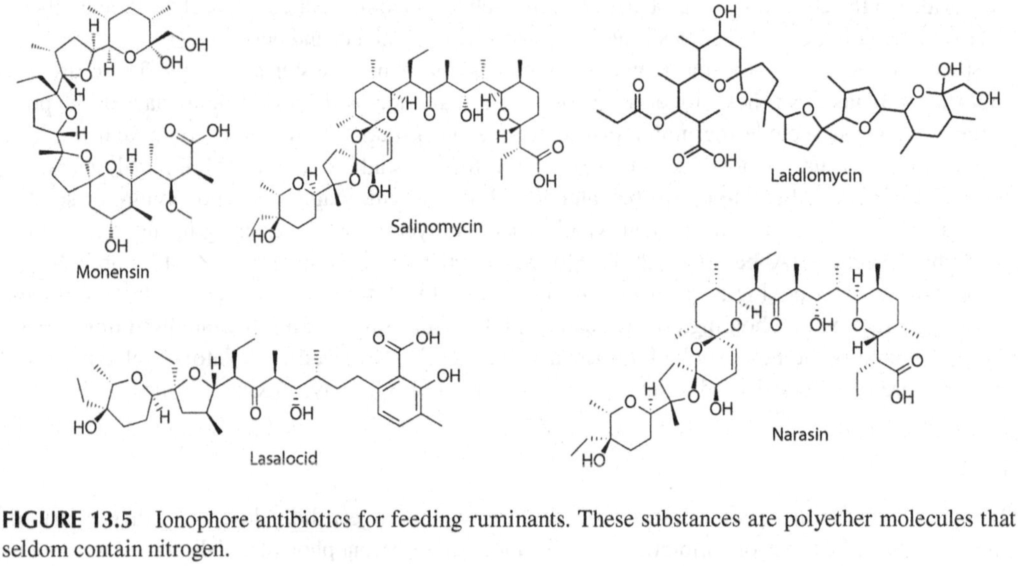

**FIGURE 13.5** Ionophore antibiotics for feeding ruminants. These substances are polyether molecules that seldom contain nitrogen.

by up to 30% at least over short durations, which lessens the irreversible loss of dietary DM (Johnson and Johnson 1995). Note that ruminal methanogens are not directly inhibited by monensin; rather, the bacteria responsible for feeding [2H] to methanogens are inhibited (Dellinger and Ferry 1984). Furthermore, these two ionophores inhibit proteolytic and deaminative enzymes, thereby increasing the amounts of dietary proteins that escape the rumen to enter the abomasum and small intestine for digestion. Thus, monensin and salinomycin have gained wide acceptance as feed additives for growing and lactating ruminants.

Monensin, which was originally used to kill coccidia in poultry as noted previously, also kills protozoa in ruminants. The contribution of protozoa to rumen digestion and ruminant productivity has long been a matter of controversy (Chapter 7). Protozoa can digest polysaccharides and aid in the absorption of several minerals (e.g., calcium, magnesium, and phosphorus). However, protozoa are largely retained in the rumen and therefore reduces the amount of microbial protein that enters the abomasum and small intestine. This means that continuous flow of protozoa from the rumen into the abomasum is required for optimal protein nutrition in ruminants. Thus, defaunation of the rumen reduces the digestion of fiber but increases the quantity of microbial protein reaching the duodenum by ~25% (Chapter 7).

### Direct-Fed Microbials

Many producers and veterinarians have long inoculated sick ruminants (especially those that do not eat well) with rumen fluid from healthy animals to stimulate normal rumen function and improve feed intake. However, there had been little scientific data to document the efficacy of dietary supplementation of microorganisms to ruminants until the 1980s. The proof of the concept of direct-fed microbials for ruminants is provided by the following examples. First, the tropical forage *Leucaena leucocephala* present in some regions of the world (e.g., Australia and India) contains mimosine (a nonprotein AA), whose metabolite (3-hydroxy-4(1H)-pyridone; DHP) is a toxic, goitrogenic agent (Thompson et al. 1969). Interestingly, the rumen of goats raised in Hawaii contains a specific organism (*Synergistes jonesii*) capable of degrading DHP and thus preventing its toxicity. When *Synergistes jonesii* is inoculated into the rumen of Australian cattle that consume the forage *Leucaena leucocephala*, this bacterium confers protection from DHP toxicity (Allison et al. 1990). Second, some plants (e.g., *Dichapetalaceae*) in certain regions of the world (e.g., Australia and South Africa) contain a toxic substance called monofluoroacetate (an inhibitor of the Krebs cycle) (Peters et al. 1960). This substance, even at a low intake level (e.g., 0.3 mg/kg BW), can kill ruminants. When several strains of *Butyrivibrio fibrisolvens*, which contain an inserted gene encoding for fluoroacetate dehalogenase, are administered into the rumen of sheep, the toxicity of monofluoroacetate is markedly reduced (Gregg et al. 1998).

To date, there are many bacteria-based direct-fed microbials for use in ruminant diets. These products often contain *Lactobacillus acidophilus*, *Bifidobacterium*, *Enterococcus*, or *Bacillus*. Young calves fed milk, weanling calves, cattle being shipped, and high-producing cows in early lactation have been shown to benefit from the use of direct-fed microbials. In addition, there is evidence that fungal direct-fed microbials are beneficial to ruminants. With the rapid development of molecular biology techniques, ruminal microorganisms and traditionally used direct-fed microbials may be modified to better improve growth performance and feed efficiency in ruminants.

## OTHER SUBSTANCES FOR RUMINANTS AND NONRUMINANTS

### Amino Acids and Related Compounds

Crystalline AAs (e.g., arginine, glutamine, glycine, lysine, DL-methionine, threonine, and tryptophan) have been supplemented to nonruminant diets to improve protein deposition, intestinal integrity, immune function, and growth performance (Chapter 7). Likewise, rumen-protected protein, lysine, and methionine are widely used as feed additives for lactating cows and, to a limited extent, beef cattle (Awawdeh 2016). There are also reports that creatine or its precursor, guanidinoacetate, can replace some arginine in poultry diets (Baker 2009; Dilger et al. 2013) and that guanidinoacetate is an effective precursor of creatine in swine (McBreairty et al. 2015). Furthermore, dietary supplementation with betaine (trimethyl glycine) may be beneficial for improving nitrogen and energy utilization in pigs and poultry (Eklund et al. 2005). This may be because betaine is a methyl donor and thus involved in many important methylation reactions in animals.

## Anti-Mold Feed Additives and Antioxidants

The water content of dry feed ingredients and formula feeds is generally <13%. However, when they are harvested wet or stored for prolonged periods during the rainy or summer seasons, their water content may exceed 15% to promote the growth of molds, such as *Aspergillus*. Some mold species produce toxic substances (e.g., aflatoxins) to cause adverse effects on livestock, poultry, and fish. To date, anti-mold feed additives include propionic acid, sodium propionate, and calcium propionate, as well as other organic acids (Chapter 12), which may be added to any type of feed at the inclusion level of <0.3% of the total diet (Jacela et al. 2010). Finally, vitamins C and E (Gostner et al. 2014), as well as butylated hydroxyanisole [a synthetic antioxidant; <1 mg/kg BW per day; Figure 13.1 (EFSA 2011)], are often used as antioxidants in animal diets.

### *Yucca schidigera* Extract (BIOPOWDER)

Heat stress reduces the feed intake and production of animals, while impairing their immune function (Morrow-Tesch et al. 1994). For example, increasing environmental temperatures from 23°C to 33°C markedly reduced feed intake, growth performance, and the efficiency of nutrient utilization in swine (Collin et al. 2001) and poultry (Hu et al. 2016). Consequently, a climate change toward global warming is expected to negatively impact animal production worldwide (Renaudeau et al. 2012). Methods to ameliorate heat stress include physical cooling systems (e.g., sprinklers and water baths) (Huynh et al. 2006), reduction in dietary levels of protein coupled with dietary supplementation with some AAs (lysine, tryptophan, and threonine; Kerr et al. 2003) or saturated fat (Spencer et al. 2005). These methods are partially effective because they can enhance heat dissipation, decrease whole-body heat production (primarily via reduced whole-body protein metabolism), and attenuate the thermal effect of feeding, but have the disadvantages of high costs, inadequate provision of most AAs, and an excess deposition of subcutaneous fat. Thus, novel means for optimal mitigation of production problems brought about by climate change are much needed. One effective method is dietary supplementation with the *Yucca schidigera* extract (Yucca; BIOPOWDER), which contains steroidal saponins (Chapter 2). They are natural structural analogues of glucocorticoids, such as corticosterone and cortisol, which are the major types of glucocorticoids in birds and mammals, respectively.

The *Yucca schidigera* plant, which is native to the southwest desert in the United States and the northern part of Baja California in Mexico, is highly resistant to drought and heat stress (Gucker 2006). Yucca is a GRAS product and approved by the U.S. Food and Drug Administration (FDA) as a natural food additive under Title 21CFR 172.510. This substance is also fed to swine and poultry to improve air quality in production barns via reducing ammonia levels (Cheeke 2000). Dietary supplementation with *Yucca schidigera* extract (120 and 180 ppm) did not affect the feed intake or growth performance of broiler chickens when they were housed at an average ambient temperature of 24°C (with the maximum value of 27°C). However, when the maximum ambient temperatures of the housing facility were naturally elevated gradually from 27°C to 37°C, the *Yucca schidigera* supplementation enhanced the BW gain of the chickens by 38%–43% and feed efficiency by 46%–52%, when compared to the control group (Table 13.9).

It was previously thought that the *Yucca schidigera* extract reduced the levels of ammonia within swine, poultry, and dairy facilities through binding ammonia in, and consequently decreasing the

**TABLE 13.9**
**Effects of Supplementing the *Yucca schidigera* Extract to the Diets of Broiler Chickens on Their Growth Performance Under the Conditions of Heat Stress[a,b,c]**

| Variable | Supplemental Dose of the Yucca Extract (ppm) | | |
|---|---|---|---|
| | 0 | 120 | 180 |
| Body weight (BW, g) | | | |
| Day 35 | 1299 ± 32 | 1271 ± 26 | 1294 ± 31 |
| Day 42 | 1563 ± 39[e] | 1636 ± 29[d] | 1672 ± 36[d] |
| Average BW gain (g/week per animal) | 264 ± 14[e] | 365 ± 11[d] | 377 ± 17[d] |
| Average feed intake (g/week per animal) | 912 ± 20 | 883 ± 18 | 876 ± 19 |
| Gain:Feed ratio (g/g) | 0.284 ± 0.013[e] | 0.416 ± 0.016[d] | 0.432 ± 0.017[d] |

*Source:* Rezaei, R. et al. 2017. *J. Anim. Sci.* 95 (Suppl. 4): 370–371.

[a] Beginning at 35 days of age, male broiler chickens had free access to the basal diet supplemented with 0, 120, or 180 ppm *Yucca schidigera* extract. The birds were assigned randomly to their treatment groups (24/group; 6/pen). Composition of the basal diet (%, as-fed basis) was: corn grain, 64.79; soybean meal, 25.91; glycine, 0.50; DL-methionine (98%), 0.21; L-lysine-HCl, 0.08; blended fat, 4.98; limestone, 1.57; BIOFOS-16 (21% phosphorus), 1.28; salt, 0.38; trace mineral premix, 0.05; vitamin premix, 0.25. The basal diet contained 3246 kcal metabolizable energy/kg and the following (%): dry matter, 90.17; crude protein, 18.4 (including lysine, 1.00; arginine, 1.18; methionine, 0.50; and glycine, 0.75); supplemental glycine, 0.50; crude fat, 7.7; calcium, 0.89; phosphorus, 0.61 (available phosphorus, 0.38); ash, 5.55; acid detergent fiber, 3.23; and NDF, 8.57. Body weights of individual chickens and the amounts of feeds/pen at the beginning and end of the study were measured.

[b] Values are means ± SEM, $n = 24$ for body weight and BW gain (based on the number of chickens per treatment group), and $n = 4$ for feed intake and gain:feed ratio (based on the number of pens per treatment group). Data were analyzed using one-way analysis of variance and the Student–Newman–Keuls multiple comparison test (Assaad et al. 2014).

[c] The maximum ambient temperatures of the chicken housing facility, which were naturally elevated gradually during a 1 week period, were 27°C, 29°C, 32°C, 35°C, 36°C, 37°C, and 37°C, respectively, on Days 1, 2, 3, 4, 5, 6, and 7 of the trial; and the average ambient temperatures of the chicken housing facility were 18°C, 21°C, 23°C, 27°C, 29°C, 31°C, and 31°C, respectively. The maximum ambient relative humidity of the chicken housing facility on Days 1, 2, 3, 4, 5, 6, and 7 of the trial was 76%, 71%, 86%, 87%, 84%, 87%, and 87%, respectively; and the average ambient relative humidity of the chicken housing facility on Days 1, 2, 3, 4, 5, 6, and 7 of the trial was 46%, 46%, 55%, 58%, 60%, 57%, and 60%, respectively.

[d,e] Within a row, means not sharing the same superscript letter differ at $P < 0.05$

release of free ammonia from, the large intestine of animals (Cheeke 2000). However, ammonia concentrations in the hindgut are at least 100-fold greater than the concentrations of the *Yucca schidigera* extract. When the circulating levels of corticosterone and cortisol in animals are markedly elevated in response to heat stress, they exhibit: (1) enhanced degradation of AAs to generate ammonia in the whole body; and (2) reduced protein synthesis and increased protein degradation in skeletal muscle (Chapter 7), resulting in growth depression. Under conditions of heat stress, the *Yucca schidigera* extract can block the binding of glucocorticoids to their receptors in cells (e.g., skeletal muscle), thereby ameliorating the adverse effects of heat stress on animal growth (Figure 13.6). Thus, the *Yucca schidigera* extract may be most effective in promoting the growth of farm animals raised in hot climates. Since global warming threatens to adversely impact animal agricultural productivity by decreasing the growth performance and feed efficiency of livestock, poultry, and fish, the use of the *Yucca schidigera* extract as a feed additive has important implications for enhancing animal-protein production worldwide.

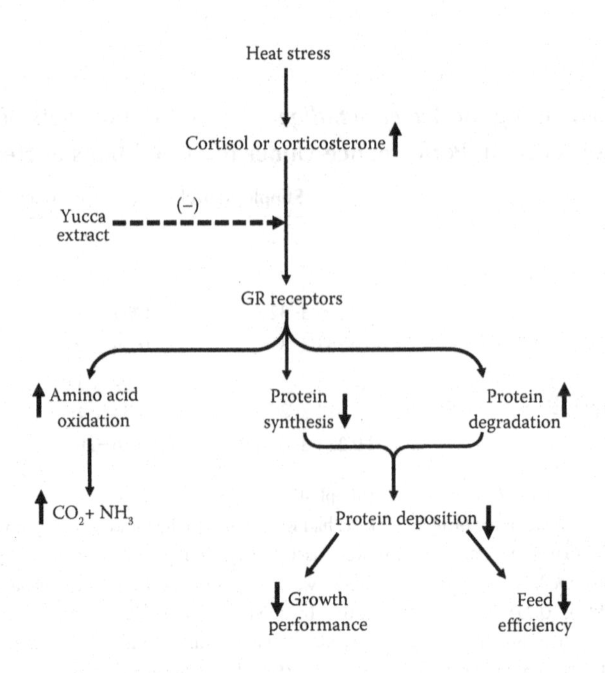


**FIGURE 13.6** Mechanisms whereby the *Yucca schidigera* extract improves the growth performance of animals under heat stress conditions. Elevated levels of glucocorticoids bind to receptors in cells (including skeletal muscle), thereby stimulating whole-body AA oxidation and muscle protein degradation, while inhibiting muscle protein synthesis. As a structural analogue of glucocorticoids, the *Yucca schidigera* extract blocks the binding of glucocorticoids (cortisol and corticosterone) to their receptors, thereby ameliorating the adverse effects of heat stress on the growth performance and feed efficiency of animals.

## SUMMARY

An important advance in animal nutrition over the past five decades is the use of feed additives to improve livestock, poultry, and fish growth and feed efficiency. An improvement in the growth performance and feed efficiency of animals will generate significant economic returns to producers. β-Glucanase, pentosanase, phytase, and a mixture of proteases may be added to nonruminant diets as feed enzymes, whereas cellulases and hemicellulases may be used in ruminant diets. The addition of a combination of carbohydrases (xylanase and β-glucanase) and phytases to corn–soybean-based diets deficient in metabolizable energy, CP, Ca, and P resulted in a significant increase in growth performance and utilization of P, DM, energy, and N in swine and broiler chickens. These enzymes can increase the digestibility and feeding value of dietary nutrients, reduce the variation in nutrient quality of ingredients, decrease the incidence of wet litter, and minimize environmental pollution. Nonenzyme feed additives in poultry and swine diets include antibiotics, probiotics, prebiotics, mycotoxin adsorbents, and crystalline AAs, which improve gastrointestinal function, nutrient absorption, and muscle protein synthesis. Of note, nearly all antibiotics used for feeding nonruminants contain nitrogen and some of them are aminoglycosides to confer or enhance their activity to kill susceptible bacteria. Since the digestive system of ruminants differs from that of nonruminants, a general inhibition of all ruminal microbes will impair the fermentation of starch, fatty acids, fiber and protein and therefore be counterproductive. Thus, the types of nonenzyme feed antibiotics (mainly ionophores) and direct-fed microbials for ruminants are different from those for nonruminants, and are used to modulate the production of short-chain fatty acids and microbial protein in the rumen. The ionophores are polyether molecules that seldom contain nitrogen, and reduce ATP synthesis by select ruminal bacteria through stimulation of their membrane ion transport. Appropriate application of ionophores (e.g., monensin) and bacteria-based direct-fed microbials can enhance the provision of metabolizable energy and a balanced mix of AAs to enhance ruminant growth, lactation, and production. Other feed additives include crystalline AAs and their metabolites, as well as anti-mold organic acids. Collectively, feed additives (e.g., AAs, anti-mold compounds, and the *Yucca schidigera* extract) hold promise for successfully improving weight gain and feed efficiency of both ruminants and nonruminants (particularly under stress conditions), while sustaining global animal agriculture.

## REFERENCES

Abbès, S., J. Salah-Abbès, M.M. Hetta, M.I. Ibrahim, M.A. Abdel-Wahhab, H. Bacha, and R. Oueslati. 2008. Efficacy of Tunisian montmorillonite for in vitro aflatoxin binding and in vivo amelioration of physiological alterations. *Appl. Clay Sci.* 42:151–157.

Allison, M.J., A.C. Hammond, and R.J. Jones. 1990. Detection of ruminal bacteria that degrade toxic dihydroxypyridine compounds produced by mimosine. *Appl. Exp. Microbiol.* 56:590–594.

Amerah, A.M., C. Gilbert, P.H. Simmins, and V. Ravindran. 2011. Influence of feed processing on the efficacy of exogenous enzymes in broiler diets. *World Poult. Sci. J.* 67:29–46.

Amerah, A.M., P.W. Plumstead, L.P. Barnard, and A. Kumar. 2014. Effect of calcium level and phytase addition on ileal phytate degradation and amino acid digestibility of broilers fed corn-based diets. *Poult. Sci.* 93:906–915.

Assaad, H., L. Zhou, R.J. Carroll, and G. Wu. 2014. Rapid publication-ready MS-Word tables for one-way ANOVA. *SpringerPlus* 3:474.

Awawdeh, M.S. 2016. Rumen-protected methionine and lysine: Effects on milk production and plasma amino acids of dairy cows with reference to metabolisable protein status. *J. Dairy Res.* 83:151–155.

Baker, D.H. 2009. Advances in protein-amino acid nutrition of poultry. *Amino Acids* 37:29–41.

Beauchemin, K.A., D.P. Morgavi, T.A. McAllister, W.Z. Yang, and L.M. Rode. 2001. The use of enzymes in ruminant diets. *Recent Adv. Anim. Nutr.* 297–322.

Beauchemin, K.A., S.D.M. Jones, L.M. Rode, and V.J.H. Sewalt. 1997. Effects of fibrolytic enzymes in corn or barley diets on performance and carcass characteristics of feedlot cattle. *Can. J. Anim. Sci.* 77:645–653.

Bedford, M.R. 2000. Exogenous enzymes in monogastric nutrition—Their current value and future benefits. *Anim. Feed Sci. Tech.* 86:1–13.

Bedford, M.R. and H. Schulze. 1998. Exogenous enzymes for pigs and poultry. *Nutr. Res. Rev.* 11:91–114.

Bedfordt, M.R., J.F. Patience, H.L. Classens, and J. Inborra. 1992. The effect of dietary enzyme supplementation of rye- and barley-based diets on digestion and subsequent performance in weanling pigs. *Can. J. Anim. Sci.* 72:97–105.

Bergen, W.G. and D.B. Bates. 1984. Ionophores: Their effect on production efficiency and mode of action. *J. Anim. Sci.* 58:1465–1483.

Bergen, W.G. and G. Wu. 2009. Intestinal nitrogen recycling and utilization in health and disease. *J. Nutr.* 139:821–825.

Biely, P. 2016. Microbial glucuronoyl esterases: 10 years after discovery. *Appl. Environ. Microbiol.* 82:7014–7018.

Brauder, R., H.D. Wallace, and T.J. Cunha. 1953. The value of antibiotics in the nutrition of swine: A review. *Antibiot. Chemother (Northfield)* 3:271–291.

Brenes, A., W. Guenter, R.R. Marquardt, and B.A. Rotter. 1993. Effect of β-glucanase/pentosanase enzyme supplementation on the performance of chickens and laying hens fed wheat, barley, naked oats and rye diets. *Can. J. Anim. Sci.* 73:941–951.

Burnett, G.S. 1966. Studies of viscosity as the probable factor involved in the improvement of certain barleys for chickens by enzyme supplementation. *Br. Poult. Sci.* 7:55–75.

Burroughs, W., W. Woods, S.A. Ewing, J. Greig, and B. Theurer. 1960. Enzyme additions to fattening 30 cattle rations. *J. Anim. Sci.* 19:458–464.

Callaway, T.R., T.S. Edrington, J.L. Rychlik, K.J. Genovese, T.L. Poole, Y.S. Jung, K.M. Bischoff, R.C. Anderson, and D.J. Nisbet. 2003. Ionophores: Their use as ruminant growth promotants and impact on food safety. *Curr. Issues Intest. Microbiol.* 4:43–51.

Cameron, A. and T.A. McAllister. 2016. Antimicrobial usage and resistance in beef production. *J. Anim. Sci. Biotechnol.* 7:68.

Campbell, G.L. and M.R. Bedford. 1992. Enzyme applications for monogastric feeds: A review. *Can. J. Anim. Sci.* 72:449–466.

CAST. 2003. Council for Agricultural Science and Technology Task Force Report 139. *Mycotoxins: Risks in Plant, Animal and Human Systems.* CAST, Ames, IA.

Castillo, M., S.M. Martin-Orue, J.A. Taylor-Pickard, J.F. Perez, and J. Gasa. 2008. Use of mannan-oligosaccharides and zinc chelate as growth promoters and diarrhea preventative in weaning pigs: Effects on microbiota and gut function. *J. Anim. Sci.* 86:94–101.

Cheeke, P.R. 2000. Actual and potential applications of *Yucca schidigera* and *Quillaja saponaria* saponins in human and animal nutrition. *Proc. Phytochem. Soc. Eur.* 45:241–254.

Choct, M. 2006. Enzymes for the feed industry: Past, present and future. *World's Poult. Sci. J.* 62:5–16.

Clicker, F.H. and E.H. Follwell. 1925. Application of "protozyme" by *Aspergillus orizae* to poultry feeding. *Poult. Sci.* 5:241–247.

Collin, A., J. van Milgen, S. Dubois, and J. Noblet. 2001. Effect of high temperature and feeding level on energy utilization in piglets. *J. Anim. Sci.* 79:1849–1857.

Cowieson, A.J. and F. Roos. 2016. Toward optimal value creation through the application of exogenous mono-component protease in the diets of non-ruminants. *Anim. Feed Sci. Technol.* 221:331–340.

Cromwell, G.L. 2000. Antimicrobial and promicrobial agents. In: *Swine Nutrition.* Edited by A.J. Lewis and L.L. Southern. CRC Press, New York, pp. 401–426.

Cromwell, G.L. 2002. Why and how antibiotics are used in swine production. *Anim. Biotechnol.* 13:7–27.

Daly, K., A.C. Darby, N. Hall, A. Nau, D. Bravo, and S.P. Shirazi-Beechey. 2014. Dietary supplementation with lactose or artificial sweetener enhances swine gut Lactobacillus population abundance. *Br. J. Nutr.* 111:S30–S35.

Dellinger, C.A. and J.G. Ferry. 1984. Effect of monensin on growth and methanogenesis of *Methanobacterium formicicum. Appl. Environ. Microbiol.* 48:680–682.

Deng, Z.Y., J.W. Zhang, G.Y. Wu, Y.L. Yin, Z. Ruan, T.J. Li, W.Y. Chu et al. 2007. Dietary supplementation with polysaccharides from semen cassiae enhances immunoglobulin production and interleukin gene expression in early-weaned piglets. *J. Sci. Food Agric.* 87:1868–1873.

Dersjant-Li, Y., A. Awati, H. Schulze, and G. Partridge. 2015. Phytase in non-ruminant animal nutrition: A critical review on phytase activities in the gastrointestinal tract and influencing factors. *J. Sci. Food Agric.* 95:878–896.

Dilger, R.N., K. Bryant-Angeloni, R.L. Payne, A. Lemme, and C.M. Parsons. 2013. Dietary guanidino acetic acid is an efficacious replacement for arginine for young chicks. *Poult. Sci.* 92:171–177.

Edney, M.J., Campbell, G.L., and H.L. Classen. 1989. The effect of p-glucanase supplementation on nutrient digestibility and growth in broilers given diets containing barley, oat groats or wheat. *Anim. Feed Sci. Technol.* 25:193–200.

EFSA. 2011. Scientific opinion on the re-evaluation of butylated hydroxyanisole—BHA (E 320) as a food additive. *EFSA J.* 9(10):2392.

Eklund, M., E. Bauer, J. Wamatu, and R. Mosenthin. 2005. Potential nutritional and physiological functions of betaine in livestock. *Nutr. Res. Rev.* 18:31–48.

Fakruddin, M.d. 2017. Thermostable enzymes and their industrial application: A review. *Discovery* 53:147–157.

Fry, R.E., J.B. Allred, L.S. Jensen, and J. McGinnis. 1957. Influence of cereal grain components of the diet on the response of chicks and poults to dietary enzyme supplements. *Poult. Sci.* 36:1120.

Gaskins, H.R., C.T. Collier, and D.B. Anderson. 2002. Antibiotics as growth promotants. *Anim. Biotechnol.* 13:29–42.

Gírio, F.M., C. Fonseca, F. Carvalheiro, L.C. Duarte, S. Marques, and R. Bogel-Lukasik. 2010. Hemicelluloses for fuel ethanol: A review. *Bioresour. Technol.* 101:4775–4800.

Gostner, J., C. Ciardi, K. Becker, D. Fuchs, and R. Sucher. 2014. Immunoregulatory impact of food antioxidants. *Curr. Pharm. Des.* 20:840–849.

Graham, H., W. Lowgren, D. Pettersson, and P. Aman. 1988. Effect of enzyme supplementation on digestion of a barley/pollard-based pig diet. *Nutr. Rep. Int.* 38:1073–1079.

Gregg, K., B. Hamdorf, K. Henderson, J. Kopecny, and C. Wong. 1998. Genetically modified ruminal bacteria protect sheep from fluoroacetate poisoning. 1998. *Appl. Environ. Microbiol.* 64:3496–3498.

Grootwassink, J.W.D., G.L. Campbell, and H.L. Classen. 1989. Fractionation of crude pentosanase (Arabinoxylanase) for improvement of the nutritional value of rye diets for broiler chickens. *J. Sci. Food Agric.* 46:289–300.

Gucker, C.L. 2006. *Yucca schidigera.* U.S. Department of Agriculture, Forest Service. https://www.fs.fed.us/database/feis/plants/shrub/yucsch/all.html. Accessed on April 12, 2017.

Halas, V. and I. Nochta. 2012. Mannan oligosaccharides in nursery pig nutrition and their potential mode of action. *Animal* 2:261–274.

Hastings, W.H. 1946. Enzyme supplements for poultry feeds. *Poult. Sci.* 25:584–586.

Hou, Y.Q., Z.L. Wu, Z.L. Dai, G.H. Wang, and G. Wu. 2017. Protein hydrolysates in animal nutrition: Industrial production, bioactive peptides, and functional significance. *J. Anim. Sci. Biotechnol.* 8:24.

Hu, H., X. Bai, A.A. Shah, A.Y. Wen, J.L. Hua, C.Y. Che, S.J. He, J.P. Jiang, Z.H. Cai, and S.F. Dai. 2016. Dietary supplementation with glutamine and γ-aminobutyric acid improves growth performance and serum parameters in 22- to 35-day-old broilers exposed to hot environment. *J. Anim. Physiol. Anim. Nutr.* 100:361–370.

Humer, E., C. Schwarz, and K. Schedle. 2015. Phytate in pig and poultry nutrition. *J. Anim. Physiol. Anim. Nutr.* 99:605–625.

Huynh, T.T.T., A.J.A. Aarnink, C.T. Truong, B. Kemp, and M.W.A. Verstegen. 2006. Effects of tropical climate and water cooling methods on growing pigs' responses. *Livest. Sci.* 104:278–291.

Iwaasa, A.D., L.M. Rode, K.A. Beauchemin, and S. Eivemark. 1997. Effect of fibrolytic enzymes in barley-based diets on performance of feedlot cattle and in vitro gas production. *Proceedings of the Joint Rowett Research Institute and INRA Rumen Microbiology Symposium*. Aberdeen, Scotland.

Jacela, J.Y., J.M. DeRouchey, M.D. Tokach, R.D. Goodband, J.L. Nelssen, D.G. Renter, and S.S. Dritz. 2010. Feed additives for swine: Fact sheets—Flavors and mold inhibitors, mycotoxin binders, and antioxidants. *J. Swine Health Prod.* 18:27–32.

Jackson, M.E., K. Geronian, A. Knox, J. McNab, and E. McCartney. 2004. A dose-response study with the feed enzyme beta-mannanase in broilers provided with corn-soybean meal based diets in the absence of antibiotic growth promoters. *Poult. Sci.* 83:1992–1996.

János Bérdy, J. 2012. Thoughts and facts about antibiotics: Where we are now and where we are heading. *J. Antibiot.* 65:385–395.

Ji, F., D.P. Casper, P.K. Brown, D.A. Spangler, K.D. Haydon, and J.E. Pettigrew. 2008. Effects of dietary supplementation of an enzyme blend on the ileal and fecal digestibility of nutrients in growing pigs. *J. Anim. Sci.* 86:1533–1543.

Jiang, J. and Y.L. Xiong. 2016. Natural antioxidants as food and feed additives to promote health benefits and quality of meat products: A review. *Meat Sci.* 120:107–117.

Jo, J.K., S.L. Ingale, J.S. Kim, Y.W. Kim, K.H. Kim, J.D. Lohakare, J.H. Lee, and B.J. Chae. 2012. Effects of exogenous enzyme supplementation to corn- and soybean meal-based or complex diets on growth performance, nutrient digestibility, and blood metabolites in growing pigs. *J. Anim. Sci.* 90:3041–3048.

Johnson, K.A. and D.E. Johnson. 1995. Methane emissions from cattle. *J. Anim. Sci.* 73:2483–2494.

Kerr, B.J., J.T. Yen, J.A. Nienaber, and E.A. Easter. 2003. Influences of dietary protein level, amino acid supplementation and environmental temperature on performance, body composition, organ weights and total heat production of growing pigs. *J. Anim. Sci.* 81:1998–2007.

Kerr, B.J. and G.C. Shurson. 2013. Strategies to improve fiber utilization in swine. *J. Anim. Sci. Biotechnol.* 4:11.

Kim, S.W., D.A. Knabe, K.J. Hong, and R.A. Easter. 2003. Use of carbohydrases in corn-soybean meal-based nursery diets. *J. Anim. Sci.* 81:2496–2504.

Kong, C., J.H. Lee, and O. Adeola. 2011. Supplementation of β-mannanase to starter and grower diets for broilers. *Can. J. Anim. Sci.* 91:389–397.

Kulkarni, N., A. Shendye, and M. Rao. 1999. Molecular and biotechnological aspects of xylanases. *FEMS Microbiol. Rev.* 23:411–456.

Kung, L. 2001. Developments in rumen fermentation—Commercial applications. *Recent Adv. Anim. Nutr.* 105:281–295.

Li, S., W.C. Sauer, R. Mosenthin, and B. Kerr. 1996. Effect of β-glucanase supplementation of cereal-based diets for starter pigs on the apparent digestibilities of dry matter, crude protein and energy. *Anim. Feed Sci. Tech.* 59:223–231.

Lu, H., S.A. Adedokun, A. Preynat, V. Legrand-Defretin, P.A. Geraert, O. Adeola, and K.M. Ajuwon. 2013. Impact of exogenous carbohydrases and phytase on growth performance and nutrient digestibility in broilers. *Can. J. Anim. Sci.* 93:243–249.

Lv, J.N., Y.Q. Chen, X.J. Guo, X.S. Piao, Y.H. Cao, and B. Dong. 2013. Effects of supplementation of β-mannanase in corn-soybean meal diets on performance and nutrient digestibility in growing pigs. *Asian-Australas. J Anim. Sci.* 26:579–587.

McBreairty, L.E., Robinson, J.L., K.R. Furlong, J.A. Brunton, and R.F. Bertolo. 2015. Guanidinoacetate is more effective than creatine at enhancing tissue creatine stores while consequently limiting methionine availability in Yucatan miniature pigs. *PLoS One* 10:e0131563.

McDonald, P., R.A. Edwards, J.F.D. Greenhalgh, C.A. Morgan, and L.A. Sinclair. 2011. *Animal Nutrition*, 7th ed. Prentice Hall, New York.

Meale, S.J., K.A. Beauchemin, A.N. Hristov, A.V. Chaves, and T.A. McAllister. 2014. Opportunities and challenges in using exogenous enzymes to improve ruminant production. *J. Anim. Sci.* 92:427–442.

Moore, P.R., A. Evension, and T.D. Luckey. 1946. Use of sulfasuxidine, streptothricin and streptomycin in nutritional studies with the chick. *J. Biochem.* 165:437–441.

Morrow-Tesch, J.L., J.J. McGlone, and J.L. Salak-Johnson. 1994. Heat and social stress effects on pig immune measures. *J. Anim. Sci.* 72:2599–2609.

Newbold, C.J., R.J. Wallace, and N.D. Walker. 1993. The effect of tetronasin and monensin on fermentation, microbial numbers and the development of ionophore-resistant bacteria in the rumen. *J. Appl. Bacteriol.* 75:129–134.

Omogbenigun, F.O., C.M. Nyachoti, and B.A. Slominski. 2004. Dietary supplementation with multienzyme preparations improved nutrient utilization and growth performance in weaned pigs. *J. Anim. Sci.* 82:1053–1061.

Patrick, G.L. 1995. *An Introduction to Medicinal Chemistry.* Oxford University Press, New York.

Perez-Muñoz, M.E., M.-C. Arrieta, A.E. Ramer-Tait, and J. Walter. 2017. A critical assessment of the "sterile womb" and "in utero colonization" hypotheses: Implications for research on the pioneer infant microbiome. *Microbiome* 5:48.

Perry, T.W., D.D. Cope, and W.M. Beeson. 1960. Low vs high moisture shelled corn with and without 14 enzymes and stilbestrol for fattening steers. *J. Anim. Sci.* 19:1284.

Peters, R.A., R.J. Hall, P.F.V., Ward, and N. Sheppard. 1960. The chemical nature of the toxic compounds containing fluorine in the seeds of *Dichapetalum toxicarium. Biochem. J.* 77:17.

Pettersson, D. and P. Aman. 1989. Enzyme supplementation of a poultry diet containing rye and wheat. *Br. J. Nutr.* 62:139–149.

Pettey, L.A., S.D. Carter, B.W. Senne, and J.A. Shriver. 2002. Effects of beta-mannanase addition to corn-soybean meal diets on growth performance, carcass traits, and nutrient digestibility of weanling and growing-finishing pigs. *J. Anim. Sci.* 80:1012–1019.

Phillips, T.D., A.B. Sarr, and P.G. Grant. 1995. Selective chemisorption and detoxification of aflatoxins by phyllosilicate clay. *Nat. Toxins* 3:204–213.

Pier, A.C. 1992. Major biological consequences of aflatoxicosis in animal production. *J. Anim. Sci.* 70:3964–3967.

Pierce, K.M., T. Sweeney, P.O. Brophy, J.J. Callan, E. Fitzpatrick, P. McCarthy, and J.V. O'Doherty. 2006. The effect of lactose and inulin on intestinal morphology, selected microbial populations and volatile fatty acid concentrations in the gastrointestinal tract of the weaned pig. *Anim. Sci.* 82:311–318.

Renaudeau, D., A. Collin, S. Yahav, V. de Basilio, J.L. Gourdine, and R.J. Collier. 2012. Adaptation to hot climate and strategies to alleviate heat stress in livestock production. *Animal* 6:707–728.

Rezaei, R., D.A. Knabe, and G. Wu. 2013. Impact of aflatoxins on swine nutrition and possible measures of control and amelioration. *Aflatoxin Control: Safeguarding Animal Feed with Calcium Smectite.* Edited by Joe B. Dixon, Ana L. Barrientos Velázquez, and Youjun Deng, American Society of Agronomy and Soil Science, Madison, WI, pp. 54–67.

Rezaei, R., J. Lei, and G. Wu. 2017. Dietary supplementation with *Yucca schidigera* extract alleviates heat stress-induced growth restriction in chickens. *J. Anim. Sci.* 95 (Suppl. 4):370–371.

Rode, L.M., W.Z. Yang, and K.A. Beauchemin 1999. Fibrolytic enzyme supplements for dairy cows in early lactation. *J. Dairy Sci.* 82:2121–2126.

Russell, J.B. and H.J. Strobel. 1989. Effect of ionophores on ruminal fermentation. *Appl. Environ. Microbiol.* 55:1–6.

Rust, J.W., N.L. Jacobsen, A.D. McGilliard, D.K. Hotchkiss. 1965. Supplementation of dairy calf 25 diets with enzymes. II. Effect on nutrient utilization and on composition of rumen fluid. *J. Anim. Sci.* 24:156–160.

Sauvage, E., F. Kerff, M. Terrak, J.A. Ayala, and P. Charlier. 2008. The penicillin-binding proteins: Structure and role in peptidoglycan biosynthesis. *FEMS Microbiol. Rev.* 32:234–258.

Shi, Y.H., Z.R. Xu, C.Z. Wang, and Y. Sun. 2007. Efficacy of two different types of montmorillonite to reduce the toxicity of aflatoxin in pigs. *New Zealand J. Agric. Res.* 50:473–478.

Spangler, M. 2013. Genetic improvement of feed efficiency: Tools and tactics. http://www.iowabeefcenter.org/proceedings/FeedEfficiencySelection.pdf. Accessed on April 10, 2017.

Spencer, J.D., A.M. Gaines, E.P. Berg, and G.L. Allee. 2005. Diet modifications to improve finishing pig growth performance and pork quality attributes during periods of heat stress. *J. Anim. Sci.* 83:243–254.

Starr, M.P. and Reynolds, D.M. 1951. Streptomycin resistance of coliform bacteria from turkeys fed streptomycin. *Am. J. Public Health* 41:1375–1380.

Sujani, S. and R.T. Seresinhe. 2015. Exogenous enzymes in ruminant Nutrition: A review. *Asian J. Anim. Sci.* 9:85–99.

Tan, B. and Y. Yin. 2017. Environmental sustainability analysis and nutritional strategies of animal production in China. *Annu. Rev. Anim. Biosci.* 5:171–184.
Thacker, P.A. 2013. Alternatives to antibiotics as growth promoters for use in swine production: A review. *J. Anim. Sci. Biotechnol.* 4:35.
Thacker, P.A., Campbell, G.L. and J.W.D. Grootwassink. 1988. The effect of betaglucanase supplementation on the performance of pigs fed hulless barley. *Nutr. Rep. Int.* 38:91–99.
Thacker, P.A., J.G. McLeod, and G.L. Campbell. 2002. Performance of growing-finishing pigs fed diets based on normal or low viscosity rye fed with and without enzyme supplementation. *Arch. Tierernahr.* 56:361–70.
Thieu, N.Q., B. Ogle, and H. Pettersson. 2008. Efficacy of bentonite clay in ameliorating aflatoxicosis in piglets fed aflatoxin contaminated diets. *Trop. Anim. Health Prod.* 40:649–656.
Thompson, J.F., C.J. Morris, and I.K. Smith. 1969. New naturally occurring amino acids. *Annu. Rev. Biochem.* 38:137–158.
Vieille, C. and G.J. Zeikus. 2001. Hyperthermophilic enzymes: Sources, uses, and molecular mechanisms for thermostability. *Microbiol Mol. Biol. Rev.* 65:1–43.
Visek, W.J. 1978. The mode of growth promotion by antibiotics. *J. Anim. Sci.* 46:1447–1469.
Wang, X.Q., F. Yang, C. Liu, H.J. Zhou, G. Wu, S.Y. Qiao, D.F. Li, and J.J. Wang. 2012. Dietary supplementation with the probiotic Lactobacillus fermentum I5007 and the antibiotic aureomycin differentially affects the small intestinal proteomes of weanling piglets. *J. Nutr.* 142:7–13.
Wang, S., X. Zeng, Q. Yang, and S. Qiao. 2016. Antimicrobial peptides as potential alternatives to antibiotics in food animal industry. *Int. J. Mol. Sci.* 17 (5) pii:E603.
Wang, X.W., Y.G. Du, X.F. Bai, and S.G. Li. 2003. The effect of oligochitosan on broiler gut flora, microvilli density, immune function and growth performance. *Acta Zoonutr. Sin.* 15:32–45.
Weaver, A.C. and S.W. Kim. 2014. Supplemental nucleotides high in inosine 5′monophosphate to improve the growth and health of nursery pigs. *J. Anim. Sci.* 92:645–651.
Woyengo, T.A. and C.M. Nyachoti. 2013. Review: Anti-nutritional effects of phytic acid in diets for pigs and poultry—Current knowledge and directions for future research. *Can. J. Anim. Sci.* 93:9–21.
Wu, G. 1998. Intestinal mucosal amino acid catabolism. *J. Nutr.* 128:1249–1252.
Wu, G., J. Fanzo, D.D. Miller, P. Pingali, M. Post, J.L. Steiner, and A.E. Thalacker-Mercer. 2014. Production and supply of high-quality food protein for human consumption: Sustainability, challenges and innovations. *Ann. N.Y. Acad. Sci.* 1321:1–19.
Wu, L., J. Li, Y. Li, T. Li, Q. He, Y. Tang, H. Liu, Y. Su, Y. Yin, and P. Liao. 2016. Aflatoxin B1, zearalenone and deoxynivalenol in feed ingredients and complete feed from different Province in China. *J. Anim. Sci. Biotechnol.* 7:63.
Yue, Y., Y.M. Guo, and Y. Yang. 2017. Effects of dietary L-tryptophan supplementation on intestinal response to chronic unpredictable stress in broilers. *Amino Acids* 49:1227–1236.
Yang, W.Z., K.A. Beauchemin, and L.M. Rode. 2000. A comparison of mentors of adding fibrolytic enzymes to lactating cow diets. *J. Dairy Sci.* 83:2512–2520.

# Index


## A

25-AA polypeptide, 580
AAs, *see* Amino acids
AASAs, *see* Synthesizable AAs
ABC, *see* ATP-binding cassette
ABCA1, *see* ATP-binding cassette transporter A1
ABC drug transporter-1 (ABCC1), *see* Multidrug resistance protein 1 (MRP1)
ABC drug transporter-2 (ABCG2), 528
ABCG2, *see* ABC drug transporter-2
Abomasum, 26
  microbial and feed proteins digestion in, 381–382
  in preruminants, 366
  in ruminants, 28
Abomomasum, lipids digestion in, 283–284
Absolute animal growth rate, 653–654
Absorption, 22
  of dietary minerals, 556–559
  of microminerals, 560
  of nucleic acids in small intestine, 382
  of protein in nonruminants, 349–366
  of protein in preruminants, 366–367
  in ruminants, 367–383
ACAT, *see* Acyl-CoA:cholesterol acyltransferase
ACC, *see* Acetyl-CoA carboxylase
Accessory factors, 479
Accessory sex glands, 35, 37
Acetate, 207, 208, 240, 299
Acetic anhydride, 177
Acetone, 314
Acetylating reagents, 177
Acetylation of α-AAs, 177–178
Acetylcarnitine, 534
Acetyl chloride, 177
Acetylcholine, 15
  parasympathetic nervous system, 16
Acetyl-CoA, 226
  ATP production and water in mitochondria, 224–225
  $C_4$ fatty acid chain formation from, 296
  cholesterol synthesis from, 306–308
  Crabtree effect in animal cells, 228
  energetics of acetyl-CoA oxidation, 225
  energetics of glucose oxidation in aerobic respiration, 225
  intracellular concentrations of, 241
  isotopic tracing of Krebs cycle, 227–228
  metabolic control of Krebs cycle, 226–227
  mitochondrial oxidation of pyruvate to, 222–223
  mitochondrial redox state, 228
  nutritional and physiological significance of Krebs cycle, 225–226
  oxidation via mitochondrial Krebs cycle and ATP synthesis, 223
  reaction of Krebs cycle, 223–224
  saturated fatty acids synthesis from, 295
Acetyl-CoA:acetoin O-acetyltransferase, 538
Acetyl-CoA carboxylase (ACC), 295, 304, 321, 498
  malonyl-CoA formation from acetyl-CoA by, 295–296
Acetyl-glyceryl-ether-phosphorylcholine, 125
Acid–base balance, 247–248, 568
  renal Gln utilization for regulation, 402
Acid detergent fiber (ADF), 6, 202
Acid hydrolysis of protein, 176, 185
Acidic AA, 153–154
Acidic phytases, 714
"Acid value" of fatty acids, 140
ACP, *see* Acyl carrier protein
Acquired immune deficiency syndrome, 6
ACS, *see* Acyl-CoA synthetase
$ACS_L$, *see* Acyl-CoA synthetase for LCFAs
$ACS_M$, *see* Medium-chain ACSs
$ACS_S$, *see* Short-chain ACSs
ACTH, *see* Adrenocorticotropic hormone
Actin, 166–167, 670
Actinomyces, 353
Action potentials in skeletal muscle, 564
Active transport, 13, 37, 277, 568
  of organic nutrients, 634
  secondary, 13, 536
Acute arsenic poisoning, 616
Acute copper toxicity, 594
Acyl-CoA
  β-oxidation of Acyl-CoA to form Acetyl-CoA, 316–318
  esters, 277–278
  fatty acid activation to, 315
  potential, 48
Acyl-CoA:cholesterol acyltransferase (ACAT), 279
Acyl-CoA synthetase (ACS), 277
Acyl-CoA synthetase for LCFAs ($ACS_L$), 315
Acyl carrier protein (ACP), 296, 493
1-Acylglycerol-3-phosphate acyltransferase, 310
Adaptive immune system, 39
Adenine nucleotides, intracellular concentrations of, 241
Adenosine triphosphate (ATP), 240, 449
  ATP synthesis, acetyl-CoA oxidation via, 223–228
  production, 57, 224–226
  synthase, 54
  synthesis in animals, 450
  synthesis in cells, 452
ADF, *see* Acid detergent fiber
Adipocytes, 329
Adipose triglyceride lipase (ATGL), 312
  ATGL activity regulation, 312–313
  intracellular lipolysis by, 312–313
  tissue distribution and function of, 312
Adrenocorticotropic hormone (ACTH), 336
Adrenoleukodystrophy protein (ALD protein), 322
Aerobic
  conditions, 220
  glucose oxidation energetics in aerobic respiration, 225
  glycolysis, 219
Afferent neurons, 16

Aflatoxins, 722, 723
selective clay, 723
Agar, 97
Agar–Agar, *see* Agar
Agaran, 97
Agaropectin, 97
Age-dependent metabolic pathways, 49–50
Agmatinase, 412
Agmatine, 152, 412
Agouti-related peptide (AgRP), 688
AgRP, *see* Agouti-related peptide
Akt signaling pathway, 656
Alanine, 239, 403
Alanyl-alanine, 179
Ala synthesis from BCAAs, 402–404
Albumen, *see* Egg white
Albumin, 169
Aldehyde group (–CHO), 69
Aldohexose, 101
Aldopentoses, 75
Aldoses, 70
dehydration, 100–101
sugar, 100
ALD protein, *see* Adrenoleukodystrophy protein
Algae, heteropolysaccharides in, 97–98
Algin, 97
Alginic acid, 97
Alkaline
carboxyl group of α-AAs reactions with, 179
Cu carbonate, 589
hydrolysis of protein, 176, 185
phytases, 714
All-*trans*-retinol, *see* Vitamin A
Allantoic fluid, 38
Allo-forms of AAs, 158–159
L-Allo-threonine, 158
Allosteric activators or inhibitors, 48
Allosteric enzymes, 47, 218
Allosteric regulation, 48
Alnine, 151
α,α-trehalose, 82
α-Amino acid (α-AAs), 149–151
acetylation, 177–178
amino group chemical reactions in, 177
carboxyl group chemical reactions in, 179–180
chemical reaction, 177
chemical reactions involving both amino and carboxyl groups, 181
chemical reactions of side chains in, 180
α-aminophenyl-acetic acid [$C_6H_5CH(NH_2)COOH$], 179
α-amylase activity, 212
α-amylase in mouth and stomach, 194
α-carbon, 150
α-D-galactopyranosyl-(1,6)-α-D-galactopyranosyl-(1,6)-α-D-galactopyranosyl-(1,6)-α-D-glucopyranosyl-(1,2)-β-D-fructofuranoside, *see* Verbascose
α-D-galactopyranosyl-(1,6)-α-D-galactopyranosyl-(1,6)-α-D-glucopyranosyl-(1,2)-β-D-fructofuranoside, *see* Stachyose
α-D-galactopyranosyl-(1,6)-α-D-glucopyranosyl-(1,2)-β-D-fructofuranoside, *see* Raffinose
α-D-Glucose, 73, 81
α-globulin, *see* Transcalciferin
α-helix, 168
α-isomer, 70
α-keto-γ-methylthiobutyrate, *see* 2-keto-4-methylthiobutanoic acid (KMB)
α-Ketoacids
synthesis of AAs from, 392–394
transamination of AAs with, 179
α-Ketoglutarate (α-KG), 227, 372, 412
α-Linolenic acid, 119, 283
α-Lipoic acid, *see* Lipoic acid
α-Melanocyte-stimulating hormone (α-MSH), 688, 689
α-*N*-Oxalyl-α, β-diamino-propionic acid (α-ODAP), 156
α-Oxidation of fatty acids, 328–329
α-Pyranose, 70
α-Tocopherol transfer protein, 524
DL-α-Tocopherol, 522
α-Dicarbonyls, 178
α-KG, *see* α-Ketoglutarate
α-MSH, *see* α-Melanocyte-stimulating hormone
α-ODAP, *see* α-*N*-Oxalyl-α, β-diamino-propionic acid
Aluminum (Al), 553, 613
absorption and transport, 613–614
maximum tolerable levels of dietary minerals for farm animals, 615
sources, 613
toxicity, 614–615
Amadori rearrangement of Schiff's base, 186
Ameliorating metabolic syndrome, peroxisomal β-oxidation role in 324
Amidation, 180
Amiloride-sensitive Na+ channels (AMSC), 562
4-Amino-1-butanol, 178
2-Amino-2-deoxy-β-D-glucose, *see* *N*-acetyl-D-glucosamine
2-Amino-2-deoxysugar, 75
Amino acids (AAs), 2, 15, 149, 152, 165, 178, 239, 274, 349, 449, 553, 633, 687, 694–697, 709
AA-mineral chelates, 182
AA-OPA-ME adduct, 178
allo-forms of, 158–159
α-, β-, γ-, δ-, or ε-AAs, 149–151
bioavailability of dietary AAs to extra-digestive organs, 385–387
chemical classification and properties, 149
chemical reactions of free AAs, 177–185
chemical stabability, 164
chemical structures, 151
composition of proteins in rumen and small-intestinal mixed bacteria, 380
configurations of AAs, 150
crystalline AAs, 164, 172–173
D-or L-configurations of, 155–158
degradation inhibition, 379
degradation of AAs in animals, 395–414
dietary requirements for AAs by animals, 428–433
differences in structures, 151–153
digestion and absorption of protein in fish, 384–385
endogenous synthesis in animals, 387–395
energetic efficiency of oxidation, 462
in enterocytes, metabolism of, 365–366
fermentation of protein in large intestine, 384
in food and animal proteins, 6
free AAs and peptide-bound AAs, 161–163
intracellular protein synthesis from, 371–372, 373
intracellular protein turnover, 414–428

metabolism of AAs in enterocytes, 365–366
metabolites and functions in animals, 415–416
in milk, 664
modified AA residues in proteins or polypeptides, 159–161
naming and chemical expression, 153
nonprotein AAs chemical structures, 151
nonruminants, digestion and absorption of protein in, 349–366
physical appppearance, melting points, and tastes of, 163–164
polarity of enterocytes in, 364–365
preruminants, digestion and absorption of protein in, 366–367
quality evaluation of dietary protein and AAs, 433–438
and related compounds, 725–726
requirements for maintenance, 636–637
R/S configurations, 158, 159
ruminants, digestion and absorption of protein in, 367–383
by small intestine of nonruminants, absorption of small peptides and, 360
solubility of AAs in water and solutions, 164
stability in water and buffers, 164–165
supplements from Rumen degradation, 378
synthesis of dipeptide from two AAs, 166
transport of di-and tri-peptides by enterocytes, 360–361
transport of free AAs by enterocytes, 361–364
Zwitterionic form, 153–155
D-Amino acid (D-AAs), 150, 156, 157
L-Amino acid, 150
4-Aminobenzoic acid, *see para*-Aminobenzoic acid
Amino group ($-NH_2$), 150
AAs transamination with α-ketoacids, 179
acetylation of α-AAs, 177–178
carboxyl group chemical reactions in α-AAs, 179–180
chelation of AAs with metals, 182
chemical reactions, 177, 180–181
deamination of AAs, 178
esterification and $N^{\alpha}$-dehydrogenation of α-AAs, 182
intramolecular cyclizazation reactions, 183
oxidative deamination of AAs, 182–183
oxymethylation of AAs, 179
peptide synthesis, 183–185
reaction of α-AAs, 177
Ammonia, 183, 382
in microbes, 371–372, 373
regulation of AA oxidation to, 405–406
Ammonia detoxification
energy requirement of urea synthesis, 407–408
energy requirement of uric acid synthesis, 410
regulation of urea cycle, 408
regulation of uric acid synthesis, 411
species differences in uric acid degradation, 410–411
urea cycle for disposal of ammonia in mammals, 406–407
as uric acid in birds, 408–411
uric acid synthesis for disposal of ammonia, 408–410
Ammonium sulfate, 168
Amniotic fluid, 38
AMP, 226
AMP-activated protein kinase (AMPK), 321
AMPK, *see* AMP-activated protein kinase
AMSC, *see* Amiloride-sensitive Na+ channels
Amylolytic bacteria, 210
Amylopectin, 87, 195
Amylose, 87, 195
Anaerobic conditions, 220
*Anaerovibrio lipolytica* (*A. lipolytica*), 283
Animal-source
chitin, 88
ingredients, 171, 174
proteins, 149, 379
Animal calorimeter, 462
Animal cells, 184
AA synthesis, 390
activity of pentose cycle in, 229–231
composition and function, 8–10
Crabtree effect in, 228
cytosolic redox state in, 219
glycolysis quantification in, 220
Pasteur effect in, 220
regulation of glycolysis, 221
structure, 8–13
syntheses of D-AAs in, 394
synthesis of AAs from α-ketoacids or analogs in, 392–394
Animal growth
β-agonists, 655–656
dietary AA intake role in, 657–658
growth-promoting agents for ruminants, 656
regulation by anabolic agents, 654
Animal nutrition, 1
biochemistry as chemical basis of nutrition, 6–7
classification of lipids in, 110
composition of foods from plants and animals, 4
composition of nutrients in feedstuffs and pigs, 5
differences between *Trans* unsaturated fatty acids and PUFAs in, 301–302
feedstuffs composition, 2–4
fundamental concepts, 2–8
modified methods for analysis of feedstuffs and animals, 6
nutrients and diets, 2
nutrition, 2
physiology as foundational basis of nutrition, 7–8
proximate or Weende analysis of feedstuffs, 4–6
systems physiology integration in nutrient utilization, 8–13
unit of energy in, 450–451
Animals, 1
age of, 635–636
BCAA degradation in, 398
composition of foods, 4
dietary protein quality evaluation for, 437
dietary requirements for AAs by, 428–433
dipeptides and tripeptides in, 184
endogenous synthesis of AAs in, 387–395
fat deposition and health in, 338–340
fatty acids oxidation in, 314–329
feeding experiments, 437–438
glucose-alanine cycle in, 404
glucose and fructose in, 73–75
glutamine degradation via phosphate-activated glutaminase pathway in, 397
glycoaminoglycans in, 95

Animals (*Continued*)
heteropolysaccharides in, 94–96
homopolysaccharides in, 88–89
interrelationships among metabolism of glucose, amino acids, and fatty acids in, 46
lipoprotein transport and metabolism in, 287–294
major products of AA catabolism in, 413–414
metabolites and functions of AAs in, 415–416
methionine degradation via transsulfuration pathway in, 399–400
modified methods for analysis of feedstuffs and, 6
monosacccharides in, 75
MUFAs synthesis in, 299–301
nervous system in, 15
nutrients requiring by, 3
nutritional and physiological effects of dietary NSPS in, 259–262
production and utilization of ketone bodies in, 324
production of ketone bodies primarily by liver, 324–325
proteins in, 166–167
regulation of hepatic ketogenesis, 325–327
secretion of hormones and major functions in, 40–41
simple aminosugars as monosacccharides in, 75–76
sources of ethanolamine and choline in, 333–335
threonine degradation in liver, 399
tryptophan degradation in, 399, 401
utilization of ketone bodies by extrahepatic tissues, 327–328
waxes in, 121
Animal system, 13
circulatory system, 16–20
digestive system, 22–34
endocrine system, 38–39
female reproductive system, 37–38
immune system, 39–42
lymphatic system, 21–22
male reproductive system, 35–37
musculoskeletal system, 34
nervous system, 14–16
respiratory system, 34
secretion of hormones and major functions in animals, 40–41
sense organs, 42
transport of sodium, glucose, AAs, $NH_3$, and $NH_4^+$ by proximal renal tubules, 37
urinary system, 35
utilization of food by animals, 14
Animal tissues, 109
fructose metabolism in, 253–256
galactose metabolism in, 256–259
glucose metabolism in, 213–253
HSL activity regulation in, 312
intracellular lipolysis by diacylglyceol lipase and monoacylglycerol lipase, 313
intracellular lipolysis by HSL, 311–312
UDP-galactose synthesis pathway from D-glucose in, 256–257
Anserine, 167
Antibiotics, 709, 719–720
antibiotic-like substances, 655
antibiotic-resistant bacteria, 719–720
Antimicrobial
effects, 591
peptides, 176
Anti-mold feed additives, 726–728
Anti-mold feed additives and antioxidants, 726–728
Anti-nutritional factors, 174, 177
Antioxidants, 726
dipeptides, 184
*Yucca schidigera* Extract, 726–728
Antioxidative
peptides, 175
reactions, 591
Antiporter, 570
Apical membrane
AA transporters, 364
disaccharidases, 194–195
of enterocytes, 197–199
Apo, *see* Apolipoproteins
ApoB, *see* Apoproteins B
ApoC2, 294
Apolipoproteins (Apo), 126–127, 271
Apoproteins B (ApoB), 278–279, 285
ApoB48, 278–279
Apparent digestibility of dietary protein, 434–436
Aquaporins (AQPs), 609, 639
Aquaporin 7, 13
Aquaporin 9, 13
classification and characteristics of AQP in animals, 640
Arabinan chain, 96
Arabinan structure, 85
Arabinase, 712–716
Arabinogalactan, 92–93, 96
Arabinose, 75
2-Arachidonoylglycerol, 313
ARC, *see* Arcuate nucleus
Arcuate nucleus (ARC), 688
Arg, *see* Arginine
Arginase, 414
Arginine (Arg), 151, 177, 666
Arginine catabolism, 414
intake, 649, 651
intestinal–renal axis for Arg synthesis, 402
metabolism, 412
synthesis, 391
L-Arginine, 412
Argininosuccinate (AS), 155, 576
Argininosuccinate lyase (ASL), 365–366
Argininosuccinate synthase (ASS), 365–366, 408
Arsenic (As), 4, 553, 615
absorption and transport, 616
poisoning, 616
sources, 616
toxicity, 616–617
AS, *see* Argininosuccinate
Ascorbate oxidase, 591
Ascorbic acid, 222, 232, 507, 579; *see also* Pantothenic acid
absorption and transport, 509
deficiencies and diseases, 510–511
functions, 510
sources, 508–509
structure, 507–508
Ash, 2–3
ASL, *see* Argininosuccinate lyase
Asparagine, 149, 151, 180
Aspartate, 151
Aspartic acid, 153

*Aspergillus*, 722, 726
 *A. oryzae*, 177
 *A. sojae*, 177
 *A. tamari*, 177
ASS, *see* Argininosuccinate synthase
Asymmetrical dimethylarginine, 155
Asymmetric carbon, 155
ATGL, *see* Adipose triglyceride lipase
Atherosclerosis, 294
Atomic mass, 555
Atomic number, *see* Proton number
ATP, *see* Adenosine triphosphate
ATP7b, *see* Copper-binding P-type ATPase
ATP-binding cassette (ABC), 501, 577, 597
 transporters, 276
ATP-binding cassette transporter A1 (ABCA1), 293
ATP-dependent carboxylases, 498
Autocrine hormones, 38
Autonomic nervous system, 16
Avian female reproductive system, 38
Avian RBCs, 9
Avian species, 197, 200
 developmental changes in extracellular proteases in small intestine, 358–359
 developmental changes of gastric proteases in, 354
Avidin, 499
Axon, 14
Azlactone, 182

**B**

Bacteria(l), 202, 282, 367–368
 bacterial proteases, extracellular proteolysis by, 368, 369
 levans, 91
 syntheses of D-AAs in, 394
 synthesis of AAs from α-ketoacids or analogs in, 392–394
Balenine, 167, 185
Basal metabolic rate (BMR), 449
 age and sex of animals, 635–636
 factors affecting, 635
 metabolic size of animals, 635
 normal living conditions of animals, 636
Basic AA, 153–154, 177
Basolateral membrane
 GLUT2 in monosaccharides, 199
 $Na^+/K^+$-ATP pump, 363
BAT, *see* Brown adipose tissue
BCAAs, *see* Branched-chain AAs
BCKAs, *see* Branched-chain α-ketoacids
Beef cattle, 657
Benedict's reagent, 100, 102
Benzaldehyde ($C_6H_5CHO$), 179
Beryllium (Be), 553
β-agonists, 655–656
β-Alanine, 152
β-Amino acids (β-AAs), 149–151
β-Aminoisobutyrate, 152
β-Cyano-L-alanine, 156
β-D-fructose, 81
β-D-glucan glucanohydrolases, *see* β-Glucanases
β-D-Glucans, 85
β-galactosidase, 196
β-Glucanases, 711–712
β-glucans, 85, 713
β-hydroxybutyrate, 328
(β-hydroxyethyl)trimethylammonium, *see* 2-Hydroxy-*N,N,N*,-trimethylethanaminium
3β-hydroxysteroid dehydrogenase (3β-HSD), 336
Betaine, 152
β-isomer, 70
β-Mannanase, 715
β-Mannosidase, *see* Microbial β-mannanase
β-Muricholic acid, 130
β-*N*-Oxalyl-α, β-diamino-propionic acid (β-ODAP), 156
β-oxidation of Acyl-CoA to form Acetyl-CoA, 316–318
β-pleated sheets, 169
β-pyranose, 70
β-strand, 169
D-β-tocopherol, 522
β-Carotene, 512, 513
β-Hydroxybutyrate dehydrogenase, 228
β-Methylcrotonyl-CoA carboxylase, 498
β-ODAP, *see* β-*N*-Oxalyl-α, β-diamino-propionic acid
*Bifidobacteria*, 722
*Bifidobacterium*, 721
Bile acids, 130, 131
Bile alcohols, 132
 structures in fish, 133
Bile salts, 130, 131, 274, 277
 bile salt-stimulated lipase, 274
Bioactive eicosanoids
 degradation, 330–332
 synthesis from PUFAs, 329–330
Bioavailability of dietary AAs to extra-digestive organs
 extraction of AAs from portal vein by liver, 385–387
 metabolism of AAs in small intestine and liver, 386
 net entry of dietary AAs from small intestine into portal vein, 385
Biochemistry
 biochemical studies, 48
 as chemical basis of nutrition, 6–7
Bioflavonoids, 541
 absorption and transport, 542
 deficiencies and diseases, 542
 functions, 542
 sources, 542
 structure, 541
Biohydrogenation, 140
 of unsaturated fatty acids, 283
Biological efficiency of animal production, 642–643
Biological half-lives of proteins, 423
Biological oxidation in mitochondria, 50
 electron transport system in mitochondria, 53–57
 Krebs cycle for oxidation of acetyl-CoA to $CO_2$, water, NADH + $H^+$, and $FADH_2$, 51
 Krebs cycle in mitochondria, 50–53
 metabolic diseases or disorders, 59–60
 uncouplers of oxidative phosphorylation, 57–58
Biomass, 260
Biomineralization, 573–574
Biotin, 497; *see also* Cobalamin
 absorption and transport, 498
 biotin-dependent enzymes in animal and microbes, 499
 chemical structure, 498
 deficiencies and diseases, 499–500
 functions, 498–499

Biotin (*Continued*)
- sources, 498
- structure, 497–498

Birds, 197
- ammonia detoxification as uric acid in, 408–411
- blood circulation in, 18
- cell-and tissue-specific catabolism of AAs, 396
- digestive systems in, 24
- feather growth and color, 675–676

2,3-Bisphosphoglycerate, 218
Biuret assay of protein and peptides, 185
Black vomit, 156
Blood, 16–17
- pressure, 563
- vessels, 17

Blood–brain barrier, 20
Blood circulation, 16
- blood, 16–17
- in fetal–placental tissues, 19
- heart and blood vessels, 17
- microcirculation, 18–20
- in microvasculature, 20
- in postnatal mammals and birds, 18

Blood flow direction
- in fetuses, 17–18
- in postnatal animals, 17

BMR, *see* Basal metabolic rate
Body weight (BW), 449, 553, 633, 687, 711–712
Bomb calorimeter, 453
Bone marrow, 34, 39, 503 507, 584, 591
Borax, *see* Sodium tetraborate decahydrate ($Na_2B_4O_7 \cdot 10H_2O$)
Boron (B), 553, 605
- absorption and transport, 606
- deficiency syndromes, 606
- excess, 606
- functions, 606
- sources, 606

Bowman's capsule, 35
Brain, 16
- synthesizing AAs, 390

Branched-chain AAs (BCAAs), 390, 666
- degradation in animals, 398
- Gln and Ala synthesis from, 402–404
- transaminase activity, 398

Branched-chain α-ketoacids (BCKAs), 372, 390, 403
Branched glucose oligomers, 195
Branched trisaccharides, 93
Bromine (Br), 141, 553, 607
- absorption and transport, 607
- deficiency syndromes, 607
- excess, 607
- functions, 607
- oxidation, 100
- sources, 607

Brown adipose tissue (BAT), 8, 57
Brown seaweeds, 97
Buffers
- buffering reactions of proteins, 187
- stability of AAs in, 164–165

Burning foot syndrome, 493
Butyrate, 113, 193, 207, 211, 299
*Butyrivibrio fibrisolvens* (*B. fibrisolvens*), 283, 368
BW, *see* Body weight


## C


C-5 epimerase, 96
$C_{16}$ fatty acids, 296–297
$C_{27}$ bile acids, 130
$C_4$ fatty acid chain formation, 296
$Ca^{2+}$/calmodulin-dependent protein kinase, 250
Cadmium (Cd), 4, 553, 617
- absorption and transport, 617
- sources, 617
- toxicity, 617

*Caesalpinia spinosa* gum, *see* Tara gum
Calbindin, 570
Calcitriol, *see* 1,25-dihydroxyvitamin $D_3$
Calcium (Ca), 553, 569
- absorption and transport, 569–570
- calcium-activated enzymes and calcium-binding proteins, 571
- deficiency symptoms, 572
- excess, 572
- functions, 571–572
- sources, 569

Calcium transporter-1 (CaT1), 569
Camphor, 6
Canavanine, 156
Cancer cells, 220
Capillaries, 18, 19
Carbamoylphosphate synthase-I (CPS-I), 395, 408
Carbanion, 485
Carbohydrases
- developmental changes, 196–197
- substrate specificity, 196

Carbohydrate(s), 4, 67, 193, 553
- chemical reactions, 99–102
- classification, 67–69
- composition of complex carbohydrates in selected feedstuffs, 92
- cyclic hemiacetals, 69
- D-and L-configuration, 68
- digestion and absorption in fish, 211–213
- digestion and absorption in nonruminants, 194–201
- digestion and absorption in pre-ruminants, 201
- digestion and absorption in ruminants, 201–210
- disaccharides, 76–82
- fermentation, 207
- fermentation in large intestine of nonruminants and ruminants, 210–211
- fructose metabolism in animal tissues, 253–256
- galactose metabolism in animal tissues, 256–259
- glucose metabolism in animal tissues, 213–253
- heteropolysaccharides, 92–99
- homopolysaccharides, 84–92
- metabolism diversity, 193
- monosaccharides, 70–76
- nutritional and physiological effects of dietary NSPS, 259–262
- nutritional, physiological, and pathological significance of fructose, 256
- oligosaccharides, 82–84
- type effects on microbial protein synthesis in Rumen, 375–376

Carbon (C), 151
Carbon dioxide ($CO_2$), 183, 225, 674
- hemoglobin binding to, 187–188

metabolism of nutrients, 642
mitochondrial β-oxidation of fatty acids to, 314–318
prododuction, 314
production of methane from, 208
regulation of AA oxidation to, 405–406
Carbon monoxide (CO), 18, 188, 608
hemoglobin binding to, 187–188
Carbonyl group (-C=O), 69
Carboxyl ester lipase, *see* Bile salt-stimulated lipase
Carboxyl group (-COOH), 149
chemical reactions involving, 181–183
chemical reactions in α-AAs, 179–180
reactions with alkaline, 179
Carcinine, 167, 185
Carnauba palm, 121
Carnauba wax, 121
Carnaubic acid, *see* Lignoceric acid
Carnaubyl, 121
Carnitine, 152, 479, 530, 534; *see also* Choline
absorption and transport, 534–535
carnitine-acylcarnitine translocase, 315
deficiencies and diseases, 535
functions, 535
sources, 534
structure, 534
Carnitine palmitoyltransferase I (CPT-I), 315, 321
CPT-1A, 316
CPT-1B, 316
Carnitine palmitoyltransferase II (CPT-II), 315
Carnivora, 1
Carnivores, 1
Carnivorous fish, 212
Carnosine, 167
Carotenemia, 518
Carotenoids, 137, 513, 675
Carrageenans, 98
Carrier-mediated transport, 12
CART, *see* Cocaine–amphetamine regulated transcript
Casein, 664
CAT, *see* Cationic AA transporters
CaT1, *see* Calcium transporter-1
Catabolism
of free AAs and small peptides by luminal bacteria, 359–360
partition of AAs into pathways for, 395–396
of substrate, 47
Cationic AA transporters (CAT), 362–363
Caudal vena cava, *see* Inferior vena cava
CCK, *see* Cholecystokinin
CCS, *see* Cytosolic superoxide dismutase
CD36 protein, 291
CDP, *see* Cytidine diphosphate
CEAAs, *see* Conditionally essential AAs
Cecum, 31
Cell, 8; *see also* Animal cells
cell-dependent metabolic pathways, 49–50
cell-specific degradation of AAs, 396–401
cell-specific syntheses of AAs, 390–392
cellular cholesterol, 308
cellular sources, 306–308
membrane, 8
metabolism, 226
proliferation, 219–220
Cellobiose, 79
Cellular retinoid-binding proteins (CRBPs), 514
Cellulolytic bacteria, 202
Cellulose, 85, 89–90
Central nervous system (CNS), 16, 576
CCK, 691–692
control centers in, 687
ghrelin, 691
GLP-1, 692
hypothalamus, 687–689
insulin, 689–691
leptin, 689–691
neuropeptides, 687–689
neurotransmitters, 687–689
peptide YY, 691
Cerebrocortical necrosis, 486
Ceruloplasmin, 590
CETP, *see* Cholesteryl ester transfer protein
Cetyl palmitate, 121
CFTR, *see* Cystic fibrosis transmembrane conductance regulator
CGI-58, *see* Comparative gene identification 58
$CH_3HgX$, *see* Methylmercury (MeHg)
Channel proteins, 12
Cheilosis, 487
Chelation
of AAs with metals, 182
drugs, 621
Chemical communications, 39–40
Chemical energy, 449
Chemical reactions of carbohydrates, 99
dehydration of aldoses and ketoses, 100–101
disaccharides and polysaccharides, 102
epimerization, 99
esterification, 101
glycosides formation, 101
Molisch test for carbohydrates, 102
monosaccharides, 99–101
nonenzymatic glycation, 101
oxidation, 100, 102
reacting with iodine, 102
reduction, 100
Chemical treatments, 379
Chemiosmosis, 56
Chemoreceptors, 42
Chirality center, 155
Chitin, 88, 90
Chloride, 567
absorption and transport, 568
deficiency symptoms, 569
excess, 569
functions, 568–569
sources, 568
Chlorine (Cl), 553, 567–568
atomic structures, 556
Cholecalciferol, 518
Cholecystokinin (CCK), 352, 691–692
Cholesterol, 130
cholesterol-derived 17α-hydroxy-pregnenolone, 336
digestion of cholesterol esters, 274–275
HDLs in cholesterol metabolism, 294
synthesis by MECs, 667
synthesis from acetyl-CoA in liver, 306–308
Cholesteryl esters formation, 279–280
Cholesteryl ester transfer protein (CETP), 293

Cholic acid, 130
Choline, 152, 479, 530, 531; *see also* Carnitine
absorption and transport, 533–534
deficiencies and diseases, 534
*De novo* synthesis, 532
functions, 534
sources, 333–335, 531–533
structure, 531
Chondroitin sulfates, 95
Chromanols, 522
Chromate, 602
Chromium (Cr), 553, 602
absorption and transport, 602
deficiency syndromes, 602
excess, 602
functions, 602
sources, 602
Chromodulin, 602
Chronic copper toxicity, 594
Chronic diseases, 287
Chronic iron toxicity, 585
Chylomicrons, 126, 279, 291, 528
assembly, 278–280
metabolism, 287–293
Cinnamaldehyde, 138
Circulatory system, 16; *see also* Digestive system; Lymphatic system; Nervous system
blood–brain barrier, 20
blood circulation, 16–20
*cis* fatty acids, 112, 116
*cis*-4-Hydroxy-L-proline, 158
Citrate, 51, 306
intracellular concentrations of, 241
Citric acid, 715
cycle, *see* Krebs cycle
Citrulline (Cit), 152, 363
CLAs, *see* Conjugated linoleic acids
Classical peroxisomal β-oxidation system, *see* Peroxisomal system I
Clay minerals, 720
Closed-circuit indirect calorimetry, 470–471
"Clubbed down" symptom, 488
CNS, *see* Central nervous system
CoA, *see* Coenzyme A
Cobalamin, *see* Vitamin $B_{12}$
Cobalt (Co), 553, 596
absorption and transport, 596–597
content in body and tissues, 597
deficiency syndromes, 597
excess, 597
functions, 597
sources, 596
Cocaine–amphetamine regulated transcript (CART), 689
Coenzyme, 48
Coenzyme A (CoA), 492, 493
Coenzyme Q (CoQ), *see* Ubiquinone $Q_{10}$
Cofactor(s), 48, 321, 561
of dopamine β-hydroxylase, 591
of protein kinase C, 571
Colipase, 275
Collagens, 168, 169–170
Colloid, 170
Colonic fermenters, 31
Colonocytes, 31
Color of birds, 675–676
Colostrum, 658
Comparative gene identification 58 (CGI-58), 312
Comparative slaughter technique for estimating heat production, 471–472
Compartmentalization of AA degradation in cells, 401–402
Compensatory growth, 656
daily gains of whole body, fat and protein and feed, 658
role of dietary AA intake in animal growth, 657–658
Competitive inhibition, 48
Complex III, *see* Cytochrome c reductase (CoQ-cytochrome c reductase)
Complex IV, *see* Cytochrome c oxidase
Complex V, *see* ATP synthase
Compound lipids, 110, 121; *see also* Derived lipids; Simple lipids
abundant sphingolipids structures in plants, bacteria, and animals, 126
composition of lipids, protein, and carbohydrates in biological membranes, 125
ether glycerophospholipids, 122, 124–126
glycolipids, 121–123
lipoproteins, 126–127
phospholipids, 122, 123
positional distribution of fatty acids in liver and brain phosphatidylserine, 123
sphingolipids, 122–124
Concentrations
of activators and inhibitors, 48
of phosphocreatine, 670
of substrates and cofactors, 48
Conceptuses, early developmental events of, 645
embryonic origins of fetal tissues, 647
functions of placenta, 647–648
stages of embryonic development, 645–647
Condensation of two AAs, 181
Condensed tannins, 98
Conditionally essential AAs (CEAAs), 429
D-Configurations of AAs, 155
in nature, 155–158
optical activity, 155
L-Configurations of AAs, 155–158
in nature, 155–158
optical activity, 155
Conjugase, 504
Conjugated carbohydrates, 67
Conjugated fatty acids, 116, 118
Conjugated linoleic acids (CLAs), 116
Connective tissue, growth and development of, 591
Constant interconversions of energy, 452
Convection direct calorimeter, 470
Conversion of Pro to Gly through Hydroxyproline, 404
Coomassie solution, 185
Copper-AA Chelate, 182
Copper-binding P-type ATPase (ATP7b), 593
Copper-zinc superoxide dismutase (Cu, Zn-SOD), 591
Copper (Cu), 553, 584, 589
absorption, 589
atomic structures, 556
content in body and tissues, 590
deficiency symptoms, 592–593
excess, 594
functions, 590–592

genetic diseases, 593
Menke's disease, 593
metalloenzymes and binding proteins, 590
sources, 589
transport in blood, 590
Wilson's disease, 593–594
Copper sulfide ($Cu_2S$), 578
CoQ-cytochrome c reductase, *see* Cytochrome c reductase
Cori cycle, conversion of pyruvate into lactate and, 219
Corn-based diet, 715
Corn oil, 119
Corticosteroids, 130
Cotransporters, *see* Symporters
Coumarin, 526
Covalent modifications, 48
COX, *see* Cyclooxygenases
CP, *see* Crude protein
CPS-I, *see* Carbamoylphosphate synthase-I
CPT-I, *see* Carnitine palmitoyltransferase I
Crabtree effect in animal cells, 228
CRBPs, *see* Cellular retinoid-binding proteins
Creatine, 152
Crude fat, 6
Crude fiber, 6
Crude protein (CP), 4, 6, 170–172, 349–350, 367–368, 696, 711
dietary and endogenous sources, 435
Crustaceans, 159, 592
Crypt of Lieberkühn, 30
Crypt–villus junction, 30
Crystalline AAs, 172–173, 725
stability of, 164
CTP, *see* Cytidine triphosphate
Cupric ions ($Cu^{2+}$), 185
Cupric oxide (CuO), 589
Cuprous ions ($Cu^{+}$), 185
Curled toe paralysis, 487
Cu,Zn-SOD, *see* Copper-zinc superoxide dismutase
Cyclic hemiacetals, 69, 70–73
Cyclooxygenases (COX), 329
CYP enzymes, *see* Cytochrome P450 enzymes
Cysteamine, 152
Cysteine, 151, 164
cysteine-rich intracellular protein, 586
Cysteinesulfinic acid, 152
Cysteinyl LTs, 135
Cystic fibrosis, 273, 569
Cystic fibrosis transmembrane conductance regulator (CFTR), 568
Cystine, 155, 165
Cytidine diphosphate (CDP), 333
Cytidine triphosphate (CTP), 450
Cytochrome $aa_3$, 582
Cytochrome $bc_1$ complex, *see* Cytochrome c reductase (CoQ-cytochrome c reductase)
Cytochrome c oxidase, 54
Cytochrome c reductase (CoQ-cytochrome c reductase), 56
Cytochrome oxidase, *see* Cytochrome $aa_3$
Cytochrome P450 enzymes (CYP enzymes), 331, 336
Cytochrome P450 monooxygenases, 329
Cytochromes, 582
Cytokines, 411
Cytoplasm, 8, 11
Cytoplasmic transcription factors, 304
Cytosolic pentose cycle, 229; *see also* Krebs cycle
activity in animal tissues and cells, 229–231
pentose cycle reactions, 229
physiological significance of pentose cycle, 231–232
quantification of pentose cycle, 232–233
regulation of pentose cycle, 233
Cytosolic redox state in animal cells, 219
Cytosolic superoxide dismutase (CCS), 589
Cytosol into peroxisome, Acyl-CoA transport from, 322


## D


DAG, *see* Diacylglycerol
DAG acyltransferase (DGAT), 310
Dalton (Da), 555
*Danio rerio. See* Zebrafish
DAPA, *see* Diaminopimelic acid
DCAM, *see* Decarboxylated 5-adenosylmethionine
DCT1, *see* Divalent cation transporter-1
DCYTB, *see* Duodenal cytochrome *b*
DDGS, *see* Distiller's dried grains with solubles
DE, *see* Digestible energy
Deamidination, 180
Deamination of AAs, 178
Debranching enzymes, 716
Decarboxylated 5-adenosylmethionine (DCAM), 412
Decarboxylation of AAs, 179–180, 182–183
Degradation
cell-and tissue-specific degradation of AAs, 396–401
comparison between urea and uric acid synthesis, 411–412
compartmentalization of AA degradation in cells, 401–402
detoxification of ammonia as urea via urea cycle in mammals, 406–408
detoxification of ammonia as uric acid in birds, 408–411
of dietary protein in rumen, 368–374
effects of type of dietary protein on, 374–375
interorgan metabolism of dietary AAs, 402–405
major products of AA catabolism in animals, 413–414
partition of AAs into pathways for catabolism and protein synthesis, 395–396
regulation of AA oxidation to ammonia and $CO_2$, 405–406
species-specific degradation of AAs, 412–413
Dehydration, 670
of aldoses and ketoses, 100–101
Dehydroascorbic acid, 508
Dehydroxylation, 131
δ-AAs, 149–151
D-δ-tocopherol, 522
$\Delta^9$ Carbon
double bonds between $\Delta^1$ Carbon and, 300–301
failure of animals to introducing double bonds, 301
$\Delta^9$ MUFAs synthesis, 299–300
Dementia, 491
*De novo* synthesis of fatty acids, 271, 296, 302
in MECs, 667
species differences in substrates for, 302–303
tissue differences in substrates for, 303–304
3-Deoxy-D-mannooctulosonic acid, 96
5′-Deoxyadenosylcobalamin, 502, 597
Deoxygenated blood, 17

Deoxygenated hemoglobin, 187–188
2-Deoxyglucose, 215
Derived lipids, 111, 127; *see also* Compound lipids; Simple lipids
  eicosanoids, 134–137
  steroids, 128–134
  terpenes, 137–139
Dermatan sulfate, 95
Dermatitis, 487, 491
Detoxification
  of ammonia as urea, 406–408
  of ammonia as uric acid in birds, 408–411
Dextrans, 90, 194
Dextrorotatory, 155, 158
DGAT, *see* DAG acyltransferase
DGL, *see* Diacylglyceol lipase
DHP, *see* 3-Hydroxy-4(1H)-pyridone
DIAAS, *see* Digestible indispensable AA score
Diaccharides, digestion of milk-and plant-source, 196
Diacylglyceol lipase (DGL), 313
Diacylglycerol (DAG), 274, 310–313
  function in protein kinase C signaling, 310
Diaminopimelic acid (DAPA), 152
Diaphragm muscle, 34
Diarrhea, 491
Diastereomerism, 158
Diastereomers, 158
Dichromate, 602
Dicumarol, 526
Dietary calcium
  content, 714–715
  requirement, 675
Dietary/diet, 2
  AAs analysis in, 433–434
  acetylcarnitine, 535
  boron, 606
  bromine, 607
  cadmium, 617
  carbohydrates, 193, 211–212
  complex carbohydrates in rumen, 201–202
  content of sweet sugars, 692
  deficiency of copper, 592–593
  dietary minerals, absorption of, 556–559
  effects concentrate and forage intake on proteolytic bacteria, 376–377
  FAD, 487
  fibers, 99, 193
  FMN, 487
  iodine, 603
  macronutrients, 42
  ME, 457, 461
  NE, factors affecting, 461
  nickel, 608
  nitrogen content, 700
  nonruminants, 701–702
  nutrients, 709
  provision of AAs and energy, 426
  ruminants, 702
  selection, 701
  sulfur, 577–578
  supplement, 172
  supplementation, 722
Dietary energy, 633
  content, 692, 700
  protein, and calcium for egg production, high requirements for, 674–675
  protein, and minerals for muscular work, high requirements for, 670–672
  requirement, 675
Dietary lipids, 286
  digestibility of, 275–276
Dietary NSPs
  nonruminants, 259–260
  nutritional and physiological effects of, 259
  ruminants, 261–262
Dietary protein, 359, 414
  degradation in Rumen, 368–374
  on degradation in rumen, 374–375
  requirement, 675
Dietary requirements for AAs by animals
  factors affecting, 432
  general considerations, 428–429
  "ideal protein" concept, 432–433
  needs for formulating, 428
  qualitative requirements, 429–430
  quantitative requirements, 430–432
Diethylmercury, 620
Differential direct calorimeter, 470
Digalacto-diglycerides, 283
Digesta flow from stomach into small intestine, 354–355
Digestibility
  measurements of feeds, 456
  of starch, 212–213
Digestible energy (DE), 454; *see also* Gross energy (GE); Metabolizable energy (ME)
  digestibility measurements of feeds, 456
  losses of fecal energy in animals, 454–456
Digestible indispensable AA score (DIAAS), 433
Digestion, 22
  digestive enzymes, 709
  digestive function of gastric HCl and gastric proteases, 352–353
  of microbial and feed proteins in abomasum and small intestine, 381–382
  in nonruminants, 349–366
  of nucleic acids in small intestine, 382
  in preruminants, 366–367
  in ruminants, 367–383
Digestive system, 22; *see also* Circulatory system; Lymphatic system; Nervous system
  bacterial species in digestive tract and feces of animals, 23
  coordination among stomach, small intestine, liver, and pancreas, 26
  in fish, 25
  large intestine, 31
  liver, 32–34
  in mammals and birds, 24
  pancreas, 31–32
  small intestine, 28–31
  stomach in nonruminants, 22–25
  stomach in ruminants, 26–28
4,5-Dihydro-4,5-dioxo-1*H*-pyrrolo-[2,3-*f*]quinoline-2,7,9-tricarboxylic acid, *see* Pyrroloquinoline quinine
Dihydrolipoamide, 223
Dihydrovitamin K, 526
Dihydroxyacetone phosphate, 218
1,25-Dihydroxyvitamin $D_2$, 520

1,25-Dihydroxyvitamin $D_3$, 518, 520, 570
3,5-Diiodotyrosine, 152
Diketopiperazine, 182
2,3-Dimethoxy-5-methyl-6-multiprenyl-1, 4-benzoquinone, *see* Coenzyme Q (CoQ)
Dimethylmercury, 620
Dipeptides
  in animals, 184
  by enterocytes, 360–361
Direct calorimetry for measurement of heat production, 469–470
Direct-fed microbials, 721–722, 725
Direct-fed microorganisms, 709
Direct-fed microorganisms, 721
Direct inhibition of proteases, 359
Disaccharides, 67, 76; *see also* Heteropolysaccharides; Homopolysaccharides; Monosaccharide(s); Oligosaccharides
  α,α-trehalose, 82
  cellobiose, 79
  chemical reactions of carbohydrates, 102
  isomaltose, 80–81
  lactose, 79–80
  maltose, 80–81
  in nature, 80
  sucrose, 81
Diseases, 650, 652
  ascorbic acid, 510–511
  of beriberi, 485
  bioflavonoids, 542
  biotin, 499–500
  carnitine, 315
  choline, 534
  cobalamin, 502–503
  folate, 506–507
  hemorrhagic, 8, 530
  Menkes', 593
  *myo*-Inositol, 537
  Niacin, 491
  pantothenic acid, 493–494
  *para*-aminobenzoic acid, 543
  pyridoxal, 496–497
  pyridoxamine, 496–497
  pyridoxine, 496–497
  pyrroloquinoline quinine, 539
  riboflavin, 487–488
  thiamin, 485–486
  ubiquinones, 540–541
  vitamin A, 516
  vitamin D, 521
  vitamin E, 525
  vitamin K, 530
  Wernicke's, 485
  Wilson's, 593–594
Distiller's dried grains with solubles (DDGS), 174, 578
Diurnal changes in intestinal lipid absorption, 280
Divalent cation transporter-1 (DCT1), 579
Divalent metal ion transporter-1 (DMT1), *see* Divalent cation transporter-1 (DCT1)
Djenkolic acid, 156
DM, *see* Dry matter
DMH, *see* Dorsomedial hypothalamic nucleus
Dopamine, 152
Dorsomedial hypothalamic nucleus (DMH), 691–692
Dried blood products, 175
Dry feed, 27
Dry matter (DM), 2, 67, 193, 210, 272, 350, 564, 633, 687
Ductus arteriosus, 18
Duodenal cytochrome *b* (DCYTB), 579
Duodenal ferric reductase, *see* Duodenal cytochrome *b* (DCYTB)
Duodenum, 28
  pancreactic pro-proteases release into lumen, 355–356
Dye-binding of protein and polypeptides, 185
Dyslipidemia, 649

## E

EAAs, *see* Essential AAs
E cadherin protein, 30
Ectoderm, 647
EDDI, *see* Ethylenediamine dihydriodide
EDTA, *see* Ethylenediaminetetraacetate
Eggs production in poultry, nutritional requirements for, 672
  composition of egg, 672–673
  feather growth and color of birds, 675–676
  formation of egg, 673–674
  high requirements for dietary energy, protein, and calcium, 674–675
Egg white, 673
Egg yolk lipids, 673
Eicosanoids, 134
  degradation of bioactive eicosanoids, 330–332
  formation, 300
  lipoxins, 136–137
  LT, 135
  metabolism and functions of, 329
  PG, 134–135
  physiological functions of eicosanoids, 332
  precursors, 134
  synthesis of bioactive eicosanoids from PUFAs, 329–330
  TX, 135–136
Eicosapentaenoic acid, 135
eIF5A, *see* Eukaryotic translation initiation factor 5A
Elastin, 168
Electron
  acceptors, 209
  carriers, 209
  configuration, 556
  configuration of nutritionally essential minerals, 557
Electron transport system in mitochondria, 53
  chemiosmosis, 56
  FMN, 55
  inhibitors of, 57–58
  reduction–oxidation reactions, 54
  role of FAD in reduction–oxidation reactions, 56
  role of $NAD^+$ and $NADP^+$ in reduction–oxidation reactions, 55
  translocation of protons in complex I, 55
Electrophile, 140
Elemental mercury, 619
Elemental sulfur, 577
Elongation of ovine conceptuses, 646
Embden–Meyerhof pathway, *see* Glycolysis pathway
Embryonic development stages, 645–647
Embryonic origins of fetal tissues, 647

Enantiomers, 68
Endocrine system, 38–39
Endoderm, 647
Endogenous nitrogen, 637
Endogenous synthesis of AAs in animals, 390
from α-ketoacids or analogs, 392–394
cell-and tissue-specific syntheses of AAs, 390–392
of D-AAs in animal cells and bacteria, 394
EAAs as precursors for synthesis of NEAAs, 388–390
metabolism of AAs, 389
need for, 387–388
regulation in animals, 394–395
species differences, 392
Endothermic reaction, 451–452
Endotoxins, *see* Lipopolysaccharides (LPSs)
Enediol, 100
Energetic efficiency
of metabolic transformations in animals, 462–467
of muscular work, 671
of oxidation of AAs, 462
Energetics
of acetyl-CoA oxidation, 225
of glucose oxidation in aerobic respiration, 225
Energy, 449
ATP synthesis, 450, 452
chemical, 449
conversion in skeletal muscle, 669–670
dietary provision, 426
expenditure, 472–473
Gibbs free energy, 451–452
and substrates use for maintenance, 641
unit of energy in animal nutrition, 450–451
utilization efficiency for milk production, 669
Energy for maintenance ($NE_m$), 458
Energy for production ($NE_p$), 458
Energy in urine (UE), 457
Energy metabolism, 449
in cells or animals, 450
energetic efficiency of metabolic transformations in animals, 462–467
energy, 449–452
heat production determination as indicator of energy expenditure by animals, 468–475
of male Sprague–Dawley rats, 475
partition of food energy in animals, 453–462
Energy requirement
for intracellular protein degradation, 423
for maintenance, 634–635
of protein synthesis, 420–421
of urea synthesis, 407–408
of uric acid synthesis, 410
Enhancers of feed efficiency, 719
Enteral feeding, 353–354
Enteral nutrients, 687
Enterocytes, 30, 385
assembly of chylomicrons, VLDLs, and HDLs in, 278–280, 285
glucose and fructose transporters in, 197–199
lipids absorption into, 276–277, 285
metabolism of AAs in, 365–366
TAGs resynthesis in, 277–278, 285
transport of di-and tri-peptides by, 360–361
transport of free AAs by, 361–364
Enteroendocrine cell, 30
Enterohepatic circulation, 277, 278
Enterokinase, 355–356
Enthalpy of reaction (ΔH), 453
Enzyme additives, 709; *see also* Nonenzyme additives
for nonruminants, 711–716
for ruminants, 716–718
special thermozymes for feeds, 710–711
use of carbohydrases and proteases, 710
Enzymes, 47, 229
amounts, 48
enzyme-catalyzed deamination of AAs, 178
enzyme-catalyzed reactions, 45–48
mixtures, 716
Epididymis, 35
Epimerization, 99
of monosaccharides, 73
Epimers, 73
Epithelial sodium channels (ENaC), *see* Amiloride-sensitive Na+ channels (AMSC)
Epithelium, 29
Epoxygenases, 329
ε-AAs, 149–151
ε-$NH_2$ group of lysine
chemical reactions involving, 180–181
Equine diets, 272
Ergocalciferol, 129–130, 518
Ergosterol, 129–130
ERK1/2, *see* Extracellular signal-regulated kinases
*Escherichia coli* (*E. coli*), 90, 124, 125, 196, 359, 699, 724
Esophageal groove, 27
Essential AAs (EAAs), 387, 429, 430
as precursors for synthesis of NEAAs, 388–390
Essential oils, 138–139, 720
Esterification, 101
with alcohols, 140
of α-AAs, 182
Estrogen synthesis, 336–338
Ethanol
conversion of pyruvate into, 219
and gluconeogenesis, 245
Ethanolamine sources in animals, 333–335
Ether glycerophospholipids, 122, 124–126
Ethyl acetate, 140
Ethylenediamine dihydriodide (EDDI), 603
Ethylenediaminetetraacetate (EDTA), 6
Eugenol, 138
Eukaryotic cells, 251
Eukaryotic translation initiation factor 5A (eIF5A), 160
Evaporation
evaporative heat loss, 470
of water from animals, 452
Excess minerals, 650, 652
Exergonic reaction, 451
Exogenous substances, 709
Exothermic reaction, *see* Exergonic reaction
Expected FI ($FI_{exp}$), 703
Extracellular
degradation of NPN into ammonia in Rumen, 368–371
osmolarity regulation, 562
pathogens, 39
proteolysis by bacterial proteases and oligopeptidases, 368, 369
Extracellular hydrolysis

of complex carbohydrates into monosaccharides, 202–203
of proteins and polypeptides in small intestine, 356–357
Extracellular proteases
developmental changes in fish intestine, 385
in small intestine of avian species, developmental changes in, 358–359
in small intestine of nonruminant mammals, developmental changes, 357–358
Extracellular signal-regulated kinases (ERK1/2), 588
Extra-digestive organs
bioavailability of dietary AAs to, 385–387
Extraembryonic membranes, 38
Extrahepatic tissues, ketone bodies utilization by, 327–328
Extruded SBMs, 174
Exudate gums, 93

## F

$F_0$ domain, 9, 54, 56
$F_1$ domain, 9, 54, 56
$F_{420}$-dependent formate dehydrogenase (FAD), 208
FABPs, *see* Fatty acid-binding proteins
Facilitated diffusion, 12–13
Factorial method for determining AA requirements, 430
FAD, *see* $F_{420}$-dependent formate dehydrogenase; Flavin adenine dinucleotide
$FADH_2$, 50, 52–53, 55–58, 221, 223–225, 262, 315, 452, 467, 468
Farm animals, 172
Farnesoid X receptor (FXR), 131
Fasting, 247
FATP1, *see* Fatty acid transport protein 1
Fat(s), 110, 119, 120, 271
deposition and health in animals, 338–340, 341
hydrolysis, 139
malabsorption, 530
synthesis by MECs, 667
Fatty acid-binding proteins (FABPs), 271
Fatty acids, 109, 111, 271, 553, 697–698, 709
β-oxidation energetics, 318
of bovine and sow's milk, 118
composition of individual fatty acids in common foodstuffs, 116
in feedstuffs and animals, 113
in foodstuffs, 117
LCFA, 114–119
from lipoproteins in MECs, 666
MCFA, 113–114
melting points and solubility in water, 114
nomenclature, 111, 112
requirements for maintenance, 637
saponification, 139–142
saturated, monounsaturated, ω3 polyunsaturated, and ω6 PUFAs, 115
SCFA, 112–113
Fatty acids oxidation in animals, 314, 321
α-oxidation of fatty acids, 328–329
energetics of Fatty Acid β-Oxidation, 318
long-chain unsaturated fatty acids oxidation, 318
measurements of fatty acid oxidation and lipolysis, 329
metabolic fate of fatty acids, 314
mitochondrial β-oxidation of fatty acids to $CO_2$ and water, 314–318
ω-oxidation of fatty acids, 329
oxidation of short-and medium-chain fatty acids, 318–320
peroxisomal β-oxidation systems I and IIII, 321–324
production and utilization of ketone bododies in animals, 324–328
regulation of mitochondrial fatty acid β-oxidation, 320–321
Fatty acid synthesis, 231
$C_4$ fatty acid chain formation from acetyl-CoA and Malonyl-CoA, 296
cholesterol synthesis and cellular sources, 306–308
differences between *Trans* unsaturated fatty acids and PUFAs, 301–302
long-term mechanisms, 306
malonyl-CoA formation from acetyl-CoA by ACC, 295–296
malonyl-CoA to $C_4$ fatty acid to form $C_{16}$ fatty acids, 296–297
measurements of, 302
measurements of fatty acid synthesis, 302
metabolic fate of palmitate, 297–298
MUFAs synthesis in animals, 299–301
nutritional and hormomonal regulation of, 304
saturated fatty acids synthesis, 299
short-chain fatty acids synthesis, 299
short-term mechanisms, 304–306
species differences in substrates for De Novo fatty acid synthesis, 302–303
synthesis of saturated fatty acids from acetyl-CoA, 295
tissue differences in substrates for De Novo fatty acid synthesis, 303–304
in tissues, 295
Fatty acid transport protein 1 (FATP1), 304
Fatty liver, 338
FDA, *see* U.S. Food and Drug Administration
Feather
feathers production, nutritional requirements for, 672
growth of birds, 675–676
Fecal energy, 454
losses in animals, 454–456
Feed additives, 709
enzyme additives, 709–718
nonenzyme additives, 718–725
peptides as, 175–177
substances for ruminants and nonruminants, 725–728
Feed ingredients
AAs analysis in, 433–434
protein digestibility measurement of, 436–437
Feed intake (FI), 703
NDF effects on, 261–262
NSPs effects on, 259
Feed(s)/feeding, 2
analysis, 271
center, 687
economic benefits of feed efficiency improvement, 702–703
feed antibiotics, alternatives to, 720
of fibrous diets, 458
processing methods, 196
proteins digestion in abomasum and small intestine, 381–382

Feedstuffs, 2
composition, 2–4
modified methods for analysis, 6
nutrients composition in, 5
proximate or Weende analysis, 4–6
Female reproductive system, 37–38
early developmental events of conceptuses, 645–648
effects of nutrients and related factors, 648–650
IUGR, 650
nutritional requirements for, 643, 650–651
Fenton reaction, 584
Fe–O–Fe, *see* Oxo–diiron
Fe–O–Zn, *see* Oxo–iron–zinc
Fermentable fiber, 99, 299
Fermentation
of carbohydrates in large intestine of nonruminants and ruminants, 210–211
of protein in large intestine, 384
Fermentative digestion of carbohydrates, 201
dietary complex carbohydrates in rumen, 201–202
entry of SCFAs from rumen into blood, 206–207
extracellular hydrolysis of complex carbohydrates, 202–203
generation and utilization of NADH and NADPH, 203–204
intracellular degradation of monosaccharides, 203
intracellular hydrolysis of complex carbohydrates, 203
methane production in rumen, 207–209
retention times of feed particles and carbohydrates, 202
ruminal metabolic disorders, 209–210
SCFAs production in rumen, 204–206
species differences in carbohydrate digestion, 210
Ferritin, 579
Ferroxidase, 591
FeS centers, *see* Iron–sulfur centers
Fetal lungs, 18
Fetal–placental tissues, blood circulation in, 19
Fetal programming, 652
Fetal tissues, embryonic origins of, 647
Fetuses direction of blood flow in, 17–18
FEX, *see* Fluoride export protein
FFAs, *see* Free fatty acids
FI, *see* Feed intake
Fibers, 85
*Fibrobacter succinogenes* (*F. succinogenes*), 202
Fibrous proteins, 169
Fish
absorption of lipids in intestine, 286
bile alcohols structures in, 133
dietary carbohydrates for, 211–212
diets, 350
digestion and absorption of carbohydrates in, 211
digestion and absorption of lipids in, 285
digestion of carbohydrates in, 212–213
digestive systems in, 25
extracellular proteases developmental changes in intestine, 385
gastric proteases developmental changes, 384
lipids digestion in intestine, 285–286
monosaccharides absorption, 213
Flavin adenine dinucleotide (FAD), 222, 487
Flavin mononucleotide (FMN), 55, 222, 487
Flavonoids, 479, 530
9-Fluorenylmethyl chloroformate (FMOC), 183
Fluoride export protein (FEX), 605
Fluorine (F), 553, 604
absorption and transport, 605
deficiency syndromes, 605
excess, 605
functions, 605
sources, 604
Fluorite, 604, 605
FMN, *see* Flavin mononucleotide
FMOC, *see* 9-Fluorenylmethyl chloroformate
Folate, 166, 503
absorption and transport, 504–505
chemical structure, 504
deficiencies and diseases, 506–507
functions, 505–506
sources, 504
structure, 503–504
Folate receptors (FRs), 505
FRα, 505
FRδ, 505
Folic acid, 503, 504
Folin Ciocalteu Reagent, 185
Follicle-stimulating hormone (FSH), 338
Folymonoglutamates, 504
Folypolyglutamates, 504
Food, 2
consumption, 687
intake regulation, 564–565
Foramen ovale, 18
Forestomach, 24, 26
Formaldehyde, 379
Formate, 208
Free amino acids (Free AAs), 161–163
amino group chemical reactions in α-AAs, 177–179
chemical reactions, 177
in milk, 666
transport by enterocytes, 361–364
Free fatty acids (FFAs), 271, 284
Free LCFAs, 271
FRs, *see* Folate receptors
D-Fructofuranose, 69
Fructofuranoside, 101
D-Fructopyranose, 69, 71
Fructose
in animals, 73–75
fructose catabolism, pathways for, 254–256
nutritional, physiological, and pathological significance of, 256
in plants, 73
synthesis from glucose in cell-specific manner, 253–254
toxicity, 200
transporters in apical membrane of enterocytes, 197–199
Fructose-1-phosphate (F-1-P), 255
Fructose-1,6-bisphosphatase, 237
Fructose-1,6-bisphosphate, 220
Fructose-2,6-bisphosphate (F-2,6-P), 242
Fructose-6-phosphate (F-6-P), 76, 218, 255
Fructose metabolism in animal tissues, 253–256
fructose synthesis from glucose in cell-specific manner, 253–254
nutritional, physiological, and pathological significance of fructose, 256
pathways for fructose catabolism, 254–256
D-Fructose, 71, 253

concentrations, 76
FSH, *see* Follicle-stimulating hormone
Functional AAs, 414
Functional groups, 182
Furanose, 67
Furfural, 100, 102
Fusarium, 722
Futile cycles, 469
FXR, *see* Farnesoid X receptor

## G

G3P, *see* Glycerol-3-phosphate
G3P pathway for TAG synthesis, 310
GABA, *see* γ-Aminobutyric acid
GAGs, *see* Glycosoamino glycans
D-Galacitol, 258
Galactan, 85
Galactoglucomannans, 93–94
Galactomannans, 93–94
Galactosan, *see* Pure galactan
Galactose
catabolism pathway, 257–258
toxicity syndrome, 259
Galactose metabolism in animal tissues, 256–259
galactose catabolism pathway, 257–258
physiological and pathological significance of galactose, 258–259
UDP-galactose synthesis pathway from D-glucose in animal tissues, 256–257
Galactosemia, 259
D-Galactose, 73, 256–257
Galactoside, 101
Galactosyl β-1, 4-linkage, 79
Gallbladder, 32
γ-Amino acids (γ-AAs), 149–151
γ-AMINOBUTYRATE, 152
γ-Aminobutyric acid (GABA), 15
γ-Glutamyl cycle, 361
γ-Glutamyl hydrolase, 504
D-γ-Tocopherol, 522
Gases, 457
Gasotransmitters, 15
Gas-6 protein, *see* Growth arrest-specific gene 6 protein
Gastric acid secretion
inhibitors, 351–352
stimuli of, 351
Gastric HCl, digestive function of, 352–353
Gastric hydrochloric acid, 568
secretion, 350–352
Gastric inhibitory peptide (GIP), 352
Gastric juice, 568
Gastric lipase activity, 272
Gastric lipid emulsions, 273–274
Gastric proteases
digestive function, 352–353
regulation of secretion, 354
Gastric proteases developmental changes
in avian species, 354
in fish, 384
in nonruminant mammals, 353–354
Gastroferrin, 579
Gastrointestinal tract, 22
GE, *see* Gross energy
Gelatin, 176
Generally recognized as safe (GRAS), 134, 378, 722–723
Gene transcription to form mRNA, 417
Gestating dams, nutrient requirements determination by, 650–651
Ghrelin, 691
Gibbs free energy, 451–452
GIP, *see* Gastric inhibitory peptide
Gizzerosine, 156
Glial cells, 14
Gln, *see* Glutamine
Glomerular filtrate, 35
Glomerular filtration, 35
GLP-1, *see* Glucagon-like peptide-1
Glu, *see* Glutamate
Glucagon-like peptide-1 (GLP-1), 259, 692
Glucagon, 166, 242
D-Glucitol, 100
Glucocorticoids, 197, 243–245, 251, 252, 304–305, 336, 353–354, 354
Glucogenic
AAs, 239
glucogenic-plus-ketogenics AAs, 239
precursors, 240
Glucokinase, *see* HK-IV
Glucomannans, 93–94
Gluconeogenesis, 234
hyperglycemia, 234–235
nutritional and physiological significance of, 248
pathway, 235–238
physiological substrates, 238–240
quantification, 245–246
regulation, 240–245
D-Glucopyranose, 69, 71
D-Glucopyranosyl uronic acid, 97
Glucosamine-6-phosphate (G-6-P), 75, 76, 218
Glucose, 67, 193, 251, 302, 666, 687, 700
in animals, 73–75
concentrations, 76, 692–694
fructose synthesis from, 253–254
homeostasis, 246–247
oxidation energetics in aerobic respiration, 225
in plants, 73
sensor, 217
transport, 215
turnover in whole body, 213–214
UDP-galactose synthesis pathway from, 256–257
Glucose-alanine cycle in animals, 404
Glucose-dependent insulinotropic peptide, *see* Gastric inhibitory peptide (GIP)
Glucose metabolism, 231
acetyl-CoA oxidation via mitochondrial Krebs cycle and ATP synthesis, 223–228
in animal tissues, 213
cytosolic pentose cycle, 229–233
gluconeogenesis, 234–248
glucose turnover in whole body, 213–214
glycogen metabolism, 248–253
glycolysis pathway, 214–222
metabolism of glucose via uronic acid pathway, 233–234, 235
mitochondrial oxidation of pyruvate to acetyl-CoA, 222–223
via uronic acid pathway, 233–234, 235

Glucose-6-phosphatase (G-6-P), 218, 237, 248, 251
dehydrogenase, 234
Glucose transporters (GLUTs), 197
in apical membrane of enterocytes, 197–199
Glucoside, 101
Glucosyl, 77
Glufosinate ammonium, 156
GLUT1, 213
GLUT2, 197
in monosaccharides, 199
GLUT3, 215
GLUT4, 215
GLUT5, 198, 200, 213
Glutamate (Glu), 151, 372
D-Glutamate, 164
L-Glutamate, 164
Glutamic acid, 153
Glutamine (Gln), 153
and Ala Synthesis from BCAAs, 402–404
synthesis from BCAAs, 402–404
synthetase, 413
Glutamine, 151, 161, 218, 239, 403
degradation via phosphate-activated glutaminase pathway, 397
Glutamyl-γ-semialdehyde, 155
Glutathione (GSH), 166, 167, 330–331, 509
glutathione-dependent dehydroascorbic acid reductase, 508
GLUTs, *see* Glucose transporters
D-Glyceraldehyde, 150
L-Glyceraldehyde, 150
Glycerides, 101
Glycerol, 238, 312
3-phosphate pathway, 278
Glycerol–glycolipids, 121–123
Glycerol-3-phosphate (G3P), 218, 309
Glyceroneogenesis, 238–239
Glycerylphosphorylcholine (GPC), 78, 533
Glycine, 151
decarboxylase complex, 538
Glycoaminoglycans, 94
in animals, 95
Glycogen, 88–90, 193
degradation, 249–250
digestion of, 194–196, 212
phosphorylase, 249, 252
synthesis pathway, 248–249
Glycogenesis, 248
determination, 253
intracellular compartmentalization, 251
regulation, 250–252
Glycogenin, 248–249
Glycogen metabolism, 248
glycogen as hydrophilic macromolecule, 248
glycogenesis regulation, 250–252
glycogenolysis regulation, 252–253
nutritional and physiological significance of, 253
pathway of glycogen degradation, 249–250
pathway of glycogen synthesis, 248–249
Glycogenolysis, 249–250
determination, 253
regulation, 252–253
Glycogen synthase, 251
kinases, 250
phosphatase, 250
Glycogen synthase phosphatase, 252
Glycolipids, 121–123
Glycolysis pathway, 214–218, 452
conversion of pyruvate into lactate and Cori cycle, 219
conversion of pyruvate into lactate or ethanol, 219
cytosolic redox state in animal cells, 219
energetics and significance, 218–219
entry of glucose into cells, 215
glycolysis and cell proliferation, 219–220
glycolysis quantification in animal cells, 220
NADH transfer from cytosol into mitochondria, 220–222
Pasteur effect in animal cells, 220
regulation of glycolysis, 220, 221
Warburg effect, 220
Glycoprotein, *see* Sodium/iodide cotransporter
Glycoside, 77, 101
Glycosoamino glycans (GAGs), 167, 168
Glycosylphosphatidylinositol-anchored ceruloplasmin, *see* Membrane-bound ceruloplasmin
GnRH, *see* Gonadotropin-releasing hormone
Goiter, 604
Golgi apparatus, 279
Gonadotropin-releasing hormone (GnRH), 643–644
GPC, *see* Glycerylphosphorylcholine
GRAS, *see* Generally recognized as safe
Green algae, 91
Gross energy (GE), 453–454
ΔH values of organic substances, 454
Growth arrest-specific gene 6 protein (Gas-6 protein), 530
Growth hormone, 166, 305
Growth performance
NDF effects on, 261
NSPS effects on, 259–260
Growth-promoting agents for ruminants, 656
Growth studies for determining dietary requirements of AAs, 430
GSH, *see* Glutathione
GTP, *see* Guanosine triphosphate
Guaiacol, 138
Guanine nucleotide-binding protein-coupled receptors (G protein-coupled receptors), 164
Guanosine triphosphate (GTP), 450
Gut, 30–31
closure, 30

## H

Halogens, 568
reaction of fatty acids with, 142
reaction of hydrogen atom in methylene and carboxyl groups, 142
Haptocorrin (HC), 501
Haworth projection, 70, 71, 72
Haworth structures of hexoses and heptoses, 75, 78
HB, *see* Hydrogen bromide
HC, *see* Haptocorrin
HCl, *see* Hydrochloric acid
$HCO_3^-$, 306
HCP1, *see* Heme carrier protein-1
HDLs, *see* High-density lipoproteins
Hearing receptors, *see* Mechanoreceptors
Heart, 17, 248
synthesizing AAs, 390

Heat increment (HI), 458
differences among energy substrates, 460
of feeding, 460
measurement, 461–462
species differences in, 460–461
Heating, 378–379
Heat of combustion, 453
Heat production as indicator of energy expenditure, 468
caution in interpretation of RQ values, 474–475
coefficients for estimating heat production, 472
comparative slaughter technique for estimation, 471–472
contributions of tissues to fasting heat production, 469
ΔH, $O_2$ consumption, and $CO_2$ production, 471
direct calorimetry for measurement, 469–470
indirect calorimetry for measurement, 470–471
lean tissues and energy expenditure, 472–473
rates of resting oxygen consumption, 468
total heat production by animals, 468–469
usefulness of RQ values in assessing substrate oxidation, 473–474
Heat-sink direct calorimeter, 470
Heme-binding protein, 583
Heme carrier protein-1 (HCP1), 579
Heme enzymes, 582–583
Heme iron (Heme-$Fe^{2+}$), 579
Heme proteins, 581
Heme sulfur center, 584
Hemiacetal, 101
Hemicellulases, 6, 716
Hemicelluloses, 93
Hemiketal form, 70–73
Hemiketals, 69
monosaccharide, 101
Hemoglobin, 169
binding to $O_2$, $CO_2$, CO, and NO, 187–188
Hemoglobins, 581–582
Hemojuvelin (HJV), 580
Hemopexin, 583
Hemorrhagic disease, 8, 530
Hemosiderin, 580
Heparan sulfate, 95
Heparin sulfate, 95–96
Hepatic
acinus, 32, 33
glycogen phosphorylase, 253
ketogenesis regulation, 325–327
lipase, 290
lobules, 32
portal circulation, 17
urea cycle, 6–7
Hepatocytes, 245
Hepcidin, 580
Hephaestin, 579–580
Herbivores, 1, 260
Herbivorous animals, 272
15(*S*)-HETE, *see* 15-Hydroxyicosatetraenoic acid
Heteropolysaccharides, 92; *see also* Disaccharides; Homopolysaccharides; Monosaccharide(s); Oligosaccharides
agar, 97
in algae and seaweeds, 97–98
algin, 97
in animals, 94–96
arabinogalactan, 92–93
carrageenans, 98
exudate gums, 93
hemicelluloses, 93
hyaluronic acid, 94
inulins, 93
mannans, 93–94
in microbes, 96–97
mucilages, 94
pectins, 94
phenolic polymers in plants, 98–99
in plants, 92–94
sulfated heteropolysaccharides, 95–96
Hexokinase (HK), 216
HK-I, 216
HK-II, 216
HK-III, 217
HK-IV, 216, 217
Hexose, 67, 77, 100
monophosphate shunt, *see* Pentose cycle
HF, *see* Hydrogen fluoride
HFE, *see* Human hemochromatosis protein
HI, *see* Heat increment
High-density lipoproteins (HDLs), 126, 272, 479
assembly, 278–280
in cholesterol metabolism, 294
metabolism, 293–294
High-performance liquid chromatography (HPLC), 157, 178, 434
Hindgut, *see* Large intestine
"Hindgut fermenters", 31
Histamine, 152
Histidine, 151
Histotroph, 37
HJV, *see* Hemojuvelin
HK, *see* Hexokinase
$H^+$-$K^+$-ATPase, 567
HMG-CoA reductase, *see* Hydroxymethylglutaryl-CoA reductase
D-HMTBA, *see* D-2-Hydroxy-4-methylthio-butanoic acid
Homeostasis regulation, 308
Homoanserine, 167
Homoarginine, 152
Homocarnosine, 167
Homocysteine, 152
Homoglycans, *see* Homopolysaccharides
Homopolysaccharides, 84; *see also* Disaccharides; Heteropolysaccharides; Monosaccharide(s); Oligosaccharides
in animals, 88–89
arabinan, 85
β-D-Glucans, 85
cellulose, 85
chitin, 88, 90
composition of nonfiber carbohydrates and SCFAs, 87
dextrans, 90
galactan, 85
glycogen, 88–89
levan, 87, 91
mannans, 87, 91–92
in microbes and other lower organisms, 89–92
in plants, 84–88
pullulan, 92
starch, 87–88

Homoserine, 152
Hormomonal regulation of fatty acid synthesis, 304–306
Hormone-sensitive lipase (HSL), 290
activities in WAT and SKM, 292
intracellular lipolysis, 311–312
Hormones, 38, 271, 304–306, 321
hormonal regulation of intracellular protein turnover, 426–428
hormone-like substances, 655
synthesis, 567
HPLC, *see* High-performance liquid chromatography
H-protein, 538
HSDs, *see* Hydroxysteroid dehydrogenases
HSL, *see* Hormone-sensitive lipase
Human civilization, 1
Human hemochromatosis protein (HFE), 580
Humoral factors, 39
Hyaluronan, *see* Hyaluronic acid
Hyaluronic acid, 94
Hydantoin, 182
Hydrated state of mucus, maintaining, 568–569
Hydrochloric acid (HCl), 25, 350–351, 568
Hydrochlorides of L-arginine (L-arginine-HCl), 164
Hydrochlorides of L-lysine (L-lysine-HCl), 164
Hydrochlorides of L-ornithine (L-ornithine-HCl), 164
Hydrogen (H), 151, 555
Hydrogenation of unsaturated fatty acids, 140
Hydrogen bromide (HB), 607
Hydrogen fluoride (HF), 557
Hydrogen gas ($H_2$), 207, 208
Hydrogen ion ($H^+$), 153
Hydrogen sulfide ($H_2S$), 15, 372
Hydrolases, 47
Hydrolysis
of peptide bond, 185
of sphingolipids, 336
of TAG, 139–142
Hydrolyzable tannins, 98
Hydrophilic macromolecule, glycogen as, 248
Hydrophobic molecule, 653
Hydrophobic peptides, 176
Hydroxocobalamin, *see* Vitamin $B_{12}$
D-2-Hydroxy-4-methylthio-butanoic acid (D-HMTBA), 393
L-2-Hydroxy-4-methylthio-butanoic acid (L-HMTBA), 393
3-Hydroxy-4(1H)-pyridone (DHP), 725
5-Hydroxy-6-S-glutathionyl-7, 9, ll-eicosatrienoic acid, 135
3-Hydroxy-L-proline, 158
2-Hydroxy-*N,N,N*,-trimethylethanaminium, 531
Hydroxy acid, 178
L-2-Hydroxy acid oxidase, 393
4-Hydroxydicoumarin, *see* Dicumarol
15-Hydroxyicosatetraenoic acid (15(*S*)-HETE), 136
Hydroxylation of aromatic AAs, 400
Hydroxyl group (–OH), 69
Hydroxyl hydrogen substitution, 140
Hydroxymethylglutaryl-CoA reductase (HMG-CoA reductase), 139
Hydroxyproline, 151
Pro conversion to Gly through, 404
4-Hydroxyproline, 152
Hydroxysteroid dehydrogenases (HSDs), 336
25-Hydroxyvitamin $D_3$, 520
Hyocholic acid, 130
Hyper-allergenic factors, 177
Hyperchloremia, 569
Hyperglycemia, 234–235
Hyperkalemic periodic paralysis (HYPP), 566–567
Hypermagnesemia, 570, 576
Hypernatremia, 565, 570
Hyperphosphatemia, 574
Hyperthermophilic enzymes, 710–711
Hypervitaminosis A, 516
Hypochloremia, *see* Deficiency of chloride
Hypoglycemia, 247
Hypokalemia, 567
Hypomagnesemia, 576
Hyponatremia, 565
Hypophosphatemia, 574
Hypothalamus, 39, 687–689
HYPP, *see* Hyperkalemic periodic paralysis
Hypusine, 160

## I

IBWM, *see* International Bureau of Weights and Measures
IDDM, *see* Insulin-dependent diabetes mellitus
Ideal AA patterns, 658
"Ideal protein" concept, 432–433
L-Iduronic acid, 96
IE, *see* Isotope enrichment
IF, *see* Intrinsic factor
IFN$\gamma$, *see* Interferon-$\gamma$
IGF-I, *see* Insulin-like growth factor I
Ileum, 28
Imino acids, 151
Immune system, 39–42, 156
Immunoglobulins, 667
Indirect calorimetry for measurement of heat production, 470
closed-circuit indirect calorimetry, 470–471
open-circuit indirect calorimetry, 471
Inferior vena cava, 32
Inhibitors of electron transport system, 57–58
Innate immune system, 39
Inner mitochondrial membrane, 9, 10
Inorganic
arsenic, 616
matter, 2
mercury, 620
nutrient, 182
Inorganic phosphate (Pi), 452, 572
Inorganic pyrophosphate (PPi), 248
Inositol-1, 4, 5-triphosphate ($IP_3$), 536–537
Inositol, 75
phosphosphingolipids, 124
Insensible perspiration, 639
Insoluble NSPs, 259, 260
Insulin, 242–243, 304, 306, 689–691
suppresses intramuscular glycogenolysis, 252
Insulin-dependent diabetes mellitus (IDDM), 220
Insulin-independent diabetes mellitus, 31
Insulin-like growth factor I (IGF-I), 658
Integumentary system, 42
Intercellular junction, 18
Interferon-$\gamma$ (IFN$\gamma$), 39
International Bureau of Weights and Measures (IBWM), 450

International Union of Pure and Applied Chemistry (IUPAC), 324
International units (UI), 479, 513
Interneurons, 14
Interorgan metabolism of AAs, 362–363
conversion of Pro to Gly through hydroxyproline, 404
Gln and Ala synthesis from BCAAs, 402–404
intestinal–renal axis for Arg synthesis, 402
NO-dependent blood flow, 404–405
renal Gln utilization for regulation of acid–base balance, 402
Intestinal/intestine
absorption of lipids, 460
absorption of lipids in, 286
developmental changes of intestinal monosaccharide transport, 200–201
diurnal changes in intestinal lipid absorption, 280
GLUT5, 200
intestinal–renal axis for Arg synthesis, 402
lipids digestion in, 285–286
NDF effects on intestinal health, 261
secretion, 568
Intracellular
degradation of NPN into ammonia in rumen, 368–371
$Fe^{2+}$, 579–580
hydrolysis of complex carbohydrates into monosaccharides ruminal protozoa, 203
Janus kinase, 304
osmolarity regulation, 566
Intracellular compartmentalization, 8, 240
of glycogenesis, 251
of metabolic pathways, 48–49
Intracellular lipolysis, 311
by adipose triglyceride lipase, 312
by diacylglyceol and monoacylglycerol lipase in, 313
by HSL in animal tissues, 311–312
by LAL, 313–314
Intracellular protein degradation
biological half-lives of proteins, 423
energy requirement for, 423
intracellular proteolytic pathways, 422–423
measurements, 423–424
proteases for, 422
ruminal fungi role in, 374
ruminal protozoa role in, 372–374
Intracellular protein synthesis, 414–417
gene transcription to form mRNA, 417
initiation of mRNA translation to generate peptides, 417–418
pathway of protein synthesis, 417
peptide chain elongation termination, 418
peptide elongation to produce protein, 418
posttranslational modifications, 418–420
from small peptides, AAs, and ammonia, 371–372, 373
Intracellular protein turnover, 414, 416
dietary protein quality and energy intake effects, 425
energy requirement of protein synthesis, 420–421
intracellular protein degradation, 422–424
intracellular protein synthesis, 414–420
nutritional and hormonal regulation, 426–428
nutritional and physiological significance, 424–426
protein synthesis in mitochondria, 420
Intracellular proteolysis, 373–374
Intracellular proteolytic pathways, 422–423
Intramolecular cyclizazation reactions, 183
Intrauterine growth restriction (IUGR), 650
Intrinsic factor (IF), 501
Inulins, 93
Invertebrates, 159
*In vitro* incubation of cells, 245–246
*In vitro* reaction, 141
*In vivo* reaction, 141
Involuntary nervous system, *see* Autonomic nervous system
Iodination
and bromination of double bonds of unsaturated fatty acids, 141
of phenol ring in tyrosine, 180
Iodine (I), 141, 553, 602
absorption and transport, 603
content in body and tissues, 603
deficiency syndromes, 604
excess, 604
functions, 603–604
reacting with, 102
sources, 602
value, 141
Iodine monochloride (Icl), 141
Iodine number, *see* Iodine value
Ion, 555
channels, 13
concentrations, 48
ion-coupled transport, 13
ionized form of AAs, 153–155
Ionophores, 209
antibiotics, 724–725
Iron (Fe), 188, 553, 578
absorption, 579–580
content in body and tissues, 581
content in hemoglobin and bodies of young pigs, 585
deficiency symptoms, 584–585
enzymes and proteins, 584
excess, 585
Fenton reaction, 584
functions, 581–584
interaction with copper, 584
metabolism, 591
sources, 578–579
transport in blood, 580–581
Iron–sulfur centers (FeS centers), 54, 578, 584
Iron–sulfur proteins, 584
Isoelectric point (pI), 153
Isoflavones, 542
Isoleucine, 151, 164, 173
Isomaltose, 80–81
Isomerases, 47
Isoprenoids, 137
2-Isopropyl-5-methylphenol, *see* Thymol
Isothermal direct calorimeter, 470
Isotope
randomization, 227
tracing of Krebs cycle, 227–228
Isotope enrichment (IE), 246
Isovaleric acid, 109
IUGR, *see* Intrauterine growth restriction
IUPAC, *see* International Union of Pure and Applied Chemistry
Ivory nut (*Phytelephas macrocarpa*), 87

## J


Janus kinase (JAK), 304
Jejunum, 28, 350


## K


κ-carrageenan, 98
Katz and Wood's equation, 232
Keratan sulfate, 95
Keratins, 188, 668, 672
2-Keto-4-methylthiobutanoic acid (KMB), 393
Keto-deoxy-octulosonate (KDO), *see* 3-deoxy-D-mannooctulosonic acid
3-Ketoacid-CoA transferase, 327
Ketogenesis, 314, 324
Ketogenic AAs, 239
Ketone bodies, 271, 697–698
 production and utilization in animals, 324
 production of ketone bodies primarily by liver, 324–325
 regulation of hepatic ketogenesis, 325–327
 utilization of ketone bodies by extrahepatic tissues, 327–328
Ketose(s), 70, 100
 dehydration, 100–101
Kidneys, 34, 35, 36
 in endogenous synthesis of AAs, 391
 Lys degradation, 398
Kjeldahl analysis of total nitrogen, 4
KMB, *see* 2-Keto-4-methylthiobutanoic acid
$K_M$ value, 48
Krebs bicarbonate buffer, 164
Krebs cycle, 6, 45, 220, 383; *see also* Cytosolic pentose cycle
 acetyl-CoA oxidation, 223–228
 isotopic tracing of, 227–228
 metabolic control of, 226–227
 in mitochondria, 50–53
 nutritional and physiological significance of, 225–226
 for oxidation of acetyl-CoA to $CO_2$, water, NADH + $H^+$, and $FADH_2$, 51
 regulation by intrinsic and extrinsic factors, 52
Kupffer cells, 32
Kynurenic acid, 152
Kynurenine, 152
Kynurenine pathway, 399–400
Kyotorphin, 167, 184


## L


*l*-carrageenan, 98
L-HMTBA, *see* L-2-Hydroxy-4-methylthio-butanoic acid
Labeled isotopes, 246
Labeled tracers, 227
Lactase-phlorizin hydrolase, *see* β-galactosidase
Lactase, 196, 197
Lactate, 238
 conversion of pyruvate into, 219
 lactate-producing bacteria, 209
L-Lactate dehydrogenase, 219
L-Lactate, 50
Lactation, 247
 lactating gland, 658–659
 NDF effects on, 261
Lactic acidosis, 209
*Lactobacillus*, 721, 722
Lactose, 67, 79–81
 in milk, 666
 synthase, 257
LAL, *see* Lysosomal acid lipase
λ-carrageenan, 98
Lamina propria, 29
 basolateral membrane GLUT2 in monosaccharides, 199
 monosaccharides trafficking from lamina propia into liver, 199–200
Lanolin, 121
Large bowel, *see* Large intestine
Large intestine, 31
 protein fermentation in, 384
Larrabee's approach, 232–233
Lateral hypothalamic area (LHA), *see* Feed(s)/feeding—center
Lauric acid, 112
Lauric arginate, 182
LCAT, *see* Lecithin:cholesterol acyltransferase
LCFAs, *see* Long-chain fatty acids; Lonvag-chain fatty acids
LDLs, *see* Low-density lipoproteins
Lead (Pb), 4, 553, 618
 absorption and transport, 618
 sources, 618
 toxicity, 618
Lean tissues, 472–473
Lecithin:cholesterol acyltransferase (LCAT), 279
Left lymphatic duct, *see* Thoracic duct
Leloir pathway, 257
Leptin, 689–691
Leucine, 151, 164
Leukocytes, 16
Leukotrienes (LTs), 111, 135
 LTA, 135
 $LTA_4$ and $LTB_4$, $LTC_4$, $LTD_4$, $LTE_4$, and $LTF_4$, $LTC_4$, 135
 LTB, 135
 $LTD_3$, 135
 $LTE_3$, 135
Levan, 87, 91
Levorotatory, 155
LH, *see* Luteinizing hormone
Lignins, 98
Lignoceric acid, 119
"Limiting AA" concept, 429–430
Linoleic acid, 109, 112, 119, 283
Linoleic acid oxidation, 320
Linolenic acid, 115
Lipid-soluble oils, 308
Lipid-soluble vitamins, 138, 511; *see also* Quasi-vitamins; Water-soluble vitamins
 absorption and transport in animals, 531
 content and β-carotene in feedstuffs, 511
 vitamin A, 512–518
 vitamin D, 518–521
 vitamin E, 522–525
 vitamin K, 526–530
Lipids, 109, 271
 chemical reactions, 139–142
 classification and structures, 109
 classification in animal nutrition, 110
 compound lipids, 121–127

derived lipids, 127–139
digestion and absorption in nonruminants, 272–280
digestion and absorption in preruminants, 280–281
digestion and absorption in ruminants, 281–285
digestion and absorption of lipids in fish, 285–287
esterification with alcohols, 140
fat deposition and health in animals, 338–340, 341
fatty acids, 111–119
fatty acid synthesis in tissues, 295–308
hydrogenation of unsaturated fatty acids, 140
hydrolysis of TAG and saponification of fatty acids, 139–142
iodination and bromination of double bonds of unsaturated fatty acids, 141
LCFAs, 272
lipid-bilayer membranes, 8
lipid micelles formation, 273–274
lipoprotein transport and metabolism in animals, 287–294
metabolism and functions of eicosanoids, 329–332
metabolism of steroid hormones, 336–338
in milk, 666
oxidation of fatty acids in animals, 314–329
peroxidation of unsaturated fatty acids, 141–142
phospholipid and sphingolipid metabolism, 333–336
products of lipid hydrolysis, 282–283
reaction of fatty acids with halogens, 142
reaction of hydrogen atom in methylene and carboxyl groups with halogens, 142
simple lipids, 119–121
substitution of hydroxyl hydrogen, 140
TAGs mobilization from tissues to release glycerol and fatty acids, 311–313
TAG synthesis and catabolism in animals, 308–310
Lipoglycans, *see* Lipopolysaccharides (LPSs)
Lipoic acid, 479, 530, 537
absorption and transport, 538
deficiencies and diseases, 538
functions, 538
sources, 537–538
structure, 537
Lipolysis, 283, 329
Lipopolysaccharides (LPSs), 96–97
Lipoprotein lipases (LPLs), 271
Lipoproteins, 126–128, 271
Lipoprotein transport and metabolism in animals, 287
HDLs in cholesterol metabolism, 294
metabolism of chylomicrons, VLDLs, and LDLs, 287–293
metabolism of HDLs, 293–294
release of lipoproteins from small intestine and liver, 287
species differences in lipoprotein metabolism, 294
Lipoxins, 136–137
Lipoxygenases, 329
Liquid-phase peptide synthesis, 183
Liquid soy flour, 366
Liver, 32–34, 248, 325
extraction of AAs from portal vein by, 385–387
glycogen phosphorylase, 253
lipoproteins release from, 287–294
Lys degradation, 398, 399
metabolism of AAs, 386
production of ketone bodies primarily by, 324–325
synthesizing AAs, 390
threonine degradation, 399
Liver isoform, *see* CPT-1A
Living conditions of animals, 636
"Local hormones", 332
Long-chain acyl-CoAs, 306
transfer from cytosol into mitochondrial matrix, 315–316
Long-chain fatty acids (LCFAs), 109, 114–119
synthesis pathway of, 298
Lonvag-chain fatty acids (LCFAs), 271–272, 278
Low-density lipoproteins (LDLs), 287, 479, 666
metabolism, 287–293
Lowry assay of protein and peptides, 185–186
LPLs, *see* Lipoprotein lipases
LPSs, *see* Lipopolysaccharides
LTs, *see* Leukotrienes
Lugol's reagent, 102
Lumen of duodenum, release of pancreactic pro-proteases into, 355–356
Luminal bacteria, catabolism of free AAs and small peptides by, 359–360
Luteinizing hormone (LH), 336, 644
Lyases, 47
Lymphatic(s), 21
capillaries, 21
ducts, 21
vessels, 21
Lymphatic system, 21–22; *see also* Circulatory system; Digestive system; Nervous system
Lymph node, 21
Lymphocytes, synthesizing AAs, 392
L-Lysine-HCl, 173
Lysine (Lys), 151, 177
degradation in liver of animals, 398–399
degradation in liver of animals, 399
ε-NHNH2 group of, 180–181
Lyso-PC, 533
Lysophosphatidic acid acyltransferase, *see* 1-Acylglycerol-3-phosphate acyltransferase
Lysophosphatidylcholine, 274
Lysosomal acid lipase (LAL), 290, 313
intracellular lipolysis by, 313–314
Lysosomal proteolytic pathway, 422–423

## M

Macrominerals, 553, 561; *see also* Microminerals
calcium, 569–572
chloride, 567–569
concentrations in serum of animals, 561
content in newborn and adult animals, 554
magnesium, 574–576
phosphorus, 572–574
potassium, 565–567
sodium, 561–565
sulfur, 576–578
Macrophages, synthesizing AAs, 392
MAG acyltransferases (MGATs), 310
Magnesium (Mg), 216, 218, 553, 574
absorption and transport, 575
deficiency symptoms, 576
excess, 576
functions, 575–576
sources, 575

MAGs, *see* Monoacylglycerols
Maillard reaction, 101, 186–187
L-Malate, 52
Male reproductive
  hormones, 35
  system, 35–37
Males reproduction, nutritional requirements for, 651
  deficiencies of minerals and vitamins, 651
  diseases, 652
  excess minerals, 652
  overall undernutrition or overnutrition, 651
  protein and arginine intake, 651
  stress, 652
  toxins, 652
Malonyl-CoA, 321
  $C_4$ fatty acid chain formation from, 296
  formation from acetyl-CoA by ACC, 295–296
  malonyl-CoA to $C_4$ fatty acid to form $C_{16}$ fatty acids, 296–297
Maltase-glucoamylase, 197
Maltose, 80–81, 195
Maltotriose, 195
Mammalian
  female reproductive system, 37
  male reproductive system, 35
Mammals
  cell-and tissue-specific catabolism of AAs, 396
  digestive systems in, 24
  urea cycle for disposal of ammonia in, 406–407
  urea synthesis from ammonia and bicarbonate, 407
Mammary epithelial cells (MECs), 658–659
  milk synthesis by, 662–668
  release of milk proteins, lactose, and fats from MECs to lumen of alveoli, 668–669
Mammary gland, 658–662
Mammary tissue, synthesizing AAs, 390
Mammogenesis, 659
Manganese (Mn), 553, 594
  absorption and transport, 595
  atomic structures, 556
  content in body and tissues, 595
  deficiency syndromes, 595–596
  excess, 596
  functions, 595
  manganese-dependent enzymes in animals, 596
  $Mn^2$, 594
  sources, 595
Manganese sulfide (MnS), 578
Mannans, 87, 91–92, 93–94
D-Mannose, 73
Manometric methods, 178
Marbling fat, 653
Marine plants, heteropolysaccharides in, 97–98
Marine teleost fish (*Siganus canaliculatus*), 301
Maternal protein, 649
Matrix Gla protein, 530
MBM, *see* Meat and bone meal
MC3R, *see* Melanocortin-3 receptors
MC4R, *see* Melanocortin-4 receptors
MCFAs, *see* Medium-chain fatty acids
ME, *see* 2-Mercaptoethanol; Metabolizable energy
Meat and bone meal (MBM), 170, 357
Mechanical stomach, *see* Ventriculus
Mechanistic target of rapamycin signaling (MTOR signaling), 256, 426–427, 636
Mechanoreceptors, 42
MECs, *see* Mammary epithelial cells
Medium-chain ACSs ($ACS_M$), 318
Medium-chain fatty acids (MCFAs), 112–114, 280
  oxidation, 318–320
MeHg, *see* Methylmercury
Melanocortin, *see* α-melanocyte-stimulating hormone (α-MSH)
Melanocortin-3 receptors (MC3R), 689
Melanocortin-4 receptors (MC4R), 689
Melatonin, 152
Melezitose, 82
Melissic acid, 112, 121
Melissyl, 121
Melitose, *see* Raffinose
Membrane-bound ceruloplasmin, 591
Menadione, 526
Menadione, 530
Menaquinone-4, 528
Menaquinone, 526
Meninges, 16
Menke's disease, 593
Menthol, 6
2-Mercaptoethanol (ME), 178
Mercury (Hg), 4, 553, 618
  absorption and transport, 619–621
  intoxication syndromes, 621
  sources, 619
  toxicity, 621
Mesoderm, 647
Metabolic BW, 635
Metabolic control of Krebs cycle, 226–227
Metabolic disorder, 259
Metabolic fate
  of fatty acids, 314
  of palmitate, 297–298
Metabolic nitrogen, 637
Metabolic pathways, 42, 452
  biological oxidation in mitochondria, 50–58
  cell-, zone-, age-, and species-dependent, 49–50
  characteristics, 45–50
  enzyme-catalyzed reactions, 45–48
  hyperbolic relationship, 47
  interrelationships among metabolism of glucose, amino acids, and fatty acids, 46
  intracellular compartmentalization, 48–49
  for nutrient metabolism and physiological significance, 43–45
  primary localization, 49
  and significance, 42–45
Metabolic rates, 633
Metabolic size of animals, 635
Metabolism of AAs in enterocytes, 365–366
Metabolism of minerals
  intestinal absorption of dietary minerals and transport in blood, 622
  macrominerals, 561–578
  macrominerals content in newborn and adult animals, 554
  microminerals, 578–621
  minerals, 555–561
  periodic table of elements, 554

Metabolism of vitamins
chemical and biochemical characteristics of vitamins, 479–481
lipid-soluble vitamins, 511–530
quasi-vitamins, 530–543, 544
water-soluble vitamins, 481–511
Metabolite of tryptophan, *see* Serotonin
Metabolite of tyrosine, *see* Norepinephrine
Metabolites, 271
AAs, 694–697
control of food intake by, 692, 700
dietary content of sweet sugars, 692
dietary energy content, 692, 700
dietary nitrogen content, 700
fatty acids, 697–698
glucose, 700
glucose concentrations in plasma, 692–694
ketone bodies, 697–698
NO, 698
norepinephrine, 698
other chemical factors, 699
protein, 694–697
serotonin, 698
short-chain fatty acids, 701
Metabolizable energy (ME), 457–458, 634; *see also* Digestible energy (DE); Gross energy (GE)
efficiency of utilization, 459
energy values of feedstuffs for animals, 459
values of feed ingredients for animals, 458
Metabolon, 49
Metal-activated enzymes, 561
Metalloenzymes, 561
Metallothionein, 586
Metals, chelation of AAs with, 182
Metal transporter protein 1 (MTP1), 617
Methane, 193, 457
production in rumen, 207–209
Methanogens, 207
*Methanosarcina* genus, 208
Methionine (Met), 151, 164, 173, 393, 412
degradation via transsulfuration pathway in animals, 399–400
synthesis, 393
synthetase, 597
Methoxatin, *see* Pyrroloquinoline quinine
2-Methyl-1,4-naphthoquinone, *see* Vitamin K
3-Methyl-histidine, 152
Methylamines, 207
Methylcobalamin, 502
Methyl cobalamin, 597
3-*O*-Methylglucose, 215
Methylmercury (MeHg), 619
Methylthioadenosine (MTA), 412
MGATs, *see* MAG acyltransferases
Mg deficiency, 576
MGL, *see* Monoacylglycerol lipase
Michaelis–Menten kinetics, 48, 428
Microbes, 371–372, 373
arabinogalactan, 96
heteropolysaccharides in, 96–97
homopolysaccharides in, 89–92
LPSs, 96–97
murein, 97
xanthan, 97
Microbial fermentation, 203
Microbial hydrolysis of protein, 177
Microbial proteins
digestion in abomasum and small intestine, 381–382
effects of type of carbohydrate on microbial protein synthesis in Rumen, 375–376
Microbial sources, 176
Microbial β-mannanase, 715
Microcirculation, 18–20
Microminerals, 578; *see also* Macrominerals
aluminum, 613–615
arsenic, 615–617
boron, 605–607
bromine, 607
cadmium, 617
chromium, 602
cobalt, 596–597
Cu, 589–594
fluorine, 604–605
iodine, 602–604
iron, 578–585
lead, 618
mercury, 618–621
$Mn^{2+}$, 594–596
molybdenum, 597–599
nickel, 608–609
selenium, 599–601
silicon, 609–610
tin, 612–613
toxic metals, 613
vanadium, 610–612
Zn, 585–589
Microorganisms, 282
Microsomal triglyceride transfer protein (MTP), 278, 280, 285
Microsomes, 356
Microvasculature, blood circulation in, 20
Midzone, 33
Milk fever, 521, 572
Milk production, nutritional requirements for, 658
efficiency of energy utilization for milk production, 669
mammary gland, 658–662
milk synthesis by MECs, 662–668
Milk protein
lactose, and fats release from MECs to lumen of alveoli, 668–669
processing in MECs, 664
Milk secretion, 660
Milk-source di-and oligosaccharides, 196
Milk synthesis by MECs, 662–668
Mimosine, 156
Mineral(s), 553
chemistry, 555–556
deficiencies, 649, 651
general functions, 559–561
in milk, 667
overall view of absorption of dietary minerals, 556–559
requirements for maintenance, 638
Mitchell's chemiosmotic theory, 225
Mitochondria(l), 10
biological oxidation in, 50
electron transport system in, 53–57
electron transport system, 590–591

Mitochondria(l) (*Continued*)
fatty acid β-oxidation, regulation of, 320–321
glycerol 3-phosphate dehydrogenase, 221
Krebs cycle in, 50–53
matrix, 10
oxidation of pyruvate to acetyl-CoA, 222–223
protein synthesis in, 420
redox state, 228
Mitochondrial β-oxidation, 314, 328
of Acyl-CoA to form Acetyl-CoA, 316–318
fatty acid activation to Acyl-CoA, 315
long-chain Acyl-CoA transfer from cytosol into mitochondrial matrix, 315–316
pathway of, 314
Mitochondrion, 9
Modes of action, 719
Molisch test for carbohydrates, 102
Molybdenosis, 599
Molybdenum (Mo), 208, 553, 597
absorption and transport, 598
content in body and tissues, 598
deficiency syndromes, 598
excess, 599
functions, 598
sources, 597
Monensin, 724, 725
Mono-glutamates, 504
Monoacylglycerol lipase (MGL), 313
Monoacylglycerols (MAGs), 271, 274, 276, 278, 310
Monoamines, 15
Monomer, 296
Monomethyl mercury, 620
Monosaccharide(s), 67, 70, 203, 258; *see also* Disaccharides; Heteropolysaccharides; Homopolysaccharides; Oligosaccharides
absorption by intestine of fish, 213
absorption by small intestine, 197, 210
basolateral membrane GLUT2 in monosaccharides, 199
chemical reactions of carbohydrates, 99–101
chemical representation, 70–73
composition, 75
concentrations of D-sorbitol, inositol, GPC, and citric acid, 78
cyclic hemiacetal or hemiketal form, 70–73
developmental changes of intestinal monosaccharide transport, 200–201
epimerization, 73
extracellular hydrolysis of complex carbohydrates into, 202–203
glucose and fructose, 73–76, 197–199
Haworth projection, 72
intracellular degradation in ruminal microbes, 203
intracellular hydrolysis of complex carbohydrates, 203
monosaccharides trafficking from lamina propia into liver, 199–200
mutarotation, 74
open-chain form, 70
in plants and animals, 75
simple aminosugars, 75–76
structural forms distributions at equilibrium in water, 72
Monounsaturated fatty acids (MUFAs), 115, 272, 318; *see also* Short-chain fatty acids (SCFAs)
$\Delta^9$ MUFAs synthesis, 299–300
double bonds between $\Delta^9$ Carbon and $\Delta^1$ Carbon, 300–301
failure of animals to introducing double bonds beyond $\Delta^9$ Carbon, 301
synthesis in animals, 299
Montmorillonites, 723
Motor neurons, 14
Mouth, 22
lipids digestion in, 272, 280–281
mRNA, 416
gene transcription to form, 417
translation initiation to generate peptides at ribosomes, 417–418
MRP1, *see* Multidrug resistance protein 1
MTA, *see* Methylthioadenosine
MTOR complex 1 (MTORC1), 426–427
MTOR complex 2 (MTORC2), 426–427
MTOR signaling, *see* Mechanistic target of rapamycin signaling
MTP, *see* Microsomal triglyceride transfer protein
MTP1, *see* Metal transporter protein 1
Mucilages, 94
Mucin-producing and mucin-secreting goblet cell, 30
Mucosa, 29–30
MUFAs, *see* Monounsaturated fatty acids
Multidrug resistance protein 1 (MRP1), 501, 528
Multinucleated muscle cells, 34
Murein, 97
Muscle cells, 329
Muscle fibers, *see* Multinucleated muscle cells
Muscle isoform, *see* CPT-1B
Muscular activity benefits in enhancing animal growth and feed efficiency, 671–672
Muscularis externa, 29–30
Muscular work production, nutritional requirements for, 669
energy conversion in skeletal muscle, 669–670
high requirements for dietary energy, protein, and minerals for, 670–672
Musculoskeletal system, 34
Mycose, *see* Trehalose
Mycotoxins in feeds, agents to remove or absorb, 722–723
Myelin, 123
Myocytes, *see* Multinucleated muscle cells
Myofibrils, 34
Myogenin, 34
Myoglobin, 582
*myo*-Inositol, 479, 530, 535
absorption and transport, 536
deficiencies and diseases, 537
functions, 536–537
sources, 536
structure, 535
Myosin, 166–167, 670
Myristic acid, 114, 116

## N

NaB, *see* Sodium bromide
$Na_2B_4O_7 \cdot 10H_2O$, *see* Sodium tetraborate decahydrate
*N*-acetyl-D-glucosamine, 76, 88
*N*-acetyl-glucosamine, 94
*N*-acetyl-*para*-aminobenzoic acid, 543
$N^1$-acetylpolyamine oxidase (PAO), 412
Na+-coupled *myo*-inositol transporter-2 (SMIT2), 536

NAD, *see* Nicotinamide adenine dinucleotide
$NAD^+$, 224
NADH-CoQ reductase, *see* NADH dehydrogenase complex I
NADH, 224, 240
dehydrogenase complex I, 54
generation and utilization in rumen, 203–204
transfer from cytosol into mitochondria, 220–222
NADP, *see* Nicotinamide adenine dinucleotide phosphate
NADPH, 253
generation and utilization in rumen, 203–204
$Na^+/H^+$ exchange, 563
$Na^+/H^+$ exchanger (NHE3), 13, 393
Na-K-ATPase, 563
$Na^+/K^+$-ATPase, *see* Basolateral membrane $Na^+/K^+$-ATP pump
NaPi2b, *see* Sodium-phosphate cotransporter
Nascent HDLs, 293
Natural killer cells (NK cells), 39
Natural resistance–associated macrophage protein–2 (NRAMP2), *see* Divalent cation transporter–1 (DCT1)
NCA, *see N*-carboxy AA anhydride
*N*-carbamoylglutamate (NCG), 395
*N*-carboxy AA anhydride (NCA), 181, 182, 183
NCG, *see N*-carbamoylglutamate
NDF, *see* Neutral detergent fiber
NE, *see* Net energy
NEAAs, *see* Nutritionally essential AAs; Nutritionally nonessential AAs
Neonatal programming, 652
Neonates, 234, 247
Nephron, 35
Nerve cell, *see* Neuron
Nerve fiber, *see* Axon
Nerves and muscle cells, functions of, 566–567
Nervous system, 14; *see also* Circulatory system; Digestive system; Lymphatic system
in animals, 15
central nervous system, 16
neuron, 14–15
neurotransmitters, 15
peripheral nervous system, 16
Net energy (NE), 458–462, 634, 636
factors affecting dietary NE, 461
Net hepatic flux
of ammonia, 388
of glucose and AAs, 387
Net portal flux
of ammonia, 388
of glucose and AAs, 387
Neuroactive dipeptide, 184
Neuron, 14–15
Neuropeptides, 687–689
Neuropeptide Y (NPY), 688
Neurotransmitters, 15, 687–689
Neutral AA, 153–154
Neutral detergent fiber (NDF), 6, 202, 375–376
effects on feed intake, 261–262
effects on intestinal health, 261
effects on lactation and growth performance, 261
effects on rumen pH and environment, 261
Neutrophil extracellular traps, 39
NFE, *see* Nitrogen-free extract
$N^G$-Monomethylarginine, 155
NHE-1, 562
NHE3, *see* $Na^+/H^+$ exchanger
Niacin, 222, 488; *see also* Riboflavin; Thiamin
absorption and transport, 490
chemical structure, 489
deficiency and diseases, 491
functions, 490
sources, 488–489
structure, 488
Nickel (Ni), 553, 608
absorption and transport, 608
deficiency syndromes, 608
excess, 608–609
functions, 608
sources, 608
Nicotinamide, 488
Nicotinamide adenine dinucleotide (NAD), 490
Nicotinamide adenine dinucleotide phosphate (NADP), 490
Nicotinamide nucleotide transhydrogenase, 232
Nicotinate, *see* Nicotinic acid
Nicotinic acid, 488, 490
NIDDM, *see* Noninsulin-dependent diabetes mellitus
Niels Bohr's prototypical model of atomic structure, 555
Niemann–Pick C1-like 1 protein (NPC1L1 protein), 276
Ninhydrin, 183
NIS, *see* Sodium/iodide (Na+/I–) symporter
Nitrate, 368–371
Nitrate reductase, 598
Nitric oxide (NO), 188, 367, 644, 698
hemoglobin binding to, 187–188
NO-dependent blood flow, 404–405
NO-dependent nervous system, 16
synthesis, 7–8
Nitrite ($NO^{2-}$), 188, 368–371
Nitrogen-free extract (NFE), 4, 6
Nitrogen (N), 149, 151
balance studies for determining dietary requirements of AAs, 430, 431
dietary and endogenous sources, 434
recycling in ruminants and nutritional implications, 382–383
Nitrous acid, 178
Nitrous oxide ($N_2O$), 582
NK cells, *see* Natural killer cells
N-Methyl-D-aspartate receptors (NMDA receptors), 576
NO, *see* Nitric oxide
Non-acetylcholine nervous system, 16
Noncompetitive inhibition, 48
Nonenzymatic glycation, 75, 101
Nonenzyme additives, 718; *see also* Enzyme additives
nonruminants, 718–723
ruminants, 723–725
Nonesterified fatty acids, *see* Lonvag-chain fatty acids (LCFAs)
Non-fiber carbohydrates, 202
Non-heme iron enzymes and proteins, 584
Noninsulin-dependent diabetes mellitus (NIDDM), 220
Nonlysosomal proteolytic pathways, 423
Non-neuronal cells, *see* Glial cells
Non-norepinephrine nervous system, 16
Non-oxidative reversible phase, 229
Nonprotein AAs chemical structures, 151

Nonprotein nitrogen (NPN), 28, 170, 367–368, 383
extracellular and intracellular degradation of NPN into ammonia, 368, 369
utilization of nucleic acids, 371
utilization of urea, nitrate, and nitrite, 368–371
Nonproteinogenic AAs, 149, 156
Nonruminant(s), 193, 259, 272, 718; *see also* Ruminants
absorption of small peptides and AAAAs, 360–366
agents to remove or absorb mycotoxins in feeds, 722–723
amino acids and related compounds, 725–726
anti-mold feed additives and antioxidants, 726–728
antibiotics, 719–720
β-glucanases, 711–712
control centers in central nervous system, 687–692
control of food intake by nutrients and metabolites, 692–699
developmental changes of carbohydrases, 196–197
developmental changes of gastric proteases, 353–354
dietary NSPs effects, 259–260
diet selection in, 701–702
digestion and absorption of carbohydrates in, 194–201
digestion of milk-and plant-source di-and oligosaccharides, 196
digestion of protein in stomach, 350–354
digestion of proteins in small intestine, 354–360
digestion of starch and glycogen, 194–196
direct-fed microbials, 721–722
EAAs in, 388
enzyme additives for, 711
fermentation of carbohydrates in large intestine of, 210–211
herbivores, 31
lipids absorption by small intestine, 276–280
lipids digestion in mouth and stomach, 272
lipids digestion in small intestine, 272–276
mammals, 196–197, 200
monosaccharides absorption by small intestine, 197–201
NSPs effects on feed intake by animals, 259
NSPs effects on intestinal and overall health, 260
NSPS effects on nutrient digestibility, growth, and feed efficiency, 259–260
other enzymes, 715–716
pentosanases, 712–716
prebiotics, 722
protein fermentation in large intestine, 384
regulation of food intake by, 687
stomach in, 22–25
substances for, 725
substrate specificity of carbohydrases in, 196
Nonspecific binding protein (NSBP), 586
Non-starch polysaccharides (NSPs), 98, 202, 357, 709
effects on feed intake by animals, 259
effects on intestinal and overall health, 260
effects on nutrient digestibility, growth, and feed efficiency, 259–260
in plants, algae, and seaweeds, 98–99
Nonstructural carbohydrates (NSCs), 202
Noradrenaline, 688
Norepinephrine-dependent sympathetic nervous system, 16
Norepinephrine, 656, 698
NPC1L1 protein, *see* Niemann–Pick C1-like 1 protein
NPN, *see* Nonprotein nitrogen
*N*-pteroyl-L-glutamate, 166
NPY, *see* Neuropeptide Y
NRC, *see* U.S. National Research Council
NSBP, *see* Nonspecific binding protein
NSCs, *see* Nonstructural carbohydrates
NSPs, *see* Non-starch polysaccharides
NTS, *see* Nucleus of tractus solitarius
Nucleic acids
digestion and absorption in small intestine, 382
utilization, 371
Nucleosides, 371
diphosphate kinase, 226
Nucleus, 8, 555
Nucleus of tractus solitarius (NTS), 689
Nutrient(s), 2, 709
AAs, 694–697
control of food intake by, 692, 700
dietary content of sweet sugars, 692
dietary energy content, 692, 700
dietary nitrogen content, 700
fatty acids, 697–698
glucose, 692–694, 700
ketone bodies, 697–698
muscular work-induced increases in nutrient metabolism, 670
NO, 698
norepinephrine, 698
NSPS effects on nutrient digestibility, 259–260
other chemical factors, 699
protein, 694–697
and related factors effects on reproductive performance, 648–650
requirements determination by gestating dams, 650–651
requiring by animals, 3
serotonin, 698
short-chain fatty acids, 701
transport systems, 562
Nutrition, 2
biochemistry as chemical basis, 6–7
physiology as foundational basis, 7–8
Nutritional copper toxicity and treatment syndromes, 594
Nutritional dilemma, 193
Nutritional implications, nitrogen recycling in, 382–383
Nutritional importance of protein digestion in Rumen, 377–378
Nutritionally essential AAs (NEAAs), 387, 388
EAAs as precursors for synthesis of, 388–390
Nutritionally nonessential AAs (NEAAs), 349, 429, 432
Nutritional physiology, 8
Nutritional regulation
of fatty acid synthesis, 304–306
of intracellular protein turnover, 426–428
Nutritional requirements for maintenance, 634
additional factors affecting BMR, 635–636
energy requirements for maintenance, 634–635
fatty acid requirements for maintenance, 637
mineral requirements for maintenance, 638
protein and AA requirements for maintenance, 636–637
total requirements of swine for nutrients, 677–678
use of energy and substrates for maintenance, 641
vitamin requirements for maintenance, 638
water requirements for maintenance, 638–641

Nutritional requirements for production, 641
compensatory growth, 656–658
fetal programming, 652
for milk production, 658–669
neonatal programming, 652
for postnatal growth of animals, 652–656
for production of eggs in poultry, 672–676
for production of muscular work, 669–672
for production of wool and feathers, 672
for reproduction of females, 643–651
for reproduction of males, 651–652
suboptimal efficiencies of animal protein production, 642–643
total requirements of swine for nutrients, 677–678
Nutritional science, 2, 42
"Nutritional wisdom" of animals, 702
Nutrition of minerals
intestinal absorption of dietary minerals and transport in blood, 622
macrominerals, 561–578
macrominerals content in newborn and adult animals, 554
microminerals, 578–621
minerals, 555–561
periodic table of elements, 554
Nutrition of vitamins
chemical and biochemical characteristics of vitamins, 479–481
lipid-soluble vitamins, 511–530
quasi-vitamins, 530–543, 544
water-soluble vitamins, 481–511
$N^{\alpha}$-dehydrogenation of α-AAs, 182

## O

$O_2$, hemoglobin binding to, 187–188
OAA, *see* Oxaloacetate
OAT, *see* Ornithine aminotransferase
OCT2, 534
OCT3, 534
Octadeca*dienoic* acid, *see* Linoleic acid
9,12-Octadeca*dienoic* acid, 112
Octadecanoic acid, *see* Oleic acid
Octadeca*trienoic* acid, *see* Linolenic acid
Octadec*enoic* acid, *see* Oleic acid
OCTs, *see* Organic cation transporters
Oleic acid, 112
Oleoyl, 121
Olfactory sensory neurons, *see* Chemoreceptors
Oligopeptidases
extracellular proteolysis by, 368, 369
from small-intestinal mucosa into intestinal lumen, 356
Oligosaccharides, 67, 82, 177, 722; *see also* Disaccharides; Heteropolysaccharides; Homopolysaccharides; Monosaccharide(s)
digestion of milk-and plant-source, 196
pentasaccharides, 82, 84
tetrasaccharides, 82
trisaccharides, 82
OM, *see* Organic matters
Omasum, 26, 28
Omega nomenclature, 112
ω-oxidation of fatty acids, 329
Omnivores, 1
Oncogene activation, 220
One joule, 451
OPA, *see* *O*-Phthalaldehyde
Open-chain form, 70
Open-circuit indirect calorimetry, 471
*O*-Phthalaldehyde (OPA), 178
Optical isomer, 155
Optical isomerism of organic molecules, 155
Optimizing dietary formulations, 643
Orbitals, 556
Organ, 8
Organelles, 8, 11
Organic cation transporters (OCTs), 533
Organic matters (OM), 2, 454
Organic mercury, 620–621
Organic solvents, 271
Organomercury compounds, 619
Ornithine (Orn), 152, 365, 412
Ornithine aminotransferase (OAT), 412
Orthophosphatase, 493
Orthophosphoric monoester phosphohydrolase, *see* Orthophosphatase
Osmosis, 11–12
Osmotic effect, 197
Osteocalcin, 530
Outer mitochondrial membrane, 9
Overnutrition, 648, 651
Ovum, 37–38
Oxaloacetate (OAA), 51, 224, 295, 372
Oxidation, 50, 100, 102
Oxidative deamination of AAs, 182–183
Oxidative nonreversible phase, 229
Oxidative phosphorylation, uncouplers of, 57–58
Oxidoreductases, 47
Oxo-diiron (Fe–O–Fe), 578
Oxo–iron–zinc (Fe–O–Zn), 578
Oxygen (O), 151
Oxyhemoglobin[Hb(Fe(II)-$O_2$)], 188
Oxymethylation of AAs, 179

## P

P5C, *see* Pyrroline-5-carboxylate
Palmitate, metabolic fate of, 297–298
Palmitic acid, 112
Palmitoylation, 313
*p*-aminobenzoic acid, 479, 530
Pancreatic/pancreas, 31–32
α-amylase, 194–195
cancer, 273
enzymes, 274
juice, 32
lipase-related protein-2, 274–275
pro-protease release into lumen of duodenum, 355–356
protease precursors, 353
TAG lipase hydrolyzes, 274
Paneth cell, 30
Pantothenate, 491–494
Pantothenic acid, 491; *see also* Ascorbic acid
absorption and transport, 493
chemical structure, 491
deficiencies and diseases, 493–494
functions, 493
sources, 492
structure, 491–492

PAO, *see* $N^1$-acetylpolyamine oxidase
Papillae, 26, 27
*Para*-Aminobenzoic acid, 542
absorption and transport, 543
deficiencies and diseases, 543
functions, 543
sources, 542
structure, 542
Paracellular transport or absorption, 558
*Paracolobactrum aerogenoides* (*P. aerogenoides*), 371
Paracrine hormones, 38
Parasympathetic nervous system, 16
Parathyroid hormone (PTH), 570
Paraventricular nucleus (PVN), 687–688
Partition of food energy in animals, 453
DE, 454–456
GE, 453–454
HI, 458–462
ME, 457–458
measurement of heat production by animals, 463
NE, 458–462
Parturient paresis, *see* Milk fever
Pasteur effect in animal cells, 220
Pathological stresses, 427–428
Paylean for swine and Optaflexx for cattle, *see* Ractopamine
PBM, *see* Poultry by-product meal
PC, *see* Phosphatidylcholine
PCAT, *see* Phosphatidylcholine acyltransferase
PCFT, *see* Proton-coupled folate transporter
PDCAAS, *see* Protein digestibility corrected AA score
PDE3B, *see* Phosphodiesterase 3B
PDH, *see* Pyruvate dehydrogenase
PDV, *see* Portal-drained viscera
PE, *see* Phosphatidylethanolamine
PEC-60, 166
Pectin, 202
Pectins, 94
Pellagra, 491
D-Penicillamine, 593
Penicillium, 722
Penis, 35
Pentasaccharides, 82, 84
Pentosanases, 712
effects of dietary supplementation, 712
effects of dietary supplementation with sources of xylanase, 713
phytase, 713–715
Pentosans [$(C5H8O4)_n$], 712
Pentose, 100
Pentose cycle, 229, 254
activity in animal tissues and cells, 229–231
physiological significance of, 231–232
quantification of, 232–233
reactions, 229
regulation of, 233
Pentose phosphate pathway, *see* Pentose cycle
Pentoses, 77
PEP, *see* Phosphoenolpyruvate
PEPCK, *see* Phosphoenolpyruvate carboxykinase
Pepsin, 176
PepT1, *see* Peptide transporter 1
Peptidases, 422
Peptide-bound AAs, 161–163
Peptide(s), 15, 165–166, 183
Biuret assay of, 185
bonds, 349
chain elongation termination, 418
chemical classifications, and properties of, 165
chemical reactions, 185
dye-binding of, 185
elongation to produce protein, 418
as feed additives, 175–177
hydrolysis of peptide bond, 185
Lowry assay of, 185–186
Maillard reaction of, 186–187
polarity of enterocytes in peptide transport, 364–365
synthesis, 183–185
Peptide transporter 1 (PepT1), 13, 360–361
Peptide tyrosine tyrosine (PYY), *see* Peptide YY
Peptide YY, 259, 691
Perchloric acid ($HClO_4$), 168
Perfused organs, 246
Peripheral nervous system, 16
Peripheral tissues, 156
Periportal hepatocytes, 32–33
Perivenous hepatocytes, 33
Peroxidation of unsaturated fatty acids, 141–142
Peroxisomal fatty acid β-oxidation, 321
Peroxisomal system I, 321–322
Peroxisomal β-oxidation regulation, 323–324
Peroxisomal β-oxidation systems I and IIII, 321
activation of very-long-chain fatty acids into very-long-chain Acyl-CoA, 321–322
regulation of peroxisomal β-oxidation, 323–324
role of peroxisomal β-oxidation in ameliorating metabolic syndrome, 324
shortening of very-long-chain fatty Acyl-CoA, 322
transport of very-long-chain Acyl-CoA from cytosol into peroxisome, 322
Peroxisome proliferator-activated receptors (PPARs), 271, 323
PPAR-α, 323
PPAR-β, 323
PPAR-γ1, 324
PPAR-γ2, 324
PPAR-γ3, 324
PPARγ proteins, 324
PFK-1, *see* Phosphofructokinase-1
PG, *see* Prostaglandins
pH, 48, 366
Phenolic polymers in plants, 98
lignins, 98
NSPs in plants, algae, and seaweeds, 98–99
tannins, 98
Phenol ring iodination in tyrosine, 180
Phenylacetic acid, 314
Phenylalanine, 151, 164
$^{14}C$-Phe radioactivity in protein, 421
Phosphate, 572
Phosphate transporter-1 (PiT1), 573
Phosphate transporter-2 (PiT2), 573
Phosphatides, *see* Phospholipids
Phosphatidic acid, 123
Phosphatidylcholine (PC), 123, 274, 335, 531
Phosphatidylcholine acyltransferase (PCAT), 279
Phosphatidylethanolamine (PE), 333, 532
Phosphatidylinositol, 536–537

Phosphatidylserine (PS), 333, 532
Phosphoarginine, 452
Phosphocreatine, 452
Phosphodiesterase 3B (PDE3B), 305
Phosphoenolpyruvate (PEP), 218, 236, 237
Phosphoenolpyruvate carboxykinase (PEPCK), 236, 237
Phosphofructokinase-1 (PFK-1), 218
Phosphoglucomutase, 255
Phosphoinositol 3-kinase (PI3K), 656
Phospholipid metabolism, 333; *see also* Steroid hormones metabolism
  sources of ethanolamine and choline in animals, 333–335
  synthesis of phospholipids, 333
Phospholipids, 111, 122, 123, 275
  digestion, 274–275
  in plants, bacteria, and animals, 124
  synthesis, 333
  synthesis by MECs, 667
4′-Phosphopantetheine, 493
5-Phosphoribosyl-1-pyrophosphate (PRPP), 231
Phosphoric acid ($H_3PO_4$), 140, 573
Phosphorus (P), 553, 572
  absorption and transport, 573
  deficiency, 649
  deficiency symptoms, 574
  excess, 574
  functions, 573–574
  sources, 573
Phosphorylase kinase, 252
Photoreceptors, 42
Phylloquinone, 526
Phyllosilicates, 723
Physical encapsulation of protein or AAs, 379
Physiological stresses, 427–428
Physiology as foundational basis of nutrition, 7–8
Phytanic acid, 328
Phytase, 557, 713–715
Phytate, 713, 714
*Phytelephas macrocarpa. See* Ivory nut
Phytol, 137
pI, *see* Isoelectric point
PI3K, *see* Phosphoinositol 3-kinase
Pigmentation, 592
PiT1, *see* Phosphate transporter-1
PKB, *see* Protein kinase B
Placenta, 38
  functions, 647–648
  synthesizing AAs, 390
Plant(s)
  composition of foods from, 4
  glucose and fructose in, 73
  heteropolysaccharides in, 92–94
  homopolysaccharides in, 84–88
  monosacccharides in, 75
  phenolic polymers in, 98–99
  plant-source carbohydrates, 202
  plant-source di-and oligosaccharides, 196
  plant-source heteropolysaccharides, 92
  plant-source homopolysaccharides, 85
  plant-source materials, 257
  plant-source proteins, 149
  protein sources, 174
  simple aminosugars as monosacccharides in, 75–76
  waxes in, 121
Plasma, 16–17
  glucose concentrations, 234, 692–694
  membrane, 8, 11
  osmolarity, 562
Plasmalogens, 125, 127
Platelet-activating factor, 125–126
Polarity of enterocytes in AA and peptide transport, 364–365
Polyamine synthesis, 412
Polyglutamates, 504
Polyhydroxy aldehydes, *see* Aldoses
Polyhydroxy ketones, *see* Ketoses
Polyneuritis, 486
Polypeptide(s), 166, 354–355
  extracellular hydrolysis of proteins and polypeptides, 356–357
  modified AA residues in, 159–161
  sequences, 153
Polyphenolic phytochemicals, 379
Polysaccharides, 67, 102
  chemical reactions of carbohydrates, 102
  glycosidic linkages in, 103
Polyunsaturated fatty acids (PUFAs), 110, 306
  bioactive eicosanoids synthesis from, 329–330
  differences with *Trans* unsaturated fatty acids in animal nutrition and, 301–302
  ω3, 115, 119, 302, 637
  ω6, 115, 119, 637
POMC, *see* Pro-opiomelanocortin
Porin protein, 9
Portal-drained viscera (PDV), 18
  metabolism of AAs, 386
Portal tracts, *see* Portal triads
Portal triads, 32
Portal vein
  extraction of AAs from portal vein by liver, 385–387
  net entry of dietary AAs from small intestine into, 385
Postnatal animals
  blood circulation in, 18
  direction of blood flow in, 17
Postnatal growth of animals, nutritional requirements for, 652
  absolute *vs.* relative rate of animal growth, 653–654
  components of animal growth, 652–653
  regulation of animal growth by anabolic agents, 654–656
Posttranslational modifications, 160
  of newly synthesized proteins, 418–420
Potassium (K), 553, 565
  absorption and transport, 566
  atomic structures, 556
  deficiency symptoms, 567
  excess, 567
  functions, 566–567
  sources, 565
Pouch, *see* Shell gland
Poultry, 711, 712
Poultry by-product meal (PBM), 170
PPAR-δ, *see* Peroxisome proliferator-activated receptors (PPARs)—PPAR-β
PPARs, *see* Peroxisome proliferator-activated receptors
PPi, *see* Inorganic pyrophosphate
PQQ, *see* Pyrroloquinoline quinine
Prebiotics, 709, 722

Precursor lipids, *see* Fatty acids
Precursors, 134
Pregastric esterase, 281
Preruminants, 27; *see also* Nonruminant(s); Ruminants
absorption of carbohydrates in, 201
absorption of protein digestion products by small intestine in, 366–367
digestion and absorption of lipids in, 280–281
digestion of carbohydrates in, 201
digestion of proteins in abomasum and small intestine in, 366
stomachs, 27
*Prevotella ruminicola* (*P. ruminicola*), 368
Primary bile acids, 130, 132
Primary structure of protein, 168–169
Pristane, 137
*Pristis* "shark", 137
Proanthocyanidins, *see* Condensed tannins
Probiotics, *see* Direct-fed microorganisms
Pro conversion to Gly through hydroxyproline, 404
Pro-colipase, 273
Progesterone synthesis, 336
Prolamines, 168
Prolidase, 176
Proline, 151, 159, 169, 412
Pronase, 176
Pro-opiomelanocortin (POMC), 689
Pro-phospholipase $A_2$, 273
Propionate, 207, 234, 239, 318–319
Propionyl-CoA carboxylase, 498
Prostaglandins (PG), 111, 134–135
Proteases, 176
for intracellular protein degradation, 422
release from small-intestinal mucosa into intestinal lumen, 356
Protein-bound 4′-phosphopantetheine, 493
Protein-bound AAs, 161–163
Protein(s), 149, 165–166, 349, 694–697
accretion, 652
acid hydrolysis of, 176
actin and myosin, 166–167
alkaline hydrolysis of, 176
in animals, 166
biological half-lives of, 423
biotinylation, 498
Biuret assay of, 185
buffering reactions of, 187
chemical classifications, and properties of, 165–172
chemical reactions, 185
in connective tissues, 167–168
crude protein and true protein, 170–172
degradation, 426
dye-binding of, 185
fermentation in large intestine, 384
hemoglobin binding to $O_2$, $CO_2$, CO, and NO, 187–188
hydrolysates, 174
hydrolysis of peptide bond, 185
ingredients, 174–175
intake, 651
Lowry assay of, 185–186
Maillard reaction of, 186–187
in milk, 664
modified AA residues in, 159–161
nonruminants, digestion and absorption of protein in, 349–366
pores, 12
preruminants, digestion and absorption of protein in, 366–367
requirements for maintenance, 636–637
ruminants, digestion and absorption of protein in, 367–383
sepaparation of peptides from proteins, 168
solubility in water, 188
structural and physiological roles in animals, 150
structures, 168–170
Protein C, 530
Protein digestibility, 359
apparent *vs.* true digestibility of dietary protein, 434–436
measurement of $AA_{EIb}$ in small intestine, 436
measurement of feed ingredient added to basal diet, 436–437
Protein digestibility corrected AA score (PDCAAS), 433
Protein kinase B (PKB), 305
Protein kinase C signaling, DAG function in, 310
Proteinogenic AAs, 156, 172, 388
Protein palmitoyltransferases, 297
Protein phosphatase-1, *see* Glycogen synthase phosphatase
Protein S, 530
Protein synthesis
energy requirement, 420–421
measurement, 421
in mitochondria, 420
partition of AAs into pathways for catabolism and, 395–396
Protein Z, 530
Proteoglycan, 93, 168
Proteolysis, digesta flow from stomach into small intestine for, 354–355
Proteolytic bacteria, dietary effects concentrate and forage intake on, 376–377
Proton-coupled folate transporter (PCFT), 504
Proton, *see* Hydrogen ion ($H^+$)
Protonation, 58
Proton number, 555
Protoplasm, 8
Protozoa, 282, 372–373, 725
turnover in rumen, 379–380
Protozymes, 711
Proventriculus, 24, 25
Provitamins, 480–481
Proximate or Weende analysis of feedstuffs, 4–6
PRPP, *see* 5-Phosphoribosyl-1-pyrophosphate
PS, *see* Phosphatidylserine
Pteroylglutamic acid, *see* Folic acid
PTH, *see* Parathyroid hormone
PUFAs, *see* Polyunsaturated fatty acids
Pullulan, 92
Pure galactan, 85
Pure mannans, 87
Putrescine, 152, 412
PVN, *see* Paraventricular nucleus
Pyranose, 67
Pyridoxal, 494
absorption and transport, 494–495
deficiencies and diseases, 496–497
functions, 495–496

phosphate, 494, 495
sources, 494
structure, 494
Pyridoxamine, 494–497
Pyridoxine, 494–497
Pyrimidine nucleotides, 231
Pyrophosphatase, 493
Pyrophosphate, *see* Thiamin diphosphate
Pyrrolidine-2-carboxylic acid, 159
Pyrroline-5-carboxylate (P5C), 231, 365, 412
synthase, 232, 402
Pyrroloquinoline quinine (PQQ), 479, 530, 538; *see also* Ubiquinones
absorption and transport, 539
deficiencies and diseases, 539
functions, 539
sources, 539
structure, 538–539
Pyruvate, 52, 236
carboxylase, 237, 498
conversion into lactate and Cori cycle, 219
conversion into lactate or ethanol, 219
kinase, 218
mitochondrial oxidation of pyruvate to acetyl-CoA, 222–223
Pyruvate dehydrogenase (PDH), 222–223, 306

## Q

Q-cycle, 56
QPRT, *see* Quinolinate phosphoribosyl transferase
Qualitative requirements of dietary AAs, 429–430
Quality evaluation of dietary protein and AAs, 433
AAs analysis in diets and feed ingredients, 433–434
animal feeding experiments, 437–438
determination of protein digestibility, 434–437
Quantitative requirements of dietary AAs, 430–432
Quasi-vitamins, 530; *see also* Lipid-soluble vitamins
bioflavonoids, 541–542
carnitine, 534–535
choline, 531–534
dietary and metabolically active forms of vitamins and, 544
lipoic acid, 537–538
*myo*-Inositol, 535–537
*para*-Aminobenzoic acid, 542–543
pyrroloquinoline quinine, 538–539
ubiquinones, 539–541
Quaternary structure of protein, 168–169
Quinolinate phosphoribosyl transferase (QPRT), 491
Quinoproteins, 539

## R

Racemization, 157
Ractopamine, 655
Raffinose, 82
Rancimat method, 142
Rapidly digested starch, 88
Rat endocrine glands, 156
RBCs, *see* Red blood cells
RDP, *see* Rumen-degraded CP
Reactive carbonyls, 178
Reactive oxygen species (ROS), 220
Receptors, 42
Red blood cells (RBCs), 8
Redox states of $CoQ_{10}$, 540
Reduced-folate carriers (RFC), 504
RFC-1, 483, 504
RFC-2, 483, 504
Reductant, 50
Reduction–oxidation reactions, 48, 54
role of FAD in, 56
role of $NAD^+$ and $NADP^+$ in, 55
Regulation
of AA oxidation to Ammonia and $CO_2$, 405–406
of AA syntheses in animals, 394–395
of activities of small-intestinal proteases in nonruminants, 359
of CCK secretion, 359
economic benefits of feed efficiency improvement, 702–703
factors affecting food intake of animals, 688
of food intake by nonruminants, 687–699
of food intake by ruminants, 699–701
of gene expression, 359
of secretion of gastric proteases in nonruminants, 354
of urea cycle, 408
of uric acid synthesis, 411
Relative rate of animal growth, 653–654
Renal capsule, 35
Renal Gln utilization
for acid–base balance regulation, 402
for regulation of acid–base balance, 402
Renal gluconeogenesis, 239
Rennin, 352
Reproduction, fructose effects in, 256
Reproductive organs, 156
RER, *see* Rough endoplasmic reticulum
Residual feed intake (RFI), 703
Resistant starch, 88
Respiratory Quotient (RQ), 471
caution in interpretation of RQ values, 474–475
usefulness of RQ values in assessing substrate oxidation, 473–474
Respiratory system, 34; *see also* Digestive system
Retention times of feed particles and carbohydrates, 202
Reticulo-rumen, 575
Reticulorumen, 26
Reticulum, 26
Retinal, 512
Retinoic acid, 515, 516
9-*cis*-Retinoic acid receptor (RXR), 323
Retinoids, 512
Retinol, 512, 514, 515
Retinol esters, 514
RF-1, *see* Riboflavin transporters
RFC, *see* Reduced-folate carriers
RFI, *see* Residual feed intake
Riboflavin, 222, 486; *see also* Niacin; Thiamin
absorption and transport, 487
deficiency and diseases, 487–488
functions, 487
sources, 486–487
structure, 486
Riboflavin transporters (RF-1), 487
Riboflavin transporters (RF-2), 487
Ribonuclease (RNAase), 32

Ribose-5-P, 231
Ribosomal protein synthesis, 183
Ribosomes, mRNA translation initiation to generate peptides at, 417–418
Right lymphatic duct, 21
Right thoracic duct, *see* Right lymphatic duct
RNAase, *see* Ribonuclease
ROS, *see* Reactive oxygen species
Rough endoplasmic reticulum (RER), 664
R-protein, *see* Haptocorrin (HC)
RQ, *see* Respiratory Quotient
*R/S* configurations of AAs, 158, 159
Rumen, 26, 27–28
  digestive function, 28
  lipids digestion in, 282–283
  NDF effects on rumen pH and environment, 261
  physical limits, 699–700
  protecting high-quality protein and supplements of AAs from rumen degradation, 378
  wall, 27
Rumen, degradation of dietary protein in, 368
  dietary effects concentrate and forage intake on proteolytic bacteria, 376–377
  effects of type of carbohydrate on microbial protein synthesis, 375–376
  effects of type of dietary protein on degradation, 374–375
  extracellular and intracellular degradation of NPN into ammonia, 368–371
  extracellular proteolysis by bacterial proteases and oligopeptidases, 368
  intracellular protein synthesis from small peptides, AAs, 371–372, 373
  major factors affecting protein degradation, 374
  nutritional importance of protein digestion, 377–378
  role of ruminal fungi in intracellular protein degradation, 374
  role of ruminal protozoa in intracellular protein degradation, 372–374
Rumen degradation, protecting high-quality protein and supplements of AAs from, 378
  chemical treatments, 379
  heating, 378–379
  inhibition of AA degradation, 379
  physical encapsulation of protein or AAs, 379
  polyphenolic phytochemicals, 379
Rumen-degraded CP (RDP), 367–368
Ruminal bacteria
  turnover in rumen, 379–380
Ruminal bloat in ruminants, 209–210
Ruminal epithelium, 557
Ruminal fungi, 202
  role in intracellular protein degradation, 374
Ruminal microbes
  extracellular hydrolysis of complex carbohydrates into monosaccharides, 202–203
  intracellular degradation of monosaccharides in, 203
Ruminal microbial ecosystems, 202
Ruminal protozoa, 203
  role in intracellular protein degradation, 372–374
Ruminants, 193, 281, 723; *see also* Nonruminant(s)
  absorption of lipids by small intestine, 285
  compartments of stomach, 26–27
  contributions of tissues to fasting heat production by, 469
  dietary NSPs effects, 261–262
  digestion and absorption of carbohydrates in, 201
  digestion of lipids in abomomasum, 283–284
  digestion of lipids in small intestine, 284–285
  digestive function of rumen and abomasum in ruminants, 28
  direct-fed microbials, 725
  enzyme additives for, 716–718
  fermentation of carbohydrates in large intestine of, 210–211
  fermentative digestion of carbohydrates in, 201–210
  growth-promoting agents for, 656
  inclusion of fats, 281–282
  ionophore antibiotics, 724–725
  lipids digestion in rumen, 282–283
  monosaccharides absorption by small intestine in, 210
  nitrogen recycling in, 382–383
  protein fermentation in large intestine, 384
  regulation of food intake by, 699–701
  rumen development, 27–28
  stomach in, 26, 27
  substances for, 725–728
Ruminants, digestion and absorption of protein in, 367
  degradation of dietary protein in rumen, 368–374
  digestion and absorption of nucleic acids in small intestine, 382
  digestion of microbial and feed proteins in abomasum and small intestine, 381–382
  flow of microbial protein from rumen into abomasum and duodenum, 379–381
  major factors affecting protein degradation, 374–377
  nitrogen recycling in ruminants and nutritional implications, 382–383
  nutritional importance of protein digestion, 377–378
  protecting high-quality protein and supplements of AAs, 378–379
Rumination, 28
*Ruminobacter amylophilus* (*R. amylophilus*), 368
*Ruminococcus albus* (*R. albus*), 202
*Ruminococcus flavefacians* (*R. flavefacians*), 202
RXR, *see* 9-*cis*-Retinoic acid receptor


## S


SA, *see* Specific radioactivity
*Saccharomyces cerevisiae* (*S. cerevisiae*), 92, 177
*S*-Adenosylmethionine (SAM), 365, 412
*S*-adenosylmethionine decarboxylase (SAMD), 412
Safflower oil, 119
Salinomycin, 724
Salivary lipase, 280–281
SAM, *see S*-Adenosylmethionine
SAMD, *see S*-adenosylmethionine decarboxylase
Saponification of fatty acids, 139–142
Sarcomeres, 34
Satiety center, 687
"Satiety hormone", 689
Saturated fatty acids, 115
  synthesis, 299
  synthesis from acetyl-CoA, 295
SBM-based diet, *see* Soybean meal-based diet
SBM, *see* Soybean meal
S-carboxymethyl-cysteine, 178
SCD, *see* Stearoyl-CoA desaturase

SCFAs, *see* Short-chain fatty acids
Schiff's base, 101, 186
Schilling test, 502
Scrotum, 35
SD, *see* Sorbitol dehydrogenase
Seaweed(s), 607
  heteropolysaccharides in, 97–98
Secondary active transport, 13
Secondary bile acids, 131, 132
Secondary bile salts, 277
Secondary functions, 34
Secondary lymphoid organs, 39
Secondary structure of protein, 168–169
Secreted glycoprotein, *see* Intrinsic factor (IF)
Secretin, 39
Secretion of gastric hydrochloric acid, 350–352
Selenates, 599
Selenites, 599
Selenium (Se), 553, 599
  absorption and transport, 599–600
  content in body and tissues, 600
  deficiency syndromes, 600
  excess, 600–601
  functions, 600
  seleno-enzymes and proteins in animals, 601
  sources, 599
  use, 621
Selenocysteine, 152, 155, 161
Selenoprotein P (Seppl), 599
Semen, 35–36, 37
Seminal plasma, 37
Sense organs, 13, 42, 60
Sensible heat, 462, 470
Sensitive heat loss, 469, 470
Sensory neurons, 14, 42
Seppl, *see* Selenoprotein P
Serine, 151, 239
Serosa, 29–30
Serotonin, 152, 698
Serum, 16–17
Sex hormones, 130
Sex of animals, 635–636
SGLTs, *see* Sodium–glucose linked transporters
Sheep, wool production in, 672
Shell gland, 38, 674
*Shiliuhuang*, 576
Short-chain ACSs ($ACS_S$), 318
Short-chain fatty acids (SCFAs), 6, 84, 112–113, 193, 203, 261, 280, 282, 314, 372, 641, 687, 701; *see also* Monounsaturated fatty acids (MUFAs)
  oxidation, 318–320
  production in rumen, 204–206
  from rumen into blood, 206–207
  synthesis, 299
Shrimp, 34
*Siganus canaliculatus*. *See* Marine teleost fish
Sigmoid curve of animal growth, 652
Signal transducer and activator of transcription proteins (STAT proteins), 304
Silages, 112–113
Silica, *see* Silicon dioxide ($SiO_2$)
Silicate minerals, 723
Silicon (Si), 553, 609
  absorption and transport, 609
  deficiency syndromes, 610
  excess, 610
  functions, 609
  sources, 609
Silicon dioxide ($SiO_2$), 609
Silicosis, 610
Simple aminosugars, 75–76, 79
Simple diffusion, 11–12
Simple lipids, 110, 119; *see also* Compound lipids; Derived lipids
  fats, 119
  waxes, 119–121
Skeletal muscle, 16, 34, 248, 325
  action potentials in, 564
  energy conversion in, 669–670
  synthesizing AAs, 390
Skin, 42
SLC, *see* Solute carrier
SLC19A1, *see* Reduced-folate carriers (RFC)
SLC46A1, *see* Proton-coupled folate transporter (PCFT)
Slowly digested starch, 88
Small-intestinal mucosa, 365
  proteases and oligopeptidases release, 356
Small intestine, 28–31, 281
  absorption of protein digestion products, 366–367
  absorption of small peptides and AAs by, 360–366
  assembly of chylomicrons, VLDLs, and HDLs in enterocytes, 278–280
  assimilation of wax esters, 278
  catabolism of free AAs and small peptides, 359–360
  developmental changes in extracellular proteases, 357–359
  digestibility of dietary lipids, 275–276
  digestion and absorption of nucleic acids in, 382
  digestion of microbial and feed proteins in, 381–382
  digestion of proteins in, 354
  digestion of TAGs, phospholipids, and cholesterol esters, 274–275
  diurnal changes in intestinal lipid absorption, 280
  extracellular hydrolysis of proteins and polypeptides, 356–357
  flow of digesta from stomach into small intestine, 354–355
  general process, 272–273
  in preruminants, 366
  lipid micelles formation, 273–274
  lipids absorption by, 276–277, 281, 285
  lipids digestion in, 272, 284–285
  metabolism of AAs in, 386
  monosaccharides absorption by, 197–201, 210
  protein digestibility measurement of $AA_{EIb}$ in, 436
  protein digestibility *vs.* dietary AA bioavailability, 359
  regulation of activities of small-intestinal proteases, 359
  release of lipoproteins from, 287–294
  release of pancreactic pro-proteases into lumen of duodenum, 355–356
  release of proteases and oligopeptidases, 356
  resynthesis of TAGs in enterocytes, 277–278
  small-intestinal contractions, 30
  small-intestinal epithelium, 30
  structure of wall, 29
  synthesizing AAs, 390

Small peptides
absorption by small intestine of nonruminants, 360–366
catabolism, 359–360
intracellular protein synthesis from, 371–372, 373
Smell receptors, *see* Chemoreceptors
SMIT2, *see* Na+-coupled *myo*-inositol transporter-2
Smooth muscle cells
synthesizing AAs, 392
*sn*-1 position, 123, 125
*sn*-2 position, 123, 125
*sn*-3 position, 123, 125
Sodium-dependent vitamin C transporters (SVCT), 509
Sodium-phosphate cotransporter (NaPi2b), 573
Sodium (Na), 553, 561
absorption and transport, 562
atomic structures, 556
deficiency, 565
deficiency symptoms, 565
excess, 565
functions, 562–565
pump activity, 563, 566–567
sources, 562
Sodium alginate, 97
Sodium bromide (NaB), 607
Sodium–glucose linked transporters (SGLTs), 199
SGLT1, 13, 197, 213, 562
SGLT2, 198
Sodium/iodide (Na+/I–) symporter (NIS), 603
Sodium/iodide cotransporter, *see* Sodium/iodide (Na+/I–) symporter (NIS)
Sodium tetraborate decahydrate ($Na_2B_4O_7 \cdot 10H_2O$), 605
Solid-phase peptide synthesis, 183
Soluble fibers, *see* β-glucans
Soluble NSPs, 259
Soluble plant proteins, 210
Solute carrier (SLC), 361
Somatic nervous system, 16
D-Sorbitol, 75
Sorbitol dehydrogenase (SD), 253
Soybean meal (SBM), 174, 357
Soybean meal-based diet (SBM-based diet), 155, 715
Soybean protein concentrates (SPC), 174
Soybean protein isolates (SPI), 174
SPC, *see* Soybean protein concentrates
SPD, *see* Spermidine
Species-dependent metabolic pathways, 49–50
Species-specific degradation of AAs, 412–413
Specific dynamic effect of foods, *see* Heat increment (HI)
Specific radioactivity (SA), 246
Sperm, 35
Spermaceti, 121
Spermidine (SPD), 152, 412
Spermine, 152, 412
Sphingoid bases, 124
Sphingolipids, 122–124
metabolism, 333, 335–336
Sphingomyelin, 124, 293, 533–534
Sphingosine, 533
SPI, *see* Soybean protein isolates
Spinal cord, 16
SREBP-1c, *see* Sterol regulatory element-binding protein-1c
Stachyose, 82
Starch, 73, 87–88, 193
α-amylase in mouth and stomach, 194
digestibility, 212–213
digestion, 212
digestion of, 194
granules, 202
pancreatic α-amylase and apical membrane disaccharidases, 194–195
structure effects of, 195–196
STAT proteins, *see* Signal transducer and activator of transcription proteins
Steam distillation, 138
Stearic acid, *see* Octadecanoic acid
Stearoyl-CoA desaturase (SCD), 299–300
Steroidal saponins, 132–134
Steroid hormones metabolism, 336; *see also* Phospholipid metabolism
synthesis of progesterone and glucocorticoids, 336
synthesis of testosterone and estrogen, 336–338
Steroid(s), 111, 128
bile acids, 130, 131
bile alcohols, 132
hormones, 130
prohormone, 518
steroidal saponins, 132–134
sterols, 128–130
Sterol regulatory element-binding protein-1c (SREBP-1c), 306
Sterols, 128–130
*Stevia rebaudiana* leaves, 92
Stimuli of gastric acid secretion, 351
Stomach, 22
developmental changes of gastric proteases, 353–354
digestion of protein in, 350
digestive function of gastric HCl and gastric proteases, 352–353
in nonruminants, 22–25
in ruminants, 26–28
lipids digestion in, 272, 280–281
regulation of secretion of gastric proteases in nonruminants, 354
secretion of gastric hydrochloric acid, 350–352
*Streptococcus bovis* (*S. bovis*), 209
*Streptomyces*, 156
*Streptomyces albus* (*S. albus*), 724
*Streptomyces cinnamonensis* (*S. cinnamonensis*), 724
Stress(es), 650, 652
physiological and pathological, 427–428
Strong acid(s), 185
reaction of α-amino group of AAs, 177
Structural carbohydrates, 202
Submucosa, 29–30
Substrates, 302, 321
species differences in, 302–303
substrate-level phosphorylation, 452
tissue differences in, 303–304
Succinate-CoQ reductase, *see* Succinate dehydrogenase complex II
Succinate dehydrogenase, 51
Succinate dehydrogenase complex II, 56
Sucrose-isomaltase, 196
Sucrose, 81
Sugar, 256, 709
Sulfate conjugates, 132

Sulfated heteropolysaccharides, 95–96
Sulfonate, 150
Sulfonic acid group (–$SO_2$–OH), 150
Sulfur (S), 372, 553, 576; *see also* Vanadium (V); Zinc (Zn)
  absorption and transport, 577
  deficiency symptoms, 577–578
  excess, 578
  functions, 577
  sources, 576
Sunshine vitamin, 519
Superoxide anion ($O2^-$), 231
SVCT, *see* Sodium-dependent vitamin C transporters
Sweet sugars, dietary content of, 692
Swine, 711–713
Swine diets, 272
  antimicrobial agents for, 718
Symmetrical dimethylarginine, 155
Sympathetic nervous system, 16
Symporters, 13
Synthesizable AAs (AASAs), 429, 430, 432–433, 439
Synthetic PPAR-α ligands, 323
System, 8
Systematic naming system, 112
Systems physiology integration in nutrient utilization, 8
  animal cell structure, 8–13
  cell, tissue, organ, and system, 8
  composition and function of animal cell, 8–10
  scheme for sucrose-based cell or tissue fractionation, 10
  transport of substances across biological membrane, 10–13

T

TAAR1, *see* Trace amine-associated receptor 1
TAGs, *see* Triacylglycerols
Tannic acids, *see* Tannins
Tannin–protein complex, 379
Tannins, 98
Tara gum (*Caesalpinia spinosa* gum), 94
Taste receptors, *see* Chemoreceptors
Taurine, 152
t-BOC, *see* t-butyloxy carbamate
t-butyloxy carbamate (t-BOC), 183
TCA, *see* Trichloroacetic acid
Tectosilicates, 723
Temperature, 48
Terpenes, 111, 128, 137
  carotenoids, 137
  CoQ, 139
  essential oils, 138–139
  lipid-soluble vitamins, 138
  phytol, 137
Tertiary structure of protein, 168–169
Testosterone, 254
  synthesis, 336–338
3,5,3',5'-Tetraiodothyronine, 152
3,7,11,15-Tetramethylhexadecanoic acid, *see* Phytanic acid
Tetrasaccharides, 82, 84
Tetroses, 77
Texas A&M University's optimal ratios of AAs, 658, 659, 660
TGN, *see* Trans-Golgi network
Theanine, 156
Thermochemical calorie (Thermochemical cal), 450
Thermoneutral Zones (TNZ), 635
Thermozymes for feeds, 710–711
Thiamin, 482; *see also* Niacin; Riboflavin
  absorption and transport, 483–485
  chemical structure, 485
  deficiency and diseases, 485–486
  functions, 485
  sources, 483
  structure, 482–483
Thiamin diphosphate, 482–483
Thiamine, 222
Thiamin pyrophosphate, 483
Thiamin transporters 1 (ThTr1), 483
Thiamin transporters 2 (ThTr2), 483
Thioctic acid, *see* Lipoic acid
Thionyl chloride ($SOCl_2$), 182
Thoracic duct, 21
Three-dimensional structures (3D structures), 149
Threonine, 149, 151, 158, 173
  degradation in liver of animals, 399
Thromboxanes (TXs), 111, 135–136
ThTr1, *see* Thiamin transporters 1
Thymol, 138
*Thymus vulgaris* (*T. vulgaris*), 138
Thyroglobulin, 603
Thyroxine, *see* 3,5,3',5'-Tetraiodothyronine
Tight junctions, 18, 619
Tin (Sn), 553, 612
  absorption and transport, 612
  deficiency syndromes, 612
  excess, 613
  sources, 612
Tissue, 8
  differences in substrates, 303–304
  distribution and function of HSL, 311
  tissue-specific degradation of AAs, 396–401
  tissue-specific syntheses of AAs, 390–392
TNZ, *see* Thermoneutral Zones
Tocopherols, 522, 524
Tocotrienols, 522
Tollens' reagent, 100
Total dietary protein, 374–375
Total heat production by animals, 468–469
Touch receptors, *see* Mechanoreceptors
Toxicity of fructose, 200
Toxic metals, 613
Toxins, 650, 652
TP, *see* True protein
Trace amine-associated receptor 1 (TAAR1), 655
Tracer studies for determining dietary requirements of AAs and protein, 430–431
Trans-Golgi network (TGN), 589
*Trans*-unsaturated fatty acids, 116
Transamination, 413
  of AAs with α-ketoacids, 179
  vitamin B6 participates in AA transamination, 495–496
Transcalciferin, *see* Vitamin D-binding protein
Transcellular transport or absorption, 558
Transcobalamin II, 502
Transcobalamins, 501–502
*Trans* fatty acids, 112, 116
Transferases, 47
Transglutaminases, 161

Transient receptor potential channel type M5 (TRPM5), 359
Transient receptor potential melastatin-related protein-6 (TRPM6), 575
Transition metals, 556
Transporters, 12
Transport of di-and tri-peptides by enterocytes, 360–361
Transport of free AAs by enterocytes, 361–364
Transport of substances across biological membrane, 10, 12
  active transport, 13
  carrier-mediated transport, 12
  facilitated diffusion, 12–13
  simple diffusion, 11–12
*Trans* unsaturated fatty acids
  differences with PUFAs in animal nutrition and, 301–302
Trehalase, 196, 197
Trehalose, 82
Tremalose, *see* Trehalose
Triacylglycerols (TAGs), 109, 110, 119, 120, 271, 286, 287, 653
  additional pathways for synthesis, 310
  DAG function in protein kinase C signaling, 310
  digestion, 274–275
  G3P pathway for, 310
  HSL activity regulation in animal tissues, 312
  hydrolysis, 139–142
  intracellular lipolysis, 311–314
  lipid-soluble oils, 308–309
  MAG pathway for, 310
  mobilization, 311
  resynthesis in enterocytes, 277–278
  storage in WAT and other tissues, 310
  synthesis in animals, 308
Tricarboxylic acid cycle, *see* Krebs cycle
Trichloroacetic acid (TCA), 165
Triglycerides, *see* Triacylglycerols (TAGs)
3,5,3',-Triidothyronine ($T_3$), 152
Triolein, 119
Trioses, 77
Tri-peptides, 167
  in animals, 184
  transport by enterocytes, 360–361
Trisaccharides, 82
  in plant-source feedstuffs, 83
Tristearin, 119
tRNA, 416
Trophectoderm, 645
TRPM5, *see* Transient receptor potential channel type M5
TRPM6, *see* Transient receptor potential melastatin-related protein-6
True digestibility of dietary protein, 434–436
True protein (TP), 170–172, 664
True stomach, *see* Proventriculus
Trypsin, 176
Tryptamine, 152, 177
Tryptophan (Trp), 151, 164, 173, 488
  degradation in animals, 399, 401
  degradation in animals, 401
Tubular fluid, 35
Tubular reabsorption of nutrients, 35
Tubular secretion, 35
Tungsten, 597
Tungstic acid, 168
TXs, *see* Thromboxanes
Type 1 diabetes mellitus, *see* Insulin-dependent diabetes mellitus (IDDM)
Type 2 diabetes mellitus, *see* Noninsulin-dependent diabetes mellitus (NIDDM)
Type I collagen, 168
Type II collagens, 168
Type III collagen, 168
Type IV collagen, 168
Tyrosine, 151, 164
  kinase, 304
  oxidase, 591
  phenol ring iodination in, 180
Tyrosine kinase, *see* Janus kinase (JAK)

## U

Ubiquinone Q, *see* Ubiquinone $Q_{10}$
Ubiquinone $Q_{10}$, 54, 139, 539–540
Ubiquinones, 479, 530, 539; *see also* Pyrroloquinoline quinine (PQQ)
  absorption and transport, 540
  deficiencies and diseases, 540–541
  functions, 540
  sources, 540
  structure, 539–540
Ubiquitin, 166
UCP-1, *see* Uncoupling protein-1
UDP-galactose 4-epimerase, *see* UDP-glucose-4-epimerase
UDP-galactose synthesis pathway from D-glucose, 256–257
UDPGlc, *see* Uridine diphosphate glucose
UDP-glucose-4-epimerase, 257
UDP-glucuronate, 234
UDP-glucuronosyltransferase, 331
UE, *see* Energy in urine
UI, *see* International units
UIP, *see* Undegraded intake CP
Ultraviolet radiation, 519
Uncompetitive inhibition, 48
Uncouplers of oxidative phosphorylation, 57–58
Uncoupling protein-1 (UCP-1), 57
Uncoupling protein-2 (UCP-2), 57
Uncoupling protein-3 (UCP-3), 57
Undegraded intake CP (UIP), 374
Undernutrition, 648, 651
Unit of energy in animal nutrition, 450–451
Unsaturated fatty acids, 276
  biohydrogenation, 283
  hydrogenation, 140
  iodination and bromination of double bonds, 141
  peroxidation, 141–142
Unsaturated LCFAs, 283
Unstable peroxyl-fatty acid radical, 141
Unstirred water layer, 29, 31
Urea, 383, 406
  ammonia detoxification as, 406–408
  comparison with uric acid synthesis, 411–412
  cycle for disposal of ammonia in mammals, 406–407
  cycle regulation, 408
  energy requirement of, 407–408
  recycling, 28
  recycling in ruminants, 383
  synthesis
  utilization, 368–371

Uric acid
ammonia detoxification as, 408–411
comparison with urea synthesis, 411–412
for disposal of ammonia in birds, 408–410
energy requirement of, 410
regulation of, 411
species differences in uric acid degradation, 410–411
synthesis
Uridine diphosphate glucose (UDPGlc), 248, 258
Uridine triphosphate (UTP), 248, 450
Urinary excretion of 3-methylhistidine, 424
Urinary system, 35
Uronic acid, 97
Uronic acid pathway, 233–234
U.S. Food and Drug Administration (FDA), 134, 599, 726
U.S. National Research Council (NRC), 349
Uterine endometrium, 645
Uteroferrin, 580
Uterus, 37
UTP, *see* Uridine triphosphate

## V

Vaccenic acid, 283, 302
Vagina, 37
Valence electrons, 556
Valeric acid, 113
Valine, 151, 164, 173
Vanadium (V), 553, 610; *see also* Silicon (Si); Zinc (Zn)
absorption and transport, 610–611
deficiency syndromes, 611
excess, 611–612
functions, 611
sources, 610
Van Slyke assay, 178
Van Soest Method, 6
forage fractions classification using, 7
Vas deferens, 35
Vegetable oils, 119
Ventriculus, 24
Ventromedial hypothalamus (VMH), *see* Satiety center
Verbascose, 82, 84
Very-long-chain Acyl-CoA
transport from cytosol into peroxisome, 322
very-long-chain fatty acids activation into, 321–322
Very-long-chain fatty acids, 321–322, 332
Very-long-chain fatty Acyl-CoA shortening, 322
Very-low-density lipoproteins (VLDLs), 272, 277, 291, 479
assembly, 278–280
metabolism, 287–293
Villus columnar absorptive cell, 30
Villus of Lieberkühn, 30
Vision receptors, *see* Photoreceptors
Vitamin A, 111, 512
absorption and transport, 513–514
deficiencies and diseases, 516
excesses, 516–518
functions, 514–516
sources, 512–513
structure, 512
Vitamin $B_1$, *see* Thiamin
Vitamin $B_2$, *see* Riboflavin
Vitamin $B_3$, *see* Niacin
Vitamin $B_5$, *see* Pantothenic acid
Vitamin $B_6$, *see* Pyridoxine
Vitamin $B_9$, *see* Folate
Vitamin $B_{12}$, 239, 500; *see also* Biotin
absorption and transport, 501–502
chemical structure, 500
Cobalamin C, 501
Cobalamin D, 501
deficiencies and diseases, 502–503
functions, 502
sources, 500–501
structure, 500
Vitamin C, *see* Ascorbic acid
Vitamin D, 130, 518
absorption and transport, 519–520
deficiencies and diseases, 521
excesses, 521
functions, 520–521
sources, 518–519
structure, 518
vitamin D-binding protein, 519
Vitamin $D_2$, *see* Ergocalciferol
Vitamin $D_3$, *see* Cholecalciferol
Vitamin E, 522
absorption and transport, 523–524
deficiencies and diseases, 525
excesses, 525
functions, 524–525
sources, 522–523
structure, 522
vitamin E-containing micelle, 524
Vitamin K, 526
absorption and transport, 528
chemical structure, 526
deficiencies and diseases, 530
excesses, 530
functions, 528–530
recycling in animal cells, 527
sources, 528
structure, 526–527
Vitamin K-dependent mechanism, 8
Vitamin $K_1$, *see* Phylloquinone
Vitamin $K_2$, *see* Menaquinone
Vitamin $K_3$, *see* Menadione
Vitamins, 149, 479, 709; *see also* Mineral(s)
chemical and biochemical characteristics, 479
deficiencies, 649, 651
general characteristics of vitamins, 479–480
general sources of vitamins for animals, 480–481
important in animal nutrition, 480
from major plant-and animal-source foods, 482
requirements for maintenance, 638
VLDLs, *see* Very-low-density lipoproteins
Voltage-dependent anion channel, *see* Porin protein
Volumetric methods, 178
Voluntary nervous system, *see* Somatic nervous system

## W

Warburg effect, 220
WAT, *see* White adipose tissue
Water ($H_2O$), 638
mitochondrial β-oxidation of fatty acids to, 314–318
protein solubility in, 188
requirements for maintenance, 638–641

Water ($H_2O$) (*Continued*)
  stability of AAs in, 164–165
  water-insoluble fiber, 211–212
  water-insoluble lipids, 275
  water-insoluble NSPs, 99
  water-insoluble peptidoglycan, 97
  water-soluble inorganic compounds, 168
  water-soluble NSPs, 98–99, 260
Water-soluble vitamins, 481; *see also* Lipid-soluble vitamins; Quasi-vitamins
  absorption and transport in animals, 531
  ascorbic acid, 507–511
  biotin, 497–500
  cobalamin, 500–503
  folate, 503–507
  niacin, 488–491
  pantothenic acid, 491–494
  pyridoxal, 494–497
  pyridoxamine, 494–497
  pyridoxine, 494–497
  riboflavin, 486–488
  thiamin, 482–486
Wax(es), 119–121
  assimilation of wax esters, 278
  in plants and animals, 121
Wernicke's disease, 485
White adipose tissue (WAT), 271, 308, 325
  synthesizing AAs, 390
  TAGs storage in, 310
Wilson's disease, 593–594
Wolff–Chaikoff effect, 604
Wool grease, *see* Lanolin
Wool production in sheep and goats, 672
Wool wax, *see* Lanolin

## X

Xanthan, 97
Xanthophylls, 137
*Xenopus laevis oocytes*, 215
Xerophthalmia, 516
Xylanase, 712–716
D-Xylan, 93
Xylose, 75
D-Xylulose, 258

## Y

*Yucca aloifolia* (*Y. aloifolia*), 132
*Yucca schidigera* (*Y. schidigera*), 132
*Yucca schidigera* Extract (BIOPOWDER), 726–728
*Yucca whipplei* (*Y. whipplei*), 132

## Z

Zebrafish (*Danio rerio*), 286
Zinc (Zn), 553, 585
  absorption and transport, 586
  atomic structures, 556
  content in body and tissues, 586
  deficiency symptoms, 588
  excess, 588–589
  functions, 587–588
  sources, 586
  zinc-dependent enzymes and binding proteins in animals, 587
  zinc finger structure in protein, 588
Zinc sulfide (ZnS), 578
ZIP4, 586
Zone-dependent metabolic pathways, 49–50
Zone I, *see* Periportal hepatocytes
Zone II, *see* Midzone
Zone III, *see* Perivenous hepatocytes
Zoosterols, 128–129
Zwitterionic form of AAs, 153–155
Zymogens, 352, 529

Printed in the United States
by Baker & Taylor Publisher Services

Printed in the United States
by Baker & Taylor Publisher Services